International Neurology

To Deena Lisak for her support over many years.

R.P.L.

To my parents, Te Truong and Cam Tran, who sacrificed for my opportunity; to my wife, Diane Truong and my children, who endured the commitments of my career; to my teachers, Stanley Fahn and Edward Hogan, who opened my door to neurology; to Victor Tsao and Suzanne Mellor, for whose support and wisdom I am grateful; finally, to all my patients from whom I've learned so much.

D.D.T.

To my beloved grandmother Pranom Chivakiat, my parents Mitr and Nisaratana Bhidayasiri, all my teachers of neurology, and lastly my patients who have taught me much about neurology.

R.B.

To my wife Kathryn and our daughters Gemma, Bonita and Laura. I thank you for your support, encouragement and forbearance.

W.M.C.

International Neurology

A Clinical Approach

EDITED BY

ROBERT P. LISAK MD FAAN FRCP
Parker Webber Chair in Neurology
Professor and Chair of Neurology
Professor of Immunology and Microbiology
Wayne State University School of Medicine;
Neurologist-in-Chief, Detroit Medical Center
Chief of Neurology, Harper University Hospital
Detroit, MI, USA

DANIEL D. TRUONG MD FAAN
Head of The Parkinson and Movement Disorder Institute
Memorial Neuroscience Institute
Orange Coast Memorial Medical Center
Fountain Valley, CA, USA

WILLIAM M. CARROLL MBBS MD FRACP FRCP(E)
Head of Neurology and Clinical Neurophysiology
Sir Charles Gairdner Hospital
Nedlands, Perth, Australia

ROONGROJ BHIDAYASIRI MD FRCP
Director
Chulalongkorn Comprehensive Movement Disorders Center
Chulalongkorn University Hospital
Bangkok, Thailand;
University of California at Los Angeles
Los Angeles, CA, USA

FOREWORD BY JOHN WALTON (LORD WALTON OF DETCHANT)

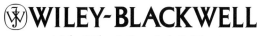
A John Wiley & Sons, Ltd., Publication

This edition first published 2009, ©2009 by Blackwell Publishing Ltd

Blackwell Publishing was acquired by John Wiley & Sons in February 2007. Blackwell's publishing program has been merged with Wiley's global Scientific, Technical and Medical business to form Wiley-Blackwell.

Registered office: John Wiley & Sons Ltd, The Atrium, Southern Gate, Chichester, West Sussex, PO19 8SQ, UK

Editorial offices: 9600 Garsington Road, Oxford, OX4 2DQ, UK

The Atrium, Southern Gate, Chichester, West Sussex, PO19 8SQ, UK

111 River Street, Hoboken, NJ 07030-5774, USA

For details of our global editorial offices, for customer services and for information about how to apply for permission to reuse the copyright material in this book please see our website at www.wiley.com/wiley-blackwell

Library of Congress Cataloging-in-Publication Data

International neurology : a clinical approach / edited by Robert P. Lisak ... [*et al.*].
  p. ; cm.
  Includes bibliographical references and index.
  ISBN 978-1-4051-5738-4
  1. Neurology. 2. Nervous system--Diseases. I. Lisak, Robert P. [DNLM: 1. Nervous System Diseases. 2. Neurology--methods. WL 140 I614 2009]
  RC346.I58 2009
  616.8--dc22

                                                                                    2008044353

A catalogue record for this book is available from the British Library.

Set in 9.25/12 pt Palatino by Newgen Imaging Systems (P) Ltd, Chennai, India
Printed and bound in Singapore by Fabulous Printers Pte Ltd

1 2009

Contents

List of contributors

Editors

Robert P. Lisak MD, FAAN, FRCP

Parker Webber Chair in Neurology,
Professor and Chair of Neurology,
Professor of Immunology and Microbiology,
Wayne State University School of Medicine;
Neurologist-in-Chief, Detroit Medical Center,
Chief of Neurology, Harper University Hospital,
Detroit, MI, USA

Daniel D. Truong MD, FAAN

Head of The Parkinson and Movement Disorder Institute,
Memorial Neuroscience Institute,
Orange Coast Memorial Medical Center,
Fountain Valley, CA, USA

William M. Carroll MBBS, MD, FRACP, FRCP(E)

Head of Neurology and Clinical Neurophysiology,
Sir Charles Gairdner Hospital,
Nedlands, Perth, Australia

Roongroj Bhidayasiri MD, FRCP

Director, Chulalongkorn Comprehensive Movement
Disorders Center, Chulalongkorn University Hospital,
Bangkok, Thailand;
University of California at Los Angeles
School of Medicine,
Los Angeles, CA, USA

Section editors

Johan A. Aarli MD

Professor, Department of Clinical Medicine, University of Bergen;
Department of Neurology, Haukeland University Hospital,
Bergen, Norway

Bruce J. Brew MBBS, MD, FRACP

Professor of Medicine (Neurology),
University of New South Wales;
Head of Neurology,
Program Director (Medicine),
Department of Neurology,
St Vincent's Hospital,
Sydney, Australia

Cynthia L. Comella MD, FAAN

Professor,
Department of Neurological Sciences/Movement
Disorders Section,
Rush University Medical Center,
Chicago, IL, USA

Josep O. Dalmau MD, PhD

Professor of Neurology, Division of Neuro-Oncology,
Department of Neurology,
Director, Center for Paraneoplastic Neurologic Disorders,
University of Pennsylvania,
Philadelphia, PA, USA

Larry E. Davis MD

Chief, Neurology Service,
New Mexico VA Health Care System;
Professor of Neurology and Molecular
Genetics and Microbiology,
University of New Mexico School of Medicine,
Albuquerque, NM, USA

Marianne de Visser MD

Neurologist, Professor of Neuromuscular Diseases,
Department of Neurology,
Academic Medical Center,
Amsterdam, The Netherlands

Oscar H. Del Brutto MD

Staff Member,
Department of Neurological Sciences,
Hospital-Clìnica Kennedy,
Guayaquil, Ecuador

Howard H. Feldman MDCM, FRCP (C)

Division of Neurology,
UBC Hospital Clinic for Alzheimer's Disease and Related
Disorders,
University of British Columbia,
Vancouver, British Columbia, Canada

Christopher C. Giza MD
Associate Professor of Neurosurgery and Pediatric Neurology,
UCLA Brain Injury Research Center,
David Geffen School of Medicine at UCLA,
Mattel Children's Hospital – UCLA,
Los Angeles, CA, USA

Chung Y. Hsu MD, PhD
Chair Professor, Graduate Institute of Clinical Medical Research,
China Medical University;
Advisory Attending Physician, China Medical University
Hospital; Chief Executive Officer, China Medical University
Health Care System,
Taichung, Taiwan

Ho Jin Kim MD, PhD
Head of Center for Clinical Supports and MS Clinic,
Department of Neurology,
Research Institute and Hospital of National Cancer Center,
Ilsan-gu, Goyang-gi, Gyeonggi-do, Korea

Sudesh Prabhakar MD, DM
Professor and Head, Department of Neurology,
Post Graduate Institute of Medical Education and Research,
Chandigarh, India

Myrna R. Rosenfeld MD, PhD, FAAN
Professor of Neurology,
Chief, Division of Neuro-Oncology,
Department of Neurology, University of Pennsylvania,
Philadelphia, PA, USA

Friedhelm Sandbrink MD
Assistant Professor in Neurology, Georgetown University;
Director EMG Laboratory and Chief, Chronic Pain Clinic,
Veterans Affairs Medical Center,
Washington, DC, USA

Raman Sankar MD, PhD
Professor and Chief of Pediatric Neurology,
Rubin Brown Distinguished Chair,
David Geffen School of Medicine at UCLA,
Los Angeles, CA, USA

Jacques Serratrice MD
Assistant Professor,
Timone Hospital,
Marseille, France

Stephen D. Silberstein MD, FAAN
Professor of Neurology,
Jefferson Medical College,
Thomas Jefferson University;
Director, Jefferson Headache Center,
Thomas Jefferson University Hospital,
Philadelphia, PA, USA

Marylou V. Solbrig MD
Professor of Internal Medicine (Neurology) and
Medical Microbiology,
Health Sciences Center,
University of Manitoba,
Winnipeg, Manitoba, Canada

Barbara E. Swartz MD, PhD
Director, The Epilepsy Clinics of S. Cal.,
Newport Beach, CA, USA;
Volunteer Faculty, Neurology,
Department of Radiology,
UCLA-West LA VA and UCI

Ann Tilton MD
Section Chair, Child Neurology,
Professor of Neurology and Pediatrics,
Louisiana State University Health Sciences Center and
Children's Hospital of New Orleans,
New Orleans, LA, USA

Einar P. Wilder-Smith MD, DTM&H,
FAMS (Neurology)
Senior Consultant and Associate Professor,
Department of Medicine,
Yong Loo Lin School of Medicine,
National University of Singapore,
Singapore

Authors

Obed Abramsky MD
Professor of Neurology,
Director of Agnes Ginges Center for
Human Neurogenetics,
Department of Neurology,
Hadassah University Hospital,
Hebrew University Hadassah Medical School,
Jerusalem, Israel

Megan Alcauskas MD
Resident, Department of Neurology and Stroke Center,
The Mount Sinai School of Medicine and Medical Center,
New York, NY, USA

Yuri Alekseenko MD, PhD
Associate Professor, Chairman of the Department of Neurology
and Neurosurgery, Vitebsk State Medical University,
Vitebsk, Republic of Belarus

Muhammad Al-Lozi MD
Professor of Neurology,
Department of Neurology,
Washington University in Saint Louis,
St Louis, MO, USA

Asmahan Alshubaili MD, FRCP
Consultant and Head of Neurology Department,
Ibn Sina Hospital, Safat, Kuwait

Monica L. Andersen PhD
Associate Professor,
Department of Psychobiology,
Universidade Federal de São Paulo (UNIFESP-EPM),
São Paulo, Brazil

Slobodan Apostolski MD, PhD
Head of the Neuromuscular Unit,
School of Medicine, University of Belgrade,
Belgrade, Serbia

Abelardo Araújo MD, PhD, FAAN
Head, The Clinical Research Laboratory on Neuroinfections,
Evandro Chagas Clinical Research Institute, FIOCRUZ,
Brazilian Ministry of Health;
Associate Professor of Neurology,
The Federal University of Rio de Janeiro, Brazil;
Visiting Professor, School of Medicine and Medical Science,
University College, Dublin, Ireland

Zohar Argov MD
Kanrich Professor of Neuromuscular Diseases,
Department of Neurology,
Hadassah-Hebrew University Medical Center,
Jerusalem, Israel

Ovidiu Bajenaru MD, PhD
Professor of Neurology,
University of Medicine and Pharmacy "Carol Davila", Bucharest;
Chairman and Head of Department of Neurology,
University Hospital of Emergency,
Bucharest, Romania

Brenda L. Banwell MD, FRCPC
Associate Professor of Pediatrics (Neurology),
Director, Pediatric Multiple Sclerosis Clinic,
Associate Scientist, Research Institute,
The Hospital for Sick Children,
University of Toronto,
Toronto, Ontario, Canada

Delwyn J. Bartlett PhD, MAPS
Co-Ordinator,
Medical Psychology,
Sleep and Circadian Group,
Woolcock Institute of Medical Research,
University of Sydney,
Sydney, Australia

Brandon Barton MD
Fellow, Movement Disorders Section,
Department of Neurology,
Rush University Medical Center,
Chicago, IL, USA

Tracy T. Batchelor MD, MPH
Executive Director, Stephen E. and Catherine Pappas Center for
Neuro-Oncology;
Associate Professor of Neurology, Harvard Medical School;
Associate Neurologist, Massachusetts General Hospital,
Boston, MA, USA

Roongroj Bhidayasiri MD, FRCP
Director, Chulalongkorn Comprehensive Movement
Disorders Center, Chulalongkorn University Hospital,
Bangkok, Thailand;
University of California at Los Angeles,
Los Angeles, CA, USA

Lia R.A. Bittencourt MD, PhD
Associate Professor,
Department of Psychobiology,
Universidade Federal de São Paulo (UNIFESP-EPM),
São Paulo, Brazil

Jed Black MD
Associate Professor of Sleep Medicine,
Department of Psychiatry and Behavioral Sciences,
Stanford University;
Medical Director, Stanford Sleep Medicine Clinic,
Stanford, CA, USA

David Blacker MBBS, FRACP
Consultant Neurologist and Stroke Physician,
Sir Charles Gairdner Hospital and
Royal Perth Rehabilitation Hospital;
Clinical Associate Professor, University of Western Australia,
Western Australia, Nedlands, Australia

Deborah T. Blumenthal MD
Co-Director of Neuro-Oncology Service,
Tel-Aviv Sourasky Medical Center,
Tel-Aviv University, Tel-Aviv, Israel;
Adjunct Associate Professor of Neuro-Oncology,
Huntsman Cancer Institute at the University of Utah,
Salt Lake City, UT, USA

Enver I. Bogdanov MD
Head of Neurology and Rehabilitation Department,
Kazan State Medical University,
Kazan, Russia

Saeed Bohlega MD, FRCPC
Chairman,
Distinguished Senior Consultant,
Department of Neurosciences,
King Faisal Specialist Hospital and Research Centre,
Riyadh, Saudi Arabia

Michael Brada BSc, MB ChB, FRCP, FRCR
Professor of Clinical Oncology,
The Institute of Cancer Research and The Royal Marsden NHS
Foundation Trust,
Sutton, Surrey, UK

Herbert Budka MD, MSc, Dhc
Professor of Neuropathology and Institute Director,
Institute of Neurology (Obersteiner Institute),
Medical University of Vienna,
Vienna, Austria

Ferdinando S. Buonanno MD
Associate Professor of Neurology,
Massachusetts General Hospital and
Harvard Medical School,
Boston, MA, USA

Bernardo Cacho Díaz MD
Neurologist,
Department of Neurology,
National Institute of Medical Sciences and Nutrition,
Mexico City, Mexico

Louis R. Caplan MD
Professor of Neurology,
Harvard Medical School;
Chief of the Division of Cerebrovascular Disease,
Department of Neurology,
Beth Israel Deaconess Medical Center,
Boston, MA, USA

Patrick Carney BMed (Hons), FRACP
Neurologist/Epilepsy Fellow,
Epilepsy Research Center,
Neuroscience Building,
Austin Health,
West Heidelberg, Victoria, Australia

Francisco Javier Carod-Artal MD, PhD
Professor of Neurology,
Neurology Department,
Sarah Network of Rehabilitation Hospitals,
Brasilia DF, Brazil

Jonathan Carr MB ChB, FCP (SA) Neurology
Head, Division of Neurology,
University of Stellenbosch,
South Africa

Ignacio M. Carrillo-Nunez MD
Neurologist, Orange Coast Memorial Medical Center,
Fountain Valley Regional Medical Center;
Fountain Valley, CA, USA

William M. Carroll MBBS, MD, FRACP, FRCP(E)
Head of Neurology and Clinical Neurophysiology,
Sir Charles Gairdner Hospital,
Nedlands, Perth, Australia

John N. Caviness MD
Professor of Neurology,
Mayo Clinic College of Medicine,
Scottsdale, AZ, USA

Stephen Cederbaum MD
Professor of Psychiatry, Pediatrics and Human Genetics,
University of California, Los Angeles (UCLA),
Los Angeles, CA, USA

Thomas C. Cesario MD
Professor and Dean Emeritus,
University California, Irvine
Orange, CA, USA

Jong-Hee Chae MD, PhD
Associate Professor,
Department of Pediatrics,
Seoul National University Children's Hospital,
Seoul National University College of Medicine,
Seoul, Korea

Marc Chamberlain MD
Professor and Chief,
Department of Neurology and Neurological Surgery,
Division of Neuro-Oncology,
Fred Hutchinson Research Cancer Center,
Seattle Cancer Care Alliance, University of Washington,
Seattle, WA, USA

Bernard P.L. Chan MB, ChB, MRCP
Senior Consultant and Director of Stroke Service,
Division of Neurology,
Department of Medicine,
National University Hospital,
Singapore

Christopher Li-Hsian Chen MD, PhD
Senior Clinician Scientist, Biomedical &
National Medical Research Councils;
Associate Professor, Dept of Pharmacology,
National University of Singapore;
Associate Staff (Senior Consultant Neurologist),
Department of Medicine,
National University Hospital,
Singapore

Olivier L. Chinot MD
Head, Unité de Neuro-Oncologie,
Professor of Oncology,
Centre Hospitalo-Universitaire Timone,
Université de la Méditerranée,
Marseille, France

Young-Chul Choi MD, PhD
Professor, Department of Neurology,
Gangnam Severance Hospital,
Yonsei University College of Medicine,
Seoul, Korea

Heng Thay Chong FRCP (Glasg)
Associate Professor,
Faculty of Medicine,
University of Malaya,
Kuala Lumpur, Malaysia

Sajeel Chowdhary MD
Department of Interdisciplinary Oncology,
H. Lee Moffitt Cancer Center,
University of South Florida,
Tampa, FL, USA

Nai-Shin Chu MD, PhD
Professor of Neurology, Department of Neurology,
Chang Gung Memorial Hospital,
Chang Gung University College of Medicine,
Taipei, Taiwan

Luis A. Chui MD
H.S. Clinical Professor,
Department of Neurology, Neuromuscular Program,
University of California, Irvine, Orange;
Neurology Section,
VA Long Beach Health Care System,
Long Beach, California, CA, USA

Anthony Ciabarra MD, PhD
Neurology Center of North Orange County,
La Habra, CA, USA

Allison Conravey MD
Neurophysiology Fellow, Child Neurologist,
Department of Neurology,
Louisiana State University Health Sciences Center,
New Orleans, LA, USA

Patricia K. Coyle MD
Professor and Acting Chair,
Department of Neurology,
Stony Brook University Medical Center,
Stony Brook, NY, USA

Esther Cubo MD, PhD
Neurologist Attending, Neurology Department,
Hospital General Yague,
Burgos, Spain

Liying Cui MD
Professor, Department of Neurology,
Peking Union Medical College Hospital,
Beijing, China

Le Quang Cuong MD, PhD
Associate Professor and Chairman,
Department of Neurology,
Hanoi Medical University of Vietnam,
Ha Noi, Vietnam

Anna Członkowska MD, PhD
Head, The Second Department of Neurology,
Institute of Psychiatry and Neurology;
Professor, The Department of Pharmacology,
Medical University,
Warsaw, Poland

Marinos C. Dalakas MD
Chair, Clinical Neurosciences, Neuromuscular Diseases,
Imperial College, London, UK;
Professor of Neurology, Chief Neuromuscular Division,
Thomas Jefferson University,
Philadelphia, PA, USA

Stephen M. Davis MD, FRCP (Edin), FRACP
Divisional Director of Neurosciences,
Director of Neurology,
Royal Melbourne Hospital, University of Melbourne,
Parkville, Melbourne, Victoria, Australia

T. De Mello PhD
Associate Professor,
Department of Psychobiology,
Universidade Federal de São Paulo (UNIFESP-EPM),
São Paulo, Brazil

Antonio V. Delgado-Escueta MD
Professor of Neurology,
University of California, Los Angeles,
Los Angeles, CA, USA

Thomas Deufel MD
Professor and Head,
Department of Clinical Chemistry and Laboratory Diagnostics,
University Hospital Jena,
Jena, Germany

Stephen Deputy MD, FAAP
Associate Professor of Neurology,
Louisiana State University School of Medicine,
New Orleans, LA, USA

Günther Deuschl MD
Professor and Head,
Department of Neurology,
Christian-Albrechts-University of Kiel,
Kiel, Germany

Salvatore DiMauro MD
Lucy G. Moses Professor of Neurology,
College of Physicians and Surgeons,
New York, NY, USA

Geoffrey A. Donnan MD, FRCP, FRACP
Director, National Stroke Research Institute, Austin Health,
Department of Neurology, University of Melbourne,
Heidelberg, Victoria, Australia

Ira J. Dunkel MD
Associate Attending Pediatrician,
Department of Pediatrics,
Memorial Sloan-Kettering Cancer Center,
New York, NY, USA

Jennifer Durphy MD
Indiana University School of Medicine,
Indianapolis, IN, USA

Jeffrey Ekstrand MD, PhD
Assistant Professor of Pediatrics and Neurology,
University of Utah School of Medicine,
Salt Lake City, UT, USA

Colin A. Espie MAppSci, PhD, CPsychol, FBPsS, FCS
Professor of Clinical Psychology,
Director of University of Glasgow Sleep Centre,
Sackler Institute of Psychobiological Research,
Faculty of Medicine,
Southern General Hospital,
Glasgow, Scotland, UK

Stanley Fahn MD, FAAN
H. Houston Merritt Professor of Neurology,
Department of Neurology,
Columbia University College of Physicians and Surgeons,
New York, NY, USA

Birgit Frauscher MD
Neurologist and Sleep Disorders Specialist,
Sleep Disorders Clinic, Department of Neurology,
Innsbruck Medical University,
Innsbruck, Austria

Karen P. Frei MD
Neurologist and Movement Disorder Specialist,
The Parkinson and Movement Disorder Institute,
Memorial Neuroscience Institute,
Orange Coast Memorial Medical Center,
Fountain Valley, CA, USA

Guillermo García-Ramos MD
Professor and Chair, Neurology Department,
National Institute of Medical Sciences and Nutrition,
Mexico City, Mexico

Ellen Gelpi MD
Researcher, Institute of Neurology,
Medical University of Vienna,
Austrian Reference Centre for Human Prion Diseases,
Vienna, Austria

Elizabeth R. Gerstner MD
Fellow in Neuro-Oncology,
Massachusetts General Hospital,
Boston, MA, USA

Nir Giladi MD
Professor of Neurology,
Sackler School of Medicine,
Tel-Aviv University;
Chairman, Department of Neurology,
Tel-Aviv Sourasky Medical Center,
Tel-Aviv, Israel

Nils Erik Gilhus MD
Professor, Department of Clinical Medicine,
University of Bergen;
Department of Neurology,
Haukeland University Hospital,
Bergen, Norway

David Gloss MD
Chief Resident,
Department of Neurology,
Tulane University School of Medicine,
New Orleans, LA, USA

Christopher G. Goetz MD
Professor of Neurological Sciences,
Professor of Pharmacology, Movement Disorders Section,
Department of Neurology, Rush University Medical Center,
Chicago, IL, USA

Alejandra Gonzalez-Duarte MD
Instituto Nacional de Ciencias Medicas y Nutricion
Salvador Zubiran,
Mexico, DF, Mexico

Marc Gotkine BSc (Hons), MBBS Lond. (Hons)
Neurologist, Department of Neurology,
Agnes Ginges Center for Human Neurogenetics,
Hadassah University Hospital,
Hebrew University Hadassah Medical School,
Jerusalem, Israel

Alla Guekht MD, PhD
Professor of Neurology,
Department of Neurology and Neurosurgery,
Russian State Medical University,
Moscow, Russia

Christian Guilleminault MD
Professor,
Stanford University School of Medicine,
Stanford University, Stanford, CA, USA

Kapila Hari MBBCh (Wits), MMed (Wits)
Lecturer, Division of Neurology,
Department of Neurosciences,
School of Clinical Medicine,
Faculty of Health Sciences,
University of the Witwatersrand,
Johannesburg, South Africa

Silvia Hofer MD
Medical Oncologist,
Departments of Neurology and Oncology,
University Hospital Zürich,
Zürich, Switzerland;
Academic Unit of Radiotherapy and Oncology,
The Institute of Cancer Research and Neuro-Oncology Unit,
The Royal Marsden NHS Foundation Trust,
London and Sutton, UK

Birgit Högl MD
Assistant Professor of Neurology,
Board Certified Sleep Specialist,
Head of the Sleep Disorders Clinic,
Department of Neurology, Innsbruck Medical University,
Innsbruck, Austria

Ahmet Höke MD, PhD, FRCPC
Associate Professor of Neurology and Neuroscience,
Director, Neuromuscular Division,
Department of Neurology, Johns Hopkins University,
Baltimore, MD, USA

Jakub Hort MD, PhD
Associate Professor of Neurology,
Department of Neurology,
Charles University,
Teaching Hospital Motol,
Prague, Czech Republic

Chin-Chang Huang MD
Professor of Neurology, Department of Neurology,
Chang Gung Memorial Hospital,
Chang Gung University College of Medicine,
Taipei, Taiwan

Marcel Hungs MD, PhD
Assistant Professor of Clinical Neurology,
Director, Center for Sleep Medicine,
Department of Neurology, University of California,
Irvine, Orange, CA, USA

Sergei N. Illarioshkin MD, PhD, DSci
Vice-Director and Professor of Neurology,
Research Center of Neurology,
Russian Academy of Medical Sciences,
Moscow, Russia

Takeshi Iwanaga MD
Stroke Fellow,
National Stroke Research Institute, Austin Health,
Heidelberg, Victoria, Australia

Regina I. Jakacki MD
Associate Professor of Pediatrics,
Director, Pediatric Neuro-Oncology Program,
Children's Hospital of Pittsburgh,
Pittsburgh, PA, USA

Andres M. Kanner MD
Professor of Neurological Sciences, Rush Medical College;
Director, Laboratory of Electroencephalography and
Video-EEG-Telemetry;
Associate Director, Section of Epilepsy and Rush Epilepsy Center,
Rush Medical College at Rush University,
Rush University Medical Center,
Chicago, IL, USA

Ronnie Karayan MD
Fellow, Clinical Neurophysiology,
Department of Neurology,
University of California, Irvine,
Orange, CA, USA

Kevin A. Kerber MD
Assistant Professor,
Departments of Neurology and Otolaryngology,
University of Michigan Health System,
Ann Arbor, MI, USA

Jee Hyun Kim MD
Post Doctoral Research Fellow,
Stanford University Sleep Medicine Program,
Stanford University,
Stanford, CA, USA

Jun-ichi Kira MD
Professor and Chairman,
Department of Neurology,
Neurological Institute,
Graduate School of Medical Sciences,
Kyushu University,
Fukuoka, Japan

Yasuhisa Kitagawa MD
Professor of Neurology,
Tokai University School of Medicine;
Senior Executive Director of Tokai University Hachioji Hospital,
Tokyo, Japan

Vladimir Kostic MD, PhD
Professor of Neurology,
Institute of Neurology, School of Medicine,
University of Belgrade,
Belgrade, Serbia

Srivicha Krudsood MD
Professor, Department of Tropical Hygiene,
Faculty of Tropical Medicine,
Mahidol University,
Bangkok, Thailand

Lee I. Kubersky MD
Resident,
Department of Neurology,
University of Virginia Health System,
Charlottesville, VA, USA

Nigel G. Laing PhD
Professor, Centre for Medical Research,
University of Western Australia,
Western Australian Institute for Medical Research,
QEII Medical Centre,
Nedlands, Western Australia, Australia

Sandi Lam MD
Chief Resident, Division of Neurosurgery,
University of California, Los Angeles,
Los Angeles, CA, USA

Phillipa J. Lamont MBBS, PhD, FRACP
Associate Professor,
Neurogenetic Unit,
Department of Neurology,
Royal Perth Hospital,
Perth, Western Australia, Australia

Dean A. Le MD, PhD
Neurology Consultant,
Saddleback Memorial Medical Center,
Laguna Hills, CA, USA

Minh Le MD
Senior Lecturer of Neurology and Consultant in Neurology,
Head, Neurology Department, University Medical Center;
Deputy Head, Neurology Department,
The University of Medicine and Pharmacy,
Ho Chi Minh City, Vietnam

Thomas W. Leung MD
Assistant Professor, Division of Neurology,
Department of Medicine and Therapeutics,
The Chinese University of Hong Kong,
Hong Kong

Steven R. Levine MD
Professor of Neurology,
Department of Neurology and Stroke Center,
The Mount Sinai School of Medicine and Medical Center,
New York, NY, USA

Richard A. Lewis MD
Professor and Associate Chair of Neurology,
Wayne State University School of Medicine,
Detroit, MI, USA

Peter LeWitt MD
Professor of Neurology, Wayne State University School of
Medicine; Director, Parkinson's Disease and Movement Disorders
Program, Henry Ford Hospital,
Detroit, MI, USA

Marco A. Lima MD, PhD
Assistant Researcher,
The Reference Center on Neuroinfections and HTLV,
Evandro Chagas Clinical Research Institute (IPEC), FIOCRUZ,
Rio de Janeiro, Brazil

Li Ling Lim MBBS, MRCP (UK), MPH (USA), Dip. ABPN, ABSM, ABEM, ABCN (USA)
Medical Director and Consultant Neurologist,
Singapore Neurology and Sleep Centre,
Gleneagles Medical Centre;
Director, Sleep Disorders Unit, Singapore General Hospital,
Singapore

Alfred Lindner MD
Professor of Neurology and Head,
Department of Neurology, Marienhospital,
Stuttgart, Germany

Robert P. Lisak, MD, FAAN, FRCP
Parker Webber Chair in Neurology,
Professor and Chair of Neurology,
Professor of Immunology and Microbiology,
Wayne State University School of Medicine;
Neurologist-in-Chief, Detroit Medical Center,
Chief of Neurology, Harper University Hospital,
Detroit, MI, USA

Mingsheng Liu MD
Associate Professor, Department of Neurology,
Peking Union Medical College Hospital,
Beijing, China

Warren P. Mason MD, FRCPC
Staff Physician, Department of Medicine,
Princess Margaret Hospital;
Associate Professor, Department of Medicine,
University of Toronto,
Toronto, Ontario, Canada

Frank L. Mastaglia MD
Director, Centre for Neuromuscular
and Neurological Disorders,
University of Western Australia,
Queen Elizabeth II Medical Centre,
Perth, Australia

Radoslav Matěj MD, PhD
Neuropathologist,
Department of Pathology and Molecular Medicine,
National Laboratory for Diagnostics of Prion Diseases,
Thomayer Teaching Hospital,
Prague, Czech Republic

Marco T. Medina MD
Professor of Neurology and Epilepsy,
Director, Neurology Training Program,
Postgraduate Direction,
National Autonomous University of Honduras,
Tegucigalpa, Honduras

Manu Mehdiratta MD, FRCPC
Fellow, Department of Neurology,
Beth Israel Deaconess Medical Center,
Boston, MA, USA

Giorgia Melli MD, PhD
Neurologist, Neuroimmunology and
Neuromuscular Diseases Unit,
National Neurological Institute "Carlo Besta",
Milan, Italy

Chokri Mhiri MD
Professor of Neurology,
Head of the Department of Neurology,
Habib Bourguiba University Hospital,
Sfax, Tunisia

Emmanuel Mignot MD, PhD
HHMI Investigator, Professor of Psychiatry and
Behavioral Sciences,
Department of Psychiatry and Behavioral Sciences,
Stanford University Center for Narcolepsy,
Howard Hughes Medical Institute,
Palo Alto, CA, USA

Andre Mochan MD (Munich), FCP (SA)
Senior Lecturer, Division of Neurology,
Department of Neurosciences,
School of Clinical Medicine,
Faculty of Health Sciences,
University of the Witwatersrand,
Johannesburg, South Africa

Girish Modi MBBCh (Wits), MSc (Lond), PhD (Lond),
FCP (SA), FRCP (Lond)
Chair of Neurology, Academic Head of Neurosciences
and Chief Neurologist,
Division of Neurology, Department of Neurosciences,
School of Clinical Medicine,
Faculty of Health Sciences, University of the Witwatersrand,
Johannesburg, South Africa

Tahseen Mozaffar MD
Associate Professor (Neurology and Orthopaedic Surgery),
University of California, Irvine;
Director, Neuromuscular Program;
Director, UC Irvine-MDA ALS and Neuromuscular Center,
Orange, CA, USA

D. Nagaraja DPM (Psych), DM (Neuro)
Professor of Neurology,
Director/Vice Chancellor,
National Institute of Mental Health and Neurosciences
(NIMHANS),
Deemed University,
Bangalore, India

Merrilee Needham MBBS
Consultant Neurologist,
Royal North Shore Hospital, Sydney, Australia;
Centre for Neuromuscular and Neurological Disorders,
University of Western Australia,
Queen Elizabeth II Medical Centre,
Perth, Australia

Tien T. Nguyen MD
Neurosurgeon,
Fountain Valley Regional Hospital and Medical Center,
Fountain Valley, CA, USA

Hirokazu Oguni MD
Professor of Pediatrics, Department of Pediatrics,
Tokyo Women's Medical University,
Tokyo, Japan

Ayman I. Omar MD, PhD
Neuro-Oncology Fellow, Department of Medicine,
Princess Margaret Hospital and the University of Toronto,
Toronto, Ontario, Canada

Björn Oskarsson MD
Assistant Professor of Clinical Neurology,
University of California,
Davis, Sacramento, CA, USA

Bruce Ovbiagele MD
Associate Professor,
Stroke Center and Department of Neurology,
UCLA School of Medicine,
Los Angeles, CA, USA

George W. Padberg MD, PhD
Professor and Chairman,
Department of Neurology,
Radboud University Nijmegen Medical Centre,
Nijmegen, The Netherlands

Chrysostomos P. Panayiotopoulos MD, PhD
Honorary Consultant,
Department of Clinical Neurophysiology and Epilepsies,
St Thomas' Hospital, London, UK

Margaret Park MD
Assistant Professor,
Departments of Behavioral Sciences and
Neurological Sciences,
Sleep Disorders Service and Research Center,
Rush University Medical Center, Chicago, IL, USA

Min Su Park MD
Clinical Professor,
Department of Neurology,
Yeungnam University
School of Medicine, Taegu, Korea;
Research Institute and Hospital of
National Cancer Center,
Ilsan-gu, Goyang-su, Gyeonggi-do, Korea

Mary Payne MD
Assistant Professor,
Pediatric Neurology,
Department of Neuroscience,
Marshall University,
Huntington, WV, USA

Alan Pestronk MD
Professor of Neurology,
Department of Neurology,
Washington University in Saint Louis,
St Louis, MO, USA

Kammant Phanthumchinda MD
Professor of Neurology,
Head, Department of Medicine,
Faculty of Medicine,
Chulalongkorn University,
Bangkok, Thailand

Claudio Sergio Podestá MD
Neurologist, Neurology Department,
Sleep Disorders Center, Fleni,
Buenos-Aires,
Argentina

Simon Podnar MD, PhD
Associate Professor of Neurology,
Division of Neurology, University Medical Centre,
Ljubljana, Slovenia

Anuchit Poonyathalang MD
Associate Professor,
Ophthalmology Department,
Ramathibodi Hospital,
Bangkok, Thailand

D.K. Prashantha MD
Senior Resident, Department of Neurology,
National Institute of Mental Health and Neurosciences
(NIMHANS),
Deemed University,
Bangalore, India

Paul B. Pritchard III MD
Professor of Neurosciences,
Director, Postgraduate Education (Neurology),
Department of Neurosciences,
Medical University of South Carolina,
Charleston, SC, USA

Leon D. Prockop MD
Founding Chairman,
Emeritus Professor of Department of Neurology,
University of South Florida,
Tampa, FL, USA;
Chair, Environmental Neurology Research Group (ENRG)/
World Federation of Neurology (WFN)

Najeeb Qadi MD
Consultant, Cognitive & Behavioral Neurology,
Director, Neurology Residency Training Program,
Department of Neurosciences,
King Faisal Specialist Hospital and Research Centre,
Riyadh, Saudi Arabia

Jan Raethjen MD
Associate Professor,
Department of Neurology,
Christian-Albrechts-University of Kiel,
Universitätsklinikum Schleswig-Holstein,
Kiel, Germany

Jeffrey Raizer MD
Associate Professor of Neurology, Department of Neurology,
Director, Medical Neuro-Oncology,
Northwestern University, Feinberg School of Medicine,
Robert H. Lurie Comprehensive Cancer Center,
Chicago, IL, USA

Kumar Rajamani MD
Assistant Professor, Department of Neurology,
Comprehensive Stroke Program,
Wayne State University,
Detroit, MI, USA

Vidosava Rakocevic-Stojanovic MD, PhD
Associate Professor,
Institute of Neurology, Clinical Centre of Serbia,
School of Medicine, University of Belgrade,
Belgrade, Serbia

Nathan J. Ranalli MD
Resident in Neurosurgery,
Department of Neurosurgery,
Hospital of the University of Pennsylvania,
Philadelphia, PA, USA

Sandeep Randhawa MD
Fellow, Neuro-Ophthalmology,
Kresge Eye Institute/Wayne State University,
Detroit, MI, USA

Didier Raoult MD, PhD
Medical doctor,
Unité des Rickettsies et Pathogènes Emergents,
Faculté de Médecine, Centre Collaborateur OMS,
Université de la Méditerranée, Marseille, France

Ivan Rektor MD
Vice-Rector for Development,
President, European Society for Clinical
Neuropharmacology;
Head, First Department of Neurology,
St Anne's Hospital,
Masaryk University,
Brno, Czech Republic

Irena Rektorová MD, PhD
Associate Professor of Neurology,
First Department of Neurology,
Masaryk University and St Anne's Hospital,
Brno, Czech Republic

Laurie Rice RN, MSN, APN-BC
Nurse Practitioner,
Department of Neurology,
Northwestern University, Feinberg School of Medicine,
Chicago, IL, USA

Steven P. Ringel MD
Professor of Neurology,
University of Colorado,
Denver, Aurora, CO, USA

John M. Ringman MD
Associate Clinical Professor,
UCLA Department of Neurology,
Mary S. Easton Center for Alzheimer's Disease Research,
Los Angeles, CA, USA

Bradley J. Robottom MD
Movement Disorders Fellow,
University of Maryland Parkinson's Disease and Movement
Disorders Center,
University of Maryland School of Medicine,
Baltimore, MD, USA

Ildefonso Rodríguez-Leyva MD
Professor of Neurology,
Facultad de Medicina,
Universidad Autónoma de San Luis Potosí,
San Luis Potosi, México

Luis C. Rodríguez-Salinas MD
Chief of Residents,
Neurology Training Program,
National Autonomous University of Honduras,
Tegucigalpa, Honduras

Yvonne D. Rollins MD, PhD
Assistant Professor of Neurology,
University of Colorado,
Denver, Aurora, CO, USA

Karen L. Roos MD
John and Nancy Nelson Professor of Neurology and
Professor of Neurosurgery,
Indiana University School of Medicine,
Indianapolis, IN, USA

Raymond L. Rosales MD, PhD
Professor of Neurology and Psychiatry,
University of Santo Tomas, Manila;
Centers for Movement Disorders and
Clinical Neurophysiology,
International Institute of Neurosciences,
Saint Luke's Medical Center,
Quezon City, Philippines

Clarisse Rovery MD
Medical doctor,
Unité des Rickettsies et Pathogènes Emergents,
Faculté de Médecine, Centre Collaborateur OMS,
Université de la Méditerranée, Marseille, France

Sabine Rudnik-Schöneborn MD, PhD
Professor, Medical Faculty, Institute of Human Genetics,
University Hospital RWTH,
Aachen, Germany

Robert Rusina MD
Neurologist, Department of Neurology,
Thomayer Teaching Hospital and Institute of Postgraduate
Education in Medicine,
Prague, Czech Republic

Sureshbabu Sachin MD, DM
Senior Research Officer (SRO),
All India Institute of Medical Sciences,
New Delhi, India

Gerard Said MD
Professor of Neurology, Hôpital de la Salpétrière,
Paris, France

Sabahattin Saip MD
Professor of Neurology,
Clinical Neuroimmunology Unit,
Department of Neurology,
Cerrahpaşa School of Medicine,
University of Istanbul,
Istanbul, Turkey

David Schiff MD
Professor of Neurology, Neurological Surgery, and
Medicine (Hematology-Oncology),
Co-Director, University of Virginia Neuro-Oncology Center,
University of Virginia Health System,
Charlottesville, VA, USA

Josef Schill MD
Attending Physician,
Department of Neurology,
Klinikum Ludwigshafen,
Ludwigshafen, Germany

Georges Serratrice FRCP
Emeritus Professor of Neurology,
Head of the Department of Neurology,
Timone Hospital, Marseille;
Past President of Aix-Marseille University;
Past President of the French Society of Neurology;
France

Samir H. Shah MD
Clinical Fellow,
Stroke Center and Department of Neurology,
UCLA School of Medicine,
Los Angeles, CA, USA

Lisa M. Shulman MD
Associate Professor of Neurology,
Co-Director, University of Maryland Parkinson's Disease and
Movement Disorders Center,
Rosalyn Newman Distinguished Scholar in Parkinson's Disease,
Department of Neurology,
University of Maryland School of Medicine,
Baltimore, MD, USA

Donald Silberberg MD
Professor of Neurology,
Department of Neurology,
University of Pennsylvania Medical Center,
Philadelphia, PA, USA

Marcus Tulius T. Silva MD, PhD
Neurologist and Senior Researcher,
The Clinical Research Laboratory on Neuroinfections,
Evandro Chagas Clinical Research Institute, Fiocruz,
Brazilian Ministry of Health,
Rio de Janeiro, Brazil

David M. Simpson MD
Professor of Neurology,
Director, Clinical Neurophysiology Laboratories,
Director, Neuro-AIDS Program,
Mount Sinai Medical Center,
New York, NY, USA

Gagandeep Singh MD, DM
Professor and Head,
Department of Neurology,
Dayanand Medical College and Hospital,
Ludhiana, India

Aksel Siva MD
Professor of Neurology,
Head, Clinical Neuroimmunology Unit,
Department of Neurology,
Cerrahpaşa School of Medicine,
University of Istanbul,
Istanbul, Turkey

Carlo Solinas MD
Research Fellow,
Monash University and Medical Centre,
Clayton, Victoria, Australia;
University of Siena,
Siena, Italy

Mark M. Souweidane MD
Professor of Neurological Surgery and Pediatrics,
Department of Neurological Surgery,
New York Presbyterian Hospital,
Weill-Cornell Medical College;
Associate Attending Neurosurgeon,
Division of Neurosurgery,
Memorial Sloan-Kettering Cancer Center,
New York, NY, USA

Mark Stacy MD
Associate Professor of Neurology,
Director of the Movement Disorders Program,
Division of Neurology,
Duke University,
Durham, NC, USA

Elka Stefanova MD, PhD
Associate Professor of Neurology,
Institute of Neurology,
School of Medicine,
University of Belgrade,
Belgrade, Serbia

Thorsten Steiner MD, PhD, MME
Vice Director, Department of Neurology,
Ruprecht Karls University Heidelberg,
Heidelberg, Germany

Rick Stell MBBS, FRACP
Director of Movement Disorders Clinic,
Australian Neuromuscular Research Unit,
Sir Charles Gairdner Hospital,
Perth, WA, Australia

Barney J. Stern MD
Professor of Neurology,
Department of Neurology,
University of Maryland,
Baltimore, MD, USA

Valerie Suski DO
Fellow, Division of Neurology,
Duke University,
Durham, NC, USA

Nijasri C. Suwanwela MD
Associate Professor of Neurology,
Director, Chulalongkorn Stroke Center,
Neurological Unit,
Department of Medicine,
Faculty of Medicine,
Chulalongkorn University,
Bangkok, Thailand

Takeshi Tabira MD, PhD
Professor, Department of Diagnosis, Prevention and
Treatment of Dementia,
Graduate School of Juntendo University,
Bunkyo-ku, Tokyo, Japan

Kay Sin Tan MBBS (Melb), FRCP (Edin)
Senior Lecturer,
Division of Neurology,
Department of Medicine,
University of Malaya Medical Centre,
Kuala Lumpur, Malaysia

Chong Tin Tan MD, FRCP
Professor, Department of Medicine,
University of Malaya,
Kuala Lumpur, Malaysia

Louis C.S. Tan MD
Senior Consultant, Neurology,
Parkinson's Disease and Movement Disorders Centre;
National Neuroscience Institute,
Singapore

Stacey K.H. Tay MBBS, MRCP (Paeds), MRCPCH
Associate Professor,
Department of Paediatrics,
Yong Loo Lin School of Medicine,
National University of Singapore,
Singapore

Hock L. Teoh MD, MRCP
Research Fellow,
National Stroke Research Institute, Austin Health,
Heidelberg, Victoria, Australia

Gaby T. Thai MD
Associate Clinical Professor,
Department of Neurology,
University of California,
Irvine, CA, USA

Mirela E. Toma MD
Resident, Albert Einstein College of Medicine,
Bronx Lebanon Hospital,
New York, NY, USA

Manjari Tripathi MD, DM
Associate Professor,
Department of Neurology,
All India Institute of Medical Sciences,
New Delhi, India

Daniel D. Truong MD, FAAN
Head of The Parkinson and Movement Disorder Institute,
Memorial Neuroscience Institute,
Orange Coast Memorial Medical Center,
Fountain Valley, CA, USA

Alexandros C. Tselis MD, PhD
Associate Professor,
Department of Neurology,
Wayne State University School of Medicine,
Detroit, MI, USA

Sergio Tufik MD, PhD
Professor of Sleep Medicine and Biology,
Department of Psychobiology,
Universidade Federal de São Paulo (UNIFESP-EPM),
São Paulo, Brazil

Frank J.E. Vajda MD, FRCP (Ed), FRACP
Professor of Clinical Neuropharmacology,
Monash University and Monash Medical Centre
Clayton, Victoria, Australia

Martin J. van den Bent MD
Neurologist, Head, Neuro-Oncology Unit,
Department of Neuro-Oncology,
Daniel den Hoed Cancer Center,
Erasmus University Medical Center,
Rotterdam, The Netherlands

Stanley van den Noort MD
Professor Emeritus,
Department of Neurology,
University of California,
Irvine, CA, USA

Anneke J. van der Kooi MD, PhD
Consultant Neurologist,
Department of Neurology,
Academic Medical Center,
Amsterdam, The Netherlands

Gregory P. Van Stavern MD
Associate Professor,
Departments of Ophthalmology, Neurology, and Neurosurgery,
Kresge Eye Institute/Wayne State University,
Detroit, MI, USA

S.M. Schade van Westrum MD
Consultant Neurologist,
Martini Ziekenhuis,
Groningen, The Netherlands

Arousiak Varpetian MD
Assistant Professor of Clinical Neurology,
Keck School of Medicine,
University of Southern California,
Clinical Director, Rand Schrader HIV-Neurology Clinic,
Los Angeles, California, USA

Bruno Estañol Vidal
Head of the Neurophysiology Laboratory,
National Institute of Medical Sciences and Nutrition,
Mexico City, Mexico

John Vissing MD, DMSci
Professor of Neurology,
Director, Neuromuscular Clinic and Research Unit,
Department of Neurology,
University of Copenhagen, Rigshospitalet,
Copenhagen, Denmark

David B. Vodušek MD, PhD
Professor of Neurology,
Medical Faculty,
University of Ljubljana;
Medical Director,
Division of Neurology, University Medical Centre,
Ljubljana, Slovenia

Melanie Walker MD
Clinical Assistant Professor,
Departments of Neurology and Neurological Surgery,
University of Washington School of Medicine,
Seattle, WA, USA

William J. Weiner MD
Professor and Chairman,
Department of Neurology,
University of Maryland School of Medicine,
Director, Maryland Parkinson's Disease and
Movement Disorders Center,
Baltimore, MD, USA

Thomas Wieser MD
Consultant and University Lecturer (Medical University Vienna),
Department of Neurology,
Krankenhaus Göttlicher Heiland,
Vienna, Austria

Polrat Wilairatana MD
Professor, Department of Clinical Tropical Medicine,
Faculty of Tropical Medicine,
Mahidol University,
Bangkok, Thailand

Ernest W. Willoughby MB ChB, FRACP
Neurologist, Department of Neurology,
Auckland City Hospital;
Clinical Associate Professor (Hon.),
Department of Medicine,
Faculty of Medical and Health Sciences,
University of Auckland,
Auckland, New Zealand

Christine Won MD
Assistant Clinical Professor,
University of California,
San Francisco, CA, USA

Eric L. Zager MD
Professor of Neurosurgery,
Department of Neurosurgery,
Hospital of the University of Pennsylvania,
Philadelphia, PA, USA

Afawi Zaid MD, MPH
Coordinator, Genetics of Epilepsy Research in Israel,
Tel-Aviv Sourasky Medical Center,
Tel Aviv, Israel

Jorge A. Zavala MD
Research Fellow,
National Stroke Research Institute, Austin Health,
Heidelberg, Victoria, Australia

Klaus Zerres MD
Head, Institute for Human Genetics,
RWTH, Aachen University,
Aachen, Germany

Stephan Zierz MD
Professor of Neurology,
Head, Department of Neurology,
University Halle-Wittenberg,
Halle/Saale, Germany

Foreword

I have known Robert Lisak for many years, not only as an outstanding neurologist, but also as the distinguished editor of the *Journal of the Neurological Sciences*. I congratulate him and his co-editors most warmly on planning and eventually launching this outstanding volume. While many notable textbooks of clinical neurology exist, there is none, to my knowledge, that deals with neurological medicine so comprehensively in an international context. It is of course true that many of the neurological disorders familiar to neurologists in the developed world also occur in the tropics and in developing countries. There are nevertheless many neurological conditions unique to different locations in the tropics and in the developing world, and this book seems to me to present the first really comprehensive coverage of international clinical neurology. The range and coverage of such diseases in this book are truly remarkable, as indeed is the team of authors whom the editors have been able to recruit, including many of the glitterati of international neurology. I cannot imagine that in the 22 sections and the 173 chapters any disorder of significance can possibly have been omitted, and I believe that this book represents an astonishing achievement. Neurologists from across the world, and indeed innumerable physicians, whatever their particular interests in medicine and neurology, will surely owe a very great debt of gratitude to Bob Lisak and his co-editors, and to the authors of the individual contributions for creating such a remarkable work of scholarship, which clearly will be consulted, quoted, and read widely. In my view this work is an outstanding volume which will stand the test of time and of which the editors and authors can justifiably be proud.

John Walton (Lord Walton of Detchant)
Kt TD MA MD DSc FRCP FMedSci

Former Professor of Neurology and
Dean of Medicine,
University of Newcastle upon Tyne, UK
Former President, World Federation of Neurology

Endorsement from the World Federation of Neurology

Neurological disorders affect as many as a billion people worldwide. They occur in all geographical regions and among all age groups and are a significant part of the global health burden. The spectre of their clinical manifestations is complex, from noncommunicable conditions such as cerebrovascular diseases, epilepsy, multiple sclerosis, Alzheimer and other dementias to deficiency disorders, brain and spinal injuries and communicable infectious diseases.

Many countries now face a double burden of a continuing high level of infections and also an increase in noncommunicable diseases. The panorama of disorders which the neurologist meets is different in various parts of the world. The progress in knowledge in clinical neurosciences is rapid and increasing. It is part of the mission of the World Federation of Neurology to encourage research and education, and it is a privilege to endorse *International Neurology*, a textbook with a true global authorship, written by neurologists who are familiar with the diagnostic problems in neurology, the treatment and the practical aspects of neurology in their part of the world.

Johan A. Aarli
President
World Federation of Neurology

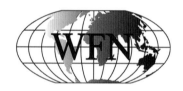

Preface

The idea for this text, *International Neurology: A Clinical Approach*, grew out of the involvement of the editors at the first two international neurology meetings held in Vietnam. It is commonplace to say that the world has contracted with international travel, a global economy, and the internet. With that change, which seems to increase with every year, there is an increased chance of travelers becoming ill when visiting or living in a foreign country and being seen by a physician who is from that country. In the instance of people from North America or Europe, they may be evaluated by a physician without significant educational experience with diseases that are not common in the country they are in at the time or perhaps they may give a somewhat different clinical presentation than the physician in the developing nation is used to observing. Even more of an issue is someone from a developing nation seeking care in a Western nation where a physician may have only read in medical school of a disease common in the nation of the visitor. These are problematic scenarios in neurologic diseases as much for any other specialty of medicine.

The authors and section editors were chosen from multiple countries to give yet another international component to the volume. In some instances chapters had authors from more than one country. When diseases have somewhat different presentations in different populations, the authors took this into account in their chapters, as well as considering differences in genetic, epidemiologic, demographic factors, and therapeutic approaches. In the latter instance, unproven treatments not based on evidence or scientific approaches were not included. Although chapters include etiology and pathogenesis, the emphasis is on clinical neurology, not basic science.

Finally, given our hope that this text would be widely available and affordable, particularly in emerging nations, and given the costs of medical publications in general, we limited the length of the chapters and bibliographies, which we chose to frame as suggested further reading lists, as well as colored figures, in an attempt to achieve these hopes.

We would like to thank the authors and sections editors for their efforts and contributions, as well as Gill Whitley, Elisabeth Dodds, Rob Blundell, and Martin Sugden of Wiley-Blackwell and Assumpta Sharon of Newgen Imaging Systems for their assistance and support in this project.

Robert P. Lisak
Daniel D. Truong
William M. Carroll
Roongroj Bhidayasiri

Chapter 1
Stroke: an overview

Christopher Li-Hsian Chen[1] and Chung Y. Hsu[2]
[1]National University of Singapore, Singapore
[2]China Medical University, Taichung, Taiwan

Stroke, whether of ischemic or haemorrhagic origin, is a major health burden globally. It is the second most common cause of death, the leading cause of disability in adults and the second most important cause of dementia worldwide. According to WHO figures, global stroke deaths were 5.8 million in 2005 and are projected to increase to 6.5 million in 2015 and 7.8 million in 2030.

Stroke mortality and incidence declined rapidly in developed countries during the 1980s and early 1990s, but this trend appears to have slowed recently. Despite the lack of reliable data on stroke statistics from several developing regions in the world, there are indications that the age-standardized mortality rate of stroke in developing nations may be substantially higher than in developed countries. The burden of stroke is accordingly greater due to larger populations in developing countries. Furthermore, as a result of epidemiological transition, rapid urbanization, and industrialization, many developing regions are exhibiting increased life expectancy, as well as a changing profile of risk factors for developing cardiovascular diseases. This may contribute to a looming epidemic of stroke in medium to low income nations as more of the population in these countries is at increased risk of cardiovascular diseases including stroke.

Fortunately, stroke is a preventable disease. Implementation of effective primary and secondary prevention strategies is likely to have an enormous effect in reducing the burden of stroke. Moreover, important advances have been made in the treatment of acute stroke and in improving recovery after stroke. Nevertheless, it is essential that more clinical studies be undertaken to understand the pathophysiology of stroke and clinical trials performed to provide a sound evidence base for effective interventions.

Of major importance are the differences in stroke etiology and pathology among various ethnic groups and the impact such differences may have on treatment strategies in selected patient populations in different parts of the world. Obvious examples are the higher incidence of intracerebral hemorrhage and intracranial atherosclerosis in non-white populations including people of Hispanic, Asian, and African origin.

Stroke is the most common disease managed by neurologists. Stroke patients constitute approximately two-thirds of the inpatient neurology ward in virtually every hospital with comprehensive neurology services in most countries around the world. With advances in evidence-based medicine, consensus on the diagnosis and treatment of selected types of strokes has gradually emerged across national boundaries. To present a global view on how practicing neurologists approach this most common neurological disorder, we have gathered a group of distinguished stroke neurologists from a number of esteemed institutions around the world to contribute chapters covering the clinical aspects of various types of stroke, including epidemiology, pathophysiology, clinical features, investigations, and treatment/management. We are grateful to these experts for their contributions and hope that readers will draw inspiration as well as knowledge from their efforts. We hope that collectively these chapters will serve as a pivotal vehicle for facilitating international exchange of expertise and experience to improve the quality of preventive and therapeutic measures for this important health care problem affecting every country in the world.

International Neurology: A Clinical Approach. Edited by Robert P. Lisak, Daniel D. Truong, William M. Carroll, and Roongroj Bhidayasiri. © 2009 Blackwell Publishing, ISBN: 978-1-4051-5738-4.

Chapter 2
Transient ischemic attacks

Samir H. Shah and Bruce Ovbiagele
UCLA School of Medicine, Los Angeles, USA

Introduction

A transient ischemic attack (TIA) is classically defined as a transient, sudden-onset neurological deficit due to brain or retinal ischemia that lasts less than 24 hours. TIAs usually involve focal loss of neurological function and typically are less than 1 hour in duration.

The 24-hour time cutoff is an historical, arbitrary time point that was chosen to distinguish patients who likely had no tissue injury from those who had brain infarction or stroke. Recent advances in neuroimaging have shown that many classically defined TIA patients have radiographic evidence of permanent ischemic brain injury. Reports on TIA patients evaluated with diffusion-weighted magnetic resonance imaging (MRI) suggest that up to 50% of classically defined TIA patients have corresponding evidence of bioenergetic failure or infarction and are more appropriately classified as stroke patients. Based on these diagnostic advances and the arbitrary nature of the 24-hour time cutoff, a group of cerebrovascular experts proposed a tissue-based, rather than time-based, definition of TIA in 2002 as follows: "Transient ischemic attack (TIA) is a brief episode of neurological dysfunction caused by focal brain or retinal ischemia, with clinical symptoms typically lasting less than one hour, and without evidence of acute infarction."

The importance of appropriate diagnosis and management of a TIA lies in its role as a harbinger of subsequent ischemic stroke, the latter of which carries a high risk of disability and death. We will outline in this chapter the epidemiology, clinical features, evaluation, and management of TIA patients.

Epidemiology

Determining the precise incidence and prevalence of TIA can be difficult. Many patients do not come to medical attention given the transitory nature of symptoms,

while for others historical details become blurred with time or the symptoms experienced are neurologically non-specific. In spite of these limitations several studies from around the world have examined the incidence and prevalence of classically defined TIAs.

A study in Rochester, Minnesota reported a crude age- and sex-adjusted incidence rate of 68 per 100000 persons per year for the years 1985 to 1989. TIA incidence increased with age, rising to 584 per 100000 persons for those aged 75–84. There were no obvious gender differences, although rates were slightly higher among men. Three-fourths of the TIAs in this study were attributable to the carotid circulation, the remainder to the vertebrobasilar circulation. Approximately 18% of the TIAs manifested as transient monocular blindness (amaurosis fugax). Lower age- and sex-adjusted incidence rates for TIA have been reported in other populations, from a low of 18 per 100000 persons per year from 1987 to 1988 in Novosibirsk, Russia, to a high of 37 per 100000 persons per year from 1970 to 1973 in Estonia. Studies from England, France, Japan, and Sweden revealed similar incidence rates. Lower incidence rates from around the world as compared to the Rochester study may reflect different methods of case ascertainment, since incidence rates for ischemic stroke are otherwise comparable. Overall, classically defined TIA incidence rates appear to have remained stable over time. It has been estimated that adopting a tissue-based definition of TIA in the United States (US) would reduce estimates of the annual incidence of TIA by 33%, from approximately 180000 to about 120000. Studies on TIA prevalence vary widely, but generally run between 1% and 6% and not surprisingly increase with age. The prevalence in the US is estimated to be 2.3%, which translates to approximately 5 million individuals.

Risk factors for TIA are similar to those of stroke. Well-established yet modifiable risk factors include hypertension, smoking, diabetes, atrial fibrillation, aortocervicocephalic atherosclerosis, and recent large myocardial infarction.

Comparisons across various studies indicate that the 90-day stroke risk is 10–20% after TIA, and that when these strokes occur they are disabling or fatal in up to

International Neurology: A Clinical Approach. Edited by Robert P. Lisak, Daniel D. Truong, William M. Carroll, and Roongroj Bhidayasiri. © 2009 Blackwell Publishing, ISBN: 978-1-4051-5738-4.

85% of patients. Unfortunately, available data suggest that an unacceptably high proportion of TIA patients (vs. stroke patients) are under-investigated and under-treated during the period of highest risk of stroke. Further delineating those TIA patients at highest stroke risk could facilitate stroke prevention. Some studies have shown that patients with transient monocular blindness have half the risk of stroke as patients with a hemispheric TIA, and patients with purely sensory symptoms likewise have a lower risk of stroke than patients with motor symptoms or aphasia. However, more recently prediction scores have been developed and validated to assist decision-making in the assessment of very early (within 48 hours) risk of stroke after TIA. The most robust of these is the ABCD score which is a seven point score based on five factors (age greater than or equal to 60 years (1 point); blood pressure greater than or equal to 140/90 mm Hg (1); clinical features: unilateral weakness (2), speech impairment without weakness (1); duration: greater than or equal to 60 minutes (2) or 10–59 minutes (1); and diabetes (1)). A high risk score (6–7) predicts a 8.1% 2-day risk of stroke, a moderate risk score (4–5) predicts a 4.1% 2-day risk of stroke, and a low risk score (0–3) predicts a 1% 2-day risk of stroke. Whether the score applies to populations outside of those studied remains to be determined.

Pathophysiology

The brain has little energy reserve and a massive metabolic rate that requires a constant supply of glucose and oxygen such that a reduction in cerebral blood flow can lead to neuronal dysfunction, which depending on the duration of insult manifests as a TIA or stroke.

The three major categories of TIA etiology are: (1) large artery atherosclerotic disease (LAA); (2) cardiac embolism; and (3) small penetrating vessel disease. There are many other less common causes of TIA (Table 2.1). LAA is probably the commonest precursor mechanism to TIA. The pathophysiology of LAA begins with atherosclerotic plaque formation and a perpetual inflammatory response, which eventually narrow cerebral vasculature, then coupled with platelet aggregation and subsequent thrombosis, can precipitate a TIA.

TIA pathophysiology is generally similar throughout the world, but it must be pointed out that with regard to LAA, intracranial atherostenosis is more common in Asians, Blacks, and Hispanics, compared to non-Hispanic whites, who are more likely to harbor extracranial large vessel disease. Furthermore, certain rare causes of TIA such as moyamoya disease and sickle cell disease are most common in Asian populations and persons of African descent respectively.

Table 2.1 Less common etiologies of transient ischemic attacks.

Thrombocytosis/polycythemia
Hypoperfusion
Arterial dissection
Patent foramen ovale or other right to left shunt
Atrial myxoma or other cardiac tumor
Antiphospholipid antibody syndrome or other hypercoagulable state
Subacute bacterial endocarditis
Non-bacterial thrombotic endocarditis
Hyperviscosity
Temporal arteritis or other type of vasculitis
Amphetamine or cocaine use
Moyamoya disease
CADASIL
MELAS
Sickle-cell disease
Fabry's disease
Homocystinuria

CADASIL: cerebral autosomal dominant arteriopathy with subcortical infarcts and leukoencephalopathy; MELAS: mitochondrial myopathy, encephalopathy, lactic acidosis, and stroke.

Table 2.2 Differential diagnostic possibilities for transient ischemic attacks.

Partial seizure
Migraine
Labyrinthitis/neuronitis
Transient global amnesia
Hypoglycemia
Hyponatremia
Severe postural hypotension
Arrhythmia
Cervical disk disease
Carpal tunnel syndrome
Cerebral venous thrombosis
Brain tumor
Subdural hematoma
Anxiety
Conversion disorder

Clinical features

TIAs can be challenging to diagnose conclusively because the symptoms are transient, often lasting less than 10 minutes, with considerable overlap of symptoms with non-ischemic etiologies (Table 2.2).

Virtually any neurologic symptom or sign is possible with a TIA depending on the site of arterial occlusion and on other factors including patient handedness, collateral blood supply, and vascular anatomic variation. Distinguishing characteristics of a TIA include: (1) abruptness; (2) focality (localization to a single vascular territory); (3) negative symptoms (weakness or numbness instead of aura and/or shaking); and (4) brevity (60% last less than 1 hour).

Transient monocular vision loss is often a hallmark of internal carotid artery disease. Although a history of a curtain or shade overcoming vision is classical for an ischemic basis to transient monocular vision loss, it is more common to have sudden monocular loss of vision that lasts 1–10 minutes, sometimes accompanied by aphasia and dysarthria. A phenomenon called "limb shaking TIA" can be mistaken for seizure activity. It occurs in patients with severe internal carotid stenosis manifesting as recurrent episodes of involuntary, irregular shaking or wavering movements of the contralateral arm or leg. Yet another TIA phenomenon named "spectacular shrinking deficit" results when an embolus lodges in the distal internal carotid artery or the proximal middle cerebral artery. Initially the patient has a full hemispheric syndrome with weakness, sensory loss, hemianopia, and aphasia or neglect. The hemiparesis and then the other deficits usually resolve within 4 hours as the embolus migrates distally.

The most common transient symptom of vertebral artery disease is vertigo, but it is usually accompanied by other symptoms such as dysarthria, diplopia, and headache. Isolated vertigo is a rare cause of TIA and if it is the only symptom usually leads to stroke within 3 weeks. Recurrent spells of isolated vertigo of greater than 6 weeks duration is unlikely to be due to cerebrovascular disease. Bilateral stenosis of the vertebral arteries usually leads to multiple stereotyped TIAs. Basilar artery disease leads to symptoms and signs similar to vertebral artery TIAs with the addition of bilateral weakness or weakness alternating between different limbs in different attacks. Posterior cerebral artery TIAs can lead to graying or darkening of vision on one side. Flashing lights and red and white lights have also been reported with posterior cerebral artery TIAs, but in contrast to migraine, the photopsias with ischemia are brief, in the order of 30 seconds or less compared to 20 minutes or more in patients with migraine. Small vessel TIAs generally present with pure motor or pure sensory symptoms without cortical signs such as aphasia. Small vessel TIAs are stereotyped. Compared to TIAs from large vessel disease, small vessel TIAs present with more attacks, have a longer duration of neurological deficit during each attack, and a shorter latency between attack and stroke. The phenomenon called "capsular warning syndrome" is used to describe repetitive, stereotyped attacks of hemiparesis due to ischemia affecting the internal capsule irrigated by small penetrating arteries that eventually leads to stroke. On rare occasions, capsular warning syndrome may be caused by large vessel diseases.

Investigations

Timeliness and extent of management for the TIA patient differs throughout the world. A major point of contention is whether a TIA patient should be hospitalized or managed on an outpatient basis. Risk stratification using tools such as the ABCD score may facilitate this decision, but a few studies have suggested that even individuals with low or moderate risk scores on these clinical scales can go on to have early stroke and should be evaluated urgently.

Current consensus guidelines on the evaluation and management of TIA recommend that patients who have had a TIA in the past 24–48 hours should be strongly considered for hospital admission to facilitate lytic therapy or other therapies should the symptoms recur and to facilitate prompt evaluation and secondary preventative therapies. If the patient cannot be admitted, speed is the key. Indeed, a recent population-based study found that urgent outpatient evaluation and management of TIA patients (i.e., clinic assessment and prescription of first treatment of no more than 1 day after initial presentation) was associated with a significant reduction in the 90-day stroke risk from 10.3% to 2.1%. Patients should have access to expedited ambulatory care and be educated on the need to return for emergency care should symptoms return. Management focus of the TIA evaluation should be on: (1) determining the etiology of the event so that appropriate stroke prevention measures may be implemented; and (2) excluding TIA mimics.

The initial evaluation should include a full blood count, serum electrolytes and creatinine, fasting blood glucose and lipids, and an electrocardiogram. Other laboratory studies may be undertaken based on the history and other clinical features. Brain imaging with computed tomography (CT) or MRI should be carried out to exclude the rare possibilities of subdural hematoma, tumor, or other TIA mimics. All patients should have Doppler ultrasonography of the neck or other vascular imaging of the extracranial vasculature with CT, MRI, or conventional angiography to assess for internal carotid artery disease. All patients in whom cardiac embolism is a possibility should have a transthoracic echocardiogram. Patients in whom a right to left shunt is considered or who do not have a clear mechanism of TIA after the above evaluation should have a transesophageal echocardiogram.

Treatment/management

The management of a TIA rests on the underlying pathophysiologic mechanism. All patients with a non-cardioembolic cause of TIA should be treated immediately and long term with an antiplatelet agent. Aspirin (30–325 mg/day) is the first-line antiplatelet agent for stroke prevention after a diagnosis of TIA has been made. Clopidogrel (75 mg/day) is an alternative antiplatelet agent for those patients who cannot tolerate aspirin. Aspirin (50 mg/day) combined with sustained release dipyridamole (200 mg twice daily) may be more efficacious for vascular risk reduction compared to aspirin alone. Patients who are thought to have a high-risk cardioembolic cause of TIA (e.g., atrial fibrillation) should be treated with long-term warfarin therapy. Aspirin should be used if anticoagulation is contraindicated.

All patients with hemispheric TIA and extracranial internal carotid artery stenosis between 70% and 99% should be treated with carotid endarterectomy by an experienced surgeon without delay, preferably within 2 weeks of the TIA. Patients with transient monocular blindness or internal carotid artery stenosis between 50% and 69% may also benefit from surgery, depending on other vascular risk factors, surgical complication rates, and available medical treatments. Angioplasty and stenting of the internal carotid artery may be considered if surgery is not available or is contraindicated.

TIA patients should be evaluated for cardiovascular risk factors and managed appropriately to prevent further vascular events. Patients with an atherothromboembolic cause of TIA and no contraindications should be: (1) treated with a statin medication for a goal LDL of less than 100 mg/dl; (2) evaluated for diabetes and treated accordingly to maintain normoglycemia; and (3) started on blood pressure-lowering medication to maintain blood pressure below 130/80 mm Hg. Most patients with hypertension and an atherothromboembolic cause of TIA should have blood pressure controlled. The key is blood pressure lowering, and appropriate blood pressure medication(s) should be started to meet goal levels. All smokers should be encouraged to stop, and appropriate lifestyle modification advice including regular exercise, diet counseling, and weight loss should be given.

A TIA should sound an alarm for the medical enterprise, signaling the need for prompt evaluation and treatment to reduce future vascular risk. Education of the medical community and public at large about the symptoms, signs, and appropriate management of this condition could help reduce stroke risk and mitigate the immense burden of cerebrovascular disease on society.

Further reading

Chaturvedi S, Levine SR. *Transient Ischemic Attacks*. Oxford: Futura, Blackwell Publishing; 2004.

Giles MF, Rothwell PM. Risk of stroke early after transient ischaemic attack: a systematic review and meta-analysis. *Lancet Neurol* 2007; 6: 1063–72.

Johnston SC, Nguyen-Huynh NM, Schwarz ME, *et al*. National stroke association guidelines for the management of transient ischemic attacks. *Ann Neurol* 2006; 60: 301–13.

Johnston SC, Rothwell PM, Nguyen-Huynh NM, *et al*. Validation and refinement of scores to predict very early stroke risk after transient ischaemic attack. *Lancet* 2007; 369: 283–92.

Ovbiagele B. The emergency department: first line of defense in preventing secondary stroke. *Acad Emerg Med* 2006; 13: 215–22.

Rothwell PM, Giles MF, Chandratheva A, *et al*. Effect of urgent treatment of transient ischaemic attack and minor stroke on early recurrent stroke (EXPRESS study): a prospective population-based sequential comparison. *Lancet* 2007; 370: 1432–42.

Chapter 3
Atherothrombotic disease

Nijasri C. Suwanwela
Chulalongkorn University, Bangkok, Thailand

Introduction

Atherosclerosis is a systemic disease that may involve various vascular beds. Atherothrombotic stroke occurs when the atheromatous process forms a thrombus and either occludes or narrows the lumen to produce low-flow or embolic stroke. Although atherosclerosis is a generalized condition involving various vascular beds, an atherosclerotic plaque tends to be a strategically focal process at the arterial branch points and bifurcations. For the arteries supplying the brain, common sites of atherosclerosis include carotid bifurcation in the neck, proximal part of intracranial arteries and carotid siphon, proximal and distal parts of the vertebral artery, and ascending aorta.

Atherosclerosis of extracranial arteries in the neck

Disease of the carotid arteries in the neck, especially at the carotid bifurcation and origin of the internal carotid artery, is very common among Caucasians. The risk of stroke depends on the degree of stenosis as well as the atherosclerotic plaque characteristics. More severe stenosis (>70%) and plaque with evidence of lipid core, intraplaque hemorrhage, or ulceration carry greater risk of ischemic stroke in the ipsilateral cerebral hemisphere.

Atherosclerosis of the intracranial arteries

Atherosclerosis of the intracranial arteries is more prevalent in Asians, blacks and Hispanics. Studies from Asia demonstrate that intracranial atherosclerosis accounts for approximately one-fourth of all ischemic strokes. The explanation for this racial difference is still unclear. The common sites of intracranial atherosclerosis are the proximal part of the middle cerebral artery, carotid siphon, midbasilar artery, and distal vertebral artery, and proximal parts of the anterior and posterior cerebral arteries.

International Neurology: A Clinical Approach. Edited by Robert P. Lisak, Daniel D. Truong, William M. Carroll, and Roongroj Bhidayasiri. © 2009 Blackwell Publishing, ISBN: 978-1-4051-5738-4.

Atherosclerosis of the ascending aorta

Atherosclerosis of the ascending aorta, especially when the plaque thickness is greater than 4 mm, has been shown to correlate with embolic stoke.

Epidemiology

Atherosclerosis is one of the major causes of ischemic stroke worldwide. Among patients presenting with acute ischemic stroke, atherosclerosis of the large vessels accounts for 20–45% of cases. Classical risk factors of atherosclerosis include advanced age, hypertension, diabetes, dyslipidemia, and smoking.

Pathophysiology and clinical features

Clinical manifestations of stroke in patients with atherosclerosis depend on the pathophysiology, which can be classified into three main categories.

Artery-to-artery embolism. This is a major mechanism of stroke among patients with atherosclerosis in the extracranial carotid artery and ascending aorta but probably of lesser pathophysiological significance with intracranial diseases. Embolic stroke occurs when a portion of thrombus that originates in the stenotic arteries, especially with irregular surface, dislodges and travels into distal arteries.

Clinically, patients with extracranial carotid stenosis with artery-to-artery embolism present with ischemic stroke in the cortical and subcortical areas of the anterior circulation, especially in the middle cerebral artery territory. Non-stereotyped repetitive transient ischemic attack (TIA) involving the same hemisphere and transient monocular blindness are common. In patients with intracranial atherosclerosis with distal embolism, ischemic stroke with fluctuating or progressive symptoms can be found. Emboli from atherosclerosis in the posterior circulation can occlude the branches of the vertebral and basilar arteries. The embolism may travel to the distal end or top of the basilar artery causing thalamic, midbrain, occipital lobe, and sometimes cerebellar infarction. Frequently, multiple small emboli that travel to distal arteries are asymptomatic. They can only be demonstrated by diffusion-weighted magnetic resonance imaging (MRI) as small bright dots or by transcranial Doppler ultrasound detection for microembolic signals.

Low-flow state secondary to severe arterial stenosis or occlusion: this mechanism of stroke and TIA is usually found in patients with severe arterial stenosis or occlusion with inadequate distal perfusion and insufficient collateral circulation. Stroke or TIA usually occurs in the distal territories or borderzone areas between the major cerebral arteries and may by aggravated by systemic hypoperfusion. Borderzone cerebral infarction is detailed in a separate chapter in this textbook. Although uncommon, very severe extracranial carotid stenosis can cause low-flow TIA with stereotypic focal limb weakness and sometimes limb shaking episodes resembling focal seizure. Low-flow stroke in patients with intracranial atherosclerosis may present with progressive or fluctuating symptoms in the affected vascular territory.

Occlusion of the perforating arteries due to atherosclerotic plaque: in patients with atherosclerosis of the intracranial arteries, the plaque may occlude the orifice of the perforating arteries, causing infarction in the deep areas of the brain such as the basal ganglia in middle cerebral artery disease and the pons and midbrain in basilar atherosclerosis. The clinical syndrome of these patients may resemble lacunar infarction, but the areas of infarction on brain imaging are usually larger.

Investigations

Diagnosis of atherosclerosis can be performed by imaging the arterial wall. Ultrasonogaphy is the most widely available non-invasive method to visualize the vascular wall of the neck arteries and has been used as a screening test for extracranial carotid disease. Using B-mode and duplex ultrasound, plaque components and surface as well as the degree of stenosis can be determined. Transesophageal echocardiogram is another ultrasound technique used for evaluation of the ascending aorta as a source of embolic stroke. Recently, high resolution MRI and multidetector computed tomography (CT) angiography have also been used to visualize the arterial wall.

In some patients, especially those with atherosclerosis of smaller arteries where details of the arterial wall cannot be visualized, diagnosis can be made by the specific site of stenotic lesions together with the presence of atherosclerotic risk factors. For this purpose, magnetic resonance angiography and CT angiography are generally used.

Using these vascular imaging techniques, localization, degree of stenosis, and collateral circulation can be evaluated. Currently, cerebral angiography should only be performed in cases with an inconclusive result from non-invasive studies and in those for whom endotravascular procedures are indicated.

Management

The management of acute ischemic stroke due to large vessel atherothrombosis consists of rapidly establishing the pathophysiology of the arterial lesion responsible for the ischemia, as well as the location and extent of infarct. In the acute phase of stroke, thrombolysis with tissue plasminogen activator (tPA) should be given in eligible patients within 4.5 hours of stroke onset. Antiplatelet therapy, most commonly with aspirin, should be given as early as possible for possible acute therapeutic effects and more importantly for secondary prevention of recurrent stroke. Anticoagulants have been used in patients with large vessel atherosclerosis who had progressive or unstable neurological symptoms. The efficacy of anticoagulants, however, has not been established based on randomized controlled trials. Special consideration must be paid to prevention of recurrent events since it has been shown that patients with large vessel atherosclerosis have poorer prognosis than those with other types of ischemic stroke. Moreover, these patients tend to have greater risk of major coronary events and vascular death. Lifestyle modification, risk factor management, and medical treatment including long-term antiplatelet therapy can reduce the risk of recurrent stroke. Moreover, prevention of further atherosclerotic plaque progression and possibly regression has been observed in patients treated with angiotensin converting enzyme inhibitors, angiotensin receptor blockers, and 3-hydroxy-3-methylglutaryl-coenzyme A (HMG-CoA) reductase inhibitors.

In patients with significant stenosis of the extracranial internal carotid artery with evidence of microemboli on transcranial ultrasound monitoring, the combination of aspirin and clopidogrel has been shown to reduce the number of emboli as well as recurrent TIA and stroke during the early phase. However, for long-term secondary prevention, revascularization procedures such as endarterectomy or angioplasty and stenting have been demonstrated to be superior to medical treatment.

For patients with intracranial atherosclerosis, there is a trend for increasing utilization of angioplasty with and without stenting. However, the procedure is technically challenging and higher risk. Valid randomized trials are needed to establish the efficacy of intracranial angioplasty and stenting.

Further reading

Fisher M, Paganini-Hill A, Martin A, *et al*. Carotid plaque pathology: thrombosis, ulceration, and stroke pathogenesis. *Stroke* 2005; 36(2): 253–7.

Lee DK, Kim JS, Kwon SU, Yoo SH, Kang DW. Lesion patterns and stroke mechanism in atherosclerotic middle cerebral artery disease: early diffusion-weighted imaging study. *Stroke* 2005; 36(12): 2583–8.

Meyers PM, Schumacher HC, Tanji K, Higashida RT, Caplan LR. Use of stents to treat intracranial cerebrovascular disease. *Annu Rev Med* 2007; 58: 107–22.

Suwanwela N, Koroshetz WJ. Acute ischemic stroke: overview of recent therapeutic developments. *Annu Rev Med* 2007; 58: 89–106.

Suwanwela NC, Chutinet A. Risk factors for atherosclerosis of cervicocerebral arteries: intracranial versus extracranial. *Neuroepidemiology* 2003; 22(1): 37–40.

Chapter 4
Occlusive disease of small penetrating arteries

Takeshi Iwanaga[1], Hock L. Teoh[1], Jorge A. Zavala[1], and Geoffrey A. Donnan[1,2]
[1]National Stroke Research Institute, Austin Health, Heidelberg, Australia
[2]University of Melbourne, Heidelberg, Australia

Introduction

Durand-Fardel named as "lacunes" small cavities seen in the core of cerebral infarcts and as "état ciblé" perivascular space dilatation. Fisher studied small, deep infarcts and described the classical lacunar syndromes as the result of penetrating artery occlusion. Most lacunar infarcts occur within the lenticulostriate, thalamoperforaters, and pontine paramedian arterial territories. Lacunar infarcts are usually due to occlusion of a single penetrating artery.

Epidemiology

In hospital-based series, the proportion of lacunar syndrome ranges from 14% to 24% of all ischemic strokes. In community-based incidence studies, lacunar strokes represent a similar proportion of all strokes except in Japan where they may form up to 50% of ischemic strokes (Table 4.1).

Hypertension is the most important modifiable risk factor for ischemic stroke, being present in more than half of patients. The risk of lacunar infarction is increased five- to nine-fold in hypertensives, which is not unexpected since microatheroma and lipohyalinosis are linked to hypertension (see below).

There is an increased risk of about two- to three-fold of lacunar stroke in diabetics. Smoking is a significant risk factor for lacunar strokes, with some suggestion that it may play a more important role as a risk factor in lacunar strokes than in other forms of ischemic stroke. Heart disease, including ischemic heart disease (IHD), is a risk factor for ischemic stroke, but may be less so for lacunar syndromes.

Pathophysiology

Lacunar infarcts occur in the territory of penetrating arteries. Table 4.2 shows their branches and territories.

Table 4.1 Incidence of lacunar stroke in community-based studies.

Study		Total number of ischemic strokes	Lacunar ischemic stroke	Incidence of lacunar stroke (per 100 000 persons per year)
South Alabama (1984)		138	20 (14.5%)	20
Oxfordshire (1991)		545	133 (24.4%)	31.7
Italy (1989)		90	26 (28.9%)	53.0
Mayo Clinic (1991)		1382	159 (11.5%)	13.4
Australia (1993)		259	25 (9.7%)	12.0
Norrving *et al.* (1991)		—	180 (12.6%)	26.6
Hisayama (2000)	M	144	81 (56.3%)	—
	F	154	86 (55.8%)	—

Fisher demonstrated in autopsy studies that lacunar infarcts are caused by two forms of arteriopathy: lipohyalinosis and microatheroma. Lipohyalinosis is a destructive small lesion in penetrating arteries (40–200 μm in diameter) characterized by fibrinoid necrosis, loss of normal wall structure, and collagenous sclerosis. It probably accounts for many of the asymptomatic smaller lacunes. Microatheroma (200–800 μm in diameter) can lead to occlusive thrombus and infarcts that tend to be larger than those associated with lipohyalinosis (5 mm or more in diameter) and are usually symptomatic (Plate 4.1).

Although the mechanism of lacunar infarction is traditionally held to be *in situ* small vessel disease, there is some evidence of an embolic causation in a small proportion of cases. Indeed, aortic arch atheroma has been demonstrated to be a risk factor for lacunar infarction. Whether this is a reflection of diffuse cardiovascular atheromatous load rather than an embolic source is uncertain.

Clinical features

Traditionally, lacunar infarction has been associated with five clinical syndromes. Pure motor hemiparesis is the

International Neurology: A Clinical Approach. Edited by Robert P. Lisak, Daniel D. Truong, William M. Carroll, and Roongroj Bhidayasiri. © 2009 Blackwell Publishing, ISBN: 978-1-4051-5738-4.

Table 4.2 Penetrating arteries, their branches and regions supplied.

Penetrating artery	Branch	Regions supplied
Lenticulostriate	Medial lenticulostriate artery	Lateral globus pallidus, medial putamen
	Lateral lenticulostriate artery	Lateral putamen, external capsule, upper internal capsule, corona radiata
Thalamoperforating	Tuberothalamic artery	Anteromedial and anterolateral thalamus
	Paramedian artery	Posteromedial thalamus
	Thalamogeniculate artery	Ventrolateral thalamus
	Posterior choroidal artery	Pulvinar and posterior thalamus
Paramedian	—	Basis pons, ventral part of tegmentum

most common syndrome (about 50% of all cases) and involves complete or incomplete facial, arm, and leg paresis. The most common site of infarction is the posterior limb of the internal capsule. Other sites are the corona radiata, pons, and medial medulla. Sensorimotor stroke is the second most common lacunar syndrome (about 20%). The combination of ipsilateral hemiparasis and hemihypoasthesia is the main distinguishing feature. The most common site is the posterior limb of the internal capsule. Pure sensory stroke is characterized by face, arm, and leg numbness on one side, with absence of weakness and higher cortical dysfunction. In 10% of cases the symptoms may be transient. The most common site of infarction is the thalamus. Ataxic hemiparesis encompasses hemiparesis combined with an ipsilateral cerebellar-like ataxia. Common infarct sites are the pons and internal capsule. Facial weakness, severe dysarthria, and dysphagia combined with mild weakness and hand clumsiness are the features of the dysarthria-clumsy hand syndrome. The site of infarction is frequently the internal capsule. Subcortical transient ischemic attacks (TIAs) comprised of transient lacunar syndromes occur in brief clusters (the "capsular warning syndrome"), and may evolve to capsular infarction.

In general, lacunar infarction carries a good prognosis. In contrast to other strokes, functional disability is relatively mild. The 5-year survival rate is over 80% and 5-year stroke-free survival rates are over 60%. Predictors of recurrent stroke are age, degree of neurological dysfunction, functional disability, diabetes mellitus, and leukoaraiosis.

Although lacunar infarcts are small, cognitive function may be affected. Indeed, cognitive function is intact in the acute phase, but may progressively decline over the long term. Cognitive impairment as measured by performance on the Mini Mental State Examination (MMSE); 1 year after stroke cognitive impairment may be 5%, rising to 11% after 3 years. Such cognitive impairment often develops in relation to recurrent stroke and presence of leukoaraiosis.

Investigations

Computed tomography (CT) is the most widely used neuroimaging diagnostic method in the acute setting. However, CT often fails to reveal lesions in the first 48 hours or those that are smaller than 10 mm. Magnetic resonance imaging (MRI) has been shown to be more sensitive than CT in the diagnosis of strokes, particularly for small, deep infarcts. Hence, MRI is the preferred method, either in the acute setting or in patient follow-up (Figure 4.1).

Treatment/management

No studies specifically address lacunar stroke. However, lacunar stroke patients represent a significant proportion of subjects in most landmark trials.

Acute stroke therapy
In the meta-analysis of large trials (IST, CAST), early aspirin significantly reduced the risk of recurrent ischemic stroke (including lacunar stroke), accompanied by a minor increase in the risk of hemorrahagic stroke or hemorrhagic transformation. Aspirin also reduces overall risk of death or dependency. Thrombolysis with intravenous recombinant tissue plasminogen activator (r-tPA) within 3 hours improves the overall clinical outcome of ischemic stroke, including lacunar strokes.

Secondary prevention
Lacunar stroke patients are often included in secondary prevention trials because their level of impairment is usually low. Indeed, they are often over-represented in these trials (this is known as "lacunarization" of secondary prevention trials). Hence, secondary prevention of stroke with antiplatelet agents (aspirin, clopidgrel,

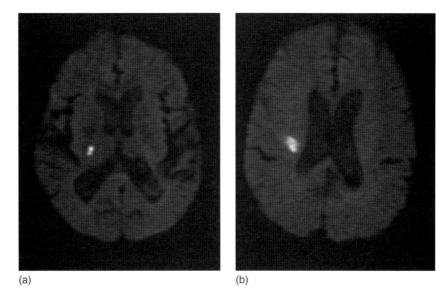

(a)   (b)

Figure 4.1 Diffusion-weighted images (DWI) showing lacunar infarcts (a) in the posterior limb of the right internal capsule and (b) in the right corona radiate.

aspirin plus dipyridamole), by blood pressure lowering with perindopril and indapamide or ramipril, and cholesterol lowering with atorvastatin is most likely effective for lacunar strokes as well as for ischaemic stroke overall. Trials are underway to more specifically study the lacunar stroke subset (SPS3).

Further reading

Donnan G, Norrving B, Bamford J, Bogousslavsky J. *Subcortical Stroke*, 2nd ed. Oxford: Oxford University Press; 2002.

Fisher CM. Lacunar strokes and infarcts: a review. *Neurology* 1982; 32: 871–6.

Chapter 5
Binswanger's disease

Dean A. Le[1] and Ferdinando S. Buonanno[2]
[1]Saddleback Memorial Medical Center, Laguna Hills, USA
[2]Massachusetts General Hospital and Harvard Medical School, Boston, USA

Introduction

In 1894 Professor Otto Binswanger (1852–1929) first described eight patients with a progressive dementia associated with episodic transient ischemic attacks and strokes. This neurological condition was subsequently called Binswanger's disease (or Binswanger's encephalopathy), and it represents one of the most common types of vascular dementia. In the Further Reading we also refer readers to two other excellent reviews of this neurological condition.

Epidemiology

The onset of Binswanger's disease is commonly after age 50, with males and females being affected equally. Although the prevalence of the disease is not known, the advance of neuroimaging techniques, especially brain magnetic resonance imaging (MRI) which demonstrates frequently the appearance of periventricular white matter lesions in demented patients, suggests that Binswanger's disease is more common than previously thought.

Pathophysiology

Hypertension and old age are likely risk factors. It is believed that the disease is caused by chronic cerebral hypoperfusion associated with arteriosclerosis of the deep penetrating arteries (cerebral medullary arteries) in the white matter. In addition, breakdown of the blood–brain barrier of these small vessels occurs and is associated with extravasation of proteases, complements, immunoglobulins, and cytokines into the perivascular parenchymal space. Consequently diffuse degeneration of white matter myelin and axons ensues.

Genetic factors may play a role in some patients with Binswanger's disease. In a study of Hungarian patients with the disease, there was an increased association of the disease with mutation of the methylenetetrahydrofolate reductase gene (MTHFR C677T) and with the presence of certain genotypes including the angiotensin-converting enzyme (ACE) D/D and APO E2/2 and APO E2/3 genotypes. Furthermore, some may argue that CADASIL (cerebral autosomal dominant arteriopathy with subcortical infarcts) is a familial form of Binswanger's disease with mutations in the *Notch3* gene located in chromosome 19q12.

The common pathological findings of Binswanger's disease are atrophy of the white matter, enlarged ventricles, multiple lacunar infarcts in the white matter and basal ganglia, loss of subcortical myelin (sparing the U fibers) and axons, and arteriosclerosis with increased arteriolar stiffness of the cerebral medullary vessels. These pathologic findings are correlated radiographically with brain MRI as periventricular white matter hyperintensities (under T2 and FLAIR sequence) or by brain computed tomography (CT) as periventricular white matter low density. These radiographic lesions, when extensive, are also called leukoaraiosis.

Clinical features

The dementia in patients with Binswanger's disease takes a slow but steadily progressive course over the years. These patients present with deficits in attention, execution, planning, information processing, conceptual reasoning, and memory function. They can be depressed, apathetic, or abulic. They also have other neurological signs including gait imbalance (parkinsonian gait), urinary incontinence, focal weakness, and pseudobulbar palsy.

Differential diagnosis should include normal pressure hydrocephalus, other types of multi-infarct dementia, CADASIL, and post-anoxic encephalopathy.

Treatment/management

At the present time, treatment for Binswanger's disease includes appropriate blood pressure control, antiplatelet therapy (aspirin, aspirin plus dipyridamole, or clopidogrel),

International Neurology: A Clinical Approach. Edited by Robert P. Lisak, Daniel D. Truong, William M. Carroll, and Roongroj Bhidayasiri. © 2009 Blackwell Publishing, ISBN: 978-1-4051-5738-4.

and dementia drugs including memantine, donepezil, galantamine, and other cholinesterase inhibitors. There have also been anecdotal reports of improvement of Binswanger's disease with ventriculoperitoneal shunt placement.

Further reading

Binswanger O. Die Abgrenzung der allgemeinen progressiven Paralyse, I–III. *Berl Klin Wochenschr* 1894; 49: 1103–5, 1137–9, 1180–6.

Fisher, CM. Binswanger's encephalopathy: a review. *J Neurol* 1989; 236: 65–79.

Patoni L, Garcia J. The significance of cerebral white matter abnormalities 100 years after Binswanger's report. *Stroke* 1995; 26: 1293–301.

Szolnoki Z, Somogyvari F, Kondacs A, *et al*. Evaluation of the roles of common genetic mutation in leukoaraiosis. *Acta Neurol Scand* 2001: 104: 281–7.

Chapter 6
Brain embolism

Bernard P.L. Chan[1] and Chung Y. Hsu[2]
[1]National University Hospital, Singapore
[2]China Medical University, Taichung, Taiwan

Introduction

Although the heart has traditionally been regarded as the major source of brain embolism, large artery disease (in the aortic arch, neck, and intracranial arteries) frequently results in artery-to-artery embolism. A new cause of brain embolism has emerged with increasing application of endovascular procedures for preventing or treating cerebrovascular diseases. This chapter focuses on brain embolism of cardiac origin, using the term cardiac embolism hereafter. Reference to other causes will be made only when comparison among different causes is deemed necessary.

Epidemiology

Cardiac embolism has consistently been noted to be a major cause of stroke in stroke registries of different countries around the world. While the incidence varies from country to country, cardiac embolism constitutes approximately one-quarter of all strokes. There is a consistent trend for the frequency of cardiac embolism to be higher among stroke patients of younger age. For age 45 and under, up to half of all strokes could be ascribed to cardiac embolism.

Pathophysiology

Established causes of cardiac embolism are listed in Table 6.1. Atrial fibrillation (AF) is the most common cause of cardiac embolism and the leading cause of ischemic stroke in the elderly population, with increasing prevalence as age advances. In developing countries, rheumatic mitral valve stenosis remains important. Cardiomyopathy resulting from Chagas' disease is prevalent in Latin America, whereas endomyocardial fibrosis

Table 6.1 Causes of cardiac embolism.

Atrial
Atrial fibrillation
Atrial flutter
Sick-sinus syndrome
Patent foramen ovale ± atrial septal aneurysm

Valvular
Prosthetic valve
Rheumatic mitral valve stenosis
Infective endocarditis
Non-bacterial thrombotic endocarditis

Ventricular
Recent myocardial infarction
Dilated cardiomyopathy/congestive heart failure
Akinetic/dyskinetic segment
Chagas' disease
Endomyocardial fibrosis/hypereosinophilic syndrome
Stress/Takotsubo cardiomyopathy
Left ventricular non-compaction

Cardiac tumors
Atrial myxoma
Papillary fibroelastoma

Iatrogenic
Cardiac surgery
Diagnostic/interventional cardiac catheterization
Intra-aortic balloon counter-pulsation
Left ventricular assist device
Inadvertent left heart pacing

related to hypereosinophilia with underlying helminthic infections is common in tropical regions of Africa. In developed countries, coronary artery disease and related cardiac surgeries are significant causes of cardiac embolism. Among young stroke patients without an established etiology (cryptogenic stroke), paradoxical embolization through patent foramen ovale (PFO) has been considered to be the cause in 40–56% of patients.

Clinical features

Presentation of cardiac embolism is frequently reported to be an abrupt onset with the worst deficit at outset followed by improvement thereafter. "Spectacular

International Neurology: A Clinical Approach. Edited by Robert P. Lisak, Daniel D. Truong, William M. Carroll, and Roongroj Bhidayasiri. © 2009 Blackwell Publishing, ISBN: 978-1-4051-5738-4.

shrinking deficit" is occasionally seen in cardiac embolism, when occlusion of a large cerebral artery (e.g., the proximal middle cerebral artery) undergoes spontaneous early recannalization, resulting in dramatic clinical improvement. However, the clinical course of embolic events does not always follow this pattern. It is not reliable to differentiate embolic strokes from thrombotic ones based on clinical course. The patient profile may be more helpful in guiding the approach toward the diagnosis of cardiac embolism. Patients with large cervicocerebral vessel diseases tend to be older, harbor multiple traditional risk factors, or have preceding transient ischemic attacks (TIAs) in the absence of overt heart disease. Elderly people with strokes secondary to cardiac embolism are likely to have clinically evident cardiac ailments including AF or coronary artery disease. However, the coexistence of risk factors for both thrombotic and embolic strokes is not rare in the elderly. Young stroke patients without apparent risk factors should raise a high index of suspicion of cardiac embolism.

Neurological symptoms and signs attributed to neuroanatomical sites have been used to predict the likelihood of cardiac embolism. However, as described below, where emboli of cardiac origin may lodge is not predictable. A traditional belief that emboli tend to cause superficial cortical branch occlusion should be balanced by the neuroimaging observations that cardiac emboli may also end in the deep penetrating cerebral arteries. In general, the middle cerebral artery and its branches carry a substantially larger load of emboli than the anterior cerebral artery or posterior circulation because of the proportion of blood flowing into the respective vascular beds. Nevertheless, embolic events causing stroke in the vertebrobasilar territory are not uncommon.

Investigations

Computed tomography (CT) and magnetic resonance imaging (MRI) are widely used to localize the ischemic sites. Like clinical presentation, neuroimaging may not be always reliable for differentiating embolic from thrombotic stroke. For instance, large vessel disease such as internal carotid artery stenosis may result in smaller cortical infarcts secondary to artery-to-artery embolism, mimicking cardiac embolism, while an embolus of cardiac origin may occlude the large proximal cerebral artery to cause a large territorial infarct. Unilateral infarcts in the watershed territories or borderzones are usually associated with hypoperfusion with ipsilateral internal carotid artery (ICA) occlusion. Diffusion-weighted MRI (DWI) can better depict the acute infarcts, and may implicate the heart or the aortic arch as the embolic source by revealing multiple infarcts in different vascular territories (Figure 6.1).

As clinical and radiological features are not specific, and multiple potential stroke etiologies and embolic sources may co-exist in individual patients, study of the neck and intracranial arteries is recommended in all ischemic stroke patients by duplex ultrasonography and transcranial Doppler (TCD), CT, or MR angiography, including those suspected of cardiac embolism.

Routine transthoracic echocardiography (TTE) is associated with a low yield, and may be omitted in selected

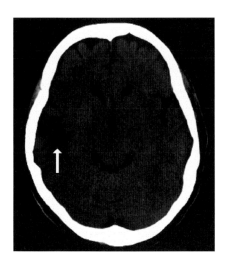 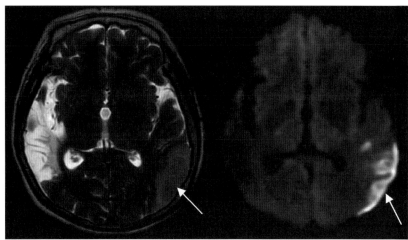

Figure 6.1 A 64-year-old woman in AF presented with acute cortical deafness but recovered over 2 months. CT of the brain (left) on admission showed an old right temporal infarct. T2 MRI (middle) 24 hours after admission revealed an additional recent left temporal infarct, confirmed by DWI (right). Bilateral cortical infarcts are typical of a cardiac source of embolism. Infarct in the territory of the posterior division of the MCA is also suggestive of embolism from a proximal source due to its more direct course from the proximal MCA. As long-term cortical deafness usually requires bilateral damages to the primary auditory cortices, sparing of the left primary auditory cortex likely accounted for the clinical recovery in this patient.

patients with normal cardiac examination, electrocardiogram (ECG) and cardiac enzyme levels, and without prior heart disease. Transesophageal echocardiography (TEE) is better than TTE in detecting PFO, aortic plaques, and left atrial appendage thrombus, and is recommended in patients with cryptogenic stroke under the age of 55. Non-invasive screening of right-to-left shunt and plaques in the ascending aorta can be performed by TCD after intravenous (IV) injection of bubble-contrast and duplex ultrasonography respectively, before confirmation by TEE.

Treatment/management

Thrombolysis or clot retrieval

Fresh emboli from the heart are susceptible to thrombolysis, and IV tPA should be considered in all cardioembolic stroke patients who present within 3 hours of onset. Intra-arterial (IA) thrombolysis can also be considered when such expertise is available, especially when patients present in the 3- to 6-hour time-window or have occlusions at sites associated with low possibilities of recannalization with IV tPA (proximal ICA and carotid T-junction), or it can be used as salvage therapy in patients with persistent major artery occlusion after IV tPA. Clot extraction using the MERCI device is an alternative or adjunctive therapy to IA thrombolysis, but these treatments should only be offered to carefully selected patients after consultation with the neurointerventional expert. Complications associated with endovascular procedures including intracranial bleeding and embolic events should be carefully assessed against the benefit to be derived in each patient.

Prevention of recurrent cardiac embolism

Anticoagulation starting with heparin followed by warfarin is a standard and acceptable therapy to prevent recurrent cardiac embolism once it has been established as the cause of stroke. There are small series studies showing the safety and benefit of early anticoagulation immediately after stroke onset that outweighed the risk of hemorrhagic transformation or intracranial hemorrhage. However, timing of anticoagulation after acute brain embolism should be individualized, taking into consideration the cause of cardiac embolism, location and size of the infarct, and the patient's condition including comorbidities and other risk factors. Early anticoagulation may be considered in selected patients with a high risk of recurrent brain embolism (early stroke recurrence, presence of intracardiac thrombus, increasing number of DWI lesions on repeat brain MRI, or robust microembolic signals on TCD) and low risk of cerebral hemorrhage (absence of large cerebral infarct, hemorrhagic transformation on neuroimaging, concomitant antiplatelet therapy, and uncontrolled

hypertension). Prevention of recurrent cardiac embolism in selected conditions is further elaborated below.

Thrombolytic and antithrombotic therapies are contraindicated in strokes secondary to infective endocarditis, due to hemorrhagic risk from mycotic aneurysms. High-dose IV antibiotic therapy is the mainstay of treatment. Urgent surgery may be indicated in patients with infective endocarditis or cardiac tumors (atrial myxoma, papillary fibroelastoma), when they are complicated with recurrent brain embolism or cardiac failure.

AF patients with a history of cerebral ischemia or peripheral embolism should be treated with long-term warfarin, unless contraindicated. Those without a prior history of embolism are risk-stratified using the CHADS$_2$ index (one point each for *C*ongestive heart failure, *H*ypertension, *A*ge more than 75 years, or *D*iabetes mellitus; and two points for prior *S*troke or TIA). Patients with scores ≥ 2 should take warfarin, but aspirin suffices for scores of 0–1. Paroxysmal AF or atrial flutter should be similarly treated, as their stroke risks are nearly as high as permanent AF. Patients with sick-sinus syndrome or pacemaker require special attention; the former is frequently associated with paroxysmal AF, whereas AF may be difficult to recognize on ECG in the latter unless the pacemaker is reprogrammed to lower ventricular rates.

Patients with mechanical heart valves should be treated with long-term warfarin. Those with bioprosthetic valves should take warfarin for 3 months after valve replacement, followed by aspirin. For rheumatic mitral valve stenosis, primary stroke prevention with warfarin may be considered in those with an enlarged left atrium, or when TTE or TEE reveals thrombus or spontaneous echo contrast in the left atrium.

Patients with acute myocardial infarct (MI) have increased stroke risks when AF, ST-elevation, anterior wall involvement, significant left ventricular (LV) dysfunction, or LV thrombus is present. Apart from global severe LV dysfunction, focal LV dyskinesia or aneurysm may also be a source of cardioembolism, especially when the apical region is involved. In patients with stroke secondary to acute MI, global, or focal ventricular dysfunction, warfarin for 3–6 months together with appropriate medical treatments for MI and heart failure is recommended, with TTE repeated to monitor the LV status. Warfarin therapy may be continued if high-risk features such as severe LV dysfunction or LV thrombus persist on TTE.

PFO is present in up to 35% of the general population. Features that increase the chance of a PFO being responsible for paradoxical embolism include: cryptogenic stroke at less than 55 years of age, concomitant venous thrombosis or pulmonary embolism, large right-to-left shunt demonstrated on TCD or TEE, co-existing atrial septal aneurysm or hypercoagulable condition, and history of cough or Valsalva maneuver before stroke onset.

Although warfarin may not be more effective than aspirin for stroke prevention, selected patients may be considered for percutaneous device closure of their PFOs.

Further reading

Adams HP Jr, Del Zoppo G, Alberts MJ, *et al*. AHA/ASA Guideline. Guidelines for the early management of adults with ischemic stroke. *Stroke* 2007; 38: 1655–711.

Caplan LR, Manning WJ, editors. *Brain Embolism*. New York: Informa Healthcare; 2006.

Goldstein LB, Adams R, Alberts MJ, *et al*. AHA/ASA Guideline. Primary prevention of ischemic stroke. *Stroke* 2006; 37: 1583–633.

Sacco RL, Adams R, Albers G, *et al*. AHA/ASA Guideline. Guidelines for prevention of stroke in patients with ischemic stroke or transient ischemic attack. *Stroke* 2006; 37: 577–617.

Chapter 7
Borderzone cerebral infarction

Thomas W. Leung
The Chinese University of Hong Kong, Hong Kong

Introduction

The borderzone (or watershed) is the junction between adjacent non-anastomosing arterial perfusion beds where the perfusion pressure is the lowest. Two distinct supratentorial borderzones have been described: (1) the cortical (or external) borderzone, which refers to the strips of brain lying between the territories of supply of the anterior cerebral artery (ACA), middle cerebral artery (MCA), and posterior cerebral arteries (PCA); and (2) the internal borderzone, which refers to the white matter alongside and above the body of lateral ventricles between the territories of ascending branches of lenticulostriate arteries and inward medullary branches of the pial-arachnoidal circulation.

Epidemiology

Borderzone infarction (BI) represents approximately 10% of all brain infarcts in autopsy series, but this might be an underestimate because unilateral BI is less likely to be fatal. BI is the most common type of infarction distal to an occluded internal carotid artery, and is evident in up to one-fourth of patients who develop ischemic stroke after cardiac surgery. In a European study that included ischemic stroke patients of all subtypes, more than two-thirds of BI identified by computed tomography was related to large artery disease.

Pathophysiology

Acute bilateral BI is classically associated with profound system hypotension, though a mild transitory hypotension may precipitate BI in patients with critical large artery disease and an exhausted perfusion reserve. Recognized causes of hemodynamic insults include an abrupt fall in blood pressure from antihypertensive drugs, heart failure induced by paroxysmal cardiac arrhythmias or cardiomyopathies,

International Neurology: A Clinical Approach. Edited by Robert P. Lisak, Daniel D. Truong, William M. Carroll, and Roongroj Bhidayasiri. © 2009 Blackwell Publishing, ISBN: 978-1-4051-5738-4.

massive acute bleeding, and hypotensive complications during cardiopulmonary bypass surgery.

BI is frequently observed in the ipsilateral cerebral hemisphere of severe carotid artery or MCA steno-occlusive disease without a preceding hypotensive event. In these patients, microembolization and chronic cerebral hypoperfusion collaborate inextricably in the pathogenesis of BI. Autopsy studies have revealed occlusion of terminal branches of leptomeningeal and pial arteries at the borderzone by small cholesterol emboli of 50–300 μm diameter. High-intensity transient signals compatible with microemboli have been consistently captured by transcranial Doppler ultrasound in patients with critical carotid stenosis and BI. It has been postulated that microemboli which might originate from unstable atherosclerotic plaques are prone to lodge at the hypoperfused borderzone where the low-flow circulation fails to wash out the emboli. The absence of effective collaterals further impedes the clearance of the microemboli.

Clinical features

The clinical presentation of BI is diverse. Small discrete BI may be clinically silent or manifest as transient ischemic attacks or lacunar syndromes. Depending on the extent of permanent ischemic injury, BI can be described as partial or confluent based on neuroimaging (see 'Investigation' below). Most patients with confluent BI develop dizziness or syncope as a prodromal symptom, followed by a fluctuating but progressive neurological deficit consisting of hemiparesis, hemisensory loss, cortical signs, or, rarely, focal limb shaking.

Investigation

BI is usually identified by computed tomography (CT) or magnetic resonance imaging (MRI). Cortical borderzone infarction (CBI) between the ACA and MCA produces a thin fronto-parasagittal wedged infarct extending from the anterior horn of the lateral ventricle to the cortex, which is termed the "anterior borderzone." CBI between

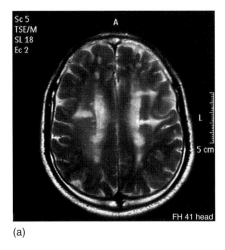
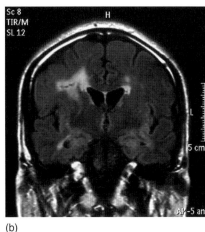

(a)   (b)

Figure 7.1 A classical "C-shaped" bilateral total cortical borderzone infarct, in which a linear chain of subcortical hyperintensity extended from the frontal pole and back along the convexity of the cerebral hemisphere in a parasagittal line to the occipital pole (a, MRI T2 axial view) and then forward again to involve the temporal lobe (b, MRI FLAIR coronal view).

the MCA and PCA causes a temporo-parieto-occipital wedged infarct extending from the occipital horn of the lateral ventricle to the cortex, referred to as the "posterior borderzone." At the level of the upper centrum semiovale, CBI between the three cerebral arteries results in a continuous strip extending from the frontal pole and back along the convexity of the cerebral hemisphere in a parasagittal line to the occipital pole, which is the so-called "superior borderzone." Internal borderzone infarction (IBI) affects the corona radiata, between the territories of the deep and medullary (or superficial) MCA perforators; or the centrum semiovale, between the superficial perforators of ACA and MCA. Considerable individual variation of cortical and internal borderzones may result from developmental anomalies (e.g., non-competent Circle of Willis or hypoplasia of intracranial arteries) or high-grade steno-occlusion of cranial arteries (e.g., critical carotid or MCA stenosis).

Compared with CT, MRI is more sensitive and reliable in the detection of BI (Figure 7.1). Diffusion-weighted MRI is useful to differentiate acute infarcts from chronic white matter hypoperfusion. Based on the extent of involvement in imaging, BI can be categorized as partial or confluent. Partial BI represents smaller, single, or multiple discrete infarcts in the corresponding borderzone. Multiple partial BI forms a linear, rosary-like chain of lesions. In its confluent form, CBI appears as a wedged infarct and IBI as a cigar-shaped infarct extending the length of the lateral ventricle at the level of the centrum semiovale.

Treatment/management

While the majority of patients with small, partial BI make an excellent recovery with minor or no residual disability, many patients with confluent BI are left with major motor disability. Bilateral watershed infarcts after cardiac surgery are associated with poor short-term outcome. Long-term prognosis and successful prophylaxis of BI depends upon identification and treatment of the underlying pathological mechanism. Without intervention, these patients are prone to repeated events. Investigations for carotid and intracranial stenosis should be performed routinely. Holter monitoring may record occult cardiac arrhythmia. Charting of erect and supine blood pressure identifies patients with orthostatic hypotension, and may prompt further investigation for autonomic failure. Calcium channel blockers and vasodilators are most commonly implicated in drug-induced hypotension. Having the least propensity to orthostatic hypotension, angiotensin-converting enzyme inhibitors or angiotensin receptor blockers can be an appropriate alternative for patients with chronic cerebral ischemia and systemic hypertension.

Further reading

Bogousslavsky J, Regli F. Borderzone infarctions distal to internal carotid artery occlusion: prognostic implications. *Ann Neurol* 1986; 20(3): 346–50.

Gottesman RF, Sherman PM, Grega MA, *et al*. Watershed strokes after cardiac surgery: diagnosis, etiology, and outcome. *Stroke* 2006; 37(9): 2306–11.

Isabelle M-M, Jean-Claude B. The pathophysiology of watershed infarction in internal carotid artery disease. Review of cerebral perfusion studies. *Stroke* 2005; 36: 567–77.

Louis RC, Michael H. Impaired clearance of emboli (washout) is an important link between hypoperfusion, embolism and ischemic stroke. *Arch Neurol* 1998; 55: 1475–82.

Paciaroni M, Silvestrelli G, Caso V, *et al*. Neurovascular territory involved in different etiological subtypes of ischemic stroke in the Perugia Stroke Registry. *Eur J Neurol* 2003; 10(4): 361–5.

Salazar JD, Wityk RJ, Grega MA, *et al*. Stroke after cardiac surgery: short- and long-term outcomes. *Ann Thorac Surg* 2001; 72(4): 1195–201.

Chapter 8
Dissection of the cervicocerebral arteries

Nijasri C. Suwanwela[1] and Chung Y. Hsu[2]
[1]Chulalongkorn University, Bangkok, Thailand
[2]China Medical University, Taichung, Taiwan

Introduction and epidemiology

Dissection of the cervicocerebral arteries is a relatively rare cause of stroke. In a population-based study, the annual incidence rate of cervical artery dissection was 2.6 per 100 000 population, with the internal carotid arteries affected more frequently than the vertebral arteries. Recurrence of dissection is rare and probably does not exceed 1%. In the younger population, however, cervicocerebral artery dissection is a common cause of stroke, constituting up to 25% of strokes in patients under the age of 45.

Pathophysiology

Trauma is a well-established cause of cervicocerebral artery dissection. Carotid and vertebral artery dissection were reported in 0.86% and 0.53% of patients with blunt trauma, respectively. It is likely that the frequency of dissection may have been under-recognized in patients with trauma. Cervical manipulation, particularly that applied in chiropractic, has been linked to vertebral and less frequently carotid artery dissection. In a systematic review of case reports of cervical artery dissection, approximately 6% of the cases were ascribed to chiropractic therapies. Most of the cases with dissection, however, were without a clear-cut cause even though trivial injury was frequently cited in the case reports. Most of the cases without obvious causes were categorized as spontaneous dissection. Among these patients, a small population (probably less than 5%) may have had hereditary disorders affecting the connective tissue. Weakening of the media and elastic tissue of the arterial wall as seen in patients with Marfan syndrome, Ehlers–Danlos, and fibromuscular dysplasia has been associated with dissection of the cervicocerebral arteries.

Tear between intima and media of the artery results in dissection of the vascular wall, leading to blood accumulation and hematoma formation. The local arterial injury causes enlargement of the arterial diameter as well as narrowing of the lumen. Luminal narrowing can alter blood flow to distal territory, and injury of endothelium may lead to intraluminal clot that may embolize distally. Less commonly, the tear is between media and adventitia resulting in aneurysm, pseudoaneursym formation, or rupture of the injured artery.

Clinical features

The dilated arteries can induce pressure effects on surrounding structures, including the adjacent nerves, which causes characteristic symptoms and signs including head, neck, and facial pain, sympathetic nerve dysfunction resulting in Horner's syndrome, and lower cranial nerve palsies. The onset of these symptoms and signs related to local arterial injury frequently precedes that caused by cerebral ischemia secondary to artery occlusion or distal emboli by hours to days. The sequence in the development of pain, ophthalmological and lower cranial nerve findings, followed by cerebral ischemia, are helpful clinical features for directing clinicians to arrive at the correct diagnosis.

Dissections are usually in the cervical and, less commonly, intracranial arteries. The clinical presentation depends on the site of dissection and the vascular territory supplied by the affected artery.

Dissection of the internal carotid artery
The presenting symptoms and signs of carotid dissection are generally based on two major mechanisms. The first is pressure effects of the dissected arterial wall on surrounding structures. The second is blood accumulation/hematoma formation/luminal stenosis/distal emboli leading to cerebral ischemia in the internal carotid artery territory.

International Neurology: A Clinical Approach. Edited by Robert P. Lisak, Daniel D. Truong, William M. Carroll, and Roongroj Bhidayasiri. © 2009 Blackwell Publishing, ISBN: 978-1-4051-5738-4.

Headache is reported in more than two-thirds of patients and is the initial symptom in up to 60%. Ipsilateral headache with a throbbing character resembling migraine or sharp pain in the face, neck, and jaw may be the presenting symptoms. The sympathetic nerves and lower cranial nerves, especially cranial nerves IX–XII, are commonly affected and dysgeusia resulting from involvement of chorda tympani or the glossopharyngeal nerve has been reported. Some patients may present with isolated Horner's syndrome, making diagnosis of carotid or vertebral artery dissection more difficult. About three-quarters of patients with carotid dissection show symptoms and signs of ischemic events including amaurosis fugax (ischemic optic neuropathy), transient ischemic attack, or ischemic stroke in the internal carotid artery territories. A small number of patients may remain asymptomatic. Dissection of the intracranial internal carotid artery does not usually present with the characteristic symptoms and signs associated with pressure effects on the cranial nerves or sympathetic nerve fibers described above.

Dissection of the vertebral artery
Vertebral artery dissection tends to involve the distal (V3) portion near the C1 and C2 vertebrae, which is highly moveable and therefore the most vulnerable segment. Dissection occurs after abrupt neck movement such as motor vehicle accident or chiropractic manipulation. Bilateral dissection of the vertebral arteries is not uncommon. Ipsilateral neck or occipital pain usually precedes neurological deficits by hours to many days. Stroke is caused by distal embolization to the posterior circulation resulting in brainstem and cerebellar infarction. In the case of intracranial dissection in the V4 segment, either primary intracranial or extension of extracranial dissection, lateral medullary syndrome can be found. Dissection of the intracranial part of the vertebral artery can extend to the basilar artery, leading to pontine and midbrain infarction. Moreover, pseudoaneurysm and rupture of this artery can cause subarachnoid hemorrhage.

Investigation

The advent of neuroimaging techniques allows us to diagnose dissection non-invasively. Moreover, new techniques provide visualization of the vascular wall, thus offering more information than conventional angiography.

For extracranial carotid dissection, B-mode ultrasound can demonstrate tapering of the arterial lumen above the carotid bifurcation and, sometimes, true and false lumens can be differentiated. Abnormal flow pattern can also be detected by Doppler study. Color duplex sonography has been reported to be of high sensitivity and specificity in spontaneous dissection of the internal carotid artery. However, in patients with isolated Horner's syndrome, ultrasound may not be a reliable method. Magnetic resonance and computed tomography can demonstrate enlargement of arterial diameter and, more importantly, blood or blood products in the arterial wall. These methods are currently used, together with information from magnetic resonance or computed tomography angiographies, as the gold standard for diagnosis. For conventional arteriography, the most distinctive feature is the string sign, which is a long, irregular filling defect due to lumen compression by blood in the vessel wall. Other rare but pathognomonic features are double-barrel lumen and mural flap. Occasionally, pseudoaneurysm can be found.

Management

There have been no randomized controlled trials for management of dissection. Patients with cervicocerebral artery dissection have been placed on intravenous or intra-arterial thrombolysis. While the efficacy of thrombolysis remains to be established, no adverse effects have been noted in a small number of patients. Within the 3-hour therapeutic window, thrombolysis probably should not be excluded as an option for managing patients with ischemic stroke secondary to cervicocerebral artery dissection. In most patients beyond the 3-hour window, anticoagulation is recommended for spontaneous extracranial dissection. Heparin in early phase followed by warfarin is generally used. Anticoagulant therapy may prevent embolization from thrombus to the distal vessels and the enlargement of the dissection. Surgery has a limited role, but angioplasty is gaining importance in patients who fail medical treatment and especially in those with major trauma who may not be treated with anticoagulants. Endovascular procedures have been tried in selected patients, but the number of patients is too small to confirm the efficacy.

For intracranial, especially vertebral artery dissection, there is a concern of arterial rupture resulting in subarachnoid hemorrhage. Therefore, anticoagulants are usually not advised.

The prognosis of patients with dissection largely depends on the location and size of the initial stroke. In general, the outcomes based on functional assessment are excellent, with a modified Rank score of 2 or less in the majority of patients. More than 70% of the stenotic lesions resolve within a few months, but recanalization of occluded vessels is less frequent. Recurrence of dissection was rare in a recent population-based survey.

Further reading

Arnold M, Baumgartner RW, Stapf C, *et al.* Ultrasound diagnosis of spontaneous carotid dissection with isolated Horner syndrome. *Stroke* 2008; 39: 82–6.

Dziewas R, Konrad C, Drager B, *et al.* Cervical artery dissection – clinical features, risk factors, therapy and outcome in 126 patients. *J Neurol* 2003; 250: 1179–84.

Fisher CM. The headache and pain of spontaneous carotid dissection. *Headache* 1982; 22: 60–5.

Grond-Ginsbach C, Debette S, Pezzini A. Genetic approaches in the study of risk factors for cervical artery dissection. *Front Neurol Neurosci* 2005; 20: 30–43.

Lee VH, Brown RD Jr, Mandrekar JN, Mokri B. Incidence and outcome of cervical artery dissection: a population-based study. *Neurology* 2006; 67: 1809–12.

Chapter 9
Coagulation disorders in stroke

Kay Sin Tan
University of Malaya Medical Centre, Kuala Lumpur, Malaysia

Introduction

Hematological diseases are uncommon causes of strokes resulting in approximately 10% of strokes in young patients and 1% of all patients with ischemic stroke.

Hyperviscosity

Sickle cell anemia contributes to hyperviscosity leading to large arterial, watershed infarcts. Intracerebral hemorrhage has also been reported. Intracerebral arteriopathy can be monitored with non-invasive imaging such as transcranial Doppler ultrasound and magnetic resonance imaging. Blood transfusion has been shown in randomized clinical trials to reduce stroke risk but has to be administered on a long-term basis. Children become vulnerable for recurrence of stroke if blood transfusion is suspended. Hydroxyurea, antiplatelet, other antithrombotic agents and bone marrow transplantation are possible treatment options but remain to be tested in valid clinical trials to confirm their efficacy in stroke prevention. Outside Africa, sickle cell anemia is most prevalent in North America, with 8.5% of African Americans carrying the sickle trait and 0.16% the disease. Sickle cell anemia is increasingly noticed in Europe because of immigration but is relatively uncommon in Asia except for the Middle East.

Polycythemia vera also causes neurovascular symptoms through hyperviscosity. Aspirin is effective in reducing stroke risk, as demonstrated in a randomized clinical trial. Thrombocytosis is associated with transient ischemic attacks or strokes and may occur with hematological malignancies. Measures to reduce platelet counts include platelet pheresis, hydoxyurea, and recombinant interferon-α.

International Neurology: A Clinical Approach. Edited by Robert P. Lisak, Daniel D. Truong, William M. Carroll, and Roongroj Bhidayasiri. © 2009 Blackwell Publishing, ISBN: 978-1-4051-5738-4.

Prothrombotic disorders

Prothrombotic coagulation abnormalities are complex and rapidly evolving. Inherited thrombophilias including deficiency in antithrombin (AT), protein C, and protein S predispose carriers to cerebral venous thrombosis, peripheral venous thrombosis and, rarely, arterial thrombosis, including stroke.

AT is an inhibitor of thrombin and other activated clotting factors. Deficiency in AT has a prevalence of 1 in 250–500 in the general population. It is inherited in an autosomal dominant pattern. The prevalence of hereditary AT deficiency is 0.5–1% among patients after a first thrombotic event. Clinical events are usually precipitated by pregnancy, surgery, infection, or oral contraceptives. Treatment of symptomatic inherited AT deficiency is with warfarin. AT deficiency is resistant to anticoagulation with heparin. Alternatively, replacement AT is available for short-term therapy or during episodes of high risk.

Protein C is an important inhibitor of plasma coagulation. It is activated when clotting is initiated on the endothelial surface. Protein S acts as a non-enzymatic cofactor for the activated protein-C (APC). APC and protein S collectively confer anticoagulant actions and also activate fibrinolysis. Most affected adult patients are heterozygous for protein C deficiency, with a prevalence of 1 in 200–500 in the general population. The prevalence of protein S deficiency is estimated at 1 in 700–3000.

Both conditions are inherited in an autosomal dominant pattern with partial expressivity. Premature stroke also affects children and young adults heterozygous for protein C deficiency when conventional stroke risk factors are also present. Acquired protein C deficiency may occur with liver disease, vitamin K malabsorption, infection, sepsis, disseminated intravascular coagulation, or malignancy. Homocystinuria (see below) in association with protein C deficiency has been recognized to cause thrombotic episodes. Acquired protein S deficiencies can also occur with nephrotic syndrome, HIV infection, and L-asparaginase chemotherapy in addition to oral contraceptive use and liver dysfunction.

Activated protein C resistance may be due to genetic mutations such as factor V Leiden G1691A. This and other point mutations such as prothrombin G20210A offer genetic insights into the pathogenesis of hypercoagulable states. It is also interesting to note the ethnic differences in the prevalence of these mutations, with the Western population suffering higher incidence than the Eastern population, which may be the basis for racial differences in thrombotic risks.

Homocysteinemia

Case-control studies and meta-analyses have demonstrated that an increase in plasma homocysteine is a significant independent risk factor for ischemic stroke. Numerous genetic errors in the metabolism of sulfur-containing amino acids produce plasma hyperhomocysteinemia and homocystinuria. Hyperhomocysteinemia may activate coagulation via endothelial injury, producing an occlusive vasculopathy. Acquired conditions such as vitamin B_{12} and folate deficiency, renal failure, hypothyroidism, and drugs including anticonvulsants predispose to hyperhomocysteinemia. Randomized controlled trials using folate and vitamin B supplements to lower homocysteinemia are ongoing, but a National Institutes of Health–National Institute of Neurological Disorders and Stroke (NIH–NINDS)-sponsored randomized trial failed to show dose-dependent effects of folate and vitamin B in reducing stroke risks.

Antiphospholipid antibodies and stroke

The presence of antiphospholipid antibodies has been associated with increased risk of strokes. Clinical features of primary antiphospholipid syndrome (APLS) include recurrent migraine-like headaches, fetal loss, mild thrombocytopenia, false-positive Veneral Disease Research Laboratory (VDRL) tests, and arterial or venous cerebrovascular events that may present with encephalopathy and seizures.

Secondary APLS occurs with lupus erythematosus, immune complex diseases, cancer, and drug reactions. These patients have either lupus anticoagulant or anticardiolipin antibody of significant titers. By contrast, low-titer APLS is found in 1–2% of the normal population. It also occurs transiently after infection, tissue trauma (including myocardial infarction or heart surgery), and secondary to drugs, and is usually not associated with thrombotic events.

To prevent recurrent stroke in patients with primary or secondary APLS is challenging. Warfarin is generally used. Immunosuppression and the addition of aspirin to anticoagulation for individuals with recurrent cerebral ischemia are therapeutic options. However, these strategies are not evidence based. Furthermore, the optimal length and intensity of anticoagulation therapy are uncertain due to the paucity of data about treatment outcomes.

Thrombotic thrombocytopenic purpura

Thrombotic thrombocytopenic purpura (TTP) is a consumptive coagulopathy characterized by microangiopathic hemolytic anemia, thrombocytopenia, and central nervous system disorders including ischemic strokes. Important pathophysiological changes occur in small arteries and include platelet microthrombi, marked intimal hyperplasia, and fibrin deposits in the subintimal parts of affected blood vessels, contributing to multiple organ damage, particularly the brain and kidney.

Clinically, TTP may present with fluctuating encephalopathic signs and seizures. Computed tomography (CT) or magnetic resonance imaging (MRI) findings may show ischemic changes, cerebral edema, or intracerebral hemorrhage. Therapeutic measures include the use of high-dose corticosteroids, repeated plasma exchanges, antiplatelet agents, and splenectomy, with varying degrees of success.

Other coagulopathies

There are other rare genetic disorders that may predispose carriers to hypercoagulable states. These hereditary diseases that affect clotting mechanisms include defect in heparin cofactor II and fibrinolysis factors such as plasminogen, tissue plasminogen activator, and excessive formation of plasminogen activator inhibitor-1. The role of these rare hereditary conditions in venous thrombosis and stroke remains to be defined.

An acquired hypercoagulopathy is frequently found in cancer patients who may have increased risk of thrombotic vascular disorders including stroke. Detailed description of the hypercoagulable state in malignancy is beyond the scope of this chapter.

Further reading

Gruppo Italiano Studio Policitemia. Polycythemia vera: the natural history of 1213 patients followed for 20 years. *Ann Intern Med* 1995; 123: 656–64.

Levine SR, Brey RL, Tilley BC, *et al.* Antiphospholipid antibodies and subsequent thrombo-occlusive events in patients with ischemic stroke. *JAMA* 2004; 291(5): 576–84.

Toole JF, Malinow MR, Chambless LE, *et al.* Lowering homocysteine in patients with ischemic stroke to prevent recurrent stroke, myocardial infarction, and death: the Vitamin Intervention for Stroke Prevention (VISP) randomized controlled trial. *JAMA* 2004; 291: 565–675.

Walters MC, Patience M, Leisenring W, *et al.* Bone marrow transplantation for sickle cell disease. *N Engl J Med* 1996; 335: 369–76.

Chapter 10
Hemorrhagic strokes

Josef Schill[1] and Thorsten Steiner[2]
[1]Klinikum Ludwigshafen, Ludwigshafen, Germany
[2]Ruprecht Karls University Heidelberg, Heidelberg, Germany

Introduction

Hemorrhagic strokes are acute bleeding events in the intracranial cavity that, in general, are more serious than ischemic strokes and have a higher mortality. In this chapter, hemorrhagic strokes will be covered in three categories based on pathological features: (1) spontaneous or primary intracerebral hemorrhage of various causes; (2) hemorrhagic events associated with arteriovenous malformations (AVM); and (3) subarachnoid hemorrhage (SAH) secondary to rupture of arterial aneurysm.

Spontaneous intracerebral hemorrhage

Epidemiology

Spontaneous intracerebral hemorrhage (ICH) constitutes 10–25% of all strokes. Ethnic differences in ICH incidence have been noted, with people of Asian and African origin showing higher frequency than the white population. In Western countries, ICH accounts for 10–17% of all strokes and in Asian countries up to 25%. In the United States, ICH incidence in the African American (32 per 100 000) or Asian American (61 per 100 000) population is higher than the white American (7–12 per 100 000) population. Among patients with atrial fibrillation who are on anticoagulant treatment, the same trend for higher incidence of ICH in the non-white population also holds.

Risk factors

The most important ICH risk factor is hypertension. The crude odds ratio (OR) for hypertension is 3.68 and the frequency of hypertension in ICH is 70–80%. Another major risk factor is age: the crude risk ratio for age (every 10-year increase) is 1.97. In the elderly, spontaneous ICH may be caused by cerebral amyloid angiopathy (CAA). For current smokers, the crude OR is 1.31 and diabetes 1.30. With regard to alcohol consumption, the

International Neurology: A Clinical Approach. Edited by Robert P. Lisak, Daniel D. Truong, William M. Carroll, and Roongroj Bhidayasiri.
© 2009 Blackwell Publishing, ISBN: 978-1-4051-5738-4.

quantity is a significant variable. High intake (>56 g/day, crude OR of 4) results in greater risk than moderate consumption (<56 g/day alcohol, crude OR of 2.05). Drug abuse (e.g., cocaine, amphetamine) is also associated with increased ICH risk as well as low cholesterol (<150 mg/dl). ICH incidence is lower among those with higher cholesterol levels. Modifying these risk factors plays an important role in lowering ICH risk. Iatrogenic causes of ICH are not uncommon. Oral anticoagulants, especially those prescribed for elderly patients with atrial fibrillation, have drawn increasing attention to a serious adverse side effect that presents with ICH. Traumatic head injury may cause acute or delayed ICH, especiallly in victims on oral anticoagulants. Traumatic ICH is beyond the scope of coverage in this chapter. Thrombolytic therapy of ischemic stroke with t-PA increases the risk of symptomatic ICH by 10-fold. Approximately 0.5% of patients who underwent carotid endarterectomy experienced ICH after surgery. Other procedures such as intracerebral electrode placement or angioplasty and stenting of the internal carotid artery or its branches may also cause ICH.

Pathophysiology

Spontaneous or primary ICH constitutes 80–85% of all hemorrhagic strokes, with secondary ICH that can be ascribed to discrete vascular lesions including AVM, and aneurysm comprising the remaining 15–20%. Secondary ICH will be reviewed in the subsequent sections on AVM and aneurysm respectively. Over 50% of primary ICH cases are attributed to hypertension, with location in the basal ganglia, the most common site of bleeding, accounting for approximately 40%. Other frequent locations of hypertensive ICH include the thalamus (30%), cerebral cortex (20%), cerebellum and brain stem (10%). The remaining cases of primary ICH are mainly those associated with CAA, which has been found to increase with age. CAA affects mainly leptomeningeal and cortical vessels, with the occipital or parietal region the common sites of hemorrhage. ICH is often caused by rupture of a small artery with subsequent hematoma formation and expansion. Miliary aneurysms (Charcot–Buchard's aneurysms) and lipohyalinosis, both associated with chronic arterial hypertension, are the key pathological features in autopsy series of ICH. CAA is characterized by amyloid deposition in the vessel walls, leading to degenerative vascular changes culminating in arterial rupture.

Following arterial rupture in ICH, the subsequent pathophysiological processes can be divided into three phases: (1) accumulation of extravascular blood leading to hematoma formation; (2) continuation or resumption of bleeding resulting in hematoma expansion; and (3) development of perihematomal edema. Hematoma expansion or enlargement secondary to continuous or re-bleeding has gained attention in recent years because of the possibility of therapeutic interventions applying hemostatic agents at a very early stage of ICH. In view of the clinical and therapeutic implications, hematoma enlargement and perihematomal edema formation are reviewed in more detail below.

Hematoma enlargement

Progressive enlargement of a hematoma is the most serious complication in patients with ICH. It is not clear whether re-bleeding or continuous bleeding is the cause of hematoma growth. Hematoma increases by about 33% in size in approximately one-third of patients within the first 4 hours of onset. In another 12% of patients the hematoma expands within the next 20 hours. Neurological deterioration follows hematoma enlargement. The following predictors of hematoma expansion have been identified: large initial blood volume, irregular bleeding contours, liver dysfunction, hypertension, hyperglycemia, and history of high alcohol consumption.

Brain edema

Brain edema can be observed in the acute and subacute stage of ICH. Edema usually progresses for up to 14 days after ICH onset. Based upon magnetic resonance imaging (MRI) and positron emission tomography (PET) studies, edema plays a minor role in the development of perihematomal ischemia, in contrast to a more significant pathophysiological role of brain edema in ischemic stroke. Brain edema following ICH is thought to involve activation of the coagulation mechanism. ICH in patients on anticoagulant therapy with iatrogenic coagulopathy is accompanied by a lesser magnitude of perihematomal edema.

An ominous pathophysiological process following ICH is bleeding into intraventricular space which is associated with higher mortality and morbidity. Intraventricular hemorrhage (IVH) is a dynamic process and is present in 38% of ICH patients at onset and in 45% 24 hours after onset.

Clinical features

Primary ICH is an acute vascular event frequently presented with sudden onset of focal neurological symptoms and signs that may not be easily distinguished from those accompanying secondary ICH caused by AVM,

SAH caused by rupture of aneurysm, or ischemic strokes. Compared to ischemic stroke, primary ICH is more likely to present with symptoms of increased intracranial pressure at onset. These include headache, nausea/vomiting, and altered consciousness. One characteristic feature of ICH is the sudden occurrence of neurological symptoms during physical activity. Symptoms may progress for hours. Hematoma enlargement plays a critical role in dictating the clinical course. Clinical presentation is dependent on the location of bleeding. Patients with basal ganglia hemorrhage usually present with contralateral sensorimotor deficit. Thalamic hemorrhage is more likely to cause sensory loss or obtundation. Lobar hemorrhage shows focal deficits characteristic of the affected cortical region. Thus patients may present with language disorders, neglect, or unilateral sensory, motor or visual deficit. Infratentorial hemorrhage presents with brainstem or cerebellar signs. Decreasing levels of consciousness and even coma are seen frequently in patients suffering from brainstem bleeding and in supratentorial ICH when mass effect or acute hydrocephalus is noted. Signs of brain herniation, especially deepening coma with dilated pupils, may be detected, some shortly after onset. Bilateral sixth nerve palsies have also been described in the context of brainstem herniation. In pontine hemorrhage, pinpoint pupils are seen.

Investigation

Non-contrast computed tomography (CT) is a sensitive procedure for detecting or excluding acute ICH. Acute bleeding presents as a hyperdense area on CT. However, in patients with low hematocrits, even an acute hematoma may appear isodense. The area of the hematoma becomes iso- and hypodense during the course of hematoma breakdown and absorption.

With the implementation of susceptibility-weighted T2* sequences, MRI has become a useful diagnostic tool to supplement CT in detecting hyperacute and acute ICH. In hyperacute hemorrhage these sequences (for a 1.5-Tesla scanner) reveal characteristic hyperintense signals. In the chronic stage, hemosiderin causes a hypointense signal on T2- and T2*-weighted sequences.

Follow-up imaging may not be necessary unless hematoma enlargement in patients with deteriorating clinical course or unusual causes of ICH (e.g., bleeding caused by a brain tumor) is suspected. In younger patients without known risk factors such as hypertension or in patients with suspected secondary bleeding (e.g., lobar bleedings or so-called "atypical ICH"), further diagnostic work-up is required to define the etiology of hemorrhage. CT angiography (CTA), MR angiography (MRA), and digital subtraction angiography (DSA) are useful in these patients. CTA is recommended as a rapid method of identifying the underlying vascular pathology when emergency surgical evacuation of the hematoma is required. Aneurysms larger than 3 mm and AVM can be detected effectively by using this technique. As larger ICH can cause hemodynamic changes in AVM, it is possible that they can no longer be detected by MRA or CTA. Under this circumstance, DSA should be performed. MRI is the best technique to reveal underlying vascular malformation of the low-pressure system or the venous system (cavernoma, hemorrhagic tumors). Using contrast-enhanced magnetic resonance venography or CTA, sinus venous thrombosis can be clearly diagnosed.

Prognosis

Prognosis of ICH depends on the extent and location of intracranial hematoma, hematoma expansion, and the presence of IVH. Complications such as enlargement of the hematoma, increasing perilesional brain edema, and hydrocephalus worsen the prognosis. The 30-day mortality is higher (43%) in patients who develop IVH than those without (9%). Both the hematoma and IVH volumes are major determinants of mortality and morbidity. IVH increases by 24 hours in 10–17% of patients who have substantially higher mortality. Risk factors for IVH expansion include baseline mean arterial pressure greater than 120 mm Hg, larger baseline ICH volume, and IVH at onset. Predictors of death or severe disability include older age, lower baseline Glasgow Coma Scale, larger baseline ICH volume, IVH presenting within 24 hours, and IVH expansion. Hydrocephalus following IVH is also an unfavorable sign for early mortality.

Treatment

Though favorable results of therapeutic interventions for ICH based on large prospective randomized clinical trials are lacking, promising insight into the development of effective treatment has been derived from a number of clinical trials. Evidence-based recommendations for managing patients with ICH have been made by the European Stroke Initiative (EUSI) and the American Heart Association/American Stroke Association (AHA/ASA).

One of the major targets in treating ICH is blood pressure control. Intracranial pressure (ICP) is an important parameter that guides the management of blood pressure. Whether the administration of hemostatic agents can prevent hematoma enlargement to improve outcomes is still the subject of clinical research. Prevention of deep vein thrombosis and pulmonary embolism in immobilized ICH patients remains a therapeutic dilemma. Surgical evacuation of hematoma is not generally recommended, but two subgroups of patients with ICH may benefit from surgery. Readers are referred to recommendations made by the EUSI and AHA/ASA and summarized in Tables 10.1 and 10.2 for management guidelines.

Treatment of ICH related to fibrinolysis

Symptomatic ICH occurs in 3–9% of patients with acute ischemic stroke treated with intravenous r-tPA. "Symptomatic" should be differentiated from "any" hemorrhage found in stroke patients treated with

Table 10.1 EUSI and AHA/ASA guidelines for major management objectives in ICH.

Recommendations	EUSI	AHA/ASA
		Monitoring and treatment in Stroke Unit or ICU
	(Level C)	(Class I, Level B)
		Mobilization and rehabilitation as soon as possible
	(Class IV)	(Class I, Level C)
Body temperature	• Temperature <37.5°C (Class IV)	• Treatment of fever (Class I, Level B)
Blood glucose	• Blood glucose levels <180 mg/dl (10 mmol/l) (Class IV)	• Blood glucose levels <185 mg/dl (10.3 mmol/l), if possible <140 mg/dl (7.8 mmol/l) (Class II b, Level C)
Blood pressure	Known HPT, SBP >180, and/or DBP >105 • <170/100 or MAP <125* Unknown HPT, SBP >160, and/or DBP >95 • <150/90 or MAP <100*	SBP >200 or MAP >150 • Aggressive reduction SBP >180 or MAP >130 Normal ICP • Modest reduction 160/90 or MAP <110
Intracranial pressure	• CPP >70 (Class IV)	SBP >180 or MAP >130 • CPP >60–80 (Class II b, Level C)
Prevention of venous thromboembolism		Compression stockings Intermittent pneumatic compression Consider low-dose subcutaneous UFH or LMWH
Anticoagulation	After 24 hours (Class IV)	After 3–4 days (Class II b, Level B)

SBP: systolic blood pressure; DBP: diastolic blood pressure; MAP: mean arterial pressure; all pressure units in mm Hg; UFH: unfractionated heparin; LMWH: low-molecular-weight heparin.
*Maximum reduction 20% of MAP on admission.

Table 10.2 EUSI and AHA/ASA guidelines for managing ICH related to oral anticoagulant treatment (OAT).

Recommendations for treatment of patients with OAT-related ICH	EUSI	AHA/ASA
Continuation of OAT in patients with high risk of thromboembolism with low risk of ICH recurrence	10–14 days after ICH (Class IV)	7–10 days after ICH (Class II b, Level B)
OAT replaced by antiplatelet agents in patients with low risk of thromboembolism with high risk of ICH recurrence		
High risk of thromboembolism	Embolic stroke + • AF • Prosthetic heart valve • Other proven cardioembolic sources	• Chronic AF and cardiogenic embolism • Prosthetic heart valve
High risk of ICH recurrence	• Lobar hemorrhage • CAA	
Recommendations for treatment of patients with heparin-related ICH Antidote of HEP: PS	• 1–1.5 mg PS/1000 IE HEP applied within last 4 hours	• HEP stopped for 30–60 min: 0.75–0.5 mg PS/100 IU HEP • HEP stopped for 60–120 min: 0.5–0.375 mg PS/100 IU HEP • HEP stopped for >120 min: 0.375–0.25 mg PS/100 IU HEP (Class I, Level B)

AF: atrial fibrillation; CAA: cerebral amyloid angiopathy; HEP: heparin; PS: protamine sulfate.

r-tPA. "Symptomatic" hemorrhage is defined as clinical deterioration attributable to hemorrhage, whereas "any" hemorrhage in acute stroke treated with r-tPA is found in 30% of patients. In cases of symptomatic hemorrhage, these tend to be serious, sometimes multifocal. The 30-day death rate can be 60% or higher. Recommended treatments include platelets and factor VIII substitution to rapidly correct the systemic fibrinolytic state.

Antiplatelet agents and ICH

Prevention of ischemic events with antiplatelet agents may be necessary in patients with ICH who have an additional risk of ischemic events (symptomatic carotid stenosis, cerebral microangiopathy) or ischemic disease (coronary artery syndrome, peripheral arterial disease). No change in bleeding risk is seen in patients with cerebral microangiopathy who are treated with aspirin. For aspirin or clopidogrel monotherapy no significant difference in the bleeding risk has been shown.

Surgical treatment
Supratentorial non-aneurysmal ICH

In prospective controlled randomized trials, surgical intervention has not been shown to offer advantages over conservative treatment. The largest group was examined in the Surgical Trial in Spontaneous Intracerebral Haemorrhage (STICH). Only in subgroup analysis was a probable benefit noted following early surgery. Thus, early evacuation of hematoma might be considered in patients showing deterioration in consciousness (Glasgow

Coma Scale (GCS) 9–12) and patients with a superficial hemorrhage (less than 1 cm from the surface). Surgical evacuation of the hematoma within 12 hours of onset, applying a less invasive approach, may be the best option until more valid results are available in future prospective controlled clinical trials. Very early craniotomy may be associated with an increased risk of recurrent bleeding.

Infratentorial non-aneurysmal ICH

Infratentorial bleeding (brainstem or cerebellar bleeding) can cause serious direct compression of functional tissue in the brainstem. Furthermore, both types of bleeding can lead to compression of the fourth ventricle or aqueduct, resulting in hydrocephalus and subsequent increase in ICP. In cases of hydrocephalus or when the cerebellar hematoma is more than 2–3 cm in size, ventricular drainage or clot evacuation should be considered even in older patients or those in coma.

ICH caused by arteriovenous malformation (AVM)

Epidemiology

In general, AVM refers to a heterogeneous group of cerebrovascular anomalies that predispose approximately half of those who harbor one of these discrete vascular lesions to bleeding events at various stages of life. In population-based studies the incidence of AVM is approximately 1 per 100 000 per year. AVM-related hemorrhage constitutes 2–4% of all hemorrhagic strokes. Bleeding caused by rupture of AVM tends to occur at an earlier age than primary ICH. The mean age of AVM hemorrhage is between age 30 and 40. Because of the relatively low incidence of AVM and lack of epidemiological studies across countries, racial or ethnic differences in AVM incidence have not been reported.

Risk factors

AVMs appear to derive from structural and functional vascular anomalies during development, with no risk factors firmly established. Age appears to be a risk factor for AVM rupture. Unlike primary ICH, however, risk factors such as hypertension and smoking have not been found to increase the risk of AVM hemorrhage. In rare cases, clusters of AVM have been reported in a small number of families. Hereditary diseases that are associated with AVM include Rendu–Osler–Weber syndrome, Wyburn–Mason's syndrome, von Hippel–Lindau disease, and Sturge–Weber disease. These rare familial cases may show features of teleangiectasia, with increasing tendency to rupture and hemorrhage.

Pathophysiology

AVMs are vascular anomalies with hetergenous vascular structures, with the most consistent findings being the lack of capillary bed between arteries and veins resulting in the evolving changes on the venous side. A–V shunting and related destruction of the vascular wall increases bleeding tendency. Brain tissue receiving blood supplies from vessels containing AVM may affect normal brain function, resulting in neurological deficits or lower threshold for seizure attacks. More superficially located AVMs may predispose to headaches. AVM may be associated with arterial aneursyms.

Clinical features

ICH caused by ruptured AVM may present with clinical features that are difficult to distinguish from those caused by primary ICH. However, the age of onset of ICH secondary to AVM is likely to be younger and common stroke risk factors such as hypertension and diabetes may be absent. Bleeding of a ruptured AVM frequently leads to the detection of the lesion. With increasing utility of new imaging tools including CT and MRI, patients with unruptured AVM may present with headache, subtle neurological deficit, or seizure disorders which lead to the neuroradiological work-up and the diagnosis of AVM.

Prognosis

In general, ICH secondary to AVM rupture bears lower mortality and morbidity than primary ICH. Patients with AVM hemorrhage also fare better in functional outcome. Among patients with AVM hemorrhages,

higher morbidity is noted in those with parenchymal than non-parenchymal hemorrhage. Recurrence of bleeding is expected in 18% of patients in the 12 months following the first AVM hemorrhage.

Investigations

Modern imaging modalities including CT and MRI are the mainstays in the diagnosis of AVM. Past bleeding events may be detected by hemosiderin deposition. Feeding arteries and shunting may be better characterized with angiography, which is useful in developing treatment strategies.

Treatment

Approximately half of all cerebral AVMs are associated with ICH. AVMs must be searched for among younger patients, particularly those with lobar or so-called "atypical" bleeding locations. The immediate short-term risk of bleeding may be relatively low. Therefore, in contrast to cerebral aneurysm, treatment is recommended within the first 4–12 weeks after the patient has been clinically stabilized. The best therapeutic results are achieved by combining the available methods (observation, endovascular embolization, radiotherapy, and surgery). Endovascular embolization and radiotherapy are often used to reduce the size in preparation for surgery or when the AVM is inaccessible. The treatment is selected according to the size of the AVM, proximity to eloquent areas, venous drainage, and accessibility.

Subarachnoid hemorrhage

Epidemiology

The incidence of subarachnoid hemorrhage (SAH) varies with region, age, and gender. In systematic studies across countries, worldwide incidence is approximately 9 per 100 000 persons per year, with Japan (21.9) and Finland (19.7) showing higher incidence and South and Central America (4.2) showing lower. An age-dependent increase in SAH incidence has been consistently noted. Gender difference is also evident, with women having a higher risk than men.

Pathophysiology

In 85% of all SAH, saccular aneurysms are found that arise from the cerebral arteries. Ten percent of the total SAHs are caused by non-aneurysmal perimesencephalic SAH. The remaining 5% are caused by AVM, dural arteriovenous fistula, dissection of intracranial arteries, septic aneurysms, or traumatic brain injuries (without contusion). SAH is frequently followed by three delayed pathophysiological processes. In view of their clinical significance, these events that complicate the initial bleeding ictus are more extensively reviewed below.

Recurrence of SAH

Re-bleeding is a common event within 2 weeks of onset. The mortality in patients who suffer rebleeding is about 50%. Thus, rebleeding of symptomatic aneurysms is a very severe complication and should therefore be prevented by early aneurysmal occlusion by surgical or endovascular measures.

Hydrocephalus

Acute, subacute, or chronic hydrocephalus is a common complication of SAH. Hydrocephalus occlusus occurs to compression of the fourth ventricle/aqueduct. Non-obstructive hydrocephalus may develop as a result of impaired absorption of CSF secondary to malfunction of pacchionian granulation. Intermittent external ventricular catheter drainage may be required for both conditions to prevent increasing ICP. In cases of chronic hydrocephalus, a ventriculo-peritoneal shunt may be necessary.

Vasospasm

Vasospasm of the cerebral basal arteries occurs mainly in the first or second week after SAH. This complication can cause a delayed ischemic neurological deficit, leading to ischemic stroke or death in one-third of patients. Transcranial sonography is a common modality for detecting and monitoring vasospasm.

Seizures, pulmonary edema, cardiovascular dysfunction secondary to increased autonomic discharges, hyponatremia, inappropriate secretion of antidiuretic hormone, or cerebral salt wasting are known pathophysiological processes complicating the management of SAH.

Risk factors

Modifiable risk factors include arterial hypertension, smoking, heavy alcohol intake, and drug consumption. Between 5% and 20% of patients have a positive familial history. There is also a known association with specific heritable disorders of connective tissue (Ehlers–Danlos disease IV, neurofibromatosis type I, Marfan's syndrome) and with polycystic kidney disease.

Clinical features

Hallmarks of SAH are acute (thunderclap) headache, nausea, vomiting, and neck stiffness. Reduced level of consciousness, hemiparesis, or other focal neurological symptoms are common in severe SAH. Seizure or confusional state may be prominent in selected cases. Preretinal hemorrhages (Terson's syndrome) indicate a more abrupt increase in ICP and are associated with higher mortality.

In the absence of classic symptoms, SAH might be misdiagnosed. In these cases patients tend to be less ill and the results of neurologic examination are normal or showing only subtle signs. In as many as 50% of cases,

complications occur later, with a higher risk of death and disability.

Sentinel or thunderclap headaches may be the only symptom of "warning leaks." It is essential to distinguish these sentinel headaches from benign headaches because of the early therapeutic options. Aneurysm can cause single or combined cranial nerve palsy, depending on the size and localization. Painful third nerve palsy is highly suspicious for aneurysm of the posterior communicating artery.

Currently, the classification of the World Federation of Neurological Surgeons (WFNS) and the classification by Hunt and Hess are mostly used for therapeutic decision-making (Table 10.3).

Prognosis

Unfavorable prognostic factors include older age, initially decreased level of consciousness, localization of the aneurysm in the posterior circulation, large amount of blood in the subarachnoid space and in cisterns, and the presence of intraventricular blood. Nearly 10–15% of patients die before reaching the hospital. One-third of surviving patients require lifelong care because of the neurological sequelae.

Investigation

Diagnosis of SAH can be made by CT in most cases. The bleeding site may also indicate the site of the aneurysm in some cases, but atypical locations have also been observed. Sensitivity of CT performed within the first 12 hours after onset is 98% but down to 50% by the seventh day after onset. Sensitivity of MRI, performed on the first day, is equal to that of CCT, but MRI has a higher sensitivity for subacute SAH.

Conventional catheter angiography is the gold standard for detecting aneurysms. Because the incidence of

Table 10.3 Clinical classification of SAH.

Grade	WFNS		Hunt and Hess
	GCS	Focal deficit*	
I	15	None	No symptoms, minor headache, minor neck stiffness
II	13–14	None	Moderate to severe headache, neck stiffness, no neurological deficit other than cranial nerve palsy
III	13–14	Present	Somnolence, confusion, minor neurological deficit
IV	7–12	Present/none	Sopor, moderate or severe neurological deficit (hemiparesis)
V	6–3	Present/none	Coma, signs of herniation

WFNS: World Federation of Neurological Surgeons; GCS: Glasgow Coma Scale.

*Cranial nerve palsies are not considered as focal deficit.

multiple aneurysms can be high (15%), all cerebral vessels should be carefully evaluated. The examination should be repeated 7–14 days after initial presentation in patients suspected of having aneurysmal hemorrhage and in whom imaging results are negative. CTA and MRA have gained popularity and are frequently used for detection of aneurysms. CTA and MRA are also helpful for planning treatment of large and complex aneurysms because of the possibility of three-dimensional visualization.

Lumbar puncture (LP) must be performed in patients with a typical clinical presentation of SAH and negative CT finding and with no contraindications for LP (e.g., signs of elevated ICP). Normal CSF excludes SAH within the prior 2–3 weeks. Signs of SAH include xanthochrome CSF. The value of the "three tube test" whereby CSF is collected in three consecutive tubes for red cell count is not clear.

Treatment/management
Patients with SAH should be evaluated and treated on an emergency basis, with close attention to airway and cardiovascular function. Further treatment should be carried out at centers where neurovascular expertise is available. Main goals of treatment are prevention and management of delayed events including re-bleeding, hydrocephalus, vasospasm, and other complications. SAH is usually managed in a neurocritical care setting. Prevention of vasospasm is a major objective in critical care of SAH patients. This topic is extensively reviewed below.

Vasospasm
To prevent vasospasm, prophylactic treatment with the calcium antagonist nimodipine is recommended in every patient with SAH (nimodipine 60 mg (oral intake) every 4 hours for 21 days). Intravenous administration is possible via a central line, but the effectiveness of this route is not known.

Triple-H therapy (hypervolemia, hypertension, hemodilution) is usually implemented to obtain adequate cerebral perfusion and oxygenation. Triple-H therapy should only be performed after an aneurysm has been occluded. To obtain a state of hypertension with systolic pressure up to 240 mm Hg catecholamines are often needed (dobutamine, norepinephrine). The central venous pressure target is 8–12 mm Hg and, when using a Swan–Ganz pulmonary artery catheter, wedge pressure should be 12–16 mm Hg.

Hemodilution can be achieved by administering hydroxethylstarch (HES) 10% 500–1000 ml/day. Cardiopulmonary function should be monitored closely because of the elevated risk of pulmonary edema, cardiac failure, cerebral edema, rupture of aneurysm, and electrolyte imbalances.

For prevention of re-bleeding, surgical or endovascular intervention is frequently needed. Early occlusion of symptomatic aneurysms by neurosurgical intervention with microsurgical clipping or by endovascular treatment with a detachable platinum coil device is commonly implemented to reduce the risk of early and fatal recurrence of hemorrhage. There is a tendency to favor neurosurgical treatment in patients who have a good clinical score (WFNS I–III), who are amenable to surgery within the first 48 hours, with the ruptured aneurysm located at a surgically accessible site, and in absence of vasospasm. Endovascular treatment may be more effective in patients with WFNS-grades IV–V who present with vasospasm or aneurysms related to the posterior circulation.

Further reading

Aguilar MI, Hart RG, Kase CS, *et al.* Treatment of warfarin-associated intracerebral hemorrhage: literature review and expert opinion. *Mayo Clin Proc* 2007; 82: 82–92.

Ariesen MJ, Claus SP, Rinkel GJ, Algra A. Risk factors for intracerebral hemorrhage in the general population: a systematic review. *Stroke* 2003; 34: 2060–65.

Ayala C, Greenlund KJ, Croft JB, *et al.* Racial/ethnic disparities in mortality by stroke subtype in the United States, 1995–1998. *Am J Epidemiol* 2001; 154: 1057–63.

Broderick J, Connolly S, Feldmann E, *et al.* Guidelines for the management of spontaneous intracerebral hemorrhage in adults: 2007 update: a guideline from the American Heart Association/American Stroke Association Stroke Council, High Blood Pressure Research Council, and the Quality of Care and Outcomes in Research Interdisciplinary Working Group. *Stroke* 2007; 38: 2001–23.

Hunt WE, Hess RM. Surgical risk as related to time of intervention in the repair of intracranial aneurysms. *J Neurosurg* 1968; 28: 14–20.

Labovitz DL, Halim A, Boden-Albala B, Hauser WA, Sacco RL. The incidence of deep and lobar intracerebral hemorrhage in whites, blacks, and Hispanics. *Neurology* 2005; 65: 518–22.

Mayer SA, Brun NC, Begtrup K, *et al.* Recombinant activated factor VII for acute intracerebral hemorrhage. *N Engl J Med* 2005; 352: 777–85.

Mendelow AD, Gregson BA, Fernandes HM, *et al.* Early surgery versus initial conservative treatment in patients with spontaneous supratentorial intracerebral haematomas in the International Surgical Trial in Intracerebral Haemorrhage (STICH): a randomised trial. *Lancet* 2005; 365: 387–97.

NINDS t-PA Stroke Study Group. Intracerebral hemorrhage after intravenous t-PA therapy for ischemic stroke. *Stroke* 1997; 28: 2109–18.

Patten J. *Neurological Differential Diagnosis*, 2nd ed. Berlin: Springer; 1995, p. 14, 53.

Rinkel GJ, Feigin VL, Algra A, van den Bergh WM, Vermeulen M, van Gijn J. Calcium antagonists for aneurysmal subarachnoid haemorrhage. *Cochrane Database Syst Rev* 2005; CD000277.

Segal AZ, Chiu RI, Eggleston-Sexton PM, Beiser A, Greenberg SM. Low cholesterol as a risk factor for primary intracerebral hemorrhage: a case-control study. *Neuroepidemiology* 1999; 18: 185–93.

Spetzler RF, Martin NA. A proposed grading system for arteriovenous malformations. *J Neurosurg* 1986; 65: 476–83.

Steiner T, Diringer MN, Schneider D, *et al*. Dynamics of intraventricular hemorrhage in patients with spontaneous intracerebral hemorrhage: risk factors, clinical impact, and effect of hemostatic therapy with recombinant activated factor VII. *Neurosurgery* 2006; 59: 767–73, discussion 773–4.

Steiner T, Kaste M, Forsting M, *et al*. Recommendations for the management of intracranial haemorrhage – part I: spontaneous intracerebral haemorrhage. The European Stroke Initiative Writing Committee and the Writing Committee for the EUSI Executive Committee. *Cerebrovasc Dis* 2006; 22: 294–316.

Steiner T, Rosand J, Diringer M. Intracerebral hemorrhage associated with oral anticoagulant therapy: current practices and unresolved questions. *Stroke* 2006; 37: 256–62.

Suarez JI, Tarr RW, Selman WR. Aneurysmal subarachnoid hemorrhage. *N Engl J Med* 2006; 354: 387–96.

Teasdale GM, Drake CG, Hunt W, *et al*. A universal subarachnoid hemorrhage scale: report of a committee of the World Federation of Neurosurgical Societies. *J Neurol Neurosurg Psychiatry* 1988; 51: 1457.

van Gijn J, Rinkel GJ. Subarachnoid haemorrhage: diagnosis, causes and management. *Brain* 2001; 124: 249–78.

Chapter 11
Strokes in children and young adults

Alfred Lindner
Marienhospital, Stuttgart, Germany

Introduction and epidemiology

Cerebrovascular diseases in children cause considerable morbidity and are among the top ten causes of death. The incidence of arterial ischemic stroke ranges from 2 to 13 per 100 000 children under the age of 18 per year in Europe and North America. Hemorrhagic and ischemic strokes account for approximately 50% of cases. The incidence of sinus venous thrombosis (SVT) in children is 0.6 per 100 000 children per year and is highest in the first year of life.

Pathophysiology

Cardiac diseases, including congenital and acquired heart diseases, are among the most common causes of stroke in children, accounting for up to 50% in case series.

Sickle cell disease (SCD) is the most common cause of stroke in black children. The strokes are associated with stenosis of large vessels such as the distal internal carotid and proximal middle cerebral artery. Stroke occurs by the age of 20 in about 11% of patients with SCD. Untreated, two-thirds of patients with a first stroke will have recurrence.

Several acquired and genetic *coagulation factor abnormalities* have been associated with pediatric stroke. Small case series and case control studies found various abnormalities, such as the prothrombin mutation G20210, the presence of the Factor V Leiden G1691A mutation, antiphospholipid antibodies, deficiency of natural anticoagulant protein C, protein S, and antithrombin III, and elevations in homocysteine and lipoprotein (a).

Overall, prothrombotic abnormalities have been identified in 20–50% of children presenting with acute ischemic stroke and 33–99% of children with cerebral SVT. Iron deficiency anemia is an important risk factor for stroke

in children because it is easy to treat. It is found in more than 25% of children with stroke and probably is due to thrombocytosis related to low iron stores. Fabry disease and homocystinuria are associated with an increased risk of ischemic stroke.

At least one-third of pediatric strokes are caused by *infectious disorders* such as meningitis, encephalitis, human immunodeficiency virus infection, *Varicella zoster* virus infection, and systemic sepsis. Underlying pathogenetic mechanisms include direct inflammation of blood vessels of the brain, hypercoagulopathy due to infection, or cardiovascular causes related to endocarditis or hypotension. Typical findings in children with post-varicella angiopathy are stenosis of the distal internal carotid and proximal cerebral arteries as well as subcortical ischemic lesions.

Abnormalities of the intracranial vessels in children with ischemic stroke have been found in almost 80% of cases in a series from the UK. The most common abnormalities were narrowing or occlusion of proximal large arteries such as the distal internal carotid artery or proximal middle cerebral artery.

Arterial dissection is found in up to 20% of children with ischemic stroke. In contrast to adults, intracranial dissection in the anterior circulation without trauma is more common than extracranial dissection in children. If diagnosis of stroke in the posterior circulation is made, vertebral artery dissection should always be considered, especially since posterior circulation stroke is rare in children. Pain is not a prominent presenting feature, with headache reported in only half of patients, and neck pain rarely noted. This contrasts to adults, in whom pain is often noted to be the most common presenting feature.

Moyamoya arteriopathy typically involves the small, fragile, basal, collateral vessels (puff of smoke). The disease is usually bilateral, but may also be unilateral and in more severe cases may involve the posterior circulation. The pathogenesis of moyamoya syndrome is unknown. Children present with ischemic stroke during the first decade of life and young adults present with intraparenchymal, intraventricular, or subarachnoid hemorrhage, as well as ischemic stroke during the third decade of life. Seizures and involuntary

International Neurology: A Clinical Approach. Edited by Robert P. Lisak, Daniel D. Truong, William M. Carroll, and Roongroj Bhidayasiri. © 2009 Blackwell Publishing, ISBN: 978-1-4051-5738-4.

movement disorders may also occur in the pediatric population.

In patients with *transient cerebral arteriopathy* typical clinical and radiological features can be found. All were previously healthy children, with acute hemiplegia as the initial symptom. Imaging studies revealed small subcortical infarcts located in the internal capsule or the basal ganglia. Conventional arteriography in the acute stage showed multifocal abnormalities of the cerebral arterial wall, with focal stenosis or segmental narrowing in the distal internal carotid and the proximal anterior, middle, or posterior cerebral arteries. Over time most of the patients had complete regression, improvement, or stabilization. The underlying condition is probably a transient inflammation of the arterial wall (angiitis) due to prior viral infection such as varicella. There are also case reports of transient cerebral arteriopathy triggered by enteroviral or HIV infection.

Fibromuscular dysplasia is a segmental, non-inflammatory, non-atheromatous angiopathy affecting small and medium sized arteries of unknown aetiology that most commonly affects the renal and internal carotid arteries but has also been described in almost every arterial bed in the body.

The incidence of *SVT* is highest in the first year of life. Most of the thromboses are located within the superior sagittal sinus with or without thrombosis of the lateral sinus. Approximately 50% of children with SVT present with seizures or focal abnormalities, but clinical presentation can also be subtle. Risk factors include neck and head infections, perinatal complications, dehydration, and coagulation disorders.

Clinical features

Clinical presentation varies from hemiparesis with or without hemisensory signs or visual field defects to unexplained altered consciousness. If headache is present, venous thrombosis or arterial dissection should be considered. Seizures, with or without focal neurological deficit, are a common presentation of cerebral venous thrombosis. If deterioration at the level of conciousness occurs, large middle cerebral territory infarcts, posterior fossa strokes, and intracranial hemorrhage should be considered, which require transfer to a pediatric neurological and neurosurgical intensive care unit.

The differential diagnosis in children presenting with an acute hemiparesis includes central nervous system infections (e.g., abscess, focal encephalitis), trauma (subdural, epidural hematoma, traumatic intracerebral bleeding, cerebral contusion), tumor, and demyelinating diseases such as acute demyelinating encephalomyelitis (ADEM). Todd's paresis and hemiparesis due to migraine must be carefully excluded.

Investigations

Intracranial hemorrhage must be excluded by emergency computed tomography (CT) or magnetic resonance imaging (MRI), since urgent neurosurgical intervention may be necessary. MRI and MRI-angiography can provide more important information about intra- and extracranial vessels, venous sinus, and other pathologies confirming vascular diseases. If arterial dissection is suspected, additional MRI of the neck with fat suppression is indicated. Standard digital subtraction cerebral angiography (DSA) should be strongly considered in cases with equivocal or negative findings on MRI or where no other explanation can be identified. Transcranial color-coded duplex sonography (TCCS) enables the reliable assessment of intracranial stenoses, occlusions, and cross-flow through the anterior and posterior communicating arteries, as well as the midline shift in hemispheric infarcts. TCCS is also useful for diagnosis and monitoring of vasospasm and detection of supratentorial hematomas and aneurysms, and may identify arteriovenous malformations.

Electroencephalography (EEG) should be urgently performed if post-ictal hemiparesis ("Todd's paresis") is assumed. On EEG, epileptic activity can be found. On the other hand, seizures may also be caused by stroke. Hemiplegic migraine usually shows unilateral slow background activity, and without MRI no clear distinction between migraine and stroke can be made.

Cardiac examinations should include transthoracic echocardiogram (TTE) with agitated saline for detection of persistent foramen ovale (PFO). TTE is the gold standard for detection of valve vegetations in endocarditis and structural cardiac abnormalities.

Laboratory evaluation includes electrolytes, liver and renal functions, HIV, Veneral Disease Laboratory Research (VDLR) test, fasting lipid profile, C-reactive protein, antinuclear antibody, and erythrocyte sedimentation rate. Lactate, plasma amino acids, urine amino, and organic acids should be quantified if homocystinuria or MELAS (mitochondrial encephalopathy, lactic acidosis, and stroke-like episodes) is suspected. Analysis of the cerebrospinal fluid is the diagnostic clue in the diagnosis of stroke caused by infections of the central nervous system due to vasculitis.

There is still controversy about the significance of laboratory evaluation for hypercoagulability in the diagnosis of childhood stroke. Screening laboratory evaluations include detection of possible underlying acquired and genetic coagulation factor abnormalities (see above).

Treatment/management

At the present time, acute management and treatment of strokes in children and young adults is based on extrapolation from the adult literature and expert opinion, as no evidence-based guidelines exist, except in sickle cell anemia. International, multicenter trials are beginning and should provide some answers over the next few years.

There is currently no evidence to support use of thrombolytic agents such as tissue plasminogen activator (tPA) in the acute treatment of arterial ischemic stroke in children.

There is only one small series in which thrombolysis showed an unclear benefit in children with acute ischemic stroke. Larger studies are needed to evaluate the safety and efficacy of this treatment for children.

The use of anticoagulation in children with cardiac embolism is controversial. It involves balancing the risk of precipitating hemorrhagic transformation of the infarct with the potential to prevent further embolic events. The decision may be influenced by several factors (time elapsed after the stroke, neurological and imaging findings, pathology of the cardiovascular system).

The efficacy and optimal dose of aspirin in the treatment of children with acute arterial ischemic stroke is not known. Aspirin therapy is commonly used at a dose of 3–5 mg/kg/day. Most experts recommend aspirin for secondary stroke prevention in children. Experience with other antiplatelet drugs such as clopidogrel hardly exists in children.

Supportive care should ensure adequate hydration, ventilation, and oxygenation. Infarct volume and outcome may be related to body temperature during the first days of the stroke. Blood glucose levels should be maintained in normal range. Seizures in the acute stage should be treated rapidly. A change in the level of arousal may be the first sign of expanding brain edema. Surgical decompression in children presenting with coma with large ischemic infarcts of the middle cerebral artery may be necessary, which are very often lethal if managed conservatively. In SCD, chronic blood transfusion is effective for secondary and primary prevention.

In patients with moyamoya-related strokes, revascularization surgery using different techniques may be helpful.

In summary, stroke in children and young adults is an important cause of morbidity and mortality. The clinical presentation varies, and adequate diagnosis requires fast multidisciplinary approaches to reduce the probability of serious neurological consequences. Clinical trials are needed to confirm the efficacy in children of selected therapies now used in adults.

Further reading

Ganesan V, Prengler M, McShane MA, Wade AM, Kirkham FJ. Investigation of risk factors in children with arterial ischaemic stroke. *Ann Neurol* 2003; 53(2): 167–73.

Giroud M, Lemesle M, Gouyon JB, Nivelon JL, Milan C, Dumas R. Cerebrovascular disease in children under 16 years of age in the city of Dijon, France: a study of incidence and clinical features from 1985 to 1993. *J Clin Epidemiol* 1995; 48(11): 1343–8.

Jordan LC, Hillis AE. Hemorrhagic stroke in children. *Pediatr Neurol* 2007; 36(2): 73–80.

Lanska MJ, Lanska DJ, Horwitz SJ, Aram DM. Presentation, clinical course, and outcome of childhood stroke. *Pediatr Neurol* 1991; 7(5): 333–41.

Lynch JK, Hirtz DG, DeVeber G, Nelson KB. Report of the National Institute of Neurological Disorders and Stroke workshop on perinatal and childhood stroke. *Pediatrics* 2002; 109(1): 116–23.

Ramaswami U, Whybra C, Parini R, *et al*. Clinical manifestations of Fabry disease in children: data from the Fabry Outcome Survey. *Acta Paediatr* 2006; 95(1): 86–92.

Sebire G, Tabarki B, Saunders DE, *et al*. Cerebral venous sinus thrombosis in children: risk factors, presentation, diagnosis and outcome. *Brain* 2005; 128(Pt 3): 477–89.

Chapter 12
Other cerebrovascular syndromes

David Blacker
Sir Charles Gairdner Hospital, Nedlands, Australia

Introduction

This chapter covers a miscellaneous collection of cerebrovascular conditions not covered elsewhere in this textbook, including stroke and migraine, stroke and substance abuse, cerebral autosomal dominant arteriopathy with subcortical infarcts and leukoencephalopathy (CADASIL) and allied conditions, hypertensive encephalopathy and posterior reversible encephalopathy syndrome (PRES), peri-procedural, post-operative and in-hospital stroke, and some rare stroke syndromes. These conditions might be encountered in a wide variety of medical settings throughout all areas of the world.

Stroke and migraine

The relationship between stroke and migraine is complex, and is strongest for migraine with aura. Migraine may be a risk for stroke or a consequence of stroke, and both conditions may share a common underlying cause, for example, as part of CADASIL, mitochondrial encephalopathy, lactic acidosis, and stroke (MELAS), or be concurrent with arterial dissection or patent foramen ovale. Migraineurs also have a higher prevalence of cardiovascular risk factors. Previously, it was thought that migraineurs harbor antiphospholipid antibodies more frequently than controls and that this may explain the migraine and stroke relationship, but recent studies have not borne this out.

Estimates of the incidence of migrainous infarction are variable, and may vary according to the rigour with which diagnostic criteria from the International Headache Society (IHS) are followed. The range is from 0.5% to 1.5% of ischemic strokes, up to 10–14% of strokes in young patients. The IHS criteria suggest that the infarction results from hypoperfusion during an aura, and thus the stroke symptoms, are similar to that of the

aura, but many cases may occur in patients with migraine without aura. Although imaging modalities measuring cerebral blood flow have demonstrated oligemia associated with spreading neuronal depression, this would appear to be less than the threshhold for ischemia, so the precise mechanism of migrainous stroke is not entirely clear. One-third of migrainous infarcts are located in the occipital lobe, the usual site of origin of the spreading depression.

Investigation should be as for all usual ischemic strokes, with migrainous infarction essentially being a diagnosis of exclusion. Secondary prevention measures include the usual antithrombotic therapies and vascular risk factor reduction. Specific concerns include cessation of oral contraceptives and other hormones, and avoidance of vasoactive migraine treatments such as ergot derivatives and triptans, based on concerns regarding hypoperfusion.

Stroke and substance abuse

A tragic and eminently avoidable stroke syndrome is stroke associated with substance abuse. Although "legal" drugs such as nicotine and alcohol probably account for a large majority of such strokes, the focus of this section will be on illicit substances such as amphetamines, cocaine, and others that may be implicated in strokes in a wide range of patients, particularly the young, in many different countries. Weight loss medications such as phenylpropanolamine are implicated in hemorrhagic stroke. A mechanistic approach to the etiology of such strokes is outlined below.

Cardiac
Cardiac mechanisms leading to substance abuse-related stroke include infective endocarditis from intravenous drug use, hypertension from stimulants, and arrhythmias and cardiomyopathy from alcohol.

Extracranial large arteries
Metamphetamine and cocaine have been associated with arterial dissection leading to stroke. It is likely that these drugs may have a direct vasculopathic effect, but it is

International Neurology: A Clinical Approach. Edited by Robert P. Lisak, Daniel D. Truong, William M. Carroll, and Roongroj Bhidayasiri. © 2009 Blackwell Publishing, ISBN: 978-1-4051-5738-4.

also possible that traumatic dissection may be related to behaviors and activities induced by the neuropsychiatric effects of the drugs.

Intracranial vessels

As noted above, metamphetamine and cocaine may have direct toxic effects on blood vessels as well as causing vasospasm, vasculitis, and hypertension. Both ischemic and hemorrhagic stroke may result.

Other

Metabolic disturbances such as hyponatremia associated with metamphetamine use may lead to stroke-like symptoms. Complications of intravenous drug use include hepatic failure with development of coagulopathy leading to hemorrhagic stroke. Heroin-related nephropathy may lead to renal failure with hypertension and its concomitant stroke risks.

CADASIL and allied conditions

CADASIL is an inherited microangiopathy characterized by migraine with aura, recurrent strokes, and cognitive impairment at an early age. The strokes are typically subcortical, often presenting with classic lacunar syndromes. Rarely, it may present as an acute encephalopathy or intracerebral hemorrhage. CADASIL is caused by a mutation in the *Notch*3 gene on chromosmome 19, the discovery of which was a major breakthrough in cerebrovascular genetics. Various differing mutations are now described, including an autosomal recessive form in a Japanese population. MRI typically shows marked periventricular and subcortical white matter T2 signal hyperintensities, which may be differentiated from hypertensive leucoareosis by predilection for the external capsule and anterior temporal lobes. Differential diagnoses also include Binswanger's disease and multiple sclerosis. No specific treatment for CADASIL is currently available.

Hypertensive encephalopathy and posterior reversible encephalopathy syndrome (PRES)

Stroke physicians may encounter patients with hypertensive encephalopathy and PRES, and also see patients with elevated blood pressure following both ischemic and hemorrhagic stroke. Hypertensive encephalopathy occurs when cerebral autoregulation is overwhelmed by a sudden rise in blood pressure, usually to extreme levels in the vicinity of 250/150 mm Hg. Vasodilatation of intracranial vessels, cerebral hyperperfusion, and exudation of fluid may lead to raised intracranial pressure.

Renal disease, pheochromocytoma, sympathomimetic drugs, systemic vasculitidies, and pregnancy may be the predisposing conditions. Previously normotensive patients may be more susceptible than chronic hypertensives (particularly if the change is abrupt), since in the latter, cerebral autoregulation is already "shifted to the right." Clinical features include headache, nausea and vomiting, visual symptoms, impaired consciousness, and seizures. Physical examination findings include retinal hemorrhages and hyperreflexia. Focal neurological deficits suggest a complicating hemorrhage or infarction. Imaging findings are similar to that seen in PRES (see below). Treatment with parenteral antihypertensive agents (e.g., sodium nitroprusside) is essential, although excessive reduction might result in hypoperfusion.

Since the first descriptions of PRES in the mid-1990s, it has become recognized that the syndrome may not necessarily be posterior in location, or reversible. The typical presentation of PRES is with headaches, seizures, and visual loss, typically with accelerated hypertension, often in patients taking immunosuppressant medications such as cyclopsorin and tacrolimus. The pathogenesis is proposed to be vasogenic edema without infarction related to disruption of normal cerebral autoregulation. The white matter of the parieto-occipital region is most commonly involved, possibly related to the degree of sympathetic innervation in the arteries supplying this area. MRI diffusion weighted (DWI) and apparent diffusion coefficient (ADC) sequences may be helpful in studying the vasogenic and cytotoxic components of the edema, and give some indication of tissue destined to either recover or infarct. Treatment includes antihypertensive and anticonvulsant agents and adjustment of immunosuppressant medications.

Hypertensive encephalopathy and PRES are distinct from the commonly encountered problem of hypertension after ischemic or hemorrhagic stroke. Excessively low and high blood pressures, along with large degrees of variability, seem to be associated with poor outcome in ischemic stroke. Higher levels of blood pressure are linked with hematoma expansion and possibly poorer outcome in hemorrhagic stroke. Previous concerns regarding a "rim" of hypoperfused tissue around a hematoma have not been demonstrated by perfusion imaging. There are little data on which to base treatment and several trials are ongoing.

Peri-procedural, post-operative and in-hospital stroke

There is an increasing literature on stroke related to medical procedures, perhaps driven by medico-legal concerns, but also by the realization that when stroke occurs in patients already in hospital, there may be an opportunity for intervention. Cardiac, carotid, and neurosurgeries carry an inherent stroke risk, due to the nature of the surgery, and the fact that such patients frequently have stroke risk factors. Additionally, other surgeries and procedures carry a stroke risk, possibly related to the interruption of antiplatelet or antithrombotic medications and other factors such as the potentially thrombogenic mileu of surgery, and hemodynamic alterations. One large series of general surgery patients found a stroke risk of 0.2%. Prospective studies of coronary artery bypass grafting show a stroke risk of 2%, but this varies greatly according to the age of the patients and whether or not valve surgery is also undertaken.

Patients on medical wards may also be at risk, particularly cardiac patients who share common risk factors, who may have atrial fibrillation and angiograms that predispose to ischemic stroke, or who may be treated with antithrombotic agents predisposing to hemorrhage. General medical patients with infections, dehydration, and renal impairment may also be at risk. Cancer patients with either hyperviscosity or coagulopathy, often with hematological malignancies, are at particular risk.

Acute therapeutic options may be limited by the potential for hemorrhage from the fresh surgical site, but intra-arterial techniques may provide a potential treatment option for ischemic stroke in this setting.

Rare stroke syndromes

A number of rare, non-inflammatory cerebral vasculopathies may lead to stroke, including those associated with Fabry's disease, the post-partum state, and several that have predominantly ophthalmological features such as Eale's and Susac's diseases.

Further reading

Blacker DJ. In-hospital stroke. *Lancet Neurol* 2003; 2: 741–6.
Bousser MG, Welch KM. Relation between migraine and stroke. *Lancet Neurol* 2005; 4: 533–42.
Stott VL, Hurrell MA, Anderson TJ. Reversible posterior leukoencephalopathy syndrome: a misnomer reviewed. *Int Med J* 2005; 35: 83–90.

Chapter 13
Diseases of the cerebral venous system

Patrick Carney[1] and Stephen M. Davis[2]
[1]Epilepsy Research Center, Victoria, Australia
[2]Royal Melbourne Hospital, University of Melbourne, Melbourne, Australia

Introduction

Diseases of the cerebral venous system lead to cerebral venous sinus thrombosis (CVST). CVST may present as a cause of stroke or chronically with symptoms of intracranial hypertension. The prevalence and cause of CVST are variable and to some extent relate to cultural and economic factors.

Epidemiology

The epidemiology of CVST is difficult to define. Previously, CVST was thought to be an uncommon serious condition, with the diagnosis predominantly made at autopsy. However, recent developments in neuroimaging have established that CVST is much more prevalent than previously thought. A Saudi Arabian study found that 7 cases per 100 000 hospitalized patients had CVST. In India CVST is believed to cause up to 30% of young strokes. A Canadian review of pediatric stroke presentations estimated a population incidence of 0.67 cases per 100 000 per year. Mortality from CVST is approximately 8%. In a substantial proportion of patients, the cause of death could be attributed to underlying diseases that led to the sinus thrombosis. Functional outcome for survivors, however, is generally excellent, with minimal disability. Furthermore, recurrence rates are very low.

CVST commonly affects young people. The mean age of onset in several series is approximately 37 years of age and younger patients with CVST often have different underlying causes and a better outcome. The condition predominantly affects women with a ratio of 3:1 and is strongly related to hormonal factors, including pregnancy and oral contraceptive use (see below).

International Neurology: A Clinical Approach. Edited by Robert P. Lisak, Daniel D. Truong, William M. Carroll, and Roongroj Bhidayasiri.
© 2009 Blackwell Publishing, ISBN: 978-1-4051-5738-4.

Pathophysiology

A variety of risk factors for the development of CVST have been identified (Table 13.1). CVST may occur due to systemic or local intracranial factors. Both acquired and inherited thrombophilic risk factors can lead to spontaneous cerebral venous thrombosis. Local processes, such as

Table 13.1 Recognised causes of dural sinus thrombosis.

1. Systemic diseases/factors
a. Hormonal
  i. Pregnancy and the puerperium
  ii. Oral contraceptive pill
  iii. Other hormone supplements
b. Coagulation disorders
  i. Inherited
    1. Factor V Leiden
    2. Prothrombin gene mutation
    3. Protein C and S deficiencies
  ii. Acquired
    1. Antiphospholipid antibodies/lupus anticoagulant
    2. Disseminated intravascular coagulation
c. Other hematological disorders
  i. Polycythemia Vera
  ii. Thrombocythemia
d. Systemic inflammatory disease
  i. Systemic lupus erythematosis
  ii. Behcet's disease
e. Malignancy
f. Other
  i. Systemic infections
  ii. Nephrotic syndrome
  iii. Any cause of dehydration

2. Local diseases/factors
a. Infection
  i. Extra-dural
    1. Mastoiditis
    2. Sinusitis
  ii. Intra-dural
    1. Meningitis
    2. Abscess
    3. Empyema
b. Neurosurgical procedures including lumbar puncture
c. Head injury
d. Tumor

infection or intracranial tumors, may also cause venous obstruction.

Spontaneous venous sinus thrombosis is particularly a disorder of women and occurs in frequent association with hormonal factors including pregnancy and the oral contraceptive pill (OCP). Increasingly, it has been recognized that inherited hypercoagulability disorders may lead to the development of CVST in isolation or more commonly in conjunction with risk factors such as pregnancy or OCP use. Commonly identified risk factors include activated protein C resistance associated with the Factor V Leiden mutation, the prothrombin gene mutation, and isolated factor deficiencies such as protein C, S, and anti-thrombin III.

Although local infection leading to venous sinus thrombosis is becoming increasingly rare, sepsis remains an important potential cause of CVST in the developing world. Infections including otitis media, mastoiditis, and paranasal sinusitis may lead to local venous sinus thrombophlebitis. Systemic sepsis also increases the risk of thrombosis, including cerebral venous thrombosis. The largest prospective study of CVST, the International Study on Cerebral Vein and Dural Sinus Thrombosis, found an increased rate of infections leading to CVST amongst African and Asian populations, although obstetric factors remain the most significant cause.

CVST may arise as a complication of traumatic brain injury and should be considered as a cause of further neurological deterioration.

Clinical features

The clinical presentation of venous sinus disease is highly variable and relates to the underlying cause and the effect of venous obstruction. Venous sinus obstruction leads to a generalized increase in intracranial pressure associated with reduced venous outflow and impaired CSF absorption. This leads to headaches, impairment of conscious state, cognitive deficits, and visual blurring due to papilledema. Symptoms relating to increased intracranial pressure may be acute, subacute, or chronic in their presentation. Chronic presentations occurred in approximately 7% of cases in the largest prospective analysis of CVST, typically with idiopathic intracranial hypertension. These patients are frequently women and have an overall better outcome.

If sinus thrombosis is complicated by occlusion of cortical veins, venous infarction, often accompanied by hemorrhage, may occur. Such patients present acutely with focal neurological deficits such as hemiplegia, hemiparesis, sensory and visual inattention, and receptive and expressive speech deficits relating to the site of stroke damage. Seizures are a common presenting symptom of venous infarction and are seen more commonly than in arterial stroke. Seizures may occur in patients with venous sinus disease without stroke, related to increased intracranial pressure or underlying causes such as infection or trauma.

Investigations

The diagnosis of CVST has been transformed by cerebral imaging. Plain CT scan is useful for identifying venous infarction. The empty delta sign of low-attenuation thrombus surrounded by a triangular area of enhancement may be seen on contrast CT scan. However, CT is not sufficiently accurate to rule out CVST. CT venography is a further advance in assessment of cerebral venous anatomy.

Traditionally, cerebral angiography with venography was the diagnostic test of choice for cerebral sinus disease. However, magnetic resonance imaging (MRI) particularly with MR venography (MRV) has largely replaced angiography and is generally the definitive investigation in the diagnosis of CVST. This modality not only enables imaging of thrombosed venous sinuses which are hyperintense on T1- and T2-weighted sequences (Figure 13.1), but also shows an absence of flow within the venous sinus. Furthermore venous infarction and hemorrhage can be clearly identified.

Cerebral angiography remains helpful for some difficult cases where MRI/MRV is not definitive. It is also used as the basis for delivery of topical thrombolysis.

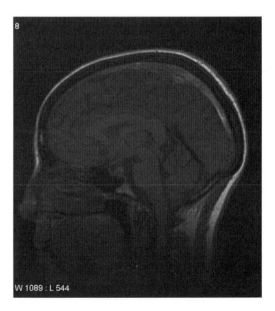

Figure 13.1 T1-weighted sagittal image of a patient with sagittal sinus thrombosis. The thrombosed sinus is hyperintense compared to the normal brain parenchymal signal. (Courtesy of Dr G. Fitt.)

Treatment/management

The approach to managing CVST involves investigation and treatment of the underlying cause and specific therapy for the sinus thrombosis. The mainstay of therapy is systemic anticoagulation. A meta-analysis performed on three small studies of anticoagulation in CVST showed a trend toward benefit with anticoagulation, although not statistically significant. In contrast, expert opinion strongly supports acute anticoagulation, based on a dramatic reduction in case fatality rates in modern case series where heparin use has been routine. Initial intravenous anticoagulation with heparin is followed by a variable period of warfarin therapy, even in the presence of parenchymal hemorrhage.

The appropriate duration of oral anticoagulation therapy remains unclear. Commonly warfarin would be used for 6 months, but longer term if there is a demonstrated persisting coagulopathy. With these guidelines, recurrence is very rare. MRI can be used to follow the progress of sinus recanalization, but this may be incomplete and is not a reliable guide to the duration of therapy.

Local thrombolysis has been employed to treat more serious cases with extensive thrombosis or poor prognostic signs. This approach may lead to a more frequent and rapid restoration of venous flow, but there are no randomized control trials of thrombolysis versus anticoagulation.

In some progressive cases with prominent pressure effects, decompressive craniectomy has been successfully employed.

Further reading

Ferro JM, Canhao P, Stam J, Bousser MG, Baringagarrementeria F. Prognosis of cerebral vein and dural sinus thrombosis: results of the International Study on Cerebral Vein and Dural Sinus Thrombosis. *Stroke* 2004; 35: 664–70.

Stram J. Thrombosis of the cerebral veins and sinuses. *N Engl J Med* 2005; 352: 1791–8.

Chapter 14
Spinal cord stroke

Manu Mehdiratta and Louis R. Caplan
Beth Israel Deaconess Medical Center, Boston, USA

Introduction

Clinicians around the world encounter vascular diseases of the spinal cord. Though relatively rare, they remain an important cause of myelopathy. It is important to become familiar with the clinical presentation of spinal cord stroke syndromes as the diagnosis is often challenging.

Epidemiology

The prevalence of spinal cord stroke in not known. A study completed in London, Ontario, Canada, found spinal cord infarcts in 52 of 4000 consecutive autopsies (4%). In another study, it was found that infarcts of the spinal cord represented only approximately 1.2% of all stroke admissions to one stroke center. In non-Western countries, spinal cord infarction is also considered uncommon. In a study conducted in India over a 2-year period it was found that spinal cord infarction was the etiology in only 3.65% of patients presenting with a non-compressive myelopathy. In contrast, transverse myelitis and post-infectious myelopathy were much more common.

Pathophysiology

The clinical approach to vascular diseases of the spinal cord depends on understanding the vascular anatomy of the spinal cord, which is unique. The anterior spinal artery (ASA) emanates from the two vertebral arteries at the base of the skull. This ASA runs on the ventral surface of the spinal cord from the foramen magnum to the filum terminale and supplies the anterior horns and white matter of the cord. Supply to the cervical region of the ASA comes from the vertebral arteries. In the lower thoracic and upper lumbar regions, supply is largely from the Artery of Adamkiewicz which usually enters between

International Neurology: A Clinical Approach. Edited by Robert P. Lisak, Daniel D. Truong, William M. Carroll, and Roongroj Bhidayasiri. © 2009 Blackwell Publishing, ISBN: 978-1-4051-5738-4.

T9 and T12. This leaves an area of relatively less supply in the upper thoracic cord known as the "longitudinal spinal cord watershed region," between T2 and T4 primarily. The paired posterior spinal arteries lie along the dorsal surface of the spinal cord and supply the dorsal columns and the posterior gray matter. The area between the anterior and posterior spinal arteries can also be a border zone or watershed area if blood supply is decreased.

A variety of different vascular diseases can affect the spinal cord including infarction, hemorrhage, and infections and each of these has a different clinical presentation depending upon the site of involvement.

Clinical features

Clinical features of spinal cord vascular disease vary depending upon the underlying etiology. Each of the major spinal cord vascular diseases are discussed below.

Ischemia and infarction

Spinal cord infarction is most commonly secondary to disease of the aorta which compromises flow through the ASA. This often occurs after surgery to repair thoracic and abdominal aortic aneurysms. Clinically, if the thoracic cord is involved, the patient develops a flaccid paraplegia with a thoracic sensory level and urinary incontinence. The lower extremities become spastic later. The posterior columns are usually spared such that the patient has intact vibration and proprioception. Other causes of this clinical picture are unruptured aneurysm, aortic dissection, and rupture of the aorta secondary to trauma. Aortic atherosclerosis can affect the origins of the radicular spinal arteries, causing infarcts as well.

Infarcts can be classified as:

1 Bilateral, predominatly anterior – these patients have bilateral motor and spinothalamic-type sensory deficits. Posterior column sensory functions (vibration and position sense) are spared.

2 Unilateral, predominantly anterior – the motor deficit is a hemiparesis below the lesion and a contralateral spinothalamic tract sensory loss – a Brown–Sequard syndrome.

3 Bilateral, predominantly posterior – posterior column type of sensory loss below the lesion with variably severe bilateral pyramidal tract signs.
4 Unilateral, mostly posterior – ipsilateral hemiparesis and posterior column sensory loss.
5 Central – bilateral pain and temperature loss with spared posterior column and motor functions. Similar to a syrinx.
6 Transverse – loss of motor, sensory, and sphincter functions below the level of the lesion.
Anterior patterns are more common than posterior especially after aortic surgery.

In pregnant and peripartum women there is a risk of fibrocartilaginous emboli in which cartilaginous material from the intervertebral discs can break off and spread through the spinal arteries and veins, resulting in infarction. Patients often present with pain in the neck or upper back followed by rapid onset of quadraparesis that can be asymmetric.

In developing countries, infectious causes of spinal cord infarction are especially important. Emboli to the brain and spinal cord can originate from bacterial endocarditis. More directly, tuberculosis, syphilis, Lyme borreliosis, and various fungi can affect the spinal arteries, resulting in spinal arteritis and infarction. Schistosoma mansoni is an important cause of spinal cord infarction and granulomatous infection in some parts of the world. Infection can also result in chronic adhesive arachnoiditis. This can result in damage to penetrating spinal arteries and infarction. Cerebrospinal fluid studies and spinal imaging are important aids to these diagnoses.

Spinal cord infarction can also occur with systemic hypoperfusion secondary to shock or cardiac arrest. The watershed areas between T4 and T8 are most commonly affected. Venous infarct are also possible due to venous thrombosis, compression of veins by epidural masses, or with spinal dural arteriovenous malformations (AVMs).

Hemorrhage
Referred to as hematomyelia, hemorrhage into the spinal cord parenchyma can occur for a number of reasons. Trauma is the most common etiology, but AVMs, anticoagulants and bleeding disorders such as hemophilia can also produce hematomyelia. The clinical picture is usually one of neck pain, weakness, areflexia, and pain and temperature loss in a cape-like distribution.

Spinal vascular malformations
Vascular malformations within the spinal cord are different from intracranial malformations because they are more likely to cause ischemia than hemorrhage. Spinal AVMs can be dural or intradural. Dural AVMs receive their vascular supply from radicular arteries and they drain intradurally via enlarged tortuous veins. The resulting venous hypertension and intermittent thrombosis of the venous system causes the myelopathic symptoms and signs. Men are preferentially affected (4:1) and usually between the ages of 40 and 70. The lower thoracic and lumbrosacral areas of the cord are most often affected. The clinical findings are usually characterized by a slow and progressive neurological decline, sometimes with acute worsening. Patients often describe leg weakness and radicular pain that can be episodic and worsened with exercise. Spinal transient ischemic attacks (TIAs) can occur.

Intradural AVMs can be located within the parenchyma of the spinal cord (intramedullary) or between the dura and the cord. They are more likely to hemorrhage, causing sudden onset of neurological symptoms, than dural AVMs because they have higher flow. Again, men are more often affected than women, but patients with intradural AVMs tend to be younger, with 65% of affected patients being less than 25 years old in one case series.

Investigations

Ideally, in all patients presenting with myelopathic symptoms, a compressive cause for myelopathy should be excluded urgently, preferably with MRI. In developing countries, this may not always be possible. A contrast CT myelogram or dye myelogram suffices to exclude spinal cord compression. If an infectious, post–infectious, or inflammatory cause of myelopathy is suspected, the next diagnostic step should be a lumbar puncture (LP). Acute spinal cord infarction can cause an elevation in protein levels but does not usually result in a pleocytosis. This can be helpful in differentiating infectious and vascular causes of spinal cord infarction.

In Western countries, especially in patients who are recently post-operative, an MRI of the cord is often done first to evaluate for infarction, though it does not reveal the infarct in all affected patients. In a recent series of 27 patients with spinal cord infarcts, only 67% of patients who underwent MRI had the infarct visualized. Infarcts are usually seen on MRI as a T2-weighted hyperintensity within a vascular distribution. Diffusion-weighted imaging has been shown to be helpful in identifying early spinal cord ischemia, but there is more artifact within the spinal column than there is intracranially, which leads to a higher incidence of false positive results.

Hematomyelia is usually evident on MRI, especially with the use of the T2* or gradient echo sequences. It can be more difficult to diagnose dural AVMs as they are often not easily seen with MRI. Myelography or spinal angiography is usually necessary if the diagnosis of spinal dural AVM is considered likely. Key to the diagnosis of spinal dural fistulas is demonstration of dilated veins along the spinal cord surface.

Treatment/management

Unfortunately, treatment of spinal cord infarction is very limited and usually consists of rehabilitation and management of vascular risk factors. For spinal cord hemorrhage, surgical approaches can be considered in selected cases only. For example, patients who have a cavernoma can have it removed surgically. It is especially important to be aware of spinal AVMs as these progress insidiously and patients can be treated surgically or via an endovascular approach to prevent the progression of symptoms.

Outcomes vary according to the etiology of spinal cord stroke. In a recently published case series of 27 patients with spinal cord infarction, the outcome was favorable in 70% of patients with complete or near complete recovery. Patients with motor deficits were more likely to recover than those with sensory or sphincter disturbances. Despite this, more research is needed in the area of spinal cord stroke to improve diagnosis, treatment, and clinical outcomes.

Further reading

Buchan AM, Barnett HJM. Infarction of the spinal cord. In: Barnett HJM, Mohr JP, Stern B, Yatsu F, editors. *Stroke: Pathophysiology, Diagnosis and Management*. New York: Churchill Livingstone; 1986, pp. 707–19.

Das K, Saha SP, Das SK, Ganguly PK, Roy TN, Maity B. Profile of non-compressive myelopathy in eastern India: a 2-year study. *Acta Neurol Scand* 1999; 99(2): 100–5.

Gilbertson JR, Miller GM, Goldman MS, Marsh WR. Spinal dural arteriovenous malformations: a comparison of dural arteriovenous fistulas and intradural AVMs in 81 patients. *J Neurosurg* 1987; 67: 795–802.

Novy J, Carruzzo A, Maeder P, Bogousslavksy J. Spinal cord ischemia. *Arch Neurol* 2006; 63: 1113–20.

Vinters HV, Gilbert JJ. Hypoxic myelopathy. *Can J Neurol Sci* 1979; 6: 380.

Chapter 15
Extracranial granulomatous arteritis (giant cell arteritis)

Sandeep Randhawa and Gregory P. Van Stavern
Wayne State University, Detroit, USA

Introduction

Giant cell arteritis (GCA) is a relatively common systemic vasculitis with a predilection for large and medium-sized arteries usually affecting patients older than 55 years. It is a necrotizing granulomatous arteritis involving the aorta and its major branches, especially the extracranial branches of the carotids.

Epidemiology

GCA is the most frequent systemic vasculitis in the elderly, predominantly affecting the Caucasian population, with the incidence being higher in Scandinavia, northern Europe, and North America (between 17 and 18 cases per 100 000 population aged more than 50 years). It rarely occurs in Asians, Blacks, or Hispanics. Women are affected twice as often as men, and the incidence increases with age (mean age at presentation is 71 years).

Pathogenesis

Converging lines of evidence suggest a genetic predisposition and emphasize the role of immune pathways in the pathogenesis of GCA. Studies have shown a higher prevalence of the major histocompatibility complex antigens HLA-DR 1, 3, 4, and 5, with expression of an HLA-DRB1*04 allele in the majority of patients. Both cellular and humoral immsunity are involved in the pathogenesis of the disease.

Cellular immunity (vascular lesion)

The vessel-wall infiltrates of GCA are a consequence of inappropriate activation of the CD4+ T-cells, macrophages, and multinucleated giant cells. T-cells enter the artery through the vasa-vasora, encounter stimulatory

signals in the adventitia, and clonally expand to release interferon-gamma. Interferon-gamma recruits macrophages into the adventitia (to produce interleukins IL-1 and IL-6) and the media (to produce metalloproteinases, causing fragmentation of the elastic lamina). The multinucleated giant cells and macrophages lining the fragmented internal lamina produce growth factors which promote smooth-cell migration towards the lumen, causing intimal hyperplasia.

GCA commonly affects the superficial-temporal, occipital, vertebral, ophthalmic, and posterior ciliary arteries (PCA), and sometimes the aorta, coronary arteries, and the carotid circulation (inflammatory involvement may be related to the amount of elastic tissue in the artery; consequently, the intracranial arteries are spared).

Histological criteria for diagnosis as defined by the American College of Rheumatology (ACR) include segmental cellular infiltrates of the vessel wall with T-helper and suppressor lymphocytes, plasma cells, and macrophages (Figure 15.1a). Presence of giant cells is not essential for pathologic diagnosis.

Humoral immunity

The systemic inflammatory response of GCA, best described as an acute-phase response, is the result of humoral immunity. Circulating monocytes produce IL-6, which stimulates production of acute-phase hepatic proteins, many of which are elevated in GCA.

Clinical manifestations

Systemic manifestations

Symptoms of systemic inflammation are present in almost all patients. New onset temporal/occipital headache (sensory-fiber stimulation within inflamed extracranial arteries) and temporal scalp tenderness are common. Jaw claudication (pain/fatigue of masticatory muscles brought on by chewing and relieved by rest) is a classic and maybe the most specific symptom of GCA. Low-grade fever and symmetric proximal myalgias around the shoulder girdle may be present in association with polymyalgia rheumatica (PMR). The temporal

International Neurology: A Clinical Approach. Edited by Robert P. Lisak, Daniel D. Truong, William M. Carroll, and Roongroj Bhidayasiri. © 2009 Blackwell Publishing, ISBN: 978-1-4051-5738-4.

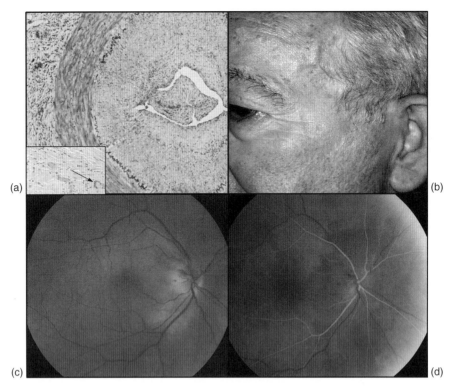

Figure 15.1 (a) Histopathological cross section of the temporal artery, showing narrowing of the arterial lumen, fragmentation of the elastic lamina, segmental cellular infiltrate, and multinucleate giant cells (arrow, inset). (b) A prominent temporal artery in a patient with GCA. (c) Fundus photograph of right eye showing pallid optic disc edema and peripapillary hemorrhage in AION secondary to GCA. (d) Fundus fluorescein angiogram of right eye demonstrating impaired choroidal perfusion (dark areas) in AION secondary to GCA.

artery may feel normal, tender, nodular, or pulseless (Figure 15.1b).

Neuro-ophthalmic manifestations

Patients with GCA may present with eye pain, diplopia, muscle paresis, or most commonly with irreversible visual loss (arteritic anterior ischemic optic neuropathy (A-AION), posterior ischemic optic neuropathy, or central retinal artery occlusion). Transient monocular visual loss (TMVL) with GCA occurs in 31% of patients and may be due to transient ischemia of the optic nerve head or retina (signifying impending blindness). The most common cause of visual loss (81.2%) in GCA is secondary to A-AION resulting from occlusive inflammation in the PCA causing optic nerve-head infarction. Fifty percent of affected eyes have hand-movement vision or worse, with a relative afferent pupillary defect, and an inferior altitudinal visual field defect. In the acute stage, optic-disk edema and pallor with peripapillary splinter hemorrhages may be seen (Figure 15.1c). It is important to differentiate A-AION from non-arteritic anterior ischemic optic neuropathy (N-AION). Patients with N-AION have no systemic symptoms, less severe visual loss, and TMVL is extremely rare. Fundus fluorescein angiography shows delayed optic-disc and choroidal filling in A-AION, whereas only optic-disc filling is delayed in N-AION (Figure 15.1d).

Neurological manifestations

Both the central and peripheral nervous systems can be involved. GCA may commonly manifest as neuropathies (14%) including mononeuropathies, peripheral polyneuropathies of the arms/legs, and rarely ischemic strokes (1%) or dementia. Patients with permanent visual loss or jaw claudication are more prone to ischemic strokes that affect the areas supplied by the carotid or vertebrobasilar arteries.

Large-vessel arteritis

Large-vessel arteritis affecting the aorta, subclavian, and axillary arteries is a recognized complication of GCA, with approximately 50% of these cases having negative temporal-artery biopsy (TAB) results; the diagnosis in these cases is made by vascular imaging. Aortic involvement has been estimated in 10–15% of patients, with aortic aneurysms (thoracic/abdominal), aortic dissection, and aortic valve insufficiency as potential complications.

Polymyalgia rheumatica

A variable portion of patients with GCA (about 50%) have PMR, a clinical syndrome characterized by pain and stiffness in the neck, shoulder girdle, and pelvic girdle. Despite a suggestion that PMR and GCA belong to the same clinical continuum, they seem to be distinct conditions, as evidenced by differences in the HLA – Class II associations. Patients with PMR aged less than 70 years without typical cranial features of GCA carry a low risk of vasculitis.

Systemic inflammatory syndrome with arteritis

Arteritis can present in the absence of intimal hyperplasia, luminal stenosis, or tissue ischemia. In these cases, the systemic inflammatory syndrome (malaise, anorexia, weight loss, fever, night sweats, and depression) dominates clinical manifestations. The risk of visual loss may be less than that in cranial arteritis. A TAB is the procedure of choice and should be performed even in the absence of arterial tenderness/nodularity.

Diagnostic approaches to GCA

Laboratory findings

Erythrocyte sedimentation rate (ESR) is usually higher than 50 mm/hour, but a lower value has been reported in <5% of GCA patients. C-reactive protein (CRP), a dynamic acute-phase protein, is usually elevated. Since either the ESR or the CRP may be normal (more commonly the ESR) in the presence of the elevation of the other, using both tests in combination provides greater sensitivity for diagnosis. Anemia of chronic disease, raised liver enzymes, and thrombocytosis are frequent. Thrombocytosis has a high specificity and positive predictive value (PPV) in diagnosis. There is evidence that IL-6 may be particularly sensitive in detecting the disease-associated acute-phase response.

Diagnosis

A definitive diagnosis of GCA requires histological examination of arterial tissue (TAB). This is important, given the low specificity of the clinical and laboratory markers and implications of prolonged corticosteroid therapy. Because vascular inflammation is discontinuous, arterial specimens of sufficient size (≥2.5 cm) with analysis of closely spaced sections (0.25–0.5 mm) is recommended. If frozen sections from the first temporal artery do not reveal inflammatory infiltrates, the contralateral side is biopsied if clinical suspicion is high. The sensitivity of TAB is not significantly affected if the biopsy is performed within 2 weeks of starting therapy. An experienced pathologist may see signs of a "healed arteritis" even after months of corticosteroid treatment. Therefore, therapy should not be postponed while awaiting the biopsy.

Imaging

Imaging may play a role in patients with large-vessel arteritis with negative TAB results. Conventional X-ray angiography, digital subtraction angiography, computerized tomography, and magnetic resonance imaging have emerged as reliable methods to assess vessel anatomy and luminal status. The distal subclavian, any portion of the axillary, and the proximal brachial artery are susceptible sites. The lesions are typically smoothly tapered. If there is clinical evidence of cerebral ischemia, evaluation of the carotid and vertebral arteries is important. However, the findings on angiography are not pathognomonic for vasculitis and should not substitute for a definitive tissue diagnosis.

The criteria proposed by ACR for diagnosis of GCA require the presence of at least three of the following: age at onset more than 50 years; new headache; temporal-artery abnormalities; ESR >50 mm/hour; and a positive TAB. However, these criteria have been found to have limitations, including a PPV of only 29%. Since patients will need to remain on corticosteroid therapy for an extended period, with the attendant risk of complications, confirming the diagnosis with tissue biopsy is recommended in even the most clear-cut cases.

Treatment

Systemic corticosteroids are the treatment of choice for GCA, though the initial dose has varied in the literature. Patients with suspected GCA should usually be started on oral prednisolone of 1 mg/kg/day. For patients with ocular or cerebrovascular symptoms of GCA, a higher dose (80–100 mg/day) is advocated. For biopsy-confirmed GCA, oral prednisolone (80–100 mg/day) or high-dose intravenous systemic corticosteroids (1 g methylprednisolone/day for 3 days) followed by high-dose oral prednisolone is recommended. Intravenous high-dose corticosteroids have especially been recommended in patients who present with a history of amaurosis fugax, marked visual loss, or early signs of involvement of the second eye. Follow-up protocol should include ophthalmic evaluation, ESR, and CRP at least once a week when patients are on high-dose oral steroids.

Tapering of steroid therapy in GCA must be individualized, guided by ESR and CRP levels (systemic symptoms may be unreliable), to be commenced only when the ESR and CRP have reached consistently low levels and remain stable, which takes approximately 2 weeks on the initial high doses of oral steroids. Subsequently, the goal should be to maintain the achieved lowest levels of ESR and CRP with the lowest possible prednisolone dose. Patients must be carefully monitored for any ocular/visual problems and systemic side effects of corticosteroids.

The total duration of steroid therapy is usually prolonged, and when patients with visual loss are being treated, a longer duration is anticipated (some requiring indefinite treatment). There is little evidence to suggest any useful role of steroid-sparing agents or aspirin in GCA.

Prognosis

The overall life expectancy of GCA patients and the general population has been reported to be similar, but there is morbidity due to the side effects of prolonged steroid use. Permanent visual loss is more common in patients who present with amaurosis, transient diplopia, or jaw claudication. The goal of treatment in cases with visual loss is to arrest further visual deterioration in the affected eye and to prevent involvement of the other eye. The visual prognosis of GCA if untreated is devastating visual loss in both eyes. Early diagnosis and prompt initiation of treatment may result in favorable visual outcomes.

Further reading

Calamia KT, Hunder GG. Clinical manifestations of giant cell (temporal) arteritis. *Clin Rheum Dis* 1980; 6: 389–403.

Hayreh SS. Acute ischemic disorders of the optic nerve: pathogenesis, clinical manifestations and management. *Ophthalmol Clin North Am* 1996; 9: 407–42.

Hayreh SS, Podhajsky PA, Raman R, Zimmerman B. Giant cell arteritis: validity and reliability of various diagnostic criteria. *Am J Ophthalmol* 1997; 123: 285–96.

Salvarani C, Cantini F, Boiardi L, Hunder GG. Polymyalgia rheumatica and giant-cell arteritis. *N Engl J Med* 2002; 347: 261–71.

Weyand CM, Goronzy JJ. Medium- and large-vessel vasculitis. *N Engl J Med* 2003; 349: 160–9.

Chapter 16
Intracranial granulomatous arteritis (primary angiitis of the CNS)/idiopathic CNS vasculitis

Donald Silberberg
University of Pennsylvania Medical Center, Philadelphia, USA

Nomenclature

The terms "intracranial granulomatous arteritis" and "primary angiitis of the central nervous system" are synonyms for CNS vasculitis of unknown etiology, perhaps better termed idiopathic CNS vasculitis (ICNSV). To further confound the situation, this category of what are surely disorders with multiple, as-yet-to-be identified causes, often includes peripheral nervous system, ocular, and sometimes systemic manifestations during the course of the illness. ICNSV is uncommon, but treatable, so its identification is very important. ICNSV is being increasingly recognized, and may account for up to 5% of cerebrovascular disease occurring below the age 50 years. No information regarding geographic distribution is available; all relevant publications are from high-income countries.

One must keep in mind that CNS, ocular, cranial nerve, peripheral nervous system, and muscle signs and symptoms are often the first manifestations of what proves to be a systemic disorder. For example, acute disseminated lupus erythematosis often begins with seizures, sarcoidosis may present as cranial nerve or diffuse cerebral dysfunction, and a vasculitis syndrome has been associated with the beginning of Hodgkin's disease.

Diagnosis and clinical course

Signs and symptoms suggestive of vasculitis in the absence of evidence for another diagnostic entity, most of which are themselves idiopathic (Table 16.1), lead to considering ICNSV. The occurrence of CNS infarcts or hemorrhages in unrelated vascular distributions should suggest the possibility of vasculitis. By definition, systemic signs such as fever, arthralgia, and myalgia, or an elevated

Table 16.1 Causes of cerebral vasculitis.

Infectious
Bacterial (e.g., tuberculosis)
Chagas' disease
Viral (e.g., Varicella zoster)
HIV
Malaria
Syphilis

Presumably non-infectious
Arthritis-associated
Juvenile rheumatoid arthritis
Rheumatoid arthritis
Relapsing polychondritis
Seronegative (HLA-B27-associated) spondyloarthropathies

Ocular
Acute posterior multifocal placoid pigment epitheliopathy
Eale's disease
Idiopathic retinal vasculitis

Other
Antiphospholipid antibody-associated vasculopathy
Behcet's disease
Churg–Strauss syndrome
Cogan's syndrome
Giant-cell arteritis
Hodgkin's disease
Polyarteritis nodosa
Sarcoidosis
Henoch–Schönlein purpura
Hypersensitivity vasculitis
Mixed cryoglobulinemia
Polymyositis, dermatomyositis
Scleroderma
Sjogren's syndrome
Systemic lupus erythematosis
Takayasu's arteritis
Thromboangiitis obliterans
Wegener's granulomatosis

**Idiopathic (intracranial granulomatous arteritis/
primary angiitis of the CNS)**

International Neurology: A Clinical Approach. Edited by Robert P. Lisak, Daniel D. Truong, William M. Carroll, and Roongroj Bhidayasiri. © 2009 Blackwell Publishing, ISBN: 978-1-4051-5738-4.

peripheral blood leukocyte count or erythrocyte sedimentation rate are not present, at least initially. However, an elevated erthrocyte sedimentation rate occurs in up to 50% of cases. Common features include those of diffuse cerebral dysfunction: headache, confusion, paresthesias, hemiplegia, seizures, ataxia, and visual disturbances. Cranial nerves are often affected, and peripheral neuropathy is present in up to 10% of cases at the time of presentation. Less commonly, ICNSV presents as an isolated mass lesion. The signs and symptoms are often long-lasting and recurrent. ICNSV is most common in adults, but also occurs in children. If untreated, ICNSV usually leads to death within 1–2 years or less. However, ICNSV affecting primarily small vessels may have a better prognosis than that involving medium-sized vessels.

Diagnostic aids include examination of the cerebrospinal fluid (CSF), electroencephalogram (EEG), CT, and MRI, including MRI angiography, fluorescein angiography where ophthalmoscopy is abnormal, intracranial arteriography, and brain and meningeal biopsy. CSF abnormalities, primarily elevated protein and lymphocytic pleocytosis, are present in 80–90% of individuals. Diffuse EEG abnormalities are very common, and may help to monitor the course of the disorder. Intracranial imaging often reveals one or more infarctions or hemorrhages, and may show evidence of perivascular inflammation or meningeal enhancement. Alternatively, imaging studies may be normal. Conventional angiography reveals occlusions, focal narrowing, beading, distal attenuation, or aneurysms in no more than 50% of those with ICNSV. MRI angiography may show the same abnormalities with no risk to the patient, but no studies are available that compare sensitivity or specificity with conventional angiography.

Brain and meningeal biopsy seek to reveal the characteristic perivascular, primarily peri-arterial, inflammation that includes a variety of lymphocytes, plasma cells, and often multi-nuclear giant cells. However, it is important to realize that even biopsy fails to reveal an abnormality in about 20% of patients who otherwise appear to have ICNSV. One explanation for negative biopsies is undoubtedly the very focal nature of the disorder in many individuals, similar to what characterizes systemic giant cell arteritis (temporal arteritis). Another reason for biopsy is to rule out the possibility of an infectious or other etiology of the vasculitis/vasculopathy.

Treatment

In the face of these uncertainties, the decision as to whether or not to treat for ICNSV often must be made despite a lack of laboratory evidence to support the diagnosis. Since ICNSV is almost uniformly fatal if not treated, and the risk of treatment is acceptable, it is usually prudent to proceed. That said, one must recognize that what informs the clinician is experience in treating vasculitis in other settings, and uncontrolled, mostly small reported series that describe the treatment of ICNSV. The small number of cases at any one institution has so far precluded organization of a randomized, controlled, clinical trial.

What has been observed is that treatment with a combination of synthetic corticosteroids with a more potent immunosuppressant agent is often effective in reducing the severity and duration of the initial episode, and in preventing recurrences. Prednisone or prednisolone are most often used (1 mg/kg/day), in combination with cyclophosphamide (2 mg/kg, maximum 150 mg/day) for the initiation of treatment. Since treatment must be maintained for at least a year in most individuals, azathioprine (2 mg/kg/day) is often substituted for cyclophosphamide for maintenance, and one seeks to use the lowest dose of steroids that seems to be effective for the long term.

Efficacy can be judged on the basis of clinical response, absence of recurrences, absence of new MRI abnormalities, and reduction in EEG abnormalities. However, one must recognize that, as is the case for many known causes of vasculitis, very long-term treatment (1–3 years or indefinitely) may be needed to limit the disorder.

Future developments

The factors that lead to the development of vasculitis in any organ system are complex and mostly poorly understood. As these are elucidated, more specific, effective, and less toxic treatments will follow. The factors that lead to the selection of a particular vascular tree, or its component parts, as the target for an inflammatory response are beginning to be unraveled, an important step along the way.

Further reading

Ferro JM. Vasculitis of the central nervous system. *J Neurol* 1998; 245: 766–76.

Hoffman GS. Determinants of vessel targeting in vasculitis. *Ann N Y Acad Sci* 2005; 1051: 332–9.

MacLaren K, Gillespie J, Shrestha S, Neary D, Ballardie FW. Primary angiitis of the central nervous system: emerging variants. *QJM* 2005; 98: 643–54.

Salvarani, C, Brown, R, Calamia, K, *et al.* Primary central nervous system vasculitis: analysis of 101 patients. *Ann Neurol* 2007; 62: 442–51.

West SG. Central nervous system vasculitis. *Curr Rheumatol Rep* 2003; 5(2): 116–27.

Chapter 17
Takayasu's arteritis

Yasuhisa Kitagawa
Tokai University School of Medicine, Tokyo, Japan

Introduction

Takayasu's arteritis is a chronic, non-specific arteritis of unknown cause characterized by stenosis and/or occlusion of the aorta and its branches. Its major features were first described by Davy in 1839 and independently by Savort and by Kussmaul in 1856. In 1905, a Japanese ophthalmologist, Takayasu, reported a case with wreath-like arterial-venous anastomosis in the central retinal artery, and based on his description, the term Takayasu's arteritis is now most commonly used worldwide.

Epidemiology

The reported incidence of Takayasu's arteritis is 2.6 cases per million per year in North America. In Japan, newly developed cases amount to more than 100 per year and the prevalence rate is 33 per million per year. It is nine times more frequent in females than males in Japan. The age at onset is from 20–40 years in females, although there is no clear age peak in males. In China, the female:male ratio is 2.9:1. Although Takayaku's arteritis affects mainly Asians, it can occur in all racial groups. The age of onset of Takayasu's arteritis in North American and European countries is later than is observed in Asian countries. The reason for the later onset could relate to two factors: (1) the slow progression of occlusive arteritis, and (2) the rarity of the disease in "western" countries which results in a longer delay in diagnosis compared with eastern countries.

Pathology

The pathologic lesion is a granulomatous angiitis. The initial involvement is characterized by mononuclear cell infiltration in the adventitia, followed by prominent fibrous proliferation in the media and intima. Inflammatory cell infiltration foci are accompanied by perinecrotic foci and Langhans-type multinucleated giant cell infiltration. Long-standing cases show fibrosis and hyalinization of intima, stenosis of the vascular lumen, and finally complete occlusion.

Pathogenesis

The etiology of Takayasu's arteritis is unknown, but its predominance in Asia and Central and South America is consistent with some involvement of genetic factors, perhaps acting in concert with environmental factors. A study of human leucocyte antigen (HLA) patterns in Japan in 1998 reported a significant correlation of HLA-B52, HLA-B39, and HLA-DR2 with Takayasu's arteritis. However, North American studies have failed to identify any association of HLA with the disease.

Clinical manifestations

The vascular manifestations arising from stenosis and occlusion of vessels vary, and the geographical variation of clinical features and prognosis as reported in Japan, North America, Europe, Asia, and South Africa is shown in Table 17.1. Characteristic findings in the upper limbs are lack of pulses and/or a difference in arterial blood pressure between the right and left radial arteries. Hypertension has been found in about half of cases. Hypertension is caused by stenosis of the renal artery and by decreased elasticity of the aorta, which induces systolic hypertension. Cardiac symptoms are shortness of breath, palpitations, and chest discomfort. Aortic valve insufficiency has been noted and the comcommitant rupture of the aortic aneurysm was associated with a poor outcome. Systemic features include fever, general malaise, arthralgias, and myalgias in the acute phase of the disease.

A survey of Takayasu's vasculitis in Japan reported that the most common initial symptoms were associated with ischemia of the extremities, including paresthesias, cold sensation, pulselessness, and claudication (73.8%), followed by systemic symptoms including fever and

International Neurology: A Clinical Approach. Edited by Robert P. Lisak, Daniel D. Truong, William M. Carroll, and Roongroj Bhidayasiri.
© 2009 Blackwell Publishing, ISBN: 978-1-4051-5738-4.

Table 17.1 Geographical variation of clinical manifestations and prognosis of Takayasu's arteritis.

	Japan	North America	Germany	Italy	China	Korea	Thailand	India	South Africa
No. of cases	1318	60	17	104	530	129	46	83	272 (8% Caucasian)
Age (mean)	31	25	23	29	25.8	29.5	7–40	5–53	25 (14–66)
Female/male ratio	9:1	29:1	3.2:1	7:1	2.9:1	6.6:1	1.9:1	1.6:1	3:1
Affected artery	Subclavian Common carotid Innominate	Subclavian Aorta Common carotid	Subclavian Common carotid	Subclavian Carotid Renal	Subclavian Abdominal Renal	Subclavian Renal Common carotid	Abdominal aorta Renal Subclavian	Renal Abdominal aorta Subclavian	Subclavian Abdominal aorta Renal
Clinical features									
Cerebral ischemic symptom	42.3%	57%	35.3%	50%	30.6%	46%	24%	8%	20%
Stroke	11.9%	9%	11.8%	4%	5.4%	3%	24%	7%	11%
Visual	23.6%	8%	35.3%	—	9.6%	20%	—	22%	—
Cardiac	41.4%	38%	—	—	23.2%	46%	28%	14%	45%
Carotid bruit	—	70%	23.5%	—	47.4%	37%	—	25%	—
Hypertension	55.7%	33%	58.8%	60%	60.0%	40%	80%	81%	77%
Ischemia of extremities	73.8%	—	—	—	—	—	—	—	—
Claudication	—	70%	88.2%	59%	24.7%	21%	—	—	30%
Dim. or no pulse	—	62%	82.4%	75%	37.2%	72%	50%	46%	—
Cause of death	Cardiac failure 23.7% Rupture of aneurysm 20.3% Cerebral hemorrhage 5.1%	—	—	—	Cerebral hemorrhage 23.6% Cardiac failure 5.5% Cerebral thrombosis 3.6% Rupture of aneurysm 1.8%	—	—	Cardiac failure 36% Renal failure 18% Cerebral hemorrhage 9%	Cardiac failure 46% Renal failure 11% Rupture of aneurysm 11% Stroke 9.5%

fatigue (60.1%). Symptoms related to cerebral ischemia, such as dizziness, headache, and syncope, sometimes orthostatic, were noted in 42.3% of 1302 cases. Cerebral infarction, transient ischemic attack, and cerebral hemorrhage were found in 5.5%, 5.7%, and 0.7% of cases, respectively. Geographical variation in the pattern of affected arteries is seen. In Japan, the most frequently involved artery is the subclavian artery, followed by the common carotid artery and innominate artery. The vertebral artery tends to be spared until the final stage. Takayasu's arteritis presents with similar cerebrovascular signs in Europe and Japan. It may present as the subclavian steal syndrome. On the other hand, the renal artery is the most common vascular involvement seen in India.

Causes of death in a series of Japanese patients included heart failure in 14 patients, rupture of aortic aneurysm in 12, cerebral hemorrhage in 2, and other cerebrovascular syndromes in 2. In a Chinese study, 23.6% of patients suffered from cerebral hemorrhage, and cerebral infarction was found in only 3.6%. The higher incidence of cerebral hemorrhage in China compared to Japan could be related to a higher rate of renal-vascular hypertension.

Diagnosis

Laboratory findings include elevated sedimentation rate (ESR), C-reactive protein (CRP), and increased serum gamma globulin in a polyclonal pattern. Angiography remains the cornerstone of diagnosis, revealing narrowing of large arteries arising from the aorta. The presence of vascular lesions and their progression can be detected by duplex ultrasonography. Homogenous circumferential intima-media thickening of the common carotid arteries in ultrasonography is highly specific, particularly in young women. Micro-embolic signals can be detected by transcranial Doppler ultrasound and have been reported to be present in 22% of patients with Takayasu's arteritis during the acute and chronic stage. Cerebrovascular disease-induced changes can be detected using functional imaging with SPECT (single photon emission computed tomography) and PET (positron emission tomography).

Therapy

Treatment of Takayasu's arteritis involves control of general inflammation and neurological complications. In the acute stage, corticosteroids are initiated (0.5–1.5 mg prednisone/kg/day), and the dosage is adjusted depending on the clinical findings and the degree of inflammatory reaction as monitored by ESR and/or CRP. Sixty percent of patients given glucocorticoids alone responded to varying degrees. If blindness seems imminent, intravenous high-dose corticosteroids should be given, employed on an urgent basis (1 g intravenous methylprednisiolone/day for 3–7 days). If corticosteroid therapy is insufficient, immmunosuppressive therapy such as methotrexate is indicated. However, immunosuppressive treatment failed to induce remission in 25% of cases, and about half of those who achieved remission later relapsed.

Antiplatelet therapy is indicated for patients with transient ischemic attack (TIA) and cerebral infarction. Strict control of hypertension is essential to reduce the incidence of cerebral infarction and cerebral hemorrhage. Indications for surgery in the chronic stage include severe aortic insuffiency, coarctation of the aorta, and renovascular hypertension. Angioplasty may be indicated for certain patients with subclavian steal syndrome or stenosis of the carotid and renal arteries.

Further reading

Deyu Z, Dijun E, Lisheng L. Takayasu arteritis in China : a report of 530 cases. *Heart Vessels* 1992; 7(Suppl): 32–6.

Johnson SL, Lock RJ, Gompels MM. Takayasu arteritis: a review. *J Clin Pathol* 2002; 55: 481–6.

Kerr GS, Hallahan CW, Gierdant J, *et al.* Takayasu's arteritis. *Ann Intern Med* 1994; 120: 919–29.

Koide K. Takayasu's arteritis *Heart Vessels* 1992; 7(Suppl): 48–54.

Ringleb PA, Strittmater EI, Loewer M, *et al.* Cerebrovascular manifestations of Takayasuarteritis in Europe. *Rheumatology* 2005; 44: 1012–15.

Chapter 18
Polyarteritis nodosa, Churg–Strauss syndrome, overlap and related syndromes

Stanley van den Noort and Gaby T. Thai
University of California, Irvine, USA

Introduction

Vasculitis covers a heterogeneous group of disorders most commonly cared for by rheumatologists, dermatologists, and internists. However, 80% of patients have involvement of either the central nervous system or the peripheral nervous system. Rarely, the nervous system may be the only affected organ.

Polyarteritis nodosa

Polyarteritis nodosa (PAN) is a necrotizing inflammation of small and medium-sized arteries, with a predeliction for branching points and vessel bifurcation. It affects many organ systems, most commonly the kidney and the viscera, and if untreated, long-term remission and survival is unusual. Arteries are affected segmentally, and there may be small aneurysms that can be seen on angiography. There are two patterns of CNS involvement: global and focal. With global dysfunction, patients most frequently present with headaches, and a smaller number would have evidence of aseptic meningitis, with CSF under elevated pressure, with increased protein concentration and lymphocytic pleocytosis. Others may have generalized cognitive impairment or psychiatric symptoms.

The vessels may occlude and lead to ischemic stroke and focal abnormalities. Intracerebral hemorrhage and subarachnoid hemorrhage may also be seen. Neuroimaging studies often show focal or multifocal areas of infarction and, less frequently, intraparenchymal hemorrhage.

The peripheral nervous system is more commonly involved in PAN than the central nervous system, with mononeuritis multiplex being the hallmark finding. Its onset may be acute or indolent, often accompanied by severe pain or dysesthesia. Several nerves may be involved simultaneously, giving rise to asymmetrical motor and sensory signs. The lower extremities are more commonly affected than the upper, involving especially the sciatic nerve and its branches. Mononeuritis multiplex may become more widespread, appearing as asymmetrical then symmetrical polyneuropathy. Symmetrical polyneuropathy may also appear de novo and is considered a separate syndrome. Multiple cranial nerves, especially the oculomotor (III), trochlear (IV), abducens (VI), facial (VII), and vestibuloacoustic (VIII), can be affected and present as cranial mononeuritis multiplex.

Spinal cord involvement is rare, and necrotizing arteritis in spinal arterial branches is seen. Patients can present acutely or subacutely with transverse myelopathy at any cord level.

The etiology of PAN is not known in most cases. Polyarteritis has been described in association with viral infections, including with hepatitis B, hepatitis C, HIV, cytomegalovirus, parvovirus B 19, and HTLV type I. Other associations include antiphospholipid syndrome, minocycline exposure, perforin deficiency, amyloid angiopathy, and mitochondrial neurogastrointestinal encephalomyopathy or MNGIE.

If untreated, the 5-year survival rate of PAN is 10–13%, with renal failure being the most common cause of death. The use of corticosteroid treatment alone improves the 5-year survival rate to approximately 55%, and the combination of corticosteroid and IV cyclophosphamide shows further improvement, attaining an 82% 5-year survival rate. Newer immunosuppressants and monoclonal agents may or may not prove superior.

Churg–Strauss syndrome

This is a syndrome of allergic angiitis and granulomatosis, described by Churg and Strauss in 1951. It is characterized by pulmonary and systemic small vessel vasculitis, intra- and extravascular granulomas, and hypereosinophilia, and is most commonly seen in relatively young adults. Pulmonary findings are the dominant clinical feature.

International Neurology: A Clinical Approach. Edited by Robert P. Lisak, Daniel D. Truong, William M. Carroll, and Roongroj Bhidayasiri. © 2009 Blackwell Publishing, ISBN: 978-1-4051-5738-4.

Patients present with severe asthma attacks, often starting in their mid-30s or 40s, later than with common asthma. Pulmonary infiltrates may be seen in up to half of cases. There is severe eosinophilia, with levels greater than 1000 cells/μl in more than 80% of patients. Two-thirds of the patients have skin lesions, purpura, and cutaneous or subcutaneous nodules. Peripheral neuropathy, usually mononeuritis multiplex, is found in up to 75% of patients. Its clinical aspects are similar to that of PAN. CNS involvement is also similar to that in PAN.

The prognosis of untreated Churg–Strauss syndrome is poor, with a 5-year survival rate of approximately 25%. The cause of death is more likely related to pulmonary and cardiac disease, as opposed to renal failure in classic PAN. Similar to PAN, the use of corticosteroid increases the 5-year survival rate to more than 50%. The combined regimen of cyclophosphamide and corticosteroid may result in even greater survival rate, similar to PAN.

Hypersensitivity angiitis

This is considered a common vasculitis. In its most severe form, it can be a life-threatening multisystem disease similar to PAN, but most commonly it presents as a more limited form. The most consistent features are cutaneous lesions, often purpura, but also petechiae, urticaria, ecchymoses, and ulcers. Rarely there is neurological involvement. The usual pathology includes leukocytoclasis and neutrophilic debris in and around the affected vessels. Commonly, there are decreases in C3 and C4 complements and increases in blood and CSF gamma globulin and variable pleocytosis. Circulating antibodies or immune complexes may aid in diagnosis. Often a relation with another disease is evident: systemic lupus erythematosus, Sjögren's syndrome, rheumatoid arthritis, scleroderma, West Nile virus infection, hepatitis B, and neoplasia.

Takayasu's arteritis

This is a rare chronic disease seen in young women, characterized by inflammation, scarring, and occlusion of the aorta and the proximal parts of its major branches. The onset is usually from age 10 to 30. Patients may initially present with systemic symptoms including fever, malaise, arthralgia, and weight loss. In the later phase, with aortitis and branch occlusion, there may be hypertension, valvular insufficiency, extremity claudication, and angina. The common neurological symptoms are headache, dizziness, and syncope. Significant neurological complications are transient ischemic attacks and ischemic strokes in the distribution of the carotid artery. Other important clinical findings include absent or diminished peripheral pulses, cardiac murmurs, and congestive heart failure.

Notable laboratory findings include mild anemia, leukocytosis, hypergammaglobulinemia, and elevated ESR. Cerebral angiography or non-invasive modalities such as CT angiography or MR angiography are fundamental in establishing the diagnosis.

The prognosis for Takayasu's arteritis is generally good, with the 5-year survival rate being approximately 83%. Causes of death usually stem from myocardial infarction, congestive heart failure, ruptured aortic aneurysm and renal failure. The treatment of choice is corticosteroids, and ESR may be used to monitor disease activity.

Polyangitis overlap syndrome

This is a subgroup of systemic necrotizing vasculitis that encompasses patients with clinicopathologic features which do not fall precisely into one of the major groups – PAN, Churg–Strauss syndrome, Wegener's granulomatosis, Takayasu's arteritis, or hypersentivity vasculitides. Rather, they have overlapping features. Multiple organ systems and vessels of all sizes, including capillaries and veins, are involved. Peripheral neuropathy is the common neurological disorder seen in this subgroup.

Vasculitis secondary to infection

Infection is a well-recognized cause of secondary vasculitis. Many agents have been identified: bacterial – mycobacterium, spirochetes; viral – herpes zoster, cytomegalovirus (CMV), hepatitis, human immunodeficiency virus (HIV), human T-cell leukemia/lymphoma virus (HTLV); mycoses; parasites; rickettsiae; and mycoplasma. Infectious vasculitis is often associated with fever, abnormal peripheral leukocyte count, and recent history of infection.

Many different mechanisms have been proposed to explain vasculitis in this setting, including direct invasion of blood vessels, immune-mediated reactions, and toxin-mediated reactions. The pathogenetic mechanism is dependent on the specific pathogen involved. With herpes zoster infection, patients may develop necrotizing angiitis affecting the carotid artery and meningeal vessels. The angiitis may lead to arterial stenosis, occlusion, and cerebral infarction.

Other vasculitides

Some other vasculitides worth mentioning include Kawasaki's disease, Susac's syndrome, and vasculitis associated with oral contraceptive use.

Kawasaki's disease is a childhood illness presumably of infectious cause, presenting with a rash on the trunk with magenta discoloration of the palms and soles. Patients have cervical adenopathy, and may develop vasculitis involving coronary arteries and cerebral vessels. Susac's syndrome is a vasculopathy of the brain, retina, and cochlea. It is usually monophasic, and diagnosis rests on demonstration of branch vessel occlusions in the retina and unusual lesions in the corpus callosum. When oral contraceptives were first approved, we began to see venous and arterial thromboses in some women, most of whom had migraines, hypertension, and were smokers. Hormone-induced hypercoagulability is thought to play an important role, but there is also evidence implicating immune-mediated vasculitis in the pathogenesis of contraceptive-related stroke.

Vasculitis in the nervous system is heterogeneous, may be uncommon, and almost certainly is underrecognized and undertreated. It is important to keep these disorders in mind when attempting to sort out nervous system disease process at any stage.

Further reading

Abad S, Kambouchner M, Nejjari M, Dhote R. Additional case of minocycline-induced cutaneous polyarateritis nodosa: comment on the article by Celver *et al*. *Arthritis Rheum* 2006; 55(5): 831; author reply 832.

Das CJ, Pangtey GS. Images in clinical medicine. Arterial microaneurysms in polyarteritis nodosa. *N Engl J Med* 2006; 355(24): 2574.

Gorson K. Vasculitic neuropathies. *Neurologist* 2007; 1: 9–12.

Saadoun D, Bieche I, Authier F-J, *et al*. Role of matrix matalloproteinases, pro-inflammatory cytokines, and oxidative stress-derived molecules in hepatitis C virus associated mixed cryoglobulinemia. *Arthritis Rheum* 2007; 56: 1315–24.

Susac J, Egan R, *et al*. Susac's syndrome. *J Neurol Sci* 2007; 257(1–2): 270–2.

Chapter 19
Wegener's granulomatosis

Gerard Said
Hôpital de la Salpétrière, Paris, France

Primary vasculitides are often classified according to the size of the vessels predominantly affected, but overlaps are common and the nomenclature of the systemic vasculitides remains enigmatic. The group of *small vessel vasculitis* of this recent classification includes *Wegener's granulomatosis (WG)*, the *Churg–Strauss syndrome (CSS)*, and what the group calls *microscopic polyangiitis* with involvement of capillaries, which is sometimes associated with polyarteritis nodosa. The prevalence of WG is about 3 in 100 000, with a slightly higher prevalence in men than in women (3:2). The peak incidence of the disease is at 50–60 years of age. The process typically affects the upper and lower airways and kidneys. The most common manifestations include upper respiratory, pulmonary, and kidney involvement. Other organ systems that can be affected include the joints, eyes, skin, central nervous system, and, less commonly, the gastrointestinal tract, parotid gland, heart, thyroid, liver, and breast.

Common manifestations include persistent rhinorrhea; purulent or bloody nasal discharge; oral or nasal ulcers; polyarthralgia or myalgias; sinus pain; earaches/hearing loss; hoarseness; hemoptysis, cough and dyspnea; nodules and opacities seen on chest radiograph; plus non-specific complaints: fevers, night sweats, anorexia, weight loss, malaise.

WG is an antibody-mediated autoimmune granulomatous vasculitis, in which antibodies against proteinase 3 and myeloperoxidase are demonstrable in the serum of patients. Serologic demonstration of these antineutrophil cytoplasmic antibodies (ANCAs) is a sensitive and specific means by which to diagnose WG, provided a positive result on a screening leukocyte indirect immunofluorescence microscopic ANCA study is followed up by enzyme-linked immunoabsorbent assay demonstration of antiproteinase 3 and antimyeloperoxidase.

Ninety percent of patients with active generalized disease are ANCA positive. However, in patients with milder, limited forms of the disease, the ANCA test may be negative up to 40% of the time. A positive perinuclear (P)-ANCA result is less specific. Other frequent but non-specific laboratory findings include leukocytosis, thrombocytosis, an elevated erythrocyte sedimentation rate, and a normocytic, normochromic anemia. A tissue biopsy is essential for the definitive diagnosis of WG.

Peripheral neuropathy has been observed in 25% of patients with WG. Peripheral neuropathy seldom is the first manifestation of the disease. In a review of 324 patients with WG by Nischino *et al.*, 109 had neurological manifestations at some stage. Fifty-three patients had peripheral neuropathy, which was multifocal in 42. Cranial nerves were involved in 21/109, and ophthalmoplegia was present in 16/21. The mean interval between the onset of WG and neurological manifestations was 8.4 months. However, in a recent study peripheral neuropathy was inaugural in a higher proportion of patients with WG than previously thought, a finding that was not accepted by all.

Treatment of WG generally consists of cyclophosphamide and glucocorticoids. This regimen is maintained until the patient is in stable remission, usually after 3–6 months. Alternative regimens include (1) intravenous monthly cyclophosphamide instead of daily, oral cyclophosphamide; and (2) methotrexate instead of cyclophosphamide in patients with mild disease, limited bone marrow reserve, or bladder toxicity. Maintenance therapy is usually given for 12–18 months after the initial remission to prevent relapse. Cyclophosphamide is continued for approximately 12 months. However, corticosteroids are not shown to have any added benefit in maintenance therapy; thus, they should be tapered rapidly after the disease stabilizes.

Further reading

De Groot K, Schmidt DK, Arlt AC, Gross WL, Reinhold-Keller E. Standardized neurologic evaluation of 128 patients with Wegener granulomatosis. *Arch Neurol* 2001; 58: 1215–21.

Duna GF, Galperin C, Hoffman GS. Wegener's granulomatosis. *Rheum Dis Clin North Am* 1995; 21: 949–86.

International Neurology: A Clinical Approach. Edited by Robert P. Lisak, Daniel D. Truong, William M. Carroll, and Roongroj Bhidayasiri. © 2009 Blackwell Publishing, ISBN: 978-1-4051-5738-4.

Morgan MD, Harper L, Williams J, Savage C. Anti-neutrophil cytoplasm-associated glomerulonephritis. *J Am Soc Nephrol* 2006; 17: 1224–34.

Nishino H, Rubino FA, DeRemee RA, Swanson JW, Parisi JE. Neurological involvement in Wegener's granulomatosis: an analysis of 324 consecutive patients at the Mayo Clinic. *Ann Neurol* 1993; 33: 4–9.

Stern GM, Hoffbrand AV, Urich H. The peripheral nerves and skeletal muscles in Wegener's granulomatosis: a clinico-pathological study of four cases. *Brain* 1965; 88: 151–164.

White ES, Lynch JP. Pharmacological therapy for Wegener's granulomatosis. *Drugs* 2006; 66: 1209–28.

Chapter 20
Cerebrovascular disease associated with antiphospholipid antibodies

Megan Alcauskas and Steven R. Levine
The Mount Sinai School of Medicine and Medical Center, New York, USA

Introduction

Antiphospholipid antibodies (aPL) are a family of autoantibodies directed against phospholipids and phospholipid-binding proteins. The most commonly identified subgroups of aPL are lupus anticoagulant (LA) antibodies, anticardiolipin antibodies (aCL), and β-2-glycoprotein I antibodies (anti-β-2).

The antiphospholipid antibody syndrome (APS) is considered to be a primary coagulopathy rather than a primary vasculopathy, in which the presence of these antiphospholipid autoantibodies creates a hypercoaguable state leading to vascular thromboses, both venous and arterial, and obstetrical complications. It is considered a secondary APS when seen in the context of systemic lupus erythematosus (SLE). APS is a complicated syndrome, the diagnosis, pathophysiology, and treatment of which remains the subject of ongoing research.

Epidemiology

In young, healthy people, the prevalence of any aPL is 1–5%. The prevalence increases with both age and illness and has been found to be as high as 12.3% in elderly patients with chronic diseases. In patients with SLE, the prevalence of aPL is significantly higher, ranging from 11% to 30% for LA and from 17% to 39% for aCL.

In healthy controls with laboratory evidence of aPL but without clinical manifestations, there are insufficient data to determine what percentage will go on to have a thrombotic event or obstetrical complication. Some risk factors, however, have been identified. A history of thrombosis, the presence of LA, an elevated level of isotype IgG aCL, or the persistence of aPL levels can increase a patient's risk of a thrombotic event by up to five times.

There is some evidence that genetic factors play a role in APS. One study that looked at relatives of patients with

aCL found that one-third of those relatives also had aCL. In addition, there is an association between the presence of aPL and certain HLA subtypes, including HLA-DR7 in Canadians, Germans, Italians, and Mexicans and HLA-DQ7 in Americans.

aPL are also associated with certain bacterial, viral, and parasitic infections (including Lyme, cytomegalovirus, mumps, and Epstein–Barr virus), neoplasms, chronic systemic illnesses (such as sickle cell disease and diabetes mellitus), and certain medications (such as procainamide). The significance of these associations is controversial and remains under investigation.

Pathophysiology

The mechanism by which the presence of aPL results in an increased risk of thrombosis is only partially understood but is thought to be heterogeneous and multifactorial, based on characteristics of the individual's aPL. There is strong evidence that aPL disrupt the coagulation pathway at several points, interfering with the regulatory functions of prothrombin, protein C, annexin V, and tissue factor, leading to a hypercoaguable state. β-2 glycoprotein I is thought to act as a natural anticoagulant, whose inhibition could promote thrombosis. In addition, aPL are thought to induce the activation of endothelial cells as well as predispose the vascular endothelium to injury, both of which can lead to thrombosis.

Clinical features

The most common manifestation of APS is venous thrombosis, especially deep venous thrombosis of the leg. Arterial thromboses are the second most likely clinical manifestations of APS, the brain and the heart being the sites most frequently affected, accounting for 50% and 23% of arterial occlusions, respectively. Thromboses in APS, however, can occur in any vessel in the body and frequently occur in vascular beds less commonly affected by other prothrombotic states. The site of thrombosis may be related to the type of aPL present, with venous

International Neurology: A Clinical Approach. Edited by Robert P. Lisak, Daniel D. Truong, William M. Carroll and Roongroj Bhidayasiri.
© 2009 Blackwell Publishing, ISBN: 978-1-4051-5738-4.

thromboses more frequent in patients with LA and arterial events more frequent in patients in aCL.

The recurrence rate of thrombotic events in APS is variable, from 9% to 31% in different studies. Risk factors for recurrence include more than one prior thrombotic event, high levels of aCL, and abnormalities on transesophageal echocardiogram. Initial arterial thrombosis tends to be followed by an arterial event whereas initial venous thrombosis is usually followed by another venous event.

APS should be suspected in cases of thromboses in young, otherwise healthy, patients without significant risk factors. In one study, aPL were found in 25% of patients under the age of 45 with a stroke of unclear etiology. aPL can be found in 5–21% of patients with venous thrombosis.

Other common manifestations of APS include thrombocytopenia (in 40–50% of patients), hemolytic anemia (in 14–23%) and livedo reticularis (in 11–22%).

Diagnosis

According to a recent Consensus Statement, the diagnosis of APS is based on both clinical and laboratory criteria. Diagnosis requires at least one clinical event, defined as either an arterial, venous, or small-vessel thrombosis in any tissue or organ, or a complication of pregnancy resulting in fetal morbidity, and evidence of aCL, LA, or anti-β-2 on laboratory testing.

aPL are detected solely via laboratory testing. Identification of LA requires prolongation of coagulation in at least one phospholipid-dependent coagulation assay. Both aCL and anti-β-2 are detected through standardized enzyme-linked immunoassays (ELISA).

Management

Whether to manage the initial arterial thrombotic event such as a first ischemic stroke or transient ischemic attack (TIA) with an antiplatelet agent or an anticoagulant is controversial and not established based on randomized clinical trials. When anticoagulant therapy is chosen, the international normalized ratio (INR) should be kept between 2.0 and 3.0 as randomized clinical trials show no benefit to higher intensity warfarin therapy. Anticoagulation is sometimes continued long term, or even lifelong, as discontinuation may be associated with an increased risk of thrombosis and death, although this is not established and remains empiric.

Prophylactic therapy for patients with laboratory evidence of aPL who have not had a thrombotic event or obstetrical complication is uncertain. Low-dose aspirin therapy has been recommended in non-pregnant patients even though it has not shown any benefit in clinical trials. Hydroxychloroquine may be beneficial in patients with SLE. In addition, patients should eliminate or control other factors, such as smoking, hyperlipidemia, diabetes, oral contraceptive use, and uncontrolled high blood pressure, all of which increase their risk of thrombosis.

Further reading

Asherson RA, Khamashta MA, Ordi-Ros J, *et al*. The "primary" antiphospholipid syndrome: major clinical and serological features. *Medicine* 1989; 68: 366–74.

Crowther MA, Ginsberg JS, Julian J, *et al*. A comparison of two intensities of warfarin for the prevention of recurrent thrombosis in patients with the antiphospholipid syndrome. *N Engl J Med* 2003; 349: 1133–8.

Giannakopoulos B, Passam F, Rahgozar S, Kulis SA. Current concepts on the pathogenesis of the antiphospholipid syndrome. *Blood* 2007; 109(2): 422–30.

Rolden JF, Brey RL. Neurologic manifestations of the antiphospholipid syndrome. *Curr Rheumatol Rep* 2007; 9(2): 109–15.

Turiel M, Sarzi-Puttini P, Peretti R, *et al*. Thrombotic risk factors in primary antiphospholipid syndrome: a five-year prospective study. *Stroke* 2005; 31: 1490–4.

Chapter 21
Thromboangiitis obliterans – Buerger's disease

Kumar Rajamani
Wayne State University, Detroit, USA

Background

Thromboangiitis obliterans (TAO) is a non-atherosclerotic idiopathic inflammatory disease of the blood vessels of the upper and lower extremities predominantly involving medium- and small-sized arteries as well as veins. There is a resultant segmental obliteration of the affected vessels. Persistent tobacco smoking has long been associated with TAO, although alternative forms of tobacco consumption such as chewing and sniffing have also been implicated. It occurs throughout the world, but higher incidences have been described from Japan, Eastern Europe, India, Israel, and the Middle East, while the incidence is lower in Western Europe and the USA. The reason for this geographic distribution is not entirely clear and has been variably attributed to local smoking habits as well as genetic predisposition. A decline in the incidence of TAO is reported in the USA and is likely due to general decline in smoking, but application of stricter diagnostic criteria could also be contributory.

Etiology

Chronic and often heavy exposure to tobacco use is implicated in the onset as well as the progression of the disease. Quiescent disease can be reactivated if the patient starts to smoke again. Patients demonstrate hypersensitivity to intradermally injected tobacco extracts. Although the target antigen is yet to be convincingly demonstrated, an autoimmune process is implicated in the vascular endothelial dysfunction and inflammatory thrombi that characterizes the endarteritis. Deposition of immunoglobulins and complement factors has been shown along the internal elastic lamina. There is increased cell-mediated sensitivity to type I and III collagen (both of which are present in vessel walls) and elevated titers of anticollagen and anti-endothelium antibodies. However, these are

International Neurology: A Clinical Approach. Edited by Robert P. Lisak, Daniel D. Truong, William M. Carroll, and Roongroj Bhidayasiri. © 2009 Blackwell Publishing, ISBN: 978-1-4051-5738-4.

non-specific and could be an epiphenomenon rather than the cause. Increased incidences of HLA-A9 and HLA-B5 antigens and reduced HLA-B12 have been described, supporting the notion of a genetic influence over the immune response.

Pathology

In the acute phase there is a highly cellular inflammatory thrombus. There is progressive organization of the thrombus and the late stage is characterized by an organized thrombus and fibrosis of the vessel wall. Differentiation from arteriosclerosis may be difficult, but intimal inflammation, characteristic preservation of the internal elastic lamina, adventitial fibrosis without affection of the media, onion-like recanalized vessels, and swelling of the endothelium of the vasa-vasorum are more characteristic of TAO.

Clinical features

Males are more affected than females (6:1) and symptoms typically start in the third and fourth decades. Claudication pain in the feet may progress to the calf. More than one limb can be affected. Isolated involvement of large proximal arteries without small vessels being affected is unusual. Rest pain, non-healing ulcers of toes and fingers, and gangrene are later features. Raynaud's phenomenon and superficial thrombophlebilitis are characteristic features which could help distinguish TAO from arteriosclerosis. Coronary, cerebral, mesenteric, and multiorgan involvement are described but are decidedly rare. There are no definite laboratory tests for the diagnosis. Tests to rule out other vasculitides include those for acute phase reactants, antinuclear antibodies, rheumatoid factor, serologic markers for the CREST syndrome (calcinosis, Raynaud's, esophageal dysmotility, sclerodactyly, and telangiectasia), scleroderma, and hypercoagubility. Angiography demonstrates more distal vascular occlusions, characteristic corkscrew collaterals without proximal lesions, but is not pathognomonic.

Management

Early treatment is important, with complete avoidance of tobacco consumption being the most effective. In spite of the role of inflammation, steroids and other anti-inflammatory medications have not been shown to be useful. Intravenous Iloprost (prostaglandin analogue) and subcutaneous Teprostilin (prostacyclin) have been shown to be useful in critical limb ischemia to heal ulcers and prevent the dreaded complication of limb amputations. Supportive care is needed for maximizing blood supply to the limb mainly by avoiding injuries and emphasizing properly-fitting footwear. Judicious and timely use of sympathectomy may alleviate pain and promote healing while avoiding amputation. Bypass vascular surgery is not generally possible or useful because of the diffuse and distal nature of the disease and problems with graft thrombosis. Gene therapy aimed at therapeutic angiogenesis holds future promise.

Further reading

Eichhorn J, Sima D, Lindschau C, *et al*. Antiendothelial antibodies in thromboangiitis obliterans. *Am J Med Sci* 1998; 315(1): 17–23.

Kurata A, Franke F, Machinami R, Schulz A. Thromboangitis obliterans: classic and new morphological features. *Virchows Arch* 2000; 436: 59–67.

Olin JW. Thromboangiitis obliterans (Buerger's disease). *N Engl J Med* 2000; 343(12): 864–9.

Olin JW, Shih A. Thromboangitis obliterans (Buerger's disease). *Curr Opin Rheumatol* 2006; 18: 18–24.

Puechal X, Fiessinger JN. Thromboangiitis obliterans or Buerger's disease: challenges for the rheumatologist. *Rheumatology* 2007; 46(2): 192–9.

Chapter 22
Systemic lupus erythematosus, rheumatoid arthritis, and Sjögren's syndrome

Marc Gotkine and Oded Abramsky

Hebrew University Hadassah Medical School, Jerusalem, Israel

Introduction

These rheumatological conditions have clinical features which in their full-blown form leave little room for diagnostic confusion. The importance of recognizing the neurological manifestations of these systemic conditions is manifold. Both psychiatric and neurological symptoms occur which may signal damage to diverse components of the nervous system from the brain and spinal cord to the peripheral nerve and muscle. Consequently, a patient with a rheumatological condition presenting, for example, with "difficulty walking" requires a neurologist to provide clinical expertise in order to localize the pathology, as management decisions invariably depend on the neuroanatomical site involved.

Furthermore, when a patient diagnosed with one of these conditions develops neurological involvement such as central nervous system (CNS) vasculopathy, the treatment regimen often involves robust immunosuppressive therapy.

The most challenging patients from the neurological perspective are those who exhibit neurological manifestations at the beginning or very early in the course of their systemic disease. In these cases recognition of the patterns of neurological involvement as well as knowledge of the non-neurological features of these conditions is critical in order to identify the systemic condition.

Systemic lupus erythematosus (SLE)

Introduction

Systemic lupus erythematosus (SLE) is a systemic autoimmune disease affecting multiple organ systems. The diagnosis is made on the basis of fulfillment of accepted clinical and paraclinical criteria, as summarized

in Table 22.1. Neurological and psychiatric symptoms occur in many patients and may reflect damage to various components of the nervous system from the cerebral cortex to the muscle, although the CNS is usually affected more often than the peripheral nervous system (PNS) (Table 22.2).

In SLE only seizures and psychosis among neurological manifestations contribute to the diagnostic criteria (Table 22.1). However, the distinction between neurological conditions said to be "associated" with SLE (such as immune-mediated myelitis or myasthenia gravis) and those contributing to the diagnosis of SLE (psychosis and seizures) may reflect statistical associations rather than a specific pathogenetic mechanism.

The issue is further complicated by the fact that drugs used in SLE and other rheumatological conditions may have a variety of neurological side effects and that neurological complications may result from derangements in other organ systems such as the liver and kidneys.

Epidemiology

The disease is most commonly encountered in women of childbearing age. Both geography and race seem to affect the distribution of SLE. The prevalence in the US population is around 40–50 cases per 100000 and prevalence rates in Europe and Australia are also high. Differences in detection methods worldwide make it difficult to obtain accurate comparative data between countries. In most countries the prevalence rate is considerably lower in Caucasians in comparison to other ethnic groups. While SLE is seen frequently in African-Americans, it is rare in blacks in West Africa.

While genetic factors seem to be important, environmental factors play a sizeable role in both the frequency and severity of the disease, and factors such as socioeconomic status often confound epidemiological studies.

Pathophysiology of neurological features of SLE

SLE is characterized by the presence of circulating autoantibodies directed against a variety of cellular components

International Neurology: A Clinical Approach. Edited by Robert P. Lisak, Daniel D. Truong, William M. Carroll, and Roongroj Bhidayasiri. © 2009 Blackwell Publishing, ISBN: 978-1-4051-5738-4.

Table 22.1 Criteria for classification of Systemic Lupus Erythematosus.

Criterion	Definition
1. Malar rash	Fixed erythema, flat or raised, over the malar eminences, tending to spare the nasolabial folds
2. Discoid rash	Erythematous raised patches with adherent keratotic scaling and plugging; atrophic scarring may occur in older lesions
3. Photosensitivity	Skin rash as a result of unusual reaction to sunlight, determined by patient history or physician observation
4. Oral ulcers	Oral or nasopharyngeal ulceration, usually painless, observed by physician
5. Arthritis	Non-erosive arthritis involving two or more peripheral joints, characterized by tenderness, swelling, or effusion
6. Serositis	Pleuritis-convincing history of pleuritic pain or rub heard by physician or evidence of pleural effusion OR Pericarditis documented by ECG or rub or evidence of pericardial effusion
7. Renal disorder	Persistent proteinuria greater than 0.5 g/day or greater than 3+ if quantitation not peformed OR Cellular casts – may be red cell, hemoglobin, granular, tubular, or mixed
8. Neurologic disorder	Seizures OR psychosis in the absence of offending drugs or metabolic derangements known to cause these features
9. Hematologic disorder	Hemolytic anemia with reticulocytosis OR Leukopenia OR Lymphopenia OR Thrombocytopenia in the absence of offending drugs
10. Immunologic disorder	Positive LE cell preparation OR Anti-DNA antibodies OR Anti-Sm antibodies OR False positive serologic test for syphilis
11. Antinuclear antibody	High antinuclear antibody titers in the absence of drugs known to be associated with "drug-induced lupus syndrome"

A diagnosis of SLE is made if any four or more of the criteria are present (not necessarily simultaneously). It should be remembered that these criteria are intended for designing inclusion criteria for clinical trials and some patients who do not fulfill these criteria may have a partial or "forme fruste" of the condition which otherwise behaves pathogenetically and clinically like SLE.

including the plasma membrane, cytoplasm, and nucleus. The neurological features may be a result of the damaging effects that these antibodies trigger directly on the various tissue components within the nervous system or the blood vessels that supply them. For example, the cerebral cortex may be damaged directly by the inflammatory process or alternatively may be damaged by multiple infarcts as a result of "cerebral vasculitis." However, there is little histological support for the pathological diagnosis of "lupus cerebritis", and cerebral vasculitis in SLE is uncommon whereas vasculopathy is often seen.

Clinical features and investigations

A wide variety of neurological symptoms may occur in patients previously diagnosed with SLE. However, patients ultimately diagnosed with SLE may initially present with neurological symptoms and have no overt systemic involvement on initial clinical evaluation. As a corollary, many patients presenting with neurological syndromes should be screened for clinical and paraclinical parameters associated with SLE (Table 22.1).

Conversely, neurological evaluation of patients with established SLE may not be straightforward, as neurological dysfunction may be a direct consequence of the disease, secondary to other organ involvement or due to therapeutic interventions. The American College of Rheumatology defined 19 neuropsychiatric syndromes (NPS) occurring

in SLE. These represent conditions directly associated with SLE and exclude conditions occurring secondary to other organ involvement or therapy. Table 22.2 summarizes the full range of neurological syndromes associated with SLE including "secondary associations." While cardiac, renal, and hematological involvement are related to the core diagnostic features of SLE, it should be remembered that SLE and the drugs used to treat it are associated with a multitude of other conditions such as liver dysfunction, endocrine derangement, and hypertension, which themselves may have neurological ramifications beyond the scope of this chapter.

The antiphospholipid antibody syndrome (APLAS) is a frequent accompaniment to SLE, and the frequency of NPS is higher in SLE patients with antiphospholipid antibodies, particularly anticardiolipin antibodies. Furthermore, neuropsychiatric syndromes frequently occur in APLAS in the absence of SLE (see Chapter 20 on APLAS). Serum antibodies to ribosomal P proteins (anti-P) have been proposed as a marker for neuropsychiatric involvement in SLE; however, low sensitivity and specificity limit its diagnostic value.

Various NPS may be causally interrelated. For example, cerebrovascular disease may lead to focal deficits, cognitive decline, seizures, and a movement disorder. Similarly, myelitis may either be isolated or a manifestation of more widespread CNS involvement. The fact that these

Table 22.2 Neurological and psychiatric features associated with systemic lupus erythematosus, rheumatoid arthritis, and Sjögren's syndrome.

System	Clinical features	SLE	Possible pathogenetic relationship with other recognized NPS	Possible relationship with core SLE systemic disorders	Rheumatoid arthritis (RA)	Sjögren's syndrome (SS)	Drug side effects
Brain	Cognitive	(1) Acute confusion (encephalopathy) (2) Dementia. Unclear whether this occurs in isolation or only in association with other NPS or drug side effects	(1) Meningoencephalitis (2) Stroke (3) Seizures (4) Demyelinating syndrome	Renal dysfunction	No clear association	Associated	Steroids Cyclosporine Methotrexate
	Psychiatric	(1) Mood disorder (2) Anxiety disorder (3) Psychosis. Psychosis included in SLE diagnostic criteria	(1) Stroke (2) Seizures	Increased incidence of affective disorders in chronic systemic disease	Increased incidence of affective disorders in all chronic systemic diseases	(1) Affective disorders (2) Psychosis	Steroids
	Seizures	Associated and included in SLE diagnostic criteria	(1) Stroke (2) Meningoencephalitis	Renal dysfunction	No clear association	Associated	TNF-α antagonists Cyclosporine Methotrexate Hydroxychloroquine Gold salts
	Stroke	Mechanisms include • Vasculopathy • Hypercoaguable state associated with APLAS • Endocarditis with thromboembolism	—	Renal dysfunction Thrombocytopenia may increase susceptibility to brain hemorrhage	Secondary to cervical spine pathology with atlanto-axial dislocation affecting vertebral arteries (rare)	Associated	Methotrexate IVIG Anticoagulant drugs (hemorrhage)
	Movement disorders	Usually chorea occurring almost exclusively in the presence of APLAS	Stroke or other focal lesions affecting basal ganglia	Uremia (usually myoclonus)	No clear association	Associated (rare)	Cyclosporine (tremor) Hydroxychloroquine (ataxia)
	Demyelinating syndromes	Includes optic neuritis and myelitis. May be related to NMO antibodies	Myelitis included as NPS in own right	—	Possible association	May be difficult to distinguish from MS	TNF-α antagonists
	Headache	Includes migraine with or without aura. May be due to idiopathic intracranial hypertension	Meningitis/ meningoencephalitis	Frequent non-specific symptom of systemic/ metabolic derangement	Secondary to cervical spine pathology/atlanto-axial dislocation	No clear association	Cyclosporine Sulphasalazine Cyclophosphamide Steroids Leflunomide Gold salts Hydroxychloroquine

(Continued)

Table 22.2 Continued.

System	Clinical features	SLE	Possible pathogenetic relationship with other recognized NPS	Possible relationship with core SLE systemic disorders	Rheumatoid arthritis (RA)	Sjögren's syndrome (SS)	Drug side effects
Brain (Continued)	Meningitis/meningoencephalitis	Aseptic meningitis may be related to vasculitis, NAIM	—	—	Pachymeningitis (rare)	Associated	IVIG (aseptic meningitis)
Spinal cord	Myelopathy/myelitis, Cord compression	May be associated with NMO antibodies; No clear association	May be part of a "demyelinating syndrome"; No clear association	No clear association	No clear association; Pannus compression; Atlanto-occipital dislocation; Vertebral collapse	Associated; No clear association	TNF-α antagonists; Steroids via osteoporotic fractures
Motor neurons (upper and lower)	Amyotrophic lateral sclerosis	—	—	—	—	Associated (rare)	—
Peripheral nerves	Cranial neuropathy	Trigeminal sensory	Demyelinating disease (fascicular involvement)	No clear association	Secondary to cervical spine pathology with atlanto-axial dislocation (rare)	Trigeminal sensory; Oculomotor; Vestibulocochlear	No clear association
	Peripheral neuropathy	(1) Polyneuropathy (distal SM); (2) MM (vasculitic); (3) GBS-like; (4) Plexopathy; (5) Autonomic	No clear association	Renal dysfunction; Musculoskeletal disorders increase compression neuropathies	(1) MM (vasculitic); (2) Polyneuropathy (distal SM); (3) Compression sites	(1) Polyneuropathy (distal SM); (2) Posterior ganglionopathy; (3) Autonomic; (4) MM (vasculitic)	Gold salts; Leflunomide
Muscle	Myopathy, myalgia, cramps	Not considered to represent an NPS; Myalgia common; Myopathy rare	No clear association	Renal dysfunction (cramps, myokymia)	Inflammatory myopathy (rare)	Myalgia common but myopathy rarely noticeable on clinical examination	Steroids; Penicillamine; Hydroxychloroquine; Gold salts; Cyclosporine; Azathioprine
NMJ	Myasthenia gravis	Associated	No clear association	No clear association	Associated	Associated (rare); SS is associated with thymus hyperplasia	Penicillamine (reversible on drug withdrawal)

The features comprising the 19 NPS are shaded; APLAS: antiphospholipid antibody syndrome; NMO: neuromyelitis-optica; NAIM: non-vasculitic autoimmune meningoencephalitis; NPS: neuropsychiatric syndromes associated with SLE; MS: multiple sclerosis; IVIG: intravenous immunoglobulin; NMJ: neuromuscular junction; SM: sensorimotor; MM: mononeuritis multiplex; GBS: Guillain–Barré syndrome; SS: Sjögren's syndrome.

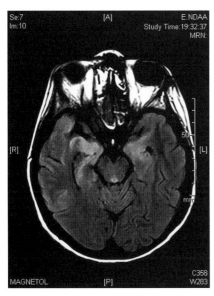

Figure 22.1 FLAIR MRI scan showing bilateral hippocampal inflammation ("limbic encephalitis") in a young woman with SLE.

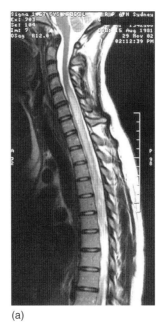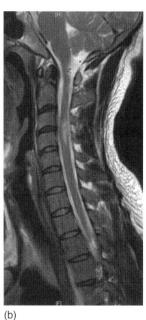

(a)   (b)

Figure 22.2 (a) T2-weighted MRI scan showing acute longitudinal myelitis spanning more than six spinal cord segments in a young woman with SLE. (Reproduced with permission from Krishnan AV, Halmagyi GM. Acute transverse myelitis in SLE. *Neurology* 2004; 62(11): 2087.) (b) T2-weighted MRI scan showing a characteristic plaque of myelitis limited to less than three cervical spinal cord segments in a woman with MS.

syndromes can occur independently of one another means they are listed as NPS of SLE in their own right. A possible exception to this is chronic cognitive decline which is invariably secondary to one or more of the other processes listed. An acute amnestic syndrome due to bilateral hippocampal inflammation known as "limbic encephalitis" may occasionally occur (Figure 22.1); however, the relationship to idiopathic autoimmune limbic encephalitis is not clear.

Of special note is a characteristic form of severe myelitis occurring in SLE. These patients present with an acute flaccid tetraparesis or paraparesis and loss of sphincter control, which usually involves multiple cord segments and is referred to as "acute longitudinal myelitis" (ALM) (Figure 22.2a). This type of myelitis is distinguished from the type that occurs in multiple sclerosis (MS), which is usually limited to less than two to three spinal segments (Figure 22.2b). ALM also occurs in Devic's syndrome, commonly referred to as neuromyelitis-optica (NMO), and antibodies to water channels known as NMO-IgG are often found in these cases. NMO may be associated with full-blown SLE, which raises the possibility that the myelitis of SLE is closely related to the spectrum of neuromyelitis-optica-related disorders.

Although headache is often considered to be one of the neurological manifestations of SLE, the association is controversial. Headache prevalence as a whole is probably similar to the general population, while migraine with aura may be more common in SLE sufferers especially with anticardiolipin antibodies. In children with SLE, headache may be associated with CNS involvement.

Rheumatoid arthritis

Introduction and epidemiology

Rheumatoid arthritis (RA) is the commonest of the rheumatic diseases with a prevalence of around 1% worldwide. Some ethnic groups such as certain native American populations have an increased prevalence, indicating a genetic component, whilst the higher rate of RA in urban as compared to rural African areas also confirms a strong environmental influence. The sex and age profile is similar to that of SLE.

Clinical features

The disease is characterized by a chronic inflammatory arthropathy. There is frequently extra-articular involvement including the skin, kidney, lung, heart, eyes, and blood components. In contrast to SLE, neurological involvement is almost exclusively confined to the PNS, manifesting primarily with peripheral neuropathy (Table 22.2). Neurological evaluation may be very difficult in patients with advanced disease who may be so severely limited by arthritis that an advanced neuropathy may remain unnoticed by patient and physician alike.

The commonest type of neuropathy is due to vasculitis affecting the vasa nervosum, and as with other vasculitic neuropathies this usually manifests as multiple mononeuropathies (mononeuritis multiplex) occurring during single or multiple episodes. It occurs in roughly 10% of all patients, but the figure rises to 50% in those RA patients with systemic vasculitis. It mainly affects patients with rheumatoid factor seropositivity and long-standing highly manifest disease.

A mild symmetrical polyneuropathy is common and is usually asymptomatic, whilst entrapment neuropathies are important to identify correctly to provide appropriate treatment aimed at decompression rather than immune suppression.

Structural derangement of the cervical spine predisposes to cervical myelopathy, and in rare instances the lower cranial nerves, brainstem, and posterior circulation may be distorted by atlanto-axial dislocation. Direct involvement of the CNS and meninges is rare, with co-existing demyelination or pachymeningitis being occasionally observed.

Sjögren's syndrome

Sjögren's syndrome (SS) may occur alone or co-exist with SLE, RA, or systemic sclerosis. The core clinical features are due to inflammation of the lachrymal and salivary glands leading to decreased saliva and tear production. Associated circulating auto-antibodies include anti-Ro (SS-A) and La (SS-B), but these are found in less than 50% of patients with neurological manifestations of SS.

The PNS and CNS are affected at roughly the same frequency (Table 22.2). A distal polyneuropathy is the commonest form of neuropathy, followed by cranial (mainly trigeminal) neuropathy and sensory ganglionopathy. The sensory ganglionopathy or neuronopathy affects all sensory modalities and is associated with lymphocytic infiltration of the dorsal root ganglia. It is frequently painful and asymmetric, affecting proximal as well as distal areas of the body including the trunk. This infrequent syndrome also occurs in other situations such as pyridoxine intoxication and a paraneoplastic syndrome associated with anti-Hu antibodies.

The CNS features may mimic MS both clinically and radiologically and this should be borne in mind when evaluating patients previously suspected of having MS, especially when atypical features are present.

Management issues (applying to SLE, RA, and SS)

Various immune therapies are employed depending on the severity of the disease, type of organ involvement, and individual patient factors. These therapies can be conveniently split into four distinct groups. Corticosteroids such as methylprednisolone may be employed for limited periods intravenously during exacerbations or orally as maintenance. Immunosuppressive drugs such as azathioprine may allow a decrease in the required steroid dose, whilst more powerful immunosuppressive agents such as cyclophosphamide are usually referred for more resistant cases. Antibody-depleting or neutralizing therapies (plasmapheresis or intravenous immunoglobulin (IVIG)) may be used for exacerbations as well as maintenance in some disorders. Finally, monoclonal antibodies directed against pro-inflammatory cytokines (such as TNF-α in the case of infliximab) or lymphocyte subpopulations (such as CD20+ B cells in the case of rituximab) or TNF-R fusion proteins are being employed more frequently; however, their promising efficacy and tolerability is offset by their prohibitive cost and rare but potentially debilitating side effects such as progressive multifocal leukoencephalopathy.

Whilst the management of these rheumatological conditions is beyond the scope of this book it should be emphasized that an accurate neurological assessment is often an essential factor in guiding appropriate therapy. For example, a seizure in a patient with SLE may occur in the context of a metabolic derangement or be due to an acute inflammatory or ischemic insult to the cerebral cortex. The former scenario should prompt correction of the metabolic problem whereas the latter may signal the need for long-term anti-epileptic medication, anticoagulation, more robust immunosuppression, or a combination of these approaches. A similar situation exists in RA in relation to the possible etiologies of peripheral neuropathy. Neurologists should be aware of the potential for neurological side effects of many of the drugs used in these conditions and the possibility of conditions occurring due to immune compromise such as opportunistic infections and malignancy.

Further reading

ACR Ad Hoc Committee on Neuropsychiatric Lupus Nomenclature. American College of Rheumatology nomenclature and case definitions for neuropsychiatric lupus syndromes. *Arthritis Rheum* 1999; 42(4): 599–608.

Delalande S, de Seze J, Fauchais AL, *et al*. Neurologic manifestations in primary Sjogren syndrome: a study of 82 patients. *Medicine* 2004; 83(5): 280–91.

Gotkine M, Fellig Y, Abramsky O. Occurrence of CNS demyelinating disease in patients with myasthenia gravis (subsequent correspondence in *Neurology* 2007; 68(16): 1326–7). *Neurology* 2006; 67(5): 881–3.

Hochberg MC. Updating the American College of Rheumatology revised criteria for the classification of systemic lupus erythematosus. *Arthritis Rheum* 1997; 40(9): 1725.

Johnson RT, Richardson EP. The neurological manifestations of systemic lupus erythematosus. *Medicine* 1968; 47(4): 337–69.

Joseph FG, Lammie GA, Scolding NJ. CNS lupus: a study of 41 patients. *Neurology* 2007; 69(7): 644–54.

Levine JS, Branch DW, Rauch J. The antiphospholipid syndrome. *N Engl J Med* 2002; 346(10): 752–63.

McLaurin EY, Holliday SL, Williams P, Brey RL. Predictors of cognitive dysfunction in patients with systemic lupus erythematosus. *Neurology* 2005; 64(2): 297–303.

Mitsikostas DD, Sfikakis PP, Goadsby PJ. A meta-analysis for headache in systemic lupus erythematosus: the evidence and the myth. *Brain* 2004; 127(Pt 5): 1200–9.

Sofat N, Malik O, Higgens CS. Neurological involvement in patients with rheumatic disease. *QJM* 2006; 99(2): 69–79.

Chapter 23
Systemic sclerosis

Ho Jin Kim[1] and Min Su Park[1,2]
[1]Research Institute and Hospital of National Cancer Center, Goyang-si, Gyeonggi-do, Korea
[2]Yeungnam University School of Medicine, Taegu, Korea

Introduction

Systemic sclerosis (scleroderma, SSc) is an acquired systemic connective tissue disease characterized by fibrosis of the skin, blood vessels, and visceral organs, including the gastrointestinal tract, lungs, heart, and kidneys, due to the overproduction and accumulation of collagen.

The disorder is referred to as *localized scleroderma* when confined to skin and as *SSc* when the visceral organs are involved. SSc is subdivided into two major forms according to the extent of skin affected. One subtype is *diffuse cutaneous scleroderma* characterized by a symmetrical widespread skin fibrosis affecting distal and proximal extremities often including the trunk and face. This type tends to progress rapidly with early involvement of the visceral organs. The other subtype is *limited cutaneous scleroderma* characterized by symmetrical, but restricted, skin fibrosis affecting distal extremities and the face. This type frequently shows features of CREST (calcinosis, Raynaud's phenomenon, esophageal dysmotility, sclerodactyly, and telangiectasia) syndrome.

Epidemiology

SSc has a worldwide distribution and affects all races. It affects all ages, but is uncommon in children. The incidence increases with age, peaking in the third to fifth decade. Women are affected about 3–4 times more often than men, and even more often during the childbearing years.

Pathophysiology

The prominent pathological features of SSc are the overproduction and accumulation of collagen and other extracellular matrix proteins, microvascular damage, and inflammation. Although the precise pathogenesis of SSc

remains to be elucidated, presumably these pathological features and their interactions can be regarded as the pathophysiological mechanisms of SSc. Environmental triggers and genetic predisposition interact to produce these features. The widespread pathologic process in SSc leads to microvasculopathy and fibrosis, which can decrease the reserve function of many organs.

Clinical features

The initial symptoms of SSc are non-specific and include Raynaud's phenomenon, fatigue, musculoskeletal complaints, and swelling of the hands. The characteristic skin thickening usually begins as swelling of the skin on the fingers and hands and is associated with tightness, deceased mobility, hyperpigmentation, and eventual atrophy and ulceration of the skin. Patients with systemic involvement frequently develop esophageal dysfunction resulting in symptoms of dysphagia and reflux. Gastrointestinal involvement results in hypomotility and malabsorption, constipation, and episodic diarrhea. Interstitial fibrosis may cause restrictive pulmonary disease, and cardiac involvement can cause arrhythmia, pericarditis, myocarditis, and myocardial fibrosis with congestive heart failure. Renal failure may result from hypertension due to renal microvascular involvement.

Neurological involvement with SSc is uncommon when compared to other connective tissue diseases and is thought to be coincidental, iatrogenic, or secondary to the involvement of other organs such as the kidney or the gastrointestinal tract, rather than the result of the disease itself. Myopathy is the most common form of neurological problem seen in SSc, usually occurring within the first year or two of the disease. It is usually non-inflammatory and characterized by proximal muscle weakness, mild increase in the level of creatine kinase, and occasionally muscle atrophy. Electromyography may show polyphasic motor unit potentials in the absence of denervation. Muscle biopsy may show histiocyte infiltration and muscle fiber atrophy, but there is no evidence of true inflammatory myositis, nor is there atrophy of the outer portions of the muscle bundles that might suggest dermatomyositis.

International Neurology: A Clinical Approach. Edited by Robert P. Lisak, Daniel D. Truong, William M. Carroll, and Roongroj Bhidayasiri. © 2009 Blackwell Publishing, ISBN: 978-1-4051-5738-4.

Although this type of muscle involvement usually tends to be mild, some patients develop severe muscle weakness and atrophy. True inflammatory myositis (sclerodermatomyositis) resembling idiopathic polymyositis is an even less common muscle complication of SSc.

Peripheral neuropathy has been regarded as uncommon in SSc. In retrospective studies, neuropathy was seen in only 1–2% of patients. However, prospective studies using electrodiagnostic methods revealed that 10–20% of SSc patients develop peripheral neuropathy during the course of their disease. The exact pathogenic mechanism is uncertain, but most neuropathies associated with SSc are thought to be ischemic in origin, resulting from either a chronic non-inflammatory vasculopathy or true vasculitis. Trigeminal sensory neuropathy represents the most common form of neuropathy seen in SSc, affecting 3% of patients. As in Sjögren's syndrome, this may be the result of inflammatory ganglionitis of the trigeminal sensory ganglia. Distal axonal polyneuropathy may develop and typically involves motor fibers. Ischemic infarction of different nerves may result in a painful mononeuropathy multiplex. Unilateral or bilateral optic neuropathy has also been observed in SSc.

Central nervous system involvement is rare in SSc, possibly because of the paucity of connective tissue and the absence of an external elastic lamina with a sparse media and adventitia in the cerebral arteries. When it occurs, cerebral ischemia is usually associated with renal failure or hypertension. Other rare manifestations described include encephalopathy, seizures, subarachnoid hemorrhage, psychosis, and anxiety disorder.

Investigations and diagnosis

Antinuclear antibodies are present in almost all patients. Antinuclear antibodies that are highly specific for SSc are antitopoisomerase 1 (Scl-70), antinucleolar, and anticentromere. Anti-RNA polymerase 1 is found in patients with diffuse cutaneous SSc. Anti-PM-Scl, formerly referred to as anti-PM1, may be found in SSc patients with polymyositis, whereas anti-Jo-1 generally is not found in SSc patients with polymyositis, but is usually found in polymyositis patients with arthritis and alveolitis. Anti-U3 nucleolar ribonucleoprotein (RNP), different from anti-U1 RNP of mixed connective tissue disease, is also highly specific for SSc and is associated with SSc with skeletal muscle disease.

The clinical picture of SSc is so distinctive that the diagnosis of SSc is not difficult, with the presence of Raynaud's phenomenon, typical skin lesions, and visceral involvement.

Treatment

No curative therapy for SSc exists. Instead, treatments for SSc focus mainly on ameliorating the organ-specific consequences of SSc. Meticulous monitoring and treatment of the pulmonary, gastrointestinal, cardiac, and renal complications are crucial in the management of the disease. Acute myositis is usually responsive to glucocorticoids; these drugs should not be used in the indolent primary form of muscle disease of SSc because steroids are risk factors for the development of scleroderma renal crisis.

Further reading

Averbuch-Heller L, Steiner I, Abramsky O. Neurologic manifestations of progressive systemic sclerosis. *Arch Neurol* 1992; 49: 1292–5.

Carpentier PH, Maricq HR. Microvasculature in systemic sclerosis. *Rheum Dis Clin North Am* 1990; 16: 75–91.

Harvey GR, McHugh NJ. Serologic abnormalities in systemic sclerosis. *Curr Opin Rheumatol* 1999; 11: 490–4.

Hietaharju A, Jaaskelainen S, Kalimo H, Hietarinta M. Peripheral neuromuscular manifestations in systemic sclerosis (scleroderma). *Muscle Nerve* 1993; 16: 1204–12.

LeRoy EC, Black C, Fleischmajer R, *et al*. Scleroderma (systemic sclerosis): classification, subsets and pathogenesis. *J Rheumatol* 1988; 15: 202–5.

Chapter 24
Mixed connective tissue disease

Ho Jin Kim[1] and Min Su Park[1,2]
[1]Research Institute and Hospital of National Cancer Center, Goyang-si, Gyeonggi-do, Korea
[2]Yeungnam University School of Medicine, Taegu, Korea

Introduction

Mixed connective tissue disease (MCTD) is an overlap syndrome characterized by the combined features of systemic lupus erythematosus (SLE), systemic sclerosis (SSc), polymyositis (PM), and rheumatoid arthritis (RA) and is associated with high titers of antibody to the U1 nuclear ribonucleoprotein (U1-RNP) antigen. Since it was first described a few decades ago, the concept of MCTD has been highly controversial. Although the original view that it is a relatively benign disease (due to the good response to corticosteroids) was invalidated by subsequent long-term follow-up studies, MCTD remains a useful concept in clinical practice.

Epidemiology

MCTD has been reported in all races and literature suggests that no specific protection or propensity based on race exists. It affects mainly women in the second and third decades. It is estimated to attack women 8 to 15 times more frequently than it attacks men. Careful epidemiological studies have not been performed, but MCTD appears to be more prevalent than dermatomyositis (1–2 cases per 100 000 population) but is less prevalent than SLE (15–50 cases per 100 000 population).

Pathophysiology

As with other autoimmune connective tissue diseases, the etiology of MCTD remains unknown. A prominent histopathological feature is a widespread proliferative vasculopathy characterized by intimal and medial proliferation resulting in the narrowing of the lumen of small arteries and large vessels. These lesions may lead to visceral involvement, particularly pulmonary

International Neurology: A Clinical Approach. Edited by Robert P. Lisak, Daniel D. Truong, William M. Carroll, and Roongroj Bhidayasiri. © 2009 Blackwell Publishing, ISBN: 978-1-4051-5738-4.

hypertension. Whether MCTD can be widely accepted as a distinct clinical entity awaits the demonstration of common pathogenic events underlying the development of U1-RNP antibodies and their associated clinical features.

Clinical features

Being an overlap syndrome, MCTD lacks any unique clinical features. The most common clinical features include a high frequency of Raynaud's phenomenon, arthritis, swollen hands, sclerodactyly, esophageal dysfunction, pulmonary involvement, and polymyositis. Cardiac, cerebral, and renal involvement occur less frequently.

Raynaud's phenomenon affects most patients and is frequently the initial symptom. Sometimes it is severe and associated with digital ulceration, a major cause of morbidity.

Cutaneous features of MCTD include a swollen, sausage-like appearance of the fingers, non-scarring alopecia, lupus-like rashes, heliotrope eyelids, erythematous patches over the knuckles, and periungual telangiectasia. SSc-like changes may be present but rarely become extensive.

Musculoskeletal abnormalities occur in most patients. Arthritis may resemble the features of RA but rarely causes deformity. Polymyositis is frequent and may be severe. Rarely, a necrotizing myopathy is associated with MCTD with muscle necrosis and "pipe-stem" vessels.

Esophageal dysfunctions, seen in 80% of MCTD patients, include reduced upper and lower esophageal sphincter pressures and decreased amplitude of peristalsis in the distal two-thirds of the esophagus.

Pulmonary involvement occurs in 85% of patients and often is clinically silent until well advanced. Reduced diffusion capacity for carbon monoxide is the most frequent functional abnormality. Occasionally this is secondary to interstitial pulmonary fibrosis, but more commonly it is a primary consequence of the intimal proliferation of pulmonary arterioles. Pulmonary hypertension is the most frequently observed serious complication and the leading cause of disease-related death.

Nervous system involvement is uncommon. Trigeminal neuropathy is the most common neurological disorder. It can be a presenting manifestation and occurs in 10–25% of patients with MCTD, observed more commonly than in SSc, SLE, and Sjögren's syndrome. The clinical features of this neuropathy include facial numbness and paresthesia; frequent bilateral involvement with the usual sparing of motor fibers is identical to that seen in other connective tissue diseases. The neuropathy does not improve with corticosteroid treatment. Headaches, often with features of migraine, are also common. Aseptic meningitis and transverse myelitis have been reported, but other neurological complications are rare. There are a few reports of symmetric sensory polyneuropathy, acute autonomic neuropathy, carpal tunnel syndrome, and chronic polyradiculoneuropathy similar to that seen in chronic inflammatory demyelinating polyneuropathy. The polyradiculoneuropathy responds to corticosteroid treatment, but the sensory polyneuropathy does not.

Investigations and diagnosis

Almost all patients have high titers of antinuclear antibody with a speckled pattern and very high titers of immunoglobulin G antibodies to U1 ribonucleoprotein (U1-RNP). The high titers of circulating U1-RNP antibodies usually persist for years, but antibody levels may decline significantly or become undetectable in those patients with prolonged remission. Rheumatoid factor is found, often at very high titers, in half of the patients. Less frequent findings include hypocomplementemia, leukopenia, anemia, and thrombocytopenia (mainly in children).

The diagnosis of MCTD is based on a combination of the typical overlapping clinical symptoms and high titers of circulating antibody to U1-RNP. MCTD usually develops slowly and is rarely obvious upon initial evaluation, making it difficult to diagnose. However, MCTD is now being recognized in an earlier phase with minimal symptoms (e.g., Raynaud's phenomenon, arthralgia, myalgia, and swollen hands). In some patients, these mild symptoms may persist for years, but a prospective long-term study showed that the majority of patients with high titers of U1-RNP antibodies and limited clinical manifestations ultimately developed signs and symptoms consistent with MCTD.

Treatment

Because of the lack of controlled studies to guide therapy and the heterogeneous clinical course of MCTD, therapy should be individualized depending on the specific organs involved and the severity of the underlying disease activity. Salicylates, other non-steroidal anti-inflammatory agents, hydroxychloroquine, vasodilators, and low doses of corticosteroids are used to treat mild forms of the disease. If the disease is severe or involves major organ systems, higher doses of corticosteroids (1 mg prednisone/kg/day) and/or cytotoxic drugs are usually required. In general, the more advanced the disease is, the greater the organ damage and the less effective the treatment will be.

Further reading

Bennett RM, O'Connell DJ. Mixed connective tissue disease: a clinicopathologic study of 20 cases. *Semin Arthritis Rheum* 1980; 10: 25–51.

Burdt MA, Hoffman RW, Deutscher SL, Wang GS, Johnson JC, Sharp GC. Long-term outcome in mixed connective tissue disease: longitudinal clinical and serologic findings. *Arthritis Rheum* 1999; 42: 899–909.

Sharp GC, Irvin WS, Tan EM, Gould RG, Holman HR. Mixed connective tissue disease: an apparently distinct rheumatic disease syndrome associated with a specific antibody to an extractable nuclear antigen (ENA). *Am J Med* 1972; 52: 148–59.

Chapter 25
Behçet's syndrome and the nervous system

Aksel Siva and Sabahattin Saip
University of Istanbul, Istanbul, Turkey

Introduction

Behçet's disease, originally described in 1937 by the Turkish dermatologist Hulusi Behçet as a distinct disease with orogenital ulceration and uveitis known as the "triple-symptom complex," is an idiopathic chronic relapsing multisystem vascular-inflammatory disease of unknown origin. As the disease affects many organs and systems, its clinical manifestations and presentations show a wide range; hence it is more appropriate to consider it as a syndrome rather than a disease.

Epidemiology

The epidemiology of the disease shows a geographic variation, seen more commonly along the Silk Road that extends from the Mediterranean region to Japan. There are also several genetic predisposing factors, such as the human leukocyte antigen HLA-B51, which might be responsible for the geographic distribution of Behçet's syndrome (BS). Its prevalence has been reported to be less than $0.5/10^5$ in the US, between 0.5 and $1/10^5$ in northern and central Europe, and up to $2.5/10^5$ in the northwestern Mediterranean region, and it increases further in the eastern Mediterranean region. Prevalence rates of up to $400/10^5$ have been found in a population-based study in Turkey and rates between 10 and $20/10^5$ have been reported in Japan, China, and Korea, countries at the other end of the ancient trade routes of the Silk Road.

The reported range of neuro-Behçet's syndrome (NBS) prevalence varies between 4% and 10% of patients with BS in large clinical series. The mean age of onset for BS and NBS is 26.7 ± 8.0 and 32.0 ± 8.7 years respectively. Although the gender distribution is almost equal in BS in general, the neurological complications occur more commonly in males, with a male to female ratio of 3–4:1.

International Neurology: A Clinical Approach. Edited by Robert P. Lisak, Daniel D. Truong, William M. Carroll, and Roongroj Bhidayasiri. © 2009 Blackwell Publishing, ISBN: 978-1-4051-5738-4.

Etiopathogenesis

Despite increased understanding of this disease, the etiology is unknown. Three major pathophysiologic changes have been reported in BS, namely excessive functions of neutrophils, endothelial injury with vasculitis, and autoimmune responses, although these findings are not always universal. BS may belong to a newly designated group of auto-inflammatory diseases.

Diagnosis

The diagnosis of BS is clinical and is made according to the criteria of the International Study Group for Behçet's disease, which states that for a clinical diagnosis, patients must have recurrent oral ulcerations, plus at least two of the following: recurrent genital ulcerations, eye inflammation (uveitis or retinal vasculitis), skin lesions, or a positive pathergy test. The pathergy phenomenon, which is positive in about half of BS patients, is the occurrence of an aseptic erythematous nodule or pustule that is more than 2 mm in diameter, developing 48 hours after pricking a sterile needle into the patient's forearm.

Nervous system involvement in Behçet's disease – "neuro-Behçet's syndrome"

Patients with BS may present with different neurological problems, related either directly or indirectly to the disease (Table 25.1). The direct effects will be reviewed here as "neuro-Behçet's syndrome" (NBS), those with cerebral venous sinus thrombosis (CVST) will be called extra-axial NBS, and cases with parenchymal-CNS involvement will be called intra-axial NBS. The diagnostic criteria for NBS in a patient that fulfills the international diagnostic criteria for Behçet's disease are the presence of neurological symptoms not otherwise explained by any other known systemic or neurological disease or treatment, and in whom objective abnormalities are detected on neurological examination, and/or with neuroimaging studies (magnetic resonance imaging (MRI) disclosing findings

Table 25.1 The neurological spectrum of Behçet's syndrome. (Modified from Siva A, Altintas A, Saip S. Behçet's disease. *Curr Opin Neurol* 2004.)

Primary neurological involvement (neurological involvement directly related to BS)
- Headache (migraine-like, non-structural)
- Cerebral venous sinus thrombosis (extra-axial NBS)
- Central nervous system involvement (intra-axial NBS)
- Neuro-psycho-Behçet's syndrome
- Peripheral nervous system involvement
- Subclinical NBS

Secondary neurological involvement (neurological involvement indirectly related to BS)
- Depression and headache
- Neurological complications secondary to systemic involvement of BS (i.e., cerebral emboli from cardiac complications of BS, increased intracranial pressure secondary to superior vena cava syndrome)
- Neurologic complications related to BS treatments (i.e., CNS neurotoxicity with cyclosporine; peripheral neuropathy secondary to thalidomide or colchicine)

Coincidental – unrelated (non-BS) neurological involvement
- Primary headaches and any other coincidental neurological problem

---

BS: Behçet's syndrome; NBS: neuro-Behçet's syndrome; CNS: central nervous system.

suggestive of NBS), and/or with abnormal cerebrospinal fluid findings consistent with NBS.

Headache in BS

The most common neurological symptom among patients with BS is headache. Headache can occur as a presenting symptom of NBS due to either CNS involvement or CVST. It can also be seen in association with ocular inflammation. Some patients with BS report a bilateral, frontal, moderate paroxysmal migraine-like pain, which is not idiopathic migraine, since it generally starts after the onset of BS and commonly accompanies the exacerbations of systemic findings of the disease, such as oral ulcerations or skin lesions, although this is not always the case. It may be explained by a vascular headache triggered by the immunologically-mediated disease activity in susceptible individuals. Finally co-exiting primary headaches such as migraine and tension-type headache occur in patients.

Extra-axial NBS

CVST is seen in 10–20% of BS patients in whom neurological involvement occurs. Thrombosis of the venous sinuses may cause increased intracranial pressure with severe headache, papilledema, motor ocular cranial nerve (sixth nerve) palsies, and mental changes, but in some patients the only manifestation may be a moderate headache. CVST in BS evolves relatively slowly in most cases, but acute onset with seizures and focal neurological signs

have also been reported. The superior sagittal sinus is most commonly involved, with a substantial number of these patients also having lateral sinus thrombosis. CVST tends to occur earlier than parenchymal-CNS disease and this difference is significant in male patients. Intracranial hypertension with initially normal neuro-imaging with subsequent findings of CVST has been reported.

Extension of the clot-causing focal venous hemorrhagic infarction is uncommon, and the occurrence of CVST simultaneously with primary CNS involvement is also extremely rare. BS patients with CVST have a better neurological prognosis than those with CNS-NBS cases, but since patients with CVST in BS are more likely to also have systemic major vessel disease, and that major vessel disease has a higher overall morbidity and mortality, a diagnosis of CVST in a patient with BS may not be always associated with a favorable outcome.

Intra-axial NBS

Parenchymal involvement in NBS may present with symptoms and signs consistent with focal or multifocal CNS dysfunction with or without headache. The most common are pyramidal weakness, brainstem and cerebellar signs, and cognitive/behavioral changes. The onset of a subacute brainstem syndrome in a young man, especially of Mediterranean, Middle-Eastern, or Asian origin, including cranial nerve findings, dysarthria, corticospinal tract signs, and a mild confusion with severe headache should raise the probability of NBS. Such a patient (if a reliable history cannot be obtained from the patient, then his/her family member/s) needs to be interviewed for the presence of systemic findings of BS. In the case of BS, it will very likely reveal a past or present history of recurrent oral aphtous ulcers and some other systemic manifestations of the disease. Hemiparesis, cognitive-behavioral changes, emotional lability, seizures, or a self-limited or progressive myelopathy may be seen but are less common, whereas isolated optic neuritis, aseptic meningitis, and extrapyramidal syndromes are extremely rare presentations. Many of the CNS-NBS patients initially follow a relapsing-remitting course, some ultimately develop secondary progression, while a few will have a progressive CNS dysfunction from the onset.

Arterial-NBS

Arterial involvement resulting in CNS vascular disease is rare, but has been reported in BS. Observations in cases with bilateral internal carotid artery occlusion, vertebral artery dissection or thrombosis, intracranial arteritis, and aneurysms with their corresponding neurological consequences suggest that arterial involvement may represent a subgroup of intra-axial NBS. Intracranial hemorrhages may occur but are extremely rare, most occurring within ischemic lesions.

Neuro-psycho-Behçet's syndrome

Some patients with BS may develop a neurobehavioral syndrome, which consists of euphoria, loss of insight/ disinhibition, indifference to their disease, psychomotor agitation or retardation, with paranoid attitudes and obsessive concerns not associated with glucocorticosteroid or any other therapy, known as "neuro-psycho-Behçet's syndrome."

Neuromuscular disease in BS

PNS involvement with clinical manifestations is extremely rare in BS. Reported PNS involvement includes mononeuritis multiplex, a distal sensory motor neuropathy, an axonal sensory neuropathy, and myositis.

Subclinical NBS

The incidental finding of neurological signs in patients with BS without neurological symptoms was reported in some studies, with a minority of patients subsequently developing mild neurological attacks. The detection of abnormalities in neurophysiological studies, as well as

by neuroimaging in asymptomatic patients, suggests that there might be a subgroup of patients with subclinical NBS. However, the clinical and prognostic value of these findings in this group of patients currently is not clear.

Diagnostic studies in NBS

Neuro-imaging

In BS patients with neurological problems consistent with intra-axial NBS, cranial MRI is generally highly suggestive of this diagnosis. The lesions are generally located within the brainstem, extending to the diencephalon and/or basal ganglia (Figure 25.1a–d). Less often they are in the periventricular and subcortical white matter. The pattern of parenchymal lesions is suggestive of small vessel vasculitis, but the pathology in NBS with CNS involvement is not always uniform and covers a wide spectrum. A definite vasculitis is not observed in all cases. Spinal cord involvement is not common, but when seen the major site involved is the cervical cord, with

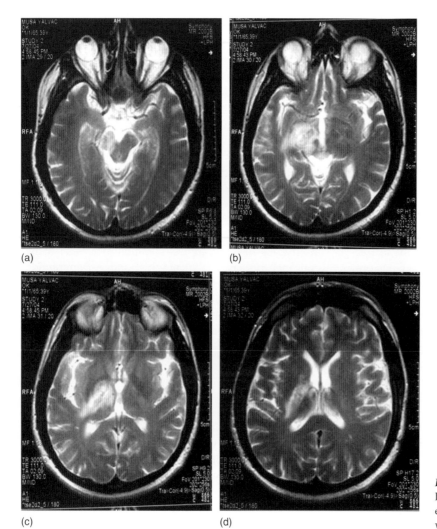

(a)   (b)

(c)   (d)

Figure 25.1(a–d) T2W MR images showing a lesion in the right meso-diencephalic region extending towards the basal ganglia in a patient with NBS.

a myelitis-like lesion continuing along more than two segments and extending to the brainstem in some patients. Gadolinium enhancement, subsequent resolution of these lesions, and thoracic cord involvement have also been reported.

MR venography (MRV) is the preferred study to diagnose or confirm CVST in Behçet's disease, but T1- and T2-weighted images also disclose the venous sinus thrombosis. In most cases cerebral arteriography is not needed in NBS, unless the patient presents with subarachnoid hemorrhage or an overt cerebral arterial lesion. Infiltration of neurtrophils, sometimes with arterial injury, may occur at the site of arteriographic puncture in patients with BS.

Cerebrospinal fluid (CSF)

During the acute stage, CSF studies usually show inflammatory changes in most cases of CNS-NBS. Oligoclonal bands can be detected, but this is an infrequent finding. CSF in patients with CVST may be under increased pressure, but the cellular and chemical composition is usually normal.

Differential diagnosis

Differential diagnosis of intra-axial (parenchymal) NBS

Patients with NBS are young and frequently present with a subacute brainstem syndrome or hemiparesis, as well as with other neurological manifestations. Hence, the possibility of BS is often included in the differential diagnosis of multiple sclerosis (MS) and in stroke in the young adult, especially in the absence of its known systemic symptoms and signs.

Optic neuritis, sensory symptoms and spinal cord involvement, which are common in MS, are rarely seen in NBS. However, sometimes the clinical presentation of NBS may be confused with MS, but the neuroimaging – MRI – findings are clearly different, with more discrete and smaller brainstem lesions seen in MS, as well as more periventricular and ovoid lesions in the hemispheres. Spinal cord involvement rarely extends more than a few vertebral segments in MS, compared to the more extensive lesions that are reported in NBS, similar to neuromyelitis optica (NMO). The CSF also reveals different patterns, with a more prominent pleocytosis and low rate of positivity for oligoclonal bands in CNS-NBS.

An acute stroke-like onset is uncommon in NBS, and MRI lesions compatible with classical arterial territories are also not expected. The absence of systemic symptoms and signs will serve to differentiate primary CNS vasculitis from NBS, and the difference in some of the systemic symptoms and signs, as well as the MRI findings and specific blood tests from the secondary CNS vasculitides.

Sarcoidosis can be confused with BS due to uveitis, arthritis, and CNS involvement, but the absence of oral and genital ulcers, and the presence of peripheral lymphadenopathy, and bilateral hilar lymph nodes on chest X-ray, as well as pathological examination of the non-caseating granulomatous lesions of sarcoidosis, help in the differential diagnosis.

Tuberculosis may resemble BS because of its multisystem involvement and its potential to affect the nervous system. Hilar lymphadenopathy and pulmonary cavities are not expected in BS, whereas its mucocutaneous manifestations are unusual for tuberculosis. Furthermore CSF and MRI findings are different.

Tumefactive lesions have been reported in NBS, but the imaging findings, the response to steroids, and the absence of systemic findings in primary CNS tumors helps to distinguish NBS from brain neoplasms.

Due to their ophthalmologic and other systemic manifestations, rare diseases such as Vogt–Koyanagi–Harada syndrome, Reiter syndrome, Eales' disease, Cogan's syndrome, and Susac's syndrome are other considerations in the differential diagnosis of BS. All may present with nervous system manifestations and therefore are included in the differential diagnosis of NBS. However, a complete ophthalmologic examination will reveal the true nature of eye involvement in each of these syndromes, which is different from the eye involvement seen in BS.

Gastrointestinal symptoms in Behçet's disease may mimic Crohn's disease or chronic ulcerative colitis. Eye disease is rare and genital ulcers are absent in inflammatory bowel diseases. The diagnosis can be confirmed by intestinal biopsy. Whipple's disease with its gastrointestinal and various nervous system symptoms may also resemble BS.

Prognosis

Neurological involvement in BS is a major cause of morbidity. Approximately 50% of NBS patients are moderately to severely disabled after 10 years of disease. Onset with cerebellar symptoms and a progressive course were found to be unfavorable factors, while onset with headache, a diagnosis of CVST, and disease course limited to a single episode were more favorable neurologically. An elevated protein level and pleocytosis in the CSF were also reported to be associated with a poorer prognosis.

Treatment

Neurological involvement in BS is heterogeneous and it is difficult to predict its course and prognosis, and assess response to treatment. Therefore it is not possible to reach a conclusion on the efficacy of any treatment unless properly designed, double-masked, placebo-controlled studies are done for each form of NBS. However, this is difficult to accomplish, as numbers of new neuro cases seen yearly are limited even in large centers. Currently we have no firm evidence for the efficacy of any treatment for any form of NBS. Empirical impressions currently create the guidelines for management.

Intra-axial NBS – acute episodes

Glucocorticoids are used to treat acute CNS involvement in BS, but their effects are short-lived and they do not prevent further attacks or progression. Acute attacks of CNS-NBS are treated with either oral prednisolone (1 mg/kg for up to 4 weeks, or until improvement is observed) or with high-dose intravenous methylprednisolone (IVMP, 1 g/day) for 5–7 days. Both forms of treatment should be followed by an oral tapering dose of glucocorticoids over 2–3 months in order to prevent early relapses. Our current practice is to give IVMP, 1 g/day for 7 days, followed by the oral regimen in patients with clinical and imaging evidence of CNS involvement.

Intra-axial NBS – long-term treatments

Colchicine, azathioprine, cyclosporine-A, cyclophosphamide, methotrexate, chlorambucil, immunomodulatory agents such as interferon-α and, more recently, thalidomide, have been shown to be effective in treating some of the systemic manifestations of BS, but none of these agents has been shown to be beneficial in NBS in a properly designed study. Cyclosporine was reported to cause neurotoxicity or to accelerate the development of CNS symptoms and therefore its use in NBS is not recommended. A common clinical practice is to add an immunosuppressant drug, such as azathioprine or monthly pulse cyclophosphamide, to glucocorticoids in progressive NBS cases. However, the efficacy of such a combination has not been proven.

Succcessful treatment of neurological manifestations of BS with monoclonal anti-TNF-α antibody (infliximab) in a few patients has recently been reported. The occurrence of neuro-relapses after stopping infliximab, formation of neutralizing antibodies, and the possibility of increased CNS auto-immunity with monoclonal anti-TNF-α antibody treatment should be kept in mind. Mycophenolate mofetil and tacrolimus are other immunosuppressant/immunomodulating agents that are used to treat ocular inflammation and significant systemic manifestations in patients with BS, but there is no information regarding the potential effects of all these drugs in preventing CNS involvement or new neurological attacks.

In our limited experience with a few cases with progressive CNS involvement, we have not observed any significant improvement with intravenous immunoglobulin. Data on the use of plasma exchange in NBS are also limited and unclear.

Cerebral aneurysms are rare in BS, but when small unruptured aneurysms are detected, medical therapy with steroids with or without cytotoxic agents may be tried. As an alternative to surgery, endovascular treatment is another option in the management of Behçet's disease-associated intracranial axial disease.

Cerebral venous sinus thrombosis (CVST) in NBS

There is no consensus on the treatment of CVST in NBS. Some authors use a combination of anticoagulation with glucocorticoids, while others administer glucocorticoids alone. Extreme caution is needed as BS patients with CVST are more likely to also have systemic large vessel disease including pulmonary and peripheral aneurysms. Therefore the use of anticoagulants should be considered only after such possibilities are ruled out. Recurrence of CVST is uncommon after the initial episode.

Further reading

International Study Group for Behçet's Disease. Criteria for diagnosis of Behçet's disease. *Lancet* 1990; 335: 1078–80.

Kantarci O, Siva A. Behçet's disease: diagnosis and management. In: Noseworthy J, editor. *Neurological Therapeutics: Principles and Practice*, Chapter 96, 2nd ed. New York: Informa Healthcare; 2006, pp. 1196–1206.

Koçer N, Islak C, Siva A, *et al*. CNS involvement in neuro-Behçet's syndrome: an MR study. *Am J Neuroradiol* 1999; 20: 1015–24.

Siva A, Altıntaş A, Saip S. Behçet's syndrome and the nervous system. *Curr Opin Neurol* 2004; 17: 347–57.

Yazıcı H, Fresko I, Yurdakul S. Behçet's syndrome: disease manifestations, management, and advances in treatment. *Nat Clin Pract Rheumatol* 2007; 3: 151–5.

Chapter 26
Sarcoidosis

Barney J. Stern
University of Maryland, Baltimore, USA

Introduction

Neurologic complications occur in approximately 5% of patients with sarcoidosis. Neurosarcoidosis is a diagnostic consideration in patients with known sarcoidosis who develop neurologic symptoms and signs, and in patients without documented sarcoidosis who present with a spectrum of neurologic findings consistent with neurosarcoidosis. Approximately 50% of patients with neurosarcoidosis present with neurologic disease at the time sarcoidosis is first diagnosed.

Epidemiology

The prevalence of sarcoidosis is approximately 40 per 100 000 population, although in certain groups the incidence and prevalence can be substantially greater.

Sarcoidosis occurs throughout the world and can develop in any racial/ethnic population. Certain areas of the world, such as Sweden, also seem to have a higher incidence of sarcoidosis, whereas it appears to be quite rare in other areas, such as China or Southeast Asia. It most commonly presents in persons in their 20s or 30s, though individuals of any age can be afflicted. A study of familial risk for sarcoidosis among siblings revealed an odds ratio of 5.8 (95% confidence interval 2.1–15.9) and in a familial multivariate model the adjusted familial relative risk was 4.7 (95% confidence interval 2.3–9.7).

Pathophysiology

Non-necrotizing granulomas, the key pathologic finding of sarcoidosis, are composed of epithelioid macrophages, lymphocytes, monocytes, and fibroblasts. The inflammation is often perivascular and there can be involvement in the outer aspect of the media and the adventitia. With time, fibrosis can develop along with thickening of the intima and media of blood vessels, leading to ischemic injury.

Moller and Chen stated that "the etiology of … sarcoidosis is linked to genetically determined enhanced Th1 immune responses to a limited number of microbial pathogens." This results in an enhanced production of interferons β and γ and select interleukins. Cytokines, such as tumor necrosis factor alpha, are expressed. With time, a Th2 response can develop and lead to fibrosis. The antigen inciting the inflammatory response remains unknown, although *Mycobacterium* and *Propionibacterium* species are implicated.

Clinical features

The neurologic manifestations of sarcoidosis and their approximate frequencies are: cranial neuropathies (overall 50–75%; facial palsy 25–50%); meningeal disease including aseptic meningitis and mass lesion (10–20%); hydrocephalus (10%); parenchymal disease (overall 50%) including endocrinopathy (10–15%), mass lesion(s) (5–10%), encephalopathy/vasculopathy (5–10%), seizures (5–10%), vegetative dysfunction, extramedullary or intramedullary spinal canal disease, and cauda equina syndrome; neuropathy (15%) including axonal, mononeuropathy, mononeuropathy multiplex, sensorimotor, sensory, motor, demyelinating, and Gullain–Barré syndrome; and myopathy (15%) including nodule(s), polymyositis, and atrophy. On rare occasions, stroke syndromes can occur. Many of the diverse presentations of neurosarcoidosis can be placed within one of these broad categories.

Patients can be classified based on the certainty of the diagnosis of multisystem sarcoidosis, the pattern of neurologic disease, and the response to therapy. The following is adapted from Zajicek *et al.*:

Possible: The clinical syndrome and neurodiagnostic evaluation are suggestive of neurosarcoidosis. Infection and malignancy have not been rigorously excluded *or* there is no pathologic confirmation of systemic sarcoidosis.

International Neurology: A Clinical Approach. Edited by Robert P. Lisak, Daniel D. Truong, William M. Carroll, and Roongroj Bhidayasiri. © 2009 Blackwell Publishing, ISBN: 978-1-4051-5738-4.

Probable: The clinical syndrome and neurodiagnostic evaluation are suggestive of neurosarcoidosis and alternative diagnoses have been excluded, especially infection and malignancy. There is pathologic evidence of systemic sarcoidosis.

Definite:
(a) The clinical presentation is suggestive of neurosarcoidosis, other possible diagnoses are excluded, and there is the presence of supportive nervous system pathology. *Or*
(b) The criteria for a "probable" diagnosis are met and the patient has had a beneficial response to therapy for neurosarcoidosis over a 1-year observation period.

Investigations

Patients with known systemic sarcoidosis who develop neurologic disease consistent with sarcoidosis should be evaluated for the reasonable exclusion of other disease entities, particularly infection and neoplasia. If the patient does not respond to treatment as expected, the diagnosis should be questioned and a more extensive evaluation pursued.

If a patient without known sarcoidosis develops a clinical syndrome consistent with neurosarcoidosis, the diagnostic challenge can be considerable. Since corticosteroid therapy can mask signs of systemic sarcoidosis or other diseases, treatment should be postponed, if possible, while a search for systemic disease is initiated.

Sarcoidosis most frequently affects intrathoracic structures, followed by lymph node, skin, and ocular disease. If the patient has impaired smell or taste, nasal or olfactory nerve disease might be present. If dry eyes or mouth are noted, lacrimal, parotid, or salivary gland inflammation is possible. Other clues to the presence of systemic sarcoidosis include an elevated serum angiotensin-converting enzyme (ACE) activity, hypercalcemia, hypercalciuria, elevated immunoglobulins, and anergy. Patients with possible CNS disease should be questioned about symptoms relating to neuroendocrinologic or hypothalamic dysfunction.

Systemic sarcoidosis can often be demonstrated if a comprehensive, but selective, approach is followed: chest X-ray, thoracic CT scan, pulmonary function tests including diffusing capacity, ophthalmologic examination, endoscopic nasal examination, whole-body gallium scan, muscle magnetic resonance imaging (MRI), and fluorodeoxyglucose positron emission tomography imaging.

The preferred imaging technique to evaluate CNS sarcoidosis is MRI without and with contrast enhancement. T1-weighted images depict hydrocephalus, the optic nerves and chiasm, and spinal cord enlargement. With T2-weighted and fluid-attenuated inversion-recovery (FLAIR) imaging, areas of increased signal intensity are visualized, especially in a periventricular distribution.

Contrast administration can demonstrate leptomeningeal enhancement as well as parenchymal abnormalities and, occasionally, cranial nerve lesions. Spinal MRI can visualize intramedullary disease, which appears as an enhancing fusiform enlargement, focal or diffuse enhancement, or atrophy. Enhancing nodules or thickened or matted nerve roots can be noted with cauda equina imaging.

The cerebrospinal fluid (CSF) pressure can be elevated and analysis can reveal an increased total protein, hypoglycorrhachia, and a predominantly mononuclear pleocytosis. The IgG index can be elevated and oligoclonal bands detected. CSF angiotensin-converting enzyme (ACE) activity can be elevated in patients with CNS sarcoidosis, although abnormalities are also seen in the presence of infection and malignancy. A normal CSF ACE assay does not exclude the diagnosis of neurosarcoidosis.

Nerve conduction studies can be of assistance in evaluating a neuropathy. However, there is nothing specific about the spectrum of findings to suggest the diagnosis of sarcoidosis. Electromyography can demonstrate denervation in appropriate muscles and myopathic changes. Peripheral nerve and muscle samples can be obtained for pathologic examination. A skin biopsy can document disease of peripheral nerve endings in patients with neuropathic symptoms and otherwise unrevealing nerve conduction and electromyographic studies.

Differential diagnostic considerations include multiple sclerosis, Sjögren syndrome, systemic lupus erythematosus, neurosyphilis, neuroborreliosis, human immunodeficiency virus infection, Behçet's disease, Vogt–Koyanagi–Harada disease, toxoplasmosis, brucellosis, Whipple's disease, lymphoma, germ cell tumors, craniopharyngioma, isolated angiitis of the CNS, primary CNS neoplasia, lymphocytic hypophysitis, pachymeningitis, cytomegalovirus (CMV) meningoencephalitis, Rosai–Dorfman disease, and low CSF pressure/volume meningeal enhancement.

Treatment/management

There have been no rigorous studies to define the optimal treatment for neurosarcoidosis. Most authorities recommend corticosteroid therapy as first-line therapy for patients, if there are no contraindications. Increasingly, adjunct therapy with other immunosuppressive and immunomodulatory agents is being utilized. Therapeutic decisions should be guided by the patient's clinical course, the expected natural history of the patient's clinical manifestations, and adverse treatment effects.

Two-thirds of patients have a monophasic neurologic illness; the remainder have a chronically progressive or remitting–relapsing course. Patients with a monophasic illness typically have an isolated cranial neuropathy, most often involving the facial nerve, or an episode of aseptic meningitis. Patients with a chronic course usually have CNS disease (parenchymal abnormalities, hydrocephalus, and multiple cranial neuropathies, especially cranial nerves II and VIII), peripheral neuropathy, and myopathy. A goal of treatment is to diminish the irreversible fibrosis that can develop as well as the tissue ischemia that might result from perivascular inflammation. With time, the inflammatory process can become quiescent, allowing therapy to be decreased, at least temporarily.

A peripheral facial nerve palsy usually responds to 2 weeks of prednisone therapy. The first week's prednisone dose is 0.5–1.0 mg/kg/day (or 40–60 mg/day), followed by a taper over the second week. This approach can also be used as initial therapy for other cranial neuropathies and aseptic meningitis. Patients with a peripheral neuropathy or myopathy can also respond to a short course of corticosteroid therapy; however, prolonged treatment is often necessary.

Asymptomatic ventricular enlargement probably does not require treatment. Mild, symptomatic hydrocephalus can respond to corticosteroid therapy, although prolonged treatment is often required. Life-threatening hydrocephalus or corticosteroid-resistant hydrocephalus require ventricular shunting. Unfortunately, patients can rapidly evolve from mild hydrocephalus to severe life-threatening disease. Patients and caregivers should be educated as to when to seek emergency care. Shunt placement is not without risk in these patients, which is why "prophylactic" shunting is discouraged. Shunt obstruction from the inflamed CSF and ependyma is common and placement of a foreign object in the CNS of an immunosuppressed host predisposes to infection.

Corticosteroid therapy can improve the status of patients with a diffuse encephalopathy/vasculopathy or a CNS mass lesion. Seizures occur most commonly in patients with parenchymal disease or hydrocephalus. Control of seizures is usually not difficult if the underlying inflammatory process can be controlled.

Corticosteroid treatment for CNS parenchymal disease and other severe neurologic manifestations of sarcoidosis usually starts with prednisone 1.0 mg/kg/day. These patients often require prolonged therapy and prednisone should be tapered slowly. The patient might be observed on high-dose prednisone for 2–4 weeks to determine the clinical response. The prednisone dose can then be tapered by 5 mg decrements every 2 weeks as the clinical course is monitored. The disease tends to exacerbate at a prednisone dose approximating 10 mg/day (or 0.1 mg/kg/day). If a low dose of prednisone can be achieved, the patient should be evaluated for evidence of subclinical worsening prior to further tapering by decrements of 1 mg every 2–4 weeks.

Patients may require multiple cycles of higher and lower corticosteroid doses. This effort is usually warranted since the disease can become quiescent and, without attempts at withdrawing medication, patients may be needlessly exposed to corticosteroid long-term side effects.

A short course of methylprednisolone 20 mg/kg/day intravenously for 3 days, followed by high-dose prednisone for 2–4 weeks, is occasionally warranted for patients with severe acute neurologic compromise. Another approach to treating severe disease is the use of infliximab, a monoclonal antibody directed at tumor necrosis factor α.

Alternative or adjunct therapies are increasingly being considered for neurosarcoidosis. Experience in this area is limited and firm recommendations are not available. Indications for the use of alternative treatments include the need to avoid corticosteroids as initial therapy, serious adverse corticosteroid effects, and disease activity in spite of aggressive corticosteroid therapy.

Immunosuppressive medications to treat sarcoidosis include mycophenolate mofetil, azathioprine, methotrexate, cyclophosphamide, cyclosporine, chlorambucil, and cladribine. Anecdotal experience suggests that these drugs, especially when used in combination with relatively low-dose corticosteroid therapy, can be effective. Patients can incrementally improve beyond that experienced with corticosteroid monotherapy or the corticosteroid dose can be decreased with the addition of an adjunct therapy. Rarely is it possible to withdraw corticosteroid treatment completely; patients tend to do best on a modest dose of corticosteroid combined with an alternative agent.

Immunomodulatory agents can also be used to treat sarcoidosis and neurosarcoidosis. These agents can be used in conjunction with corticosteroids or corticosteroids and immunosuppressive agents. Hydroxychloroquine, pentoxyfillin, thalidomide, minocycline, and infliximab, adalimumab, and etanercept are reported in case reports and case series to be beneficial.

If a patient with CNS disease fails or cannot tolerate alternative agents, consideration should be given to radiotherapy. Patients may stabilize, though corticosteroids and alternative agents often need to be continued.

Patients require close attention to their general medical condition. Adverse effects of treatment should be sought. Prescribed exercise and dietary programs are often beneficial. Rehabilitation services should be utilized as appropriate. Depression is common and treatable.

Hypothyroidism and hypogonadism should be treated. Since patients are often on protracted, low-dose corticosteroid regimens, supplemental corticosteroids are appropriate during surgery or intercurrent illness. Treatment of osteoporosis is often a challenge since sarcoidosis itself can cause hypercalcemia and hypercalciuria; appropriate consultation is suggested.

Fatigue can be due to a variety of conditions including exercise intolerance, depression, obesity, hypothyroidism, hypogonadism, corticosteroid myopathy, occult neuromuscular disease, sleep apnea, and primary hypersomnia. "Idiopathic" fatigue can be responsive to modafinil therapy.

Further reading

Allen RKA, Sellars RE, Sandstrom PA. A prospective study of 32 patients with neurosarcoidosis. *Sarcoidosis Vasc Diffuse Lung Dis* 2003; 20: 118–25.

Baughman RP. Therapeutic options for sarcoidosis: new and old. *Curr Opin Pulm Med* 2002; 8: 464–9.

Gal AA, Koss MN. The pathology of sarcoidosis. *Curr Opin Pulm Med* 2002; 8: 445–51.

Moller DR, Chen ES. What causes sarcoidosis? *Curr Opin Pulm Med* 2002; 8: 429–34.

Olugemo OA, Stern BJ. Stroke and neurosarcoidosis. In: Caplan L, editor. *Uncommon Causes of Stroke*, 2nd ed. New York: Cambridge University Press; 2008, pp. 75–80.

Pritchard C, Nadarajah K. Tumour necrosis factor (alpha) inhibitor treatment for sarcoidosis refractory to conventional treatments: a report of five patients. *Ann Rheum Dis* 2004; 63: 318–20.

Stern BJ, Krumholz A, Johns C, *et al.* Sarcoidosis and its neurological manifestations. *Arch Neurol* 1985; 42: 909–17.

Tikoo RK, Kupersmith MJ, Finlay JL. Treatment of refractory neurosarcoidosis with cladribine. *N Engl J Med* 2004; 350: 1798–9.

Zajicek JP, Scolding NJ, Foster O, *et al.* Central nervous system sarcoidosis – diagnosis and management. *QJM* 1999; 92: 103–17.

Chapter 27
Inflammatory spondyloarthropathies

Asmahan Alshubaili
Ibn Sina Hospital, Safat, Kuwait

Introduction

Inflammatory spondyloarthropathies are a heterogeneous group of disorders characterized by axial skeletal involvement with inflammatory back pain and enthesitis (an inflammation at sites where tendons join bones and joint capsules). They are also linked by their association with HLA-B27 antigen, which is present in more than 90% of cases of ankylosing spondylitis (AS), a prototype of this group of diseases.

Spondyloarthropathies include AS, Reiter's syndrome (reactive arthritis), psoriatic arthritis, inflammatory bowel disease-associated arthropathy, and undifferentiated spondyloarthropathy.

Epidemiology

AS is the commonest form of spondyloarthropathies and is two to three times more common in males than in females. In females, joints away from the spine are more frequently affected than in men. AS commonly occurs during adolescence, but it can affect any age group including children. The global prevalence of AS appears to be related to the presence of HLA-B27 in specific populations.

Pathogenesis

The etiology of these spondyloarthropathies is unknown and may vary depending on the different disorders.

Clinical features

The clinical symptoms of AS are insidious in onset, with stiffness and low back pain which progresses later to immobility due to fibrosis and ossification of entheses around the spine. The entire spine may be affected and patients may develop bamboo spine.

Extra-articular manifestations of AS and its related group of disorders can involve almost any organ system and significantly increase the disease-associated morbidity. Constitutional symptoms include fatigue, anorexia, and mild fever. Anterior uveitis is the most frequent extra-articular manifestation, occurring in 25–30% of patients. Cardiac manifestations include aortic and mitral root dilatation. Fibrosis may develop in the upper lobes of the lungs in patients with long-standing disease.

The most relevant complications to neurologists are spinal complications. The immobile spine can be easily fractured by minor trauma. The commonest site of fracture is the cervical spine around C5, and it may result in gross instability leading to compression of the spinal cord or vertebral arteries. These fractures, which represent an emergency, may be easily missed on plain radiographs and require CT scans to visualize them. Another spinal complication is cauda equina syndrome, which may present with insidious pain in the lower back, buttocks, or legs associated with bowel and bladder symptoms. The MRI of lumbar spine may demonstrate lumbar diverticuli and compression. Finally, AS may be complicated by spinal stenosis due to bone overgrowth and ligamental hypertrophy leading to nerve compression and neurogenic claudication.

Diagnosis

There are no specific diagnostic tests; hence the diagnosis of inflammatory spondyloarthropathies is mainly based on the patient's history and physical examination. Supportive laboratory tests may include an elevation of erythrocyte sedimentation rate or C-reactive protein, anemia, and non-specific inflammatory synovial fluid. There may be evidence of sacroiliitis or spondyloitis in the lumbar spine or pelvis on radiologic studies.

International Neurology: A Clinical Approach. Edited by Robert P. Lisak, Daniel D. Truong, William M. Carroll, and Roongroj Bhidayasiri. © 2009 Blackwell Publishing, ISBN: 978-1-4051-5738-4.

Treatment

Traditionally non-steroid anti-inflammatory drugs (NSAIDs) have been used to control the symptoms of spondyloarthropathies. The selective cyclo-oxygenase-2 inhibitors may be less ulcerogenic, but they have not been shown to be more effective than conventional NSAIDs. Patients in whom NSAID therapy failed are often treated with disease-modifying antirheumatic drugs. However, the efficacy of these drugs has not been well established in placebo-controlled trials. Recently antitumor necrosis factor α (TNF-α) therapy has become available and etanercept, a soluble fusion protein of the p75 TNF receptor, is approved in the United States for treatment of AS and psoriatic arthritis. Mobility exercise is an important adjunct to medications to prevent fusion and consequently complications.

Further reading

Davis JC, Dougados M, Braun J, Sieper J, van der Heijde D, van der Linden S. Definition of disease duration in ankylosing spondylitis: reassessing the concept. *Ann Rheum Dis* 2006; 65: 1518–20.

Harrop JS, Sharan A, Anderson G, *et al*. Failure of standard imaging to detect a cervical fracture in a patient with ankylosing spondylitis. *Spine* 2005; 30: E417–19.

Reveille JD. The genetic basis of spondyloarthritis. *Curr Opin Rheumatol* 2006; 18: 332–41.

Smith MD, Scott JM, Murali R, Sander HW. Minor neck trauma in chronic ankylosing spondylitis: a potentially fatal combination. *J Clin Rheumatol* 2007; 13: 81–4.

Chapter 28
Epilepsy: overview

Andres M. Kanner
Rush University Medical Center, Chicago, USA

Introduction

Epilepsy is a neurological disorder characterized by recurrent and unprovoked epileptic seizures. While 8–10% of people are at risk of experiencing a single epileptic seizure in the course of their life, the lifetime risk of developing epilepsy is 3.2%. The diagnosis of epilepsy is established after the occurrence of at least two unprovoked seizures, though a diagnosis of epilepsy after a first seizure can be made if epileptiform activity can be demonstrated in electrographic (EEG) recordings.

Classification

In 1981, the International League against Epilepsy (ILAE) introduced a classification that separated seizures as partial (i.e., of focal origin) or generalized. Partial seizures were further classified as either simple partial, complex partial, or partial with secondary generalization, also known as secondarily generalized tonic–clonic (GTC) seizures. Simple partial seizures do not involve an alteration in consciousness, while complex partial seizures do. Simple partial seizures were subdivided into four subcategories: with motor symptoms, with somatosensory or special sensory symptoms, with autonomic symptoms, and with psychic symptoms. Complex partial seizures were subdivided as those preceded by simple partial seizures and those with impairment of consciousness at onset. Generalized seizures include both convulsive and non-convulsive events and include: absence seizures (typical and atypical), myoclonic, clonic, tonic–clonic, atonic, and unclassified.

In 1989 the ILAE published the classification of the epilepsies: (1) localization-related (focal, local, or partial), (2) generalized, (3) undetermined whether focal or generalized, and (4) special syndromes.

International Neurology: A Clinical Approach. Edited by Robert P. Lisak, Daniel D. Truong, William M. Carroll, and Roongroj Bhidayasiri. © 2009 Blackwell Publishing, ISBN: 978-1-4051-5738-4.

Epidemiology

The worldwide incidence of epilepsy ranges from 50 to 120 cases per 100 000 per year, with a prevalence rate of 4–10 cases per 1000 people and higher rates in underdeveloped countries as well as in lower socioeconomic classes. The rates are similar between different ethnic groups, and slightly higher for men than women. Across age, there is a bimodal distribution, with higher incidence at the extremes of age, specifically before the age of 1 year and in the elderly. In studies conducted in Rochester, Minnesota, the proportion of incident epilepsy cases in those 65 years of age or older approximately doubled from 14% to 29% over the period from 1935 to 1984. With the aging of the US population, this trend is expected to continue. In fact, epilepsy is the third most frequent neurologic disorder of elderly people in the US.

Age and seizure types
Seizure types vary with age. Patients can experience more than one seizure type, and wide variation in prevalence of the various seizure types is reported in the literature. There is a consensus that generalized seizures account for approximately half of seizures in patients younger than 15 years. The incidence of partial seizures, particularly complex partial seizures, increases with age. In individuals 35–64 years old, complex partial seizures have been found to be present in close to 40–50% of new cases of epilepsy. Absence seizures, which account for approximately 13% of seizures in pediatric patients younger than 15 years, are rare after adolescence. In elderly patients seizures of focal onset account for the most frequent seizures.

Mortality
Epilepsy is associated with a higher risk of mortality. The standardized mortality ratio (SMR), which expresses the number of observed deaths per number of expected deaths, is two to three times higher than that in the general population. The causes of mortality include causes related to seizures such as drowning, aspiration, burns, status epilepticus, and suicide. Nevertheless, the cause of death may often be undetectable, in which case it is referred as sudden unexpected death in epilepsy

(SUDEP). Death related to SUDEP has been estimated to account for 17% of all deaths in patients with epilepsy. Its incidence ranges between 0.35 and 10 per 1000 patients per year, with patients with persistent seizures having a higher risk of SUDEP.

Pathophysiology

The etiology of epileptic seizure disorders varies with age. Thus, 70% of seizure disorders are idiopathic among children and young people, while 90% of incident cases in adults have localization-related epilepsy, with 80% of seizures being of temporal lobe origin. Provoked seizures result from acute, reversible systemic, or neurological conditions, including but not limited to metabolic or toxic disturbances.

Risks

Any animal and human brain is susceptible to the development of epileptic seizures. Hauser investigated the relative risk (RR) of various causes of epilepsy. Relative risks of 1 imply that the relative risk of exposed and unexposed are equal, while a risk less than 1 suggests a protective effect of the exposure. Relative risks greater than 10 can be considered definite and clinically detectable. Those between 4 and 10 are considered likely risks, those between 2.5 and 3.9 probable, and those between 1.1 and 2.4 possible. Among the variables with relative risks greater than 10, Hauser identified: cerebral palsy (RR: 17.9–34.4), mental retardation (RR 22.6–31), cerebral palsy with mental retardation (RR: 53.7–92.5), severe head trauma (RR: 25–580), stroke (RR: 22), and CNS infections (RR: 10.8), of which viral encephalitis had the highest RR (16.2).

Investigations

In the evaluation of patients with an epileptic seizure disorder, clinicians must answer the following questions in order to develop a rational and comprehensive treatment plan: (1) Is it possible that these paroxysmal events may not be epileptic seizures? (2) If they are epileptic seizures, what is the epileptic syndrome and seizure type? (3) Are there comorbid medical, neurologic, and psychiatric disorders? (4) Is the patient taking any concomitant medications that need to be factored in the treatment plan? (5) How will the age and gender of the patient impact on the choice of the pharmacologic treatment?

Differential diagnosis

One out of every 4–5 patients referred to an epilepsy center with a diagnosis of epilepsy does not suffer from epilepsy. These paroxysmal events can mimic epileptic seizures and are therefore referred to as non-epileptic events, non-epileptic seizures (NES), or pseudoseizures, though the use of this latter term is discouraged. NES are grouped into two types: organic and psychogenic. A detailed history is pivotal to reach the proper diagnosis.

The following types of organic NES events (ONES) are among the most commonly misdiagnosed as epileptic seizures.

Convulsive syncope
Convulsive syncope is the most frequent type of ONES to be misdiagnosed as epilepsy. The clonic and/or tonic activity associated with the transient drop of blood perfusion in the CNS accounts for the confusion. The short duration of the period of loss of consciousness (less than 30 seconds) and the rapid re-orientation in all spheres upon recovery of consciousness are key in differentiating the syncopal episode from a generalized convulsion in which the ictus can last up to 2 minutes followed by a postictal period of unresponsiveness (several minutes) and confusion (up to several hours duration). In elderly people with an underlying dementia or mild cognitive impairment, the syncopal episode can be longer and can be followed by a prolonged period of confusion. This frequently causes a false positive diagnosis of epilepsy.

Sleep disorders
Sleep disorders include the cataplectic events in narcolepsy, automatic behavior seen in obstructive sleep apnea, and parasomnias.

Complicated migraines and basilar migraines
The transient focal symptoms in the former and the confusional state that is typical of the latter account for the misdiagnosis.

Movement disorders
Acute dystonic reactions, hemifacial spasms, non-epileptic myoclonus, and hyperekplexia are movement disorders misdiagnosed as epileptic seizures. Acute dystonic reactions can present as dystonic movements of cervical, pharyngeal, and cranial muscles or oculogyric crisis, typically triggered by certain drugs 1–4 days after their ingestion (neuroleptics, lithium, trazodone, illicit drugs). Hemifacial spasms typically involve peri-orbital muscles initially but may propagate to other facial muscles. Non-epileptic myoclonus may affect any muscle group in the body and usually occurs associated with toxic, metabolic, and degenerative encephalopathies.

Psychogenic NES are the most frequent type of NES identified in patients misdiagnosed as epileptics.

These include panic disorders, conversion disorders, dissociative disorders, and malingering. The correct diagnosis requires the recording of a typical event in the course of a video-electroencephalogram (V-EEG) monitoring study.

Treatment/management

The treatment of an initial unprovoked epileptic seizure has been the source of continuous debate among epileptologists. The following principles can be used in guiding the decision of whether or not to treat: (1) immediate or delayed treatment after a first seizure does not impact on the long-term outcome of the seizure disorder. On the other hand, immediate treatment prolongs the time to a first breakthrough seizure and increases the percentage of patients that reach an immediate 2-year remission; (2) the following parameters are suggestive of an increased risk of seizure recurrence: (a) partial seizure, (b) remote symptomatic seizure, (c) any abnormal EEG findings in children and epileptiform activity in adults, and (d) first seizure occurring out of sleep.

The success of antiepileptic drugs (AEDs) varies according to the epileptic syndrome, age of onset of the seizure disorder, and cause of epilepsy. Total seizure remission in the entire population of patients with epilepsy is 60–70%. About 80–90% of patients with idiopathic generalized epilepsy are expected to enter remission with the appropriate AED. In the case of partial epilepsy, about 50% of patients will become seizure-free. However, these expectations vary according to the type of focal epileptic syndrome. For example, almost every child with benign focal epilepsy of childhood is expected to become seizure-free, and often these children do not need to be treated with AEDs. Partial seizure disorders beginning after the age of 65 have a significantly better prognosis than those beginning at younger age. Seizure-freedom with AEDs may range from 11% to 50% when the cause of partial epilepsy is mesial temporal sclerosis and is lower than 5% in the case of double pathology in the temporal lobe (mesial temporal sclerosis and a structural lesion, such as a tumor, hamartoma). Finally, the likelihood of seizure-freedom in secondary generalized epilepsy (Lennox–Gastaut syndrome) is virtually zero.

Special populations

Epilepsy in the elderly

Epilepsy in the elderly is the third most frequent neurologic disorder, after stroke and Alzheimer's dementia. Most patients suffer from a partial seizure disorder presenting as simple partial, complex partial, and secondarily generalized tonic–clonic seizures. The most frequent causes of epilepsy in this age group are stroke, dementia, and head trauma. In fact stroke increases the risk of seizures by 23-fold within a year, relative to the general population. Conversely, a seizure disorder after the age of 60 increases the risk of stroke (RR 2.89 (95% CI 2.45–3.41)).

Elderly patients have a five- to ten-fold higher frequency of status epilepticus than younger adults, and mortality in this age group is significantly higher, reaching 48% in the elderly group and 35% in the adult group.

Comorbid medical and psychiatric disorders are common in this age group. In a recent multicenter study, 65% of patients with epilepsy beginning after the age of 60 were being treated for hypertension, 49% for cardiac disease, 27% for diabetes, and 23% had a history of cancer. The average nursing-home patient on an AED is on five other drugs. The addition of an enzyme inducing AED can result in the loss of efficacy of concomitant medications metabolized in the liver. Slower metabolic rate results in greater toxicity in this population. Thus, the AED should be devoid of any pharmacokinetic interaction with other pharmacologic agents, and should be used at the lowest possible doses to avert adverse events.

Epilepsy in women

In addition to the identification of the epileptic syndrome and seizure type, the planning of the treatment of seizure disorders in women must encompass the following considerations: (1) catamenial occurrence and/or exacerbation of seizures and impact of menopause on seizures; (2) reproductive disorders; (3) contraception; (4) pregnancy, including obstetric aspects and teratogenic risks of AEDs; and (5) breast feeding. Epilepsy per se may affect these functions. For example, women with epilepsy have a significantly higher risk of having polycystic ovaries than the general population. They are more likely to suffer from a variety of menstrual dysfunctions, including anovulatory cycles, which, in turn, have been associated with an increase in seizure frequency. Women with epilepsy have a lower sexual drive and lower birth rates than women in the general population. These menstrual and reproductive disturbances can be worsened with AEDs, particularly the older AEDs. Valproic acid facilitates the development of polycystic ovarian syndrome (PCO) in those exposed to this AED between the time of menarchy and the age of 25. Enzyme-inducing AEDs may interfere with sexual drive by decreasing the free fraction of estrogens and testosterone through increased synthesis of binding globulins.

Approximately 30–40% of women experience their seizures around the time of their menstrual cycle or of their ovulation, in which case they are considered to suffer from catamenial epilepsy. The use of hormone therapy with progesterone can decrease the seizure frequency in approximately 60% of women.

The use of AED in women of child-bearing age is of concern, as there is no AED that is completely safe to date. A woman with epilepsy on AED has in general twice the risk of giving birth to a baby with major malformations (e.g., 4–8%) compared to a healthy woman. This risk increases with polytherapy, high doses of AED, and family history of genetic disorders. In addition, certain AEDs are known to increase the risk of teratogenic effects. Finally, women with epilepsy have twice the risk of experiencing obstetric complications as healthy women, and their pregnancy has to be managed by high-risk obstetricians whenever possible.

Psychiatric comorbidities

Psychiatric disorders can be identified in 25–50% of patients with epilepsy, with higher prevalence among patients with poorly controlled seizures. These disturbances include depression, anxiety, psychotic disorders, attention deficit disorders, and cognitive and personality changes occurring in the interictal or ictal/postictal states. The prevalence rates of these major psychiatric disorders are presented in Table 28.1.

Depression and anxiety disorders are among the most frequent psychiatric comorbidities identified in adults. Attention deficit disorders (ADHD) are the most frequently reported in children, but recent studies carried out in pediatric populations have identified a significant prevalence of anxiety and mood disorders that are often misdiagnosed as ADHD. Despite the high prevalence of these psychiatric disorders, they are usually unrecognized and untreated. Only 25–66% of patients with a depressive disorder severe enough to warrant pharmacotherapy are recognized and properly treated early in the course of the condition.

There is evidence of a bidirectional relationship between some psychiatric disorders and epilepsy. Thus, patients with a history of major depressive disorders or

suicidality (independent of a major depressive disorder) have a four- to seven-fold greater risk of developing epilepsy, while children with a history of ADHD of the inattentive type have a 3.7-fold higher risk of developing epilepsy. In a recent study of pre-adolescents and young people with new onset epilepsy, 45% met criteria for an axis I diagnosis according to the DSM-IV-TR classification at the time of the evaluation of the seizure disorder. In a separate study, children with a psychiatric comorbidity were almost three times more likely to develop epilepsy than those without. Clearly, the relationship between psychiatric disorders and epilepsy is complex: not only patients with epilepsy at greater risk of developing a psychiatric disorder but patients with certain psychiatric disorders are at greater risk of developing epilepsy.

Conclusions

Epilepsy is a disorder of the CNS that occurs at all ages and has multiple causes and clinical expressions. Its course is benign in two-thirds of patients. The management of seizure disorder is not limited to the abolition of epileptic seizures, but requires the consideration of comorbid medical, neurologic, psychiatric disorders, some of which may precede the onset of the epilepsy, and of the concomitant medications.

Further reading

Commission on Classification and Terminology of the International League Against Epilepsy. A revised proposal for the classification of epilepsy and epileptic syndromes. *Epilepsia* 1989; 24: 502–14.

Engel J Jr. Epileptic seizures. In: Engel J Jr, editor. *Seizures and Epilepsy.* Philadelphia: FA Davis; 1989, pp. 137–78.

French JA, Kanner AM, Bautista J, *et al.* Efficacy and tolerability of the new antiepileptic drugs II: treatment of refractory epilepsy. *Neurology* 2004; 62: 1261–73.

Hauser WA, Hesdorffer DC. Risk factors. In: Hawser WA, Hesdorffer DC, editors. *Epilepsy: Frequency, Causes and Consequences.* New York, NY: Demos; 1990, pp. 53–100.

Hauser WA, Annegers JF, Kurland LT. Incidence of epilepsy and unprovoked seizures in Rochester, Minnesota: 1935–1984. *Epilepsia* 1993; 34: 453–68.

Herzog AG, Harden CL, Liporace J, *et al.* Frequency of catamenial seizure exacerbation in women with localization-related epilepsy. *Ann Neurol* 2004; 56(3): 431–4.

Hitiris N, Mohanraj R, Norrie J, Sills GJ, Brodie MJ. Predictors of pharmacoresistant epilepsy. *Epilepsy Res* 2007; 75(2–3): 192–6.

Kanner AM. Psychogenic seizures and the supplementary sensory motor area. In: Luders HO, editor. *The Supplementary Sensory Motor Area. Advances in Neurology*, Vol 70. Philadelphia, PA: Lippinkott, Raven; 1996, pp. 461–6.

Table 28.1 Prevalence of psychiatric disorders in epilepsy and the general population.

Psychiatric disorder	Prevalence rates	
	Epilepsy	General population
Depression	11–80%	3.3%: Dysthymia 4.9¯17%: Major depression
Psychosis	2–9.1%	1%: Schizophrenia 0.2%: Schizophreniform disorder
Generalized anxiety disorders	15–25%	5.1–7.2%
Panic disorder	4.9–21%	0.5–3%
Attention deficit disorders	12–37%	4–12%

La France W, Kanner AM. Epilepsy. In: Jeste DV, Friedman JH, editors. *Psychiatry for Neurologists.* Totowa, NJ: Humana Press; 2006, pp. 191–208.

Marson A, Jacoby A, Johnson A, Kim L, Gamble C, Chadwick D, on behalf of the Medical Research Council MESS Study Group. Immediate versus deferred antiepileptic drug treatment for early epilepsy and single seizures: a randomised controlled trial. *Lancet* 2005; 365: 2007–13.

Rowan AJ, Ramsay RE, Collins JF, *et al.*, VA Cooperative Study 428 Group. New onset geriatric epilepsy: a randomized study of gabapentin, lamotrigine, and carbamazepine. *Neurology* 2005; 64(11): 1868–73.

Tomson T, Walczak T, Sillanpaa M, Sander JW. Sudden unexpected death in epilepsy: a review of incidence and risk factors. *Epilepsia* 2005; 46(Suppl 11): 54–61.

Chapter 29
Cryptogenic and symptomatic generalized epilepsies and syndromes

Marco T. Medina[1], Antonio V. Delgado-Escueta[2], and Luis C. Rodríguez-Salinas[1]

[1]National Autonomous University of Honduras, Tegucigalpa, Honduras
[2]University of California, Los Angeles, USA

Introduction

Cryptogenic and symptomatic epilepsies are common during infancy and childhood. While cryptogenic epilepsies have an unknown cause, the etiology of symptomatic epilepsies is clearly recognized and may include head injury, infection (such as meningitis), perinatal brain lesions, etc.

Severe myoclonic epilepsy in infancy (SMEI)

Introduction
SMEI, also known as Dravet's syndrome, is characterized by febrile and afebrile, generalized, and unilateral clonic or tonic–clonic seizures that occur in the first year of life in an otherwise normal infant. Myoclonus, atypical absences, and partial seizures later develop.

Epidemiology
SMEI is a rare disorder, with an incidence of less than 1 per 40 000. The syndrome affects males more frequently than females, at a ratio of 2:1.

Etiology
SMEI is not associated with previous significant brain pathology; there is usually no history of abnormal CT scan or MRI. In 25–53% of cases there is a family history of either epilepsy or febrile seizures. Recent clinical genetic studies suggest that SMEI is at the most severe end of the spectrum of generalized epilepsy with febrile seizures (GEFS+), which has been associated with molecular defects in three sodium channel subunit genes and a γ-aminobutyric acid (GABA) subunit gene. Defects of these genes have been identified in patients with SMEI as well.

International Neurology: A Clinical Approach. Edited by Robert P. Lisak, Daniel D. Truong, William M. Carroll, and Roongroj Bhidayasiri.
© 2009 Blackwell Publishing, ISBN: 978-1-4051-5738-4.

Clinical features
Febrile clonic seizures, either generalized or unilateral, are the first seizures seen in SMEI. These often recur in 6- to 8-week intervals and may lead to status epilepticus. These seizures may recur later without fever. Myoclonic seizures are the second type of seizure to occur. These are typically generalized and present as generalized spike-waves and polyspike-waves on electroencephalogram (EEG). Borderline SMEI patients do not experience myoclonic seizures but nonetheless follow the same clinical course as those who do. Absence seizures are the third type of seizure to present. These are atypical and brief, with rhythmical generalized spike-waves on EEG. Lastly, complex partial seizures occur. These are atonic or adversive and include autonomic phenomena as well as automatisms. Status epilepticus is frequent, either convulsive or as obtundation status; obtundation status includes impairment of consciousness with the presence of fragmentary and segmental erratic myoclonias. The disorder progresses to psychomotor retardation in the second year of seizure onset; neurologic deficits such as ataxia and corticospinal tract dysfunction later develop.

Diagnostic approach
EEG shows generalized spike- and polyspike-waves. Periodic photic stimulation as well as drowsiness may increase the appearance of EEG paroxysms. Interictal background activity is generally *normal at onset and has a tendency to deteriorate afterwards*. EEG spikes tend to be absent when the patient is awake and rather marked when the patient is sleeping. CT scan and MRI are usually normal.

Treatment
All seizure types are resistant to anti-epileptic drugs (AEDs). Valproate and benzodiazepines are the most useful drugs. Other treatments that can be used are: stiripentol, topiramate and ketogenic diet. Lamotrigine, carbamazepine and phenytoin are reported to exacerbate seizures in this condition and should not be used.

Table 29.1 Cryptogenic/symptomatic generalized epilepsies and syndromes: main features.

Epileptic syndrome	Age at onset (latest)	Initial seizure type	Continued seizure type	EEG: wake (W)/sleep (S)	Therapy	Cognitive prognosis
Dravet's syndrome	3–12 (18) months	"FS"/unilateral TCS	GTCS > MS > CS > atypical AB	W: theta, sw, poly sw	VPA, TPM, Bromide, Benzo, Stiri, KD	Unfavorable (50% with severe mental retardation)
West syndrome	3–7 (24) months	TS	MS > CS > Aka	W: hypsa / S: reduced hypsa, s, poly sw	High-dose ACTH, steroids, VPA, NTZ, VGB, surg, KD	75–80% with psychomotor retardation
Lennox–Gastaut syndrome	3–10 years	FS, TS	AB > AS > GTCS > mixed types	S: more HSA / W: diffuse slsw	Difficult: polytherapy, VPA, CLB, LMT, FBM, surg	Mental retardation present in 78–96% of patients
Epilepsy with myoclonic absences	11–12 months	MA	TS > GTCS > mixed types	Symmetrical slsw at 3 Hz	VPA, Etho, LMT, TPM, LVT, ZNS	Variable, but often unfavorable

AB: absences; ACTH: adrenocorticotropine hormone; Aka: akinetic attacks; AS: atonic seizures; Benzo: benzodiazepines; CLB: clobazam; CS: clonic seizure; Etho: ethosuximide; FBM: felbamate; FS: febrile seizure; GTCS: generalized tonic–clonic seizure; HSA: generalized hypersynchronous activity; hypsa: hypsarrhythmia (involves high-voltage slow waves, spikes, and sharp waves; KD: ketogenic diet; LMT: lamotrigine; LVT: levetiracetam; MA: myoclonic absences; MS: myoclonic seizure; NTZ: nitrazepam; poly sw: polyspike wave; s: spikes; slsw: slow spike wave; Stiri: stiripentol; Surg: Surgery; Sw: slow waves; TCS: tonic–clonic seizure; sw: slow waves; TPM: topiramate; TS: tonic seizure; VGB: vigabatrine; VPA: valproate; ZNS: zonisamide

Prognosis

Seizures continue throughout childhood, leading to an unfavorable outcome. Fifty percent of patients are severely cognitively impaired, and all have some level of impairment. Many also have behavioral disorders. The mortality rate is high, ranging from 16% to 18%.

West syndrome (WS)

Introduction

WS is characterized by infantile spasms (IS), mental retardation, and a hypsarrhythmic EEG pattern. While 85–91% of cases are symptomatic, the remaining cases are of unknown origin.

Epidemiology

The incidence of WS ranges from 2.9 to 4.5/100 000 live births.

Etiology

Symptomatic WS is associated with several prenatal, perinatal, and postnatal factors including prenatal infections; neonatal ischemia; postnatal encephalitis due to herpes virus; several brain dysgeneses; tuberous sclerosis complex; chromosomal mutation (Down syndrome); or single gene (ARX or STK9) mutation, etc. A family history of epilepsy or febrile seizures is found in 7–17% of patients with WS, although familial incidence of WS ranges from only 3% to 6%. Several authors have proposed a polygenic mode of inheritance combined with environmental factors. Two novel genes, ARX and CDKL5, have been found to be responsible for cryptogenic WS. Both are located in the human chromosome Xp22 region and are crucial for the development of GABAergic interneurons. Abnormal interneurons appear to play an essential role in the pathogenesis of WS, which can be considered an interneuronopathy.

Clinical features

Fifty to 80% of cases begin between the ages of 3 and 7 months. Previously normal infants may have behavioral regression with the onset of WS. Spasms are often the first manifestation, but cognitive deterioration may precede the spasms by weeks. Spasms consist of repetitive clusters of sudden, briefly sustained movements of the axial musculature. The flexor spasm, although not the most common, is most characteristic of WS. Extensor spasms involve abrupt extension of the neck and lower extremities with extension and abduction of the arms. Forty to 50% of patients exhibit mixed flexor-extensor spasms. In some cases, no spasms are apparent, although they may be present on polygraphic recording. Myoclonic, clonic, and akinetic seizures also occur. Contraction, which is common during wakefulness and awakenings, is often

followed by a cry. Some patients continue to have normal intellectual development. Absence of psychomotor regression is the best prognostic factor of favorable outcome.

Diagnostic approach

EEG during spasms shows either generalized low-amplitude fast activity or a generalized high-amplitude slow wave activity; however, 13% of patients show no EEG abnormalities during spasms. A hypsarrhythmic pattern,which is most common in early stages of infancy spasms, involves high-voltage slow waves, spikes, and sharp waves that seem to occur randomly from all cortical regions, giving the impression of chaotic disorganization of cortical electrogenesis. This pattern is almost continuous in the waking state. During drowsiness, spikes increase and polyspikes may appear. In REM sleep, hypsarrhythmia is clearly reduced. Spasms in clusters may occur without a hypsarrhythmic pattern, as it represents a refractory subtype of IS. MRI is more sensitive at detecting focal lesions, including abnormal or delayed myelination areas, and cortical dysplasias. In some children, positron emission tomography (PET) scans have revealed focal areas of hypometabolism, which often correlate with the dysplastic cortex and white matter.

Treatment

Treatment of IS with high-dose adrenocorticotropic hormone often results in cessation or amelioration of seizures and disappearance of the hypsarrhythmic EEG pattern (90%). There is no consensus regarding the exact dose of steroids or duration of treatment. Among other treatments valproic acid, nitrazepam, vigabatrin, kitogenic diet, etc. have been reported to be effective. Some infants with medically intractable IS and focal lesions may benefit from surgical resection. Persistent spasms not amenable to focal resection may benefit from total callosotomy.

Prognosis

Spasms and hypsarrhythmic EEG tend to disappear spontaneously before 3 years of age. However, the majority of survivors suffer from partial epilepsy (10–32%), generalized epilepsy (42–90%), or various motor, sensory, and mental defects. Only 5–12% of patients have normal mental and motor development. Forty to 60% of patients later develop Lennox–Gastaut syndrome (LGS). Evolution to completely normal EEG pattern is the least common outcome. After steroid treatment, more than one-third of patients relapse 3–12 months after remission. Different types of seizures, prior neurologic and developmental deficits, asymmetric spasms, gross asymmetry on EEG tracings, and abnormal neuroradiologic findings prior to steroid treatment all predict an unfavorable outcome. Overall long-term outcome remains grim, with a 20% mortality rate. Risk of death is six times higher in symptomatic cases than in cryptogenic patients.

Lennox–Gastaut syndrome (LGS)

Introduction
The characteristic features of LGS are (1) generalized seizures, typically tonic, atonic, myoclonic, and atypical absence; (2) interictal EEG characterized by abnormal background, diffuse slow spike-and-wave complexes, and paroxysmal fast rhythms approximately 10 Hz in sleep; and (3) diffuse cognitive dysfunction, which often becomes apparent only later in the disorder.

Epidemiology
Although incidence of LGS is low, the intractable nature accounts for 5% of epileptic patients of all ages and about 10% of epileptic patients under 15 years of age.

Etiology
Approximately 30% of cases are cryptogenic. These cases have been reported to have a higher incidence of epilepsy or febrile seizures, although there is no evidence of genetic predisposition. The remaining 70% of patients have pre-existing brain damage, usually acquired in the prenatal or neonatal period or in infancy. Pre- and perinatal factors include ABO blood group incompatibility, prematurity, prolonged labor, cord prolapse, respiratory depression, and several cerebral malformations. With the advent of high-resolution MRI, cortical dysplasias are being identified as an increasingly common substrate. Postnatal factors include neuroinfections, degenerative or neurometabolic disorders, head injury, anoxic encephalopathy, stroke, and hypoglycemia. Approximately one-third of patients with symptomatic LGS represent evolution from WS. Neuroimaging studies occasionally demonstrate an underlying cause for LGS, but non-specific abnormalities are more common.

Clinical features
LGS usually presents in early childhood, although onset in early adult life has been described. The first seizure occurs between 1 and 8 years of age, with a peak between 3 and 5 years. Tonic seizures are the most common, particularly in patients with seizure onset at an early age, and have a reported prevalence between 74% and 90% in sleep EEG recordings. These are often associated with sudden falls and may be difficult to distinguish from astatic episodes. Atypical absence seizures have a gradual onset/offset and are not precipitated by hyperventilation and/or photic stimulation. Associated myoclonic jerks may be observed. The prevalence of non-convulsive status epilepticus has ranged from 54% to 97%, with lower rates observed in atypical LGS. Tonic seizures and confusion are the most common ictal manifestations and may be precipitated by intravenous administration of benzodiazepines. EEG during status epilepticus may be difficult to distinguish from interictal EEG. Diffuse cognitive dysfunction may not be evident at seizure onset but becomes more marked with time. Mental retardation is present eventually in 78–96% of patients. Behavioral and personality disturbances complicate social adjustment; motor development is less affected.

Diagnostic approach
Diagnosis is based on the combination of several types of generalized seizures. Tonic and atypical absences may need ictal EEG recording to be properly identified. Interictal EEG background demonstrates a lower-than-normal frequency at all ages, as well as an increased amount of slow activity. The waking record is dominated by 2–2.5 Hz spike-and-wave and polyspike-and-wave discharges, which are usually diffuse. During slow wave sleep, discharges are more obviously bisynchronous and are often associated with polyspikes. Paroxysmal fast rhythms (>10 Hz), particularly during slow wave sleep, are an integral feature of LGS. During tonic seizures, EEG demonstrates bilaterally synchronous (10–25 Hz) activity that is maximal in the anterior and vertex regions, or attenuation of the background rhythm, which may be preceded by polyspikes. Atypical absence seizures appear as irregular, diffuse, slow spike-wave discharges approximately 2–2.5 Hz which may be difficult to distinguish from the interictal slow spike-wave pattern.

Treatment
Treatment, which includes both seizure control and management of associated cognitive and behavioral issues, has been difficult and disappointing. Lamotrigine, benzodiazepines, valproic acid, and felbamate appear to be the most effective drug therapies. Corticosteroid and corticotrophin (adrenocorticotropic hormone, ACTH) treatment has resulted in seizure control, particularly if started shortly after onset of cryptogenic LGS. The ketogenic diet may be effective as well. Corpus callosotomy can reduce or abolish drop attacks in many patients, with no major diffuse brain malformation. Total versus anterior callosotomy depends on the age at which the epilepsy started. Patients with cryptogenic LGS have a better prognosis than do those with symptomatic LGS.

Prognosis
Only a minority of patients achieve seizure control. Seizure onset before 3 years of age, a history of WS, symptomatic LGS, severe cognitive dysfunction, and difficulty achieving control are predictive of refractory seizures. Atypical absence myoclonic seizures carry a more hopeful prognosis, as does the coexisting fast and

slow spike-wave activity and precipitation of spike-wave activity by hyperventilation.

Epilepsy with myoclonic absences (EMA)

Introduction

In 1969, myoclonic absences (MA) were recognized as a specific seizure type and proposed as the essential feature of a distinct syndrome. There are two forms of EMA: a pure form in which myoclonic absences are the single or predominant type of seizures and another form in which MA are associated with other seizures types, particularly with generalized tonic–clonic seizures (GTCSs).

Epidemiology

In some specialized centers, MA is an uncommon syndrome, accounting for 0.5–1% of all epilepsies observed in selected populations. Seventy percent of EMA cases are male.

Etiology

The etiology of EMA is unknown. Although a family history of seizure disorders can be found in about one-fourth of cases, genetic factors and hereditary mechanisms are not known. Some published cases have been described relating etiologic factors such as prematurity, perinatal damage, consanguinity, congenital hemiparesis, and chromosomal abnormalities, such as trisomy 12p and Angelman's syndrome.

Clinical features

The average age of onset of EMA is 7 years (range: 11 months to 12.5 years). Approximately half of affected children are normal and half are mentally retarded prior to the onset of seizures. Manifestations include abrupt onset of absences accompanied by bilateral rhythmic myoclonic jerks of severe intensity. Loss of consciousness during the absence may be complete or partial. Movements may be associated with tonic contraction, which is maximal in shoulder and deltoid muscles. Hyperventilation, awakening, and intermittent photic stimulation may precipitate the attack. During sleep, however, myoclonic seizures decrease in frequency. Episodes of MA status, although rare, have been described. Association with other seizures, such as GTCS, pure absence, and falling seizures, occurs in two-thirds of cases.

Diagnostic approach

Ictal EEG shows synchronous and symmetrical discharges of spike-waves at 3 Hz, similar to that of childhood absences. Polygraphic recording of MA reveals bilateral myoclonias at the same frequency as spikes and waves, followed by a tonic contraction. Interictal EEG findings include normal background activity with superimposed generalized spikes-waves or, more rarely, focal or multifocal spikes and waves.

Treatment

A combination of valproate and ethosuximide at high doses with appropriate plasma level control can lead to rapid remission of MA. Lamotrigine, levetiracetam, topiramate, or zonisamide may also be useful.

Prognosis

EMA has a variable but often poor prognosis. MA seizures may persist into adulthood in about half of patients. Patients with "refractory" MA seizures have a high incidence (85%) of associated seizures, mostly tonic–clonic and falling seizures. The duration of MA is likely to play a significant role in the appearance of mental deterioration.

Further reading

Aicardi J, Ohtahara S. Severe neonatal epilepsies with suppression-burst pattern. In: Roger J, Bureau M, Dravet Ch, Genton P, Tassinari CA, Wolf P, editors. *Epileptic Syndromes in Infancy, Childhood and Adolescence*, 4th ed. London: John Libbey; 2005, pp. 39–52.

Bureau M, Tassinari CA. Myoclonic absences: the seizure and the syndrome. In: Delgado-Escueta A, Guerrini R, Medina MT, Genton P, Bureau M, Dravet Ch, editors. *Advances in Neurology: Myoclonic Epilepsies*, Vol. 95. Philadelphia, PA: Lippincott Williams & Wilkins; 2005, pp. 175–84.

Dravet C, Bureau M, Oguni H, Fukuyama Y, Cokar O. Severe myoclonic epilepsy in infancy (Dravet syndrome). In: Roger J, Bureau M, Dravet Ch, Genton P, Tassinari CA, Wolf P, editors. *Epileptic Syndromes in Infancy, Childhood and Adolescence*, 4th ed. London: John Libbey; 2005, pp. 89–114.

Dulac O, N'Guyen T. The Lennox–Gastaut syndrome. *Epilepsia* 1993; 34(Suppl 7): S7–17.

Dulac O, Plouin P, Schlumberger E. Infantile spasms. In: Wyllie E, editor. *The Treatment of Epilepsy: Principles and Practice*, 2nd ed. Baltimore, MD: Williams & Wilkins; 1997, pp. 540–72.

Elia M, Guerrini R, Musumeci SA, Bonanni P, Gambardella A, Aguglia U. Myoclonic absence-like seizures and chromosome abnormality syndromes. *Epilepsia* 1998a; 39: 660–3.

Farrell K. Symptomatic generalized epilepsy and Lennox–Gastaut syndrome. In: Wyllie E, editor. *The Treatment of Epilepsy: Principles and Practice*, 2nd ed. Baltimore, MD: Williams & Wilkins; 1997, pp. 530–9.

Ohtahara S, Yamatogi Y. Epileptic encephalopathies in early infancy with suppression-burst. *J Clin Neuro* 2003; 20(6): 398–407.

Scheffer IE, Wallace R, Mulley JC, Berkovic SF. Clinical and molecular genetics of myoclonic–astatic epilepsy and severe myoclonic epilepsy in infancy (Dravet syndrome). *Brain Dev* 2001; 23(7): 732–5.

Vigevano F, Bartuli A. Infantile epileptic syndromes and metabolic etiologies. *J Child Neurol* 2002; 17(3): S9–13.

Chapter 30
Genetic (primary) idiopathic generalized epilepsy (IGE)

Afawi Zaid

Tel-Aviv Sourasky Medical Center, Tel Aviv, Israel

Introduction

Since genetic structure gives us an important opportunity to unravel etiology and pathogenesis of disease, genetics has become an important field in epileptology. Many new techniques have become available for studying brain processes. Major advances in neuroimaging, electroencephalography, and neurochemistry, in addition to the ability to perform DNA testing, are greatly contributing to understanding symptomatic epilepsy and the molecular basis of generalized and idiopathic seizure disorders.

Epilepsy is an interesting field for geneticists because hereditary factors are generally present. Indeed, modern syndrome-orientated epileptology has identified numerous individual phenotypes that provide improved access for geneticists to the wide and heterogeneous panorama of epilepsy.

Absence seizures

Absence seizures, also known as petit mal seizures, refer to the seizure semiology described below, with abnormal interictal electroencephalogram (EEG) patterns and multiple seizure types. The heterogeneity of absence epilepsies has been recognized by the Commission on Classification of the International League Against Epilepsy.

Childhood absence epilepsy (CAE) (pyknolepsy)

The age of onset of CAE is most often between 4 and 8 years, and a peak occurs at 6–7 years. Seizures are accompanied by upward deviation of the eyes and retropulsion of the head and trunk. Forty percent of patients with CAE develop generalized tonic–clonic seizures (GTCS). The incidence rate has been reported at 6–8 per 100 000 persons. Females are more commonly affected than males and there is a strong multifactoral genetic predisposition.

CAE is characterized by absence attacks with stereotyped 3 Hz generalized spike-wave discharges. The EEG pattern is a classic 3 cycles/second (c/s) generalized polyspike-wave frontal maximum. Ethosuximide and sodium valproate are equally effective in treating the absence of CAE, achieving a total suppression in over 70% of patients. Lamotrigine, zonisamide, and levetiracetam can be used as well. Absence becomes less frequent through adolescence and approximately 80% of patients remit by adulthood.

Juvenile absence epilepsy (JAE)

JAE represents approximately 20% of idiopathic generalized epilepsies (IGEs). Prevalence is estimated at 0.1 per 1000 persons, with age of onset at 9–13 years. GTCS occur in most patients; myoclonic jerks occur in about one-fifth of all patients, but tend to be mild. There are no significant differences in sex distribution. JAE has a strong genetic component; linkage to chromosomes 5, 8, 18, and 21 has been noted. The EEG background is normal, but bursts of generalized spike- or polyspike-wave discharges occur at 3–5 Hz. Medication choices are similar to those of CAE, with the exception of ethosuximide.

Epilepsy with grand mal seizures on awakening (EGMA)

EGMA is characterized by GTCS occurring predominantly on awakening (independent of the time of day) or at leisure time (just before evening). Sleep deprivation and alcohol can increase the seizures. There is a wide range of presentation, from 6 years of age to middle age, and it is slightly more prominent in men than women. Rates of EGMA vary from 22% to 37%. Interictal EEG shows fast 3–4 c/s generalized spike- and polyspike-wave discharges.

Patients should be advised to avoid excessive fatigue and alcohol. Sodium valporate is the drug of choice except in women of child-bearing age. Lamotrigine can also be effective. Other options are zonisamide, levetiracetam, and topiramate. Seizures are controlled with medication in 65% of patients.

International Neurology: A Clinical Approach. Edited by Robert P. Lisak, Daniel D. Truong, William M. Carroll, and Roongroj Bhidayasiri. © 2009 Blackwell Publishing, ISBN: 978-1-4051-5738-4.

Myoclonic epilepsy

Myoclonic seizures generally cause abnormal movement on both sides of the body simultaneously. Myoclonic activity presents itself in many disorders; below are some of the epileptic presentations. See Table 30.1 for a summary.

Juvenile myoclonic epilepsy (JME)

JME is a common form of IGE, comprising 5–10% of all epilepsies. The age of onset is 12–18 years, with an average of 15 years of age; however, it may begin or become clinically identifiable in adult life. Both sexes are equally affected.

JME is characterized by the following triad: (1) myoclonic jerks on awakening (all patients); (2) GTCS (more than 90% of patients); (3) typical absences (about 33% of patients). It may vary in severity from mild myoclonic jerks to frequent and severe falls and GTCS if not appropriately diagnosed and treated.

JME is genetically determined: between 50% and 60% of probands with JME report seizures in first- or second-degree relatives. Inheritance is probably complex. Autosomal dominant, autosomal recessive, two locus, and multifactorial models have been proposed. EEG shows 4–6 Hz polyspike and slow-wave generalized discharges that last up to 20 s, with normal background activity (Figure 30.1).

Seizures are generally well controlled with appropriate medication in up to 90% of patients. Valproate is unquestionably the most effective anti-epileptic drug for JME, although it is contraindicated in women; levetiracetam may be substituted in such cases. Lamotrigine is well tolerated and effective, with the occasional exacerbation of myoclonus; topiramate and zonisamide are also effective. All seizure types in JME appear to be lifelong, although improvement is seen after the fourth decade of life.

Myoclonic–astatic epilepsy (Doose syndrome)

Originally referred to as myoclonic–astatic petit mal, myoclonic–astatic epilepsy or Doose syndrome, as it is now called, accounts for approximately 1–2% of all childhood epilepsies. Age of onset is between 7 months and 6 years. Febrile convulsions are the first symptom seen in the majority of cases. These are characterized by symmetric myoclonic jerks that last less than 100 ms and are often followed by equally long periods of absent muscle tone. Absence seizures are seen in about half of patients, sometimes in association with myoclonus, and usually are not long-lasting.

Genetic causes are probably polygenic. EEG shows bursts of brief generalized spike- or polyspike-wave discharges with a repetition rate of 2–4 Hz. Pharmacologic treatment includes valproate, and possibly the other broad-spectrum AEDs, with the exception of lamotrigine. The ketogenic diet may be remarkably effective as well. Prognosis is variable, with at least half of patients doing well and ultimately going into remission. A minority will have profound defects.

Lafora's disease

Lafora's disease is characterized by epilepsy, myoclonus, dementia, and Lafora bodies, which are periodic acid-Schiff-positive intracellular polyglycosan inclusion bodies found in neurons, heart, skeletal muscle, liver, and sweat gland duct cells.

Table 30.1 Molecular genetics of progressive myoclonic epilepsy (PME).

Disease	Age at onset (years)	Inheritance	Location	Gene	Protein
Lafora's disease	12–17	AR	Ch6q24, Ch6p22	EPM2A, NHLRC1	Laforin
ULD	6–12	AR	Ch21q22.3	CSTB	Cystine B
MERRF	Any age		Mitochondrial DNA	MTTK	tRNALys
NCLs	Variable				
Classical late infantile	2.5–4	AR	Ch11p15	TPP1	Tripeptidyl peptidase 1
Juvenile	4–10	AR	Ch6p	CLN3	Unknown
Adult (Kufs' disease)	11–50	AR/AD	NA	ND	Unknown
Finnish-variant late infantile		AR	Ch13q21–q32	CLN5	Unknown
Variant late infantile		AR	Ch15q21–23	CLN6	Unknown
Sialidoses	Variable				
Type I	8–20	AR	Ch6p21.3	NEU1	Sialidase
Type II	10–30	AR	Ch20	NEU1	Sialidase

ULD: Unverricht–Lundborg disease; MERRF: myoclonic epilepsy with ragged red fibers; NCLs: neuronal ceroid lipofuscinoses; AR: autosomal recessive; AD: autosomal dominant; NA: data not available; D: data undetermined.

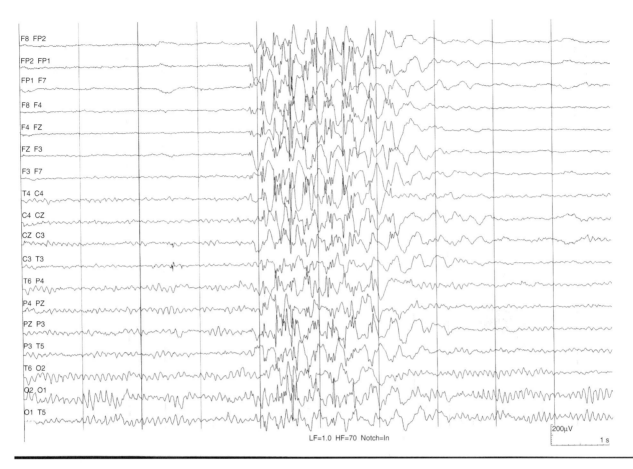

F8 FP2
FP2 FP1
FP1 F7
F8 F4
F4 FZ
FZ F3
F3 F7
T4 C4
C4 CZ
CZ C3
C3 T3
T6 P4
P4 PZ
PZ P3
P3 T5
T6 O2
O2 O1
O1 T5

LF=1.0 HF=70 Notch=In

200μV

1 s

Figure 30.1 Generalized spike and polyspike activity.

The onset of seizures occurs at 12–17 years of age. Types of seizures in Lafora's disease include myoclonus, occipital seizures with transient blindness and visual hallucinations, atypical absences, and atonic and complex partial seizures. Cognitive decline, dysarthria, and ataxia appear early.

Lafora's disease is an autosomal recessive disorder. Up to 80% of patients with the disorder have a mutation in the EPM2A gene on chromosome 6q at locus 24. The gene encodes Laforin, a dual-specificity protein tyrosine phosphatase, primarily associated with ribosomes. More recently, a new Lafora's disease locus, NHLRC1 (formerly PM2B), has been mapped to a 2.2 Mbp region at 6p22, a region that codes for several proteins.

EEG may have a well-organized background activity with multiple spike and wave discharges and photo-sensitivity is common to low frequency (1–6 Hz) stimuli. The spike-and-wave pattern changes from a frequency of 3 Hz in the early stages to faster frequencies of 6–12 Hz as the disease progresses and the background becomes less organized with time (Figure 30.2). Treatment for Lafora's disease remains palliative.

Other myoclonic disorders
Unverricht–Lundborg disease (ULD)

ULD is the most common progressive myoclonic epilepsy. The age of symptom onset is 6–12 years. GTCS are the presenting features in many patients; other symptoms may include myoclonus, ataxia, incoordination, intention tremor, and dysarthria. ULD is an autosomal recessive disorder linked to chromosome 21q22.3, cystatin B (CSTB) gene mutation, known as EPM1. EEG shows generalized spike or polyspike-wave discharges at 2.5–4 Hz and the background may become progressively disorganized over decades. Treatment choices are valproate and other broad-spectrum AEDs. Phenytoin is contraindicated, as it has been associated with increased dementia and death rates.

Myoclonic epilepsy with ragged red fibers (MERRF)

MERRF is characterized by myoclonus, generalized epilepsy, ataxia, and ragged red fibers in muscle biopsy. EEG shows generalized spike-and-wave discharge at 2–5 Hz with background slowing that progresses as the

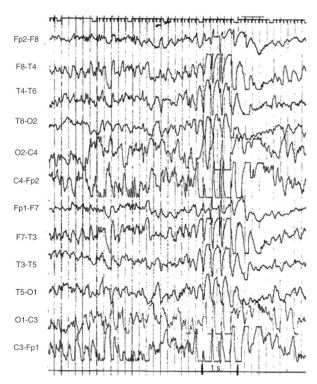

Fp2-F8

F8-T4

T4-T6

T8-O2

O2-C4

C4-Fp2

Fp1-F7

F7-T3

T3-T5

T5-O1

O1-C3

C3-Fp1

1 s

Figure 30.2 A weak EEG of a 26-year-old patient with Lafora disease showed generalized spike and polyspike activity, slowing of background activity.

disease advances. The molecular defect is an adenosine to guanine, protein tRNALys, gene MTTK of mitochondrial DNA, which can be both maternally and paternally inherited. There is no specific therapy for MERRF.

Neuronal ceroid lipofuscinoses (NCLs)

NCLs, also referred to as Kufs' disease, are characterized by the accumulation of abnormal amounts of lipopigment in lysosomes. There are five types of NCLs (see Table 30.1).

Sialidoses

Two types of sialidoses cause progressive myoclonic epilepsy (PME). Sialidosis type I (cherry-red spot myoclonus syndrome) is caused by a deficiency of α neuraminidase. Sialidosis type II is caused by a deficiency of both N-acetyl neuraminidase and β galactosialidase. The sialidoses are autosomal recessive disorders, linked to gene NEU1 mutation on chromosome ch6p21.3 (type I) and chromosome ch20 (type II) (Table 30.1).

Further reading

Delanty N, Farrell M, Shahwan A. Progressive myoclonic epilepsies: a review of genetic and therapeutic aspects. *Lancet Neurol* 2005; 4: 239–48.

Douglas R, Nordil J. Idiopathic generalized epilepsies recognized by the International League Against Epilepsy. *Epilepsia* 2005; 46(Suppl 9): 48–56.

John SD. Idiopathic generalized epilepsies with typical absences. *J Neurol* 1997; 244: 403–11.

Panayiotopoulos CP. *Juvenile Myoclonic Epilepsy*. Updated and reprinted from *The Epilepsies: Seizures, Syndromes and Management*. Chipping Norton: Bladon Medical Publishing; 2005.

Pierre J, Patrick L. Epidemiology of idiopathic generalized epilepsies. *Epilepsia* 2005; 46(Suppl 9): 10–14.

Chapter 31
Localization-related epilepsies

Hirokazu Oguni[1] and Chrysostomos P. Panayiotopoulos[2]
[1]Tokyo Women's Medical University, Tokyo, Japan
[2]St. Thomas' Hospital, London, UK

Introduction

Localization-related (focal, local, partial) epilepsies (LRE) are disorders whose seizures originate in a circumscribed locus in one cerebral hemisphere regardless of etiology.

Historically, LRE were believed to develop from an abnormal pathological cortical region giving rise to epileptic seizures (symptomatic or cryptogenic LRE). However, it is now known that idiopathic (presumably genetically determined) and familial syndromes of LRE with gene mutations exist.

Idiopathic LRE

Benign childhood focal seizures are the most common idiopathic LRE, affecting 25% of children with non-febrile seizures. Seizures are infrequent, usually nocturnal, and remit within 1–3 years. Febrile seizures occur in around one-third of patients, particularly in patients of Japanese descent. Affected children have normal physical and neuropsychological development, but some may experience mild and reversible cognitive and linguistic problems during the active stage of the disorder. Brain imaging is normal, as is resting background electroencephalogram (EEG). Severe EEG abnormalities evince as high-amplitude focal spikes which are disproportionate to the frequency of seizures. A normal EEG is rare and should provoke a sleep EEG study. Similar EEG features resolving with age are frequently found in normal school-age children (2–4%) and children having an EEG for reasons other than seizures.

Rolandic epilepsy

Rolandic epilepsy (RE), officially designated as benign childhood epilepsy with centrotemporal spikes, accounts for 15% of all LRE in children 1–15 years of age. The age

of seizure onset ranges from 3 to 14 years and peaks at 5–8 years, with 1.5 male predominance. The cardinal features of RE are infrequent, often single, focal seizures consisting of unilateral facial sensorimotor symptoms, oro-pharyngo-laryngeal manifestations, speech arrest, and hypersalivation. They sometimes spread to the ipsilateral arm or arm and leg. Consciousness may be retained throughout the seizures. Secondary generalization to convulsions occurs in 1/3–2/3 patients. Three-quarters of the seizures occur during non-REM sleep, most often soon after sleep onset and just before awakening.

High-amplitude biphasic sharp or sharp-slow wave discharges appear in the centrotemporal regions (rolandic spikes). They are markedly enhanced by sleep, and shift from one side to the other or appear bilaterally. Multifocal epileptic foci including an occipital or frontal spike may appear. Onset of ictal EEG is unilateral from the rolandic region (Figure 31.1, bottom).

Etiology

The high incidence of familial antecedents for epilepsy (18–36%) suggests that a genetic trait is playing a major role. Linkage to chromosome 15q14 has been reported, but no responsible gene mutation has been identified.

Prognosis and treatment

Seizure recurrence is usually limited to a few times, though around 10–20% of patients may have many seizures. Although the seizures themselves remit in 80% of patients by 2 years, the rolandic spikes tend to persist up to age 16. Early onset of RE, especially under age 5, is a risk factor for frequent seizure recurrences. Treatment with prophylactic anti-epileptic drugs (AED) may not be needed because of the excellent prognosis. Carbamazepine or oxcarbazepine are choices of AED for recurrent seizures, although they will respond to any other narrow or broad-spectrum AED.

Panayiotopoulos syndrome

Panayiotopoulos syndrome (PS) is an idiopathic LRE accounting for 6% of all non-febrile childhood epilepsies. The age at onset ranges from 1 to 14 years with a peak

International Neurology: A Clinical Approach. Edited by Robert P. Lisak, Daniel D. Truong, William M. Carroll, and Roongroj Bhidayasiri. © 2009 Blackwell Publishing, ISBN: 978-1-4051-5738-4.

at 4–5 years. The cardinal features of PS are infrequent or often a single focal seizure with autonomic symptomatology and prolonged duration, occurring mostly during sleep. In one-third of cases, the seizures last longer than 30 min (autonomic status epilepticus). Typically, the children are initially fully conscious and complaining of nausea, retching, or vomiting followed by deviation of eyes and progressive cloudiness of consciousness. One-third of seizures may evolve to hemiconvulsions or generalized convulsions. In one-fifth of seizures, the patient remains flaccid and unresponsive (ictal syncope).

Interictal EEG shows multifocal spikes predominating in the posterior regions. Single occipital, centrotemporal, or frontopolar spikes occur. Ictal onsets are unilateral from posterior or anterior regions (Figure 31.1, top).

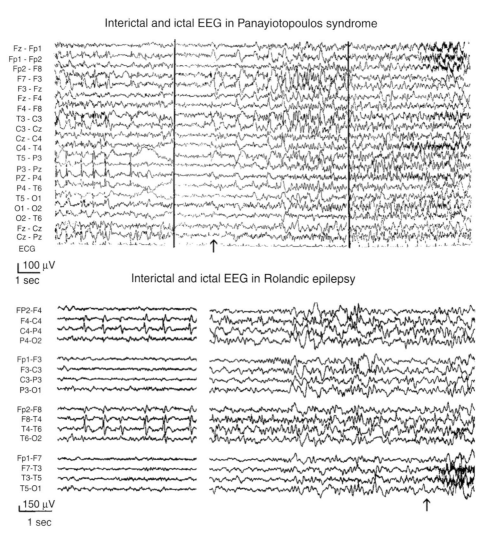

Interictal and ictal EEG in Panayiotopoulos syndrome

100 µV
1 sec

Interictal and ictal EEG in Rolandic epilepsy

150 µV
1 sec

Figure 31.1 Top: Interictal (left) and ictal (right) EEG of a lengthy autonomic seizure of non-occipital onset in a child with Panayiotopoulos syndrome. Interictal EEG showed cloned-like repetitive multifocal spike-wave complexes that were mainly bifrontal, left more than right, midline, and occipital. Clinically, while asleep, the child suddenly got up with both eyes open, vomited several times, and then showed a prolonged atonic state with cyanosis and irregular respiration for 3 min. The first EEG change (arrow) consisted of periodic slow waves from the left frontotemporal region (F3) for 3 s followed by rhythmic generalized discharge of mainly monomorphic rhythmic slow waves intermixed with spikes. Electrocardiogram (ECG) showed significant tachycardia during the ictus (see ECG trace). (Modified from Oguni *et al.*, *Epilepsia* 1999; 40: 1020–30, with permission of the Editor.)

Bottom: Interictal (left) and ictal EEG (right) of a child with Rolandic epilepsy. Interictal EEG showed high-amplitude right-sided centrotemporal spikes. Ictal EEG discharge started in the right centrotemporal region during sleep. The first clinical manifestations (arrow) consisted of contractions of the left facial muscles (note muscle artefacts on the left), progressing to a prolonged generalized clonic seizure, which lasted for 5 min. (Modified from Panayiotopoulos CP. *A Clinical Guide to Epileptic Syndromes and Their Treatment*, 2nd ed. London: Springer; 2007, with permission from Springer.)

Etiology

Etiology may be genetically determined as suggested by its association with RE and febrile seizures. A case with *SCN1A* mutation has been reported.

Prognosis and treatment

Prognosis is excellent, although rarely autonomic seizures may cause cardiorespiratory arrest. One-third of patients have only one seizure and most patients experience less than five seizures during the clinical course. The other 10–20% may have frequent seizures. AED treatment is usually not recommended for isolated seizures. Carbamazepine or valproic acid are generally used for recurrent attacks.

Idiopathic childhood occipital epilepsy of Gastaut

This is a pure form of idiopathic occipital epilepsy with onset at a peak age of 8–9 years (range 3–15 years). Patients have frequent visual seizures of mainly elementary visual hallucinations, blindness, or both (see symptomatic occipital epilepsy). Spreading to temporal lobe involvement is exceptional and may indicate a symptomatic cause.

Interictal EEG shows occipital spikes or occipital paroxysms. Ictal onset with fast spikes is unilateral from the occipital regions.

Prognosis and treatment

Prognosis is unpredictable. Half of the patients will remit within 2–4 years from onset. The others will continue having seizures, particularly if not appropriately treated with carbamazepine.

Monogenic focal epilepsies

Monogenic (single gene) focal epilepsies have been identified in large families with an epileptic trait segregating in the absence of environmental factors. In these families, phenotypes are determined by mutations in susceptibility genes, some of which have been identified or localized. Most of the genes discovered code for either voltage-gated or ligand-gated ion channel subunits. Genetic polymorphisms have been identified that result in marked ethnic and interindividual differences in response to treatment.

Benign familial neonatal seizures

Seizures mainly start in the first week of life of full-term normal neonates. Seizures are brief, usually 1–2 min, and may be as frequent as 20–30 per day. Most seizures start with tonic motor activity and posturing with apnea followed by vocalizations, ocular symptoms, other autonomic features, motor automatisms, chewing, and focal or generalized clonic movements. Pure clonic or focal seizures are rare.

Etiology

It is an autosomal dominant disorder with 85% penetrance. Mutations in the voltage-gated potassium channel subunit gene *KCNQ2* on chromosome 20q13.3 and *KCNQ3* on chromosome 8q24 produce the same phenotype.

Prognosis and treatment

Prognosis is good with normal development. Seizures remit between 1 and 6 months from onset, but 10–14% may later develop other types of seizures. Development occurs. AED may not be needed.

Benign familial infantile seizures

These seizures start at 3–20 months (peaking at 5–6 months) in otherwise normal infants. Seizures consist of motion arrest, decreased responsiveness, staring, eye and head deviation, simple automatisms, and mild clonic movements. They may progress to generalized convulsions. Alternating from one side to the other side is common. Duration is usually short, from 30 s to 3 min. They occur in clusters of a maximum of 8–10 per day for 1–3 days and may recur after 1–3 months.

Etiology

It is probably an autosomal dominant disorder with genetic heterogeneity (chromosomes 19q, 16, or 2). Non-familial infantile seizures are common.

Prognosis and treatment

Prognosis is excellent, with normal development and complete seizure remission. In the active seizure period, empirical drug treatment is usually effective.

Autosomal dominant nocturnal frontal lobe epilepsy (ADNFLE)

The age at seizure onset ranges from 1 to 50 years, but most cases (85%) start earlier than 20 (mean age = 8–11.5 years). Most patients are intellectually and neurologically normal. The clinical seizures are mainly nocturnal and are characterized by brief, less than 1 min, hyper-motor attacks occurring in clusters. Typically, patients wake up by non-specific aura and manifest with vocalization, grasping, or grunting and hyperkinetic–dystonic attacks of the extremities lasting less than a minute. Consciousness is usually intact. The attacks are often misdiagnosed as nocturnal parasomnias, night terror, or nightmares. Infrequent secondarily generalized convulsions occur in 60% of cases.

Etiology

ADNFLE is an autosomal dominant disorder with 70% penetrance. Mutations have been identified in two genes encoding neuronal nicotinic acetylcholine receptor α_4 or β_2 protein subunits.

Prognosis and treatment

The seizure frequency and prognosis are different amongst patients even in the same family. With carbamazepine or other sodium channel blockers, two-thirds of the patients become seizure-free. The other third have poor seizure outcome.

Familial mesial temporal lobe epilepsy (FMTLE)

Seizures typically start after the age of 10 with a median in the mid-30s. They mainly manifest with déjà vu, other mental illusions and hallucinations, fear, and panic. Consciousness is usually (90%) intact. Ascending epigastric sensation does not occur. Two-thirds of patients also have infrequent secondarily generalized tonic-clonic seizures.

Etiology

FMTLE is an autosomal dominant disorder with 60% penetrance. The genetic locus is probably on chromosome 4q.

Prognosis and treatment

The prognosis is usually good and seizures are easily controlled with carbamazepine or other narrow- or broadspectrum AED. The phenotype can be variable, with some cases becoming refractory, but with good response to surgical therapy.

Familial lateral temporal lobe epilepsy (FLTLE)

FLTLE and "autosomal dominant focal epilepsy with auditory features" are the same disorder, caused by defects in the same gene. The age at seizure onset ranges from 11 to 40 years with an average of 24 years. The seizures are characterized by simple elementary auditory hallucinations arising from the lateral temporal lobe. EEG and single photon emission computed tomography (SPECT) tests show epileptic foci in the temporal lobe.

Etiology

FLTLE is of autosomal dominant inheritance with high penetrance of about 80%. It is the first non-ion-channel familial epilepsy to have been discovered. Mutations have been identified in the leucine-rich, glioma-inactivated 1 (*LGI1*) epitempin gene on chromosome 10q.

Prognosis and treatment

Prognosis and response to carbamazepine or other AED is excellent.

Familial partial epilepsy with variable foci

The defining feature of this syndrome is that different family members have focal seizures emanating from different cortical locations, including temporal, frontal, centroparietal, and occipital regions. Each individual patient has the same electroclinical pattern of single location focal epilepsy. Seizures are often nocturnal, and there is great intra-familial variability.

Age at onset of seizures varies markedly (range from months to 43 years), although the mean age at onset is 13 years.

Etiology

Familial partial epilepsy with variable foci is of autosomal dominant inheritance with 60% penetrance and genetic heterogeneity. It has been mapped to chromosome 22q11–q12, but also linkage to chromosome 2q has been reported.

Prognosis and treatment

Severity varies among family members: some are asymptomatic manifesting with only an EEG spike focus, and most are easily controlled with AED, but a few may be intractable to medication.

Symptomatic and cryptogenic LRE

Symptomatic LRE are of known pathology and are largely classified according to anatomical localization into temporal, frontal, parietal, and occipital lobe epilepsies. Cryptogenic epilepsy, a term used for probably symptomatic epilepsy for which the etiology has not been identified, is included in this section. LRE may further be classified into limbic or neocortical epilepsy.

Etiology

Structural causes include malformations of brain development, hippocampal sclerosis, tumors, vascular, traumatic, viral and other infectious and parasitic disorders, and cerebrovascular disease.

Diagnostic procedures

MRI provides in vivo visualization of the abnormal brain tissue in nearly all patients with symptomatic LRE.

The interictal EEG usually demonstrates focal slow wave activity and EEG spikes. The yield of interictal EEG abnormalities varies from around 30% in temporal lobe epilepsy (TLE) to as little as 5–10% in frontal lobe epilepsy (FLE).

Temporal lobe epilepsy (TLE)

TLE constitutes nearly two-thirds of symptomatic LRE in adolescence and adulthood. It is divided into mesial and lateral TLE. Mesial TLE is the more common form and includes hippocampal epilepsy. Most of the patients follow a characteristic clinical course, often starting with febrile convulsions during infancy, and developing simple and complex focal seizures several years later. The seizures manifest with ascending epigastric sensation and fear, followed by oral or gestural automatisms. They usually last 1–2 min and leave short-lasting confusional state.

Lateral TLE manifests with simple and complex focal seizures with auditory hallucinations or illusions, vestibular phenomena, experiential symptoms, complex visual hallucinations, and illusions. Motor ictal symptoms include clonic movements, dystonic posturing, and motor automatisms. Impairment of consciousness is not as pronounced as with mesial TLE.

Frontal lobe epilepsy (FLE)

FLE is the most common localization-related epilepsy after TLE. The clinical seizure manifestations differ significantly according to the localization of the epileptogenic focus within the frontal lobe, although they tend to show abrupt onset, short duration, rapid secondary generalization, and minimal or no postictal confusional state, and to occur in clusters. Nocturnal attacks are relatively common. There are three broad categories of seizure types: focal clonic motor seizures, asymmetrical tonic seizures, and frontal lobe complex focal seizures.

The focal clonic motor seizures arise from the motor cortex and involve the oro-facial and/or ipsilateral arm or both arm and leg, and at times spread with jacksonian march.

Asymmetrical tonic/dystonic seizures arise from the supplementary sensory-motor cortex and manifest with one arm being flexed and the other extended, the legs being flexed or extended (see ADNFLE). Consciousness is frequently preserved during the attacks.

Frontal complex partial seizures (CPS) are associated with screaming or bizarre violent behaviour, previously misdiagnosed as hysterical attacks. Typical frontal lobe automatisms originate in the cingulate cortex.

Parietal lobe epilepsy (PLE)

The seizures of PLE are usually difficult to identify prior to their spreading to adjacent brain areas and manifesting with more overt ictal symptoms there. In PLE, simple focal seizures predominate. Subjective ictal symptoms are somatosensory (paresthetic, dysesthetic, and painful sensations), disturbances of body image, vertiginous, visual illusions, or complex visual hallucinations.

Occipital lobe epilepsy (OLE)

OLE, accounting for 5–10% of all SLRE, is much easier to locate by symptoms than other SLRE. Seizures develop in seconds and they are usually brief (seconds to a minute) and consist of the elementary visual hallucinations which are mainly circular and multicolored. Postictal headache occurs in half of visual seizures. Blindness may occur from onset. The seizures of OLE are entirely different from visual aura of migraine for which they are commonly misdiagnosed. The seizures may spread to temporal or frontal lobes, generating TLE or FLE seizures and secondary generalizations.

Prognosis and treatment

The natural history of symptomatic TLE is variable, with as many as 30–40% of patients continuing to have seizures despite appropriate medical treatments. In other SLRE, known cause, congenital neurological deficits, frequent secondarily generalized convulsions, need for multiple medications, and epileptic EEG abnormality all reduce the likelihood of remission.

The first-line AED are oxcarbazepine or carbamazepine, levetiracetam, and lamotrigine, followed by topiramate, zonisamide, and phenytoin. Recent progress in epilepsy surgery has enabled 70–90% of patients with MTLE to become seizure-free. In patients with refractory extratemporal lobe epilepsies, the surgical result is not always satisfactory, especially without well-circumscribed MRI lesions.

Further reading

Commission on Classification and Terminology of the International League Against Epilepsy. Proposal for revised classification of epilepsies and epileptic syndromes. *Epilepsia* 1989; 30: 389–99.

Cossette P, Rouleau GA. Monogenic epilepsies in humans: molecular mechanisms and relevance for the study of intractable epilepsy. *Adv Neurol* 2006; 97: 381–8.

Covanis A, Ferrie CD, Koutroumanidis M, Oguni H, Panayiotopoulos CP. Panayiotopoulos syndrome and Gastaut type idiopathic childhood occipital epilepsy. In: Roger J, Bureau M, Dravet C, Genton P, Tassinari CA, Wolf P, editors. *Epileptic Syndromes in Infancy, Childhood and Adolescence*, 4th ed. with video. Montrouge, France: John Libbey Eurotext; 2005, pp. 227–53.

Ferrie C, Caraballo R, Covanis A, *et al.* Panayiotopoulos syndrome: a consensus view. *Dev Med Child Neurol* 2006; 48(3): 236–40.

Ferrie CD, Caraballo R, Covanis A, *et al.* Autonomic status epilepticus in Panayiotopoulos syndrome and other childhood and adult epilepsies: a consensus view. *Epilepsia* 2007; 48(6): 1165–72.

Gourfinkel-An I, Baulac S, Nabbout R, *et al.* Monogenic idiopathic epilepsies. *Lancet Neurol* 2004; 3(4): 209–18.

Grosso S, Orrico A, Galli S, Di Bartolo R, Sorrentino V, Balestri P. SCN1A mutation associated with atypical Panayiotopoulos syndrome. *Neurology* 2007; 69(6): 609–11.

Neubauer BA, Fiedler B, Himmelein B, *et al.* Centrotemporal spikes in families with rolandic epilepsy: linkage to chromosome 15q14. *Neurology* 1998; 51(6): 1608–12.

Oxbury JM, Polkey CE, Duchowny M, editors. *Intractable Focal Epilepsy.* London: W.B. Saunders; 2000.

Panayiotopoulos CP. *A Clinical Guide to Epileptic Syndromes and Their Treatment*, 2nd ed. London: Springer; 2007.

Scheffer IE. The role of genetics and ethnicity in epilepsy management. *Acta Neurol Scand Suppl* 2005; 181: 47–51.

Wyllie E, Gupta A, Lachhwani D, editors. *The Treatment of Epilepsy. Principles and Practice*, 4th ed. Philadelphia: Lippincott Williams & Wilkins; 2006.

Chapter 32
Neurodiagnostic tools for the paroxysmal disorders

Barbara E. Swartz
The Epilepsy Clinics of S. Cal., Newport Beach, USA

Electrophysiology

Although neuroimaging has greatly enhanced our understanding of the epilepsies, electrophysiological techniques remain the gold standard diagnostic tool, simply because they actually measure the brain electrophysiologic function in real time. These techniques are rapidly changing with the almost universal reliance on digital systems.

Electroencephalography (EEG)

The brain's electrical activity can be directly recorded with proper filtering and amplification. Analogue recording systems have been available commercially since the mid-1900s, but the size of the components limited the number of channels. Nevertheless, using machines with 8 or 12 channels, the early EEG pioneers made contributions to the understanding of brain function that are nearly unparalleled by other disciplines. The filter settings of the standard Grass EEG machine were based on the mechanical characteristics of pens. The frequencies that could be detected were divided into delta (0.5–3 Hz), theta (3.5–7.5 Hz), alpha (8–12 Hz), and beta (12.5–30 Hz) (sometimes broken into low and high beta) and are simply artificial descriptions of a continuum that starts at DC and extends into the 500 Hz range. Today, 32–40 channels of EEG is routine; the 10–10 system proposed by the International League Against Epilepsy (ILAE) in 1994 to replace the 10–20 system has 65 positions, and high-density EEG (128 or more channels) can provide increasingly precise information.

The parameters used to interpret an EEG are spatial, temporal, frequency, and amplitude. In diagnosing epilepsy one looks for epileptiform sharps (75–250 ms), spikes (20–75 ms), and spike wave bursts. Focal polymorphic delta slowing or focal rhythmic theta in the temporal area are highly correlated with the seizure focus. The EEG pattern can indicate the epilepsy syndrome: focal spikes in localization-related epilepsy; multifocal independent spike waves in epileptic encephalopathies; 4–6 Hz frontal maximum polyspike waves in juvenile myoclonic epilepsy; and so on. High-frequency continuous spike bursts (continuous epileptiform discharges, CEDS) are highly indicative of cortical dysplasia.

A routine EEG is usually 20 min long and has a limited sensitivity of about 30% in focal epilepsy and 50% in generalized epilepsies. Sleep deprivation and prolongation of the record (to 40–60 min) increase the sensitivity greatly. Three routine EEGs will pick up 80–85% of focal epilepsy discharges. When doubt persists, ambulatory recording can be useful (24–48 hours).

The analysis of EEG is based on pattern recognition, with some attempt at quantification of the frequencies, amplitudes, and electrical fields done by the reader. Montages and all other parameters can now be changed with a mouse click. Additional analysis of surface current densities, dipole source localization, power spectra, and wave form correlations are readily performed with commercially available systems and a determined reader. These are quite powerful when combined with a neuroimaging tool (Plate 32.1).

Video-EEG (v-EEG)

This is the gold standard for epilepsy diagnosis and should be carried out for 72 hours to achieve specificity as well as sensitivity for the location of the seizure focus and clarification of the epilepsy syndrome. Numerous other paroxysmal disorders can be indicated by a v-EEG study, including heart block, syncopal convulsions, restless legs syndrome, and non-epileptiform seizures. v-EEG can be done with the 10–20 placement, the 10–10 system, high-density EEG, or intracranial EEG. The video recording of the behavioral characteristics under consideration (seizure semiology) is time-locked to the digital EEG recording. Detection is by the patient, seizure and spike detection programs, and direct observation by trained staff, which should always be available if medications will be withdrawn. Numerous researchers are making promising advances in the area of seizure prediction models.

International Neurology: A Clinical Approach. Edited by Robert P. Lisak, Daniel D. Truong, William M. Carroll, and Roongroj Bhidayasiri. © 2009 Blackwell Publishing, ISBN: 978-1-4051-5738-4.

Intracranial recordings

If EEG is recorded from the surface of the brain during surgery it is called electrocorticography (ECoG). Intracranial EEG recordings can be made on a more prolonged basis as discussed in Chapter 34. The video is again time-locked to EEG to correlate the seizure semiology with the seizure onset zone. In general, a low voltage fast pattern associated with high frequency discharges (up to 500 Hz) can occur at the seizure focus at onset, gradually slowing and increasing in amplitude as spread to neighboring locations occurs. Evaluating the semiology is itself a demanding technique. Some attempt to standardize semiology with epilepsy classification has been published by the ILAE.

Magnetoencephalography (MEG)

This is a relatively new technique for analyzing brain function. It measures the tangential magnetic fields that are generated by the radial electrical fields of the brain, and is less affected than EEG by sources or artifact like the skull, other electrical devices in the vicinity, movement of wires, etc. The best studies comparing MEG, which is always a high-density recording, with high-density recording EEG show comparable but complementary sensitivities (Plate 32.1). One exciting new application is the ability to do functional mapping with MEG without the need for intracranial EEG recordings.

Neuroimaging

Computerized axial tomography (CT) and magnetic resonance imaging (MRI)

These are the work horses of epilepsy imaging. Numerous studies have shown the superiority of MRI to CT, but CT remains in use in many underdeveloped countries and is used in most emergency rooms in developed nations. Sensitivity of the CT scan to a lesion leading to epilepsy is approximately 50%, but there are few false negatives with an intracranial bleed, and it can be superior to MRI when calcification is present. Sensitivity of MRI is

about 85%. The standard sequences are both T1 and T2 with thin slices (1–2 mm) sagittal, axial, and coronal, with additional fluid-attenuated inversion recovery (FLAIR) axial and coronal studies. Other techniques such as contrast and various sequences (proton density, diffusion/perfusion) can improve detection. Surface coils or high Tesla magnet MRI can show areas of cortical dysplasia that are not demonstrated in a routine scan (Figure 32.1), and have led to a new classification of pathology.

Functional imaging

This usually refers to [18]FDG-PET (18-fluorodeoxyglucose-positron emission tomography) or SPECT (single photon emission computerized tomography). The former measures glucose uptake into cells (which has been shown to be highly correlated with synaptic activity), while the latter is a measure of cerebral blood flow. Both are used in the presurgical evaluation of focal epilepsies. FDG-PET is a sensitive interictal test, and spatial resolution is improved by MRI coregistration (Plate 32.2). Ictal SPECT can be useful for identifying foci and planning intracranial recordings, particularly if performed with subtraction ictal SPECT co-registered to MRI. The latter is more cumbersome to arrange, and therefore less practical than FDG-PET. Some institutions have access to ligand-PET. The ligands that appear most useful in epilepsy diagnosis at this time are flumazenil-PET and PET that marks presynaptic serotonin receptors.

Functional MRI

Functional MRI dominates the field for imaging of cognitive brain function. It takes advantage of the fact that localized cerebral blood flow increases are associated with increased neuronal activity and this shifts the ratio of oxy- to deoxy-hemoglobin, which changes the paramagnetic signal produced by hemoglobin. It is quite useful for presurgical mapping of sensory-motor cortex. Mapping of visual cortex and auditory cortex is possible although rarely used clinically. Mapping of language cortex is possible and quite reliable for lateralization, although it tends to be overly sensitive for localization. Mapping of

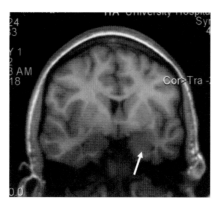 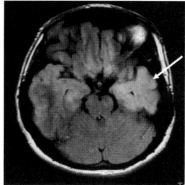

Figure 32.1 MRI with surgical protocol (left) shows no clear abnormality, while surface coil (right) shows cortical dysplasia of the temporal pole (arrow). (Courtesy of Barbara Swartz and Jonathon Lewin.)

declarative memory (medial temporal function) is not yet standardized but will some day replace the Wada test for presurgical evaluation.

Magnetic resonance spectroscopy
This technique produces a spectrum that is unique for any given chemical which has free protons in its outer electron orbit. N-acetyl acetate (NAA), a neuronal marker, and choline (Cho) and creatnine (Cr; glial markers) are usually measured and presented as a ratio (NAA/(Cr+Cho)). Abnormalities have been shown (decreased ratio) in scarring, tumors, and dysplasias. Other substances can be measured, but are for research only at this time.

Other techniques
Other techniques such as optical imaging are under investigation.

Summary

Multimodal tools exist today for the evaluation of epilepsy or its imitators. Increasing use of more complex analytic tools is changing many of our old concepts about epilepsy and its syndromes.

Further reading

Flink R, Pedersen B, Guekht AB, *et al.* Commission of European Affairs of the International League Against Epilepsy: Subcommission on European Guidelines. *Acta Neurol Scand* 2002; 106(1): 1–7.

Niedermeyer E, Lopes da Silva F. EEG. *Basic Principles, Clinical Applications and Related Fields*, 4th ed. Baltimore: Williams & Wilkins; 1999.

Ruben I, Kuzniecky MD, Robert C, Knowlton MD. Neuroimaging of epilepsy. *Semin Neurol* 2002; 22(3): 279–88.

Scherg M, Ille N, Bornfleth H, Berg P. Advanced tools for digital EEG review: virtual source montages, whole head mapping, correlation and phase analysis. *J Clin Neurophys* 2002; 19(2): 91–112.

Swartz BE, Patell A, Thomas K, *et al.* The use of 18-FDG (PET) positron emission tomography in the routine diagnosis of epilepsy. *J Mol Imag Biol* 2002; 4(3): 245–52.

Chapter 33
Antiepileptic drugs

Paul B. Pritchard III
Medical University of South Carolina, Charleston, USA

Introduction

Antiepileptic drugs (AEDs) are the cornerstone of epilepsy treatment. The goal of therapy is complete control of seizures (effectiveness), while avoiding side effects and enabling normal activities (efficacy) (Table 33.1). Selection of the appropriate AED is imperative for optimal outcome. Selection factors include cost, dosing, clinical spectrum of AED effectiveness, side-effect profile, and consideration of co-morbidities. Whenever possible, patients should be treated with a single AED, reserving polytherapy for refractory cases.

Spectrum of effectiveness

Animal models provide a screening tool for the development of AEDs and also have predictive value for narrow-versus broad-spectrum effectiveness. To some extent the maximum electroshock (MES) model is predictive of effectiveness for partial epilepsy (narrow spectrum), whereas the pentylenetetrazol model suggests a broad-spectrum effect for humans. Table 33.2 lists commonly used AEDs according to spectrum of effectiveness.

Narrow-spectrum AEDs
Absence seizures
Ethosuximide
Ethosuximide effectively combats absence seizures. Although ethosuximide effectively blocks pentylenetetrazol-induced seizures, it does not have broad-spectrum application in human epilepsy. It is available as a liquid-filled capsule or as a syrup. In most children, the optimal dose is 20 mg/kg/day, given in divided doses. Ethosuximide may exacerbate generalized tonic–clonic seizures. Common side effects are gastrointestinal upset, hiccoughs, and dizziness.

Valproate and lamotrigine are alternative drugs for absence seizures. Assuming purely absence attacks, ethosuximide is generally preferred in younger children, who are more vulnerable to the hepatotoxicity of valproate.

Partial seizures
Phenytoin
The effectiveness of phenytoin against partial seizures is predicted by the MES model. Randomized controlled trials support both phenytoin and carbamazepine as initial monotherapy for partial epilepsy.

The non-linear pharmacokinetics of phenytoin can make it difficult to secure stable levels. Phenytoin may exacerbate primary generalized epilepsy, particularly absence and myoclonic seizures. It may contribute to osteoporosis with long-term use.

The half-life of phenytoin ranges from 7 to 48 hours, with a mean value around 24 hours. The maintenance dose is 4–8 mg/kg/day. Phenytoin is available in liquid suspension, chewable tablets, capsules, extended-release forms, and intravenous (IV) preparations. Fosphenytoin, the phosphate ester prodrug version, can be given IV more rapidly and may be given by intramuscular injection.

Carbamazepine
Carbamazepine is more effective than valproate for partial seizures, with or without secondary generalization. It is available as a chewable tablet, liquid suspension, and in extended-release tablets and capsules, permitting twice daily dosage.

Carbamazepine has an initial half-life of 25–65 hours, which drops to 12–17 hours over the first 3–4 weeks through self-induction of hepatic enzymes. Like oxcarbazepine, carbamazepine may induce hyponatremia, particularly in older adults. Surveillance for blood dyscrasias and hepatic dysfunction is warranted.

Oxcarbazepine
Oxcarbazepine is a 10-keto analog of carbamazepine. The mechanism of action is uncertain but is exerted largely by the 10-monohydroxy metabolite, probably through

International Neurology: A Clinical Approach. Edited by Robert P. Lisak, Daniel D. Truong, William M. Carroll, and Roongroj Bhidayasiri. © 2009 Blackwell Publishing, ISBN: 978-1-4051-5738-4.

Table 33.1 Antiepileptic drugs.

Drug	Indications and mechanism	Dosing and therapeutic range (µg/ml)	Metabolism	Side effects and complications	Teratogenicity
Carbamazepine	Partial ↓ Polysynaptic responses Blocks voltage-dependent sodium channels	2–3× daily 4–12 µg/ml	Hepatic: isoenzyme P450 CYP3A4 Auto-induces metabolism	Hyponatremia Aplastic anemia Diplopia Drowsiness Nausea Vomiting	Craniofacial defects Neural tube defects
Ethosuximide	Absence Mechanism: possible inhibition of motor cortex; blocks calcium channels	3× daily 40–100 µg/ml	Hepatic: primarily via CYP3A4, or perhaps CYP2E1	Aplastic anemia Neutropenia Hiccoughs Nausea Drowsiness	No strong evidence in humans
Felbamate	Partial Generalized Mechanism: *N*-methyl-D-aspartate (NMDA) antagonist	3× daily 18–83 µg/ml	Hepatic	Aplastic anemia Hepatic necrosis Weight loss	Unknown
Gabapentin	Partial Mechanism unknown	3× daily Therapeutic range not established	Renal excretion	Weight gain Cognitive impairment	Unknown
Lamotrigine	Partial Generalized Mechanism unclear: blocks voltage-sensitive sodium channels	2× daily Therapeutic range not established	Hepatic	Skin rash Stevens–Johnson and toxic epidermal necrolysis, sometimes fatal	Cleft lip
Levetiracetam	Partial Generalized Mechanism unclear: binds to synaptic vesicle protein (SV2A)	2× daily Therapeutic range not well established	Primarily renal excretion; insignificant hepatic metabolism	Fatigue Behavioral problems	No strong evidence in humans
Oxcarbazepine	Partial Mechanism: blocks voltage-sensitive sodium channels	2× daily Therapeutic range not well established	Hepatic conversion to 10-monohydroxy metabolite	Hyponatremia Abdominal pain Nausea Diplopia	No strong evidence in humans

Drug	Indication / Mechanism	Dosing / Therapeutic range	Metabolism	Adverse effects	Teratogenicity
Phenobarbital	Partial Generalized Mechanism: blocks sodium-dependent action potentials; ↓ neuronal Ca^{2+} uptake	1× daily 15–40 µg/ml	Hepatic conversion to *p*-hydroxyphenobarbital	Cognitive impairment Sedation Paradoxical excitability	Four-fold increase
Phenytoin	Partial Mechanism: inhibits sodium-dependent action potentials	Once daily 10–20 µg/ml	Hepatic, primarily via P450	Skin rash Aplastic anemia Ataxic gait Dizziness Gingival hyperplasia	Fetal hydantoin syndrome
Tiagabine	Partial Mechanism: GABAergic – inhibits GABA uptake into neurons	3× daily Therapeutic range not established	Hepatic	Somnolence Dizziness Tremor Abdominal pain	No strong evidence in humans
Topiramate	Partial Generalized Mechanism: blocks voltage-dependent sodium channels, augments GABA effects	2× daily Therapeutic range not established	Hepatic hydroxylation Much excreted unchanged in urine except in presence of enzyme-inducing drugs	Renal stones Weight loss Somnolence	No strong evidence in humans
Valproate	Partial Generalized Mechanism: enhances GABA effects, ↓ sodium-dependent action potentials	3× daily (2× daily with extended-release forms) 50–125 µg/ml	Hepatic oxidation and glucuronidation	Weight gain Hair loss Hepatic necrosis Pancreatic necrosis	Neural tube defects Cognitive impairment
Zonisamide	Partial Generalized Mechanism not known	Once daily Therapeutic range not established	Hepatic conjugation	Renal stones Anhidrosis	No strong evidence in humans

Table 33.2 Classification of most AEDs.

Broad-spectrum AEDs	Narrow-spectrum AEDs
Felbamate	Carbamazepine
Lamotrigine	Ethosuximide
Levetiracetam	Gabapentin
Phenobarbital	Oxcarbazepine
Topiramate	Phenytoin
Valproate	Tiagabine
Zonisamide	

blockade of voltage-sensitive sodium channels. The metabolite has an elimination half-life of 9 hours, versus 2 hours for oxcarbazepine. Oxcarbazepine offers a more favorable side-effect profile. Either may induce hyponatremia, perhaps more often with oxcarbazepine. Approximately 1/3 of patients who have hypersensitivity reactions to carbamazepine cross react to oxcarbazepine.

Meta-analysis shows similar seizure control for oxcarbazepine and phenytoin. Oxcarbazepine is available as tablets and as a suspension, administered twice daily. The dose is proportionally higher in children, requiring up to a 50% higher dose per body weight.

Gabapentin
Gabapentin is effective in the treatment of partial seizures but is used more widely for neurogenic pain. Although the name implies a γ-aminobutyric acid (GABA)-ergic mechanism, the mechanism of action is unknown. It offers few drug interactions because it is excreted renally without significant hepatic metabolism. The drug is available in tablet form in multiple dosage strengths. It is given in three divided doses, and the dose must be adjusted for renal impairment.

Tiagabine
Tiagabine inhibits the uptake of GABA into neurons and glia. Administered in three divided doses, it is adjunctive therapy for partial seizures.

Broad-spectrum AEDs
Broad-spectrum AEDs are effective in primary generalized epilepsy and also for partial epilepsies, with or without secondary generalization.

Felbamate
Felbamate is one of few AEDs that has substantial benefit for Lennox–Gastaut syndrome. It carries the risk of aplastic anemia and hepatic necrosis. The number of cases of aplastic anemia is too few to reliably predict the fatality rate or the underlying factors that pose special risk. Felbamate should be considered only after all other reasonable alternatives, and the clinician should obtain informed consent. It is available in tablet or suspension forms. Monitoring of hepatic and hematologic parameters is mandatory.

Lamotrigine
Lamotrigine has one of the most appealing side-effect profiles of currently available AEDs. The risk of serious skin rash is increased, more in children than in adults. To limit the increased risk of toxic epidermal necrolysis (TEN) and the Stevens–Johnson syndrome (SJS), the dosage must be titrated slowly. Skin rash requires urgent dermatology consultation and discontinuation of the drug. The elimination half-life of lamotrigine ranges from 13 to 59 hours in adults and 7 to 66 hours in children, shorter with enzyme-inducing drugs and longer with simultaneous valproate. Lamotrigine, available in multiple tablet strengths, is administered in two divided doses.

Levetiracetam
Like gabapentin, levetiracetam has the advantage of minimal interactions with other drugs, a desirable attribute in patients who require antineoplastic agents. The elimination half-life is 7 hours. Dosage must be adjusted in patients with renal insufficiency. Sedation at higher doses and psychogenic side effects occur occasionally. Levetiracetam is available in multiple dose tablets and as a liquid for oral administration, given in two divided doses. Titration is usually carried out over a period of several weeks. Levetiracetam is now available for IV administration.

Topiramate
Topiramate may potentiate the activity of GABA and has a weak inhibitory effect on carbonic anhydrase isozymes, but the exact mechanism of action is unknown. Topiramate is effective in the treatment of partial and generalized seizures. The elimination half-life is 21 hours, and twice-daily dosage is used. The drug is available as sprinkle capsules and tablets. Slow titration is vital to minimize side effects.

Valproate
Valproate has a GABAergic effect, which is believed to be the basis for its antiepileptic action. The standard and new antiepileptic drugs (SANAD) study demonstrated that valproate is more efficacious than lamotrigine for generalized or unclassified seizures and better tolerated than topiramate. The drug is available as valproic acid or the sodium salt, and as an elixir, liquid-filled capsule, tablets, or IV formulation.

Zonisamide
Approved as adjunctive treatment for partial seizures, zonisamide is effective in the treatment of generalized seizures, including myoclonic and generalized tonic–clonic

events. Although zonisamide is a weak inhibitor of carbonic anhydrase, the mechanism of the antiepileptic effect is not known. The drug may be given once daily. There are few drug–drug interactions for zonisamide because it is predominantly renally excreted. Like topiramate, it can cause hypohidrosis and therefore hyperthermia.

Choosing the appropriate AED

Spectrum of effectiveness
The first consideration is the type(s) of seizures and the likely epilepsy syndrome. With absence seizures alone, ethosuximide is a reasonable choice. Ethosuximide lacks sufficient spectrum to be used in juvenile myoclonic epilepsy (JME). Ethosuximide may exacerbate generalized convulsive seizures, making valproate a more appropriate choice for JME.

Dosing requirements
Compliance with the AED regimen is critical, and the required daily doses are inversely proportional to the degree of compliance. Dosing requirements also impact institutional staffing costs. Longer drug half-lives enable once-daily administration of phenytoin, phenobarbital, and zonisamide for most patients. An extended-release preparation of valproate allows once-daily dosage. Most of the remaining AEDs should be given twice daily for epilepsy.

Consideration of co-morbidities
Migraine
Migraine is more common among patients with epilepsy. Valproate and topiramate have won Food and Drug Administration (FDA) approval for anti-migraine prophylaxis. Levetiracetam and zonisamide also provide effective dual therapy.

Obesity
AEDs associated with weight gain – valproate, gabapentin, pregabalin, and occasionally carbamazepine – can exacerbate or initiate obesity. Topiramate, zonisamide, and felbamate are often associated with weight loss. Most other AEDs are weight neutral.

Psychiatric disorders
Valproate, carbamazepine, and others are used for bipolar affective disorder. Sedating AEDs may exacerbate depression and are best avoided in depressed patients. Levetiracetam should be used cautiously with co-existing psychosis because it may exacerbate psychiatric symptoms.

Pain
Phenytoin and carbamazepine benefit trigeminal neuralgia. Gabapentin, topiramate, zonisamide, and pregabalin also are effective for neurogenic pain.

Side-effect profile
The search for less sedating AEDs lead to the development of phenytoin. Modification of the chemical structure of carbamazepine to oxcarbazepine was done to lower side effects. A favorable side-effect profile is the major advantage of the newer AEDs. Most common side effects are proportional to serum drug levels. Side effects can be avoided or minimized by starting with low doses and escalating slowly: "start low and go slow."

Proconvulsant effects of AEDs
Paradoxically, AEDs may exacerbate seizures. An obvious mechanism is drug–drug interaction. In the combination of phenytoin and carbamazepine, each induces the hepatic metabolism of the other. Another mechanism by which AEDs lower seizure threshold is by inducing drowsiness. Barbiturates may aggravate seizures in this way.

Drug cost
Economics limit access to some of the modern AEDs. Cost limits the availability to phenobarbital and phenytoin in many developing countries. The newer AEDs may prove too costly in developed countries as well, depending on health insurance or government health benefits.

Further reading

Camfield P, Camfield C. Childhood epilepsy: what is the evidence for what we think and what we do? *J Child Neurol* 2003; 18(4): 272–87.

Glauser T, Ben-Menachem E, Bourgeois B, *et al.* ILAE treatment guidelines: evidence-based analysis of antiepileptic drug efficacy and effectiveness as initial monotherapy for epileptic seizures and syndromes. *Epilepsia* 2006; 47(7): 1094–120.

Muller M, Marson MG, Williamson PR. Oxcarbazepine versus phenytoin monotherapy for epilepsy. *Cochrane Database Syst Rev* 2006; (2): CD003615. DIO:10.1002/14651858.CD003615.pub2.

Rogawski MA. Diverse mechanisms of antiepileptic drugs in the development pipeline. *Epilepsy Res* 2006; 69(3): 273–94.

Chapter 34
Surgical treatment of epilepsy

Ivan Rektor[1] and Barbara E. Swartz[2]
[1]Masaryk University, St. Anne's Hospital, Brno, Czech Republic
[2]The Epilepsy Clinics of S. Cal., Newport Beach, USA

Introduction

Epilepsy surgery is the most efficient therapy for patients with pharmacoresistant epilepsy. Patients with epilepsy refractory to pharmacotherapy should receive consultation about the suitability of a surgical solution.

Indications for epilepsy surgery

Prior to surgery, all relevant information is evaluated by a multidisciplinary team. The diagnostic process leads to the elimination of some candidates as unsuitable for epileptic surgery, or to the determination of the optimal surgical method for those suitable candidates who elect to have surgery. The results of electroencephalography (EEG), especially of ictal video-EEG, are compared with those of imaging and metabolic methods as well as neuropsychological findings. All data are considered together with individual anamnesis, including the subjective description of the aura or seizure and psychosocial impact of surgery. Surgical treatment is determined mainly by the detection and location of the seizure onset zone (SOZ; i.e., the brain area that generates epileptic seizures), as well as by the presence or absence of a detectable brain lesion, the biological nature of the lesion, relation of the SOZ to the lesion and to the location of the eloquent cortex, and, of course, by the decision of the patient.

The following questions should be answered:

1 Where is the SOZ located and how large is it?

2 Is the SOZ the only source of habitual seizures?

3 Is there an identified lesion that causes the seizures? Could the lesion be removed entirely or partially?

4 What are the risks of removal of the SOZ? What is the relation between the epileptogenic cortex and the localization of brain functions?

5 Which operation is more suitable: curative (resection) or palliative?

International Neurology: A Clinical Approach. Edited by Robert P. Lisak, Daniel D. Truong, William M. Carroll, and Roongroj Bhidayasiri. © 2009 Blackwell Publishing, ISBN: 978-1-4051-5738-4.

Semi-invasive and invasive video-EEG

The cornerstone of epilepsy diagnostics is video-EEG recordings of seizures. Intracranial video-EEG is necessary in a small portion of epilepsy surgery candidates if scalp and semi-invasive recordings do not yield enough information about the location and extent of the epileptogenic zone. Electrodes are implanted intracranially for 1 or 2 weeks while data are gathered. Electric stimulation via implanted electrodes may provoke seizure activity and also enables precise functional diagnosis of the localization of the eloquent cortex (which must be avoided during surgery). Intraoperative recording (electrocorticography, ECoG) is the main method in some centers; in others, it is complementary to long-term recordings. The invasive exploration is carried out through surgically inserted intracranial electrodes. There are two main approaches to ECoG: intracerebral recording and subdural recording. In the first, thin-depth electrodes with 5–18 contacts are stereotactically inserted into the brain (stereoencephalography, SEEG), providing for exploration of deep structures. SEEG does not require craniotomy. In order to obtain subdural recordings, subdural electrodes in the form of

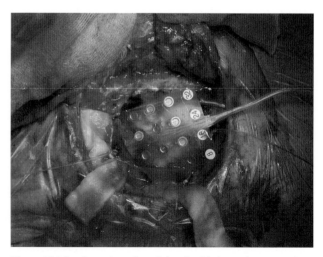

Figure 34.1 Implantation of a subdural grid electrode.

strips or grids (20–128 contacts) are placed on the surface of the brain after craniotomy. This method is less accurate than intracerebral recording, but easier. The risk for both approaches is similar, and most centers combine both methods depending on the targeted structure. Complications are headache and cerebrospinal fluid (CSF) leakage with infrequent cerebral infection or bleeding (≤5%). Generally, SEEG exploration is used for mesiotemporal structures. Extratemporal explorations are carried out subdurally or by SEEG, depending on the location of the lesion and the preference of the center. In some centers, epidural electrodes are also used; foramen ovale electrodes are used for mesial foci (Figures 34.1 and 34.2).

Operations

Epilepsy surgery can be curative or palliative. The goals of surgery are to remove the epileptogenic lesion and epileptogenic zone, to halt disease progression, to prevent the spread of seizure activity, and to inhibit seizures via neuromodulatory techniques.

Curative procedures

Amygdalohippocampectomy/temporal lobectomy

Tissue removal can be limited to mesial structures or extended to the temporal neocortex. In patients with temporal epilepsy with mesial (hippocampal) sclerosis, anteromedial temporal resection (i.e., amygdalohippocampectomy with removal of the parahippocampal gyrus and the temporal pole) is the most frequent and most successful surgical method (Figure 34.3). It can be performed on the more active side of the brain for bitemporal epilepsies if memory functions are sufficient on the opposite side. Patients showed significant improvement following surgery in 75% (bilateral foci), 80% (dominant), and 90% (non-dominant) of cases. According to a recent meta-analysis, the median long-term (more than 5 years) seizure-free outcome for patients was 66% in temporal lobe resections, 46% in parietal resections, and 27% in frontal resections. In our center, 75% of patients were seizure-free 2 years after surgery, with significant improvement in over 90%. In extratemporal operations, freedom from seizures was achieved in 63% of patients.

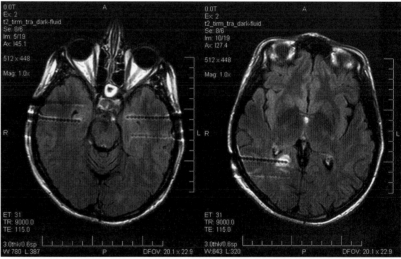

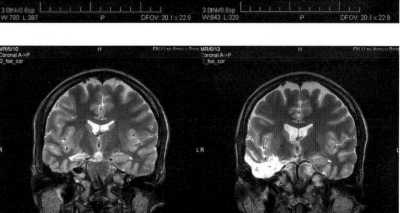

Figure 34.2 Multicontact depth electrodes implanted in a lesion and in the temporal lobes. The post-placement MRI visualized exact localization of individual contacts. The diameter of an electrode (0.8 mm) represents approximately 10% of the diameter of the displayed artefact.

Figure 34.3 Hippocampal sclerosis, before and after anteromedial temporal resection.

Complications of surgery are usually minimal; mortality is <0.1%. Hemiparesis, infections, hematomas, and cranial nerve palsies are <5%, and quandrantanopsia is 25–30%. Recent memory may be worsened (25%) or improved (75%) and is IQ-dependent. Global memory impairment is rare (≤1%). Postoperative memory impairment can be prevented by careful selection of patients (Wada test, neuropsychology). Significant dysphasia is seen in 1–3% of patients; transient, medication-responsive mood swings occur in 2–20%. Patients continue with medical treatment after surgery for 1–2 years. If patients are seizure-free, medications can be gradually and carefully reduced over time.

Lesionectomy

Removal of an epileptogenic lesion is most frequently performed in dysplasias, low-grade tumors, cavernomas, and other vascular malformations. Even in seemingly simple cases, such as with tumors, it is necessary to carry out an anatomic-electro-clinical correlation of the seizures, as the SOZ may not be identical with the lesion. Lesionectomy is successful in reducing the majority of seizures 85% of the time. Freedom from seizures (15–50%) depends on the type of lesion and extent of resection.

Sometimes the lesion itself is epileptogenic, for example, in the case of some dysplasias, while in other cases its surroundings or more distant structures are epileptogenic. Therefore, SEEG may be required to explore the SOZ.

Between 50% and 85% of patients respond favorably to lesionectomy. Complications vary with the site of surgery and the degree of cortical reorganization. Severe complications such as stroke or aphasia are less than 5%.

Topectomy/cortectomy of the SOZ

The most common site for this procedure is the frontal lobe. In non-lesional epilepsies, the SOZ identified by prior examination, often including intracranial exploration, is removed. Neuropathological examination of removed tissue often shows malformation of cortical development. Freedom from seizures ranges from 15% to 50% with significant improvement in 60–90%. The most frequent complications are due to perioperative ischemia (2.7%) and hemianopsia (2.1%).

Palliative procedures

Multilobar resections

With large lesions, lobar or multilobar resections may be performed. No outcome study has specifically assessed these. Evaluation is the same as in other cortical epilepsies. Complications such as pyramidal signs or hemianopsia are expected more frequently; however, these large resections are surprisingly well tolerated.

Hemispherectomy

Hemispherectomy is performed in extreme childhood epileptic disorders, as in cases of hemimegencephaly, perinatal common carotid occlusion, Sturge–Weber syndrome, and advanced Rasmussen syndrome. The Wada test should be performed prior to surgery. It is common to remove only the temporal lobe and surgically disconnect the other structures (hemispherotomy). Outcome of hemispherectomy is surprisingly good, with 80–95% of patients showing significant improvement. Some may become seizure-free, although EEG remains malignant in the case of hemispherotomy. Complications depend on the degree of dysfunction in the offending hemisphere and include weakness, speech impairment, and perioperative complications.

Multiple subpial transactions (MSPT)

The epileptogenic cortex is not removed but is isolated from surrounding tissue to prevent the seizure from spreading, allowing for operations in the eloquent or motor cortex. This is done for palliation or to improve outcome in conjunction with a cortectomy. Outcomes vary, with up to 50% of patients seizure-free and significant improvement in 30–90%. Complications include monoparesis, visual field defect, sensory loss, and dysphasia; less than 6% of these are persistent.

Callosotomy

In this procedure, one-half to two-thirds of the callosum is transected. The main indications for this surgery are atonic seizures of secondary generalized and multifocal epilepsies. Control depends on the type of seizure: 75–100% decrease in drops; 60–75% in generalized tonic–clonic (GTC); 50% in complex partial seizures; and no change or increase in focal motor seizures. Complications include transient mutism, hemiparesis, and apraxias, which rarely persist.

Vagal nerve stimulation (VNS)

VNS, a relatively expensive option, is carried out mainly in patients for whom resection is contraindicated or where surgery has failed. An electrode is fixed to the left vagus nerve and a generator is placed under the skin, usually under the collar bone. Patients can block a seizure as it starts by extra stimulation. While in some patients the number of seizures can be reduced by up to 90%, a realistic target is approximately 50% reduction. Fifty percent to 60% of patients are responders with a 2-year follow-up. As with other palliative techniques, the character of the seizure may be mitigated. Positive influences on mood and cognitive functions are reported. Complications are minor, including hoarseness and cough.

In practice, various operations can be combined (e.g., a lesionectomy with an amygdalohippocampectomy, a subtotal lesionectomy with MSTP) and surgery may be planned in two phases. Other methods are being developed, including gamma knife radiosurgery and thermolesioning using inserted depth electrodes. Several intracerebral targets for chronic electrical stimulation are also under investigation.

Acknowledgments

This chapter was prepared with the support of Research Project MSM 0021622404. The authors thank M. Brázdil, J. Chrastina, P. Daniel, Z. Fanfrdlová, P. Krupa, R. Kuba, Z. Novák, M. Pažourková, I. Tyrlíková, and colleagues from the Brno Epilepsy Center.

Further reading

Bancaud J, Talairach J. Séméilogie clinique des crises du lobe temporal. In: *Crises épileptiques et épilepsies du lobe temporal.* Documentation médicale LABAZ, Rennes; 1991.

Chauvel P, Delgado-Escueta AV, Halgren E, Bancaud J, editors. Frontal lobe seizures and epilepsies. In: *Advances in Neurology,* Vol. 57. New York: Raven Press; 1992.

Lüders HO, Noachtar S. Epileptic seizures: pathophysiology and clinical semiology. *Cleveland: Churchill Livingstone*; 2000.

Rektor I, Kalina M, Brázdil M, *et al*. Epilepsy surgery in the Czech Republic. *Epilepsia* 2005; 46(Suppl 6): 160.

Telezz-Zenteno JF, Dhar J, Wiebe S. Long-term seizure outcomes following epilepsy surgery: a systematic review and meta-analysis. *Brain* 2005; 128: 1188–98.

Williamson PD, Engel J Jr, Munari C. Anatomic classification of localization-related epilepsies. In: *Epilepsy: A Comprehensive Textbook*, Engel J Jr, Pedley TA, editors. Philadelphia: Lippincott-Raven; 1997, pp. 2045–426.

Chapter 35
The dementias: an overview

Howard H. Feldman[1] and Najeeb Qadi[2]
[1]University of British Columbia, Vancouver, British Columbia, Canada
[2]King Faisal Specialist Hospital and Research Centre, Riyadh, Saudi Arabia

Introduction

Within our current epoch, there has been an unprecedented increase in longevity, not only within the developed Western countries but also across the developing world. Indeed the implications within the developing world of this trend will likely exceed those within the Western world. The most recent 2001 global estimates were that 24.3 million individuals are affected by dementia, with close to 5 million incident cases each year. The projections indicate that these numbers will increase by 1.7 times by 2020 and then double again by 2040. A major public health challenge is then apparent across societies worldwide, with the intense social, economic, and health resources that dementia care demands. Care for individuals afflicted with dementia is expected to touch the clinical practice of neurologists globally, irrespective of their area of specialization or interest.

Definitions

See Table 35.1 for a glossary of dementia terminology.

Epidemiology

Across the countries of the Western world it has been generally estimated that 70–80% of the population over the age of 65 can be classified as being cognitively normal while 15–20% have mild cognitive impairment (MCI)/ cognitive impairment no dementia (CIND), and 5–10% have dementia with a variety of etiologies.

MCI/CIND

Beyond the recognition of the magnitude and the defining clinical criteria of MCI/CIND there has been emerging

interest in its etiological classification. There is potential to both modify risk factors and intervene before dementia is fully established. This would represent the most important therapeutic potential for this condition. Figure 35.1 provides a classification scheme of etiologies of CIND that can be applied in the clinic and which covers most clinical presentations.

There is converging evidence that a diagnosis of CIND/MCI does impart an increased risk of progression to dementia ranging from 10% to 15% per annum over 5 years. Considerable recent research attention has been directed at investigating the efficacy of the acetylcholinesterase inhibitors (AChEIs) in delaying the time to diagnosis of Alzheimer's disease (AD) in individuals with MCI. Unfortunately, these randomized controlled clinical trials (RCTs) have not demonstrated a significant long-term benefit on this outcome. They have also underscored the heterogeneity of the condition with progression rates in the RCTs that have fallen much lower than expected.

Dementia

There is an exponentially increasing prevalence of dementia over the age of 65, to a peak over age 85 where more than 35–45% of individuals are estimated to be affected. There are upwards of 50 medical, neurologic, and psychiatric diseases associated with dementia. As shown in Figures 35.2 and 35.3, neurodegenerative diseases account for the majority.

Across the full adult lifespan AD is the most common etiology of dementia, with other diseases having differential frequencies across age-stratified samples. In general, those with an autosomal dominant pattern of inheritance have a propensity for midlife age of onset while sporadic cases dominate in the older ages. Those dementias that occur in familial form with gene mutations are presented in Table 35.2.

Considerable clinical attention is given by neurologists to the differential diagnosis of dementia particularly in the identification of treatable or modifiable causes. However, most systematic studies of outcomes of dementia workup have reported that the percentage of reversible causes of dementia is very low. Table 35.3 provides a list of potentially reversible/modifiable causes of dementia.

International Neurology: A Clinical Approach. Edited by Robert P. Lisak, Daniel D. Truong, William M. Carroll, and Roongroj Bhidayasiri. © 2009 Blackwell Publishing, ISBN: 978-1-4051-5738-4.

Table 35.1 Glossary of dementia terms.

Term	Definition
Mild cognitive impairment (MCI)	MCI describes a state of cognitive function with aging that is below defined norms yet falls short of meeting dementia in severity. Individuals with MCI are recognized to be at an increased risk of progressing to dementia. A variety of other terms have been applied to this state including cognitively impaired not dementia (CIND), age associated cognitive decline (AACD), and age associated memory impairment (AAMI)
Dementia	Dementia describes a more severe condition than MCI, where there is a loss of prior intellectual capacity within a variety of cognitive domains including memory, language, executive functioning, and visuospatial skills. This impairment is sufficiently severe to interfere with social functioning. Neuropsychiatric symptoms are often an important part of the clinical phenomenology. Rather than representing a single disease, dementia describes a syndrome with more than 50 diseases with which it can be associated
Alzheimer's disease (AD)	AD is a neurodegenerative disease that is recognized clinically through a core amnestic disorder, with other cognitive domains affected within executive function, language, praxis, and visuospatial skills. This disease is the largest single cause of dementia across the age continuum
Frontotemporal lobar degenerations (FTLD)	FTLD include a grouping of neurodegenerative diseases that are manifest clinically by either disordered social conduct and behavior, and/or progressive aphasia, and/or executive dysfunction, and/or motor impairment
Parkinson's disease dementia (PDD)/ dementia with Lewy bodies (DLB)	PDD/DLB includes motor parkinsonism, dementia, and frequently other features including visual hallucinations, fluctuations, autonomic problems, and falls
Vascular dementia	This condition results from multifocal cerebrovascular injury either through strategic infarction or by the cumulative effects of multifocal cerebral infarctions
Mixed dementia	A dementia that results from multiple contributing factors (e.g., AD with cerebrovascular disease). This condition remains poorly defined operationally

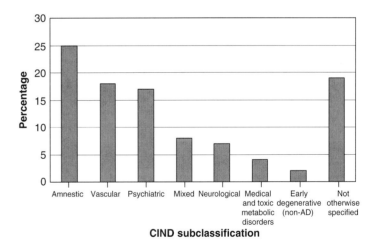

Figure 35.1 CIND etiological subclassification as determined in the Canadian Cohort Study of Cognitive Impairment and Related Dementias (ACCORD). (Modified from Feldman H, *et al.* for the ACCORD Study Group. A Canadian Cohort Study of Cognitive Impairment and Related Dementias (ACCORD): study methods and baseline results. *Neuroepidemiology* 2003; 22: 265–74.)

Infectious and inflammatory causes will generally require lumbar puncture. They are very important treatable conditions, while normal pressure hydrocephalus can sometimes have excellent treatment response to cerebrospinal fluid (CSF) shunting. While treatment of the metabolic causes identified in the workup of dementia, including vitamin B_{12}, calcium, and thyroid, can be associated with some improvement, more often it does not reverse the dementia. It can, however, reduce unnecessary comorbid decline in cognitive functioning.

Treatment

For neurologists worldwide, the treatment approach to dementia irrespective of etiology should be broad, addressing not only pharmacological therapies but also psychosocial, legal, and vocational ones. Early diagnostic disclosure should be provided to allow for the appropriate future planning that will be needed during the course of the dementia. The designation of a legal guardian for financial management and health decision making can spare significant economic and social crisis later. Future

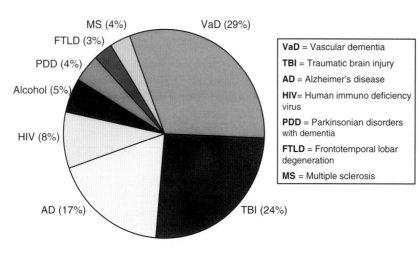

[Categories with <3% or miscellaneous are not included]

Figure 35.2 Dementia etiologies: early onset dementia (<65 years). (Modified from McMurtray A, *et al*. Early-onset dementia: frequency and causes compared to late-onset dementia. *Demen Geriatr Cogn Disord* 2006; 21: 59–64.)

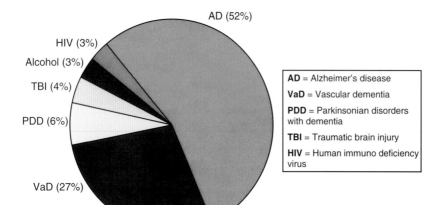

[Categories with <3% or miscellaneous are not included]

Figure 35.3 Dementia etiologies: late onset dementia (>65 years). (Modified from McMurtray A, *et al*. Early-onset dementia: frequency and causes compared to late-onset dementia. *Demen Geriatr Cogn Disord* 2006; 21: 59–64.)

Table 35.2 Genetic forms of dementia.

Disease	Chromosome	Gene
Familial Alzheimer's disease (AD)	21	Amyloid precursor protein (APP)
	14	*Presenilin 1*
	1	*Presenilin 2*
Vascular dementias (VaD)	19	*Notch 3*
Cerebral autosomal dominant arteriopathy with subcortical infarcts and leukoencephalopathy (CADASIL)		
Hereditary cerebral hemorrhage with amyloidosis of the Dutch type (HCHWA-D)	21	Amyloid precursor protein
Frontotemporal lobar degenerations (FTLD)	17	*Tau (MAPT)*
	17	*Progranulin (GRN)*
	9	Valosin containing protein (VCP)
	3	*CHMP 2B*
Parkinson's disease dementia (PDD)	4	Alpha synuclein (gene dose related)
	12	Leucine rich repeat kinase 2 (*LRRK2*)
Huntington's disease (HD)	4	*IT-5*
Prion diseases		
Familial Creutzfeldt–Jakob disease	20	Prion protein
Familial fatal insomnia	20	Prion protein
Gerstmann–Sträussler–Scheinker	20	Prion protein
Familial British dementia	13	*BR12*
Familial Danish dementia	13	*BR12*

Table 35.3 Potentially reversible/modifiable causes of dementia. (Modified from American Academy of Neurology. *Neurology* 1994; 44: 2203–6.)

Category	Cause
Intracranial	Normal pressure hydrocephalus
	Subdural hematoma
	Abscesses
	Tumors
	CNS infections
	• Bacterial (syphilis)
	• Fungal
	• Tuberculosis
Psychiatric	Depression
	Mania
	Schizophrenia
Endocrine	Hypothyroidism
	Hyperthyroidism
	Hypoparathyroidism
	Hyperparathyroidism
	Hypoadrenalism
	Hypercalcaemia
	Hypoglycemia
Autoimmune	Systemic lupus erythmatosis
	Temporal arteritis
	CNS vasculitis
	Hashimoto's encephalopathy
Metabolic	Liver disease
	Renal disease
	Cardiac insufficiency
	Respiratory insufficiency
	Wilson's disease
Nutritional	Severe malnutrition (Marasmus)
	Vitamin B_{12} deficiency
	Folate deficiency
	Thiamine deficiency
Toxic	Excess alcohol intake
	Medications or drug interactions
	Heavy metals

directives of care can be developed at an earlier dementia stage. The planning for the loss of driving fitness and provision for assessment of such fitness draws on the availability of local resources and driving legislation. At present, the pharmacological treatments that are available are directed at the symptoms of the disease. There are no approved disease-modifying treatments, though these are actively being investigated. The available symptomatic medications, including AChEIs and memantine, provide effect sizes that can favorably impact social functioning and merit at least a trial of 6–12 months to judge their efficacy. The rapid pace of basic neuroscience progress supports an optimistic view that treatments for dementia will be significantly approved in the next 5 years.

Further reading

Bachman DL, Wolf PA, Linn RT, *et al*. Incidence of dementia and probable Alzheimer's disease in a general population: the Framingham Study. *Neurology* 1993; 43(3 Pt 1): 515–9.

Busse A, Bischkopf J, Riedel-Heller SG, *et al*. Mild cognitive impairment: prevalence and incidence according to different diagnostic criteria: results of the Leipzig Longitudinal Study of the Aged (LEILA75). *Br J Psychiatry* 2003; 182: 449–54.

Feldman HH, Ferris S, Winblad B, *et al*. Effect of rivastigmine on delay to diagnosis of Alzheimer's disease from mild cognitive impairment: the InDDEx study. *Lancet Neurol* 2007; 6(6): 501–12.

Ferri CP, Prince M, Brayne C, *et al*. Global prevalence of dementia: a Delphi consensus study. *Lancet* 2005; 366(9503): 2112–7.

Graham JE, Rockwood K, Beattie BL, *et al*. Prevalence and severity of cognitive impairment with and without dementia in an elderly population. *Lancet* 1997; 349: 1793–6.

Jelic V, Kivipelto M, Winblad B. Clinical trials in mild cognitive impairment: lessons for the future. *J Neurol Neurosurg Psychiatry* 2006; 77(4): 429–38.

Jorm AF, Korten AE, Henderson AS. The prevalence of dementia: a quantitative integration of the literature. *Acta Psychiatr Scand* 1987; 76(5): 465–79.

Palloni A, Pinto-Aguirre G, Pelaez M. Demographic and health conditions of ageing in Latin America and the Caribbean. *Int J Epidemiol* 2002; 31: 762–71.

Petersen RC, Doody R, Kurz A, *et al*. Current concepts in mild cognitive impairment. *Arch Neurol* 2001; 58: 1985–92.

Petersen RC, Thomas RG, Grundman M, *et al*. Vitamin E and donepezil for the treatment of mild cognitive impairment. *N Engl J Med* 2005; 352(23): 2379–88.

Tuokko H, Frerichs R, Graham J, *et al*. Five-year follow-up of cognitive impairment with no dementia. *Arch Neurol* 2003; 60(4): 577–82.

United Nations. *World Population Prospects: The 2004 Revision*. New York, NY: UN; 2005.

Zeng Y, Vaupel JW, Zhenyu X, Chunyuan Z, Yuzhi L. The Healthy Longevity Survey and the Active Life Expectancy of the oldest old in China. *Popul Engl Sel* 2001; 13(10): 95–116.

Chapter 36
Isolated memory disorders

Elka Stefanova and Vladimir Kostic
Institute of Neurology, School of Medicine, University of Belgrade, Belgrade, Serbia

A clinical approach to memory disorders

Memory is a rather complex cognitive domain that can be viewed for clinical purposes in several phases: registration, storage, and retrieval. The disorders could be presented as disturbed episodic short-term memory and an inability to form new memories, or difficulties in long-term memory. Some patients may attempt to fill in gaps in memory with false recollections (confabulations), as temporal misplacement of genuine memories, or newly elaborated events and facts. The longest standing and most deeply ingrained memories, such as one's own name and other very personal memories, may be prominently and exclusively impaired in dissociative (psychogenic) amnesia. A disorder of memory may occur as one feature of an acute confusional state or dementia or as an isolated abnormality as shown in Table 36.1.

Transient global amnesia (TGA)

TGA most commonly occurs in the middle-aged or elderly, with an estimated incidence in persons older than 50 years of 23.5–32 per 100 000 per year. Most patients with TGA have only one single attack and the recurrence rate is 2.5–5% per year for at least 5 years. TGA is a well-defined disorder characterized by a temporary relatively isolated amnesic syndrome with sudden onset of severe memory impairment, including both anterograde and retrograde amnesia, lasting for several hours before resolving gradually over several hours to a day. The patient does not lose personal identity, is often aware that something is the matter, and may complain spontaneously of memory impairment. The mean duration of amnesia is 4 hours (ranging

International Neurology: A Clinical Approach. Edited by Robert P. Lisak, Daniel D. Truong, William M. Carroll, and Roongroj Bhidayasiri. © 2009 Blackwell Publishing, ISBN: 978-1-4051-5738-4.

Table 36.1 Classification of amnesic states.

Acute
Head trauma
Hypoxia or ischemia
Bilateral posterior cerebral artery occlusion
Transient global amnesia
Alcoholic blackouts
Temporal lobe seizures
Dissociative (psychogenic) amnesia
Accompanying confusional state

Chronic
Wernicke–Korsakoff amnesic syndrome
Postencephalitic amnesia
Brain tumor
Paraneoplastic limbic encephalitis
Accompanying dementia

from 2 to 12 hours). Neuropsychological investigation in patients during an episode of transient amnesia has shown a profound episodic memory impairment on tests of both verbal and non-verbal memory, but retrograde amnesia was variable, usually being relatively brief but occasionally prolonged, and worse for recall of episodes than of facts.

In 60–70% of cases the underlying aetiology is unclear. In 25% there was a past history of migraine, with a possible aetiological role. In a minority of cases epilepsy appears to be the underlying cause. There was no association with either a past history of risk factors for vascular disease or clinical signs indicating a vascular pathology. In particular, there was no association with transient focal ischemic attacks. The general consensus is that the amnesia results from transient dysfunction in limbic-hippocampal circuits, crucial to memory formation. Severe bitemporal hypoperfusion has been reported during TGA using single photon emission computed tomography/fluorodeoxyglucose positron emission tomography (SPECT/FDG PET) and after recovery from the episode cerebral perfusion usually returned to normal.

Traumatic amnesia

Memory is commonly the last cognitive function to show improvement following acute trauma, and patients can show the characteristic features of an amnesic syndrome. Studies show that recovery from mild head injury is typically expected 1–3 months post-injury. Head injury may result in either transient or persisting amnesia. It is important to distinguish between retrograde amnesia (RA), which is usually (but not necessarily) relatively brief and post-traumatic amnesia (PTA). Occasionally, PTA may exist without any RA and this is more common in cases of penetrating lesions. The PTA can be assessed with reasonable reliability; the length of PTA is predictive of eventual cognitive, psychiatric, and social outcome. PTA needs to be distinguished from persisting antero-grade memory impairment, which may be detected clinically or by cognitive testing long after the period of PTA has ended and characterized by accelerated forgetfulness of learned information, whereas after PTA, rates of forgetfulness were normal. Patients with PTA seen shortly after the head injury may be in a confused state in which they are unable to incorporate new memories although they may behave in an apparently normal automatic fashion.

Direct trauma can damage the frontal and anterior temporal lobes resulting in contusion, hematoma, and hemorrhage. Rotational and acceleration–deceleration forces may produce shearing or tensile stretching of axons with subsequent gliosis. The resulting intra-axonal changes lead to a failure in axoplasmic transport, axonal swelling, and, ultimately, disconnection, deafferentation, and loss of synaptic connections over a matter of hours or days.

Korsakoff's amnesia

Many cases of Korsakoff's syndrome are diagnosed after acute Wernicke's encephalopathy (WE), which is characterized by confusion, ataxia, nystagmus, and ophthalmoplegia. However, the disorder can also have an insidious onset, and these cases are more likely to come to the attention of psychiatrists: in such cases, there may be either no or only a transient history of WE. Autopsies of adults reveal a higher prevalence of WE lesions (0.8–2.8%) than is predicted by clinical studies (0.04–0.13%). It is estimated that clinical diagnosis has been missed in 75–80% of cases. About 80% patients with WE who survive develop Korsakoff's amnesia known as Wernicke–Korsakoff syndrome (WKS). It is more common in males (M:F ratio 1.7:1). Mortality is about 17%.

Short-term memory is intact in the sense of recall over a matter of seconds, but learning and retention over longer periods are severely impaired, and there is usually a retrograde memory loss. However, patients may question repetitively and have a particular problem in remembering the temporal sequence of events, associated with severe disorientation in time. Whilst it is unlikely that patients with established WKS make a complete recovery, the experience is that a substantial improvement does occur over a matter of years with alcohol abstention. Up to 75% of Korsakoff's patients may show variable degrees of improvement.

The WKS is unusual among memory disorders in that there is a distinct neurochemical pathology with important treatment implications. Thiamine (vitamin B_1) depletion was established as the mechanism giving rise to the acute WE, and the subsequent Korsakoff's amnesia. The effect of thiamine deficiency may be population specific: Asians develop mainly a cardiovascular (wet) beriberi whereas Europeans tend to develop a dry beriberi and WKS. While there is a genetic factor in the form of the transketolase gene mutation predisposing certain heavy drinkers to develop this syndrome (because transketolase is an enzyme that requires thiamine pyrophosphate (TPP) as a co-factor), it does not account for all the properties of transketolase and only very weakly for predisposition to Korsakoff's syndrome. Moreover, it remains unclear how thiamine depletion produces the particular neuropathology found in WKS patients, even though six neurotransmitter systems (including acetylcholine, γ-aminobutyric acid (GABA), and glutamate) are affected by thiamine depletion, either by reduction of TPP-dependent enzyme activity or by direct structural change.

The known neuropathology is characteristic and consists of neuronal loss, micro-hemorrhages, and gliosis in the paraventricular and periaqueductal gray matter, suggesting that the lesions described might disconnect a critical memory circuit running between the temporal lobes and the frontal cortex. MRI studies have indicated more specific atrophy in diencephalic and frontal structures.

Treatment of WKS

Whatever the precise mechanism, treatment as soon as possible with high doses of parenterally administered multivitamins is essential. The Wernicke features respond well to high doses of vitamin B_1 (50–100 mg/day) and such treatment can prevent the occurrence of a chronic Korsakoff's state. The small risk of anaphylaxis is completely outweighed by the large risk of severe brain damage if such treatment is not administered.

Other causes of amnesia

Focal vascular disorders, both infarction and hemorrhage in thalamic, medial temporal, or retrosplenial regions and subarachnoid hemorrhage, can particularly affect memory, while sparing general cognitive function. Severe hypoxia can give rise to an amnesic syndrome following carbon monoxide poisoning or cardiac or respiratory arrest. Herpes simplex encephalitis can give a particularly severe form of amnesic syndrome. Drug overdose, including heroin abuse, may precipitate prolonged unconsciousness and cerebral hypoxia, leading to an amnesic state.

Further reading

Kopelman M. Disorders of memory. *Brain* 2002; 125: 2152–90.
Kritchevsky M, Zouzounis J, Squire LR. Transient global amnesia and functional retrograde amnesia: contrasting examples of episodic memory loss. *Philos Trans R Soc Lond B* 1997; 352: 1747–54.
Sechi GP, Serra A. Wernicke's encephalopathy: new clinical settings and recent advances in diagnosis and management. *Lancet Neurol* 2006; 6: 442–55.

Chapter 37
Mild cognitive impairment

Elka Stefanova and Vladimir Kostic
Institute of Neurology, School of Medicine, University of Belgrade, Belgrade, Serbia

Introduction

The extended average life expectancy over the past 50 years has resulted in a substantial increase in the numbers of individuals over 65 years of age. Careful cross-sectional examination of cognitive function among elderly people, however, reveals a range of cognitive impairment, including deficits in various domains in the absence of clinically defined dementia. The concept of mild cognitive impairment (MCI), given by Petersen (1999) and later revisited (2004), as an intermediate transitional zone between two states, was developed as an attempt to recognize those individuals who are not normal because of deficits in at least one cognitive domain (usually recent memory), but who appear to function independently in daily affairs. Other terms that have been used to define the range of cognitive and functional states that occur between normal and demented include cognitively impaired not demented, possible dementia prodrome, age-associated memory impairment, and age-associated cognitive impairment.

Epidemiology

Prevalence studies show MCI and its subtypes ranging from 3% to 17% of elderly people (over 65 years). The age-specific prevalence of MCI has universally been found to be greater than that of dementia, and MCI is about four times more common than dementia when based on community assessment of non-institutionalized individuals. Despite the range of definitions used, older individuals with any cognitive impairment are at significantly increased risk of future conversion to dementia. The proportion of non-demented elders with isolated memory deficits (1/3) is smaller than the proportion with deficits in multiple cognitive domains (2/3). The risks of developing MCI include apolipoprotein (Apo)E genotype

(for the amnestic form of MCI), depression, racial and constitutional factors, and the presence of cerebrovascular disease. When proper normative values are used, only age and education, and not race or ethnicity, are associated with higher frequency of MCI.

The studies generally show a yearly incidence of dementia of 10–15% within the MCI population, in contrast to a rate of 1–2% per year among normal elderly persons. Conversely, community-based studies tend to show lower rates of conversion (closer to 5–10% per year). Approximately 80% of those who meet the criteria for amnestic MCI will have Alzheimer's disease (AD) within 6 years, and the presence of one or more ApoE4 alleles is associated with a more rapid rate of progression.

Clinical features

The concept of MCI refers to individuals who have some cognitive impairment but are not sufficiently handicapped as to warrant the diagnosis of dementia. The first established criteria for amnestic MCI that have been most widely adapted for use in clinical trials include the following: (1) memory complaint (preferably corroborated by an informant), (2) memory impairment for age and education, (3) generally normal cognitive function except for the memory impairment, (4) normal or only minimally impaired activities of daily living (ADL), and (5) non-demented in the opinion of the investigator and not meeting clinical criteria for dementia. As the field of MCI research has matured, it has become apparent that other clinical patterns of MCI are likely to exist. From a clinical perspective there are at least three presentations, as shown in Table 37.1. The first type is amnestic MCI, and this is the typical MCI with prominent memory impairment; these subjects progressed to AD. The second type, termed multiple-domain MCI, is characterized by slight cognitive impairment in more than one cognitive domain but of insufficient severity to constitute dementia. The third type, single-non-memory domain MCI, refers to cognitive impairment in a single domain such as executive, visuospatial, or language, with preservation of other cognitive skills and insufficient impairment in

International Neurology: A Clinical Approach. Edited by Robert P. Lisak, Daniel D. Truong, William M. Carroll, and Roongroj Bhidayasiri. © 2009 Blackwell Publishing, ISBN: 978-1-4051-5738-4.

123

Table 37.1 The heterogeneous presentation of MCI and possible outcomes.

MCI subtypes	Progression to
Amnestic	Alzheimer's disease
Multiple-domain	Alzheimer's disease
	Vascular dementia
	Normal aging
Single non-memory domain	Frontotemporal dementia
	Lewy body dementia
	Primary progressive aphasia
	Alzheimer's disease

ADL to constitute dementia. These prodromal states may progress to non-AD dementias such as frontotemporal dementia or primary progressive aphasia.

In addition to this clinical heterogeneity, there is also etiological heterogeneity: degenerative, vascular, metabolic, trauma, and psychiatric.

MCI as a clinical diagnosis should correspond to cognitive complaints coming from patients and/or their families, reporting a decline in cognitive functioning relative to previous abilities during the past year, and should be evident by clinical evaluation (impairment in memory or in another cognitive domain). The emphasis should be on the absence of major repercussions on daily life activities and social independence; mild difficulties in complex day-to-day activities should be accepted. The major clinical criterion is absence of dementia.

Pathophysiology

Neuropathological and neurochemical studies are slowly aiding the definition of the brain's status during the earliest stages of symptomatic cognitive impairment as well as presymptomatic AD. Among autopsies of patients who have died in the MCI phase, more than 2/3 have typical AD pathology. Initial conclusions suggest that significant amyloid deposition, neurofibrillary tangle (NFT) formation (especially in the mesial temporal lobe), and some loss of trophin receptors are present in MCI. Recent investigation of the larger cohorts supports the idea that the neuropathology of MCI is somewhere in the middle on a continuum between normal aging and AD dementia. In addition, the synaptic and cholinergic plasticity, which may differ from individual to individual, no doubt contributes to the variability of the pathological findings. Based upon the multiple markers thus far explored, variability in MCI cases is going to be multidimensional, and there is no indication thus far that one specific pathological or biochemical variable will be an absolute quantitative marker of MCI.

Investigations

The doctor makes the diagnosis and evaluation, but a neuropsychological expert may complete the clinical procedure. Because MCI represents a change from normal functioning, patients with MCI should undergo the same screening laboratory studies that other patients with dementia undergo. Additional tests such as brain imaging and cerebrospinal fluid (CSF) biomarkers are becoming more important in the prediction of progression to dementia state.

CSF biomarkers
Several recent studies have specifically addressed the value of CSF biomarkers in identifying prodromal AD. Combinations of abnormal markers (low Aβ42, high t-tau, and high p-tau 181) reached a hazard ratio of 17:20 for predicting AD in a follow-up of 4–6 years. Sensitivities and specificities in this study were >90% and >85%, respectively, which agreed with those in a similar study with a much shorter follow-up (1 year).

Neuroimaging
Overall, MRI/PET studies indicate the current potential of hippocampal formation atrophy measures to predict stage transitions related to AD as well as to describe disease progression from normal elderly to MCI to AD levels of impairment.

It suggests that the earliest changes occur in the anterior medial temporal lobe and fusiform gyrus, and that these changes occur at least 3 years before progression to the diagnosis of AD. Additional recent findings show that reduced entorhinal cortex (EC) size can discriminate between MCI and elderly normal controls and accurately predict future conversion of MCI subjects to AD. In a large prospective study of amnestic MCI patients, the proportion of individuals converting to dementia within 5 years was four times the normal when hippocampal size was 2.5 standard deviations below norms defined for age and sex. There is also evidence to show that size of glucose metabolism (METglu) in temporal neocortex and posterior cingulate gyrus can predict the MCI conversion to AD. In conclusion, the combined use of MRI and CSF diagnostic measures for MCI promises to improve the early and specific diagnosis of MCI as well as our understanding of the course of MCI on both brain and behavior.

Treatment

A pharmacological treatment of MCI would be considered successful if it prevented progression of cognitive and functional deficits and the development of dementia. However, to date there is no proven treatment.

In randomized clinical trials cholinesterase inhibitors, rofecoxib, non-steroidal anti-inflammatory drugs (NSAIDs), and vitamin E have failed to prevent progression of MCI to dementia. Donepezil was found to have a transient preventive effect at 1 year, with a larger and sustained effect in subjects who had at least one ApoE4 allele. With rivastigmine, there was no significant benefit on the progression rate to AD or on cognitive function over 4 years. The evidence is not strong enough for a recommendation for its routine use.

Further reading

Jisha GA, Parisi JE, Dickson DW, *et al*. Neuropathologic outcome of mild cognitive impairment following progression to clinical dementia. *Arch Neurol* 2006; 63(5): 674–81.

Petersen RC. Mild cognitive impairment. *Continuum* 2004; 10: 9–28.

Portet F, Ousset PJ, Visser GB, *et al*. Mild cognitive impairment (MCI) in medical practice: a critical review of the concept and new diagnostic procedure. Report of the MCI Working Group of the European Consortium on Alzheimer's disease. *J Neurol Neurosurg Psychiatry* 2006; 77: 714–18.

Chapter 38
The degenerative dementias

Irena Rektorová[1], Robert Rusina[2], Jakub Hort[3], and Radoslav Matěj[4]

[1]Masaryk University and St. Anne's Hospital, Brno, Czech Republic
[2]Thomayer Teaching Hospital and Institute of Postgraduate Education in Medicine, Prague, Czech Republic
[3]Charles University, Teaching Hospital Motol, Prague, Czech Republic
[4]National Laboratory for Diagnostics of Prion Diseases, Thomayer Teaching Hospital, Prague, Czech Republic

Alzheimer's disease

Introduction

The demographic composition of the world's population is changing considerably, with a marked increase in elderly people. This population aging is accompanied by a growing incidence and prevalence of dementia. Alzheimer's disease (AD) is the most common cause of dementia representing 50–70% of all dementia cases. It is not an inevitable consequence of aging, but its prevalence in the population increases as the number of people over age 65 increases. The neurodegenerative processes in AD precede the onset of dementia. Affected individuals may already have objectively detectable cognitive impairment while still functioning socially and occupationally. This transitional stage between normal aging and dementia is known as "mild cognitive impairment."

Epidemiology

AD affects up to 5% of the population at the age of 65, and the prevalence increases to exceed 40% at the age of 85.

Well-identified risk factors of AD include age, sex (women are at greater risk), and the presence of cerebrovascular disease (CVD). Other putative risk factors may include a history of head trauma and a low level of education. The presence of apolipoprotein ε 4 (Apoε4) provides a genetic risk factor for late onset AD. Inherited AD is rare and accounts for early onset of disease in patients in their 40s or 50s. It is transmitted in autosomal dominant fashion and may be caused by mutations in the *presenilin 1* gene on chromosome 14, the *presenilin 2* gene on chromosome 1, or the amyloid precursor protein gene on chromosome 21.

International Neurology: A Clinical Approach. Edited by Robert P. Lisak, Daniel D. Truong, William M. Carroll, and Roongroj Bhidayasiri. © 2009 Blackwell Publishing, ISBN: 978-1-4051-5738-4.

Pathophysiology

The amyloid precursor protein (APP) is believed to be central to the pathophysiology of AD due to the abnormal cleavage of it leading to the deposit of amyloid β 1–42 fragments. This happens when APP is not cleaved by α-secretases, but by β- and γ-secretases. These insoluble aggregates form neuritic plaques in the brain with a subsequent inflammatory response and cell destruction. Another pathologic feature of AD involves the abnormal processing of τ protein and tangle formation. These neuropathological changes are accompanied by a decrease in cholinergic and other neuromediator transmitters, a reduction in synaptic density, and a loss of neurons.

Clinical features

AD manifests as slowly progressive dementia typically lasting 7–15 years from onset to death. Structures in the medial temporal lobe, particularly the hippocampus and the entorhinal cortex, which are essential for normal memory function, are preferentially affected in early AD. Impairment of episodic memory or spatial orientation is one of the earliest hallmarks of the disease. Patients have difficulties recalling recently learned information, with no improvement after cuing. If they are provided clues or offered a list of items from which they are forced to choose the learned material, they do not perform better. Recent memory is more impaired than remote memory, which deteriorates later as the disease progresses. For the same reason, impairment of other non-memory cognitive domains emerges when the disease spreads beyond the hippocampus. Non-declarative memory, such as of motor skills, is usually spared. Developed AD features impairment of memory, visuospatial, language, and executive function. If non-memory domains are disproportionately impaired, it may reflect a frontal variant of AD or posterior cortical atrophy. If so other causes of dementia should be considered.

In addition to the cognitive disability, there is an evident decrease in functional capacity as the disease progresses. Neuropsychiatric symptoms depict the typical clinical manifestation. Therefore, in clinical evaluation, the history from both patient and informant is an essential element of the diagnostic process.

Investigations

The general neurological examination of a patient with AD is usually normal except for the mental status evaluation. In addition to the routine work-up, measurement of thyroid function and vitamin B_{12} levels can disclose common comorbidities in the elderly. HIV and syphilis serology can be tested. Cranial imaging, preferably MRI, should be performed on all patients to exclude other contributions to the cognitive deficit, some of which are treatable. Cortical atrophy of variable degree is commonly revealed. The presence of mild-to-moderate vascular changes does not exclude the diagnosis of AD. Functional imaging with single photon emission computed tomography (SPECT) or fluorodeoxyglucose positron emission tomography (FDG PET) typically demonstrates hypoperfusion or hypometabolism in the temporal and parietal lobes. Cerebrospinal fluid (CSF) examination is optional except in cases with a differential diagnosis of inflammatory disease and the identification of the 14-3-3 protein is helpful in diagnosis of Creutzfeldt–Jakob disease (CJD). Genetic testing can be considered in those with early onset or who have a familial occurrence of dementia. In such cases Apoε4 brings more confidence to the diagnosis, rather than being predictive in asymptomatic "at risk" individuals.

Neuropsychological testing can elucidate the pattern and topical characteristics of the cognitive deficit. However, the most commonly employed screening test, the Mini Mental State Examination (MMSE), is not appropriate to diagnose early dementia as it is age and education dependent and oversimplified for mnestic assessment. Further, it does not evaluate frontal function, which devalues its use in differential diagnosis of AD. Therefore a thorough neuropsychological assessment is more beneficial. It should always include evaluation of attention, memory, language, visuospatial skills, and executive functions. Some of the widely used instruments include the Wechsler Adult Intelligence Scale-Revised (WAIS-R) for assessment of general intellectual function, and there are many tests targeting specific domains. Executive functions may be assessed by verbal fluency, the Trail Making Test (A or B), Wisconsin Card Sorting Test, digit-symbol test, or Stroop Test. Visuospatial skills are assessed by the Rey–Osterrieth Complex Figure. The Boston Naming Test examines language. Mnestic function can be evaluated by the Wechsler Memory Scale, Rey Auditory Verbal Learning Test, California Verbal Learning Test, Grober–Bushke Memory Test, or Benton Visual Retention Test. Attention can be evaluated by means of digit span, and motor skills by finger tapping.

An assessment of the Instrumental Activities of Daily Living (IADL) is an inevitable part of the rating. Global opinion on patient cognition and functioning may be expressed by the Clinical Dementia Rating (CDR) Scale. Neuropsychiatric symptoms can be assessed by the Geriatric Depression Scale, Cornell Scale for Depression, or Neuropsychiatric Inventory (NPI). Neuropsychiatric symptoms, present in most patients with AD, are distressing, and may affect the quality of life of both patients and their caregivers. They may be valuable in distinguishing Lewy body (early hallucinations) and frontotemporal (deliberation, apathy) dementia. Depression may worsen or even mimic dementia.

Clinical diagnosis

Since being first diagnosed in 1906, many clinical and neuropathological tools have been used to identify AD. Currently the widely used DSM IV criteria for dementia and those National Institute of Neurological and Communicative Disorders and Stroke and the Alzheimer's Disease and Related Disorders Association (NINCDS–ADRDA) criteria for possible, probable, or definite AD lag behind the latest knowledge in some aspects. Most importantly the diagnosis of AD is one of exclusion despite having typical clinical features derived from its underlying pathology. The DSM V criteria should indeed reflect these facts.

The episodic memory impairment criterion together with application of various biomarkers is likely to be used for AD diagnosis in the future. The ideal biomarker for AD should detect the fundamental neuropathological features of AD, with sufficient diagnostic sensitivity, and should have specificity for distinguishing other dementias. It should be reliable, reproducible, non-invasive, simple to perform, and inexpensive. Promising biomarkers reflecting the underlying AD pathology comprise the still experimental and not readily accessible Pittsburgh Compound B (PIB) PET with *in vivo* amyloid imaging as well as structural (MR volumetry) or functional (SPECT) imaging and the clinically growing experience of CSF biomarkers. Increased levels of total τ or phosphorylated-τ protein and decreased levels of β-amyloid in CSF are suggestive of AD, with sensitivity and specificity over 90% when used together. The role of platelet APP-derived protein levels in the assessment of AD has been evaluated favourably. Neuropsychological testing should cover all the major cognitive domains mentioned above with special attention to memory function.

Treatment

Current treatment options are limited to the acetylcholinesterase inhibitors (donepezil, galantamine, and rivastigmine) for mild to moderate AD and memantine for moderate AD. Since these compounds are symptomatic only, there is a significant effort to develop disease-modifying medication. Experimentally these endeavours attempt to interfere with the underlying pathological processes represented mainly by amyloidogenesis and are expected to reduce the progression of AD. Other available medications only temporarily reduce the rate of decline. Vitamin E failed to prove effective, as did anti-inflammatory medications. Oestrogen replacement therapy may even worsen AD by interfering with concomitant vascular pathology. Cholinesterase inhibitors all have similar treatment potential, but may differ in the rate of side effects and individual patient response. This variability arises from their different pharmacological profile.

Pharmacotherapy of AD also includes management of neuropsychiatric symptoms. In this field, selective serotonin reuptake inhibitor (SSRI) antidepressants are preferred, and atypical neuroleptics are used to cope with agitation, aggression, delusions, or hallucinations. Treatment of neuropsychiatric symptoms behaviorally or pharmacologically ameliorates the caregiver's burden and improves quality of life for both patients and caregivers.

Non-pharmacological management, including cognitive training, is an underlying part of the treatment approach. Working with caregivers and health care and social services providers is part of building an alliance for optimal patient care.

Dementia with Lewy bodies and Parkinson's disease dementia

Introduction

Parkinson's disease (PD) and dementia with Lewy bodies (DLB) are both "synucleinopathies," that is neurodegenerative disorders that are characterized by fibrillary aggregates of α-synuclein protein in the cytoplasm of selective populations of neurons and glia. α-synuclein accumulates in Lewy bodies (LB) and dystrophic neurites that constitute the pathological hallmark of PD/DLB. While cortical LB density is not robustly correlated with either the severity or duration of dementia, extrastriatal dopaminergic and particularly cholinergic deficits play a central role in mediating dementia in both conditions. Clinically, PD dementia (PDD) is similar to DLB in terms of the main clinical symptoms (fluctuating cognition, visual hallucinations, and parkinsonian features). The difference between PDD and DLB is in the temporal sequence in which symptoms occur and therefore some authors refer to them as a disease spectrum.

Epidemiology

DLB is the second most common cause of degenerative dementia after AD. DLB is responsible for 15–20% of all dementia in old age. The prevalence of PDD in community-based PD cohorts is between 20% and 40%, reaching up to 78% over longer follow-up. The risk of developing dementia in PD is 1.7–5.9 times higher than in the age-, gender-, and education-matched populations.

Dementia in PD is associated with a twofold increase in mortality, reduced quality of life, and nursing home placement.

Pathophysiology and neurochemistry

Cortical and subcortical LB pathology is sufficient to cause dementia, although Alzheimer-type pathology may be present as well (although to a degree insufficient to cause dementia). A neuropathological staging protocol (six stages) has been proposed for sporadic PD according to the topographic distribution of PD-related pathology. According to this staging, the disease begins in the lower brainstem and progresses through the basal forebrain until it reaches the cerebral cortex. The problem of the staging is that LB pathology is not correlated with neuronal losses in the relevant regions. While cognitive decline between stages 3 and 6 indicates that the risk of developing dementia increases with disease progression, in some individuals cognitive impairment can develop in the presence of mild cortical pathology changes; conversely, widespread cortical lesions do not necessarily equate with the degree of dementia.

Although an abnormal degeneration of the dopamine-producing cells in the substantia nigra (A9) may be less extensive in DLB than in PDD, striatal dopamine concentrations are reduced to an equivalent level. In PD, cognitive impairment, in particular executive deficits, has been related to the dysfunction of the dorsolateral striatoprefrontal loop consecutive to the loss of dopaminergic nigral neurons. Extrastriatal dopaminergic systems have also been implicated (degeneration of dopamine-producing cells in ventral tegmentum (A10) and deficient mesocortical projections to the frontal cortex). However, dementia develops in part due to concomitant widespread brain pathology, including predominantly cholinergic cell losses (in the nucleus basalis of Meynert, tegmental pedunculopontine, and laterodorsal nuclei) projecting to the thalamus, basal ganglia, and prefrontal cortex. Extensive neocortical cholinergic deficits are present in both DLB and PDD; choline acetyltransferase reductions in DLB correlate with cognitive impairment and visual hallucinations.

Clinical features of DLB and PDD

For a clinical diagnosis of DLB, see Table 38.1. If one or more suggestive features in addition to one or more core features is present, a diagnosis of probable DLB is made. Two core features are sufficient for a diagnosis of probable DLB, while the absence of core features excludes the diagnosis of probable DLB. One or more suggestive features are sufficient for the diagnosis of possible DLB. Disproportionate early visual impairment and visuo-constructive dysfunction are characteristics of this disease.

In contrast to DLB, widely accepted definitions of PDD are still lacking. Motor slowing and depression

Table 38.1 Revised criteria for the clinical diagnosis of DLB. (Adapted from McKeith IG, Dickson DW, Emre M, *et al*. Diagnosis and management of dementia with Lewy bodies: third report of the DLB Consortium. *Neurology* 2005; 65: 1863–72.)

Central feature: dementia (deficits on tests of attention, executive function, and visuospatial ability may be prominent)

Core features
- Fluctuating cognition
- Recurrent visual hallucinations
- Spontaneous features of parkinsonism

Suggestive features
- REM sleep behavior disorder
- Severe neuroleptic sensitivity
- Low dopamine transporter uptake in the basal ganglia demonstrated by SPECT or PET imaging

Supportive features
- Repeated falls and syncope
- Transient, unexplained loss of consciousness
- Severe autonomic dysfunction
- Hallucinations in other modalities
- Delusions
- Depression
- Relative preservation of medial temporal lobe structures on CT/MRI scans
- Low uptake on SPECT/PET perfusion scan with reduced occipital activity
- Prominent slow EEG waveforms with temporal lobe transient sharp waves
- Abnormal MIBG myocardial scintigraphy

REM: rapid eye movement; SPECT: single photon emission computed tomography; PET: positron emission tomography; CT: computed tomography; MRI: magnetic resonance imaging; EEG: electroencephalogram; MIBG: metaiodobenzyl guanidine.

may confound testing. The neuropsychological profile of PDD is characterized by a progressive "dysexecutive" syndrome together with memory deficits and impaired abstract reasoning in the absence of higher cortical function deficits such as aphasia, apraxia, or agnosia that are typical of AD dementia. Neuropsychological studies have provided evidence that executive functions are usually affected in non-demented patients with PD. However, daily functioning is not compromised. Executive processes are involved in the planning and allocation of attentional resources to ensure that goal-directed behavior is initiated, maintained, and monitored adequately to achieve goals. According to this definition, executive processes are also an integral part of tasks for which appropriate response generation requires the suppression of habitual responses (as examined, e.g., by the Stroop Test). Recent findings have indicated that selective frontal dysfunction early in the course of the disease (as measured, e.g., by the picture completion subtest of the Wechsler Adult Intelligence Scale, a verbal fluency test, or the interference section of the Stroop Test), might be an indicative factor

for the development of dementia later in the course of the disease. Risk factors include patient age, lack of education, severe motor deficits, rigidity/bradykinesia/axial symptoms dominance, postural instability, family history of dementia, male gender, therapy-induced psychiatric disturbances, and depression.

It has to be pointed out that PDD symptoms are very similar to those in DLB. The motor phenotype of postural instability and gait difficulty with repeated falls are common for both disorders. According to the DLB consensus criteria, DLB and PDD differ with respect to the temporal evolution of the disease process. DLB should be diagnosed if dementia occurs before, concurrently, or within 12 months of the onset of parkinsonian symptoms. Conversely, PDD should be diagnosed when dementia develops in fully established PD, but at least 12 months after the onset of parkinsonian features. The 12-month cut-off is arbitrary, and therefore "LB disease" may be a preferable term according to some authors.

Differential diagnosis

The main differential diagnoses of DLB/PDD are AD (usually an early amnestic syndrome), vascular dementia (VaD) (usually step-wise cognitive deterioration, pyramidal signs, and relevant CVD changes on brain MRI), PD plus syndromes (progressive supranuclear palsy, multiple system atrophy, corticobasal degeneration), and CJD (rapid progression of dementia, characteristic electroencephalogram (EEG) changes), but sometimes it is difficult to distinguish between PDD/DLB and these other illnesses, particularly in less typical cases. This may be due to some overlapping features. MRI may be helpful and dopamine transporter imaging (SPECT or PET) may be useful in differentiating AD and DLB/PDD, in particular since it reveals the integrity of presynaptic dopamine neurons. It is also important to distinguish Wilson's disease, the rigid-akinetic Westphal variant of Huntington's disease, and other conditions such as AIDS–dementia complex, hypoparathyroidism, or carbon monoxide (CO) intoxication.

Treatment

From a practical point of view, it is important to realize that dementia in PD and DLB limits the drug treatment of extrapyramidal motor symptoms, since all antiparkinsonian drugs may exacerbate psychotic features and confusion. When addressing cognitive impairment, anticholinergic drugs particularly should be discontinued, since these agents may lead to a deterioration of memory and executive functions. Furthermore, blockade of muscarinic cholinergic receptors in PD has been associated with increased Alzheimer-type pathology.

Conversely, and in line with the described neurochemical changes in PDD/DLB, the positive effects of acetylcholinesterase inhibitors (ACHEIs) have been demonstrated by several open-label studies, but (to date) most placebo-controlled data are available for rivastigmine. Rivastigmine produced moderate but significant improvements in global ratings for dementia, cognition, and behavioral symptoms; the magnitude of effects was similar to that observed in AD patients treated with ACHEIs. The most frequent adverse effects were nausea, vomiting, and tremor.

If ACHEIs are ineffective, or if more acute symptom control of behavior is required, a cautious trial of atypical antipsychotics is recommended (clozapine, quetiapine, and aripiprazole in low doses), but clinicians should be vigilant to the possibility of a sensitivity reaction. Nonpharmacologic intervention has the potential to ameliorate many symptoms (e.g., coping strategies for visual hallucinations), but none has been systematically studied.

Vascular dementia

Introduction

Vascular dementia (VaD), AD, and DLB are the most frequent causes of dementia in the elderly. Epidemiological data suggest that at least 15–20% of all dementia cases in patients over the age of 65 are of vascular origin. There are important differences in the epidemiological risk factors for VaD worldwide.

Pure VaD is considered to be relatively rare in comparison to AD. There is, however, increasing evidence that many patients may in fact suffer from mixed dementia, for example coexistent AD and VaD or vascular involvement in AD.

The relationship between CVD (represented typically by white matter lesions on neuroimaging and/or cerebral amyloid angiopathy (CAA)) and cognitive impairment remains controversial. Sporadic CAA, a largely underestimated cause of VaD, has been found to occur more often than previously believed with the advent of T2-gradient echo MRI. It is associated with a significant risk of recurrent brain hemorrhage in patients treated with aspirin or warfarin. Genetic disorders leading to VaD are rare, but represent an interesting model of pure VaD enabling a better understanding of the pathophysiology and clinical features of VaD.

Current diagnostic criteria and therapeutic options for VaD are listed in Table 38.2.

Epidemiology

Dementia markedly increases with age, from around 5% at age 65, doubling every 5 years, to reach about 30% at age 80 to 40–70% at age 95. In Europe and North and South America, AD is estimated to be more common than VaD, whereas the ratio is inverted in Asia. In Africa, dementia of both types seems to be rare, but this low prevalence has yet to be confirmed by incidence data.

Table 38.2 Diagnostic criteria for VaD. (Adapted from Pohjasvaara T, Mantyla R, Ylikoski R, *et al*. Comparison of different clinical criteria (DSM-III, ADDTC, ICD-10, NINDS-AIREN, DSM-IV) for the diagnosis of vascular dementia. *Stroke* 2000; 31: 2952–7.)

Californian criteria (Alzheimer's Disease Diagnosis and Treatment Center, ADDTC)
Evidence of at least two ischemic strokes by history or neurological signs
and/or
neuroimaging studies (CT or T1-weighted MRI),
or
occurrence of a single stroke with a clearly documented temporal relationship to the onset of dementia
and
evidence of at least one infarct outside the cerebellum by CT or T1-weighted MRI

NINDS–AIREN (National Institute of Neurological Disorders and Stroke–Association Internationale pour la Recherche et l'Enseignement en Neurosciences) criteria
CVD defined by the presence of focal signs on neurological examination
and
evidence of relevant cerebrovascular disease by brain imaging (MRI) including
multiple large-vessel infarcts
or single strategically placed infarct (angular gyrus, thalamus, basal forebrain, posterior cerebral artery, or anterior cerebral artery)
or multiple basal ganglia and white matter lacunes
or extensive periventricular white matter lesions
or combinations thereof.
A relationship between the above two disorders manifested or inferred by the presence of at least one of the following:
Onset of dementia within 3 months after a recognized stroke
Abrupt deterioration in cognitive functions or fluctuating, stepwise progression of cognitive deficits

These differences could be attributed to difficulties in dementia diagnosis in areas with high rates of illiteracy and to different life expectancies throughout the world.

Pure vascular and mixed dementia

The term "vascular dementia" is quite heterogeneous and may refer to the following conditions:

1 Involvement of an important ("strategic") brain area, with subsequent cognitive impairment. For example, anterior cerebral artery infarction may cause apathy, behavioral changes, aphasia, or apraxia; bilateral anterior thalamic destruction leads to a severe dysexecutive syndrome with personality changes because of interruption of subcortical pathways; temporal hematoma may present with aphasia and memory loss.

2 Multiple lesions (corresponding to the term "multi-infarct dementia"). Typically, there is a sudden onset after stroke with a fluctuating or stepwise course. The cognitive impairment depends on the size, number, and distribution of the lesions, often has a subcortical profile, and may be accompanied by focal neurologic signs, such as gait disturbance, extrapyramidal features, or incontinence.

3 Widespread subcortical ischemia in many cases exhibits a decline that is not necessarily rapidly progressive. The development of large and often confluent lesions in the white matter leads to subcortical VaD (historically known as Binswanger's disease), with pronounced executive dysfunction, forgetfulness, and attention and working memory deficits, but relatively preserved autobiographical memory. Mood changes, dysarthria, and gait disturbances are frequent.

Besides these "pure" forms of VaD, the coincidence of vascular involvement and primary neurodegenerative dementia (AD in most cases) may be seen, corresponding to the term mixed dementia. Clinically there is a mixture of subcortical features, correlating with white matter changes and/or multiple vascular lesions on MRI and cortical dementia with predominant episodic memory loss due to degenerative hippocampal involvement.

Cerebrovascular disease and cognitive impairment

The term subcortical ischemic vascular disease (SIVD) has been proposed for small-vessel diseases (such as arteriosclerosis, lipohyalinosis, and CAA) causing diffuse, often confluent changes in cerebral white matter on MRI. The interpretation of such neuroimaging findings remains controversial. SIVD is probably one of the most common causes of cognitive decline in elderly people, with a clinical profile characteristic of the dysexecutive profile of subcortical dementia. However, many patients with leukoencephalopathy remain relatively cognitively unaffected or only slightly impaired.

Sporadic CAA is caused by the deposit of fibrils of amyloid-beta peptide in cortical and leptomeningeal blood vessels. This disease increases with age (being rare under 50 years, it is present in up to 50% of people over age 90 years). CAA is usually asymptomatic, but can present with lobar hemorrhage, white matter lesions, and progressive cognitive decline. Neuroimaging is very helpful in the diagnosis, using a specific sequence – T2-gradient echo MRI – able to show asymptomatic cerebral microbleeds. The diagnosis of CAA microbleeds is important for two reasons. CAA may cause cognitive decline in its own right and often manifests as recurrent intracerebral hemorrhage. Therefore, in any elderly patient presenting with cognitive impairment and white matter lesions, the diagnosis of CAA should be tested by T2-gradient echo MRI, to avoid the increased risk of further brain hemorrhage if aspirin or warfarin treatment is being suggested.

The term poststroke dementia (PSD) refers to all types of dementia that occur after stroke. The most common causes of PSD are VaD, AD, and mixed dementia. Stroke is a major risk factor for dementia – cognitive impairment is three times more common and dementia is twice as frequent in individuals who have had a stroke than in the general population. This tendency increases with age.

Genetic disorders

The most frequent hereditary VaD is cerebral autosomal dominant arteriopathy with subcortical infarcts and leukoencephalopathy (CADASIL), caused by mutations in the *Notch 3* gene on chromosome 19 resulting in silent lacunar infarcts or typical anterior temporal white matter changes on neuroimaging.

The clinical picture typically includes migraine with aura, repetitive strokes, and dementia with psychomotor slowing, executive, and visuospatial deficits. Psychiatric features and seizures may occur. Working and short-term memory defects appear insidiously, but with a long-lasting relative preservation of the encoding process in episodic memory impairment.

CADASIL reflects a pure subcortical ischemic vascular cognitive impairment and it is therefore a suitable pure VaD model for research and clinical trials for management of this type of dementia.

A possible mixed dementia model is the autosomal dominant familial British dementia with amyloid angiopathy (FBR), caused by a point mutation in the BRI gene. It is characterized by spastic tetraparesis, ataxia, and progressive dementia with impaired recognition and recall memory, delayed visual recall, and dysexecutive features.

MRI may show atrophy, white matter hyperintensities tending to confluence, lacunar infarcts, and extensive hemorrhages. Neuropathological hallmarks are amyloid deposits in leptomeningeal and brain vessels, neuronal cell loss, amyloid plaques, and τ-positive neurofibrillary tangles. Therefore, unlike hereditary hemorrhages with pure amyloid angiopathies (the Danish, Dutch, or Icelandic type) or sporadic CAA, FBR is considered to be a primary degenerative dementia involving severe hippocampal pathology unrelated to the vascular involvement alone.

Clinical diagnosis

The existence of multiple diagnostic criteria makes the diagnosis of dementia quite difficult to establish. The criteria differ by the time of their elaboration, their specificity, and their sensitivity, and may not be mutually compatible. The most frequently used criteria worldwide are summarized in Table 38.2.

The diagnosis of VaD in general requires: (1) the presence of dementia; (2) signs of CVD on clinical examination and neuroimaging (CT/MRI); and (3) a relationship between the two preceding points. This can be defined either by the time of onset (e.g., dementia develops within 3–6 months after stroke) or by the evolution (abrupt onset and/or stepwise progression and fluctuating course). The size and topography of vascular brain lesions may also play a role.

Treatment

At the present time, no proven causative treatment is available for vascular cognitive impairment. Therefore, primary and secondary prevention of cerebrovascular events is crucial.

Vascular risk factors – primary and secondary prevention

As in stroke management, it is essential to aggressively treat vascular risk factors, including arterial hypertension in particular, dyslipidemia, ischemic heart disease, atrial fibrillation, diabetes, atherosclerosis, and smoking.

Secondary prevention, like stroke management and prevention, again concentrates on the usual well-established treatments of rigorous treatment of hypertension and diabetes, and the administration of statins and antiplatelet agents as well as warfarin for atrial fibrillation and carotid endarterectomy.

Symptomatic treatment of VaD

Meta-analyses of studies of several drugs used in VaD, including vasodilators, nootropics, and antioxidants, remain disappointing. Only a few drugs, such as propentofylline and memantine, have shown some promising effect. As with AD, there is some evidence suggesting a decrease in acetylcholine transmission in VaD. Results from recent trials using cholinesterase inhibitors in the treatment of VaD are also promising, but their routine use in VaD management is not accepted in most countries.

Frontotemporal dementia

Introduction

Frontotemporal dementia (FTD), also referred to as frontotemporal lobar degeneration (FTLD), is the third most common dementia of degenerative origin after AD and DLB. The disease onset is usually before 65 years of age, but ranges from 35 to 75 years. When compared with AD, patients with FTLD tend to have a faster progression of cognitive and functional deficits and a shorter survival time (median survival of 8 years). Nevertheless, the reported range of disease duration varies widely (from 2 to 20 years) and depends on the clinical subtype. FTLD with symptoms of motor neuron disease (FTLD-MND) seems to have the poorest prognosis. Early alteration in personality and social conduct, dysexecutive syndrome, and speech problems are dominant features of FTLD. Conversely, an early severe amnesia, deficits in visuospatial function, and spatial disorientation contradict a clinical diagnosis of FTLD. FTLD is recognized by three main clinical syndromes: behavioral-dysexecutive (frontal) variant (fvFTLD), progressive non-fluent aphasia (PNFA), and semantic dementia (SD).

Epidemiology

FTLD accounts for 5–20% of all patients with dementia. The disease has a high familial incidence (positive family history has been found in up to 40% of patients) and in some families an autosomal dominant pattern of inheritance has been suggested. Mutation in tau (MAPT) gene encoding for the microtubule-associated protein tau has been demonstrated with a linkage to chromosomes 17 and 3. Familial FTD with parkinsonism linked to chromosome 17 (FTD-17) may be a possible phenotypic presentation with either parkinsonism or MND, or with both. Recently, a mutation in the progranulin (PGRN) gene has been identified in patients with τ-negative and ubiquitin-positive pathology. The clinical syndrome is variable, and has included dysphasia, disinhibition, and parkinsonism (see also Pathology below).

Clinical features and diagnosis

The course of FTLD is one of gradual evolution. The clinical criteria of the three FTLD variants (core diagnostic features) are listed in Table 38.3. It is noteworthy that clinical features of the three variants may combine during the course of the illness. To fulfil the criteria for the clinical diagnosis of probable FTLD, all core features must be present. Physical signs are few in contrast to prominent mental changes; for example, parkinsonian symptoms usually emerge during the late phase of the illness. Supportive features common to each of the

Table 38.3 Frontotemporal lobar degeneration: core features. (Adapted from Neary D, Snowden JS, Gustafson L, *et al.* Frontotemporal lobar degeneration: a consesnsus on clinical diagnostic criteria. *Neurology* 1998; 51: 1546–54.)

Frontal (behavioral-dysexecutive) variant (fvFTD)
- Insidious onset and gradual progression
- Early decline in social interpersonal conduct
- Early impairment in regulation of personal conduct
- Early emotional blunting
- Early loss of insight

Progressive non-fluent aphasia (PNFA)
- Insidious onset and gradual progression
- Non-fluent spontaneous speech with at least one of the following:
- Agrammatism
- Phonemic paraphasias (sound-based errors; e.g., "cap" for "cat")
- Anomia (difficulty in naming)

Semantic dementia (SD)
- Insidious onset and gradual progression
- Language disorder characterized by:
- Progressive, fluent, empty spontaneous speech
- Loss of word meaning with impaired naming and comprehension
- Semantic paraphasias (semantically related words replace correct nominal terms; e.g., "animal" for "elephant") and/or
- Perceptual disorder characterized by:
- Prosopagnosia (impaired recognition of familiar faces) and/or
- Associative agnosia (impairment of object identity)
- Preserved drawing reproduction
- Preserved single-word repetition
- Preserved ability to read aloud and write to dictation orthographically regular words (words with regular spelling-to-sound correspondence)

three clinical subtypes include disease onset before 65 years, a positive family history in a first-degree relative, and physical signs of motor neuron disease (MND) or parkinsonism. Formal neuropsychological assessment, brain imaging, and electroencephalography (EEG) usually provide support for the clinical diagnosis and help to differentiate other conditions associated with dementia. Major exclusion features are an early amnestic syndrome, spatial disorientation, myoclonus, and speech with a loss of train of thought.

Frontal (behavioral-dysexecutive) variant (fvFTD)

Behavioral features are mostly characterized by a profound alteration in personality and in social conduct, social disinhibition with impulsive and inappropriate behavior, loss of volition, distractibility, emotional blunting, and loss of empathy and insight. "Dysexecutive" syndrome refers to impaired attention, abstraction, planning, and problem solving.

Progressive non-fluent aphasia (PNFA)

Progressive non-fluent expressive aphasia is a dominant feature of this variant. It is particularly characterized by phonological and grammatical errors and word retrieval problems. Writing and reading difficulties develop as well (Figure 38.1). In contrast, word and sentence comprehension is relatively well preserved. In addition to the "telegraphic" speech, drawing may also be simplistic and organic (Figure 38.2).

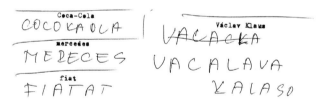

Figure 38.1 Phonemic paragraphia while copying internationally known words and the name of the president of the Czech Republic.

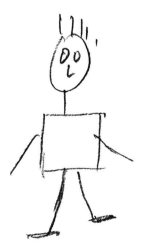

Figure 38.2 Drawing of a man.

Semantic dementia (SD)

In this type of FTLD, a severe naming and word comprehension impairment develops, while the speech is fluent and grammatically correct. Copying, writing, reading, and repetition are relatively spared. An inability to recognize the meaning of visually presented items is characteristic and is referred to as associative agnosia. Patients who possessed sketching skills provide an insight into the nature of the deficit. For example, they may draw trucks on legs or chairs atop cars. It appears that these patients lack knowledge of the intrinsic properties of things, and the loss of meaning is present for both verbal and non-verbal concepts. In contrast, they are able to remember recent events, and computing abilities and visuo-spatial skills are spared.

Investigations

Assessing behavioral and symbolic functions is necessary. A detailed neuropsychological examination is often needed to assess executive function. Addenbrooke's Cognitive Examination is a bedside screening test that may be helpful in distinguishing FTLD and AD. Executive and behavioral deficits may be tested by the Frontal Assessment Battery (FAB), Frontal Behavioral Inventory (FBI), Frontal Behavioral Score (FBS), or Neuropsychiatric Inventory (NPI).

The EEG may be normal or reveal mild non-specific slowing of waveforms (useful in differentiating CJD). Single photon emission computed tomography (SPECT) or positron emission tomography (PET) usually shows symmetrical or asymmetrical hypoperfusion/hypometabolism in the frontal and/or temporal lobes depending on the clinical subtype. MRI may demonstrate similar lobar atrophy but is less sensitive than functional imaging and may often be normal. New MRI techniques (voxel-based morphology, 1H MR spectroscopy, functional MRI, diffusion tension imaging) can be more sensitive but are to date used only for research purposes. Routine CSF examination is not helpful for diagnosis. Recent studies have shown that evaluation of specific CSF markers such as τ protein, $A\beta_{1-42}$, and isoprostane may be of help in differentiating FTLD and AD.

Pathology

Grossly there is atrophy of the frontal and anterior temporal lobes. A complicated classification has been developed based on classic neuropathological findings, immunohistochemical analysis of τ protein and ubiquitin, and biochemical studies into the isoform composition of the insoluble τ deposits. To simplify, we talk about "tauopathies" (with intracellular inclusions that contain insoluble τ protein and are therefore τ-positive) or "ubiquitinopathies" (with protein aggregates that contain ubiquitin and are therefore τ-negative but ubiquitin-positive). A typical (although rather rare) example of a tauopathy is Pick's disease, whereas FTLD-MND is a typical example of ubiquitinopathy. Interestingly, ubiquitinopathies are the most common type of FTLD, accounting for approximately 60% of all FTLD. They may present with or without clinical and pathological evidence of MND. Recently, transactive response DNA-binding protein 43 (TDP-43) was shown to be the major component of the ubiquitinated inclusions and this finding supports the new concept of TDP-43 proteinopathies. If no pathological protein aggregates are found, the term dementia lacking distinctive histopathologic features (DLDH) has been used.

Arnold Pick (who was born in the homeland of the authors) first described a clinical picture of dementia with frontotemporal brain atrophy. Pick neurons (argyrophilic intraneuronal inclusions) and Pick bodies (swollen achromatic cells) characteristic of Pick's disease were identified later by Alois Alzheimer. Nowadays, some authors prefer the term "Pick complex," which comprises a heterogeneous group of disorders from the clinical, genetic, and pathological point of view (FTD spectrum; in addition to described entities it also includes progressive supranuclear palsy or corticobasal degeneration).

Based on clinicopathological studies, it has been suggested that τ-positive pathologies, particularly Pick's disease, are the most common substrate of primary progressive aphasia, while ubiquitin-positive pathologies are the most common substrate of SD and FTLD-MND. Nevertheless, the clinical picture may vary widely and, for example, progranulin gene mutation cases may have a typical phenotype of both tauopathies (such as PNFA, extrapyramidal features) and ubiquitinopathies.

Differential diagnosis

It is essential to distinguish particularly between AD (severe amnestic syndrome, spatial disorientation), VaD (occurrence of ictal events, physical signs, MRI correlate of cerebrovascular lesions), DLB (visual hallucinations, fluctuations in cognition, REM sleep behavioral disorder), and Huntington's disease (typically occurrence of chorea). It is very difficult to differentiate FTLD from CJD disease or the frontal variant of AD.

Therapy

Patients with FTLD show deficiencies in the serotonin and dopamine neurotransmitter systems, while the acetylcholine system appears relatively intact. Antidepressant treatment (serotonergic medication) significantly improves behavioral symptoms but not cognitive deficits in FTLD. To date, only trazodone has been tested in a blinded randomized placebo-controlled trial.

Prion diseases

Introduction

Prions (proteinaceous infectious particles) are unique infectious agents lacking nucleic acids and represented only by a self-replicating protein molecule. Prion protein (PrP) is encoded by the PRNP gene, located on the short arm of chromosome 20. PrP molecules have been found on the outer surface of neuronal cell membranes, but also in other tissues, indicating that they may have different functions depending on their location.

The essential pathophysiological process is a conformational transition of PrP^C ("normal" prion protein) into PrP^{Sc} ("infectious" prion protein). PrP^C has a higher α-helical content (about 40%), whereas PrP^{Sc} contains 45% β-sheets and 30% α- helix and therefore shows remarkable amyloidogenic properties. Prion theory has recently increased in popularity, and a Nobel Prize was awarded for the discovery of prions; however, some scientists still believe the transmissible agent is virus-like and that it contains DNA.

Human prion diseases are called "transmissible spongiform encephalopathies" (TSE) because of experimental transmissibility to animals and their characteristic neuropathology, involving spongiform change. CJD is the prototype of a fatal human neurodegenerative disorder.

The human TSEs, of which CJD is by far the most common, appear to occur sporadically in about 85% of cases. Another 5–15% are inherited, and the remaining cases are iatrogenic. Gerstmann–Sträussler–Scheinker disease (GSS) and fatal familial insomnia (FFI) are extremely rare human transmissible neurodegenerative disorders and could be considered as familial variants of CJD. In the 1950s, another human TSE, kuru, was found to be endemic in the Fore tribe of Papua New Guinea with a prevalence as high as 2% in some tribes due to ritualistic cannibalism.

Creutzfeldt–Jakob disease (CJD)

Epidemiology

CJD is thought to occur worldwide, but systematic surveillance has been established only in a minority of countries. The real incidence of the disease in most of the world is unknown. A recent large study of CJD in the European Union suggests an annual incidence of 0.5–1.5 cases per million; both sexes are affected equally, and no distinct pattern of socioeconomic incidence prevails. The mean age at onset is 65 years, with a range from 14 to 92 years. The cause of sporadic CJD (sCJD) remains unknown despite extensive study.

Clinical features of sCJD

The classical diagnostic triad of CJD is a rapidly progressive dementia, myoclonus, and a characteristic EEG pattern. Diagnostic criteria are summarized in Table 38.4. The median and mean duration of illness is 4.5 and 8 months respectively; only 4% of patients survive longer than 2 years.

Patients usually present with cognitive decline, ataxia, and visual disturbance, either alone or in combination.

Table 38.4 Diagnostic WHO criteria for sporadic CJD. (Adapted from *WHO Manual for Surveillance of Human Transmissible Spongiform Encephalopathies*, 2003.)

Possible diagnosis
- Progressive dementia and
- EEG atypical or not known and
- Duration less than 2 years and
- At least two out of the following clinical features:
  ○ myoclonus
  ○ visual or cerebellar disturbance
  ○ pyramidal/extrapyramidal dysfunction
  ○ akinetic mutism

Probable diagnosis (in the absence of an alternative diagnosis from routine investigation)
- Progressive dementia and
- At least two of the following four clinical features:
  ○ myoclonus
  ○ visual or cerebellar disturbance
  ○ pyramidal/extrapyramidal dysfunction
  ○ akinetic mutism and
- A typical EEG, whatever the clinical duration of the disease, and/or
- A positive 14-3-3 assay for CSF and a clinical duration to death of less than 2 years

Definite diagnosis
- Neuropathological confirmation and/or
- Confirmation of protease-resistant prion protein (immunohistochemistry or Western blot) and/or
- Presence of scrapie-associated fibrils (SAF)

Less common presenting features include behavioral disturbances or a stroke-like illness. Myoclonus is probably the most important clinical sign. Visual abnormalities include non-specific blurring, visual field defects, perceptual abnormalities, and occasionally hallucinations.

The prime differential diagnosis for CJD and sCJD is AD. Many other neurodegenerative, infectious, and tumorous entities may mimic sCJD, for example, multiple system atrophy, gliomatosis cerebri, primary CNS non-Hodgkin's malignant lymphoma, subcortical VaD, or frontotemporal lobar degeneration.

Familial TSEs

Familial (hereditary) TSEs are inherited as an autosomal dominant trait. They represent approximately 10–15% of all known TSE cases, although some countries (Slovakia and Israel) have much higher rates of familial disease. The disorder may manifest as familial Creutzfeldt–Jakob disease (fCJD), Gerstmann–Sträussler–Scheinker disease (GSS), or fatal familial insomnia (FFI).

The clinical and neuropathologic spectrum of hereditary TSEs is extremely diverse. fCJD phenotypically may often resemble sCJD; to a significant extent, the phenotype depends upon the causative mutation. Identification of the causative mutation in the PRNP gene is an important diagnostic test that should be performed in suspected TSE cases. To date, more than 40 PRNP alleles associated with distinct phenotypes of hereditary TSEs have been reported.

Accidentally transmitted (iatrogenic) CJD

More than 300 cases of iatrogenic CJD have been identified since its first description in 1974. These cases have been related to transmission of the infectious agent during the use of contaminated human pituitary-derived growth hormone or gonadotropin, dura mater grafts, neurosurgical instruments, and corneal transplantation. Increased awareness has raised concern about the risk that human TSEs are transmissible by transfusion.

New variant CJD (vCJD)

As of May 2007, about 200 vCJD cases have been reported, the majority in the UK. vCJD was first described in 1996. It is very probably closely related to the epidemic of animal-TSE in affected cows – BSE. vCJD is characterized by a younger age of onset and by longer illness duration.

vCJD characteristically affects persons in their mid-teens to early 40s. It usually presents with non-specific psychiatric symptoms. Less often, it begins with sensory or other neurological disturbances. It progresses over months with increasing ataxia, global cognitive impairment, and involuntary movements. Finally, the disease culminates in a state of incapacity and mutism.

Although a minority of patients suffer from forgetfulness or mild unsteadiness of gait from an early stage, clear neurological signs are not apparent for many months after disease onset (range 4–25 months). During this time, the most prominent clinical features are limited to only psychiatric disturbance or sensory symptoms or both, until various neurologic dysfunction develops.

Investigations

14-3-3 level in the CSF has been examined as a laboratory marker of sCJD. 14-3-3 is a neuronal protein involved in cell signaling and is present in high concentrations within the CNS. It may be released into the CSF in a number of neurological and pathological conditions affecting neurons. Its presence in the CSF is not specific for CJD. However, in the appropriate clinical setting, the detection of 14-3-3 in CSF has a high degree of sensitivity and specificity for the diagnosis of sCJD.

The EEG was first recognized as an important aid to the diagnosis of CJD in 1954. The presence of periodic sharp-wave complexes is reported to have a sensitivity of 67% and a specificity of 86% for sCJD. The sensitivity partly depends on the number of recordings undertaken in any given case and the stage of illness at which they are carried out. The specificity depends on the context of testing. EEG recordings in vCJD usually show only non-specific slow-wave abnormalities.

MRI in sCJD typically shows hyperintense signal changes in the putamen and caudate head (relative to the thalamus and cerebral cortex with 67% sensitivity and 93% specificity). The putamen and caudate nucleus hyperintensity are usually symmetrical on long time resolved (TR) imaging, although asymmetrical involvement of the corpus striatum occurs in 20% of cases.

On MRI of vCJD, a characteristic distribution of symmetrical hyperintensity of the pulvinar nucleus (posterior nucleus) of the thalamus is seen in over 90% of patients with subsequently pathologically confirmed vCJD. These changes have been named the "pulvinar sign," and it has been shown to be a highly sensitive marker of disease.

Pathology

Definite diagnosis is made on the basis of the morphological investigation of CNS tissue. sCJD is neuropathologically characterized by the classical triad: spongiform changes, neuronal loss, and reactive astrogliosis (see Plate 38.1). Amyloid plaques, similar to those found with AD but composed of PrP, appear in about 10% of sCJD cases, but are much more common in kuru, iatrogenic CJD, and some fCJD. Spongiform changes consist of diffuse or focally clustered small round or oval vacuoles from 2 to 20 μm in size in the neuropil of the whole depth of the cerebral cortex, cerebellar cortex, or in the subcortical gray matter. The vacuoles may become confluent to form irregular cavities.

The neuropathology of vCJD is significantly different from sCJD. In particular, a large number of amyloid plaques surrounded by a halo of spongiform changes are seen, particularly in the cerebral and cerebellar cortical gray matter. The "florid plaques" are not specific for vCJD, but their widespread distribution is characteristic of the disease.

Immunohistochemistry for PrP is a very useful tool for CJD neuropathologic diagnosis. Immunohistochemical reactions with specific monoclonal antibodies prove the presence of a pathological form of prion protein.

Consequently, immunohistochemistry of lymphoreticular tissue samples can be used to diagnose vCJD. Various lymphoreticular tissues can be utilized, but tonsils are the best candidate.

Therapy of TSEs

Prion disorders are invariably fatal, and there is currently no available treatment for the underlying disease process. Palliation therapy, such as clonazepam or sodium valproate for myoclonus, is frequently successfully administered.

Further reading

Braak H, Del Tredici K, Rub U, de Vos RA, Jansen Steur EN, Braak E. Staging of brain pathology related to sporadic Parkinson's disease. *Neurobiol Aging* 2003; 24: 197–211.

Cali I, Castellani R, Yuan J, *et al.* Classification of sporadic Creutzfeldt–Jakob disease revisited. *Brain* 2006; 129(Pt 9): 2266–77.

Cordonnier C, Al-Shahi Salman A, Wardlaw J. Spontaneous brain microbleeds: systematic review, subgroup analyses and standards for study design and reporting. *Brain* 2007; 130: 1988–2003.

Cummings JL. Alzheimer's disease. *N Engl J Med* 2004; 351: 56–67.

de Leon MJ, Mosconi L, Blennow K, *et al.* Imaging and CSF studies in the preclinical diagnosis of Alzheimer's disease. *Ann N Y Acad Sci* 2007; 1097: 114-45.

Growdon JH, Rossor MN, editors. *The Dementias 2.* Philadelphia, PA: Butterworth Heinemann Elsevier; 2007.

Ironside JW, Head MW. Neuropathology and molecular biology of variant Creutzfeldt–Jakob disease. *Curr Top Microbiol Immunol* 2004; 284: 133–59.

Kertesz A, McMonagle P, Blair M, Davidson W, Munoz DG. The evolution and pathology of frontotemporal dementia. *Brain* 2005; 128: 1996–2005.

Mott RT, Dickson DW, Trojanowski JQ, *et al.* Neuropathologic, biochemical, and molecular characterization of the frontotemporal dementias. *J Neuropathol Exp Neurol* 2005; 64: 420–8.

O'Brien JT, Erkinjuntti T, Reisberg B, *et al.* Vascular cognitive impairment. *Lancet Neurol* 2003; 2: 89–98.

Chapter 39
Other dementias

John M. Ringman[1] and Arousiak Varpetian[2]
[1]Mary S. Easton Center for Alzheimer's Disease Research, Los Angeles, USA
[2]University of Southern California, California, USA

Introduction

Relatively isolated cognitive impairment due to normal pressure hydrocephalus or metabolic, infectious, genetic, or inflammatory causes is uncommon. Nonetheless, these entities are important to recognize in order to prognosticate accurately and at times treat effectively. Due to their rarity, a high index of suspicion and a knowledge of appropriate diagnostic tests are crucial. Careful attention to other signs and symptoms that accompany dementia is key in the differential diagnosis. The purpose of this chapter is to describe neurological conditions in which cognitive impairment is a common or predominant feature.

Normal pressure hydrocephalus

Normal pressure hydrocephalus (NPH) was first described by the Columbian neurosurgeon Salomón Hakim in the 1960s and is thought to account for about 2–5% of dementia cases. NPH is an important entity to recognize due its potential reversibility. The classic triad suggestive of NPH includes a gait disorder, urinary incontinence, and cognitive impairment. Among these elements, the gait disorder is most critical because it is present in nearly all cases and can be helpful in making the diagnosis. Gait in NPH is characterized by reduced speed, decreased step height and stride length, and, when advanced, by *en bloc* turning (requiring an abnormally increased number of steps to turn). However, it should be noted that even the classic gait is not specific for the presence of NPH as it can be seen in the presence of bilateral subcortical ischemic injury as well. The cognitive deficits are not always dramatic and when present typically take the form of "subcortical" impairment. Deficits are manifested in tasks of divided attention, psychomotor speed, and impaired recall, while recognition and other forms of cued memory are relatively intact. Despite the classic triad, NPH can be a challenge to diagnose considering how common these problems are in the elderly and therefore how frequently they co-exist by chance. Because of this, the presence of NPH is best judged as an estimate of the degree to which the hydrocephalus contributes to an individual patient's disability. Accordingly, published guidelines recommend cases be classified as either probable NPH, possible NPH, or unlikely NPH.

The demonstration of enlarged cerebral ventricles with neuroimaging is necessary to make the diagnosis of NPH. The pathophysiology underlying ventricular enlargement is incompletely understood but it is thought to be due to decreased reabsorption of cerebrospinal fluid (CSF) into the venous sinuses. This might occur as a result of known prior neurological illness (e.g., subarachnoid hemorrhage, trauma, or meningitis) as *secondary* NPH, or without a known causative insult as *idiopathic* NPH. The excess of CSF is transmitted to the intracerebral ventricular system, at least transiently increasing the pressure there. "Normal" pressure hydrocephalus is therefore a misnomer and many specialists prefer the term adult hydrocephalus.

Management of NPH is a challenge as not all persons who have the syndrome respond well to treatment. Enlarged ventricles seen on computerized tomography (CT) or magnetic resonance imaging (MRI) are insufficient in predicting who has NPH or who will be respond to surgical shunting of the ventricles. Relatively large cerebral ventricles are common in the elderly on an *ex-vacuo* basis due to cerebral atrophy from neurodegenerative disease, cerebral ischemia, or nutritional deficiencies. It is common practice for clinicians to attempt to differentiate hydrocephalus from *ex-vacuo* ventricular enlargement due to atrophy by estimating the disparity between ventricular size and the extra-axial subarachnoid space. However, this approach has not been validated in a controlled fashion and therefore conclusions based on such an apparent disparity should be drawn with caution.

More sophisticated neuroimaging techniques based on ways of measuring CSF flow and hemodynamics are also sometimes employed. These include estimating the rate of CSF flow through the aqueduct of Sylvius with MRI, perfusion imaging with single-photon

International Neurology: A Clinical Approach. Edited by Robert P. Lisak, Daniel D. Truong, William M. Carroll, and Roongroj Bhidayasiri.
© 2009 Blackwell Publishing, ISBN: 978-1-4051-5738-4.

emission computerized tomography (SPECT), SPECT/ acetazolamide challenge, resting metabolic imaging with positron emission tomography, and nuclear cisternography. Data supporting their utility are limited, however, and their use cannot be recommended as a standard of practice.

At some point in the evaluation of a patient with suspected NPH, an estimate of intracranial pressure (ICP) should be obtained. Though we have said that "normal" pressure hydrocephalus is a misnomer, ICPs above 240 mm H_2O suggest an alternative diagnosis such as secondary hydrocephalus. Such a measurement may be obtained during a lumbar puncture in which CSF is drained in an effort to predict outcome from shunting. Diagnostic lumbar punctures in which a large volume of CSF (40–50 ml) is removed to determine if a patient's symptoms (usually gait) improve are commonly used in the assessment of NPH. Such an approach has been demonstrated to have specificity for predicting a good outcome to shunt surgery (positive predictive value of 73–100%) but lacks sensitivity. In order to increase the sensitivity with which shunt responders might be detected, continuous external lumbar drainage (ELD) should be employed. Patients are admitted to the hospital and a lumbar catheter is placed with the goal of removing 10 ml of CSF per hour for 72 hours during which clinical changes are monitored. This has been demonstrated to improve the sensitivity in identifying shunt responders from 43–62% with lumbar puncture alone to 50–100%. However, the benefits of this procedure must be weighed against the substantial risks of infection, over-drainage with the consequent development of subdural hematoma, catheter removal in a confused patient, as well as the financial costs of hospitalization. Though a systematic review of existing data by a consensus panel failed to identify standards of practice regarding the diagnosis of NPH, a suggested algorithm (guideline) for the assessment of patients with suspected NPH can be found in Marmarou *et al.*

Depending on the method of patient selection and how a favorable response to shunting is defined, the rate of positive outcomes to ventricular shunting in NPH has been found to be in the range of 61–75%. Even when the presentation is classic and the preoperative assessment is consistent with NPH, it is still difficult to predict which patient will benefit from shunting. Lack of response in such cases can be due to the presence of concurrent illness (e.g., cerebrovascular ischemia) or to operative considerations such as inadequate shunting or complications (e.g., infections or subdural fluid collections). The duration of the condition is also important, as persons with symptoms of greater than 2 years' duration are less likely to benefit. When the long-term prognosis of patients is considered, a favorable outcome appears to be substantially less common, with one study showing a decrease in persons with improvement from 64% at 3 months to 26% at 3 years. This is due, at least in part, to death and disability from pre-morbid conditions that are common in this population (e.g., complications of atherosclerosis) and therefore each patient's overall health status needs to be taken into account when considering ventricular shunting.

Toxic and metabolic disorders
Alcohol
Alcohol is by far the most widely available and widely consumed neurotoxin. Though epidemiological studies suggest a mildly protective effect of low doses of alcohol (particularly red wine) in relation to the development of dementia and Alzheimer's disease, chronic alcoholism has been repeatedly shown to be associated with cognitive deficits. The pathology underlying these deficits is more controversial, however, as co-morbid conditions such as thiamine (see below) and other nutritional deficiencies, hepatic encephalopathy, head injury, cerebrovascular disease, and concurrent Alzheimer's changes may be contributing to varying degrees in a given case. The cognitive deficits associated with chronic alcoholism include amnesia, disorientation, and in some cases emotional lability and perseveration. The underlying neuropathological substrate is controversial, though studies of uncomplicated alcoholics tend to support a more significant decrement in white matter volume than of neuronal count. As many cases of dementia associated with alcohol consumption may represent Korsakoff's syndrome in which the Wernicke's encephalopathy is subclinical (see Chapter 109) the existence of a distinct category of dementia associated with alcohol consumption *per se* is contentious.

Wernicke–Korsakoff's syndrome
Wernicke's encephalopathy is an acute or subacute syndrome characterized by delirium, ophthalmoplegia, and gait ataxia and can lead to coma and death. Autopsy series suggest that it is underdiagnosed, possibly due to absence of the classic triad in many cases. Caused by thiamine deficiency, it is most frequently diagnosed in chronic alcoholics but can occur in any condition in which malnutrition is present. Neuropathology reveals areas of hemorrhagic necrosis in periventricular areas of the diencephalon and mesencephalon. As rapid treatment is essential, parenteral administration of 100 mg thiamine should be routine in the acutely confused patient for which the etiology is uncertain. As the acute condition resolves with treatment, patients may be left with Korsakoff's syndrome – a dense amnestic disorder in which confabulation is a classic (though variably present) feature. It has been argued that supplementation of food with thiamine is a public health measure that might decrease the prevalence of this condition.

Vitamin B$_{12}$ deficiency

The association of neurological disorders including cognitive impairment, depression, signs attributable to the corticospinal tract and dorsal column pathways (subacute combined degeneration), and peripheral neuropathy with megaloblastic anemia and vitamin B$_{12}$ deficiency has an illustrious history and led to the award of two Nobel prizes. In an English series of 50 patients presenting with megaloblastic anemia, 26% had cognitive decline, 40% had peripheral neuropathy, and 16% had subacute combined degeneration. The syndrome was due to pernicious anemia in 64%, dietary or other gastrointestinal causes in 30%, and was unexplained in 6%. Despite its relative rarity, this diagnosis should be considered in most persons presenting with memory impairment due to the potential for reversibility with treatment. Vitamin B$_{12}$ levels in the low normal range are not incompatible with the diagnosis and the deficiency can be confirmed by identifying elevated levels of methylmalonic acid in plasma. A thousand micrograms of cyanocobalamin administered intramuscularly weekly for 3 months followed by monthly maintenance injections is recommended, with the ultimate duration of treatment depending in part on the original cause. With this treatment, 90% of patients will demonstrate significant improvement, with the most advanced cases being less likely to have complete recovery. Lack of a response should lead one to consider alternative diagnoses (e.g., distinct or concurrent folate deficiency, nitrous oxide abuse, an inherited disorder of B$_{12}$ metabolism, or multiple sclerosis).

Hypo- and hyperthyroidism

Cognitive impairment can accompany the systemic symptoms of either hypo- or hyperthyroidism. Though rarely if ever a cause of an isolated dementia syndrome, thyroid disorders are common and treatable, and therefore routine screening in a person presenting with a cognitive complaint is recommended.

Infectious causes

Infectious disease is a major cause of neurological morbidity worldwide and the following review focuses on the most common infectious illnesses for which cognitive or behavioral changes may be a predominant feature.

Dementia associated with HIV infection

Human immunodeficiency virus (HIV) can cause neurological disease, including cognitive deterioration directly, by way of susceptibility to opportunistic infections, secondarily through damage to other organs, or as an effect of the medications used to treat it. Here we will focus on cognitive decline due to HIV itself.

Neurocognitive disorders in individuals infected by HIV are heterogeneous. Before the era of highly active antiretroviral treatment (HAART), dementia typically presented with advanced acquired immune deficiency syndrome (AIDS) when CD4 counts were below 200/µl. Now dementia with advanced AIDS occurs in countries where HAART is not widely used. With the use of HAART, cognitive impairment has declined in incidence but has increased in prevalence. It no longer correlates with low CD4 count or with high plasma or CSF viral load. In some patients, neurocognitive disorders manifest as asymptomatic to mild cognitive impairment which advances to dementia. In others, the course may reverse and patients return to baseline. In yet another group, the cognitive symptoms may accompany motor symptoms.

Neurocognitive testing shows early impairments in attention, psychomotor speed, and recall memory consistent with a "subcortical" dementia. T2-weighted MRI reveals bilateral and symmetric white matter hyperintensities in early disease and atrophy later.

HIV encephalitis (HIVE) is a pathological diagnosis and is found in the brains of approximately 16% of persons dying with HIV disease. The pathological features of HIVE consist of inflammation with microglia, macrophages, and multinucleated giant cells predominantly in subcortical gray and white matter structures.

Neurosyphilis (syphilitic dementia)

Syphilis is caused by *Treponema pallidum* with about 12 million new infections worldwide annually. The number of infections in South and Southeast Asia and Sub-Saharan Africa is 40 times that of North America. Syphilis is a sexually transmitted infection and facilitates transmission of HIV. If left untreated, after a 10- to 20-year incubation period, the central nervous system (CNS) can become affected, leading to dementia, psychiatric disease, and mobility problems. General paralysis of the insane, as dementia due to neurosyphilis was once called, was among the most frequent causes of hospitalization in psychiatric units in the nineteenth and twentieth centuries. The prevalence of dementia associated with syphilis is not as high with the use of penicillin. However, treatment, if not started early, does not restore normal cognitive function in affected persons. The cognitive impairment starts with memory loss and apathy and therefore may be misdiagnosed as Alzheimer's disease. Eventually language and behavior become impaired, with delusions and disinhibition sometimes being present. On neuropathological examination neuronal loss, glial proliferation, and atrophy are observed. Although the American Academy of Neurology no longer recommends serological screening for syphilis in the routine evaluation of persons presenting with dementia it should be considered in the context of local epidemiological factors.

Progressive multifocal leukoencephalopathy (PML)

Progressive multifocal leukoencephalopathy (PML) is a progressive demyelinating disorder of the human brain caused by reactivation of latent infection with JC virus, a member of the polyomavirus family. PML usually occurs as a late complication of diseases associated with impaired immunity such as AIDS and lymphoproliferative disorders such as Hodgkin's disease and chronic lymphocytic leukemia. Recently, occasional cases of PML have developed in association with the use of monoclonal antibody therapies such as Rituximab and Natalizumab. PML presents with focal CNS symptoms including limb weakness, visual symptoms, gait ataxia, incoordination, language disturbances, and general cognitive impairment. Focal non-enhancing hyperintensity of white matter on T2-weighted MRI without swelling or mass effect is characteristic. Currently, mortality from PML is 30–50% in the first 3 months after diagnosis. Starting HAART in previously treatment-naïve patients with a CD4 count greater than 100/μl carries a more favorable prognosis. Patients are usually left with neurologic sequelae because of oligodendrocyte death. Patients can present with the clinical and radiologic findings of PML without detectable JC virus in the CSF by polymerase chain reaction (PCR) if CSF viral load is low.

Whipple's disease

Whipple's disease is a systemic infection caused by *Tropheryma whippelei*, a Gram positive bacillus. Approximately 1000 cases of Whipple's disease have been reported, but its recognition is nonetheless important due to the existence of effective treatment. Whipple's disease commonly affects middle-aged white men, with symptoms of diarrhea, weight loss, and arthritis. Neurological symptoms occur in up to 63% of patients and cognitive changes occur in 71% of those with neurological signs. Cognitive symptoms include decreased attention, orientation, impaired memory, and abstract thinking. Aphasia and behavioral changes have also been reported. Other neurological signs include ophthalmoplegia and ataxia. Whipple's disease is diagnosed by detecting para-aminosalicylic acid (PAS)-positive inclusions in macrophages from small bowel biopsy specimens. Treatment with doxycycline and hydroxychloroquine is recommended. Patients should also be tested for neurological involvement using a PCR assay on CSF and if positive should also receive high-dose sulfamethoxazole or sulfadiazine for 12–18 months. With treatment, two-thirds of those infected recover. Without treatment, the infection is fatal.

Viral encephalitides

The viral encephalitides cause a greater burden of disease in tropical and developing countries. Though they usually present acutely with a general encephalopathy accompanied by various combinations of fever, headache, seizures, and other neurological manifestations, etiological agents that can cause a more indolent form of progressive cognitive decline include measles virus (subacute sclerosing panencephalitis), rubella, arboviruses, and picornaviruses. Encephalitis due to herpes simplex usually causes fulminant illness but should be mentioned here because it is the most common cause of viral encephalitis and treatment is effective particularly if begun early. Patients present with signs of frontal and temporal lobe dysfunction such as memory loss, psychiatric disorder, and seizures. The diagnosis is supported by the finding of focal slowing or spike and wave activity on electroencephalogram (EEG), edema and infarct of one or both temporal lobes on MRI, CSF examination showing lymphocytosis, and PCR demonstrating the presence of herpes simplex virus (HSV).

Other infectious agents

CNS infections with other bacteria and fungi usually manifest with focal or other non-cognitive neurological signs and symptoms. Though rarely presenting with isolated cognitive impairment, CNS infections with coccidioidiomycosis, cryptococcus neoforman, and mycobacteria have been reported to cause a dementing syndrome. Infection with *Borrelia burgdorferi* and related spirochetes (Lyme disease) can cause various neurological manifestations including meningitis, radiculitis, cranial neuropathies, and even secondary NPH, but whether chronic active infection can cause cognitive impairment is an area of controversy.

Genetic causes

Though illnesses with well-defined genetic bases most commonly manifest in childhood, a number of adult-onset neurodegenerative disorders that feature progressive cognitive impairment have genetic origins. Autosomal dominant Alzheimer's disease is described elsewhere in this book. Mitochondrial genome (mtDNA) disorders are also included in other chapters. Dementia occurs in later stages of such illnesses in adults.

Though typically presenting in childhood, a number of genetically determined storage disorders can present in adulthood with cognitive impairment. Most such illnesses are inherited in an autosomal recessive fashion and are typically accompanied by other neurological (seizures, myoclonus, movement disorders) or systemic signs and symptoms. Please see Chapter 157 for discussion of Niemann–Pick type C disease, neuronal ceroid lipofuscinosis (NCL, or Kuf's disease), and hexosaminidase A deficiency.

Huntington's disease

Huntington's disease (HD) is a gradually progressive neurodegenerative condition classically consisting of the triad of choreiform movements (see also Chapter 45), dementia, and psychiatric changes that is inherited in an autosomal dominant manner. In populations of Western European descent the frequency is between

3 and 7 per 100 000 persons and it is more rare in Japan, China, Finland, and African Blacks. Chorea is usually the most obvious manifestation of HD, but rigidity and the attendant impairment in mobility as well as the cognitive and behavioral changes have the greatest impact on quality of life and ultimately survival. The dementia tends to be of a frontosubcortical variety, with distractibility and deficits in psychomotor speed and response inhibition being evident. Recall memory is especially impaired and memory for recent and remote material can be equally affected. The behavioral changes can run the gamut from social withdrawal and depression to disinhibited behavior and overt psychosis and vary more between patients than within a given patient across time. Though the median age of onset is around 40, it can begin at any point in the lifespan, with childhood-onset HD being well characterized. Through efforts focused on an extended kindred in the Lake Maracaibo region of Venezuela, HD was linked to chromosome 4 in 1983 and the Huntington gene identified in 1993. An expanded trinucleotide repeat sequence (CAG_X) in an exonic portion of the Huntington gene gives rise to an abnormally long glutamine repeat in the corresponding *huntingtin* protein. There is a negative correlation between the length of the CAG repeat and the age of onset of HD, a feature also seen in other trinucleotide repeat disorders (see below). As these trinucleotide repeats tend to be unstable and may lengthen from one generation to the next, the age of onset of disease may be younger in successive generations, a phenomenon known as *anticipation*. The exact mechanism through which this causes neurodegeneration is an active area of investigation. In very early disease, hypometabolism in the caudate nuclei can be seen with fluorodeoxyglucose positron emission tomography, and in more advanced disease atrophy of the caudate nuclei is evident bilaterally with structural imaging. Given the appropriate clinical context, the definitive diagnosis is made through genetic testing. No disease-altering medications have yet been identified and therefore treatment is symptomatic. Lifespan from the onset of symptoms until death from inanition is typically between 10 and 20 years, though considerable variability exists.

Dementia associated with ataxia
The genetic bases of an increasingly large number of conditions that feature progressive ataxia and other neurological signs (e.g., corticospinal tract and peripheral nerve involvement, visual loss) are being revealed. Almost all involve cognitive impairment in their advanced stages, but this chapter focuses on those for which it is a relatively early or predominant feature. Many classifications of these disorders exist including a distinction between those that are inherited in an autosomal dominant fashion (spinocerebellar ataxias, or

SCAs), those that are recessively inherited, and those that are maternally inherited.

The SCAs have an incidence of about 1–5 per 100 000 persons. At least 22 different clinical subtypes of SCAs have been defined, with reclassification common as the corresponding gene defects are identified. In a manner similar to that occurring in HD, an abnormally long polyglutamine repeat underlies some of these disorders (SCA 1-3, 7, and 17), whereas others are due to alterations in genes encoding for ion channels (the "channelopathies," SCA 6) and others are due to nucleotide repeat expansions occurring in intronic sequences (SCA 8, 10, and 12). Intellectual impairment of a subcortical variety is most common in SCA 1 (20% of patients) and SCA 2 (20–25% of patients).

Dentato-rubral-pallido-luysian atrophy (DRPLA) is an autosomal dominant progressive neurological syndrome caused by a polyglutamine repeat that is most common in persons of Japanese descent. Also subject to anticipation, the disease is characterized principally by myoclonic epilepsy, mental retardation, and ataxia when the age of onset is early, and by choreoathetosis, psychiatric features, and dementia similar to that of HD with later onset disease.

Dementia associated with other movement disorders
Wilson's disease is an autosomal recessive disorder characterized by hepatic, neurologic, and psychiatric abnormalities. Onset can be from childhood but is typically in young adulthood, and onset as late as age 60 has been described. Neurological manifestations are diverse, with dysarthria being present in 97% of patients followed in frequency by dystonia, cerebellar signs, tremor, and bradykinesia. Motor impersistence and other elements of frontal lobe dysfunction are present in 19% of affected persons. It is characterized by the deposition of copper in various organs including the liver and brain, and in 1993 was found to be due to alterations in the *ATP7B* gene that encodes a protein involved in copper transport. It is an important entity to recognize in light of the efficacy of copper chelation with *D*-penicillamine in stopping and in some cases reversing neurological and other symptoms. The large number of mutations in the ATP7B gene that have been described as causing Wilson's disease, in addition to the possibility of any given patient being a compound heterozygote, preclude simple genetic testing of suspected cases. The diagnosis is therefore supported by the presence of rusty-brown deposition of copper in the outer rim of the iris (Kayser–Fleischer rings), abnormal liver function tests, low serum levels of ceruloplasmin, elevated levels of copper in the urine, or a liver biopsy demonstrating elevated copper content.

Hallervorden–Spatz syndrome is the former name for an autosomal recessive degenerative disorder consisting of progressive and severe dystonia and ridigity, choreoathetosis, and dementia. Intellectual impairment is present at birth in some cases. The identification of genetic alterations in the pantothenate kinase gene (PANK2) on chromosome 20 as being causative in some cases has led to a renaming of the syndrome as pantothenate kinase-associated neurodegeneration or PKAN. T2-weighted MRI reveals characteristic bilateral hyperintensities in the globus pallidus (caused by gliosis, demyelination, and axonal swelling) surrounded by hypointensities (from iron deposition), the so-called "eye of the tiger" sign. Treatment of PKAN is symptomatic with vigilance for myelopathy that can occur as a result of chronic cervical dystonia.

Autoimmune disorders

Immunological reactions against self-antigens are thought to be the underlying cause of dementia in a small percentage of cases. Significant cognitive impairment is common in primary autoimmune disease of the CNS such as multiple sclerosis (see Chapter 100). Cognitive impairment may also occur in the context of identifiable systemic autoimmune diseases, as distinct illnesses primarily affecting the nervous system that may respond to treatment with corticosteroids, or as paraneoplastic syndromes. As is the case with autoimmune disorders in general, the frequency of autoimmune diseases causing cognitive impairment is higher in females. In addition to mental status changes, other neurological symptoms such as seizures or systemic symptoms (e.g., fever, insomnia, dysautonomia) are frequently present in these disorders.

Systemic autoimmune disorders

Some degree of cognitive impairment is the most common neuropsychiatric manifestation of systemic lupus erythematosus (SLE) followed by psychosis and seizures. In one series, only 21% of SLE patients performed within normal limits on neuropsychological testing, with most (42%) having mild impairment and fewer having moderate (30%) or severe impairment (6%). The exact mechanism mediating cognitive impairment in SLE may be difficult to isolate, with the presence of antibodies against CNS antigens, cerebral ischemia due to cardiac emboli, antiphospholipid antibodies, and vasculitis, as well as the effects of the medications used to treat the illness, or intercurrent infection all potentially playing roles.

Steroid-responsive autoimmune encephalopathies

Steroid-responsive encephalopathy associated with autoimmune thyroiditis, also called "Hashimoto's encephalopathy," presents subacutely with altered mental status, tremor, myoclonus, and sometimes transient aphasia. It is associated with the presence of antithyroperoxidase

and antithyroglobulin antibodies in the serum. These antibodies are common in the general population, particularly in the elderly, and are unlikely to be the direct cause of CNS symptoms. Non-specific serological evidence of inflammation and elevated liver function tests may be seen. Brain MRI is normal or has non-specific changes. In this context empiric treatment with high-dose corticosteroids (1 g methylprednisolone/day) is recommended as many patients have marked improvement in cognition and other symptoms. Long-term immunosuppression may be required to prevent relapse.

In 1870 the French physician Augustin Marie Morvan described an illness consisting of myokymia, insomnia, hyperhidrosis, and encephalopathy consisting in part of hallucinations. Morvan's syndrome is more common in males and it sometimes occurs in association with myasthenia gravis or with cancer (e.g., thymoma or small-cell lung cancer). Antibodies against voltage-gated potassium channels (VGKC) may be seen and the syndrome frequently responds to immunosuppressive treatments. VGKC antibodies can also be seen in encephalopathy without muscular hyperexcitability. In this context it presents in a manner similar to paraneoplastic limbic encephalitis (see Chapter 141) with seizures, hyponatremia, and changes in the medial temporal lobes seen on T2-weighted and fluid-attenuated inversion-recovery (FLAIR) brain MRI. It is distinguished from paraneoplastic limbic encephalitis in that it usually responds to treatment with corticosteroids.

Conclusion

The conditions described in this chapter are only a partial list of the non-degenerative, non-vascular causes of dementia. Despite the vast number of diagnostic tests at our disposal, it is sometimes difficult to completely rule out a treatable cause of dementia with confidence. In such circumstances, brain biopsy may be a useful diagnostic tool. In a retrospective review of 90 brain biopsies undertaken to rule out an inflammatory or infectious process at a major referral center in London, England, 57% of cases were diagnostic with 11% of biopsies affecting subsequent treatment. The potential benefit of brain biopsy must be weighed against the risks, with institution-dependent factors (e.g., experience of the neuropathologist and neurosurgeon with the procedure) taken into account.

Further reading

Antinori A, Arendt G, Becker JT, *et al.* Updated research nosology for HIV-associated neurocognitive disorders. *Neurology* 2007; 69(18): 1789–99.

Geschwind MD, Shu H, Haman A, Sejvar JJ, Miller BL. Rapidly progressive dementia. *Ann Neurol* 2008; 64(1): 97–108.

Hulse GK, Lautenschlager NT, Tait RJ, Almeida OP. Dementia associated with alcohol and other drug use. *Int Psychogeriatr* 2005; 17(Suppl 1): S109–27.

Kent ME, Romanelli F. Reexamining syphilis: an update on epidemiology, clinical manifestations, and management. *Ann Pharmacother* 2008; 42(2): 226–36.

Marmarou A, Bergsneider M, Relkin N, Klinge P, Black PM. Development of guidelines for idiopathic normal-pressure hydrocephalus: introduction. *Neurosurgery* 2005; 57(3 Suppl): S1–3, discussion ii–v.

Vernino S, Geschwind M, Boeve B. Autoimmune encephalopathies. *Neurologist* 2007; 13(3): 140–7.

Chapter 40
Movement disorders: an overview

Roongroj Bhidayasiri[1,2,3] *and Daniel D. Truong*[3]
[1]Chulalongkorn University Hospital, Bangkok, Thailand
[2]David Geffen School of Medicine at UCLA, Los Angeles, USA
[3]The Parkinson and Movement Disorder Institute, Fountain Valley, USA

In the field of neurology, involuntary movements of hypokinesia, hyperkinesia, or abnormal execution of movements in the presence of clear consciousness are termed movement disorders. We use this term nowadays in a different way from the term "extrapyramidal disorder," which is a rather older classification referring to central motor disturbances not involving the corticospinal pathway. Used interchangeably, the term "dyskinesias" or unnatural movements implies a paucity of movements (bradykinesia and hypokinesia), loss of movements (akinesia), or an excess of spontaneous movements (hyperkinesias), including tremor, chorea, tics, myoclonus, ballism, dystonia, and ataxia (Table 40.1). However, the term "dyskinesia" is frequently used in clinical practice in the context of iatrogenic disorders caused by exposure to dopamine antagonists or levodopa.

The first step when assessing a patient with a movement disorder is to establish whether or not involuntary movements are present, which are sometimes indistinguishable from exaggerated purposeful movements, such as gestures and mannerisms. With the above operational definition, abnormal motor behavior during alteration of consciousness, for example epileptic phenomena, should not be considered as a movement disorder. This is in contrast to patients with psychiatric diseases who often exhibit a range of abnormal movements in the presence of abnormal thoughts or contents, but not at the conscious level. Once involuntary movements have been established, the next step is to determine the nature of such movements. To do so, one should evaluate the main features, including speed, rhythmicity, duration, pattern, and suppressibility as well as the key character – an important distinguished feature of that movement (Table 40.2). Furthermore, the examiner should observe which body parts are involved; whether it is focal, segmental, hemibody, or generalized. As a rule, abnormal movements usually increase with demanding conditions or anxiety, but decrease or subside during relaxation or sleep.

Table 40.1 Classification of movement disorders.

Hyperkinesias	Hypokinesias
Tremor	Parkinsonism
Dystonia/athetosis	Catatonia
Chorea/ballism	"Stiff muscles"
Tics	"Freezing"
Myoclonus	
Stereotypy	
Akathisia	
Ataxia	

Table 40.2 Definitions and key features of different types of movement disorders.

Definitions	Key character
Akathisia: a feeling of inner, general restlessness that is reduced or relieved by moving about	Restlessness
Ataxia: incoordination in the performance of a motor task	Incoordination
Athetosis: slow, writhing movements (probably a form of dystonia)	Slow, writhing movements
Ballism: large amplitude, irregular, purposeless, non-rhythmic rapid movements	Unpredictable, large amplitude (usually proximal) movements
Chorea: irregular, unpredictable, brief jerky movements that are usually of low amplitude	Unpredictable brief jerky movements
Dystonia: twisting movements that tend to be sustained at the peak of the movement, frequently resulting in abnormal postures	Sustained contractions resulting in abnormal postures
Myoclonus: brief, sudden, shock-like involuntary movements	Shock-like, brief movements
Parkinsonism: a tetrad of bradykinesia, rigidity, tremor, and postural instability	A tetrad of bradykinesia, rigidity, tremor, and postural instability
Stereotypy: coordinated movements that repeat continually and identically	Stereotypic movements
Tics: Spontaneous, purposeless, simple and complex movements or vocalizations that abruptly interrupt normal motor activity	Simple or complex movements or vocalizations
Tremor: an oscillatory, rhythmical, and regular movement that affects one or more body parts	Oscillatory rhythmical movements

International Neurology: A Clinical Approach. Edited by Robert P. Lisak, Daniel D. Truong, William M. Carroll, and Roongroj Bhidayasiri.
© 2009 Blackwell Publishing, ISBN: 978-1-4051-5738-4.

Therefore, it is important for the examiner to thoroughly evaluate patients during both rest and action. The next step is to determine the etiology of abnormal movements and perform ancillary investigations. Treatment can then be decided based on a diagnosis and the extent/severity of abnormal movements.

The field of movement disorders has rapidly expanded during the past 20 years. Nowadays, there are at least two peer-reviewed journals dedicated to the study of abnormal movements, including *Movement Disorders*, a monthly publication of the Movement Disorder Society (www. movementdisorders.org), and *Parkinsonism & Related Disorders*, an official publication of the World Federation of Neurology research group on parkinsonism and related disorders (www.wfneurology.org). In addition, the World Health Organization has issued the ICD-10 neurological adaptation in extrapyramidal and movement disorders.

Further reading

Bhidayasiri R, Waters MF, Giza CC. *Neurological Differential Diagnosis: A Prioritized Approach*. Oxford: Blackwell; 2005.

Fahn S, Jankovic J. *Principles and Practice of Movement Disorders*. Philadelphia: Churchill Livingstone Elsevier; 2007.

Wolters E, van Laar T, Berendse HW. *Parkinsonism and Related Disorders*. Amsterdam: VU University Press; 2007.

Chapter 41
Tremor

Jan Raethjen and Günther Deuschl
Christian-Albrechts-University of Kiel, Kiel, Germany

Introduction

Tremor is the most common movement disorder and denotes a rhythmic involuntary movement of one or several regions of the body. A low-amplitude, physiologic action tremor can be detected in healthy subjects and may be of functional relevance for normal motor control. Conversely, pathologic tremors can be severely disabling and often pose diagnostic problems.

Clinical features

Clinical appearance is the most important clue for the correct diagnosis of tremors, and it should be documented in a systematic way.

Clinical approach to the tremor patient

Tremor topography should always be documented first. Tremors can occur in any joint or muscle that is free to oscillate. By far the most common locations are the arms and hands, often accompanied by tremor in other regions. The degree of symmetry between the two sides of the body can provide an important diagnostic hint (Table 41.1).

Different states of muscle activity can lead to tremor. Resting tremors occur when the muscles of the affected body part are not voluntarily activated; its amplitude typically increases during mental stress (counting backwards, Stroop test, etc.) and markedly decreases during voluntary activation, especially of the affected limb. Action tremor is any tremor that is produced by a voluntary contraction of muscles. Its subgroups are postural tremor (while voluntarily maintaining a position against gravity or additional weight) and kinetic tremor (during any voluntary movement). A simple kinetic tremor is present during simple voluntary movements such as slow up and down movements of the hands. Intention tremor only occurs during movements directed at a certain target (target reaching movements); it increases while approaching the target, but amplitude and velocity may fluctuate from beat to beat. Rarer are forms of action tremor that only occur during certain positions or certain tasks (task specific, position-specific tremor, or isometric tremor).

With some experience, the three main frequency ranges can be separated on inspection: high (>7 Hz), medium (4–7 Hz), and low (<4 Hz). Although there is a large overlap between the frequency ranges of different tremors, it can be an important clinical hint (see Figure 41.1). For exact frequency measurement, a signal analysis of accelerometer or electromygram (EMG) recordings of the affected body part is necessary.

Although not strictly related to the tremor syndrome itself, additional signs and symptoms are important considerations. For example, a parkinsonian syndrome, cerebellar ataxia, and dystonia in the region of the tremor are important diagnostic and etiologic hints.

Clinical presentation of pathological tremors
Enhanced physiologic tremor (EPT)
Normal physiological tremor is an action tremor. It is usually not visible, but can be measured with sensitive accelerometers. An increase of the amplitude leads to EPT. The pathological tremor amplitudes are typically short lived and reversible once the cause is removed. Other neurological symptoms or diseases that could cause tremor must be excluded. The majority of drug-induced or toxic tremors are EPTs.

Essential tremor (ET)
Essential tremor is a slowly progressive tremor disorder typically following an autosomal dominant pattern of inheritance. It causes severe disability but is not life limiting. It is defined by the following core criteria:
• Bilateral tremor of the hands or forearms with predominant kinetic tremor, and resting tremor only in advanced stages of the disease
• Or isolated head tremor without evidence of abnormal posture (dystonic signs)
• And absence of other neurological signs with the exception of cogwheel phenomenon and slight gait disturbances.

International Neurology: A Clinical Approach. Edited by Robert P. Lisak, Daniel D. Truong, William M. Carroll, and Roongroj Bhidayasiri. © 2009 Blackwell Publishing, ISBN: 978-1-4051-5738-4.

146

Table 41.1 Differential diagnosis of tremors.

Diagnosis	Clinical clues	Helpful investigations
Essential tremor (ET) vs. enhanced physiologic tremor (EPT)	Family history (ET), duration of tremor (ET > EPT), medical history (ET), concomitant medication (EPT)	Neurophysiology (EMG frequency below 8 Hz in early ET)
Essential tremor (ET) vs. orthostatic tremor (OT)	Tremor only during stance (OT)	Neurophysiology (polygraphic EMG is pathognomic)
Essential tremor (ET) vs. parkinsonian tremor (type I)	Rest tremor (PD), unilateral beginning (PD), other PD symptoms (PD), alcohol responsivity (ET), kinetic tremor (ET), family history (ET), leg tremor (PD > ET), face tremor (PD > ET), head tremor (ET > PD), voice tremor (ET>PD)	Neurophysiology (subclinical low frequency rest tremor (PD) inhibition (PD) vs. activation (ET) of tremor amplitude during movement) Neuroimaging (DAT-Scan positive in PD)
Essential tremor (ET) vs. dystonic tremor (DT)	Family history (ET), alcohol response (ET), geste antagonistique (DT), focal (DT), further dystonic symptoms (DT)	Neurophysiology (frequency (DT ≤ ET), geste maneuver in DT) Neuroimaging (rarely lesions in DT)
Essential tremor (ET) vs. cerebellar tremor (CT)	Alcohol response (ET), intention tremor (CT > ET), ataxia (CT > ET), eye movements (CT)	Neurophysiology (frequency: CT < ET) Neuroimaging (MRI lesions/degeneration)
Cerebellar tremor (CT) vs. Holmes's tremor (HT)	Rest tremor (HT), low frequency (HT), irregularity (HT), parkinsonian symptoms (HT), ataxia (CT > HT)	Neurophysiology (frequency: HT < CT) Neuroimaging (MRI lesions/degeneration)
Organic tremor (OrT) vs. psychogenic tremor (PsT)	Distractibility (PsT), variable presentation (PsT > OrT), selective disabilities (PsT), entrainment (PsT), coactivation (PsT > OrT), somatizations (PsT > OrT)	Neurophysiology (entrainment, quantitative assessment of distractibility Left–right coherence, variable frequency)

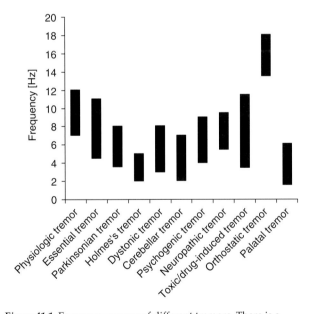

Figure 41.1 Frequency ranges of different tremors. There is a large overlap between frequency ranges. Nevertheless, frequency of tremors can be helpful for differential diagnosis. Especially the very low frequencies occurring in patients with Holmes's and cerebellar tremors can be important clues; the very high frequencies in orthostatic tremor are pathognomic.

Experts believe the following criteria support a diagnosis, although prospective studies on their diagnostic value are not yet available:

- Duration longer than 3 years
- Alcohol responsiveness
- Family history.

ET usually starts with a postural and kinetic tremor and can be suppressed during goal-directed movements. In advanced stages, an intention tremor can develop. This has been found in roughly 50% of outpatient populations and is accompanied by signs of cerebellar dysfunction of hand movements, such as movement overshoot and slowness of movements. In more advanced stages, tremor at rest can develop. Also, a mild gait disorder prominent during tandem gait is frequently found. Oculomotor disturbances are found with subtle electrophysiological techniques but cannot be detected by clinical assessment. The condition may begin very early in life. The incidence increases in those over 40 years, with a mean onset of 35–45 years and an almost complete penetrance by age 60. The topographic distribution shows hand tremor in 94%, head tremor in 33%, voice tremor in 16%, jaw tremor in 8%, facial tremor in 3%, leg tremor in 12%, and tremor of the trunk in 3% of patients. In some of the topographic regions (head, voice, and chin), tremor may occur in isolation. About 50–90% of patients improve after ingesting alcohol, which is an important feature of medical history.

The few data available on the progression of essential tremor show a decrease of tremor frequency and a tendency to develop larger amplitudes. Intention tremors develop at various intervals between 3 and 30 years after the onset of postural tremors. The disease-related disability varies significantly and depends on the severity of intention tremor. Up to 25% of the patients seeking medical attention must change jobs or retire from work.

Presence of the following features argues against a diagnosis of ET (see also Table 41.1):

- Isolated tremor in the voice, tongue, chin, or legs
- Unilateral tremor or leg tremor
- Presence of known causes of EPT (e.g., drugs, anxiety, depression, or hyperthyroidism)
- History of recent trauma preceding the onset of tremor
- History or presence of psychogenic tremor
- Sudden onset or stepwise progression
- Isolated head tremor with abnormal postures (dystonia)
- Drugs
- Other systemic disorders (endocrine, renal)
- Primary orthostatic tremor
- Isolated position-specific or task-specific tremors, including occupational tremors and primary writing tremor.

Orthostatic tremor (OT)

Primary OT is characterized by a subjective feeling of unsteadiness during stance and, rarely, during gait. Patients do not appear to experience problems while sitting or lying. There may be visible but mostly only palpable fine-amplitude rippling of leg muscles. This is the clinical correlate of the pathognomonic 13–18 Hz EMG bursts that can be recorded from the leg muscles in all OT patients.

Tremor in Parkinson's disease (PD) (parkinsonian tremor)

The most common forms of parkinsonian tremor are as follows.

Classical parkinsonian tremor (type I) is a tremor at rest, with a typical frequency of 4–6 Hz, which increases in amplitude under mental stress and is suppressed on initiation of movement and during its course. It may also be seen in the hands during walking or when sitting as a typical pill-rolling tremor of the hand. The postural/kinetic tremor (with similar frequencies for rest and postural/kinetic tremors) seems to be a continuation of the resting tremor under postural and action conditions ("re-emergent tremor"). Unilateral tremor and leg or face tremor are often seen and are typical for type I tremor.

A clinical variant of Parkinson's disease is the so-called monosymptomatic tremor at rest or benign tremulous parkinsonism, a classical PD type I tremor with otherwise no symptoms sufficient to diagnose PD.

In some patients, a second form of postural and action tremor with a higher (>1.5 Hz) non-harmonically related frequency may occur (type II tremor). In rare cases (less than 15% of patients with PD), this postural tremor can predominate. Lower amplitude, high frequency action tremors are often found in PD (type III tremor).

Dystonic tremor

Typical dystonic tremor occurs in the body region affected by dystonia. It is a postural/kinetic tremor, usually undetectable during complete rest. These are focal tremors with irregular amplitudes and variable frequencies (mostly below 7 Hz). Some patients exhibit focal tremors even before they develop overt signs of dystonia. Like dystonia, the tremor can often be inhibited by sensory tricks (geste antagonistique), which is an important clue for differential diagnosis (see Table 41.1).

Tremor associated with dystonia is a more generalized form of tremor at higher frequencies (6–10 Hz) in extremities not affected by the dystonia and can be difficult to distinguish from ET.

Cerebellar tremor

The classical cerebellar tremor is an intention tremor which may occur uni- or bilaterally, depending on the underlying cerebellar abnormality. The tremor frequency is almost always below 5 Hz. Simple kinetic and postural tremor may also be present. Some patients with a mild cerebellar ataxia present with an isolated postural and simple kinetic tremor above 5 Hz, resembling essential tremor. Titubation is a low-frequency oscillation (around 3 Hz) of the head and trunk, often occurring in cerebellar disease.

Holmes's tremor

This rare, symptomatic tremor is due to a lesion (2 weeks to 2 years delay) in the region of the midbrain, damaging nigrostriatal and cerebellar pathways. It has been labelled differently in the past (rubral tremor, midbrain tremor, myorhythmia, and Benedikt's syndrome) and is often irregular at low frequencies (<4.5 Hz) with resting, postural, and intentional components. The tremor following thalamic damage (thalamic tremor) often resembles this type of tremor.

Palatal tremor

These rare tremor syndromes affect the soft palate and can be symptomatic following brainstem lesions, with a variable delay or idiopathic presentation (essential palatal tremor). The most important symptom of the idiopathic form is a disturbing rhythmic ear-click.

Neuropathic tremor

Several peripheral neuropathies regularly present with tremors. These postural and action tremors can be difficult to distinguish from essential tremor. The frequency in hand muscles can be lower than in proximal arm muscles. Abnormal position sense need not be present.

Psychogenic tremor

Psychogenic tremors have diverse clinical presentations. Most of them are action tremors, but many remain during rest and often show unusual combinations of rest/postural and intention tremors. Typical clinical features are sudden onset and sometimes spontaneous remissions, decrease of tremor amplitude, variable frequency during distraction, and selective disability. Many patients have a positive "coactivation sign" (this is tested similarly to rigidity testing at the wrist). Variable, voluntary-like force exertion can be felt in both movement directions. Others show an entrainment of the tremor rhythm by contralateral rhythmic voluntary movements (tremor assumes the voluntary movement frequency). Some patients have a history of somatizations or additional, unrelated (psychogenic) neurologic symptoms and signs.

Epidemiology of tremors

Apart from the common, short-lived transient enhanced physiologic tremor, which most people have experienced on stressful or frightening occasions, essential tremor is the most common pathological tremor (prevalence 1.3–5.1%). Conversely, orthostatic tremor is a rare condition (less than 200 published cases) occurring only in patients above 40 years of age. Rest tremor is a very common feature of idiopathic PD. The occurrence of classical tremor at rest in a patient with parkinsonism has a likelihood of more than 95% of reflecting idiopathic PD. Cerebellar tremor, as a whole, is relatively common as it can be caused by cerebellar insults of various etiologies (demyelination in multiple sclerosis, strokes, hereditary and toxic, alcoholic degeneration). Dystonic tremor is relatively rare, but has been estimated to account for up to 20% of all tremor-patients presenting with non-parkinsonian and non-cerebellar tremors. Neuropathic tremor occurs in 70–80% of patients with dysgamaglobulinemic polyneuropathy or chronic Guillain–Barré syndrome. It is seen regularly but less commonly in hereditary polyneuropathy (40% of patients). Psychogenic tremor is the most common psychogenic movement disorder (~50%).

Pathophysiology of tremors

Physiological tremor mainly emerges from mechanical resonant mechanisms of the oscillating limb. This resonant oscillation can be enhanced by reflex mechanisms likely representing one mechanism of enhanced physiological tremor. Conversely, the majority of pathological tremors are caused by an enhancement or emergence of oscillations within the central nervous system (CNS) that are transmitted to the peripheral muscles. There is converging evidence that these oscillations originate from several oscillating loops within the motor system, rather than from one single oscillating structure. Subcortical structures (olivocerebellar circuits in ET, basal ganglia circuits in PD tremor, and brainstem circuits in OT) seem to be important pacemakers of pathological tremors. Studies of ET and PD tremors have convincingly shown that the oscillations are projected to the thalamus and motor cortex, which in turn transmits the oscillations via fast corticospinal pathways to the spinal motor centers and peripheral muscles. However, the involvement of

different loops and levels of the motor system seems to be dynamically organized and highly variable over time. Nevertheless, the notion that the oscillations converge in the motor nuclei of the thalamus is clearly supported by the efficacy of thalamic (VIM) surgery in the majority of pathological tremors.

The pathophysiology of the classical cerebellar intention tremor seems to be distinct from the mechanisms underlying most of the other central tremors. It is most likely due to altered characteristics of feed-forward or feed-back loops. An alteration of peripheral feed-back to central tremor-generating structures has also been postulated to be the basis for the tremor enhancement in peripheral neuropathies.

Voluntary-like rhythmic movements and physiological, involuntary oscillations (clonus-like mechanisms) are the most important mechanisms in psychogenic tremor.

Investigations in tremors

Blood tests are useful for excluding symptomatic tremors in general medical diseases (e.g., hyperthyreosis, Wilson's disease), as well as toxic- and drug-induced tremors.

Structural neuroimaging (magnetic resonance imaging (MRI) or computed tomography (CT)) is indispensable for diagnosing symptomatic tremors in structural brain lesions (cerebellar degeneration, lesions in cerebellar tremors, lesions in the midbrain or thalamus in Holmes's and thalamic tremors) (Table 41.1). The main functional neuroimaging technique that aids differential diagnosis in pathological tremors is single photon emission computed tomography (SPECT), after radioactive labelling of the dopamine transporter (DAT-Scan) to detect a dopaminergic deficit in the striatum. As a positive DAT-Scan is unique to parkinsonian syndromes, it is of great value in distinguishing between tremor-dominant parkinsonism and essential tremor (Table 41.1).

Clinical neurophysiology in tremors consists of surface EMG and acclerometric recordings from the affected limbs. Fourier/spectral analysis of these data can determine the exact tremor frequency – an important diagnostic hint (Figure 41.1). A highly synchronized 13–18 Hz rhythm in both leg muscles, appearing upon standing, is a pathognomonic finding for orthostatic tremor and the only way to achieve a definitive diagnosis. The pattern and rhythmicity (or lack of rhythmicity) of EMG bursts can also help distinguish between myoclonus and tremor. The coupling (coherence) between lower frequency oscillations in different limbs is unique to psychogenic tremor and is typically absent in lower-frequency organic tremors. Also, the entrainment of the psychogenic tremor rhythm by voluntary rhythmic movements of the contralateral hand, or the distraction from psychogenic tremor by such maneuvers, can be quantified neurophysiologically.

Treatment of tremors

The exact origins of, and the neurotransmitter systems involved in, pathological tremors are largely unknown and treatments are mainly symptomatic. Selection of a pharmacotherapy is typically based on the clinical appearance of the tremor (rest, postural, or intention tremor) and empirical knowledge. The mechanisms of action of most antitremor drugs are often only poorly understood. The allocation of drug treatment according to the clinical characteristics of the tremor is shown in Table 41.2. There is an improvement in 70–80% of patients with PD and essential tremor with adequate drug treatment. The most effective drugs for parkinsonian tremor are dopaminergic agents (levodopa and dopamine agonists) and anticholinergics. In essential tremor, beta blockers and primidone alone or in combination are regarded as most efficacious, although some of the new antiepileptic drugs (topiramate, gabapentin) seem to be good alternatives. Benzodiazepines can be helpful in primarily kinetic tremors. Detailed treatment strategies for these tremors are summarized in Tables 41.3 and 41.4. In focal dystonic tremor, the treatment of first choice is botulinum toxin injections. Cerebellar tremor is extremely difficult to treat. Although there are case reports of successful drug treatments with a number of different substances (cholinergics, 5-HTP, clonazepam, carbamazepine), hardly any systematic studies are available and no single substance can be recommended as first choice. Treatment of Holmes's tremor is similarly difficult; few patients respond to levodopa, anticholinergics, or clonazepam.

The most effective treatment in severe tremors is stereotactic surgery. However, the rate of severe complications is as high as 2–3% in bilateral procedures; therefore, this option is reserved for severely disabled and drug-resistant patients. The ventrolateral thalamus (VIM-nucleus) is the surgical target of choice for the majority of tremors. It can be lesioned, but deep brain stimulation is currently favored as it has less complications and may

Table 41.2 Symptomatic drug efficacy in relation to clinical presentation of tremors.

	Activation of tremor		
	Rest	Posture	Intention
Beta blockers	–	+	(+)
Primidone	–	+	+
Clonazepam/alprazolam	–	(+)	+
Topiramate/gabapentine	–	+	(+)
Anticholinergics	+	(+)	–
Levodopa	+	–	–
Dopamine agonists	+	–	–
Amantadine	+	–	(+)
Clozapine	+	+	–
Carbamazepine	–	–	(+)

Table 41.3 Drugs and their dosages for essential tremor.

	Drug	Dosage	Remarks
1st choice	Propranolol	30–320 mg, 3 doses, standard or long acting	Contraindications: cardial, pulmonal, diabetes, etc. Hand and head tremor
1st choice	Primidone	62.5–500 mg, single dose in the evening	Hand and head tremor Preferentially for patients aged more than 60 years
1st choice	Combination: propranolol/primidone	Maximum dosage for each	Try always before using 2nd and 3rd choice drugs
2nd choice	Arotinolol	10–30 mg	Crossover study with propranolol
2nd choice	Topiramate	<400 mg	So far small double-blind study only
2nd choice	Gabapentine	1800–2400 mg/day	Conflicting results of three double-blind studies: one without, two with benefit!
2nd choice	Alprazolam	0.125–3 mg/day	Two positive double-blind studies
2nd choice	Clonazepam	0.75–6 mg	For predominant kinetic tremor
3rd choice	Clozapine	Test: 12.5 mg, 30–50 mg/day	Less well-documented effect than for Parkinson's disease. Often ineffective
3rd choice	Botulinum toxin		Double-blind study with a significant result, but weakness as a significant side effect
3rd choice	Pregabalin	Max. 600 mg/day	1 case report, one positive double-blind study
3rd choice	Levetiracetam	Max. 3000 mg/day	1 positive/1 negative double-blind study
3rd choice	Sodium-oxybate	1–2 g single dose	1 positive single dose open-label trial
If 1st (+2nd and possibly 3rd) choice drug options fail	Surgery		VIM stimulation or thalamotomy

Table 41.4 Treatment strategies for tremors in Parkinson's disease.

Tremor type	First step	Second step	Third step
Classical parkinsonian tremor or monosymptomatic rest tremor	L-Dopa Dopamine agonists Anticholinergics	Amantadine Propranolol Clozapine	STN stimulation
Rest and postural tremor with different frequencies	Propranolol Primidone	Dopamine Dopamine agonists Anticholinergics Clozapine	STN stimulation
Isolated action tremor	Propranolol Primidone Anticholinergics	Amantadine	

STN: subthalamic nucleus.

be more effective (tremor nearly disappears in 80–90% of patients). However, stimulation is more expensive as it requires more equipment and ongoing support. Thus, in developing countries with limited resources, stereotactic lesioning of the VIM often is the more realistic option. In patients with parkinsonian tremor, the subthalamic nucleus is the target of choice as it has a similar effect on tremor and also alleviates the akinesia. However, lesions in this region are dangerous as they can lead to highly disabling ballism. Therefore, it is mainly a target for deep brain stimulation. For essential and parkinsonian tremors, the excellent efficacy of stereotactic surgical procedures is well documented in large studies. In cerebellar tremors, this invasive treatment seems to be less successful and careful patient selection is very important. In Holmes's tremor, neuropathic, and orthostatic tremors, there are only case reports or small case series documenting at least some efficacy of thalamic surgery.

Further reading

Bain PG, Findley LJ, Thompson PD, *et al*. A study of hereditary essential tremor. *Brain* 1994; 117(Pt 4): 805–24.

Deuschl G, Bain P, Brin M, and Adhoc-Scientific-Committee. Consensus statement of the Movement Disorder Society on Tremor. *Mov Disord* 1998; 13(Suppl 3): 2–23.

Elble RJ. Essential tremor frequency decreases with time. *Neurology* 2000; 55(10): 1547–51.

Kim YJ, Pakiam AS, Lang AE. Historical and clinical features of psychogenic tremor: a review of 70 cases. *Can J Neurol Sci* 1999; 26(3): 190–5.

Louis ED, Ford B, Wendt KJ, Cameron G. Clinical characteristics of essential tremor: data from a community-based study. *Mov Disord* 1998; 13(5): 803–8.

Marsden CD, Gimlette TM, McAllister RG, Owen DA, Miller TN. Effect of beta-adrenergic blockade on finger tremor and Achilles reflex time in anxious and thyrotoxic patients. *Acta Endocrinol* 1968; 57: 353–62.

Raethjen J, Govindan RB, Kopper F, Muthuraman M, Deuschl G. Cortical involvement in the generation of essential tremor. *J Neurophysiol* 2007; 97(5): 3219–28.

Stolze H, Petersen G, Raethjen J, Wenzelburger R, Deuschl G. The gait disorder of advanced essential tremor. *Brain* 2001; 124(Pt 11): 2278–86.

Timmermann L, Gross J, Dirks M, *et al*. The cerebral oscillatory network of parkinsonian resting tremor. *Brain* 2003; 126(Pt 1): 199–212.

Zesiewicz TA, Elble R, Louis ED, *et al*. Practice parameter: therapies for essential tremor: report of the Quality Standards Subcommittee of the American Academy of Neurology. *Neurology* 2005; 64(12): 2008–20.

Chapter 42
Parkinsonism

Bradley J. Robottom, William J. Weiner, and Lisa M. Shulman
University of Maryland School of Medicine, Baltimore, USA

Parkinsonism

Parkinsonism is a clinical syndrome characterized by tremor, bradykinesia, rigidity, and postural instability. It is not a single disease, but a common clinical presentation of a variety of disease processes that cause brain dopaminergic dysfunction. Etiologies include Parkinson's disease (PD), Parkinson's plus syndromes, other neurodegenerative diseases, toxins, vascular disease, and a variety of infections. This chapter reviews parkinsonism, excluding PD.

Progressive supranuclear palsy (PSP)

PSP was first described in the early 1900s. However, it was not until 1963 that Steele, Richardson, and Olszewski reported a series of patients with pathological confirmation of "heterogeneous system degeneration." The syndrome has been called PSP because of its distinctive clinical finding of supranuclear ophthalmoplegia.

Epidemiology
Onset of symptoms is usually in the sixth or seventh decade of life. PSP progresses more quickly than PD. Median survival ranges from 5 to 9 years and the 10-year survival rate is only 30%. The disease has no gender preference and is sporadic, although there are case reports of familial clustering with suggestion of an autosomal dominant inheritance pattern.

Prevalence ranges from 1.39 per 100 000 persons in the United States to approximately 6 per 100 000 in the United Kingdom and in Japan. Annual incidence in Rochester, Minnesota, was 1.1 per 100 000 persons in 1976 through 1990.

Neuropathology
PSP is characterized by neuronal loss, neurofibrillary tangles, and gliosis in the basal ganglia, brainstem, and cerebral cortex. The neurofibrillary tangles of PSP are primarily "globose" or rounded rather than the "flame-shaped" tangles of Alzheimer's disease (AD). As with AD, the tangles are composed of abnormally phosphorylated tau proteins.

Cortical pathology of PSP is seen most prominently in the primary motor strip and the ocular motor association area. The prefrontal cortex is largely spared, despite prominent clinical manifestations of frontal lobe and cognitive dysfunction. Behavioral changes and dementia of PSP are thought to be the result of subcortical pathology, leading to secondary cortical dysfunction.

Basal ganglia pathology is unique, involving extensive astrocytic involvement with inclusions in oligodendrocytes and neurons. Prominent midbrain atrophy is a hallmark of PSP. The gaze palsy is supranuclear and spares the cranial nerve nuclei directly responsible for control of vertical gaze.

Clinical features
Gait disturbance with falls is the presenting feature in the majority of PSP cases. This is in stark contrast to PD and should be the first clue that the patient has an atypical parkinsonism syndrome. The gait of PSP is stiff, slightly broad-based, and often accompanied by "unheralded falls" which the patient may ascribe to tripping or uneven ground. Symmetric rigidity is seen and is often prominent axially, particularly at the neck. Neck posture in PSP may be retrocolic, in contrast to the stooped, flexion posture of PD. Bradykinesia is common. Resting tremor is not common. Patients are often described as looking "surprised" or "anguished" due to tonic contracture of facial musculature. Accompanying the characteristic facial expression is a unique dysarthria that can be described as "growling."

Vertical supranuclear ophthalmoplegia is not an early finding. Early eye dysfunction is subtle, consisting of impaired vertical optokinetic nystagmus, slow saccades, and the presence of saccadic intrusions (square wave jerks). There should be an oculocephalic response even if a supranuclear ophthalmoplegia is present.

Frontal lobe dysfunction is the predominant cognitive finding. Patients have decreased verbal fluency; abstract thought becomes concrete, and set switching is severely

International Neurology: A Clinical Approach. Edited by Robert P. Lisak, Daniel D. Truong, William M. Carroll, and Roongroj Bhidayasiri.
© 2009 Blackwell Publishing, ISBN: 978-1-4051-5738-4.

impaired. Frontal release signs including grasp or palmomental reflex may be present. Motor perseveration is often present, demonstrable as the "applause" sign.

Investigations

Diagnosis is based on clinical findings. There are no available biomarkers. CT or MRI may demonstrate midbrain atrophy. Clinical diagnosis is based on National Institute for Neurological Disorders and Stroke–Society for Progressive Supranuclear Palsy (NINDS–SPSP) criteria (Table 42.1). Differential diagnosis includes other neurodegenerative disorders such as PD, corticobasal ganglionic degeneration (CBGD), multiple system atrophy (MSA), dementia with Lewy bodies (DLB), and vascular parkinsonism.

Management

Management is supportive. There are no treatments available that alter the natural course of the disease. No medication provides sustained symptomatic benefit. Some PSP patients will initially respond to levodopa replacement therapy; however, the response is usually transient. Adverse effects from dopaminergic therapy, especially visual hallucinations, are common in PSP. Treatment should include a multidisciplinary approach. Speech pathologists can recommend treatment for dysarthria and dysphagia, although percutaneous gastrostomy tubes may be needed in advanced cases. Occupational and physical therapy may be helpful in maintaining independence in activities of daily living. Physical therapists are involved in balance and gait training. Most patients eventually require a walker or some other assistive device for safety.

Corticobasal ganglionic degeneration (CBGD)

CBGD, initially termed corticodentatonigral degeneration with neuronal achromasia, was first described in 1967 in three patients with asymmetric motor symptoms who evolved over 6–8 years. At autopsy, the pathology was unique, with a pattern of asymmetric frontoparietal atrophy and neuronal loss.

Epidemiology

Symptoms usually begin after age 60, but cases have been reported with symptom onset as early as 40 years of age. The disease is progressive, with a survival of 5–10 years. There is no known hereditary component. Prevalence and incidence are unknown.

Neuropathology

CBGD is characterized by asymmetric frontoparietal and perirolandic cortical atrophy. Deep structures, including the caudate and thalamus, are atrophic, and there is pallor of the substantia nigra. White matter is affected, with thinning of the corpus callosum and asymmetric atrophy

Table 42.1 NINDS–SPSP criteria for the diagnosis of PSP.

PSP	Mandatory inclusion criteria	Mandatory exclusion criteria	Supportive criteria
Possible	• Gradually progressive disorder • Onset at age 40 or later • *Either* vertical (upward or downward) supranuclear palsy or both slowing of vertical saccades and prominent postural instability with falls in the first year of disease onset • No evidence of other diseases that could explain the foregoing features, as indicated by mandatory exclusion criteria	• Recent history of encephalitis • Alien limb syndrome, cortical sensory deficits, focal frontal or temporoparietal atrophy • Hallucinations or delusions unrelated to dopaminergic therapy • Cortical dementia of Alzheimer's type (severe amnesia and aphasia or agnosia, according to NINCDS–ADRA criteria) • Prominent, early cerebellar symptoms or prominent, early unexplained dysautonomia (marked hypotension and urinary disturbances)	• Symmetric akinesia or rigidity, proximal more than distal • Abnormal neck posture, especially retrocollis • Poor or absent response of parkinsonism to levodopa therapy • Early dysphagia and dysarthria • Early onset of cognitive impairment including at least two of the following: apathy, impairment in abstract thought, decreased verbal fluency, utilization or imitation behavior, or frontal release signs
Probable	• Gradually progressive disorder • Onset at age 40 or later • Vertical (upward or downward) supranuclear palsy and prominent postural instability with falls in the first year of disease onset • No evidence of other diseases that could explain the foregoing features, as indicated by mandatory exclusion criteria	• Severe, asymmetric parkinsonian signs, bradykinesia • Neuroradiologic evidence of relevant structural abnormality (i.e., basal ganglia or brainstem infarcts, lobar atrophy) • Whipple's disease, confirmed by polymerase chain reaction, if indicated	
Definite	• Clinically probable or possible PSP *and* histopathologic evidence of typical PSP		

NINCDS–ADRA: National Institute of Neurological and Communicative Disorders and Stroke – Alzheimer's Disease and Related Disorders Association.

of the deep white matter, internal capsule, and cerebral peduncles.

"Ballooned" achromatic neurons are found in the atrophied cerebral cortex, particularly in the fronto-parietal cortex. Swollen axons, demyelinated axons, and a spongiform appearance to the neutropil are present in the white matter underlying the atrophied cortex. In the substantia nigra, pigmented nerve cell loss and gliosis is seen. Neurofibrillary tangles may be observed in all of the affected areas. Pathologic diagnosis of CBGD is confirmed by the presence of cortical and striatal tau-positive neuronal and glial lesions.

Clinical features

CBGD is an asymmetric akinetic-rigid syndrome. Rigidity of the affected limb is generally more prominent than that of PD. There is usually no response to dopaminergic therapy. The most common presentation is of unilateral loss of dexterity and the feeling that the hand has become useless.

Motor symptoms spread to the contralateral side within several years and begin to affect midline structures with resultant dysphagia, dysarthria, postural instability, and hypomimia. Tremor may be present, but it should not be confused with that of PD. The tremors of CBGD are faster (6–8 Hz) and have an irregular, jerky quality. It is more prominent with action and maintenance of posture as opposed to the rest tremor of PD. As the disease progresses, patients may develop stimulus-sensitive and action-induced myoclonus. Other common motor findings include asymmetric limb dystonia, particularly flexion of the upper extremity. Some patients will have pain in the dystonic limb.

Higher cortical function eventually is impaired. Many CBGD patients develop "alien limb" phenomenon in which there is an inability to recognize ownership of an extremity with associated autonomous movements of the limb, which often manifest as levitation. Cortical sensory loss, such as extinction to double simultaneous stimuli and difficulty with two-point discrimination, may be present early. Ideomotor and limb-kinetic apraxias are frequently encountered and can be an early clue to diagnosis. Dementia may be present as well.

Eye movement abnormalities are common. Saccadic eye movements are affected early, with increased latency to the initiation of horizontal saccades, slowing of smooth pursuit movements, and saccadic intrusions. Patients may lose the ability to generate saccades although spontaneous saccades and optokinetic nystagmus are intact. Blepharospasm and eyelid-opening apraxia have been reported.

Investigations

Diagnosis can be difficult, but there are important clues that distinguish CBGD from PD. Lack of response to dopaminergic therapy and the presence of cortical dysfunction in the form of apraxia or cortical sensory loss indicate CBGD. No biomarker is available for diagnosis. Neuroimaging with CT or MRI is usually normal, but as the disease progresses, asymmetric frontoparietal cortical atrophy may be apparent.

Management

Early and continued involvement in rehabilitation services is helpful to maximize function and maintain independence. Pharmacologically, no effective treatment is available, although benzodiazepines may be useful for tremor and myoclonus.

Multiple system atrophy (MSA)

MSA was originally described as three distinct disorders: olivopontocerebellar atrophy (OPCA), Shy Drager syndrome (SDS), and striatonigral degeneration (SND). Because most of these patients eventually developed parkinsonism, autonomic dysfunction, and cerebellar dysfunction, these syndromes were determined to be manifestations of the same disease process and are now known as MSA. MSA is composed of two subtypes based upon presentation: MSA-P (parkinsonism) and MSA-C (cerebellar dysfunction).

Epidemiology

MSA presents on average at age 54 and median survival after diagnosis is approximately 6 years. Both sexes are affected equally. Prevalence estimates range from 2 to 5 per 100 000 persons. Incidence is less than 1 per 100 000 persons.

Neuropathology

Neuronal loss and gliosis is seen in the striatum, substantia nigra, locus ceruleus, Edinger–Westphal nucleus, middle cerebellar peduncles, cerebellar Purkinje cells, inferior olives, intermediolateral cell columns, and Onuf's nucleus. The involvement of these nuclei and tracts correlates with the clinical findings of parkinsonism, cerebellar dysfunction, and autonomic failure.

Microscopically, MSA is characterized by glial cytoplasmic inclusions (Papp–Lantos inclusions), seen primarily in the nuclei of oligodendrocytes. Inclusions stain heavily for α-synuclein, marking MSA as a synucleinopathy. The mechanism of cell loss is unknown.

Clinical features

MSA-P, the more common presentation of MSA, is characterized by parkinsonism and symmetric onset of motor signs; tremor is not a prominent feature. Dyskinesias are reported earlier than in PD. Initially, MSA-P may be difficult to distinguish from PD; however, with the passage of time, autonomic and cerebellar signs emerge.

MSA-C is more common than MSA-P in Japan, although the reasons for this are unclear. Gait ataxia appears first, followed by limb dysmetria, dysarthria, and eye movement abnormalities, including nystagmus, ocular dysmetria, slow saccades, and interruption of smooth pursuit. Essentially all patients develop some evidence of autonomic dysfunction. Urinary symptoms are common, with incontinence (71%) being more common than retention (27%). Urogenital symptoms often present early. Men develop impotence (96%) and women may experience reduced genital sensitivity and a variable decrease in libido. Orthostatic hypotension occurs in 43–88% of patients. Most patients experience mild postural symptoms and approximately 15% have severe orthostatic hypotension leading to recurrent syncope. Other manifestations of autonomic dysfunction include constipation, disordered breathing, and problems with thermoregulation.

Investigations
Diagnosis is clinical (Tables 42.2 and 42.3), but ancillary testing may be useful. Diagnosis of possible MSA requires one criterion (b) plus two features (a) from separate domains (see Table 42.2). Probable MSA requires autonomic failure/urinary dysfunction plus poorly levodopa-responsive parkinsonism or cerebellar dysfunction. Definitive diagnosis of MSA is pathologically confirmed by the presence of glial cytoplasmic inclusions (GCI) in association with a combination of degenerative changes in the nigrostriatal and olivopontocerebellar pathways. Tilt table testing may reveal subtle autonomic dysfunction. Electromyography/nerve conduction studies may show a subclinical polyneuropathy and denervation of the external anal sphincter. Neuroimaging with MRI is more useful than CT, as MRI may show cerebellar and brainstem atrophy as well as characteristic T2 abnormalities in the putamen.

Management
There is no therapy to slow progression of the disease. Thirty percent of patients have a sustained clinical response to levodopa for parkinsonism symptoms. If there is no response to 1000 mg levodopa/day, then the drug should be titrated down and discontinued. If orthostatic symptoms are not adequately managed by increased sodium intake and fluids, pharmacologic therapy with fludrocortisone (mineralocorticoid) or midodrine (α-agonist) may be employed. Incontinence may respond to anticholinergics.

Dementia with Lewy bodies (DLB)

DLB by definition is a disorder characterized by dementia and parkinsonism that begin within 1 year of each other. The disease is named after the proteinaceous intraneuronal inclusions. Whether or not DLB is a distinct entity or simply a subset of patients with PD and dementia remains to be seen.

Epidemiology
DLB is the second most common cause of dementia after AD, accounting for 20% of all cases of dementia in the United States. Typical onset of symptoms is in the seventh or eighth decade of life, later than that for most PD. The cognitive decline is more rapid than that of AD; however, life expectancy is similar to that of AD.

Neuropathology
The pathologic hallmark of DLB, as with PD, is the presence of Lewy bodies. Unlike PD, there is a significant

Table 42.2 Clinical domains, features, and criteria used in the diagnosis of MSA.

I. Autonomic and urinary dysfunction
 a. Autonomic and urinary features
  1. Orthostatic hypotension (by 20 mm Hg systolic or 10 mm Hg diastolic)
  2. Urinary incontinence or incomplete bladder emptying
 b. Criterion for autonomic failure or urinary dysfunction in MSA – orthostatic fall in blood pressure (by 30 mm Hg systolic or 15 mm Hg diastolic) or urinary incontinence (persistent, involuntary, partial or total bladder emptying, accompanied by erectile dysfunction) or both

II. Parkinsonism
 a. Parkinsonian features
  1. Bradykinesia (slowness of voluntary movement with progressive reduction in speed and amplitude during repetitive actions)
  2. Rigidity
  3. Postural instability (not caused by primary visual, vestibular, cerebellar, or proprioceptive dysfunction)
  4. Tremor (postural, resting, or both)
 b. Criterion for parkinsonism in MSA – bradykinesia plus at least one of items 2–4 above

III. Cerebellar dysfunction
 a. Cerebellar features
  1. Gait ataxia (wide-based stance with steps of irregular length and direction)
  2. Ataxic dysarthria
  3. Limb ataxia
  4. Sustained gaze-evoked nystagmus
 b. Criterion for cerebellar dysfunction in MSA – gait ataxia plus at least one of items 2–4 above

IV. Corticospinal tract dysfunction
 a. Corticospinal tract features
  1. Extensor plantar responses with hyperreflexia
 b. Corticospinal tract dysfunction in MSA – no corticospinal tract features are used in defining the diagnosis of MSA

A feature (a) is a characteristic of the disease and a criterion (b) is a defining feature or composite of features required for diagnosis.

Table 42.3 Exclusion criteria for the diagnosis of MSA.

I. History
Symptomatic onset under 30 years of age
Family history of a similar disorder
Systemic diseases or other identifiable causes for features listed in Table 42.2
Hallucinations unrelated to medication

II. Physical examination
DSM criteria for dementia
Prominent slowing of vertical saccades or vertical supranuclear gaze palsy*
Evidence of focal cortical dysfunction such as aphasia, alien limb syndrome, and parietal dysfunction

III. Laboratory investigation
Metabolic, molecular genetic, and imaging evidence of an alternative cause of features listed in Table 42.2

---

*In practice, MSA is most frequently confused with PD or PSP. Mild limitation of upward gaze alone is non-specific, whereas a prominent (>50%) limitation of upward gaze or any limitation of downward gaze suggests PSP. Before the onset of vertical gaze limitation, a clinically obvious slowing of voluntary vertical saccades is usually easily detectable in PSP and assists in the early differentiation of these two disorders.

burden of cortical Lewy bodies rather than brainstem inclusions. Since α-synuclein is one of the main components of Lewy bodies, DLB is considered one of the synucleinopathies, along with PD and MSA.

Clinical features

The hallmark feature is the emergence of both cognitive dysfunction and parkinsonism within 1 year. Either may appear first. In contrast, dementia in PD typically occurs many years after the onset of parkinsonism. Patients have bradykinesia, rigidity, and postural instability. Tremor is usually absent or minimal. Cognitive symptoms appear early, are progressive, and tend to wax and wane. Decline is quicker than that seen in AD, with the Mini-Mental State Examination declining an average of 4–5 points per year. Fluctuations in attention and arousal are common and may span days or even weeks.

Neuropsychiatric symptoms are common in DLB; hallucinations occur in 50% of patients. The visions are fully formed, often of people or animals. A majority of DLB patients have psychiatric disturbances in addition to hallucinations. These range from depression, apathy, insomnia, anxiety, and paranoia to elaborate delusions built around hallucinations.

Investigations

Diagnosis of DLB is clinical. Whether DLB can be distinguished from AD by its motor features or from PD due to dementia symptoms is a difficult nosologic problem. Definitive diagnosis is made post-mortem. No laboratory markers are available. Neuroimaging with CT or MRI may demonstrate generalized atrophy.

Management

Dopaminergic therapy may decrease bradykinesia and rigidity. Although DLB patients may respond to levodopa, the response is less robust than that seen in PD with a narrower therapeutic window. DLB patients are more prone to developing side effects (such as hallucinations and orthostasis) than patients with PD. Cholinesterase inhibitors such as tacrine, rivastigmine, and donepezil are beneficial for cognition and behavior. Hallucinations and delusions tend to be medically refractory, and neuroleptic drugs should be used with caution. If neuroleptic medication is necessary, atypicals are a better choice than typicals. Physical therapy, occupational therapy, and speech therapy may be useful.

Frontotemporal dementia and parkinsonism linked to chromosome 17 (FTDP-17)

FTDP-17 is a distinct and rare disease characterized by personality changes, deterioration of memory and executive functions, and parkinsonism.

Epidemiology

Symptom onset is usually in the fifth decade of life and often there is a positive family history. The disease is slowly progressive with disease duration averaging 10–12 years. The condition is linked to chromosome 17q21–22, with autosomal dominant transmission. Families with the disease have been identified.

Neuropathology

FTDP-17 is characterized by atrophy of the frontal and temporal lobes, basal ganglia, and substantia nigra. Microscopic examination reveals neuronal loss and gliosis with intraneuronal and glial tau protein deposits. The tau deposits are different than those seen in AD, PSP, CBGD, and Pick's disease.

Clinical features

Clinical characteristics are variable. The earliest manifestations are often behavioral, consisting of disinhibition, poor impulse control, impaired social interactions, or even psychosis. Cognitive impairment follows, affecting judgement and planning, but gradually becoming a more global dementia. Motor disturbances such as bradykinesia, axial and limb rigidity, and postural instability evolve later. In addition to parkinsonism, some patients have upper motor neuron signs.

Investigations

EEG, CT, and MRI are normal, but in later stages neuroimaging shows symmetric or asymmetric frontal and temporal atrophy.

Management
Parkinsonism in FTDP-17 is unresponsive to levodopa.

Parkinsonism–dementia complex of Guam (PDC)

PDC was first described in 1961 as a fatal neurodegenerative disease pathologically characterized by neurofibrillary tangles comprised of tau proteins. The Chamarro of Guam are at highest risk for the disease.

Epidemiology
Average age of onset of PDC is 59 years, with cases reported starting in the fifth to seventh decade of life. Approximately 60% of PDC patients are men. There is a rapid progression of disease, with a mean duration of illness of 5 years.

Clinical features
PDC may present with symptoms of symmetric parkinsonism, dementia, or both. Gait disturbance is seen in most patients at presentation. Tremor is rare. Cognitive deficits always develop and begin with difficulty with attention, recent memory, and behavioral changes. PDC patients become severely demented and bedridden.

Investigations
While there has been speculation that PDC is related to a motor neuron disease found in Guam in the 1950s known as the Parkinsonism–ALS Complex of Guam, the prevalence of the earlier motor neuron disease has markedly declined compared to that of PDC, leading to speculation that the former may have been caused by an unidentified environmental factor. More recent autopsy studies demonstrate separate pathology for the diseases and suggest that PDC and the motor neuron disease found on Guam are unrelated.

Vascular parkinsonism

Vascular parkinsonism is a syndrome characterized by subacute evolution of a levodopa-unresponsive, akinetic rigid syndrome in a patient with vascular risk factors. Clinical features include shuffling gait, tremor, symmetric rigidity with or without cogwheeling, and sometimes pseudobulbar palsy. Neuroimaging shows severe white matter disease, often with additional infarcts in the basal ganglia.

Normal pressure hydrocephalus (NPH)

The clinical picture of NPH is a triad of gait dysfunction, urinary incontinence, and gradual onset of dementia, although all symptoms are not always present. Parkinsonism may accompany this picture. Neuroimaging demonstrates ventricular enlargement out of proportion to cortical atrophy. Clinical improvement should be demonstrable hours to days after lumbar puncture with removal of 40–50 ml of CSF. Surgical shunting is the definitive treatment, although careful patient selection is necessary, due to a high complication rate.

Toxin-induced parkinsonism

MPTP
Since its discovery, 1-methyl-1-4-phenyl-4-proprion-oxypiperidine (MPTP) has been used in animal models of parkinsonism. Humans may be exposed through illicit drug use, as MPTP is sometimes found as a contaminant in intravenous drugs of abuse. Exposure in humans may lead to an acute, moderately severe parkinsonism in as little as 7 days. Neurologic damage is permanent. MPTP patients may have a dramatic response to levodopa, but tend to develop complications such as dyskinesias, "wearing off," and psychiatric side effects more rapidly than those with PD.

Methanol
Acute ingestion of methanol may lead to severe anion gap metabolic acidosis and death. The most common deficit in survivors is blindness due to retinal degeneration. Parkinsonism may develop within weeks of intoxication. Patients may exhibit hypophonia, hypomimia, rigidity, bradykinesia, gait abnormalities, and limb dystonia. MRI reveals bilateral damage in the putamen. Symptoms may respond to dopaminergic therapy.

Cyanide
Acute cyanide toxicity has a mortality rate of 95%. In those who survive, parkinsonism, characterized by gait abnormalities, rigidity, and hypomimia, develops within days. Unique characteristics of cyanide-induced parkinsonism include dystonia and dementia. Response to dopaminergic therapy is poor.

Manganese
Chronic manganese exposure leads to atypical parkinsonism. People who work in the manufacture of steel, those on long-term total parenteral nutrition, and those taking herbal supplements containing manganese are at greatest risk. First manifestations are often psychiatric, including insomnia, memory disturbance, and hallucinations. Several months after onset of psychiatric manifestations, parkinsonism and dystonia develop, affecting the limbs and trunk. Symptoms may continue to worsen after removal of the exposure. Patients have poor response to therapy. Chelation with ethylenediaminetetraacetic acid (EDTA) has been attempted, with no apparent benefit.

Carbon monoxide

Parkinsonism may develop as a delayed complication of carbon monoxide poisoning, appearing up to 4 weeks after the initial insult. MRI shows bilateral globus pallidus lesions. Some patients may recover spontaneously; however, residual parkinsonism responds poorly to levodopa.

Carbon disulfide

Carbon disulfide is used as a fumigant for grains, in the production of cellophane, and as a solvent for resins, fats, and rubber. Neurotoxicity includes acute and chronic encephalopathy, peripheral and cranial neuropathies, and parkinsonism. There is no response to dopaminergic therapy.

Infectious and post-infectious parkinsonism

Parkinsonism can develop within the context of viral encephalitis. Symptoms are often transient and rarely result in permanent parkinsonism. Causative agents include Japanese encephalitis, Western equine encephalitis, Epstein–Barr virus, coxsackie B, West Nile virus, and poliomyelitis.

Postencephalitic parkinsonism is a known consequence of encephalitis lethargica, an epidemic encephalitis that started in Europe during World War I. Encephalitis lethargica may have accounted for two-thirds of parkinsonism cases worldwide in the 1920s. This syndrome is now of historical interest. Other infections associated with the development of parkinsonism include HIV/AIDS, fungal infections, and syphilis.

Further reading

Gilman S, Low P, Quinn N, *et al.* Consensus statement on the diagnosis of multiple system atrophy. *Clin Auton Res* 1998; 8(6): 359–62.

Graham JG, Oppenheimer DR. Orthostatic hypotension and nicotine sensitivity in a case of multiple system atrophy. *J Neurol Neurosurg Psychiatry* 1969; 32: 28–34.

Litvan I, Agid Y, Caine D, *et al.* Clinical research criteria for the diagnosis of progressive supranuclear palsy (Steele–Richardson–Olszewski syndrome): report of the NINDS-SPSP international workshop. *Neurology* 1996; 47: 1–9.

Rebeiz JJ, Kolodny EH, Richardson EP Jr. Corticodentatonigral degeneration with neuronal achromasia. *Arch Neurol* 1968; 18(1): 20–33.

Steele JC, Richardson JC, Olszewski J. Progressive supranuclear palsy: a heterogeneous degeneration involving the brain stem, basal ganglia, and cerebellum with vertical gaze and pseudobulbar palsy, nuchal dystonia and dementia. *Arch Neurol* 1964; 10: 333–59.

Chapter 43
Parkinson's disease

Daniel D. Truong[1] and Roongroj Bhidayasiri[2]
[1]The Parkinson and Movement Disorder Institute, Fountain Valley, USA
[2]Chulalongkorn University Hospital, Bangkok, Thailand

Introduction

In 1817, James Parkinson first described a clinical presentation consisting of rest tremor, lessened muscular power, abnormal truncal posture, and festinant, propulsive gait. Parkinson's disease (PD) is now a common, progressive neurodegenerative disorder that can cause significant disability and decreased quality of life. In a study in the Netherlands, an estimated incidence rate of 0.3 per 1000 person-years in subjects aged 55–65 years was reported and this rate increases to 4.4 per 1000 person-years for those aged 85 or higher. The incidence is 0.11–0.12 in studies in the United States and United Kingdom, 0.045 in Libya, and 0.015 in China. The incidence increases with age.

Neuropathology

Pathological findings of PD include depigmentation and neuronal loss in the pars compacta of the substantia nigra and the presence of Lewy bodies (LBs) and pale bodies. These cells contain neuromelanin and produce dopamine. Therefore the hallmark of PD is the deficit of dopamine at the striatum, the site of its axonal projection. PD develops when the level of dopamine cell loss reaches 80%. LBs are concentric hyaline cytoplasmic inclusions, containing accumulations of α-synuclein protein and ubiquitin. In PD, α-synuclein is deposited in neuronal cell bodies and processed as LBs and Lewy neurites, respectively. Recently, Braak *et al.* devised a staging system of LB pathology in PD with six stages that characterize a progression from the medulla oblongata, through the pontine tegmentum, into the midbrain, and then the basal prosencephalon and mesocortex, and finally through the neocortex. Before the immunohistochemical demonstration of α-synuclein as a component of LBs,

it was commonly assumed that LBs cause neuronal cell death. Recent studies have indicated that LBs may represent a cytoprotective mechanism in PD. There are different hypotheses as to the cause of PD, which include oxidative stress, mitochondrial dysfunction, excitotoxicity, glial cell activation, and apoptosis. The role of toxins in the etiology of PD is not well defined, but MPTP (1-methyl-4-phenyl-1,2,3,6-tetrahydropyridine) has been known to cause Parkinson's syndrome.

The majority of PD cases are sporadic. Abnormal gene mutations have been discovered to cause or be associated with the familial form of PD. Thirteen gene loci have been identified for PD (PARK 1–13). Different genes have been linked to rare familial forms of disease (encoding *α-synuclein, parkin, DJ-1, PINK1,* and *LRRK2*) (see Table 43.1).

Rare cases of PD have been identified to occur in association with gene mutations, but they do not account for the large number of sporadic cases. Abnormal gene mutations have been discovered to cause or be associated with the familial form of PD. A large Italian American family (the Contursi kindred) was discovered to have a PD syndrome linked to PARK 1 at the q21–23 region of chromosome 4. Sequence analysis revealed a mutation in the gene that encodes α-synuclein.

PARK 2 or parkin functions as an E3 ubiquitin protein ligase by targeting misfolded proteins to the ubiquitin proteasome pathway for degradation. The loss of its E3 ligase activity due to mutation leads to autosomal recessive early onset PD.

In PARK 7 there is a loss of function mutation in the DJ-1 locus and this is associated with rare forms of autosomal recessive early onset parkinsonism. DJ-1 may function as an antioxidant protein. Overexpression of wild-type DJ-1 protects against a wide variety of toxic injury due to oxidative stress. Familial PD-linked mutations in DJ-1 are considered to cause nigral degeneration through a loss of function mechanism consistent with the recessive inheritance.

PARK 6 is caused by mutation in the *PINK1* (phosphatase and tensin homolog-induced putative kinase1) gene and is associated with early onset familial PD. Little is known about the precise function of *PINK1*, but it may

International Neurology: A Clinical Approach. Edited by Robert P. Lisak, Daniel D. Truong, William M. Carroll, and Roongroj Bhidayasiri.
© 2009 Blackwell Publishing, ISBN: 978-1-4051-5738-4.

Table 43.1 Gene loci identified for Parkinson's disease.

Locus	Gene	Chromosome	Inheritance	Probable function
PARK 1 and PARK 4	*α-Synuclein*	4q21	AD	Presynaptic protein, Lewy body
PARK 2	*Parkin*	6q25.2–27	AR	Ubiquitin E3 ligase
PARK 3	Unknown	2p13	AD	Unknown
PARK 4	Unknown	4p14	AD	Unknown
PARK 5	*UCH-L1*	4p14	AD	Ubiquitin C-terminal hydrolase
PARK 6	*PINK1*	1p35–36	AR	Mitochondrial kinase
PARK 7	*DJ-1*	1p36	AR	Chaperone, antioxidant
PARK 8	*LRRK2*	12p11.2	AD	Mixed lineage kinase
PARK 9	*ATP*	13A2 1p36	AR	Unknown
PARK 10	Unknown	1p32	AD	Unknown
PARK 11	Unknown	2q36–37	AD	Unknown
PARK 12	Unknown	Xq21–q25	Unknown	Unknown
PARK 13	*HTRA2*	2p12	Unknown	Mitochondrial serine protease

AD: autosomal dominant; AR: autosomal recessive.

have a role in mitochondrial dysfunction, protein stability, and kinase pathway.

PARK 8 is associated with mutation in the leucine-rich repeat kinase 2 (*LRRK2*) and causes autosomal dominant PD. *LRRK2* mutations present beyond familial cases and with a high frequency in patients of European, Ashkenazic Jewish, and North African Arabian origin.

Clinical presentation

The cardinal clinical features of PD consist of slowness, stiffness, rest tremors, and postural imbalance. Initially the postural imbalance symptom may not be obvious, as it is mild at the beginning. The symptoms present mostly in one part of the body and slowly spread to other extremities on the same side before spreading to the other side of the body. Shuffling gait and stooped posture are characteristic of PD. Besides slowness, there is also paucity of movements and difficulty in initiating movements. The tremors are present at rest, asymmetrical, and disappear with movements. Tremor is distal and has a frequency of 3–5 Hz. It is typically a pronation-suppination tremor of the forearm or a pill-rolling motion of the fingers. Tremors can occur in the leg or in the chin, but head or voice tremors are seldom seen. When the tremors are severe, some patients may have action tremors as well. Rigidity may occur throughout the body but is more pronounced on one side. Other symptoms include masked face, decreased blinking, increased drooling, stooped posture, difficulty walking and getting in and out of a chair, micrographia, and decreased olfaction. The patient's speech is hypophonic, rapid, and monotone. The patient often stammers and has palilalia. Drooling is a bothersome feature and is due to decreased swallowing rather than to increased saliva production. Loss of olfactory function occurs early in the disease. Dementia occurs in PD and is more often seen with older age of onset, with hallucinations, lower

mini-mental status score at baseline, early appearance of bilateral motor involvement, and early development of confusional states or psychotic symptoms with levodopa administration. The type of dementia seen in PD represents a combination of cortical and subcortical neuropsychological impairments with dysexecutive, attentional, and visuospatial deficits, and often prominent behavioral disturbances. The memory deficit is typically an impairment of retrieval with relatively preserved mnemonic function. Other cognitive disturbances, such as apraxia, aphasia, or agnosia, are often absent.

After an initially smooth response to therapy, the treatment is complicated by the emergence of variations in motor response in the majority of PD patients. These variations can occur in different forms, as early 'wearing off' during the initial stage of motor complications, dyskinesias in the intermediate stage, and complex fluctuations in the advanced stage. There are also non-motor complications. These are often neglected and include autonomic dysfunctions, sleep disorders, neuropsychiatric disorders, pain, and fatigue. The list of autonomic dysfunctions includes constipation, urinary incontinence, heat or cold intolerance, orthostatic hypotension, sexual dysfunction, and abnormal sweating. Blood pressure may fluctuate with motor impairment in patients with wearing off. Sweating disturbance can be either hyperhydrosis or hypohydrosis. Sweating problems tend to occur predominantly in off periods or in on periods with dyskinesia. Sexual dysfunction is relatively common, and some patients suffer from hypersexuality. Insomnia, hypersomnia, and parasomnia may all occur and contribute to daytime sleepiness. All Parkinson's medications may cause drowsiness. Dopamine agonists and levodopa can cause sleep attacks. Furthermore, sleep disturbances may take the form of difficulty falling asleep or more commonly fragmentation of nocturnal sleep, with frequent and prolonged awakening. This may be due to PD-specific motor phenomena, such as nocturnal immobility, resting tremor, dyskinesias, or nocturia, as well as coexisting sleep disorders, such as restless leg syndrome, periodic limb movements in sleep, or sleep-disordered breathing. PD patients may also have rapid eye movement (REM) sleep behavior disorder, which has a strong association with PD and is characterized by excessive nocturnal motor activity that usually represents attempted enactment of vivid, action-filled, and violent dreams.

Depression also occurs in PD, but the profile is not the same as in patients with primary depression. Distinct features of depression in PD include elevated levels of dysphoria, irritability, guilt or feelings of failure, and a low suicidal rate despite a high frequency of suicidal ideation. Impulse control disorders occur in a subset of patients with PD. This spectrum of disorders, characterized by excessive or poorly controlled preoccupations, urges, or behaviors, includes not only punding, pathological gambling, and hypersexuality, but also compulsive shopping and binge eating. In a small percentage of patients, these behavioral abnormalities are associated with overuse of dopamine replacement therapy (DRT) and are referred to as a homeostatic hedonistic dysregulation called dopamine dysregulation syndrome (DDS).

Differential diagnosis

The differential diagnosis of PD includes other causes of parkinsonism such as essential tremors, multiple system atrophy, progressive supranuclear palsy, corticobasal ganglionic degeneration, diffuse Lewy body disease, normal pressure hydrocephalus, and other parkinson plus entities. Essential tremor is associated with a positive family history in many family members. Essential tremor is characterized by postural tremors, but no extrapyramidal symptoms and no response to levodopa. Patients with progressive supranuclear palsy have vertical gaze paralysis or slowed vertical saccadic movements, nuchal rigidity, and marked postural rigidity. Multiple system atrophy patients may have other symptoms such as fainting, ataxia, and failure to respond to adequate doses of levodopa. Diffuse Lewy body disease patients have memory problems and hallucinations. Corticobasal ganglionic degeneration patients have apraxia, aphasia, sensory disorders, dystonia, alien hand, and myoclonus. In alien hand, the patient does not recognize his or her hand as his/hers when it rises spontaneously. MRI shows asymmetric atrophy of frontal and parietal regions. Drug-induced parkinsonism has a history of previous use of a causative drug such as an antipsychotic, reserpine, or metoclopramide. Vascular parkinsonism has stepwise progression, with the symptoms fixed from previous events. A patient with normal pressure hydrocephalus has ataxia, dementia, and incontinence. MRI would show hydrocephalus. In dementia with Lewy bodies, there are cognitive impairments, hallucinations, and episodes of

delirium in addition to parkinsonism. Patients also have impaired attention and visuospatial disabilities.

Treatment

Despite the rapid expansion in knowledge of its neurodegenerative process, the mainstay of treatment of PD remains symptomatic. Therapeutic options, including pharmacotherapy such as levodopa and other dopaminergic agents (Table 43.2), and surgical approaches such as deep brain stimulation, have been markedly improved over the past decades, resulting in better motor function, activities of daily living, and quality of life for PD patients. The principle of PD management should be individualized and the selection of treatments should aim to control symptoms as well as to prevent or delay motor complications. The authors also reviewed the clinically most important practical decision in the pharmacologic treatment of PD, provided in the form of treatment algorithm in the Appendix on page 681.

Management of early PD

Pharmacotherapy for neuroprotection
Although many agents have appeared promising based on laboratory studies, the symptomatic effects of the study

Table 43.2 Therapeutic options for motor symptoms in Parkinson's disease. (Availability is determined by the time of publication of this book, which may differ in some countries.)

Levodopa
- Levodopa/carbidopa
- Levodopa/benserazide
- Levodopa/carbidopa/entacapone
- Duodopa

Dopamine agonists
a. Non-ergot derivatives
  - Pramipexole
  - Ropinirole
  - Piribedil
  - Rotigotine
b. Ergot derivatives
  - Bromocriptine
  - Pergolide
  - Cabergoline

Indirect agonist
- Amantadine

Catechol-*O*-methyltransferase inhibitors
- Entacapone
- Tolcapone

Monoamine oxidase B inhibitors
- Selegiline
- Rasagiline

Anticholinergics
- Trihexiphenidyl
- Biperiden

medications commonly confound the clinical endpoints for clinical trials. Studies in early PD have suggested that selegiline postpones the need for dopaminergic treatment by more than 6 months, and may reduce the risk of gait freezing, indicating a delay in disability progression. Rasagiline, when tested in a delayed start design in both the TEMPO and in the ADAGIO studies, showed that the difference in disease progression between comparable early, drug-naïve, PD patient groups during double-blind placebo-controlled treatment in the first phase persisted when both groups were treated with this MAO-inhibitor in the second phase. While these findings may suggest a neuroprotective effect of selegiline and rasagiline, symptomatic effects of these agents cannot be entirely excluded.

Two studies have examined the potential neuroprotective properties of pramipexole and ropinirole using β-CIT single photon emission computed tomography (SPECT) and ^{18}F-dopa positron emission tomography (PET) to measure dopamine markers in the brain. Patients initially treated with pramipexole demonstrated a 16% reduction in the percentage loss from baseline of striatal β-CIT uptake versus a 25.5% reduction in those initially treated with levodopa during the 46-month evaluation period ($p < 0.05$). Similar results were obtained in the ropinirole study. The neuroprotective effect of dopamine agonists cannot be confirmed by these imaging studies because of the lack of placebo controls. Furthermore, the binding of these drugs with neuroimaging ligands may confound the findings.

Pharmacotherapy for symptom control
Dopamine agonists
Dopamine agonists have diverse physical and chemical properties, but they share the ability to directly stimulate dopamine receptors. This contrasts with levodopa, which needs to be transformed into *L*-dopamine in presynaptic terminals. This D_2-like receptor agonistic activity of the dopamine agonists produces their antiparkinsonian effects. There are currently five dopamine agonists marketed in the United States: two are ergot derivatives (bromocriptine and pergolide) and the other three are non-ergot derivatives (pramipexole, ropinirole, and recently rotigotine). Cabergoline and piribedil are the other two dopamine agonists which are available in Europe and some countries in Asia. With the exception of rotigotine, all the aforementioned dopamine agonists are taken orally.

The efficacy of dopamine agonists used as monotherapy in early PD has been demonstrated in numerous studies involving pramipexole, ropinirole, pergolide, and, recently, rotigotine. In the early stage, the clinical benefit of dopamine agonists is usually sufficient, but, when the disease progresses, it becomes necessary to add levodopa, which has a better effect on symptoms. Delaying the introduction of levodopa by using a dopamine agonist postpones and reduces the occurrence of motor fluctuations seen with levodopa treatment. Long-term follow-up studies indicate that approximately 85%, 68%, 55%, 43%, and 34% of PD patients initiated on pramipexole or ropinirole are still controlled on monotherapy at 1, 2, 3, 4, and 5 years later, respectively.

There are no data to suggest that one agonist is more efficacious than another. However, an association has been reported between treatment with pergolide and the development of fibrotic valvular heart disease. Similar findings have also been observed with bromocriptine and cabergoline, suggesting a preferential activation of the 5-HT$_{2B}$ receptor on heart valves. Most published studies have concluded that treatment with ergot dopamine agonists (pergolide and cabergoline in most cases), particularly at high daily doses and for periods of 6 months or longer, is associated with a substantially increased risk of newly diagnosed cardiac-valve regurgitation. As a result, pergolide has been voluntarily withdrawn from the US market and current recommendations suggest that non-ergot derivatives should be considered first when dopamine agonists are indicated.

Levodopa
Levodopa is firmly established as the gold standard in the treatment of PD from over 40 years of use in clinical practice. It remains the most reliable and effective treatment for PD symptoms. A recent placebo-controlled study confirmed a dose-dependent efficacy of levodopa to reduce Unified Parkinson's Disease Rating Scale (UPDRS) scores. Levodopa has also been proven to be better at improving symptoms than dopamine agonists in numerous studies. However, patients will develop motor complications with long-term levodopa therapy. After 5 years of treatment, about 50% of patients taking levodopa develop motor fluctuations, and 30% develop dyskinesias; these numbers may be higher in patients with young-onset PD. Levodopa is now routinely coadministered with a decarboxylase inhibitor, either carbidopa or benserazide. They block peripheral degradation of levodopa to dopamine, allowing more levodopa to cross the blood–brain barrier. The gastric mucosa is another site of action; thus decarboxylase inhibition also increases duodenal levodopa absorption.

Prevention of motor complications
A number of strategies have been developed to prevent or delay the occurrence of motor complications. First, the evidence that the early use of dopamine agonists can reduce the incidence of motor complications (versus levodopa) has influenced most neurologists to start dopamine agonists as symptomatic monotherapy in early PD patients. Second, the mechanism of levodopa-induced motor complications is probably related to the abnormal pulsatile stimulation of striatal dopamine receptors,

which does not mirror the normal continuous activation of these receptors that occurs physiologically. The concept of continuous dopaminergic stimulation (CDS), either by using long-acting dopamine agonists or continuously delivering levodopa, has been proposed as a method of preventing motor complications. Whether employing CDS therapy by continuous levodopa delivery can actually delay dyskinesias or motor fluctuations in early PD patients is not known. A few studies are ongoing to address these questions.

Management of advanced (complicated) PD

Long-term dopaminomimetic therapy, not limited to levodopa, is often complicated by the emergence of variations of motor response in the majority of PD patients. "Advanced disease" is defined as PD with progressive motor impairment despite levodopa therapy and an unstable medication response leading to motor complications. Advanced disease typically develops after 5 years of levodopa treatment in up to 50% of PD patients. Motor complications can be simply divided into motor fluctuations and dyskinesias. Typically, patients may begin to experience a wearing-off (end-of-dose) effect because the motor improvement after a dose of levodopa becomes reduced in duration and parkinsonism reappears. Subsequently, dyskinesias emerge at peak-dose levels and are classically choreiform. Eventually, patients may experience rapid and unpredictable fluctuations between on and off periods, known as the on–off phenomenon.

Treatment of end-of-dose wearing off
End-of-dose wearing off is the most common and usually the first sign of motor complications. Patients develop a loss of response to a dose of medication before taking the next dose, usually within 4 hours of the earlier dose. If they take their next dose of medication, their symptoms will improve again until the next dose begins to wear off. Treatment depends on the severity of the problem and on how dopaminergic therapy was initiated in the early stage of the disease. The predictability is somewhat reassuring to patients and this may allow simple interventions to be made. Some treatment options are suggested as follows:
• *Add a catechol-O-methyltransferase (COMT) inhibitor.* If the patient already takes stable doses of levodopa, this is an option. Entacapone is a peripheral COMT inhibitor, while tolcapone inhibits both peripheral and central a COMT. Several controlled studies have demonstrated that adding a COMT inhibitor is useful and has been shown to reduce "off" time by approximately 1.3 hours/day with entacapone and 2–3 hours/day with tolcapone (another COMT inhibitor available in the US). Patients should be advised

that they may develop dyskinesia within 1 or 2 days of adding a COMT inhibitor and that a 20–30% reduction in levodopa dose may be required. Side effects of tolcapone include diarrhea occurring in 5–6% of patients and the possibility of developing fulminant hepatitis.
• *Manipulate the dose of levodopa by shortening the interval between levodopa doses.* The next dose should be administered just before the beneficial effects from the previous dose have worn off.
• *Add a dopamine agonist.* Dopamine agonists are useful in reducing "off" time because their half-lives are longer than that of levodopa. The dose of levodopa should be maintained until a clinical response to dopamine agonist is achieved. Later, the levodopa dose can be gradually lowered. Several controlled studies confirmed the efficacy of dopamine agonists as adjunctive treatment to levodopa in reducing total daily "off" time by about 2 hours with a reduction of levodopa dose of about 19–25%.

Treatment of dyskinesia
To treat dyskinesia, the pattern of dyskinesia needs to be determined. A patient's history and PD diary are the primary source of information. While dyskinesia appears to be debilitating as considered by caregivers, most PD patients prefer to be "on" with dyskinesia rather than to be "off." Therefore, in the management of advanced PD patients, the balance between reductions in dyskinesia and the potential for deteriorating parkinsonism is critical. It is also important for advanced PD patients to be aware that it is often difficult to delineate a dose of medication that provides stable "on" time without inducing dyskinesia. A compromise to achieve "balance" is probably the goal of management. The following steps are recommended for treating patients with disabling dyskinesias:
• *Review the patient's drug regimen.* Determine if there are any drugs that may alleviate dyskinesia without reducing the antiparkinsonian effect. Examples of options are selegiline and anticholinergics.
• *Examine other adjunctive therapies.* If patients are receiving sustained-release levodopa, better symptom control may be achievable if they are switched to an immediate-release preparation, particularly if dyskinesia occurs late in the day. If a COMT inhibitor is used, dose reduction may be necessary. Alternatively, a reduction in levodopa dose may be considered, but this may result in the inability to induce an "on" response in some patients. Some authors suggest the addition of a dopamine agonist coupled with a reduction in the levodopa dose may reduce dyskinesia while sustaining motor benefit.
• *Add amantadine or clozapine.* Amantadine is the only agent that suppresses dyskinesia through its action at the *N*-methyl-*D*-aspartate (NMDA) receptor. The anti-dyskinetic effect of amantadine is effective at 300 mg/day, but it generally only lasts about 5 months, with many patients experiencing a rebound in dyskinesia after drug

discontinuation. Alternatively, clozapine may be considered. However, it lacks definite evidence in reducing dyskinesia, and its potential toxicity, such as agranulocytosis, has limited its use.

Treatment of "off" dystonia

Dystonia can be caused by levodopa or PD itself so it can occur during both the "on" and "off" state. Therefore, careful history, noting the relationship between the timing of dystonia and the timing of levodopa administration, is critically important. Generally, "off" dystonia is much more common than "on" dystonia and frequently occurs in the morning, manifested as painful dystonic cramping of the toes and feet on wakening. This symptom, termed early morning dystonia, probably occurs as a result of the wearing off of the levodopa overnight. Several treatment options are available as follows:

• Add a bedtime dose of sustained-release levodopa or long-acting dopamine agonist to increase plasma concentrations of levodopa throughout the night and early morning.

• Have the patient take the first dose of levodopa before rising from bed. This strategy can be used with water-soluble levodopa, which has an onset of action of between 10 and 15 minutes.

Treatment of dose failures, or no "on" response and delayed "on"

In some patients with advanced PD, taking a dose of levodopa may not result in any improvement in symptoms; this is known as a dose failure. If the occurrence of these symptoms is not related to a reduction in levodopa dose or appears suddenly after additional medication has been prescribed, drug interactions should be suspected. Certain medications have been reported to reduce levodopa bioavailability, including oral iron, aluminum-/ magnesium-containing antacids, pyridoxine, and cholesterol-lowering drugs. Recently, PD patients who received *Helicobacter pylori* eradication therapy showed a significant increase in levodopa absorption, which was coupled with a significant improvement in clinical disability and a prolonged "on-time" duration. If drug interactions are excluded, it is likely that these symptoms are due to inadequate absorption of levodopa, whether as a result of an inadequate dose, slowing of gastrointestinal transit time, or competition for levodopa absorption from dietary protein. The following strategies are recommended to augment levodopa absorption:

• Withdraw anticholinergic agents.

• Relieve constipation using laxatives, for example high-fiber and fruit diet and lactulose.

• Instruct the patient to take the medication sufficiently in advance of meals. A high-protein meal may reduce levodopa absorption due to large neutral amino acids competing with levodopa for transfer across the intestinal mucosa and the blood–brain barrier. If this option fails, reducing any fat intake close to the time medication is taken may be helpful.

• Add domperidone (not available in the United States): domperidone is a prokinetic D_2 receptor antagonist that does not cross the blood–brain barrier. Therefore, the incidence of extrapyramidal symptoms is rare. Domperidone therapy significantly reduces upper gastrointestinal symptoms and accelerates gastric emptying of a solid meal, and does not interfere with response to antiparkinsonism treatment.

• Switch to water-soluble levodopa or immediate-release levodopa to help shorten the delay in "on" response. The sustained-release formulation often results in a more delayed "on" response and is generally not recommended in this particular situation. Dissolving immediate-release levodopa in an ascorbic acid solution or fizzy drink may improve uptake from the gut.

The on–off phenomenon (unpredictable on–off)

As PD progresses, patients may develop an unpredictable "on–off" response to medication such that motor function does not follow levodopa dosing cycles. The typical example is that the medication may kick in, but well before the time of the next dose, there is an abrupt "off" period (without warning), unlike the gradual "off" time that develops in the wearing-off response. There is a complete loss of predictability and, therefore, patients will not know when they will be able to perform activities. Usually they have severe akinetic "off" periods, accompanied by severe dyskinesias during the "on" stage.

This is one of the most difficult fluctuations to treat. Patients at this stage are very sensitive to manipulations of even small doses of levodopa. The fine tuning of medications at this stage has to be individualized. However, sustained-release formulations are best avoided because their bioavailability is unpredictable. Other approaches to consider are as follows:

• *Add a COMT inhibitor*. It is recommended that a COMT inhibitor be gradually titrated, for example, initially 100 mg of entacapone to avoid disabling dyskinesias.

• *Try a different dopamine agonist* if the current one is not helpful.

• *Implement a protein redistribution diet*. Because patients at this stage have a decreased capacity to store dopamine centrally, a minor reduction in levodopa transport into the brain can lead to a dramatic reduction in striatal dopamine levels, resulting in an "off" episode.

• *Consider surgical procedures such as DBS*. Both globus pallidus interna and subthalamic nucleus (STN) are common surgical targets for DBS. However, STN has been proposed as the preferred surgical target site for treating motor complications. Bilateral STN DBS has been shown to provide patients with a full range of antiparkinsonian benefits, including improvements in tremor, bradykinesia, and rigidity. In addition, stimulation of the STN may allow levodopa doses to be lowered, thereby reducing the severity of levodopa-related dyskinesias.

Conclusion

Due to the improvement of medical and surgical treatments for PD, there are several therapeutic options for physicians to consider for their patients. However, the most important principle in the management of PD is to customize therapy to the needs of individual patients. The selection should be based on scientific rationale and evidence-based information. The aim should be not only to control motoric symptoms but also to prevent or delay motor complications if possible. There are no proven neuroprotective drugs, but several agents have been found to have at least levodopa-sparing effects or to reduce the risk of freezing. Surgical interventions should be reserved for patients with intractable motor complications. Because certain symptoms, for example dysarthria, dysphagia, and axial symptoms, may not respond to dopaminergic therapy, other neurochemicals may be involved and could be targets of future research. With continued research in the therapeutics of PD, it is anticipated that more pharmacologic agents and new surgical techniques will be discovered, leading to better treatments in the future.

Further reading

Bhidayasiri R, Truong DD. Motor complications in Parkinson disease: clinical manifestations and management. *J Neurol Sci* 2008; 266(1–2): 204–15.

Braak H, Del Tredici K, Rub U, de Vos RA, Jansen Steur EN, Braak E. Staging of brain pathology related to sporadic Parkinson's disease. *Neurobiol Aging* 2003; 24: 197–211.

Goetz CG, Poewe W, Rascol O, Sampaio C. Evidence-based medical review update: pharmacological and surgical treatments of Parkinson's disease: 2001 to 2004. *Mov Disord* 2005; 20: 523–39.

Horstink M, Tolosa E, Bonuccelli U, *et al*. Review of the therapeutic management of Parkinson's disease. Report of a joint task force of the European Federation of Neurological Societies and the Movement Disorder Society-European Section. Part I: early (uncomplicated) Parkinson's disease. *Eur J Neurol* 2006; 13: 1170–85.

Lang AE, Lozano AM. Parkinson's disease. First of two parts. *N Engl J Med* 1998; 339: 1044–53.

Horstink M, Tolosa E, Bonuccelli U, *et al*. Review of the therapeutic management of Parkinson's disease. Report of a joint task force of the European Federation of Neurological Societies (EFNS) and the Movement Disorder Society-European Section (MDS-ES). Part II: late (complicated) Parkinson's disease. *Eur J Neurol* 2006; 13: 1186–202.

Lang AE, Lozano AM. Parkinson's disease. Second of two parts. *N Engl J Med* 1998; 339: 1130–43.

Miyasaki JM, Shannon K, Voon V, *et al*. Practice parameter: evaluation and treatment of depression, psychosis, and dementia in Parkinson disease (an evidence-based review): report of the Quality Standards Subcommittee of the American Academy of Neurology. *Neurology* 2006; 66: 996–1002.

Pahwa R, Factor SA, Lyons KE, *et al*. Practice parameter: treatment of Parkinson disease with motor fluctuations and dyskinesia (an evidence-based review): report of the Quality Standards Subcommittee of the American Academy of Neurology. *Neurology* 2006; 66: 983–95.

Suchowersky O, Gronseth G, Perlmutter J, Reich S, Zesiewicz T, Weiner WJ. Practice parameter: neuroprotective strategies and alternative therapies for Parkinson disease (an evidence-based review): report of the Quality Standards Subcommittee of the American Academy of Neurology. *Neurology* 2006; 66: 976–82.

Suchowersky O, Reich S, Perlmutter J, Zesiewicz T, Gronseth G, Weiner WJ. Practice parameter: diagnosis and prognosis of new onset Parkinson disease (an evidence-based review): report of the Quality Standards Subcommittee of the American Academy of Neurology. *Neurology* 2006; 66: 968–75.

Truong DD, Bhidayasiri R, Wolters E. Management of non-motor symptoms in advanced Parkinson disease. *J Neurol Sci* 2008; 266(1–2): 216–28.

Chapter 44
Dystonia

Stanley Fahn

Columbia University College of Physicians and Surgeons, New York, USA

Clinical features

Dystonia refers to twisting movements that tend to be sustained at the peak of the movement, are frequently repetitive, and often progress to prolonged abnormal postures. In contrast to chorea, dystonic movements repeatedly involve the same group of muscles, that is, they are patterned. Agonist and antagonist muscles contract simultaneously (co-contraction) to produce the sustained quality of dystonic movements. The speed of the movement varies widely from slow (athetotic dystonia) to shock-like (myoclonic dystonia). Pain is uncommon in dystonia except in cervical dystonia. Rhythmical movements (dystonic tremor) can be present in the dystonic arms and neck; there is usually a null point in positioning the affected body part in which the tremor may disappear. This feature may help in differentiating dystonic tremor from other types of tremor.

When dystonia first appears, the movements typically occur when the affected body part is carrying out a voluntary action (*action dystonia*) and are not present when that body part is at rest. With progression of the disorder, dystonic movements can appear at distant sites when other parts of the body are voluntarily moving (overflow). With further progression, dystonic movements become present when the body is "at rest." Even at this stage, dystonic movements are usually more severe with voluntary activity. Whereas primary dystonia often begins as action dystonia and may persist as the kinetic (clonic) form, symptomatic dystonia often begins as fixed postures (tonic form).

One of the characteristic and almost unique features of dystonic movements is that they can often be diminished by tactile or proprioceptive "*sensory tricks*" (geste antagoniste). Thus, touching the involved body part or an adjacent body part can often reduce the muscle contractions. For example, patients with torticollis will often place a hand on the chin or side of the face to reduce nuchal contractions, and orolingual dystonia is often helped by touching the lips or placing an object in the mouth.

Classification

Dystonia is classified in three ways: age at onset, affected body distribution, and etiology (Table 44.1). Classification by age at onset is useful because this is the most important single factor related to prognosis of primary dystonia, with earlier onset usually progressing faster, and late (adult) onset remaining more static and focal. If onset is in the legs, this also indicates a more progressive course leading to generalized dystonia.

When a single body part is affected, the condition is referred to as *focal dystonia*. Common forms of focal dystonia are spasmodic torticollis (cervical dystonia), blepharospasm (upper facial dystonia), and writer's cramp (hand and arm dystonia). Involvement of two or more contiguous regions of the body is referred to as *segmental dystonia*. *Generalized dystonia* indicates involvement of one or both legs, the trunk, and some other parts of the body. *Multifocal dystonia* involves two or more regions, not conforming to segmental or generalized dystonia. *Hemidystonia* refers to involvement of the arm and leg on the same side.

The etiologic classification divides the causes of dystonia into four major categories: primary (or idiopathic), secondary (environmental causes or symptomatic), dystonia-plus syndromes, and heredodegenerative

Table 44.1 Classification of dystonia.

1. By age at onset
   a. Early onset: ≤26 years
   b. Late onset: >26 years
2. By distribution
   a. Focal
   b. Segmental
   c. Multifocal
   d. Generalized
   e. Hemidystonia
3. By etiology
   a. Primary (also known as idiopathic) dystonia
   b. Dystonia-plus
   c. Secondary dystonia
   d. Heredodegenerative dystonia (usually presents as dystonia-plus)
   e. A feature of another neurologic disease (e.g., dystonic tics, paroxysmal dyskinesias, PD, PSP)

International Neurology: A Clinical Approach. Edited by Robert P. Lisak, Daniel D. Truong, William M. Carroll, and Roongroj Bhidayasiri. © 2009 Blackwell Publishing, ISBN: 978-1-4051-5738-4.

diseases in which dystonia is a prominent feature. Primary dystonia is characterized as a pure dystonia (with the exception that tremor can be present) and excludes a symptomatic cause; primary dystonia can be genetic or sporadic. Dystonia-plus syndromes are non-degenerative (i.e., biochemical) diseases that are highlighted by dystonia and another feature, such as dopa-responsive dystonia (DRD) (incorporates features of parkinsonism)

and myoclonus dystonia (myoclonus can even predominate). Secondary dystonias are those due to environmental insult, while heredodegenerative dystonias are due to neurodegenerative diseases that are usually inherited. Other neurologic diseases in which dystonia is often present are dystonic tics, paroxysmal dyskinesias, Parkinson's disease, and progressive supranuclear palsy. Table 44.2 lists the etiologic classification of dystonia.

Table 44.2 Principal dystonic disorders by etiology. (Adapted from Fahn S, Jankovic J, *Principles and Practice of Movement Disorders*. Philadelphia: Churchill Livingstone Elsevier; 2007.)

A. Primary (also known as idiopathic) dystonia

1. Oppenheim dystonia (also called DYT1)
   Autosomal dominant inheritance of mutated *TOR1A* gene
   Early onset (age <40), affecting limbs first
2. Childhood and adult onset familial cranial and limb (DYT6)
   Autosomal dominant inheritance of mutated *THAP1* gene at 8p21-q22
   Childhood and adult onset affecting the Mennonite and Amish populations
3. Adult onset familial torticollis (DYT7)
   Autosomal dominant inheritance mapped to 18p
4. Adult onset familial cervical-cranial predominant (DYT13)
   Autosomal dominant inheritance mapped to 1p36
5. Other familial types not yet labeled as distinct entities
6. Sporadic, usually adult onset, usually focal or segmental

B. Dystonia-plus syndromes

1. Dystonia with parkinsonism
   a. Dopa-responsive dystonia (DRD) (DYT5)
      i. GTP cyclohydrolase I deficiency
         Autosomal dominant inheritance located at 14q22.1
         Childhood onset with leg and gait disorder, may be diurnal
         Adult onset with parkinsonism
      ii. Tyrosine hydroxylase deficiency
         Autosomal recessive inheritance
         Infantile onset
   b. Rapid-onset dystonia–parkinsonism (RDP) (DYT12)
      Autosomal dominant inheritance of mutated Na-K-ATPase gene (*ATP1A3*)
      Adolescent and adult onset progresses over hours to a few weeks, then plateaus
2. Dystonia with myoclonic jerks that respond to alcohol
   Myoclonus-dystonia with childhood, adolescent, and adult onset
   Autosomal dominant inheritance of the epsilon-sarcoglycan gene on chromosome 7q21 (DYT11)
   Autosomal dominant inheritance on 18p11 (DYT15)

C. Secondary dystonia

1. Perinatal cerebral injury
2. Encephalitis, infectious and postinfectious
3. Head trauma
4. Basal ganglia, thalamus, or cortical lesions
5. Hypoxia
6. Peripheral injury
7. Drug induced – levodopa, dopamine D2 receptor blocking agents
8. Toxins – Mn, CO, cyanide
9. Metabolic – hypoparathyroidism
10. Immune encephalopathy: Sjögren's syndrome, Rasmussen's syndrome
11. Psychogenic

D. Heredodegenerative diseases (typically not pure dystonia)

1. X-linked recessive
   a. Lubag (X-linked dystonia-parkinsonism) (DYT3)
      TAF1 gene, Filipino males, steadily progressive → disabling
      Parkinsonism can appear at onset and be only feature or develop after and replace dystonia
      Pathology: mosaic gliosis in striatum
2. Autosomal dominant
   a. Juvenile parkinsonism (presenting with dystonia)
   b. Huntington's disease (usually presents as chorea)
      Gene: IT15 located at 4p16.3 for huntingtin protein
   c. Neuroferritinopathy
3. Autosomal recessive
   a. Wilson's disease
      Gene: Cu-ATPase located at 13q14.3
   b. Niemann–Pick type C (dystonic lipidosis) (sea-blue histiocytosis)
      defect in cholesterol esterification; gene mapped to chromosome 18
   c. Juvenile neuronal ceroid-lipofuscinosis (Batten disease)
   d. GM1 gangliosidosis
   e. GM2 gangliosidosis
   f. Metachromatic leukodystrophy
   g. Lesch–Nyhan syndrome
   h. Homocystinuria
   i. Glutaric acidemia
   j. Neurodegeneration with brain iron accumulation type 1 (formerly called Hallervorden–Spatz syndrome), recently renamed as pantothenate kinase-associated neurodegeneration (PKAN)
   k. Neuroacanthocytosis
4. Probable autosomal recessive
   a. Familial basal ganglia calcifications
   b. Progressive pallidal degeneration
5. Mitochondrial
   a. Leigh disease
   b. Leber disease

E. Dystonia present in other neurologic syndromes

1. Parkinsonism – Parkinson's disease, progressive supranuclear palsy, multiple system atrophy, cortical-basal ganglionic degeneration
2. Tourette syndrome (dystonic tics)
3. Paroxysmal dyskinesias

Genetics

In the past decade there has been an explosion of new discoveries in the genetics of dystonia. They have been assigned the DYT label (Table 44.3). The DYT label has been applied to most of these in chronologic order of their discoveries. Of those with specific gene identifications or mapping, most are primary dystonias (DYT1, DYT6, DYT7, DYT13) or dystonia-plus syndromes (DYT5, DYT11, DYT12). One is a degenerative disorder (DYT3), and three are clinically part of the paroxysmal dyskinesia disorders (DYT8, DYT9, DYT10). DYT14 was initially misidentified, and the family in question is actually DYT5. DYT1 or Oppenheim dystonia has been the one most well studied, and represents the prototypic primary dystonia. DYT5 or DRD is most easily treated. Both are discussed below.

Oppenheim dystonia

Named after Hermann Oppenheim who coined the term dystonia in 1911 to describe Jewish children with what he called dystonia musculorum deformans; following genetic studies, it is now known as DYT1. The gene (*TOR1A*) codes for the protein torsinA, found in neurons in the endoplasmic reticulum. TorsinA is an ATPase of the heat-shock type that functions in restoring damaged proteins particularly in membranes. The abnormal torsinA becomes more prominently located in the nuclear

Table 44.3 Monogenic forms of dystonia.

Designation	Dystonia type	Inheritance	Gene name and locus	Gene product
DYT1	Early onset Limb onset Progresses Oppenheim dystonia	Autosomal dominant	*TOR1A* 9q34	TorsinA
DYT2	Early onset Generalized	Autosomal recessive	Unknown	Unknown
DYT3	Filipino males Dystonia evolves into parkinsonism	X-linked recessive	*TAF1* Xq13.1	Multiple transcript system
DYT4	Whispering dysphonia	Autosomal dominant	Unknown	Unknown
DYT5	Dopa-responsive dystonia Segawa syndrome Childhood onset	Autosomal dominant	*GCH1* 14q22.1	GTP cyclo hydrolase 1
	Tyrosine hydroxylase	Autosomal recessive	11p11.5	Tyrosine hydroxylase
DYT6	Adolescent onset dystonia Mennonite/Amish	Autosomal dominant	*THAP1* 8p21-q22	THAP1
DYT7	Familial torticollis	Autosomal dominant	18p	Unknown
DYT8	Paroxysmal non-kinesigenic dyskinesia Mount-Rebak syndrome	Autosomal dominant	*MR-1* 2q34	Myofibrillogenesis regulator 1
DYT9	Paroxysmal dyskinesia with spasticity	Autosomal dominant	1p21	Unknown
DYT10	Paroxysmal kinesigenic dyskinesia	Autosomal dominant	16p11.2-q12.1	Unknown
DYT11	Myoclonus-dystonia	Autosomal dominant	*SGCE* 7q21	Epsilon-sarcoglycan
DYT12	Rapid-onset dystonia-parkinsonism	Autosomal dominant	*ATP1A3* 19q12-q13.2	Na-K-ATPase
DYT13	Cranial-cervical-brachial dystonia	Autosomal dominant	1p36	Unknown
DYT15	Myoclonus-dystonia	Autosomal dominant	18p11	Unknown
Neurodegeneration with brain accumulation type 1		Autosomal recessive	*PANK2* 20p12.3-p13	Pantothenate kinase
Neurodegeneration with brain accumulation type 2 (neuroferritinopathy)		Autosomal dominant	*FTLI* 19q13.3	Ferritin light iron polypeptide

envelope, which is continuous with the endoplasmic reticulum. The abnormal protein loses ATPase activity, with a resultant decrease as a chaperone protein. The universal mutation in this disorder, most common in the Ashkenazi Jewish population due to a founder effect introduced about 360 years ago, is a deletion of one of an adjacent pair of GAG triplets (codes for glutamate) near the functional domain. The penetrance rate is only 30%. The *TOR1A* gene can be tested commercially for the mutation, and this is recommended for all patients with onset of primary dystonia below the age of 26.

The disorder usually begins in childhood, but sometimes in adulthood, and it almost always starts in either an arm or a leg. It tends to spread contiguously and in many cases (especially if it begins in a leg) becomes generalized and disabling.

Dopa-responsive dystonia (DRD)

DRD usually begins in childhood with a peculiar gait (walking on toes). Adult onset cases tend to resemble Parkinson's disease. Even in childhood, one can detect parkinsonian features of bradykinesia and loss of postural reflexes, a feature that distinguishes this from Oppenheim dystonia. It can resemble, therefore, childhood onset Parkinson's disease with dopamine nigrostriatal neuronal degeneration. The latter condition shows a depletion of F-DOPA uptake or dopamine transporter in positron emission tomography (PET) and single photon emission computed tomography (SPECT) scanning, whereas these studies are normal in DRD, which does not show neuronal degeneration.

The disorder is due to a mutation in the gene for the guanosine triphosphate (GTP) cyclohydrolase 1, which is the rate-limiting step for synthesis of tetrahydrobiopterin, the cofactor for tyrosine hydroxylase and other hydroxylases, required for the synthesis of biogenic amines, such as dopamine. The dopamine deficiency in the striatum accounts for the symptoms, and the patients respond extremely well to low doses of levodopa. They can respond after years of no treatment, and they do not develop the fluctuations or dyskinesias so commonly seen in patients with Parkinson's disease. Interestingly, these patients also respond to low dosages of anticholinergic medications, such as trihexyphenidyl. Some patients show a diurnal pattern of symptoms, being almost normal in the morning and markedly dystonic at the end of the day. These patients obtain benefit from sleep.

Adult-onset focal dystonias

These are the most common forms of dystonias. Their appearance varies depending on the body part affected.

Although most cases remain focal, dystonia can spread to a contiguous, neighboring segment, thus becoming segmental myoclonus. The most common focal dystonia involves the neck musculature, known as *spasmodic torticollis* or *cervical dystonia*. The head can turn (rotational torticollis), tilt, or shift to one side, or bend forward (anterocollis) or backwards (retrocollis). Any combination of head positions can be found in individual patients. About 10% have a remission within a year, but relapses usually occur, even many years later. The age at onset is usually between 20 and 50 years. The muscles involved are innervated by cranial nerve (CN) XI and the upper cervical nerve roots. Some cervical dystonias are manifested as a static pulling of the head into one direction, but most have a jerky, irregular rhythmic feature. Some patients try to fight the pulling of the neck muscles and the physician can be misled by seeing or feeling contracted muscles, thinking that these are the dystonic muscles, when, in fact, they could be the compensatory muscles contracting. To distinguish between involuntary and compensatory/voluntary contractions, the patient should be told to let the movements occur without trying to overcome them. Then the true direction of which muscles are involved in the dystonia is revealed. This is especially important when deciding which muscles to inject with botulinum toxin (BTX). Common sensory tricks to reduce dystonia are touching the face or the back of the head. Mechanical devices to place cutaneous pressure on the occiput can sometimes be used to advantage.

Bleparospasm usually affects elderly individuals and is more prevalent in women than men. It begins as excessive blinking, and many patients complain of eye irritation or dryness, although dry eyes from Sjögren's disease are usually ruled out. This blinking phase then leads to some longer closing of the eyes, even to very long durations. Usually there is a combination of eyelid closing and blinking. The muscles involved are the orbicularis oculi innervated by CN VII, and the movements are symmetrical in the two eyes, quite distinct from hemifacial spasm, which is unilateral. One interesting difference is that in blepharospasm the eyebrows may elevate due to simultaneous contractions of the frontalis muscles, while in hemifacial spasm the eyebrows come down. Dystonia can spread from the upper face causing blepharospasm to the lower face with movements around the mouth. Common sensory tricks to reduce blepharospasm are touching the corner of the eye, coughing, and talking. Bright light notoriously aggravates blepharospasm and patients have difficulty being in sunlight or bright light and they typically wear sunglasses most of the time. Driving at night is very difficult because of oncoming headlights.

Ormandibular dystonia (OMD) (jaw muscles innervated by CN V) is often associated with lingual dystonia (tongue muscles by CN XII) and is less frequent than blepharospasm. Jaw-opening dystonia is where the jaw is pulled down by the pterygoids; in jaw-clenching dystonia the masseters and temporalis muscles are the prime movers. The jaw can also be moved laterally. It is important to distinguish the latter from facial muscle pulling the mouth to one side, which is often due to psychogenic etiology. OMD can markedly affect chewing and swallowing. Some OMDs appear only with action and are not present at rest. Such actions can involve talking or chewing. Often a patient attempts to overcome jaw-opening and jaw-closing dystonias by purposefully moving the jaw in the opposite direction. This maneuvering has often led to a misdiagnosis of tardive dyskinesia because the movements superficially appear rhythmic. To distinguish between OMD and tardive dyskinesia, the patient should be told to let the movements occur without trying to overcome them. In this manner, the true direction of where the dystonia wants to take the jaw is revealed, and the rhythmic movements stop in OMD. Sensory tricks that have been useful are the placing of objects in the mouth or biting down on an object, such as a tongue blade or pencil. Dental implants have sometimes helped by the physical application of a continual sensory trick.

Embouchure dystonia is an action dystonia involving the muscles around the mouth (embouchure) that may develop in professional musicians who play woodwinds and horn instruments. More common are *musician's cramps* involving the fingers of instrumentalists such as pianists, guitarists, violinists, and other string instruments. This is a form of occupational cramp, the most common being *writer's cramp*. These are task-specific dystonias. In writer's cramp, only the action of writing brings out the dystonic tightening of the finger, hand, forearm, and arm muscles, such as the triceps. If the dystonia progresses, it may be brought out by other actions of the arm, like finger-to-nose maneuver, buttoning, and sewing. Dystonia at rest can ultimately develop, but usually does not. In about 15% of patients with writer's cramp, the dystonia spreads to the other arm. Otherwise, the patient can learn to write with the uninvolved arm. Sensory tricks that have been useful include placing of the pen/pencil between other fingers, using specially designed larger writing implements, and placing the non-writing hand on top of the writing hand.

Dystonia of the vocal cords comes in two varieties: adduction and abduction of the cords with speaking. The former produces a tight, constricted, strangulated type of voice with frequent pauses breaking up the voice, and it takes longer to complete what the patient is trying to say. The latter produces a whispering voice. With dystonic adductor dysphonia, the patient is still able to whisper normally, and may present this way to the physician who needs to be aware that this is a compensating mechanism. A major differential diagnosis is vocal cord tremor, seen fairly commonly in patients with essential tremor.

Focal trunk dystonia can present in adults, both as primary dystonia and as tardive dystonia. The dystonia is usually absent when the patient is lying or sitting, and appears on standing and walking. This is an uncommon form of adult-onset focal dystonia.

Secondary and heredodegenerative dystonias

In examining patients with dystonia, features of a neurologic insult in the medical history such as exposure to drugs, toxins, trauma, or presence of neurological abnormality on examination would suggest that the patient's dystonia is secondary rather than primary. Table 44.3 lists the major causes of secondary dystonia and also the heredodegenerative dystonias. The most common secondary dystonias seen in a busy movement disorder center are the drug-induced dystonias, especially tardive dystonia, induced by dopamine receptor blocking agents. Tardive dystonia can affect all ages, but as in classic tardive dyskinesia, older people are most susceptible. In children and young people, it can manifest as generalized dystonia, but it is usually reversible after a long period of being without the offending drugs. Older people are more likely to have a focal form of tardive dystonia, usually OMD, cervical dystonia, or blepharospasm. Tardive dystonia resembles primary dystonias unless there is an accompanying tardive akathisia or classic tardive dyskinesia, which allows the diagnosis to be made quite readily. When these other forms of the tardive syndromes are not present, one clinical feature of tardive dystonia that is fairly common to allow this diagnosis is the posture of hyperextension of the neck and trunk with pronated arms, extended elbows, and flexed wrists. The diagnosis of tardive dystonia may also be suspected if the patient has had a recent exposure to dopamine receptor blocking agents.

Prevalence, pathology, neuroimaging, and physiology

Many studies on the prevalence of dystonia have been conducted, with varying results. Generalized dystonia is about one-tenth as frequent as focal dystonias. In Olmstead County, Minnesota, generalized dystonia occurred in about 1 in 30000 individuals, while focal dystonias were found in about 1 in 3000.

Post-mortem examination of patients with primary dystonia and dystonia-plus syndrome reveals no consistent gross or microscopic pathological changes, with the exception of one paper on Oppenheim dystonia that showed perinuclear inclusions using a special immunostaining technique. On the other hand, secondary and degenerative dystonias typically have pathology in the basal ganglia or its connections (thalamus and cortex). Pallidal and thalamic stereotaxic surgical targets that can ameliorate dystonia also support a basal ganglionic pathophysiologic mechanism. Pharmacologic observations (acute and tardive dystonia, dopa-induced dystonia, DRD, treatment with anticholinergics) also support involvement of the basal ganglia.

Although routine MRI fails to show any abnormalities in primary dystonia, voxel-based morphometry has revealed an increase in the size of sensorimotor structures. Diffusion tensor MRI indicates a reduced axonal integrity in the subgyral white matter of the sensorimotor cortex in those carrying the DYT1 mutation. Fluorodeoxyglucose (FDG) PET techniques show lenticular-thalamic dissociation and dystonia network patterns. These indicate reduced pallidal inhibition of the thalamus with consequent overactivity of medial and prefrontal cortical areas and underactivity of the primary motor cortex during movements. PET scans assessing dopamine D2 receptor binding show a reduction in the striatum in primary dystonia, including non-manifesting DYT1 gene carriers. There is reduced spinal cord and brainstem inhibition in many reflex studies (long-latency reflexes, cranial reflexes, and reciprocal inhibition) in primary dystonia. Physiologic studies of the cerebral cortex show reduced preparatory activity in the electroencephalogram (EEG) before the onset of voluntary movements, enhanced premotor and supplementary motor cortical excitability, and reduced primary motor cortex activity. These studies suggest that there is defective "surround inhibition" in the basal ganglia and cerebral cortex in primary dystonia.

Treatment

Treatment of the dystonias continues to evolve, but certain principles remain fundamental. Although there are agents that can often reduce the severity of dystonia, it is most important to identify specific disorders that are treatable, for example, Wilson's disease and drug-induced and infectious diseases, and treat them. Of course, as in all diseases, one needs to educate the patient and family, and provide genetic counseling. The focal dystonias of eyelids, vocal cords, jaw, neck, and limbs are more easily treated with BTX, and this is the preferred approach. Segmental and generalized dystonias require systemic pharmacologic therapy, but residual focal involvement can be treated with BTX. Surgical therapy is reserved for disabling dystonia resistant to medications and/or BTX injections. To increase the potential for successful outcomes, the current strategy is to move to surgery before the patient develops fixed dystonic postures. The usual surgical target is the internal segment of the globus pallidus, and stimulation by implanted electrodes has replaced ablative surgery. The surgery usually does not provide immediate relief. Rather, improvement develops after several weeks and steadily increases until a plateau of benefit is reached. This delay in response suggests a plastic change is taking place in the brain. The abnormal firing pattern in the pallidum is affected and modified by the stimulation, and that supposedly leads to the gradual benefit.

Pharmacologic therapy, as applied in generalized dystonia, should start with a trial of levodopa to make sure DRD is not overlooked. If that fails, the drugs with the most success are high dosages of anticholinergics (e.g., trihexyphenidyl and benztropine), baclofen, and benzodiazepines. The sooner treatment is started, the better the chance for avoiding progressive, disabling dystonia. Other medications with some reported benefit are carbamazepine, a dopamine depletor (tetrabenazine or reserpine), dopamine receptor blockers, and a combination of dopamine depletor, dopamine receptor blocker, and anticholinergic medication. Because these drugs can produce intolerable side effects, they should be started at low doses and built up gradually until either therapeutic benefit or intolerable side effects are seen. Work with one drug first to determine what it can accomplish. If there is some benefit, a second drug could be added when the final dosage of the first drug is reached. Adding multiple drugs this way may provide benefit not seen with just a single drug. Peripheral side effects of anticholinergics can usually be controlled by employing pilocarpine eye drops (for blurred vision due to dilated pupils), pyridostigmine for urinary hesitation and constipation, and artificial saliva for dry mouth. Central side effects, like impaired memory, are the major limitation in reaching the high therapeutic doses needed for benefit, particularly in adults, who cannot tolerate these drugs as well as children.

Where deep brain stimulation (DBS) was once reserved for generalized dystonia, there is increasing evidence that this type of surgery is helpful for the focal dystonias as well, and is increasingly being utilized when these dystonias are not adequately relieved by BTX or medications. Even secondary and heredodegenerative dystonias have improved with DBS, particularly tardive dystonia, but also those in which the pallidum shows neurodegeneration, such as pantothenate kinase-associated neurodegeneration (PKAN). In general, though, the primary dystonias, including Oppenheim dystonia, have a more favorable outcome. These surgical procedures are best performed at specialty centers with an experienced team of a neurosurgeon, neurophysiologist to monitor the target during the operative procedure, and neurologist to program the stimulators. The patient needs close follow-up to adjust the stimulator settings to their optimum settings. Patients with cognitive decline should not have DBS because cognition can be further impaired. Adverse effects include surgical complications (especially cerebral hemorrhage), mechanical problems with the stimulator and leads to the electrodes, infections attacking any of the inserted hardware, and neurologic and behavioral changes, such as troubles with speech.

Further reading

Defazio G, Berardelli A, Hallett M. Do primary adult-onset focal dystonias share aetiological factors? *Brain* 2007; 130(Pt 5): 1183–93.

Fahn S, Jankovic J. *Principles and Practice of Movement Disorders.* Philadelphia: Churchill Livingstone Elsevier; 2007.

Vidailhet M, Vercueil L, Houeto JL, *et al.* Bilateral, pallidal, deep-brain stimulation in primary generalised dystonia: a prospective 3 year follow-up study. *Lancet Neurol* 2007; 6(3): 223–9.

Chapter 45
Chorea and related disorders

Roongroj Bhidayasiri[1,2,3] *and Daniel D. Truong*[3]
[1]Chulalongkorn University Hospital, Bangkok, Thailand
[2]David Geffen School of Medicine at UCLA, Los Angeles, USA
[3]The Parkinson and Movement Disorder Institute, Fountain Valley, USA

Introduction

Chorea is defined as irregular, flowing, non-stereotypic, random, involuntary movements of random muscle contractions. When chorea is proximal and of large amplitude, it is called ballism. Current neurophysiologic studies confirm the overlap between chorea and ballism. Chorea is usually worsened by anxiety and stress and subsides during sleep. Most patients attempt to disguise chorea by incorporating it into a purposeful activity. "*Athetosis*" refers to sinusoidal, slow movements affecting distal limbs, particularly in the arms. Therefore, the term "*choreoathetosis*" is often employed to describe the pattern of generalized chorea that involves the whole body, particularly distal extremities. Pseudoathetosis refers to slow writhing movements in the distal limbs, caused by a lack of proprioception.

In this chapter, we summarize the current understanding of the pathophysiology of chorea, its classification, common causes of chorea in different regions of the world, and principles of diagnostic work-up and management.

Classification of chorea

Chorea is a manifestation of a number of diseases, both acquired and inherited. Although not completely understood, current evidence suggests that chorea results from the imbalance in the direct and indirect pathways. The disruption of the indirect pathway causes a loss of inhibition on the pallidum, allowing hyperkinetic movements to occur. In addition, enhanced activity of dopamine and its receptors in the striatum are proposed mechanisms for the development of chorea. Based on current knowledge, it is possible to understand chorea and ballism as manifestations of a common pathophysiological chain of events, so that classification of choreic syndromes are increasingly based on etiology, while phenomenologically

International Neurology: A Clinical Approach. Edited by Robert P. Lisak, Daniel D. Truong, William M. Carroll, and Roongroj Bhidayasiri. © 2009 Blackwell Publishing, ISBN: 978-1-4051-5738-4.

based distinctions between chorea and ballism are becoming less important.

Chorea is characterized as primary when idiopathic or genetic in origin and secondary when related to infectious, immunological, or other medical causes (Table 45.1). Huntington's disease (HD) is a choreic prototypic disorder of inherited origin. Other inherited causes are discussed later in this chapter. In secondary chorea, stroke and tardive syndromes are among the most common causes of sporadic chorea. A number of metabolic conditions, particularly non-ketotic hyperglycemia, may also cause chorea, especially in Asians. Choreiform movements can also result from structural brain lesions, mainly in the striatum, although most cases of secondary chorea may not demonstrate any specific structural lesions.

Hereditary causes of chorea

Huntington's disease (HD)

HD, the most common cause of hereditary chorea, is an autosomal dominant disorder caused by an expansion of an unstable trinucleotide repeat near the telomere of chromosome 4. Each offspring of an affected family member has a 50% chance of having inherited the fully penetrant mutation. There are three classical peculiarities in this disease: (1) hereditary nature; (2) tendency for insanity and suicide; (3) manifestation as a grave disease only in adult life. However, in his early descriptions, George Huntington failed to mention cognitive decline, which is now recognized as a cardinal feature of the disease.

Epidemiology

HD has a worldwide prevalence of 4–8 per 100000 persons, with no gender preponderance. HD has the highest prevalence in the region of Lake Maracaibo in Venezuela, with approximately 2% of the population affected, and the Moray Firth region of Scotland. HD is notably rare in Finland, Norway, and Japan, but data for Eastern Asia and Africa are inadequate. It is believed that the mutation for HD arose independently in multiple locations and does not represent a founder effect. New mutations are extraordinarily rare.

Table 45.1 Classification of chorea (only selected causes listed).

Primary chorea	Secondary chorea	Others
1. Huntington's disease	1. Sydenham's chorea	1. Metabolic disorders
2. Neuroacanthocytosis	2. Drug-induced chorea	2. Vitamin deficiency: vitamins B_1 and B_{12}
3. Dentatorubralpallidoluysian atrophy	3. Immune-mediated chorea	3. Toxins exposure
4. Benign hereditary chorea	4. Infectious chorea	4. Paraneoplastic syndromes
5. Wilson's disease	5. Vascular chorea	5. Postpump choreoathetosis
6. Pantothenate kinase-associated neurodegenration (PKAN or formerly Hallervorden–Spatz syndrome)	6. Hormonal disorders	
7. Paroxysmal choreoathetosis		
8. Senile chorea		

Genetics

Although the familial nature of HD was recognized more than a century ago, the gene mutation and altered protein (Huntingtin) was described only recently. HD is a member of the growing family of neurodegenerative disorders associated with trinucleotide repeat expansion. The cytosine–adenosine–guanidine (CAG) triplet expansion in exon 1 encodes an enlarged polyglutamine tract in the Huntingtin protein. In unaffected individuals, the repeat length ranges between 9 and 34, with a median normal chromosome length of 19. Expansion of a CAG repeat beyond the critical threshold of 36 repeats results in disease, and forms the basis of the polymerase chain reaction-based genetic test. This expanded repeat is somewhat unstable and tends to increase in subsequent offspring, termed "anticipation." Expansion size is inversely related to age at onset, but the range in age at onset for a given repeat size is so large (with a 95% confidence interval of ±18 years for any given repeat length) that repeat size is not a useful predictor for individuals. It is likely that other genetic or environmental factors have a significant role in determining age at onset. With the exception of juvenile-onset cases, there has been poor correlation between phenotype and CAG repeat length. Because of meiotic instability with a tendency to increasing expansion size during spermatogenesis, juvenile onset cases with very large expansions usually have an affected father. Predictive genetic testing of asymptomatic at-risk relatives of affected patients is currently available and governed by international guidelines.

Clinical features

HD is a progressive disabling neurodegenerative disorder characterized by the triad of movement disorders, dementia, and behavioral disturbances. Illness may emerge at any time of life, with the highest occurrence between 35 and 40 years of age. Although the involuntary choreiform movements are the hallmark of HD, it is the mental alterations that often represent the most debilitating aspect of the disease There is also a large variability in the clinical presentation, some of which is predictable; for example,

the juvenile onset form may present with parkinsonism (the so-called Westphal variant), while the late onset form may present with chorea alone.

Chorea is the prototypical motor abnormality in HD, exhibited by 90% of affected patients. Chorea usually starts with slight movements of the fingers and toes and progresses to involve facial grimacing, eyelid elevations, and writhing limb movements (Figure 45.1). Motor impersistence is another important associated feature, whereby individuals are unable to maintain tongue protrusion or eyelid closure. Other motor manifestations also common in HD include eye movement abnormalities (slowing of saccades and increased latency of response), parakinesias, rigidity, myoclonus, and ataxia. Dystonia tends to occur when the disease is advanced or is associated with the use of dopaminergic medications. While dysarthria is common, aphasia is rare. Dysphagia tends to be the most prominent in the terminal stage and aspiration is a common cause of death.

Cognitive impairment seems to be inevitable in all HD patients. Typically, the impairment begins as selective deficits involving psychomotor, executive, and visuospatial abilities and progresses to more global impairment, although higher cortical language tends to be spared.

A wide range of psychiatric and behavioral disturbances are recognized in HD, with affective disorders among the most common, thought to be secondary to the disruption of the frontal-subcortical neural pathway. Depression occurs in up to 50% of patients. The suicide rate in HD is fivefold that of the general population. Psychosis is also common, usually with paranoid delusions. Hallucinations are rare. Apathy and aggressive behavior are commonly reported by caregivers.

Differential diagnosis

A variety of hereditary and acquired neurological disorders may mimic HD. Benign hereditary chorea is a clinically distinct condition. Although inherited in an autosomal dominant fashion, the symptoms are nonprogressive with no alterations in cognitive or behavioral functions. The onset is usually before the age of 5 years.

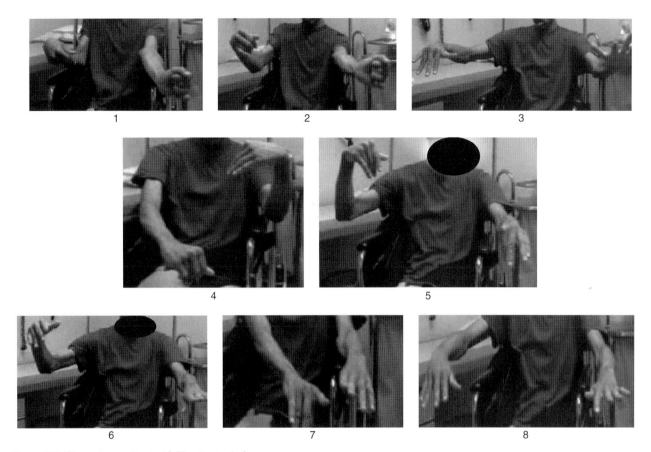

Figure 45.1 Chorea in a patient with Huntington's disease.

The presence of sensorimotor neuropathy may suggest alternative diagnosis of neuroacanthocytosis. The diagnosis is supported by the presence of acanthocytes on a peripheral smear in the context of appropriate clinical presentation. Spinocerebellar ataxias are distinguishable from HD by the prominent cerebellar dysfunction. Wilson's disease should be considered in all patients with movement disorders who are less than 40 years of age, although patients with Wilson's disease rarely exhibit chorea.

Dentatorubralpallidoluysian atrophy (DRPLA) is a triplet repeat polyglutamine disorder with profound clinical heterogeneity. It is rarely reported in North America and Europe, but is more common than HD in Japan. Symptoms vary and may include chorea, myoclonus, ataxia, epilepsy, and dementia. Although its pathology is reminiscent of HD, the involvement of the dentate nucleus of the cerebellum differentiates the disorder.

Several other distinct genetic disorders have been identified that can present with a clinical picture indistinguishable from that of HD, referring to Huntington's disease-like (HDL) syndromes. So far, four conditions have been described, namely disorders attributable to mutations in the prion protein gene (*HDL1*), the junctophilin 3 gene (*HDL2*), the gene encoding the TATA box-binding protein (*HDL4/SCA17*), and a recessively inherited HD phenocopy in a single family (*HDL3*) in which the genetic

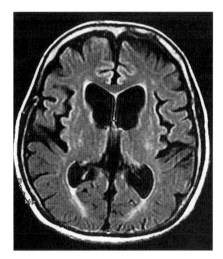

Figure 45.2 MRI of the brain in a patient with Huntington's disease disclosed predominant caudate atrophy.

is still poorly understood. While the list of HDL genes is set to grow, these disorders still account for only a small proportion of cases with the HD phenotype.

Neuropathology

Grossly, the HD brain shows significant atrophy of the head of caudate (Figure 45.2) and putamen and, to a lesser extent, the cortex, globus pallidus, substantia nigra, subthalamic nucleus, and locus coeruleus. Microscopically, medium spiny neurons are the vulnerable population in HD. Indirect projections to the external globus pallidus are the first to degenerate. The cytopathological hallmarks of HD are intranuclear inclusions, consisting of amyloid-like fibrils that contain mutant huntingtin, ubiquitin, synuclein, and other proteins.

Treatment

Current treatments in HD are largely symptomatic, aimed at reducing the motor and psychological dysfunction of individual HD patient. In general, treatment of chorea is not recommended unless it is causing disabling functional or social impairment. Clozapine, an atypical antipsychotic, has been found to reduce chorea without the extrapyramidal side effects of the typical agents. Other agents including riluzole, tetrabenazine, and amantadine have been shown to improve chorea. Traditional neuroleptics such as haloperidol can improve chorea but are associated with increased risk of tardive dyskinesia, dystonia, difficulty swallowing, and gait disturbances, and should not be considered as first-line agents.

The selective serotonin reuptake inhibitors (SSRIs) have become the first-line agents in the treatment of depression in HD. SSRIs may also suppress chorea and reduce aggression in HD. A brief course of benzodiazepines may be useful for co-occurring anxiety. The new antipsychotic agents, such as clozapine, quetiapine, and olanzapine, are often required to treat psychosis in HD. Valproic acid may be useful in the long-term management of aggression and irritability.

Neuroacanthocytosis
Clinical features

Neuroacanthocytosis is a rare, multisystem, degenerative disorder of unknown etiology that is characterized by the presence of deformed erythrocytes with spicules known as acanthocytes and abnormal involuntary movements. The disorder seems to be particularly common in Japan and can be transmitted by autosomal recessive, dominant, or X-linked inheritance. The mean age of onset is around 30 years and tends to be progressive, with death occurring within 15 years of diagnosis. Involuntary choreic and dystonic movements of the orofacial region, as well as tongue and lip biting are virtually diagnostic, although a full spectrum of movement disorders may be seen. Other clinical features include chorea of the limbs (predominantly the legs) that can mimic HD, axonal neuropathy (50% of cases), areflexia, and elevated plasma creatine kinase level. Seizures are also common and can be a presenting feature. Psychiatric symptoms are typical and include apathy, depression, anxiety, and obsessive-compulsive syndrome. However, in contrast to HD, mental deterioration is minimal.

Diagnosis and treatment

Diagnosis is usually made on the basis of family history, morphological analysis of erythrocytes, and an elevated plasma creatine kinase level. Magnetic resonance imaging (MRI) has shown degeneration of the caudate and more generalized cerebral atrophy. Increased signal on T2-weighted MRI in the caudate and putamen is a common feature. However, these findings are non-specific. The most consistent neuropathological finding is extensive loss of predominantly small and medium-sized neurons and gliosis in the caudate, putamen, pallidum, and substantia nigra with relative sparing of the subthalamic nucleus and cerebral cortex. Treatment is largely supportive.

Dentatorubralpallidoluysian atrophy (DRPLA)

DRPLA is a triplet repeat polyglutamine disorder with the gene defect localized to chromosome 12. Development of clinical phenotypes is associated with CAG repeat lengths exceeding 53. Atrophin-1 is a mutant protein and its function is not known. The condition is rarely reported in North America and Europe, but it is more common in Japan. It is inherited in an autosomal dominant fashion and clinical features include chorea, myoclonus, ataxia, epilepsy, and cognitive decline. Neuroimaging studies have revealed atrophy of the cerebellum, midbrain tegmentum, and cerebral hemispheres with ventricular dilatation. Pathologically, there is neuronal loss and gliosis in the dentate nucleus, red nucleus, globus pallidus, and subthalamic nucleus.

Benign hereditary chorea (BHC)

BHC or essential chorea is another disorder inherited in an autosomal dominant fashion and characterized by choreiform movements. The onset of choreiform movements in BHC is in early childhood; severity of symptoms peaks in the second decade and the condition is non-progressive. Life expectancy is normal and the disease may improve with age. The condition is not associated with other neurological deficits, although some authors believe that BHC is a heterogeneous syndrome that may have a variety of causes. BHC is considered to be a distinct disease of early-onset, non-progressive, uncomplicated chorea with a locus on 14q.

Others

There are other inherited neurological disorders that can present with prominent chorea. These conditions are rare and the details are not included in this chapter. Examples include paroxysmal choreoathetosis, familial chorea-ataxia-myoclonus syndrome, pantothenate kinase-associated neurodegeneration (PKAN or Hallervorden–Spatz syndrome), intracerebral calcification with neuropsychiatric features Wilson's disease, multisystem degeneration, olivopontocerebellar atrophy, and spinocerebellar degeneration (Sanger Brown type).

Sydenham's chorea

Sydenham's chorea (SC) is a delayed complication of group A β-hemolytic streptococcal infections and forms one of the major criteria of acute rheumatic fever. It is characterized by chorea, muscular weakness, and a number of neuropsychiatric symptoms. It is considered to be an autoantibody-mediated disorder, suggesting that patients with SC produce antibodies that cross-react with streptococcus, caudate, and subthalamic nuclei. However, documented evidence of previous streptococcal infection is found in only 20–30% of cases.

The age of presentation is usually between 5 and 15 years, with female preponderance. Chorea is usually generalized, consisting of finer and more rapid movements than those seen in HD. It occurs at rest or with activity but remits during sleep. The condition is self-limiting within 5–16 weeks, but recurs in 20% of patients. However, symptomatic treatment with neuroleptics, tetrabenazine, or valproic acid can be considered in severe cases with generalized chorea. Previously affected females are at increased risk of developing chorea during pregnancy (chorea gravidarum) and during sex hormonal therapy. Evidence of striatal dysfunction in SC is supported by MRI findings in the caudate and putamen in some patients and reversible striatal hypermetabolism on brain single photon emission computed tomography during the acute illness.

Other immune-mediated chorea

Although central nervous system involvement in systemic lupus erythematosus (SLE) is common, chorea has been reported in less than 2% of these patients. It usually appears early in the course of the disease and is characteristically generalized. It is often difficult to recognize chorea as a manifestation of a systemic autoimmune disease because it can simulate Sydenham's and Huntington's chorea and not infrequently appears in childhood long before other manifestations of SLE or antiphospholipid syndrome have emerged. The use of estrogen-containing oral contraceptives or pregnancy may precipitate the appearance of chorea. In addition, chorea can occur not only in patients with well-defined SLE, but also in patients with "probable" or "lupus-like" SLE and in patients with primary antiphospholipid antibody without clinical features of SLE. Some reports suggest that steroid therapy can lead to resolution.

Drug-induced chorea

Drug-induced chorea may be an acute phenomenon or the consequence of long-term therapy. Multiple drugs

Table 45.2 Drugs known to cause chorea (in addition to antipsychotic medications).

1. Anticonvulsant medications: common causative agents include
   a. Phenytoin
   b. Carbamazepine
   c. Valproate
   d. Gabapentin
2. CNS stimulants
   a. Amphetamines
   b. Cocaine
   c. Methylphenidate
3. Benzodiazepines
4. Estrogens
5. Lithium
6. Levodopa
7. Dopamine agonists
8. Catechol-*O*-methyl transferase (COMT) inhibitor in conjunction with levodopa
9. Antihistamines: H1 and H2
10. Others, for example, baclofen, cimetidine, aminophylline

including dopamine agonists, levodopa therapy, oral contraceptives, and anticonvulsants have been implicated in the acute chorea (Table 45.2). Details of drug-induced chorea are provided in Chapter 49 on Drug-induced movement disorders.

Vascular chorea

Chorea is the most common movement disorder following stroke but is a rare complication of acute vascular events. The subthalamic nucleus is the most common location of ischemic or hemorrhagic damage in patients with post-stroke chorea, especially when the chorea is severe and proximal (called hemiballismus). Chorea can also occur in polycythemia vera although it manifests in less than 1% of cases.

Metabolic causes of chorea

Metabolic alterations such as hyperglycemia, hypoglycemia, hypernatremia, hyponatremia, hypomagnesemia, hypocalcemia, and hepatic and renal failure have been implicated in the development of chorea. Recently, a combination of chorea, non-ketotic hyperglycemia, and a high signal basal ganglia lesion on T1-weighted brain MRI has been recognized to affect predominantly elderly Asian women. Characteristically, T1-weighted brain MRI shows hyperintense basal ganglia lesions (Figure 45.3), but T2-weighted MRI findings vary. The clinical course is usually benign and most patients gradually recover with medical treatment, particularly correction of hyperglycemia.

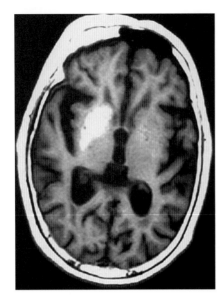

Figure 45.3 T1-weighted MRI of the brain in a patient with non-ketotic hyperglycemia chorea revealed high signal intensity lesions in the right basal ganglia, especially the putamen.

Chorea gravidarum

Chorea gravidarum or chorea occurring during pregnancy is an increasingly rare disorder. Affected patients usually have previous episodes of chorea associated with the use of oral contraceptives or a history of rheumatic fever. The movements usually remit after the delivery but may recur in the subsequent pregnancy.

Infectious chorea

Multiple infectious agents that affect the CNS have been associated with chorea. Chorea can occur in the setting of acute manifestation of bacterial meningitis, encephalitis, tuberculous meningitis, or aseptic meningitis. Movement disorders are also encountered in 2–3% of all patients with acquired immunodeficiency syndromes (AIDS). In the setting of AIDS, hemichorea and hemiballismus are relatively common due to toxoplasmosis abscess; however, direct HIV invasion and injury to the basal ganglia resulting in chorea can occur. Less commonly, Lyme disease has been reported to cause chorea.

Diagnosis and management

Although there are numerous causes of chorea, careful history and a concomitant neurological and psychiatric review of systems will guide the individual work-up. A detailed medical history is important to rule out, in particular, prior streptococcal infections or rheumatic fever, as a history of rheumatic fever predisposes individuals to the development of paroxysmal movement disorders under the influence of different agents. A family history of choreic or degenerative illness should be noted, as well as a medication history of potential causative agents. Genetic testing, neuroimaging, and laboratory investigations will help confirm the suspected diagnosis. Despite the above careful workup in most patients, causes are unidentified in 6% of cases.

For primary chorea, dopaminergic antagonists such as neuroleptic medications are effective treatments; however, their use is limited due to the side effects of mainly parkinsonism and tardive syndromes. Dopamine-depleting agents such as tetrabenazine, which inhibits presynaptic dopamine release and blocks postsynaptic dopamine receptors, show favorable results compared to other medications used to treat chorea, especially in HD, and may have synergistic effects when used in combination with the dopamine antagonist pimozide. For secondary chorea, the treatment objective should focus on the primary causative factor. If chorea is due to an exogeneous agent, the offending agent should be withdrawn. Infectious process should be treated accordingly. The drug used to treat primary chorea can be used to symptomatically treat secondary chorea.

Further reading

Bhidayasiri R, Truong DD. Chorea and related disorders. *Postgrad Med J* 2004; 80(947): 527–34.

Cardoso F. Chorea: non-genetic causes. *Curr Opin Neurol* 2004; 17(4): 433–6.

Fernandez M, Raskind W, Matsushita M, Wolff J, Lipe H, Bird T. Hereditary benign chorea: clinical and genetic features of a distinct disease. *Neurology* 2001; 57(1): 106–10.

Harper PS. The epidemiology of Huntington's disease. *Hum Genet* 1992; 89(4): 365–76.

Koide R, Ikeuchi T, Onodera O, *et al.* Unstable expansion of CAG repeat in hereditary dentatorubral-pallidoluysian atrophy (DRPLA). *Nat Genet* 1994; 6(1): 9–13.

Oh S-H, Lee K-Y, Im J-H, Lee M-S. Chorea associated with non-ketotic hyperglycemia and hyperintensity basal ganglia lesion on T1-weighted brain MRI study: a meta-analysis of 53 cases including four present cases. *J Neurol Sci* 2002; 200: 57–62.

Schneider SA, Walker RH, Bhatia KP. The Huntington's disease-like syndromes: what to consider in patients with a negative Huntington's disease gene test. *Nat Clin Pract* 2007; 3: 517–25.

Schrag A, Quinn NP, Bhatia KP, Marsden CD. Benign hereditary chorea – entity or syndrome? *Mov Disord* 2000; 15(2): 280–8.

The Huntington's Disease Collaborative Research Group. A novel gene containing a trinucleotide repeat that is expanded and unstable on Huntington's disease chromosomes. *Cell* 1993; 72: 971–83.

Vital A, Bouillot S, Burbaud P, Ferrer X, Vital C. Chorea-acanthocytosis: neuropathology of brain and peripheral nerve. *Clin Neuropathol* 2002; 21(2): 77–81.

Chapter 46
Myoclonus

John N. Caviness[1] and Daniel D. Truong[2]
[1]Mayo Clinic College of Medicine, Scottsdale, USA
[2]The Parkinson and Movement Disorder Institute, Fountain Valley, USA

Introduction

Myoclonus is defined as sudden, brief, shock-like, involuntary movements caused by muscular contractions (positive myoclonus) or inhibitions (negative myoclonus). It refers to a *symptom* or *sign* and it does not constitute a diagnosis. Myoclonus may have a variety of etiologies and physiological mechanisms. Accurate characterization of the individual patient presentation of myoclonus has strong implications for diagnosis and treatment.

The only study of myoclonus epidemiology in a defined population is from Olmsted County, Minnesota. The average annual incidence of pathologic and persistent myoclonus between 1976 and 1990 was 1.3 cases per 100 000 person-years. The lifetime prevalence of myoclonus, as of January 1, 1990, was 8.6 cases per 100 000 population. Little information is available about diseases that commonly manifest myoclonus in specific regions of the world. The incidence of idiopathic progressive myoclonic epilepsy (Unverricht–Lundborg, EPM1) in Finland is 5 in 100 000 births.

Classification

Characterization of the type of myoclonus present in a given patient is based on three types of classification methods: examination findings, neurophysiology, and clinical etiology. These methods complement each another.

Examination findings
The basic parts of a myoclonus examination should include distribution, temporal profile, and activation characteristics of the movement. The distribution can be focal, multifocal, segmental, or generalized. A multifocal myoclonus distribution may have bilaterally synchronous movements as well. The temporal profile can

be continuous or intermittent, as well as rhythmic or irregular. If intermittent, the myoclonus can occur sporadically or in trains. Myoclonus may be activated at rest (spontaneous), induced by various stimuli (reflex myoclonus), or induced by voluntary movement (action myoclonus), or some combination of these. The above activation characteristics should be noted as absent or present. Patients may exhibit more than one pattern of myoclonus and all distributions and temporal patterns should be described.

Clinical neurophysiology
Clinical neurophysiology yields information about myoclonus pathophysiology. These findings support a source for the origin of the myoclonus, which in turn assists with both diagnosis and treatment. The methods employed should include multichannel surface electromyography (EMG) recording with testing for long latency EMG responses to nerve stimulation, electroencephalography (EEG), EEG-EMG polygraphy with back-averaging, and evoked potentials (such as median nerve stimulation somatosensory evoked potential (SEP)). Positive and negative findings from these methods can then be used to provide evidence for determining the physiological type of myoclonus. For example, a back-averaged focal cortical EEG transient (Figure 46.1), enlarged cortical SEP, and enhanced long EMG responses suggest cortical-origin myoclonus. The main physiological categories for myoclonus classification are as follows:

- *Cortical*: most common; has been reported for various neurodegenerative diseases, toxic-metabolic conditions, post-hypoxic state (Lance–Adams syndrome), storage disorders, and other conditions.
- *Cortical-subcortical*: corresponds to the myoclonus in myoclonic and absence seizures. The physiology is believed to involve interactions of cortical and subcortical centers, such as the thalamus.
- *Subcortical*: seen in essential myoclonus and reticular reflex myoclonus, among others.
- *Segmental*: arises from segmental brainstem (palatal) and/or spinal generators.
- *Peripheral*: except for hemifacial spasm, peripheral myoclonus is rare.

International Neurology: A Clinical Approach. Edited by Robert P. Lisak, Daniel D. Truong, William M. Carroll, and Roongroj Bhidayasiri.
© 2009 Blackwell Publishing, ISBN: 978-1-4051-5738-4.

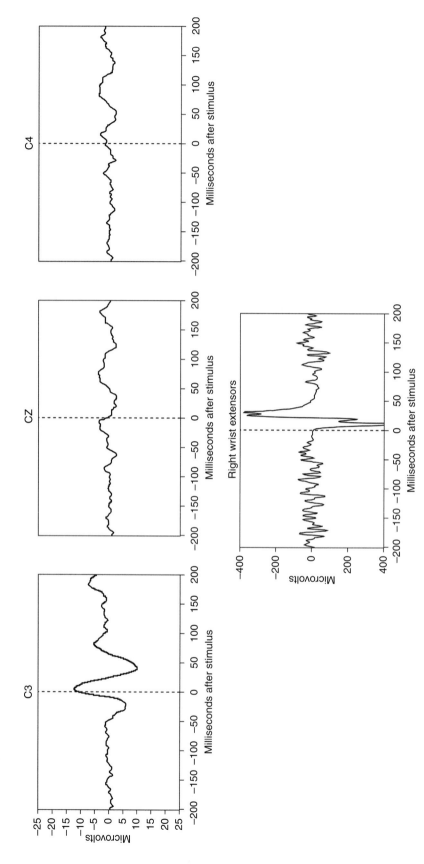

Figure 46.1 EEG back-averaging of 80 myoclonus EMG discharges recorded over right wrist extensors during muscle activation. There is a focal EEG transient present at the C3 electrode (over left sensorimotor cortex) about 20 ms before the averaged myoclonus EMG discharge.

Clinical etiology classification

The major categories of the myoclonus etiological classification scheme are physiologic, essential, epileptic, and symptomatic (secondary). Each of the major categories is associated with different clinical circumstances. Physiologic myoclonus occurs in neurologically normal people. Physical examinations do not reveal relevant abnormalities and there is minimal to no associated disability present. Jerks during sleep are the most familiar examples of physiologic myoclonus. Essential myoclonus refers to idiopathic myoclonus that progresses slowly or not at all, and the jerks represent the most prominent or only clinical finding. Epileptic myoclonus refers to the presence of myoclonus in the setting of epilepsy, a chronic seizure disorder. Myoclonus can occur as only one component of a seizure, the only seizure manifestation, or one of multiple seizure types within an epileptic syndrome. Symptomatic (secondary) myoclonus manifests in the setting of an identifiable, underlying disorder – neurologic or non-neurologic. Most cases of myoclonus are in the symptomatic category, followed by the epileptic and essential categories.

Features of major myoclonic disorders

Post-hypoxic myoclonus

Myoclonus is known to occur in post-hypoxic patients after anesthesia incidents, post cardiac arrest, near drowning, or pulmonary embolism, or following respiratory failures. Not all patients develop myoclonus after hypoxic incidents; myoclonus often occurs only following a sufficient duration of hypoxia. Spontaneous, action-induced, and stimulus-induced myoclonus may occur. Action myoclonus dominates the clinical picture. Action jerks can spread to involve other body parts early on (bilateral or generalized jerks) and later become multifocal. Myoclonus can present in facial muscles, affecting speech and swallowing. Some patients also have cerebellar ataxia and negative myoclonus, which lead to sudden falls. Epilepsy is normally not a striking feature and seizures are typically generalized tonic clonic. Most patients show some improvement in myoclonus with time. Recently, an animal model of post-hypoxic myoclonus has been developed based on systematic prolongation of cardiac arrest. In this model, meaningful myoclonus persists only after duration of hypoxia of about 7 minutes, although transient myoclonus may occur in animals with as little as 3 minutes of hypoxia.

Progressive myoclonus epilepsy

Various storage diseases fall under the clinical syndrome of progressive myoclonic epilepsy (PME). PME is a chronic, progressive, neurologic syndrome that contains some combination of myoclonus, seizures, ataxia, and dementia. These disorders usually affect individuals less than 30 years of age and are often fatal. Several clinical differences exist between individual storage diseases as to their age of onset, rate of progression, details of clinical expression, other clinical manifestations, and patterns of stimulus sensitivity. The neuropathology in the brain is widespread. Tissue biopsy and enzyme activity measurements are useful for diagnosis.

Essential myoclonus

Cases of sporadic essential myoclonus are heterogeneous with regard to distribution, what exacerbates the jerks, and other examination findings. Sporadic essential myoclonus probably consists of various heterogeneous yet undiscovered causes of myoclonus and cases with false-negative family histories. Hereditary-essential myoclonus is associated with dominant inheritance and variable severity. The myoclonus is usually distributed throughout the upper body, exacerbated by muscle activation, and dramatically decreased by alcohol ingestion. The term "myoclonus-dystonia syndrome" has been introduced because of the common occurrence of dystonia in these cases. Mutations in the ε-sarcoglycan gene have had the strongest association with the myoclonus-dystonia syndrome.

Neurodegenerative disorders

Multiple system atrophy manifests as varying degrees of parkinsonism, ataxia, and autonomic dysfunction, but a stimulus-sensitive distal limb myoclonus was found in 31% of patients in one series. Myoclonic jerks, both action and stimulus sensitive, commonly occur in corticobasal degeneration. The distribution of myoclonus in corticobasal degeneration is either asymmetric or focal, and is similar to the other clinico-pathologic manifestations of the disease. The usual presentation of myoclonus in Alzheimer's disease is small multifocal distal jerking, although more widespread or generalized jerks can be seen. The myoclonus in Creutzfeldt–Jakob disease is a clinical hallmark of the disorder and can occur at rest and/or is exacerbated by action or stimuli. When myoclonus in Alzheimer's disease is large and widespread, it may be confused with Creutzfeldt–Jakob disease. Cortical myoclonus occurs across the spectrum of Lewy body disorders. Myoclonus in Parkinson's disease is less common than in dementia with Lewy bodies, where it occurs in at least one-third of cases. Myoclonus in dementia with Lewy bodies is of larger amplitude and much more likely to occur at rest than the myoclonus in Parkinson's disease.

Metabolic disorders

In metabolic conditions, myoclonus often occurs in the hospital setting, frequently with mental status changes. The myoclonus may be multifocal and subtle, or generalized and almost constant, as in the entity "myoclonic status epilepticus." Prognosis in such cases depends on the severity and reversibility of the underlying process. Asterixis, which is known as "negative myoclonus," is a well-known accompaniment of toxic and metabolic encephalopathies. It is characterized by brief lapses in postural tone and is particularly common in kidney and liver failure. Usually, the effects are improved or reversed when use of the agent is discontinued or the metabolic condition is reversed.

Drugs

The literature on drug-induced myoclonus continues to grow. Such myoclonus is potentially fully treatable since it is almost always reversible upon withdrawal of the offending agent(s). It must be emphasized that all drugs, either in isolation or combination, must be scrutinized for a potential causative role in myoclonus. A spectrum of lithium-induced myoclonus exists with regards to different clinical manifestations of motor cortex hyperexcitability. At therapeutic levels, or mild lithium toxicity, isolated cortical action myoclonus can be associated with EEG background rhythm changes. Instances of greater lithium toxicity can demonstrate motor seizures and/or generalized convulsions. The synergistic relationship between myoclonus-causing drugs in the setting of polypharmacy in complex psychiatric cases has become very apparent.

Evaluation

Both the presence of the myoclonus and the other aspects of the clinical presentation determine what type of testing should be done. For example, if an infectious or inflammatory syndrome is present, a cerebrospinal fluid examination should be carried out. Knowledge of the various diagnostic entities will facilitate the proper diagnostic confirmation. The following minimal testing should be done in all unexplained cases of myoclonus:

Electrolytes   Drug and toxin screen
Glucose   Brain imaging
Renal function tests   Electroencephalography
Hepatic function tests

If these basic tests do not reveal the diagnosis, then more advanced testing should be considered. Additional testing may include clinical neurophysiology testing, cerebrospinal fluid examination, enzyme activity, paraneoplastic testing, and other metabolic testing. In some cases, genetic testing may be considered. Before genetic testing is begun, the patient should be fully aware of the implications for both positive and negative results. If appropriate, genetic counseling is recommended.

Treatment

General principles

The best strategy for the treatment of myoclonus is to treat the underlying disorder; however, this is not always possible. Some causes of myoclonus can be reversed partially or totally, such as an acquired abnormal metabolic state, a medication or toxin, or an excisable lesion. The general principle of the treatment of myoclonus is to control it to a level that is tolerable by the patient. The treatment of myoclonus can be effective, but is often unsatisfactory and mostly empirical (Table 46.1). Anticonvulsants may be used to treat myoclonus. In contrast to epilepsy, antimyoclonic agents for myoclonus are usually used in combination; rarely can one agent achieve complete control of myoclonus. The treatment is dictated by the underlying diagnosis, the likely origin of the myoclonus, and the side-effect profile of the antimyoclonic agents. Levitiracetam, valproic acid, and clonazepam are commonly used agents for the treatment of myoclonus.

Levitiracetam is effective in patients with cortical myoclonus, especially posthypoxic myoclonus. The standard initial dose for epilepsy is 500 mg twice daily. Because drowsiness may occur, it is wise to begin initially with 250 or 500 mg/day and gradually titrate upward. The maximum recommended dose is 3000 mg/day. Pediatric doses are 20–40 mg/kg/day. Levetiracetam is minimally protein-bound and excreted in the urine. It has virtually no interactions with other drugs. It is considered the drug of choice in the treatment of myoclonus.

Table 46.1 Common dosage of agents for the treatment of myoclonus.

Drug	Dosage (mg/day unless specified otherwise)
Baclofen	15–100
Benztropine	15–100
Carbamazepine	Up to 2000
Clonazepam	Up to 15
Diazepam	5–30
γ-Hydroxybutyric acid	Up to 6.125*
5-Hydroxytryptophan	Up to 3*†
Levetiracetam	750–3000
Phenobarbital	50–100
Phenytoin	250–325
Piracetam	2.4–16.8*
Primidone	500–750
Tetrabenazine	50–200
Trihexyphenidyl	Up to 35
Valproic acid (sodium valproate)	1200–2000

*g/day.
†In combination with a peripheral aromatic amino acid decarboxylase inhibitor (such as carbidopa 100–300 mg/day).

Valproic acid is effective in cortical and subcortical myoclonus. Valproic acid is usually begun at 125 mg twice daily, and titrated to clinical response. For the treatment of myoclonus, doses of 750–1000 mg/day are usually required. It is contraindicated in patients with significant hepatic dysfunction and urea cycle disorders. It may cause neural tube defects, craniofacial defects, and cardiovascular malformations if taken during pregnancy. Valproic acid may increase levels of warfarin, lamotrigine, phenobarbital, and phenytoin. Fatal hepatic failure and pancreatitis may occur in patients taking valproic acid requiring frequent monitoring.

Clonazepam is used in cortical, subcortical, and spinal myoclonus. It is the drug of choice for spinal myoclonus. Clonazepam is typically begun with 0.5 mg three times a day and titrated until symptoms are controlled or side effects appear. Doses of at least 3 mg/day are generally required. Most common side effects are drowsiness, but ataxia and personality changes may occur. It is contraindicated in patients with narrow angle glaucoma or with hepatic dysfunction.

Other drugs that may also be used in myoclonus are primidone, piracetam, and γ-hydroxybutyric acid (GBH).

Piracetam is available in Europe and many other parts of the world. The usual dosage for myoclonus is 16–24 mg/day. It is contraindicated in patients with renal insufficiency and hepatic dysfunction. GBH has been approved in the United States for the treatment of cataplexy in patients with narcolepsy. It is used in other countries for the treatment of alcohol withdrawal and in maintaining its abstinence. A dosage of 6.125 g/day has been reported to be effective in alcohol-sensitive myoclonus-dystonia.

Further reading

Caviness JN. Clinical neurophysiology of myoclonus. Movement disorders. In: Hallett M, editor. *Handbook of Clinical Neurophysiology*, Vol. 1. Amsterdam: Elsevier; 2003, Chapter 32, pp. 521–48.

Caviness JN. Myoclonus and neurodegenerative disease – what's in a name? *Parkinsonism Relat Disord* 2003; 9: 185–92.

Caviness JN, Brown P. Myoclonus: current concepts and recent advances. *Lancet Neurol* 2004; 3: 598–607.

Tai KK, Bhidayasiri R, Truong D. Myoclonus: post-hypoxic animal model of myoclonus. *Parkinsonism Relat Disord* 2007; 13: 377–81.

Chapter 47
Tics and Tourette

Valerie Suski and Mark Stacy
Duke University, Durham, USA

Introduction

Because Tourette syndrome (TS) is often not recognized in many patients with mild symptoms, it was once believed to be a rare disorder. TS has a prevalence of 1–2/2000 and usually occurs between the ages of 2 and 15. Simple tics occur in 0.4% to 1.76% of children aged 5–8 years and as high as 28% of children in the special education setting.

Clinical presentation

Tics are abrupt, intermittent, recurrent, and stereotypical movements or sounds that occur in the background of normal behavior. Severity may fluctuate throughout the day. Tics are difficult to categorize as voluntary or involuntary because certain patients have the ability to suppress the tic; however, this is a temporary phenomenon. There is often a buildup of an urge to tic that eventually leads to behavior that is associated with a "release of tension" to tic. In the last decade, increasing emphasis has been placed on sensory phenomena that precede tics in some patients. These premonitory stimuli are often vague, may be difficult for patients to define, and may not be recognized for years. They are most often described as an "itch-like" sensation of the skin or an uncomfortable urge to move that increases until a motor behavior provides temporary "relief." Recognition of the sensory and cognitive components in TS is important since these sensory symptoms may be more troublesome to the patient than actual tic performance.

Tics are classified as simple or complex. Simple motor tics involve a single movement with a limited number of muscle groups, lasting seconds or less. Examples include eye blinking, head jerking, or shoulder shrugging. Severity may vary and be associated with physical or emotional distress. Complex motor tics involve multiple muscle groups, are coordinated into a sequence of movements, and may be slower or more deliberate than simple motor tics. Examples include punching oneself, jumping, or performing obscene gestures (copropraxia). Simple vocal tics are described as meaningless sounds or noises, such as throat clearing, yelping, and sniffing. Complex vocal tics are usually meaningful words, phrases, or sentences (i.e., uttering words or phrases out of context and stuttering). More dramatic complex vocal tics are coprolalia (uttering obscene words), palilalia (repeating oneself), or echolalia (repeating others' words).

In addition to location, tics may be classified by duration of the symptoms. Transient tics occur for 1 month to 1 year. Chronic tics occur longer than 1 year without a period of remission greater than 3 months. The current diagnostic criteria for TS, according to the DSM-IV-TR, is (1) presence of both motor and vocal tics at some time during the course of the illness, (2) occurrence of multiple tics nearly every day through a period of more than 1 year, without a remission of tics for a period of greater than three consecutive months, (3) symptoms not due to medications or drugs and not related to another medical condition, and (4) age of onset prior to 18 years of age.

Although motor and vocal tics are the predominant feature of the disorder, it can be accompanied by a variety of behavioral comorbidities. Approximately half of TS patients report symptoms of obsessive compulsive disorder (OCD). Children with OCD often describe a system of rituals associated with retiring to bed, playing sports or musical instruments, or collecting objects. Common examples include compulsive checking, counting, touching surfaces, and obsessive worrying. Symptoms of attention deficit hyperactivity disorder (ADHD) are reported in 15–80% of TS, including impulsivity, inattention, distractibility, and hyperactivity. Although not as prevalent as OCD and ADHD symptoms, patients with TS may also manifest behavioral disturbances such as mania, affective/personality disorders, learning disabilities, and self-injurious behavior.

Epidemiology

The etiology of TS remains unknown. Although a gene for TS has not been identified, familial studies suggest an

International Neurology: A Clinical Approach. Edited by Robert P. Lisak, Daniel D. Truong, William M. Carroll, and Roongroj Bhidayasiri. © 2009 Blackwell Publishing, ISBN: 978-1-4051-5738-4.

autosomal dominant disorder with variable penetrance. Males are more commonly affected, with a predominance of 3:1. If OCD is included as an alternative expression of TS, the gender ratio is nearly equal. Besides gender influence, environmental factors affect tic severity and neuropsychological function.

Ten to fifteen percent of cases do not appear to have a familial association. Some studies suggest that increased amounts of dopamine or serotonin neurotransmitters can cause tics in areas of the brain responsible for voluntary movements. Non-genetic risk factors evaluated include prenatal (i.e., maternal smoking, drug use, toxin exposure) and perinatal (i.e., jaundice, infections) events. Most of the studies show that these factors may not necessarily cause TS, but may correlate with the severity of symptoms.

Differential diagnosis

Secondary causes of tics are commonly referred to as tourettism. They may accompany other general medical conditions such as Huntington's disease, neuroacanthocytosis, Wilson's disease, and Syndenham's chorea. Acquired causes of tics include medication side effects, head trauma, postviral encephalitis, stroke, and carbon monoxide poisoning. Tics can be associated with chromosomal disorders (i.e., Down syndrome, Klinefelter's syndrome, XYY syndrome, fragile X syndrome) and other conditions such as developmental disorders, autism, and stereotypic movement disorders. Medications can exacerbate tics including stimulants, caffeine, carbamazepine, and corticorsteroids. Group A beta-hemolytic streptococcal infection may be an extremely rare form of tourettism with sudden onset of an autoimmune neuropsychiatric disorder.

Diagnostic evaluation

There are no confirmatory tests for TS. Diagnosis is made from clinical observation, determining potential triggers, and assessing comorbidities. Given the voluntary suppressibility and the fluctuating nature of the disorder, tics may be absent at the time of an examination. It may take several visits before the tics may be witnessed.

Treatment

Most children with mild tics can avoid pharmacologic treatment. One-third of children have tics that often remit or greatly improve as they approach adulthood. General education regarding the nature of the symptoms is often highly effective as a treatment. In many instances, neuropsychological evaluation may identify ways to reconstruct the school environment and provide supportive counseling.

Medications are considered if the symptoms of TS are functionally disabling and not improved by non-pharmacologic interventions. Dopamine receptor antagonist (neuroleptic) medications are most useful for suppressing tics. The most frequently used drugs are fluphenazine, haloperidol, pimozide, sulpiride, and tiapride. Common side effects of dopamine receptor antagonists include sedation, cognitive difficulties, dysphoria, depression, dystonia, weight gain, and social phobias. Before beginning any neuroleptic drug, the patient and family should be warned of the low potential for the development of tardive dyskinesias and the rare potential for acute dystonic reaction.

Other medications with different mechanisms of action may suppress tics in certain TS patients. Clonidine and guanfacine (α-receptor agonists) may be useful medications for children with mild tics and ADHD. Clonazepam, reserpine, tetrabenazine, and calcium channel blockers also have tic-suppressing effects. Treatment of TS with stimulants remains controversial due to exacerbation of tics (in 25%), but may be tolerable if symptoms of inattention and hyperactivity are improved. A combination of clonidine plus stimulant may have an additive benefit on ADHD symptoms without worsening tics.

Antidepressant medications, particularly serotonin reuptake inhibitors, may alleviate OCD symptoms in TS. Currently available drugs include selective serotonin reuptake inhibitors (i.e., fluoxetine, fluvoxamine, paroxetine, sertraline) and tricyclic antidepressants (i.e., clomipramine, desipramine). With the overlap of complex tics and OCD, these drugs may be particularly useful in this setting, avoiding the potential risk associated with neuroleptic agents.

Alternative therapies are emerging. Habit-reversing training is the substitution of one tic for a more socially acceptable tic. Behavior modification helps with poor impulse control. Relaxation techniques and biofeedback alleviate stress, reducing tics. Botulinum toxin injections in muscles that are responsible for particular movements or vocalizations (i.e., trapezius for shoulder shrugging, vocal cords for copralalia) may be effective. Botulinum toxin may be effective by weakening the muscle, changing proprioceptive feedback, and potentially modifying the premonitory urge for movement. Deep brain stimulation surgery has been attempted for refractory TS in a small number of cases. The surgical target is still controversial; however, the most common site is the thalamus.

Prognosis

TS is not neurodegenerative; therefore, patients have a normal life span. In general, 10% of TS patients have severe tics, 30% will experience a decrease in frequency and severity, 30–40% completely resolve by late adolescence, and the other 30–40% will continue to exhibit moderate to severe symptoms in adulthood. Patients with severe tics and comorbidities appear to be more likely to become socially isolated.

Further reading

American Psychiatric Association. *Diagnostic and Statistical Manual of Mental Disorders*, 4th ed. Text revision (DSM-IV-TR). Washington, DC: American Psychiatric Association; 2000.

Bruun RB, Budman CL. The natural history of Tourette syndrome. In: Chase TN, Friedhoff AJ, Cohen DJ, editors. *Advances in Neurology*, Vol. 58. New York, NY: Raven Press; 1992, pp. 1–6.

Kadesjo B, Gillberg C. Tourette's disorder: epidemiology and comorbidity in primary school children. *J Am Acad Child Adolesc Psychiatry* 2000; 39: 548–55.

Peterson B, Riddle MA, Cohen DJ, *et. al*. Reduced basal ganglia volume in Tourette's syndrome using three-dimensional reconstruction technique from magnetic resonance images. *Neurology* 1993; 43: 941–9.

Shapiro AK, Shapiro ES, Young JG, Feinberg TE, editors. *Gilles de la Tourette Syndrome*, 2nd ed. New York, NY: Raven Press; 1988, pp. 61–193.

Chapter 48
Ataxia

Sergei N. Illarioshkin
Research Center of Neurology, Russian Academy of Medical Sciences, Moscow, Russia

Introduction

From the historical viewpoint, the term "ataxia" means "dysarray," that is any unspecified motor clumsiness. However, our present understanding of this term refers to *poorly coordinated movements* resulting mainly from lesions of the cerebellum and/or cerebellar connections. In addition to cerebellar ataxia (accounting for the majority of ataxic cases seen in clinical practice), there are also cases of so-called sensory and vestibular ataxia caused, respectively, by lesions of spinal proprioceptive pathways and the vestibular system.

Clinical presentation of different types of ataxia

Cerebellar ataxia

Clinically, cerebellar ataxia manifests by imbalanced stance and unsteady, broad-based gait, as well as by limb incoordination, clumsy movements, slurring dysarthria (scanning speech, staccato), and saccadic ocular dysmetria and oscillations. Patients stand with their legs farther apart than is normal, sway or fall in attempts to stand with the feet together, and, because of poor balance, need support or want to hold onto objects in the room. Mild gait ataxia may be exaggerated when patients attempt tandem-walking in a straight line. Ataxia may be generalized or affect predominantly gait, upper or lower extremities, speech, or eye movements; it may be unilateral or may spread to both sides of the body. It is frequently accompanied by muscle hypotonia, slowness of movements, intention tremor (action tremor with increased amplitude of oscillations upon approaching the target), abnormal control of multijoint movements (asynergia), exaggerated postural reactions, nystagmus (usually horizontal in cerebellar disease), and some alterations in mental processes and cognitive functions (so-called

"cerebellar cognitive–affective syndrome", usually caused by large and acute ischemic lesions of the posterior lobe). One should stress that motor problems in ataxic patients typically are not related to muscle weakness, hyperkinesias, spasticity, and so on, although all these and other additional symptoms may complicate clinical phenotype. Severe ataxia may become an important cause of physical disability and social disadaptation.

Relatively isolated trunk ataxia with abnormal stance and gait is seen when the disease is restricted to vermal portions of the cerebellum (patients tend to sway or fall forward with rostral-vermal lesions and backward with caudal-vermal lesions). Limb ataxia is usually attributed to diseases of the cerebellar hemispheres. Saccadic ocular dysmetria is seen with dorsal vermis involvement. With a unilateral cerebellar hemisphere lesion, ipsilateral disturbances of gait, posture, and movement are evident: such patients stand with the shoulder on the affected side lower than the other, they stagger and deviate to the side of the lesion on walking, and the affected extremities show marked ataxia in all tests of motor coordination. Although in humans there is no strict correspondence between cerebellar hemisphere subregions and locomotion of particular segments of the body, it is believed that diseases of antero-superior parts of the hemispheres manifest predominantly as lower limb ataxia (the pattern frequently seen in alcoholic cerebellar degeneration), while lateral-posterior parts of the cerebellum are responsible for upper limbs, face, and speech. Ataxia may be caused also by lesions in cerebellar pathways; these disorders are sometimes manifested by very characteristic phenotypes, such as coarse high-amplitude "rubral" tremor seen in attempts to hold hands in an upright position (the feature typical of lesions in the dentato-rubral loop, for example, in multiple sclerosis or Wilson's disease).

Sensory ataxia

Compared to cerebellar ataxia, sensory ataxia is relatively rare. It usually results from disease of the posterior columns (Friedreich's ataxia, deficiency of vitamins E and B_{12}, neurosyphilis) leading to proprioceptive deafferentation. Sensory ataxia can be diagnosed in the presence of clear proprioceptive deficit in the "ataxic" body part and

International Neurology: A Clinical Approach. Edited by Robert P. Lisak, Daniel D. Truong, William M. Carroll, and Roongroj Bhidayasiri. © 2009 Blackwell Publishing, ISBN: 978-1-4051-5738-4.

a significant worsening of clumsiness with eye closure. In addition, a phenomenon of "pseudoathetosis" is occasionally seen in affected limbs.

Vestibular ataxia

Vestibular dysfunction may cause a rare syndrome designated as "vestibular" (or "labyrinthine") ataxia; in fact, this syndrome may be regarded as a specific subtype of sensory ataxia. Patients with vestibular ataxia exhibit serious stance and gait difficulties (vestibular disequilibrium) but no incoordination of limbs or speech. With a unilateral labyrinthine lesion, "flank walking" in the direction of the lesioned side is predominantly affected. This type of ataxia is frequently associated with dizziness, vomiting, and hearing loss.

This chapter focuses on cerebellar ataxia as a major type of ataxia.

Pathophysiology

Pathophysiologically, cerebellar ataxia represents a failure to maintain normal *anti-inertia* mechanisms that ensure smoothness, evenness, and accuracy of movements.

In normal conditions, any voluntary movement is regarded as the result of precisely coordinated, "orchestrated" activity of a variety of antagonistic and synergistic muscles. This temporally and spatially ordered interplay between different muscles is being realized through extensive bilateral connections of the cerebellum, with different levels of the central nervous system participating in motor functions (motor cortex, basal ganglia, brainstem nuclei, reticular formation, spinal motor neurons, proprioceptive neurons and pathways). The cerebellum as a main "motor coordinator" receives advance information about any changes of muscle tone and postures of body segments, as well as about any planned movement. Using this advance information, the cerebellum "prepares" correct activity of voluntary muscles, organizes fine motor control, and ensures accurate execution of the movement. Therefore, cerebellar disorders result in desynchronization of muscle contractions, which clinically manifests as confused irregular "jolts" leading to scanning speech, intention tremor, dysmetria, body titubation (a coarse fore-and-aft tremor of the trunk), and other cerebellar phenomena.

Cerebellar ataxic disorders

The cerebellum and cerebellar pathways are affected in a variety of acute and chronic conditions (Table 48.1).

Acute ataxia

Acute ataxia is typically seen in ischemic (lacunar, cardioembolic, and atherothrombotic infarcts) or hemorrhagic stroke affecting cerebellar hemispheres, as well as in multiple sclerosis, head trauma, infectious cerebellitis or cerebellar abscess, parasitic invasion, MELAS (mitochondrial encephalopathy, lactic acidosis, and stroke-like episodes) syndrome, acute drug toxicity and poisonings (ethanol, neuroleptics, anticonvulsants), Arnold–Chiari malformation, and other conditions. In these disorders ataxia is frequently associated with headache, vomiting, vertigo, brainstem signs, and cranial nerve involvement. One should remember that even small cerebellar infarcts and hemorrhages are regarded, due to limited volume of the posterior fossa, as potentially life-threatening conditions in view of the high risk of obstructive hydrocephalus upon the development of brain edema and remote pressure effects. Therefore, in patients with acute cerebellar ataxia, emergency neuroimaging examinations (CT or MRI) must be performed and necessary decompression surgery (ventriculostomy or posterior craniectomy) must be promptly undertaken. The same is true for any other disorders characterized by large acute cerebellar lesions with rapidly progressive edema of the posterior fossa structures. Because of risk of herniation in these patients, lumbar puncture is strongly contraindicated.

Repeated paroxysms of acute ataxic symptoms are seen in periodic (episodic) ataxias. These hereditary diseases are caused by genetic defects of ion channels (calcium, potassium) that result in abnormalities of neuronal membrane excitability. Some patients with ataxic paroxysms may benefit from administration of acetazolamide (acetazolamide-responsive forms of periodic ataxias). Periodic ataxias belong to a group of so-called "channelopathies".

Chronic ataxia

Chronic ataxia may be caused by a number of different disorders (see Table 48.1), both genetic and non-genetic in origin. Chronic or subacute cerebellar ataxia, especially at a young age, is a typical manifestation of multiple sclerosis, for which a relapsing-remitting course and presence of multiple demyelinating lesions on brain and spinal MRI facilitate the diagnosis. One should always remember that chronic or subacute cerebellar ataxia may result from tumors (typical cerebellar tumors are cerebellopontine schwannoma, medulloblastoma, and hemangioblastoma), normal-pressure hydrocephalus (Hakim–Adams syndrome), and paraneoplastic cerebellar degeneration (lung cancer and other systemic malignancies); all these conditions require appropriate and timely surgery. Cerebellar degenerative disorder also may be caused by chronic alcoholism, hypothyroidism, gluten disease, vitamin B_{12} deficiency, heat shock, and abuse of some medications with anxiolytic, soporific, and anticonvulsant action.

Chronic progressive ataxia is a key feature of idiopathic degenerative ataxic syndromes, both hereditary and sporadic.

Table 48.1 Etiologies of acute and chronic ataxia.

Acute ataxia	Chronic ataxia
Stroke:	Multiple sclerosis
• ischemia	Cerebellar tumors
• hemorrhage	Chronic cerebral ischemia
Multiple sclerosis	Normal-pressure hydrocephalus
Head trauma	(Hakim–Adams syndrome)
Infections:	Paraneoplastic cerebellar degeneration
• cerebellitis	Cerebellar dysgenesis or hypoplasia (congenital
• cerebellar abscess	ataxia, usually non-progressive)
• neurosyphilis	Prion disease (ataxic form)
• HIV	Chronic alcoholism
• parasitic invasion	Hypothyroidism
Acute drug toxicity and poisonings:	Vitamin B_{12} deficiency
• ethanol	Hyperthermia (heat shock)
• neuroleptics, antidepressants	Abuse of medications with anxiolytic, soporific,
• anticonvulsants	and anticonvulsant action
• soporific medications	Gluten ataxia
• chemotherapeutic medications	Hereditary ataxias with autosomal dominant,
• thallium	autosomal recessive, and X-linked recessive
• methylmercury	inheritance
• bismuth	Sporadic idiopathic degenerative ataxias:
• zinc	• parenchymatous cortical cerebellar atrophy
MELAS, Leigh disease, and other	• olivopontocerebellar atrophy
mitochondrial encephalomyopathies with acute	Genetic metabolic diseases:
onset	• mitochondrial encephalomyopathies with
Tumors and malformations with acute and	chronic ataxic symptoms (NARP, etc.)
subacute manifestations	• Refsum's disease
Thiamine deficiency (Wernicke's	• Gaucher's disease type III
encephalopathy)	• Niemann–Pick disease
Periodic ataxias	• Tay–Sachs disease
Paraneoplastic cerebellar degeneration	• hexosaminidase B deficiency
Hyperthermia (heat shock)	• neuraminidase deficiency
Hypoglycemia (insulinoma)	• vitamin E deficiency (AVED)
Inborn metabolic abnormalities:	• adrenoleukodystrophy and other
• maple syrup disease	leukodystrophies
• Hartnup disease	• Wilson's disease
• mevalonic aciduria and other acidurias	• neuroacanthocytosis
• hereditary hyperammonemias	• cerebrotendinous xanthomatosis

MELAS: mitochondrial encephalopathy, lactic acidosis, and stroke-like episodes; AVED: ataxia with vitamin E deficiency; NARP: neuropathy, ataxia, and retinitis pigmentosa.

Hereditary ataxias are a clinically and genetically heterogeneous group of disorders transmitted, most frequently, as autosomal dominant or autosomal recessive traits; each of these major subtypes of hereditary ataxias also demonstrates striking genetic heterogeneity.

For *autosomal dominant spinocerebellar ataxias* (SCAs), at least 28 loci have been mapped to different chromosomes, and 14 causative genes and their protein products have been identified. In the majority of autosomal dominant SCAs, mutations represent pathological expansions of intragenic trinucleotide repeats ("dynamic" mutations). Most frequently, coding CAG repeat expansion leads, at the protein level, to proportional expansion of the polyglutamine chain (the so-called "polyglutamine disorders" with a very specific mechanism of neurodegeneration).

There is an inverse correlation between the copy number of trinucleotide repeats in the mutant gene and the age at disease onset; moreover, the longest expanded alleles are associated with the most severe phenotypes. In addition to dynamic mutations, autosomal dominant SCAs can be caused by point mutations in several genes encoding for protein kinase gamma, fibroblast growth factor, and other essential proteins. The frequencies of particular forms of autosomal dominant SCAs in different populations are strikingly different. For example, in Russia more than 40% dominant SCAs families are associated with the *ATXN1* gene mutation on chromosome 6p (SCA1), while in the majority of Western European countries, the *ATXN3* gene mutation is most prevalent (SCA3 or Machado–Joseph disease).

Among *autosomal recessive* and *X-linked recessive ataxias*, the most common form is Friedreich's ataxia caused by GAA repeat expansion in the non-coding region of the *FRDA* gene on chromosome 9q. A protein product of this gene, frataxin, is thought to be involved in the homeostasis of mitochondrial iron, and Friedreich's ataxia thus represents a Mendelian form of mitochondrial cytopathies. Typically, the disease presents with early onset (before age 20), "mixed" sensory/cerebellar ataxia, dysarthria, muscle weakness, cardiomyopathy, skeletal deformities, diabetes, and a relentlessly progressive course. There is strong correlation between the length of the GAA repeat chain and the type of clinical presentation of Friedreich's ataxia, with the oldest and relatively "benign" cases being associated with mild GAA repeat expansion.

Sporadic (idiopathic) degenerative ataxia is a heterogeneous entity comprising parenchymatous cortical cerebellar atrophy and oliovopontocerebellar atrophy. The latter is now regarded as a form of multiple system atrophy, a severe neurodegenerative disorder characterized by involvement of many cerebral and spinal systems (cerebellum, basal ganglia, brainstem, spinal autonomic nuclei, and motoneurons) and the presence of specific alpha-synuclein-positive glial cytoplasmic inclusions.

Diagnosis

The diagnosis in patients with ataxic disorders is based, first of all, on neuroimaging (CT, MRI) and neurophysiological examinations (evoked potentials, nerve conduction studies, etc.), which provide important information about structural and functional characteristics of the central and the peripheral nervous system. In many cases of hereditary ataxias, DNA diagnosis is currently available both for affected individuals and for clinically healthy relatives from the "risk group." Genetic counseling and prenatal DNA testing may be offered to prevent new cases of the disease in affected families.

In patients with sporadic ataxia, detailed search for possible somatic disorders that may cause cerebellar dysfunction (malignancies, endocrine and hepatic disorders, etc.) is needed. Since ataxia may be a major presentation of a variety of metabolic diseases (see Table 48.1), appropriate biochemical screening should be undertaken in unclear cases.

Management

Management and prognosis of ataxic syndromes are determined by the primary cause of ataxia. If radical therapy is possible (such as surgery of cerebellar tumor or vitamin supplementation in specific vitamin deficiency), one can expect complete or partial recovery or, at least, cessation of further disease progression.

There is no therapy uniformly beneficial for ataxia itself. Limited positive effects have been reported in degenerative ataxias with amantadine, buspirone, L-5-hydroxy-tryptophan, thyrotropin-releasing hormone, and pregabalin, but these have not been confirmed in randomized studies. Cerebellar tremor was reported to be successfully treated with isoniazid and some anticonvulsants (clonazepam, carbamazepine, and topiramate); stereotaxic thalamic surgery may also be a good option in some cases.

Physical therapy is important in the management of ataxic patients. It is directed towards preventing various complications (such as contractures or muscle atrophy), maximizing strength and conditioning, and improving coordination and gait. Special complexes of "cerebellar" or "sensory" exercises as well as biofeedback with stabilography are strongly recommended.

The very first approaches to gene or stem cell therapy of hereditary ataxic disorders are currently under development; hopefully, in the future these technologies will have serious advantages over any traditional therapy.

Further reading

Diener HC, Dichgans J. Pathophysiology of cerebellar ataxia. *Mov Disord* 1992; 7: 95–109.

Harding AE. *Hereditary Ataxias and Related Disorders*. Edinburgh: Churchill Livingstone; 1984.

Lechtenberg R, editor. *Handbook of Cerebellar Disease*. New York: Marcel Dekker; 1993.

Massaquoi SG, Hallet M. Ataxia and other cerebellar syndromes. In: Jankovic J, Tolosa E, editors. *Parkinson's Disease and Movement Disorders*. Baltimore: Williams & Wilkins; 1998, pp. 623–86.

Taroni F, DiDonato S. Pathways to motor incoordination: the inherited ataxias. *Nat Rev Neurosci* 2004; 5: 641–55.

Chapter 49
Drug induced movement disorders

Rick Stell
Sir Charles Gairdner Hospital, Perth, Australia

Introduction

Drugs are a frequent, though underrecognized, cause of movement disorders, and the list of potential agents is steadily increasing. The most common drugs are those that block or stimulate dopamine receptors. Though movement disorders related to antipsychotic medication were probably seen earlier, the causative effects of these drugs were not recognized until 1956 when the first report of chlorpromazine-induced movement disorder was made by Hall. Though initially thought to be rare, it is now estimated to occur in up to 20% of patients exposed to these drugs.

Clinical presentations may be acute, subacute, or delayed for months, and may mimic virtually every known hyper- and hypokinetic movement disorder, either alone or in combination.

This chapter focuses on several movement disorders caused by commonly prescribed drugs excluding the neuroleptic malignant syndrome.

Acute syndromes

Acute dystonic reactions (ADR)
The incidence of ADR has been reported to range between 2.3% and 63%, the wide range probably indicating that it is often not recognized or is misdiagnosed. Ninety percent of acute dystonic reactions occur within 5 days of exposure, and usually within 2–24 hours, lasting from hours to days. Clinical manifestations vary with age: children often develop generalized spasms, sometimes with an axial emphasis (e.g., opisthotonos), whereas adults involvement is usually segmental with a craniocervical emphasis such as blepharospasm, oculogyric crises, trismus, and torticollis.

Dystonic spasms and postures tend to have an abrupt onset and are frequently painful and may fluctuate in

International Neurology: A Clinical Approach. Edited by Robert P. Lisak, Daniel D. Truong, William M. Carroll, and Roongroj Bhidayasiri. © 2009 Blackwell Publishing, ISBN: 978-1-4051-5738-4.

their distribution. Proposed risk factors include male sex, age less than 30 years, high neuroleptic dosage, potency of the drug, and possibly a familial predisposition – several families have been reported to include a number of affected individuals. In addition to high potency neuroleptics, ADR may also be seen with the benzamide antiemetic metoclopramide, as well as domperidone and sulpiride.

The pathophysiology of ADR has been linked to a sudden imbalance between striatal dopamine and cholinergic systems, causing a relative preponderance of acetylcholine. ADR resolves spontaneously upon drug withdrawal, but may take hours. The treatments of choice are parenteral anticholinergics (biperiden, benztropine) or antihistamines (diphenhydramine); benzodiazepines are occasionally effective.

Acute akathisia
Acute akathisia is a very common and early dose-related side effect of neuroleptics and other dopamine receptor blocking drugs, though it is less frequently seen with atypical neuroleptics. There have been reports of cases in association with selective serotonin reuptake inhibitors (SSRIs). Patients present with an aversion to keeping still and a subjective sensation of restlessness, accompanied by complex or stereotyped movements, including pacing, marching on the spot, picking at clothes, rocking, and crossing/uncrossing legs. The prevalence varies widely between studies, but is estimated to affect 40% of exposed patients, though this may be an underestimate. Fifty percent of affected individuals develop the condition within the first month, and 90% within 3 months of drug exposure.

The pathophysiology of acute akathisia is not well understood, but may result from a blockage of the mesocortical dopamine receptors.

Treatment should comprise dose reduction, switching to a less potent drug, or, if possible, drug withdrawal, as this is the most effective treatment. If not possible or not effective, the addition of various drugs including anticholinergics, amantadine, propranolol, clonidine, benzodiazepines, and, more recently, opioid agonists (such as propoxyphene) have been reported to be effective.

Acute choreoathetosis

A wide variety of commonly used drugs have been reported to cause choreoathetosis, raising the question of individual susceptibility as a consequence of prior basal ganglia damage. Individual susceptibility has been well established for contraceptive-induced chorea, as affected women often present a past history of Sydenham chorea or rheumatic fever. By blocking presynaptic dopamine reuptake and also by altering post-synaptic receptor sensitivity, cocaine may cause or trigger chorea and other hyperkinetic movements. Choreoathetosis and, less frequently, tremor, asterixis, and myoclonus have also been reported with phenytoin and anticonvulsants such as carbamazepine, felbamate, and gabapentin.

Acute tics

Drug-induced tics are indistinguishable from those seen in Tourette syndrome and are caused by drugs that enhance dopaminergic transmission (e.g., amphetamines, SSRIs, and cocaine). Because tics are not always exacerbated or caused by central stimulants, undefined predisposing factors may also be important to this drug effect.

Subacute syndromes

Drug-induced parkinsonism (DIP)

Of the subacute, drug-induced movement syndromes, DIP is the most common. DIP, related to dopamine blocking agents, occurs in 10–15% of exposed patients; however, if subtle signs are included, the incidence may be as high as 90%. Fifty to seventy percent of patients develop signs or symptoms within 1 month, and 90% by 3 months, although symptoms may occur after long-term drug exposure when the dose of the drug is increased and may co-exist with typical tardive dyskinesias. Most cases of DIP follow exposure to dopamine receptor blockers, especially the piperazine class of phenothiazines and butyrophenones. The risk is smaller for atypical neuroleptics, olanzapine, and clozapine – the latter almost only occurring at doses above 250 mg. The role of the SSRIs fluoxetine and, to a lesser extent, paroxetine and fluvoxamine in DIP is controversial as in most reports there has been concomitant use of other potentially relevant drugs.

A diagnosis of DIP requires a history of neuroleptic or other potentially relevant drug exposure and cannot be entertained otherwise. The clinical features of DIP are often indistinguishable from Parkinson's disease (PD). Though it is said some patients present symmetrical akinetic rigid parkinsonian syndrome without tremor, these represent the minority. Other clues to the diagnosis include early age of onset, presentation with gait disturbance, dominant postural, kinetic tremor, and the coincidence of other well-recognized drug-related movements.

Prognosis in DIP is uncertain. Klawans and colleagues reported that patients may take 18 months or more to recover. Others have suggested that up to 20% never recover, or recover only to later develop typical PD. This suggests that certain drugs may unmask subclinical PD in a significant proportion of patients. In support of this assertion is the report of Rajput in which two patients whose DIP resolved within 3 weeks of stopping neuroleptics were later found to have pathological evidence of PD. Additionally, Burn and Brooks found that 30% of DIP patients showed abnormal F-DOPA positron emission tomography (PET) scans, 75% of whom went on to develop PD.

Treatment of DIP includes withdrawal of the offending drug, if possible, or replacement by an atypical neuroleptic. If symptomatic treatment is necessary, levodopa may help in up to 30% of cases, though at the risk of aggravating the underlying psychiatric disorder. Some patients respond well to anticholinergics and amantadine, though these may worsen psychotic symptoms or result in confusion in elderly patients.

Chronic or tardive syndromes

Chronic or tardive syndromes are those that occur after long-term exposure to drugs, requiring exposure of at least 3 months and usually 1–2 years. They have been reported most often in association with drugs that impair dopaminergic transmission, though seldom with drugs that act presynaptically, such as reserpine or tetrabenazine. Prevalence rates vary widely, probably reflecting the differences in patient samples and diagnostic criteria. A meta-analysis of 56 surveys indicates an average prevalence rate of 20%.

Risk factors for tardive dyskinesia include advanced age, duration of drug exposure, and duration of the psychiatric disease. There are several clinical subtypes of tardive dyskinesia, which may occur alone or in combination. The orobuccoliguomasticatory syndrome is the most common and first described subtype, representing 40% of patients in one study. It is characterized by stereotyped movements of tongue twisting and protrusion, along with facial grimacing. The clue to the diagnosis (apart from the history of drug exposure) is the not-infrequent co-existence of other typical tardive movement syndromes, such as tardive tics, myoclonus, and tremor. Risk factors for developing tardive dyskinesias include chronic neuroleptic therapy (especially polypharmacy), age greater than 40, chronic schizophrenia, female sex, and the indiscriminate use of anticholinergic medication.

The pathophysiology of tardive dyskinesias is only partly understood. The most enduring hypothesis is that of denervation blockade. This leads to dopamine receptor supersensitivity, in which amounts of dopamine normally too small to induce dyskinesias are able to do so.

Prevention remains the best treatment. Dopamine receptor blockers should be used for as short a time as possible and in the lowest dosage possible. Once tardive dyskinesia has developed, the offending drug should be withdrawn, although this is often not possible without relapse of the psychiatric illness. Improvement occurs in most cases, but complete and persistent resolution is seen in only 2%. The switch to atypical dopamine receptor blockers such as clozapine has been proposed as a desensitization technique and may be helpful in up to 40% of patients based on uncontrolled studies (controlled studies are lacking). Withdrawal of anticholinergics is recommended for orofacial dyskinesias, though they may help in the treatment of tardive dystonia.

Further reading

Burn DJ, Brooks DJ. Nigral dysfunction in drug-induced parkinsonism: an 18F-DOPA PET study. *Neurology* 1993; 43: 552–6.

Kane JM, Smith JM. Tardive dyskinesia: prevalence and risk factors, 1959 to 1979. *Arch Gen Psychiatry* 1982; 39: 473–81.

Klawans HL, Gegen D, Bruyn GW. Prolonged drug-induced parkinsonism. *Confin Neurol* 1973; 35: 368–77.

Rajput AH, Rodzilsky B, Hornykiewicz O, *et al*. Reversible drug-induced parkinsonism: clinicopathologic study of two cases. *Arch Neurol* 1982; 39: 644–6.

Chapter 50
Gait disorders

Nir Giladi[1,2]
[1]Tel-Aviv University, Tel-Aviv, Israel
[2]Tel-Aviv Sourasky Medical Center, Tel-Aviv, Israel

Introduction

The basic requirements for walking are the ability to stand up and maintain adequate balance and to initiate and maintain locomotion while interacting with the internal and external environments. It is essential to possess a good mechanical support system and to have a good physical state. The basic human motor skill of walking is learned at about 1 year of age, whereupon it becomes an automated function throughout the individual's lifetime.

Classification of gait disturbances

There are many ways to classify gait disturbances, but the easiest to understand and use clinically is based on clinical syndromes and pathophysiology (Table 50.1). The basic principle behind this classification is to identify the primary system from which the gait disturbance originates. The two main groups of gait problems are peripheral disturbances and those originating in the central nervous system (CNS).

Peripheral systems that cause gait disturbances are the musculoskeletal system, peripheral nerves, or the senses that are fundamental to walking (such as the vestibular system, vision, and sense of position, such as proprioception). A common form of gait disturbance orginating in the peripheral system involves the musculoskeletal system, frequently causing pain and leading to an antalgic gait. Most peripheral gait disturbances are easy to diagnose after detailed observation and a thorough neurological examination.

Normal gait is the product of harmonious functioning of almost all parts of the CNS. As a result, gait disturbances are caused by many CNS disturbances, at all levels, and have specific features that are related to the system involved. Most centrally originating gait disturbances of central origin can be diagnosed after a detailed

Table 50.1 System-oriented classification of gait syndromes.

Gait syndromes of peripheral origin
- Musculoskeletal – peripheral nerves
  - Joints, bones, ligaments, tendons, or muscles
  - Peripheral nerves, neuromuscular junction
- Senses
  - Proprioceptive, vestibular, visual

Gait syndromes of central origin
- Spinal
  - Spastic paraparetic
  - Sensory ataxic
- Pyramidal
  - Spastic
  - Paretic
- Cerebellar
  - Ataxic
- Extrapyramidal
  - Bradykinetic/hypokinetic
  - Rigid
  - Dyskinetic
  - Episodic
- Higher level gait disorders (frontal)
  - Dysequilibrium
  - "Apractic"
  - Psychogenic

neurological examination. Additional neurological signs that are associated with walking problems can also help locate the system involved. For example, a gait disturbance of spinal origin will always be accompanied by additional spinal signs. Similarly, spasticity or weakness will accompany the walking difficulty if pyramidal dysfunction is the primary cause of gait disturbances. It is important to note that the functional disturbance affecting the skill of walking is sometimes much more pronounced during the act of walking than while the patient is at rest, and so the evaluation should be structured accordingly. This is especially pertinent to disorders in which gait is the main function that is disturbed, as in cerebellar ataxia, dyskinetic, and episodic gait disturbances – as well as in higher-level gait disorders where the entire syndrome manifests itself only during walking. In some

International Neurology: A Clinical Approach. Edited by Robert P. Lisak, Daniel D. Truong, William M. Carroll, and Roongroj Bhidayasiri. © 2009 Blackwell Publishing, ISBN: 978-1-4051-5738-4.

instances, the picture becomes even more complicated when the gait disturbance is manifested only while walking in specific situations, or when using specific modes of walking. For example, involuntary dystonic movements can appear while walking forward and disappear while running or walking with different shoes, or while walking backwards. Episodic gait disturbances, such as freezing of gait, are classically experienced at step initiation, while turning, or while walking through tight quarters. Furthermore, freezing of gait is highly variable in its appearance: it can be frequently experienced at home and then disappear at the doctor's office or the gait laboratory, and it can be provoked or relieved by stress. These task- or situation-specific associated gait disturbances are special challenges in terms of assessment, diagnosis, and treatment.

The gait disorders that are most complex and difficult to characterize, diagnose, and treat are probably those caused by disturbances in the gait network at the level of the frontal lobe and its connections with subcortical structures such as the basal ganglia, thalamus, and limbic system. In general, these are the high level gait disorders (HLGD), a term coined by Nutt, Thompson, and Marsden to stress the cortical involvement. One major feature of HLGD is the feeling of disequilibrium, associated with increased anxiety in the form of fear of falling. Another common feature is the loss of regular rhythmic, synchronized, and harmonic stepping, giving the observer the impression that the person "forgot" how to walk correctly. When associated with the high level of anxiety that inevitably accompanies it, this "apractic" behavior frequently creates the impression of a psychogenic gait disorder, which can be included as an HLGD in a category by itself.

Mental aspects of gait

Many patients with gait disorders walk cautiously in order to avoid falling. This is usually a normal protective response, but can be a psychological overreaction to a previous fall experience or an overwhelming fear of some unknown origin. A cautious gait, however, demonstrates the potential role played by the mental state in locomotion. There are several mental modalities that influence gait. The executive control system is the cognitive-behavioral system that decides why, when, where, and how one will reach a goal or destination in the quickest, most efficient, and safest way. In other words, this is the system that integrates the information in the environment and leads to a decision about taking action before step initiation. Once the decision has been made, it is the cognitive response to the environment that is responsible for the continuous monitoring of walking and of the changing environment to maintain safe and efficacious walking in real time. Cognitive functions, such as working memory, attention, processing speed, reaction time, risk assessment, prioritization, navigation, visual-spatial, and visual perception all contribute to safe walking patterns. The third mental aspect is the response to internal circumstances in relation to affect and social desirability. The subject's specific mood at any given moment, the current level of anxiety, as well as the attitude toward risk-taking influence the way he/she walks. The mental state can affect all types of walking and is frequently a major contributing factor to the development of gait disturbances.

Most gait disturbances are usually caused by dysfunction of more than one of the above-cited systems. It is good practice to take a comprehensive multilevel and multisystem approach to both diagnosis and treatment for best results.

Assessment

Gait should be assessed as part of the regular general and neurological examination. A simple but very informative office assessment is the Timed Up and Go (TUaG) test where the subject is asked to get up from a chair, walk at a comfortable pace for a distance of 3–10 m, turn around, and return to a sitting position on the same chair. It is easy to perform and does not need more equipment than a chair and some open space. In most instances, observing or timing the subject while he/she is performing the TUaG will provide the necessary information for indicating (or ruling out) the presence of a gait disorder. Sophisticated gait laboratories are mainly required for planning surgical procedures and research purposes.

Treatment

The existing pathophysiology is the first decisive factor in planning treatment of a gait disorder. Once the underlying cause of the gait disturbance has been established, treatment can be initiated either with specific medications, physical therapy, or surgical intervention. It is always better to treat the cause, but if this is not possible, compensatory mechanisms should be taught and rehabilitation should be implemented. The goal should be independent, effective, efficient, and safe mobility, initially without walking aids and then with them or with a wheelchair when indicated.

Further reading

Giladi N, Bloem BR, Hausdorff JM. Gait disturbances and falls. In: Schapira AHV, editor. *Neurology and Clinical Neuroscience.* Philadelphia: Mosby Inc (Elsevier Inc); 2007, pp. 455–70.

Giladi N, Herman T, Reider-Groswasser I, Gurevich T, Hausdorff JM. Clinical characteristics of elderly patients with a cautious gait of unknown origin. *J Neurol* 2005; 252: 300–6.

Giladi N, Nieuwboer A. Gait disorders. In: Factor S, Weiner W, editors. *Parkinson's Disease: Diagnosis and Clinical Management*, 2nd ed. New York, 2008, pp. 55–63.

Nutt JG, Marsden CD, Thompson PD. Human walking and higher-level gait disorders, particularly in the elderly. *Neurology* 1993; 43: 268-79.

Snijders AH, van de Warrenburg BP, Giladi N, Bloem BR. Neurological gait disorders in elderly people: clinical approach and classification. *Lancet Neurol* 2007; 6: 63–74.

Yogev G, Hausdorff JM, Giladi N. The role of executive function and attention in gait. *Mov Disord* 2008; 15: 329–42.

Chapter 51
Psychogenic movement disorders

Brandon Barton[1], Esther Cubo[2], and Christopher G. Goetz[1]
[1]Rush University Medical Center, Chicago, USA
[2]Hospital General Yague, Burgos, Spain

Introduction

Psychogenic movement disorders (PMDs) form a heterogeneous group of clinical phenomena that have been described by a variety of terms: non-organic, functional, and, in early literature, hysterical. They have in common a manifestation of hypo- or hyperkinetic movements that cannot be accounted for by a known neural lesion or biochemical cause. Rather, PMDs are thought to result from an underlying psychiatric or psychological disturbance, and may be associated with somatization or conversion disorder, factitious disorder, or malingering.

Clinical features

Most categories of movement disorders can be simulated by PMDs. Several clinical and historical features are associated with PMDs and may strongly suggest the diagnosis. These include an abrupt onset of maximal symptoms, association with precipitating events, and sudden remissions or exacerbations. "Entrainment," where the abnormal movement takes on the rhythm of a volitional movement performed simultaneously, is also frequently seen. PMDs are often unresponsive to treatments for organic movement disorders, may improve with placebo, and can display distractibility and variability. Patients frequently display give-away weakness, fatigue that is outside the realm of the activity observed, unexplained pain, and non-physiological sensory loss.

Diagnosis

Diagnosis is often difficult given the lack of "gold standard" tests and absolute criteria. Categories of diagnostic certainty have been proposed. High confidence is established when symptoms improve by suggestion, psychotherapy, or placebo, or when the patient is observed outside the clinical context without abnormal movements. Observation of movements incongruent with known movement disorders, inconsistencies over time, multiple somatizations, or signs of psychiatric disturbance also increase diagnostic certainty. Neurophysiologic testing can support the diagnosis of PMD by documenting of unusual patterns of movements, particularly with tremor or myoclonus. In many instances, the diagnosis of PMD remains provisional even after an exhaustive search for other diagnoses.

Epidemiology

PMDs account for more than 3% of diagnoses in movement disorder clinics, but community prevalence is unknown. Compiled data from multiple movement disorder clinics show the most common PMD to be tremor (40%), followed by dystonia (31%), myoclonus (13%), gait disorders (10%), and parkinsonism (5%). Tics, chorea, and other movements were less frequent. Whereas some prevalence variations are likely due to the methods of data collection, the overall frequency of movement type in PMDs is similar between multiple US centers and those in Canada, France, and Spain.

Few studies have specifically addressed transcultural comparisons of PMDs. One study compared the characteristics of PMD patients in two countries. Eighty-eight US patients and 48 Spanish patients were videotaped and graded using a standardized PMD rating scale. Women predominated in both groups, but Spanish patients were older and less racially diverse. Consistent with previous series, the most frequently observed PMD was tremor in both populations (48%), with a significantly higher prevalence of resting tremor (vs. action tremor) among US patients (40% vs. 21%). Dystonia, myoclonus, and bradykinesia were the other most frequent forms of PMDs in both countries. No significant differences occurred between the two populations in scores for duration, incapacity, or severity of PMD. However, 64% of Spanish patients demonstrated a single movement type, compared to only 43% of US patients, who more frequently displayed multiple

International Neurology: A Clinical Approach. Edited by Robert P. Lisak, Daniel D. Truong, William M. Carroll, and Roongroj Bhidayasiri. © 2009 Blackwell Publishing, ISBN: 978-1-4051-5738-4.

motor phenomena. The anatomic locations of PMDs were similar, with the upper extremities most frequently involved, followed by the lower extremities, and then the neck; however, a higher frequency of shoulder involvement occurred in the US patient group (17% vs. 4%). This study suggests that PMDs were markedly similar across two Western populations, though some significant phenomenological differences existed.

Only case reports and small patient series exist from non-Western cultures. Research films (1957–1976) related to the prion-transmitted disease Kuru in 251 patients from New Guinea captured one case of probable PMD. The patient was reported to be a convicted murderer, and his flamboyant gait disorder was felt to be malingering in order to avoid discipline. His videotape revealed "characteristic staggering, small-spaced, elaborated gait... that never led to a fall, reminiscent of astasia-abasia." In contrast, affected Kuru patients demonstrated gait disturbances (with a wide base, high step, and truncal instability) and other concomitant movements, including tremor and dystonia. Long-term follow-up on this case was not available, and the diagnosis of PMD remains provisional. The case emphasizes the diagnostic dilemma for the clinician who must remain open to other diagnoses even after PMD is suggested, especially in the case of unusual disorders where the full clinical spectrum may not have yet been fully defined.

Treatment

Treatment of PMDs is challenging and few trials specifically address therapeutic guidelines. Although a consensus as to the best mode of treatment is lacking, individualized and interdisciplinary treatment strategies are recommended, with a team approach between mental health professionals (including psychiatrists and psychologists), the patient's family and caregivers, and neurologists. Treatment modalities may include psychotherapy, stress management, relaxation techniques, pharmacotherapy with antidepressants or anxiolytics for comorbid psychiatric disease, and physical and occupational rehabilitation. A small, single-blind trial of psychotherapy with ten patients demonstrated improvement on objective clinical scales.

Prognosis

Detailed studies of long-term outcomes have not been performed. The presence of depression or anxiety is a positive predictor for good outcomes in conversion disorders in general, while length of PMD (greater than 6 months), insidious symptom course, diagnosis of factitious disorder, malingering, and hypochondriasis are reported as poor outcome predictors. The patient's willingness to accept the diagnosis and participate in treatment as well as the physician's ability to convey a clear diagnosis and plan are important factors.

Further reading

Cubo E, Hinson VK, Goetz CG, *et al*. Transcultural comparison of psychogenic movement disorders. *Mov Disord* 2005; 20(10): 1343–5.

Jankovic J, Cloninger CR, Fahn S, Hallett M, Lang AE, Williams DT. Therapeutic approaches to psychogenic movement disorders. In: Hallett M, Fahn S, Jankovic J, Lang AE, Cloninger CR, Yudofsky SC, editors. *Psychogenic Movement Disorders*. Philadelphia: Lippincott Williams & Wilkins; 2006, pp. 323–8.

Kompoliti K, Goetz CG, Gajdusek DC, Cubo E. Movement disorders in Kuru. *Mov Disord* 1999; 14(5): 800–4.

Lang AE. General overview of movement disorders: epidemiology, diagnosis, and prognosis. In: Hallett M, Fahn S, Jankovic J, Lang AE, Cloninger CR, Yudofsky SC, editors. *Psychogenic Movement Disorders*. Philadelphia: Lippincott Williams & Wilkins; 2006, pp. 35–41.

Williams DT, Ford B, Fahn S. Phenomenology and psychopathology related to psychogenic movement disorders. *Adv Neurol* 1995; 65: 231–57.

Chapter 52
Amyotrophic lateral sclerosis

Björn Oskarsson,[1] Yvonne D. Rollins,[2] and Steven P. Ringel[2]
[1]University of California, Davis, USA
[2]University of Colorado, Denver, USA

Introduction

Amyotrophic lateral sclerosis (ALS) is a fatal neurodegenerative disease affecting upper and lower motor neurons. Several other names for ALS are used in different regions of the world including *maladie de Charcot*, named after the great French neurologist Jean Martin Charcot who described the disease in 1874, and *Lou Gehrig's disease*, after a famous US baseball player who succumbed to the disease in 1941. In the UK and commonwealth countries, the more generic term *motor neuron disease* (MND) is often used and refers to the group of neurodegenerative disorders which includes ALS. Three of these motor neuron disorders have more restricted involvement but may progress to ALS, and are sometimes considered variants of ALS:

• progressive muscular atrophy (PMA), a pure lower motor neuron condition
• primary lateral sclerosis (PLS), a pure upper motor neuron condition
• progressive bulbar palsy, which is restricted to the brainstem.

Other less common diseases that make up the MND group are as follows:
• ALS–parkinsonism–dementia complex, a disease seen in Guam and southern Japan
• monomelic amyotrophy, a disease seen mostly in young men
• familial Madras motor neuron disease, found in south India.

Although ALS primarily involves upper and lower motor neurons, it is a multisystem disorder that to a varying degree involves cognition, behavior, affect, and autonomic function. There is a clinical and pathological overlap between ALS and the most common subgroup of frontotemporal dementia, frontotemporal lobar degeneration with MND-type inclusions.

International Neurology: A Clinical Approach. Edited by Robert P. Lisak, Daniel D. Truong, William M. Carroll, and Roongroj Bhidayasiri. © 2009 Blackwell Publishing, ISBN: 978-1-4051-5738-4.

Epidemiology

The incidence of ALS varies between 0.4 and 8.3 per 100 000 person years. The prevalence is only 3–4 times higher, due to the short duration of the disease. The disease is gradually progressive, with death occurring on average 3–5 years after the occurrence of the first symptoms.

Reliable demographic data are lacking for many parts of the world, but in several studies there is a suggestion that Caucasians have a higher incidence than Africans, Asians, and Amerindians. A large part of the variation in crude incidence rates can be explained by variations in age between populations: the highest incidence of the disease is seen in the mid-70s so that prevalence is higher in countries with older populations. Men are slightly more likely than women to develop the disease, and there is some evidence that athletes, farmers, and soldiers may have a higher risk of developing ALS.

ALS can be either familial (inherited) or sporadic. Autosomal dominant familial ALS accounts for 10% of all ALS cases. Approximately 20% of familial cases are due to mutations in the copper/zinc super oxide dismutase 1 (SOD1) gene. SOD1 familial ALS (ALS1) is virtually identical clinically to sporadic ALS.

Pathophysiology

The hallmark finding in ALS is degeneration of both upper and lower motor neurons. Extra-ocular motor neurons and the motor neurons of urethral and rectal sphincters in the nucleus of Onufrowicz are largely spared, but all other motor neurons can be affected. Clinical symptoms only appear after the majority of the motor neurons have died.

The cause of sporadic ALS remains unknown, and much of the knowledge that we have regarding the pathophysiology of motor neuron degeneration is derived from transgenic animal models incorporating mutated *SOD1* genes. Motor neuron toxicity in these models appears to be caused by a toxic gain rather than a loss of SOD1 function. As in many other neurodegenerative diseases, abnormal accumulations/aggregates of proteins are seen including neurofilament, peripherin, and ubiquitin. In SOD1 models, there is also accumulation of the SOD1 protein. More recently, a protein labeled TAR DNA binding protein (TDP) 43 has been found to be a component of inclusions in all sporadic ALS and some familial cases. It is not clear that any of these accumulations are directly toxic, but protein aggregation and misfolding may be important steps in the pathogenesis of ALS. There are several proposed mechanisms for how aggregates could have a detrimental effect on cells including inhibition of proteasome activity, loss of protein function through co-aggregation, depletion of chaperone proteins, and dysfunction of mitochondria and other organelles.

Structural changes have been noted in mitochondria in both sporadic and familial ALS and in several SOD1 mouse models. Mitochondria supply vital energy production functions in the cell and also play an important role in programmed cell death. Impaired axonal transport may also be involved in the development of the disease. Inflammatory markers are increased, but it is not clear if inflammation is part of the pathogenesis or a response to the degenerating neurons. There is even some suggestion that inflammation may be beneficial.

ALS pathology is not completely limited to motor neurons; microglia and macrophages also play a role in the development of disease, particularly in the SOD1 mouse. Astrocytes are vital support cells for motor neurons and play an important role in protecting motor neurons from exitotoxicity. In both sporadic ALS and SOD1 mutant-caused ALS there is reduced ability of astrocytes to remove glutamate, which is the major inducer of excitotoxicity.

Clinical features

Typically the disease begins with focal or asymmetric weakness in any region along the neuroaxis. About one-third of patients are first affected in each of the bulbar, cervical, or lumbosacral regions. A few percent of patients have their first symptoms in the form of respiratory distress or truncal weakness ("dropped head" or "bent spine"). Progression is usually relentless. Although periods of clinical stability may occur, improvement of symptoms is very rare. The spread of symptoms is normally contiguous, extending initially to the other side of the same spinal segment before progressing to the next region. Either upper or lower motor neuron signs and symptoms can dominate in any region. Upper motor neuron signs and symptoms include spasticity, weakness, dysarthria, dysphagia, laryngospasm, increased tone, hyperreflexia, pathological reflexes, and clonus. Lower motor neuron signs and symptoms are weakness, cramps, fasciculations, atrophy, dysarthria, and dysphagia.

In addition to corticospinal motor neurons, other cerebral frontal lobe neurons are commonly affected. About half of patients may exhibit inappropriate emotional expression disorder (IEED), also called pseudobulbar effect. This takes the form of excessive or completely unprovoked crying or laughing, lasting only for a few seconds to minutes. IEED is often under-recognized and sometimes confused with depression. Cognitive frontal lobe functions are frequently impaired, especially verbal fluency and executive function. Behavioral changes such as apathy, disinhibition, and irritability are also common.

Respiratory weakness is the most common cause of death, unless mechanical ventilation is implemented. Symptoms of respiratory weakness and hypercapnia are shortness of breath with mild exertion, orthopnea, morning headache, and confusion.

Dysphagia, especially for thin liquids or mixed consistencies, often limits food intake. Poor nutritional status and weight loss contribute to shorter survival. Normal individuals produce between 1 and 1.5 liters of saliva per 24 hours. If swallowing is impaired, sialorrhea or drooling results from the inability to swallow saliva efficiently.

Investigations

Since there is no reliable diagnostic test, ALS remains a clinical diagnosis. The clinical criteria used to establish the diagnosis of ALS were first established at a meeting at the Spanish El Escorial palace/monastery. These modified El Escorial clinical criteria separate the body into four regions, bulbar, cervical, truncal, and lumbosacral, and quantify the certainty of diagnosis:
- *Clinically Definite ALS* – presence of upper and lower motor neuron signs in three regions.
- *Clinically Probable ALS* – upper and lower motor neuron signs in at least two regions, with some upper motor neuron signs rostral to the lower motor neuron signs.
- *Clinically Probable – Laboratory-supported ALS* – either (1) upper and lower motor neuron dysfunction are in only one region, or (2) when upper motor neuron signs alone are present in one region and there are lower motor neuron signs defined by electromyography (EMG) criteria in at least two limbs, along with proper application of neuroimaging and clinical laboratory protocols to exclude other causes.
- *Clinically Possible ALS* – either (1) upper and lower motor neuron dysfunction are found together in only one region, or (2) upper motor neuron signs are found alone in two or more regions, or (3) lower motor neuron signs are found rostral to upper motor neuron signs.

Diseases that can mimic ALS by causing upper and lower motor neuron symptoms alone or in combination with other conditions include cervical and lumbar radiculopathies or stenosis, myasthenia gravis, multifocal motor neuropathy (MMN), inclusion body myositis, lead and dapsone neuropathies, and spinal tuberculosis.

Diseases with more acute onset that can mimic ALS include poliomyelitis (from West Nile virus, polio virus, or other enterovirus), acute axonal motor neuropathy, and porphyria.

Depending on particular clinical features in individual patients, diagnostic studies are used to exclude other conditions. EMG is normally indicated and can show acute and chronic denervation changes from the death of lower motor neurons and decreased activation from upper motor neuron dysfunction. The EMG can also identify other diseases which could potentially mimic ALS, for example, conduction block in MMN or a neuromuscular junction defect in myasthenia.

Imaging the brain and the spinal regions that are clinically affected is frequently helpful. With modern MRI techniques subtle frontal atrophy or changes in the cortico-spinal tracts can sometimes be detected, but as a rule imaging mainly excludes other diseases mimicking ALS.

Analysis of the *SOD1* gene should be considered in familial cases and is helpful in establishing an earlier diagnosis. Testing of asymptomatic family members should be undertaken with great caution and only if resources are available to deal with the psychosocial consequences of a positive test.

No other laboratory studies identify ALS, but many studies can be of use to help exclude other conditions. Serum creatine kinase activity is often increased in ALS, and cannot be used to differentiate ALS from a myopathy. Antibodies against muscle specific receptor kinase (MuSK) and acetylcholine receptors may be useful in patients with bulbar symptoms, to help identify myasthenia gravis. In pure lower motor neuron disease, antibodies directed against GM1 ganglioside can indicate an immune-mediated neuropathy. Cerebrospinal fluid analysis is usually normal in ALS and abnormalities can suggest infection, malignancy, or nerve root inflammation.

Treatment/management

After establishing the diagnosis, the results should be shared with the patient in an unhurried and calm environment without interruptions and with time for questions. It is important to bring family members or friends to this visit, as they will help the patient deal with the diagnosis in between clinic visits and may have many questions of their own. Experienced clinicians try to be as positive as the situation allows, focusing on the many things that can be done to sustain quality of life. Handing out written material, web-links, and contact information to local support organizations is often appreciated. A multidisciplinary team that includes physicians and therapists has been shown to improve survival and quality of care in the disease. If a local ALS clinic is available, a referral there is appropriate.

Treatment remains largely supportive for this progressive fatal condition. Riluzole, a glutamate antagonist, is the only effective medication. The effect of riluzole is modest, prolonging life in ALS by 2–3 months, without having an effect on quality of life, muscle strength, or respiratory function. Antioxidant vitamins such as vitamins C and E are often recommended, but no clinical evidence supports their use.

Cramps can be effectively treated with quinine; other possible remedies include hydration, magnesium, potassium, and phenytoin. Gabapentin is also effective, but it may speed the deterioration of respiratory weakness in ALS. Fasciculations can be bothersome especially early in the disease, and are typically treatment resistant. Spasticity can be reduced by muscle relaxants including baclofen, cyclobenzaprine, and tizanidine.

Physical therapy with range of motion exercises to prevent joint contractures (e.g., frozen shoulders) is beneficial. Physical exercise is likely beneficial, at least for less disabled patients. A multitude of different devices such as ankle foot orthoses, augumentative speech devices, wheelchairs, and lifts improve the daily function of patients.

Adequate nutrition improves quality of life and prolongs survival. Many patients experience an increased calorie need and energy-rich foods are often needed to maintain a stable weight. When significant dysphagia is present, eating may lead to aspiration pneumonia. Aspiration is normally noticed by the patient as choking; silent unnoticed aspiration is rare. The severity of dysphagia can be screened by watching the patient drink a glass of water, a barium swallow study offers more details. Inability to feed oneself due to hand and arm weakness also frequently leads to reduced food intake.

Feeding tubes can be placed by several techniques. The least invasive method is to manually insert a nasogastric tube to temporarily provide nourishment. If one anticipates the need for tube feeding for more than a few weeks then a gastrostomy is a better option. Gastrostomy tubes can be positioned using gastroscopy, fluoroscopic guidance, or open surgery. The risk of anesthesia is great in ALS especially when the forced vital capacity is less than 50% of predicted. Minimizing sedation and maximizing local anesthesia is important in more debilitated patients.

It is very important to assist patients in maintaining communication. If dysarthria becomes a significant problem, writing boards, and electronic assistive communication devices can increase quality of life.

Sialorrhea can be treated with anticholinergic medications, including amitriptyline or glycopyrrolate. If swallowing is severely impaired and no feeding tube is in place, then transdermal scopolamine or oral atropine drops can be used. If anticholinergic therapy fails there are other options. Botulinum toxin A or B injections in the salivary glands reduce salivary production and are effective for several months. Radiation or surgical intervention on the salivary glands or ducts offers a more permanent solution.

While these treatments lead to reduced production of secretions, the secretions that are produced often become more viscous. If the secretions are thick, hydration and guaifenesin can make saliva more liquid. Adrenergic beta blocker drugs also reduce thick secretions. Suction devices and bibs can be helpful for oral secretions. A mechanical insufflator/exsuflator can facilitate coughing to expel secretions lodged deeper in airways.

Non-invasive positive pressure ventilation (NIPPV) should be used when signs of nocturnal hypercapnia occur in the form of morning headache and confusion or when the forced vital capacity (FVC) falls to 50% of predicted. The respiratory weakness may not be obvious and monitoring of the FVC should be performed on a scheduled basis. Supplemental oxygen can lead to depression of respiratory drive and is in general not indicated. Invasive long-term mechanical ventilation can extend life by several years but does not prevent further physical and cognitive decline. The rate of use varies greatly between countries dependent on physician preference, culture, and healthcare insurance. Japan probably has the highest proportion of ALS patients choosing this intervention at approximately 36%.

Pain due to physical immobility or other causes is often a feature of ALS, especially late in the disease. Identifying the cause of pain and managing it appropriately is important to sustain quality of life. Physical therapy with a range of motion exercises can prevent and reduce pain.

Involuntary emotional expressive disorder (IEED) can be treated when it causes social difficulties for the patient. A combination of dextromethorphan and quinidine is effective. Treatment with antidepressants (mostly tricyclic antidepressants, but also selective serotonin reuptake inhibitors) is also effective.

Appropriate recognition and aggressive treatment of depression is important and should not be overlooked. Patients can benefit from counseling as well as from trials of antidepressants.

The timing of end of life care discussions requires that the physician be familiar with a patient and family; there is no standard formula as to when such discussions should be initiated. Different patients have different needs and concerns regarding their death. Fear of pain and air hunger should be addressed with reassurance of effective treatment. The vast majority of ALS patients have a peaceful and dignified death and this should be emphasized.

A minority of patients do wish to die when the disease is severe and debilitating and this is only in part explained by depression. The choices of these patients depend on local legal and cultural norms. It is unusual for ALS patients to actively commit suicide other than by refusing food and water. In the Netherlands, where euthanasia is legal, a considerable portion of patients at least consider this option and about 20% use it.

Most patients complement the care that they receive from their physician with alternative treatments. It is important to encourage the patient to share the information on what alternative treatments he or she chooses and to advise against treatments that are clearly harmful, while not robbing the patient of hope.

Many patients find hope and comfort in participating in a clinical trial to increase our understanding of this disease.

Further reading

Bensimon G, Lacomblez L, Meininger V. A controlled trial of riluzole in amyotrophic lateral sclerosis. *N Engl J Med* 1994; 330: 585–91.

Boillee S, Vande Velde C, Cleveland DW. ALS: a disease of motor neurons and their nonneuronal neighbors. *Neuron* 2006; 52: 39–59.

Cronin S, Hardiman O, Traynor BJ. Ethnic variation in the incidence of ALS: a systematic review. *Neurology* 2007; 68: 1002–7.

Forshew DA, Bromberg MB. A survey of clinicians' practice in the symptomatic treatment of ALS. *Amyotroph Lateral Scler Other Motor Neuron Disord* 2003; 4: 258–63.

Miller RG, Rosenberg JA, Gelinas DF, et al. Practice parameter: the care of the patient with amyotrophic lateral sclerosis (an evidence-based review): report of the Quality Standards Subcommittee of the American Academy of Neurology. *Neurology* 1999; 52: 1311–23.

Morrison RS, Meier DE. Clinical practice. Palliative care. *N Engl J Med* 2004; 350: 2582–90.

Newrick PG, Langton-Hewer R. Pain in motor neuron disease. *J Neurol Neurosurg Psychiatry* 1985; 48: 838–40.

Ravits J, Laurie P, Fan Y, Moore DH. Implications of ALS focality: rostral-caudal distribution of lower motor neuron loss postmortem. *Neurology* 2007; 68: 1576–82.

Ringholz GM, Appel SH, Bradshaw M, Cooke NA, Mosnik DM, Schulz PE. Prevalence and patterns of cognitive impairment in sporadic ALS. *Neurology* 2005; 65: 586–90.

Veldink JH, Wokke JH, van der WG, et al. Euthanasia and physician-assisted suicide among patients with amyotrophic lateral sclerosis in the Netherlands. *N Engl J Med* 2002; 346: 1638–44.

Chapter 53
Primary lateral sclerosis

Yvonne D. Rollins,[1] Björn Oskarsson,[2] and Steven P. Ringel [1]
[1]University of Colorado, Denver, USA
[2]University of California, Davis, USA

Introduction

Within the spectrum of motor neuron diseases, primary lateral sclerosis (PLS) is defined as a primary upper motor neuron (UMN) disorder. Originally described by both Charcot and Erb, it accounts for 3–5% of cases of motor neuron disease. With the advent of modern imaging and laboratories, other causes of UMN dysfunction are more readily excluded, stimulating recent efforts to define PLS as a distinct entity. Controversy still exists regarding whether PLS has a separate pathophysiologic cause from amyotrophic lateral sclerosis (ALS), as it is well known that PLS can convert to ALS with the development of lower motor neuron (LMN) involvement. The absence of LMN involvement is an important prognostic indicator of improved survival.

Epidemiology

The clinical syndrome of PLS is rare, accounting for 1–3% of all patients with motor neuron disease. PLS has a younger average age of onset than ALS (mean 53 years vs. 60 years). Epidemiology studies of motor neuron diseases have not delineated between PLS and ALS. No familial cases are known in adults. Conversion to ALS has been reported up to 27 years after onset. Considered a disease of middle age, rare juvenile cases have recently been associated with a mutation in the ALS2 gene encoding alsin, a protein with cell-signaling domains.

Pathophysiology

The etiology of motor neuron degeneration remains unknown including why different forms present with exclusively UMN or LMN signs and symptoms. Pathologic tissue examination in PLS consistently reports loss of Betz cells in layer 5 of the motor cortex, with atrophy in the corticospinal tracts. Spinal anterior horn cells appear spared. The typical pathologic features of ALS including Bunina bodies and ubiquinated inclusions have been described in autopsy cases of PLS; unfortunately, most of the autopsied cases had evidence of mild LMN involvement so that technically these cases may not be PLS.

Clinical features

Progressive lower extremity spasticity without significant loss of strength is the classic initial symptom. Dysarthria frequently develops. Bladder dysfunction is rare and usually occurs late in the course of the disease. Examination reveals increased tone with a spastic gait, hyperreflexia, spastic dysarthria, and extensor plantar reflexes with relative sparing of strength, coordination, and sensation. Clinical diagnostic criteria were proposed in 1992 based on a series of eight patients and include the following:
- insidious onset of spastic paresis, usually beginning in the lower extremities but occasionally bulbar or upper extremities
- adult onset in the fifth decade or later
- absence of family history
- gradually progressive without step loss of function
- duration greater than 3 years
- symmetric distribution.

The usefulness of these criteria has been debated. A pure PLS syndrome distinct from a UMN-dominant ALS based on a cohort of 29 patients with only UMN signs and a normal electromyography (EMG) on initial evaluation was recently described. Thirteen of the 29 patients developed evidence of denervation by EMG or clinical examination within 4 years of follow-up. Disability rating, respiratory function, and life expectancy were superior in the pure PLS syndrome, while the UMN-dominant ALS group retained a better life expectancy compared to an ALS control group.

Although initially thought to spare cognition, detailed neuropsychological testing showed mild deficits in frontal lobe dysfunction and memory in eight of nine patients. Involuntary emotional expression (pseudobulbar effect)

International Neurology: A Clinical Approach. Edited by Robert P. Lisak, Daniel D. Truong, William M. Carroll, and Roongroj Bhidayasiri. © 2009 Blackwell Publishing, ISBN: 978-1-4051-5738-4.

with episodes of unprovoked crying or laughing has been described in approximately half of cases.

Investigations

PLS remains a diagnosis of exclusion. Other disorders that need to be considered include ALS, hereditary spastic paraplegia (HSP), foramen magnum lesions, cord compression, multiple sclerosis (MS), spinocerebellar atrophy, dentatorubral-pallidoluysian atrophy, adrenomyeloneuropathy, subacute combined degeneration, syphilis, neuroborreliosis, tropical spastic paraparesis, copper deficiency, vitamin E deficiency, hexosaminidase A deficiency, HIV, dystonia, and paraneoplastic syndromes. In addition, two UMN syndromes have been described with food consumption: on the Indian subcontinent, ingestion of the seed of *Lathyrus sativus* (chickling or grass pea) is associated with lathyrism and in sub-Saharan Africa, consumption of cassava root is associated with konza.

EMG is useful to distinguish PLS from ALS based on the absence of diffuse chronic denervation, although mild denervation with PLS has been reported. Laboratory studies include brain and spinal MRIs, vitamin B_{12}, rapid plasma reagin (RPR), *Borrelia* antibodies, HTLV-1 antibodies, and very long-chain fatty acids. Cerebrospinal fluid (CSF) analysis is usually unremarkable. No biomarker is currently available for definitive diagnosis.

Atrophy of the frontoparietal region of the brain, predominantly in the precentral area, with degeneration of the underlying white matter and selective T2 hyperintensity of the pyramidal tract is seen with brain MRI. In four PLS patients, cortical positron emission tomography (PET) scan showed decreased metabolism in the motor cortex and right parietal lobe similar to that seen in ALS,

with further decrease in the left superior temporal gyrus and the anterior cingulate gyrus. Cortically evoked motor potentials are often absent or prolonged in PLS, while in ALS they are often normal or mildly delayed.

It is problematic to distinguish PLS from HSP. In HSP, a dominant family history is usually present, and x-linked and recessive forms are less common. HSP tends to present at a younger age (mean 39) and is not associated with spastic dysarthria or pseudobulbar effect. Genetic testing is available for some forms of HSP.

Treatment/management

No curative treatment is available for PLS. Treatment is symptomatic and includes muscle relaxants such as baclofen, tizanadine, or dantrolene for spasticity, augmentive speech devices for dysarthria, feeding tubes for dysphagia, and walker or wheelchair for gait impairment.

Further reading

Casselli RJ, Smith BE, Osborne D. Primary lateral sclerosis: a neuropsychological study. *Neurology* 1995; 45: 2205–9.

Eymard-Pierre E, Lesca G, Dollet S, *et al.* Infantile-onset of ascending hereditary spastic paralysis is associated with mutations in the alsin gene. *Am J Hum Genet* 2002; 71: 518–27.

Gordon PH, Cheng B, Katz I, *et al.* The natural history of primary lateral sclerosis. *Neurology* 2006; 66: 647–53.

Pringle CE, Hudson AJ, Munoz DG, Kiernan JA, Brown WF, Ebers GC. Primary lateral sclerosis. Clinical features, neuropathology and diagnostic criteria. *Brain* 1992; 115: 495–520.

Tartaglia MC, Rowe A, Findlater K, Orange JB, Grace G, Strong MJ. Differentiation between primary lateral sclerosis and amyotrophic lateral sclerosis. *Arch Neurol* 2007; 64: 232–6.

Chapter 54
Hereditary spastic paraplegia

Ildefonso Rodríguez-Leyva
Universidad Autónoma de San Luis Potosí, San Luis Potosi, México

Introduction

Hereditary or familial spastic paraplegia (HSP, FSP, Strümpell–Lorraine syndrome, Strümpell's syndrome) is a group of inherited disorders characterized by progressive spasticity and to a lesser extent weakness of the legs associated with hyperreflexia and extensor plantar responses. In addition, various other neurological symptoms and signs may be observed. HSP may be inherited as an autosomal dominant, autosomal recessive, or X-linked recessive trait.

These disorders may be classified based on mode of inheritance, with various subtypes as determined by the locus of the disease gene and whether it occurs alone or is accompanied by additional neurological or systemic abnormalities.

HSP may be caused by mutations of several different genes (genetic heterogeneity). Loci for autosomal dominant, autosomal recessive, and X-linked recessive HSP have been identified in various affected families.

Epidemiology

The prevalence of HSP varies in different studies, probably due to the use of different diagnostic criteria and geographical factors. A prevalence of 1.27/100 000 was found for autosomal dominant HSP in Ireland and of 9.6/100 000 in Cantabria, Spain.

Pathophysiology

The basic underlying defect(s) in HSP remain unknown. However, the disorder is known to be associated with deterioration or degenerative changes of certain spinal cord tracts, consisting of bundles of myelinated axons.

HSP is associated with degeneration that is most severe at the ends of the longest nerve fibers in the central nervous system (CNS). These include descending (corticospinal) and ascending (gracilis) tracts. There are usually less marked degenerative changes of corticospinal tracts that convey motor and sensory impulses to and from (cuneatus) the arms; as a result, most patients do not experience associated symptoms of the upper limbs. Involvement of spinocerebellar tracts is seen in about 50% of cases.

The analysis of HSP genes provides insight into its pathogenesis by permitting pathophysiological molecular and cellular studies of the disorder. These should help to understand the molecular functions of the corticospinal tract and the design of strategies to prevent and treat spasticity of more common causes. The proteins encoded by these genes have roles in development, signal transduction between axons and myelinating cells, and particularly axonal trafficking and energy metabolism. A biochemical classification of HSP is therefore emerging.

Clinical features

The onset of stiffness and weakness of hip and leg muscles and associated gait disturbance tends to be insidious, with symptoms typically becoming progressively severe over time. The age at onset is extremely variable even among affected members of the same family. Symptoms have been known to develop as early as infancy to as late as the ninth decade of life. Up to 25% of affected patients are asymptomatic. In some kindreds symptoms appear to occur at a younger age with successive generations. This apparent anticipation may result from increased awareness and earlier detection of the disease.

In those who suffer from HSP without other associated neurological features, often described as uncomplicated or "pure" HSP, initial findings include the following:
• Spasticity of leg muscles, including the adductors, hamstrings, quadriceps femoris, and calf muscles causing the characteristic gait of scissoring, circumduction, and toe walking
• Weakness of leg muscles with a pyramidal distribution include the ankle extensors, hip flexors, and to a lesser extent the hamstrings. A characteristic feature of HSP is

International Neurology: A Clinical Approach. Edited by Robert P. Lisak, Daniel D. Truong, William M. Carroll, and Roongroj Bhidayasiri. © 2009 Blackwell Publishing, ISBN: 978-1-4051-5738-4.

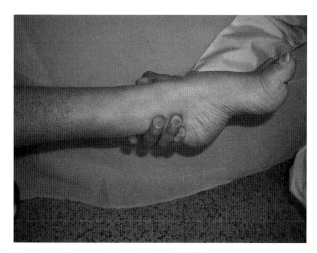

Figure 54.1 Pes cavus in a patient with HSP.

the marked discrepancy between the often severe spasticity and the mild or absent muscle weakness
• Delayed walking (a relatively rare finding that may occur in childhood-onset HSP)
• Hyperreflexia of the lower limbs and commonly also of the upper limbs, and extensor plantar responses.

Uncomplicated HSP may also be associated with additional symptoms and findings such as:
• Highly arched feet (pes cavus; see Figure 54.1)
• Muscle spasms and leg cramps
• Diminished vibration sense, paresthesia, and less often diminished joint position sense in the feet. Sensory impairment is seen in 10–65% of cases of pure HSP, especially in cases with longstanding disease
• Mild terminal dysmetria
• Loss of ankle jerks
• Relatively mild muscle atrophy. Atrophy is usually confined to the small muscles of the feet and the tibialis anterior muscles, usually in patients late in the disease course who have become dependent on wheelchairs
• Bladder control problems, such as a urinary urgency that may progress into incontinence. Such symptoms can be found in up to 50% of patients and develop as a late manifestation.

As with the age of onset, the rate of the disease progression, symptom severity, and degree of associated disability vary greatly. For example, in some patients with uncomplicated HSP, particularly those with childhood onset, symptoms may become apparent, gradually worsen over a number of years, and eventually stabilize following adolescence. In such cases, patients often maintain an ability to walk with assistive devices. In other cases, once symptoms develop, they slowly become increasingly severe throughout the patient's life. HSP patients rarely experience a complete loss of leg mobility.

Less commonly, families suffering from HSP in association with additional neurological features or "complicated HSP" have been described, including mental retardation,

dementia, epilepsy, peripheral neuropathy, thin corpus callosum, retinopathy, optic neuropathy, deafness, ataxia, dysarthria, nystagmus, disturbances of the extrapyramidal system, characterized by changes in muscle tone, postural abnormalities, impairments in the execution of voluntary actions, and/or the development of abnormal involuntary movements, and ichthyosis.

In the past, classification of HSP was based primarily on whether the symptom onset was before age 35 (type I or early onset HSP) or after age 35 (type II or late onset HSP). However, both the early and late onset type may occur in the same family, and therefore categorization into uncomplicated ("pure") and complicated HSP has been considered a more specific and useful distinction. Such classifications based upon clinical findings are gradually being revised as more is learned about the specific underlying genetic mechanisms of HSP.

Up to 70% of cases of uncomplicated HSP are transmitted as an autosomal dominant trait. Multiple genetic loci have been identified in families with autosomal dominant HSP, in chromosomes: 2p (known as *SPG4* (i.e., "spastic paraplegia gene 4")), 8q (*SPG8*), 12q (*SPG10*), 14q (*SPG3A*), 15q (*SPG6*), and 19q (*SPG12*). Mutations in the spastin gene located on the short arm (p) of chromosome 2 (2p22-p21) are by far the most common cause of uncomplicated autosomal dominant HSP and are responsible for about 40% of cases. There may be reduced expression (reduced penetrance) and, as a result, some individuals who inherit a gene mutation for HSP may be asymptomatic or unaware of symptoms. HSP linked to the *SPG3A* locus represents approximately 10% of dominantly inherited HSP cases.

Classification by mode of inheritance and genetic loci is important to answer some questions that have been raised upon observed clinical features. For example, cognitive impairment – such as learning difficulties, deficits in visuospatial function, memory disturbance, or dementia – has been reported in members of a few families with the most commonly described form of uncomplicated HSP (i.e., caused by mutations in the spastin gene). However, the development of cognitive impairment in kindreds with this form of HSP is extremely rare, and therefore its expression might depend upon additional genetic mechanisms.

Complicated autosomal dominantly inherited HSP includes SPG 9 (locus on chromosome 10q, associated with cataracts and amyotrophy), SPG 10 and 12 (loci on chromosomes 12 and 19, respectively, associated with cerebellar signs), and SPG 29 (locus on chromosome 1p, associated with hearing loss).

Autosomal recessive HSP is far less common than the dominant form. Both pure and complicated phenotypes are seen. Genetic loci have been identified on chromosome 8 (*SPG5A*), 15q (*SPG11*), and 16q (*SPG7*). The latter is caused by mutations in the paraplegin gene and may manifest as pure or complicated HSP. SPG7 mutations account for less than 5% of HSP families compatible with autosomal recessive inheritance.

Two X-linked recessive forms of HSP have also been identified. In one form, the disorder appears to result from mutations in a gene that regulates production of the L1 cell adhesion molecule (L1CAM). This gene has been mapped to chromosome Xq28 (*SPG1*). A second X-linked form of HSP is thought to be caused by mutations in a gene that regulates production of a myelin protein (proteolipid protein or PLP). The PLP gene is located on chromosome Xq22 (*SPG2*). A gene duplication is the most common mutation in the Pelizaeus–Merzbacher syndrome.

In many kindreds with HSP, linkage has not been established, suggesting that there are other, currently unknown genetic loci.

Investigations

The diagnosis of HSP is typically based on a careful patient and family history, a thorough clinical evaluation, and assessment of the characteristic symptoms and findings. Diagnostic evaluation may also include various specialized tests.

Although DNA analysis may assist in diagnosing certain forms of HSP (e.g., due to known gene mutations in certain families), such testing is not widely available. As more is learned about the different genetic causes of HSP, it is hoped that such information will lead to additional laboratory studies to help confirm the diagnosis. Thus, in most instances, there is currently no definitive test for HSP.

Spastic paraplegia may also result from various other disorders, such as cervical spondylosis, spinal cord injury, or neoplasms; certain infectious diseases (HTLV-1-associated myelopathy, neurosyphilis, HIV-AIDS, neuroborreliosis), multiple sclerosis, vitamin B$_{12}$ deficiency, vitamin E deficiency, hereditary diseases including adrenomyelopathy and other leukodystrophies, distal hereditary motor neuropathy type V, Charcot–Marie–Tooth syndrome type 2 presenting with predominant hand involvement, and Silver syndrome, motor neuron disease, neurolathyrism, arteriovenous malformations, Arnold–Chiari malformation, syringomyelia, mitochondrial disorders, spinocerebellar ataxia, and dopa-responsive dystonia. Therefore, the differential diagnosis of HSP must include certain tests to discard such conditions particularly if a family history of HSP is not present.

Recommended diagnostic studies may include the following:
• Extensive laboratory tests
• Electromyography, nerve conduction tests, and electroencephalography
• Neuroimaging studies (CT, MRI) of the brain and spinal cord
• Lumbar puncture
• Other tests to help confirm HSP or to verify or eliminate other disorders including genetic analysis.

Treatment/management

The treatment consists of symptomatic and supportive services, including physical therapy. Symptomatic treatments used for other forms of chronic paraplegia are sometimes helpful and physical therapy is important to improve muscle strength and range of motion.

Although no available treatment may prevent, slow, or alter the disease progression, therapy with baclofen, a skeletal muscle relaxant, delivered orally or intrathecally, may reduce spasticity in some patients. Another muscle relaxant, dantrolene, may also improve spasticity. Other medications that may prove beneficial include tizanidine, and benzodiazepines such as diazepam or clonazepam, although the latter may be associated with more excessive daytime sleepiness. For bladder control problems, treatment with oxybutynin, a smooth muscle relaxant and spasmolytic agent, may help relieve bladder spasticity.

Some patients may be candidates for chemodenervation. This therapeutic approach may help reduce muscle overactivity without systemic side effects. For example, patients may benefit from botulinum toxin type A injections into the hip adductors or ankle plantar flexors. In selected candidates, injections of phenol into the obturator nerve may be of some benefit. In patients with slowly progressive symptoms, neuro-orthopedic surgery to lengthen the ankle plantar flexors or hip adductors may be appropriate.

The prognosis for individuals with HSP varies. Some cases are seriously disabled while others are less incapacitated and can lead a life without limitations. The majority of individuals with HSP have a normal life expectancy.

Further reading

Fink JK. The hereditary spastic paraplegias. Nine genes and counting. *Arch Neurol* 2003; 60: 1045–9.

Harding AE. Hereditary "pure" spastic paraplegia: a clinical and genetic study of 22 families. *J Neurol Neurosurg Psychiatry* 1981; 44: 871–83.

http://neuromuscular.wustl.edu/synmot.html

McDermott CJ, White K, Bushby K, Shaw PJ. Hereditary spastic paraparesis: a review of new developments. *J Neurol Neurosurg Psychiatry* 2000; 69: 150–60.

Chapter 55
Spinal muscular atrophies

Sabine Rudnik-Schöneborn[1] *and Klaus Zerres*[2]
[1]University Hospital RWTH, Aachen, Germany
[2]Aachen University, Aachen, Germany

Introduction

The term spinal muscular atrophy (SMA) comprises a clinically and genetically heterogeneous group of diseases characterized by degeneration and loss of the anterior horn cells in the spinal cord, and sometimes also in the brainstem nuclei, resulting in muscle weakness and atrophy.

The criteria used for the subdivision of the SMAs into separate entities (Table 55.1) are age of onset, severity, distribution of weakness, inclusion of additional features, and different modes of inheritance.

Epidemiology

Proximal SMAs can be divided into autosomal recessive and rare autosomal dominant types. Less than 2% of cases with disease onset before 10 years of age show a parent-to-child transmission. Autosomal dominant transmission occurs in about two-thirds of the hereditary adult-onset proximal SMA.

Data for the most severe SMA type I suggest that the birth incidence among Caucasians varies between 1:25 000 and about 1:10 000. The incidence is much higher in certain inbred communities. Variants of early onset SMA are very rare, contributing to about 2% of all SMA cases in childhood and infancy. The more benign forms of the disease (SMA types II and III) have a prevalence among children as high as 1:18 000 and around 1:20 000 in the general population. Assuming an incidence of about 1:10 000 for all types of autosomal recessive SMA, a heterozygosity frequency of 1:50 can roughly be estimated as a basis for genetic counseling. Adult SMA accounts for 8% of all SMA cases, with a prevalence of 0.32 per 100 000 of the population.

Distal SMA accounts for about 10% of all SMAs, while the definition of scapuloperoneal syndromes is still under

Table 55.1 Classification of spinal muscular atrophies.

1. Proximal SMA (80–90%)
1.1 Autosomal recessive SMA
- infantile and juvenile SMA (SMA I–III)*
- adult SMA (SMA IV) (mostly sporadic)†
1.2 Autosomal dominant SMA (juvenile and adult onset forms) †
1.3 Spinobulbar neuronopathy type Kennedy (XL)*

2. Non-proximal SMA (10–15%)
2.1 Distal SMA†
- juvenile distal SMA/hereditary motor neuronopathy (AD, AR, XL)
- monomelic juvenile SMA type Hirayama (mostly sporadic)
- with spasticity (AD)
- with pyramidal signs (AD, AR)
- with vocal cord palsy (AD)
- with diaphragmatic palsy (AR)
- segmental SMA or benign monomelic amyotrophy (mostly sporadic)
2.2 Scapuloperoneal SMA (AD, AR)

3. Variants of infantile SMA (<2%)
3.1 Diaphragmatic SMA (AR)*
3.2 SMA plus pontocerebellar hypoplasia (AR)
3.3 SMA plus arthrogryposis and bone fractures (AR, XL)
3.4 SMA with myoclonus epilepsy (AR)

4. Bulbar palsy (very rare)
4.1 Progressive bulbar palsy of childhood type Fazio–Londe (AR)
4.2 Bulbar palsy with deafness and distal pareses (Brown–Vialetto–van Laere syndrome) (AR)
4.3 Adult onset bulbar palsy (AD)

AR: autosomal recessive; AD: autosomal dominant; XL: X-linked.
*Genetic diagnosis available.
†Genetic diagnosis possible in some cases.

debate. Progressive bulbar palsy is extremely rare, while spinobulbar neuronopathy type Kennedy has a prevalence of about 1:40 000.

Clinical features and investigations

It is still unclear whether SMA is primarily a disease of the anterior horn cells, albeit postmortem studies show a variable degeneration of motor neurons in the spinal cord and in the brain stem. Progressive muscle weakness and atrophy and reduced tendon reflexes are present in most of

International Neurology: A Clinical Approach. Edited by Robert P. Lisak, Daniel D. Truong, William M. Carroll, and Roongroj Bhidayasiri.
© 2009 Blackwell Publishing, ISBN: 978-1-4051-5738-4.

the SMAs. Serum creatine kinase (SCK) activity is normal or only mildly elevated. Electromyography (EMG) and muscle biopsy studies reveal a neurogenic lesion. Nerve conduction is generally normal which helps to differentiate SMA from clinically similar motor neuropathies.

Genetic screening is now replacing invasive neurologic tests in the diagnosis of SMA types I–III, the rare diaphragmatic type of SMA, and bulbospinal neuronopathy (Kennedy syndrome). However, the majority of genes responsible for the non-proximal SMAs and autosomal dominant forms of SMAs are as yet unidentified.

Proximal SMA

The infantile- and juvenile-onset proximal SMAs (SMA types I–III) are caused by defects of the *SMN1* gene on chromosome 5q13. The clinical picture indicates a continuous spectrum with ages of onset ranging from before birth to adulthood. SMA types I–III follow an autosomal recessive mode of inheritance, and more than 90% of patients show homozygous deletions of the *SMN1* gene, enabling a fast and reliable molecular diagnosis. The situation is different for SMA IV, where the genetic basis is largely unknown, and most patients are sporadic. However, there are some patients with SMA IV with *SMN1* gene deletions. Kennedy syndrome is X-linked and easily diagnosed by the presence of a CAG repeat expansion in the androgen receptor gene.

SMA type I

The clinical signs of the most severe SMA type I (Werdnig–Hoffmann disease, acute SMA), are evident at birth or soon thereafter; nearly all patients present by 6 months of age. Symptoms are profound hypotonia and generalized weakness. The infants are never able to sit unaided. The tongue fasciculates, and the infant lies in the "frog" position. In the final stages of the disease the child is practically immobile (Figure 55.1a), has a bell-shaped chest with paradoxic breathing, and is tachypneic, indicating imminent respiratory insufficiency. Death occurs at a median age of 7–8 months due to weakness affecting bulbar and respiratory muscles. However, 8–10% of patients show an arrested disease course and survive for several years or exceptionally into adulthood.

The differential diagnosis of early onset SMA type I comprises the whole spectrum of the *floppy infant syndrome*.

SMA type II

The clinical course of SMA type II, also known as chronic childhood SMA or intermediate type SMA, is marked by periods of apparent arrest in the clinical progression. The children fail to pass motor milestones because of proximal weakness and hypotonia within the first 18 months of life. There is wide variability of clinical severity, ranging from children who have early difficulties in sitting (Figure 55.1b) and rolling over to patients who walk with

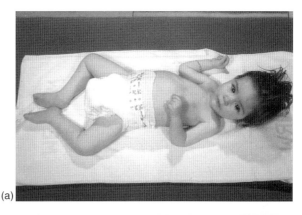

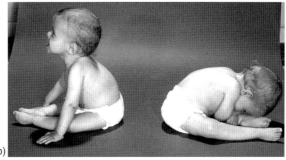

Figure 55.1 (a) Girl with end-stage SMA type I who died at the age of 10 months. (b) Twin brothers with early onset SMA type II. A sitting position is maintained only for several minutes, followed by a "pocket knife" phenomenon.

support. For practical purposes, this group is defined by the ability to sit independently, as the children never learn to stand or walk unaided. Hand tremor and fasciculations are characteristic features. Pronounced weakness of trunk muscles gives rise to spine deformities and also causes a reduced lung capacity. Contractures of all major joints occur in the disease course. Most patients survive into adulthood, but life span can vary considerably.

SMA type III

SMA type III (Kugelberg–Welander disease) is a mild form of childhood and juvenile onset disease. The age of onset varies widely from the first year of life to the third decade. Patients with SMA type III learn to walk without support. For prognostic reasons, we separate SMA types IIIa and IIIb. In SMA type IIIa, the children have early walking difficulties and often fail to pass further motor milestones within the first 3 years. Since many patients are nonambulatory by school age (50% are wheelchair-bound 14 years after onset), there is a considerable handicap in comparison to those whose walking difficulties start in youth or adulthood. Spine deformities and contractures are frequent complications, mainly in the chairbound patients. In SMA type IIIb, onset is between 3 and 30 years of age. About 50% of these patients are still ambulatory after a 45-year disease following the onset of symptoms, and life expectancy is not much reduced.

The clinical picture is often indistinguishable from *Becker's muscular dystrophy* or *limb girdle muscular dystrophy*. If cardiomyopathy is seen in patients with proximal weakness, *Emery–Dreifuss muscular dystrophy* should be taken into account. *Facioscapulohumeral muscular dystrophy (FSHD)* can also present like SMA III and can be easily diagnosed by DNA analysis. Rarely, *hexosaminidase A deficiency* may produce a clinical picture resembling SMA type III.

SMA type IV

SMA type IV (adult SMA) comprises a clinically and genetically heterogeneous condition. Usually, onset ranges from 30 to 60 years, with pronounced proximal weakness, particularly of the lower limbs. Progression is mostly slow, and life span is normal. In contrast to SMA types I–III, recurrence of SMA IV within a sibship is an exception.

The term "spinal muscular atrophy of the Finkel type" refers to a late-onset autosomal dominant SMA (mean age of onset 48.8 years), with cramps and early respiratory failure, almost exclusively found in Portuguese descendants. Two large pedigrees have been reported from Brazil, caused by a founder mutation of the *VAPB* gene.

The most important differential diagnosis of SMA type IV is *Kennedy syndrome* and progressive spinal muscular atrophy, an exclusively lower motor neuron variant of *amyotrophic lateral sclerosis*. *Adult acid maltase deficiency* shows a similar clinical picture and glycogen accumulation is not always apparent on the muscle biopsy. *Proximal myotonic myopathy (myotonic dystrophy type 2)* has also to be considered, but the presence of myotonia and CTTG repeat expansions on chromosome 3 should clarify the diagnosis. *Postpoliomyelitis muscular atrophy* can cause diagnostic confusion.

Spinobulbar neuronopathy type Kennedy

Spinobulbar neuronopathy type Kennedy is characterized by pronounced muscle cramps and fasciculations accompanying predominantly proximal and symmetrical weakness, in legs more than arms. Mean age at onset is 30 years (range 15–60). Patients often show signs of partial androgen insensitivity with gynecomastia, impotence, testicular atrophy, and reduced fertility. Frequently, facial and perioral contraction fasciculations and a postural tremor of the hands are observed. Dysarthria, dysphonia, and dysphagia are caused by progressive death of spinal and bulbar motor neurons. The disease is X-linked and caused by a CAG expansion in the androgen receptor gene.

Non-proximal SMA
Distal SMA

Distal SMA accounts for about 10% of all SMA cases, and comprises a group of genetically and clinically heterogeneous disorders with a broad spectrum of clinical manifestations. Distal SMAs, also denoted as distal hereditary motor neuronopathies, are frequently listed among the Charcot–Marie–Tooth (CMT) neuropathies. Both autosomal dominant and recessive genes cause childhood- and adult-onset forms, and the course is usually chronic and benign. The early childhood form of distal SMA starts soon after birth with distal hypotonia and wasting, but most patients show a clinical picture of distal weakness and atrophy similar to *CMT neuropathy*. Therefore, it is important to exclude peripheral nerve involvement by electroneurography before diagnosing distal SMA. In non-familial cases, *intraspinal pathology* has to be excluded. *Distal myopathies* can normally be distinguished by elevated SCK, muscle biopsy, or DNA studies.

Juvenile segmental spinal muscular atrophy, also known as "monomelic juvenile SMA of the Hirayama type" or "benign monomelic amyotrophy", deserves a separate mention. It was first reported in Japanese literature and later in other populations as well. The onset is insiduous and usually between 15 and 25 years of age. The cardinal features are asymmetric wasting and weakness confined to a single upper limb (hand and forearm), which might spread to the contralateral upper or to a lower limb. The condition is benign in most cases, with the initial progressive phase coming to a halt within 2–4 years. Sporadic occurrences have been reported in more than 200 cases, with a large predominance of males.

Scapuloperoneal SMA

The clinical manifestations of scapuloperoneal SMA are variable, affecting foot and toe extensors first, and then spreading to the shoulder girdle and proximal muscles of lower limbs. Autosomal dominant and recessive inheritance has been reported. The autosomal dominant form with adult onset was first described by Stark and Kaeser. Meanwhile, the original family has been shown to be due to a mutation of the *DES* gene, thus enlarging the clinical spectrum of the desminopathies.

Since *FSHD* can be clinically indistinguishable, it is reasonable to exclude this condition by DNA analysis before diagnosing scapuloperoneal SMA.

Future prospects

The identification of genes involved in the different forms of SMA will help to define and better differentiate these entities. Moreover, it will provide us with further insights into the pathogenic mechanisms of motor neuron degeneration and might open the way for therapeutic strategies. Since no cure for SMA is yet available, genetic counseling, prognostic assessments, and referral to a rehabilitation physician to adjust to disabilities, surgery (Achilles' tendons and scoliosis), and the preservation of respiratory function are of great importance.

Further reading

Irobi J, Dierick I, Jordanova A, *et al.* Unraveling the genetics of distal hereditary motor neuropathies. *Neuromol Med* 2006; 8: 131–46.

Monani U. Spinal muscular atrophy: a deficiency in a ubiquitous protein; a motor neuron-specific disease. *Neuron* 2005; 48: 885–96.

Ogino S, Wilson RB. Genetic testing and risk assessment for spinal muscular atrophy (SMA). *Hum Genet* 2002; 111: 477–500.

Zerres K, Davies KE. International SMA Consortium: Workshop report. *Neuromuscul Disord* 1999; 9: 272–8.

Zerres K, Rudnik-Schöneborn S. Natural history in proximal spinal muscular atrophy (SMA): clinical analysis of 445 patients and suggestions for a modification of existing classifications. *Arch Neurol* 1995; 52: 518–23.

Chapter 56
Post-polio syndrome

Nils Erik Gilhus[1,2]

[1]Department of Clinical Medicine, University of Bergen, Bergen, Norway
[2]Department of Neurology, Haukeland University Hospital, Bergen, Norway

Introduction

Acute polio is a generalized virus infection. However, paralytic polio with muscle weakness combined with meningitis and signs of generalized disease accounts for only 1% of cases. Until approximately 100 years ago, the polio virus was endemic. Due to improved hygienic standards the virus was then no longer continuously present among Western populations. When the polio virus reappeared, large and dramatic epidemics occurred. Acute polio was a dominating health issue in Europe and North America in the 1940s and early 1950s.

The inactivated polio vaccine was introduced by Salk in 1955 and the attenuated, oral vaccine by Sabin in 1961. The epidemics diminished rapidly in the Western world immediately after introduction of vaccination programs.

A polio survivor is usually left with sequelae manifesting as stable muscle weakness. However, many years after the infection new pareses may appear. Post-polio syndrome (PPS) or post-polio muscular atrophy is used as a term for this condition. It may be difficult to distinguish new primary muscle weakness from a wide variety of physical and psychosocial problems experienced by former polio patients. Gradual or abrupt onset of new neurogenic weakness should be regarded as the hallmark for PPS.

Epidemiology

In 2006, acute polio was regarded as endemic in four countries (Afghanistan, India, Nigeria, Pakistan) and there were case reports from another 13 countries accounting for 1988 new cases all together. When the World Health Organization (WHO) global polio eradication initiative was launched in 1988, the polio virus was endemic in more than 125 countries worldwide, and the estimated yearly number of acute polio cases was around 400 000,

the great majority being children. America was declared polio-free by WHO in 1994, the Western Pacific in 2000, and Europe in 2002. The vaccination program is regarded as the largest public health initiative ever.

During the epidemics in Western countries the number of new patients each year could be very high. In Norway, the number varied between 1 and 60 per 100 000 total population per year (Figure 56.1). Two-thirds were younger than 10 years old. In the United States, 640 000 people were estimated to have a history of polio in 1987, in the Netherlands 13 000 in 1999, and in Norway at least 5000 in 2008.

The prevalence and incidence of PPS depend on the definition. Most reports consist of selected hospital cases. The frequency of the key complaint, "new weakness," usually ranges from 20% to 60% of all patients with polio paresis. If adding the more distinct criterion of "new neurogenic weakness," or even "new muscular atrophy," 10–40% of patients fulfill the criteria for PPS. Even patients with non-paralytic acute polio can develop polio-related motor weakness after many years, it being found in 7% of such patients in a small cohort study. These frequencies combined with a large number of polio survivors makes the PPS by far the most prevalent motor neuron disease not only in Africa and Asia but also in Europe and America.

Pathophysiology

The polio virus is a single-stranded RNA enterovirus which multiplies in the lymphoid tissue along the gastrointestinal tract. Persistent viremia is required for entry into the central nervous system, leading to inflammation. The polio virus has a predilection for the spinal cord motor neurons. Mortality during the acute infection is partly due to the meningo-encephalitis, and partly due to muscle weakness with respiratory failure. Immediate recovery after the acute phase is due to disappearance of inflammation and recovery of motor neurons. Later improvement is due to motor unit enlargement with branching of surviving neurons, combined with adaptation and training.

International Neurology: A Clinical Approach. Edited by Robert P. Lisak, Daniel D. Truong, William M. Carroll, and Roongroj Bhidayasiri. © 2009 Blackwell Publishing, ISBN: 978-1-4051-5738-4.

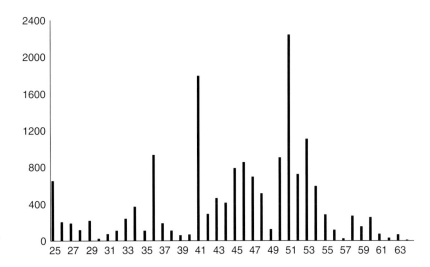

Figure 56.1 Total number of new polio cases per year in Norway, 1925–1964.

The new functional deterioration in PPS is focal and slowly progressive. There is an imbalance between degeneration and regeneration of enlarged motor units, and some motor neurons cannot maintain all nerve terminals. Muscle overuse may contribute.

Immunological and inflammatory signs have been reported in the cerebrospinal fluid and central nervous tissue of PPS patients. An increased level of cytokine expressing cells has been reported in the cerebrospinal fluid. The polio virus should be cleared by the immune system in the acute phase of the disease. However, polio virus genomic sequences have been reported in the cerebrospinal fluid decades after the acute infection.

Clinical features

Acute paralytic polio includes muscle weakness, muscle pain, meningitis, and sometimes meningo-encephalitis, and signs of general infection. Peripheral paresis, often asymmetric, more often in legs than in arms, is characteristic. Respiratory muscles can be affected. Improvement in muscle strength may occur for up to 2 years after the acute infection.

Several sets of criteria have been suggested for PPS. Those recently recommended by the European Federation of Neurological Societies are as follows:
1 A confirmed history of polio.
2 Partial or fairly complete neurological and functional recovery after the acute episode.
3 A period of at least 15 years with neurological and functional stability.
4 Two or more of the following health problems occurring after the stable period: extensive fatigue, muscle and/or joint pain, new muscle atrophy, functional loss, cold intolerance.
5 Gradual or abrupt onset of new neurogenic weakness.
6 No other medical cause.

The most common symptoms are new weakness, fatigue, and pain. Fatigue is probably the most disabling symptom, both muscular and general. New weakness occurs most frequently in muscles known to have been involved in the acute phase but can also involve muscles that were subclinically affected. New atrophy is required to fulfill the criteria for post-polio muscle atrophy. In a prospective study, muscle strength was found to be reduced by 1–2% per year in polio survivors, corresponding to the slow deterioration experienced by the patients.

Respiratory function is compromised in a minority of patients, usually in those with impaired ventilation in the acute phase. Respiratory complaints are common, as is subnormal ventilatory capacity. However, hypercapnia and sleep apnea due to previous polio are rare.

Degenerative joint disease, skeletal deformities, inactivity osteoporosis, and fractures are common in polio survivors. Radiculopathy, entrapment neuropathies, and myelopathy may occur. Such disorders will contribute to the functional disability and can be difficult to distinguish from a true PPS. Life-long morbidity and mortality is slightly increased in polio patients, especially in those with severe pareses.

Investigations

Exact information about the acute disease is helpful to confirm the polio diagnosis. Clinical neurophysiology is used to establish typical lower motor neuron involvement, to exclude non-polio causes, to find concomitant nerve or muscle disorders such as entrapment, and to assess the degree of motor neuron loss. Neurophysiological parameters cannot be used to define PPS. A thorough examination of respiratory function is often important. Muscle imaging may be helpful to detect abnormalities in subclinically affected muscles. In those with fatigue and loss of function, unrelated neurological and non-neurological disorders represent important differential diagnoses and need to be excluded. There is no specific test for the diagnosis of PPS.

Treatment/management

Two double-blind and placebo-controlled studies showed a positive effect of intravenous immunoglobulin on PPS. The effect was modest, more on pain than on muscular weakness and fatigue. The long-term effectiveness and cost-effectiveness is unknown.

Studies have shown no significant effect of acetylcholinesterase inhibitors, corticosteroids, or amantadine.

Patients with PPS benefit from a management program. This is probably more important for functions of daily living and social life than for muscle weakness. It has been claimed that muscle overuse and training may worsen the weakness in PPS, but this is unproven in prospective studies. On the contrary, patients with regular physical activity report fewer symptoms and a higher level of function than inactive patients. Significant improvement has been reported from muscular training programs. Both isokinetic and isometric training are safe and effective in PPS. Periods of rest between exercises are important.

Use and adaptation of assistive devices are important. Orthoses, walking sticks, and a wheelchair may facilitate daily life. Weight control is important. Lifestyle modifications regarding work, physical activity, and diet should be discussed.

Muscle weakness and chest deformities can lead to hypoventilation, especially during the night. Fatigue, somnolence, and morning headache are more indicative of hypoventilation than shortness of breath. Early introduction of non-invasive ventilatory support delays further decline.

Joint and soft-tissue abnormalities should be treated, if necessary, by orthopedic intervention. Non-steroid anti-inflammatory drugs may be helpful. Treatment by a multidisciplinary rehabilitation team is often advantageous.

Further reading

Farbu E, Gilhus NE, Barnes MP, *et al*. EFNS guideline on diagnosis and management of post-polio syndrome. *Eur J Neurol* 2006; 13: 795–801.

Farbu E, Rekand T, Vik-Mo E, Lygren H, Gilhus NE, Aarli JA. Post-polio syndrome patients treated with intravenous immunoglobulin. A double-blinded randomised controlled pilot study. *Eur J Neurol* 2007; 14: 60–5.

Gonzalez H, Sunnerhagen KS, Sjöberg I, Kapanides G, Olsson T, Borg K. Intravenous immunoglobulin for post-polio syndrome: a randomised controlled trial. *Lancet Neurol* 2006; 5: 493–500.

Grimby G, Stålberg E, Sandberg A, Sunnerhagen KS. An 8-year longitudinal study of muscle strength, muscle fiber size, and dynamic electromyogram in individuals with late polio. *Muscle Nerve* 1998; 21: 1428–37.

Chapter 57
Limb girdle muscular dystrophies

Ignacio M. Carrillo-Nunez[1], Anneke J. van der Kooi[2], and Marianne de Visser[2]
[1]Orange Coast Memorial Medical Center, Fountain Valley, USA
[2]Academic Medical Center, Amsterdam, The Netherlands

Introduction

The earliest cases of limb girdle weakness are ascribed to Leyden and Möbius in 1876 and 1879, respectively. They described adult patients with a pelvic and femoral distribution of weakness and atrophy with a benign course. In 1884, Erb reported a juvenile form characterized by shoulder-girdle weakness and atrophy, with sparing of other muscles of the body and a relatively benign course. In 1954, the nosological entity of limb girdle dystrophy was formally established by Walton and Nattrass who described the disease as manifesting with progressive muscle weakness and atrophy involving predominantly proximal muscles. In addition they reported a variable age of onset in the late first, second, third, fourth, or fifth decade of life; a slow clinical progression; and an autosomal recessive or autosomal dominant form of inheritance.

Development of sophisticated diagnostic tools of histology, histochemistry, electron microscopy, electrophysiology, and genetics has challenged the concept of limb girdle muscular dystrophy (LGMD) and revealed that within the entity as originally described, a variety of neuromuscular disorders (e.g., spinal muscular atrophy, polymyositis, endocrine disorders, metabolic conditions, congenital myopathies, myofibrillar myopathies) could be distinguished.

It was not until the 1990s that linkage studies and the identification of the group of proteins associated with dystrophin at the sarcolemma began to demonstrate the heterogeneity of LGMD. Initially, by using linkage analysis, autosomal-recessive cases were found to be linked to chromosome 15q, and in autosomal-dominant LGMD, an association to chromosome 5q was identified. Subsequently other LGMD phenotypes were mapped to other chromosomes. These findings led to a new nomenclature designating autosomal-dominant LGMD as LGMD1 and autosomal-recessive LGMD as LGMD2. As each distinct gene locus was identified, it received a unique letter – the first dominant LGMD linked to chromosome 5 was termed *LGMD1A*, the next *LGMD1B*, and so on (Table 57.1). In recessive LGMD the first gene locus was mapped to chromosome 15q and designated *LGMD2A*, the next 2B, and so on (Table 57.1).

Epidemiology

There are always some reservations in accepting figures about prevalence and incidence because until not long ago diagnostic criteria were too imprecise for reliable epidemiologyy. In 1985, a prevalence of at most 7×10^{-6} for adult onset cases was calculated in the Lothian region in Scotland. In 1991, a world survey of population frequencies of inherited neuromuscular disorders was undertaken. The prevalence and incidence rates for mainly adult onset cases of LGMD lie between 20×10^{-6} and 40×10^{-6}.

Autosomal recessive (Duchenne-like) LGMD appeared to be a rare disorder with a prevalence of less than 5×10^{-6}. It is, however, more common in certain Arabic communities in North Africa, in Switzerland, in certain inbred communities in North America, and in Brazil. In the Netherlands a prevalence rate of 8.1×10^{-6} was calculated for all cases and 5.7×10^{-6} for autosomal recessive and sporadic cases. *LGMD2A* seems to be the most frequent type of LGMD worldwide with a frequency of 12–33% (USA 12%, the Netherlands 21%, Italy 25%, and Brazil 33%). The reported frequency of *LGMD2B* varies; it is believed to be rare in the Netherlands and other Western countries, but is reported to be as high as 33% in Brazil and 18% in the USA, Italy, and Japan. The reported frequency of sarcoglycanopathies is 0–35%. *LGMD2I* was diagnosed in 8% of Dutch patients and 6.4% of Italian patients, whereas in the United Kingdom *LGMD2I* is considered a frequent cause of LGMD. *LGMD2G–J* are rare forms described in specific areas.

Pathophysiology

The muscle biopsy demonstrates a dystrophic pattern, which in itself is a rather non-specific pathologic

International Neurology: A Clinical Approach. Edited by Robert P. Lisak, Daniel D. Truong, William M. Carroll, and Roongroj Bhidayasiri.
© 2009 Blackwell Publishing, ISBN: 978-1-4051-5738-4.

Table 57.1 Classification of limb girdle muscular dystrophy.

Subtype	Gene product	Gene localization	Characteristic feature
Autosomal dominant			
1A	Myotilin	5q31	Dysarthria
1B	Lamin A/C	1q21	Cardiac abnormalities
1C	Caveolin-3	3p25	Childhood onset, rippling
1D		7q	
1E		6q23	Cardiomyopathy
1F		7q32	
1G		4q21	Limited flexion of fingers and toes
Autosomal recessive			
2A	Calpain-3	15q15	Scapular winging
2B	Dysferlin	2p12	Little shoulder girdle involvement, calf involvement
2C	γ-Sarcoglycan	13q12	Scapular winging, calf hypertrophy
2D	α-Sarcoglycan	17q21	Scapular winging, calf hypertrophy
2E	β-Sarcoglycan	4q12	Scapular winging, calf hypertrophy
2F	δ-Sarcoglycan	5q33	Scapular winging, calf hypertrophy
2G	Telethonin	17q11-12	Including anterior distal weakness, rimmed vacuoles
2H	TRIM32	9q31-q33	Slowly progressive
2I	FKRP	19q13.3	Calf hypertrophy, dilated cardiomyopathy
2J	Titin	2q31	
2K	POMT1	9q34	
2L		11p13	
2M	Fukutin	9q31	
2N	POMT2	19q13	

Table 57.1 Classification of limb girdle muscular dystrophy.

reaction of muscle. Various groups of LGMD-associated proteins can be described based on association with the sarcolemma, the so-called dystrophin–glycoprotein complex (LGMD 2C–F). Most of the mutations in the genes encoding these proteins destabilize the whole complex at the membrane, resulting in an inability to counteract the mechanical stress generated by contractile activity. Other proteins have a role within the contractile apparatus of muscle, for example, titin (LGMD2J) and myotilin (LGMD1A). Myotilin plays an indispensable role in the stabilization and anchorage of thin filaments, hence participating in the organization of the Z-disc. Another protein implicated in LGMD includes calpain-3 (LGMD2A), a muscle-specific calcium-dependent protease which is localized in the sarcomere and the nucleus and potentially involved in the regulation of sarcomere plasticity. Proteins involved in glycosylation may give rise to several LGMD types, that is, fukutin-related protein (LGMD2I) and rarely POMT1 (LGMD2K) and fukutin (LGMD2M). In LGMD2B dysferlin is located at the plasma membrane and may be involved in membrane fusion or repair. Caveolin-3, the causative gene of LGMD1C, is a transmembrane protein implicated in signal transduction. In LGMD1B there is involvement of a protein of the inner nuclear membrane, lamin A/C, which provides a framework for the nuclear envelope and may interact with chromatin. Its deficiency is therefore associated not only with LGMD1B but also with considerable phenotypic variability. Clinical heterogeneity is also present in LGMD1A, 1C, and 2B.

Clinical features

LGMD is a heterogeneous group of disorders characterized by progressive, usually rather symmetric, weakness and atrophy of the proximal limb muscles. Involvement of the distal muscles may also occur in due course. Symptoms commonly begin during the first two decades of life (predominantly in childhood in autosomal recessive LGMD) and the age of onset may vary both between and within subtypes and even between patients with the same mutation. Symptoms gradually worsen, resulting in loss of ambulation 10 or 20 years after onset. Some patients with sarcoglycanopathies and LGMD2I may be as severely affected as patients with Duchenne muscular dystrophy.

Some of the subtypes of LGMD show specific clinical features. Features such as muscle hypertrophy can be observed quite frequently in caveolinopathy (LGMD1C), sarcoglycanopathies (LGMD2C–F), and LGMD2I. The calf muscle is most commonly hypertrophic (Figure 57.1), but other limb muscles and the tongue may also be involved. Scapular winging is most characteristically seen in LGMD2A and 2C–F. Features such as spinal rigidity, scoliosis, limb contractures, and rippling should be asked about and looked for. Early contractures are not common in LGMD1B but may occur in a subtype of LGMD2A. Spinal rigidity is often a feature in LGMD1B, and occasionally in LGMD2A. Scoliosis is most often seen in LGMD2C–F, particularly when wheelchair dependency

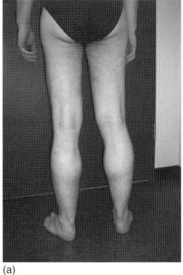

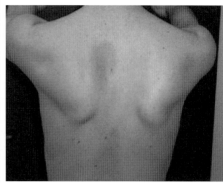

Figure 57.1 Patient with LGMD2I showing firm calves (a) and scapulae alatae (b).   (a)   (b)

occurs. Rippling muscles can be seen in LGMD1C. Intellectual impairment and facial weakness are not characteristically seen. Macroglossia is seen in LGMD2C–F and in 2I on occasion. Myoglobinuria is not uncommon in LGMD2I.

Autosomal recessive LGMD (type 2) is more frequent than dominant forms (LGMD1), the latter representing only about 10–15% of cases (Table 57.1).

Cardiac involvement is common in LGMD1B, 2C–F, and 2I. In LGMD1B rhythm and conduction disturbances are predominantly found, whereas in the other forms dilated cardiomyopathy is part of the clinical spectrum. Respiratory muscle weakness is seen most often in 2C–F and 2I.

Prognosis for LGMD is not uniform and thus timely intervention through identification of potential complications such as imminent respiratory insufficiency or cardiac involvement may improve survival. Nearly 70% of patients are still ambulatory at age 40 years.

Investigations

Serum creatine kinase (SCK) activity is usually markedly elevated in LGMD2 forms and normal to moderately elevated in LGMD1 types.

Neurophysiological studies are of little value in the diagnosis of LGMD, since electromyography usually shows a myopathic pattern.

Muscle MRI, or CT can detect patterns of muscle involvement which may not be pathognomonic but can be of help in guiding the genetic analysis and may be useful in selecting a muscle for biopsy.

Muscle biopsy sections usually show a non-specific pattern, consisting of variation in the size of muscle fibers,

de- and regeneration, an increase in the number of fibers with internal nuclei, and an increase in endomysial connective tissue. In some LGMDs such as dysferlinopathy and calpainopathy, lymphocytic mononuclear inflammatory cells can be seen. Rimmed vacuoles are observed in LGMD1A and 2J. Immunohistochemical staining for sarcoglycans, caveolin, and -dystroglycan and immuno-biochemical analysis of calpain-3 and dysferlin in muscle tissue are useful to direct genetic analysis specifically to the underlying genetic defect.

Specific clinical characteristics (see Table 57.1) can sometimes help to differentiate among the LGMDs, but a definitive diagnosis is made only by molecular identification of the specific abnormal gene or protein product. At present a classifying diagnosis can be made in about half to three-quarters of patients and families.

Awareness of symptoms of respiratory insufficiency such as frequent chest infections, morning headache, and excessive daytime sleepiness is important. Forced vital capacity (FVC) measurements should be carried out in sitting and supine (involving the diaphragm) positions. If FVC is less than 60%, overnight pulse oximetry is recommended. Serial monitoring of cardiac function using electrocardiography, echocardiography, and Holter cardiography, is advised in patients at risk of developing cardiac involvement.

Differential diagnosis

As mentioned in the Introduction, a large number of disorders share the presenting phenotype of weakness in the limb girdle. "Red flags" to an alternative diagnosis include ptosis, external ophthalmoplegia, facial involvement, or mainly distal muscle weakness. Skin rash, sensory symptoms, or subacute onset and rapid progression also suggest another diagnosis.

Idiopathic inflammatory myopathies, chronic spinal muscular atrophy (SMA), and metabolic myopathies such as mitochondrial disorders, glycogen storage diseases, and disorders of lipid metabolism should be differentiated readily from LGMD by histological, enzyme-histochemical, and biochemical investigation of a muscle biopsy specimen. If SMA is in the differential diagnosis, survival motor neuron (*SMN*) gene screening can be performed. Dystrophinopathies such as Duchenne (DMD) and Becker (BMD) muscular dystrophies and carriership of these disorders are identified by dystrophin analysis and DNA-Xp21 screening. Facioscapulohumeral muscular dystrophy (FSHD) is inherited as an autosomal dominant trait and characteristically has early involvement of facial muscles, but there are patients in whom facial weakness is absent. It can be diagnosed by showing a deletion at the telomere of chromosome 4q. Congenital muscular dystrophy (CMD) differs from LGMD by the occurrence of hypotonia or generalized muscle weakness often associated with joint contractures. X-linked Emery–Dreifuss muscular dystrophy (EDMD) is characterized by a scapulohumeral-peroneal distribution of weakness. It can be diagnosed by the absence of emerin on immunohistochemical stain, and mutation analysis of the emerin (STA) gene.

Treatment/management

There is no proven treatment to cure or significantly delay the disease progression for any LGMD. Several experimental treatments have reached preclinical proof-of-principle tests in rodent models at the level of gene, cell, and pharmacological therapies, especially for the autosomal recessive forms of the disease. Creatine monohydrate has been shown to have a modest effect on muscle strength. Corticosteroids have been used empirically in some sarcoglycanopathy patients. Treatment of heart failure is undertaken on general principles with early use of angiotensin-converting enzyme inhibitors and beta-blockers. In laminopathies implantable defibrillators are used to prevent sudden cardiac death. Annual influenza vaccination and prompt treatment of respiratory infections are recommended. Nocturnal home ventilation can be instituted in the case of nocturnal respiratory insufficiency.

Genetic counseling is advised when patients have concern for themselves, relatives, or descendants. Delineation of the LGMD subtype permits appropriate genetic counseling.

A number of the principles of general care for patients with DMD also apply to LGMDs. Supportive treatment remains the standard presently. Prevention of contracture development and splinting orthoses are important in maximizing functional ability. This treatment is best provided by a multidisciplinary team approach, including a clinical neuromyologist, physical and occupational therapists, an orthopedist for management of contractures and scoliosis, a pulmonologist for respiratory complications that may cause nocturnal hypoventilation and eventually require ventilator assistance, a cardiologist for detecting and treating the associated cardiomyopathy, a social worker to help with employment opportunities, a psychologist to help the patient adjust to his/her environment, a geneticist for genetic counseling, and patient support groups.

The care of these patients can be complex and costly, requiring help from the family and community. Even animals can be care givers, such as assistance dogs that can learn to retrieve dropped items or carry light groceries.

Further reading

Laval SH, Bushby KMD. Limb-girdle muscular dystrophies – from genetics to molecular pathology. *Neuropath Appl Neurobiol* 2004; 30: 91–105.

Lo HP, Cooper ST, Evesson FJ, *et al*. Limb-girdle muscular dystrophy: diagnostic evaluation, frequency and clues to pathogenesis. *Neuromusc Disord* 2008; 18: 34–44.

Norwood F, de Visser M, Eymard B, Lochmüller H, Bushby K, and members of the EFNS Guideline Task Force. EFNS guideline on diagnosis and management of limb girdle muscular dystrophies. *Eur J Neurol* 2007; 14: 1305–12.

van Berlo JH, de Voogt WG, van der Kooi AJ, *et al*. Meta-analysis of clinical characteristics of 299 carriers of LMNA gene mutations: do lamin A/C mutations portend a high risk of sudden death? *J Mol Med* 2005; 83: 79–83.

van der Kooi AJ, Frankhuizen WS, Barth PG, *et al*. Limb-girdle muscular dystrophy in the Netherlands: gene defect identified in half the families. *Neurology* 2007; 68: 2125–8.

Chapter 58
Dystrophinopathies

S.M. Schade van Westrum[1] and Marianne de Visser[2]
[1]Martini Ziekenhuis, Groningen, The Netherlands
[2]Academic Medical Centre, Amsterdam, The Netherlands

Introduction

Isolated cases of what almost certainly represent Duchenne muscular dystrophy (DMD), that is, boys showing progressive muscle weakness in combination with hypertrophy of the calves, were initially described in the first half of the nineteenth century. However, these cases lacked pathology reports. The first pathological examination of a patient with DMD was probably by Richard Partridge who described a case to the Pathological Society of London at a meeting on November 15, 1845. The clinical features of the same case and his siblings were described more extensively by Edward Meryon a few years later who ascribed the progressive weakness to "granular degeneration of the voluntary muscles." Despite the fact that the French neurologist Duchenne de Boulogne was aware of Meryon's cases the disease was named after him.

In 1934, Kostakow described an X-linked recessive family with similar clinical aspects but with a much more benign course compared to DMD. One-third of the patients were still ambulant after 10–20 years, which is highly unusual in DMD. The German geneticist Becker describing another family with a similar clinical picture recognized the uniqueness of this benign familial X-linked disease.

For many years, Duchenne type and Becker type muscular dystrophy (DMD and BMD, respectively) were considered distinct genetic entities. However, Becker who strongly believed that the newly discovered muscular dystrophy was allelic to DMD was proven to be right when both disorders were shown to be caused by mutations in the same gene located in the Xp21 chromosomal region. The dystrophin gene is the largest gene described in human beings, spanning more than 2.5 million bp of genomic sequence. Ninety nine percent of the gene for dystrophin is made of introns, and the coding sequence is 86 exons (including seven promoters linked to unique first exons). The dystrophin gene encodes the protein dystrophin.

Epidemiology

Most studies on the incidence and prevalence of DMD have concerned Caucasian populations. The incidence of DMD ranges from 1 in 3500 to 1 in 4215 male live births, with a prevalence of 2–9.5/100000 males. One study observed that in the West Midlands region of Britain, DMD is twice as common as expected in Asiatic Indians and less common than expected in Pakistanis. In BMD the incidence ranges from 1 in 14000 to 1 in 31000. The prevalence of BMD is 2.5 per 100000 males.

Pathophysiology

With the identification of the dystrophin gene, genetic testing for DMD and BMD became available. Deletions can happen anywhere in the dystrophin gene and account for about 60–65% of the mutations in DMD and BMD. There are two hotspot regions for deletions: at the proximal 5' end of the gene (exons 2–19) and in the center of the gene (exons 45–52). The remaining cases are thought to be caused by a combination of small mutations (most commonly point mutations resulting in nonsense or frame-shift mutations), pure intronic deletions, or exonic insertion of repetitive sequences.

In DMD the protein dystrophin is absent (<5%), whereas in BMD the dystrophin function is altered in a variable way but nearly always present.

The genetic basis for this difference is explained by the reading frame hypothesis. In DMD the mutations are "out-of-frame," leading to an early stop of the transcription resulting in a protein that is not functional or only minimally so. The mutations in BMD are usually "in-frame," so transcription leads to an altered but still functional dystrophin. Usually the reading frame hypothesis leads the way to the correct diagnosis, but otherwise prediction of the clinical phenotype on the basis of the genotype should be done with great caution, since large

International Neurology: A Clinical Approach. Edited by Robert P. Lisak, Daniel D. Truong, William M. Carroll, and Roongroj Bhidayasiri.
© 2009 Blackwell Publishing, ISBN: 978-1-4051-5738-4.

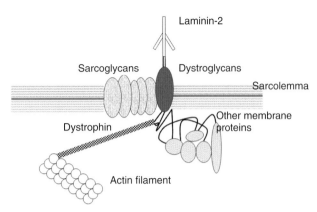

Figure 58.1 Simplified diagram of proteins of the dystrophin–glycoprotein complex and related proteins.

centrally located mutations might be nearly asymptomatic, whereas strategically located small (micro) deletions might lead to severe phenotypes. In about 10% there are exceptions to the reading frame hypothesis including patients with BMD who carry frame-shift deletions or duplications and patients with DMD with in-frame deletions or duplications.

The dystrophin protein is associated with the plasma membrane of cardiac and skeletal muscle (sarcolemma) and its main role at the sarcolemma is to interact with the membrane proteins that are assembled in the dystrophin–glycoprotein complex (DGC; Figure 58.1) including sarcoglycans, dystroglycans, syntrophin, and dystrobrevin complexes. Furthermore, dystrophin interacts with the sarcomeric network by binding to F-actin. Muscle fibers are protected from damage and necrosis following life-long contractions by the DGC. In addition to this mechanical function of stabilizing the sarcolemma there is cellular communication by acting as a transmembrane signaling complex. Although it is clear that the disrupted DCG leads to damaged myocytes it is still unknown why certain muscle groups are more prone to weakness than others and why the weakness becomes manifest after several years while the dystrophin is already altered in fetal muscle.

Clinical features

Duchenne muscular dystrophy
The criteria proposed by Duchenne in his description of "hypertrophic paraplegia of infancy" are still pivotal in the clinical diagnosis of DMD and include (1) weakness beginning in the proximal lower extremities, (2) lumbar lordosis and wide-based gait, (3) hypertrophy of some muscles, in particular the calves and deltoids, and (4) progressive course.

Starting to walk at a late age, peculiar running with toe-walking or waddling gait, and frequent falls with nevertheless firm or hypertrophic muscles are the first symptoms of DMD. With a relentlessly progressive course, boys lose their ability to climb stairs, rise from the ground, and walk short distances roughly between 7 and 11 years of age. Usually by the age of 12 they are confined to a wheelchair. The loss of ambulation increases the risk of contractures. In due course, progressive weakness leads to a kyphoscoliosis which contributes to a decrease in lung capacity which has been already deteriorating since the age of 8 due to weakness of the respiratory muscles.

Until the introduction of assisted ventilation most patients died between the ages of 15 and 20. Life span has been increased by 10 years since the introduction of ventilatory support (see below). With the increasing life expectancy the cause of death might shift from respiratory to cardiac dysfunction.

Cardiac involvement is present in ultimately all patients. Degeneration starts in mainly the posterolateral portion of the left ventricle and first leads to electrocardiographic (ECG) changes including an increased R-wave in V1 (>4 mm), increased R–S ratio in V1 or V2 in the absence of a complete or incomplete right bundle branch block, pathological Q waves (>0.2 mV) in lateral or inferior leads (II, III, AVF), and a complete or incomplete left bundle branch block or complete right bundle branch block. Subsequently, rhythm disturbances occur and finally a dilated cardiomyopathy develops.

The brain is involved in a proportion of DMD (30%) and BMD (10%) patients. In particular the verbal IQ seems to be impaired.

Although affected boys have normal visual acuity, abnormal electroretinography in patients with both DMD and BMD is found.

Becker muscular dystrophy
In patients with BMD the signs and symptoms are highly variable, with a wide range in age of onset (1–70 years), albeit generally the first symptoms are noticed between 6 and 18 years of age with a mean of 11 years. The nature of the first symptoms is usually comparable with those seen in DMD, even including delayed motor milestones. Other symptoms include exertion-related myalgia or cramps in the calf muscles or rhabdomyolysis. Sometimes BMD is revealed during or after anesthesia complicated by rhabdomyolysis, malignant hyperthermia, succinylcholine-induced arrhythmias, or cardiac arrest.

Muscle weakness starts at the proximal muscles of the pelvic girdle, that is, the gluteal musculature, and gradually progresses to the proximal muscles of the legs, the dorsal muscles of the trunk, and proximal muscles of the arms. Muscle (pseudo) hypertrophy due to fat replacement is usually but not always present and may precede symptoms of weakness (Figure 58.2). Cardiac involvement which is similar to that in DMD is also frequent and might ultimately be present in all BMD patients.

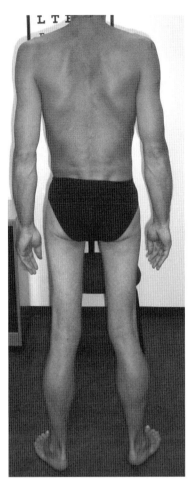

Figure 58.2 Scapular winging, atrophy of the thighs and calf hypertrophy in a patient with Becker muscular dystrophy.

Table 58.1 Differential diagnosis of limb girdle muscular dystrophy.

Autosomal recessive limb girdle muscular dystrophy
   Sarcoglycanopathies
   Dysferlinopathy
   LGMD2I (due to mutations in the fukutin-related protein)
   Merosinopathy (associated with leuoco-encephalopathy and epilesy)
   LGMD2K (due to POMT1 mutations, associated with mental retardation)
   LGMD2M (due to fukutin mutations)
Autosomal dominant limb girdle muscular dystrophy
   Caveolinopathy
Emery–Dreifuss muscular dystrophy
Congenital muscular dystrophy and congenital myopathies
Polymyositis and inclusion body myositis
Acid maltase deficiency and other glycogen storage disorders
Myofibrillar myopathies
Myotonic dystrophy type 2
Mitochondrial myopathies
Limb girdle myasthenia gravis
Hereditary spinal muscular atrophy

DMD/BMD carriers

Since DMD and BMD are X-linked diseases, related females can be carriers of a mutated dystrophin gene. Carriers may be symptomatic (manifesting carriers) due to skewed X-inactivation or, rarely, Turner syndrome patients with an XO karyogram, or with X-chromosome–autosome translocation. One fifth of the carriers experience symptoms ranging from muscle cramps or myalgia to frank – often asymmetric – weakness. A small proportion of DMD/ BMD carriers may have cardiac abnormalities ranging from ECG alterations to a dilated cardiomyopathy.

X-linked cardiomyopathy

Rare mutations cause an almost exclusive cardiac involvement usually associated with a high serum creatine kinase (CK) but no muscle weakness.

Investigations

CK is invariably elevated, usually more than ten-fold in DMD, especially in the early stages of the disease and diminishing over the years. In BMD CK is usually more than five times the upper limit of normal. A very high CK can be the only indication of BMD.

On electromyography (EMG) myopathic changes are found, that is, short duration and low amplitude motor unit potentials (MUPs). If the CK is markedly elevated, as in DMD, EMG is unnecessary. In BMD, EMG may sometimes yield non-specific findings, that is, polyphasic MUPs, sometimes erroneously leading to the diagnosis of autosomal recessive spinal muscular atrophy (Kugelberg–Welander disease).

Needle or open muscle biopsy is usually performed in the diagnostic work-up. When the pre-test likelihood of the diagnosis of DMD or BMD is very high, for example, when a case of dystrophinopathy is present in the family, one can choose to confirm the diagnosis with genetic testing. However, muscle biopsy can be of help if there is a differential diagnosis (Table 58.1) in a sporadic patient with progressive limb girdle muscle weakness (associated with hypertrophic calves) and a moderately to markedly elevated CK. Morphological changes usually include an increased variation in fiber size, fiber necrosis, phagocytosis, signs of regeneration, and endomysial fibrosis. Rarely in BMD, clumps of atrophic muscle fibers are noted which may erroneously lead to a diagnosis of spinal muscular atrophy. Most informative is immunocytochemical staining of the muscle biopsy. In DMD the sarcolemmal dystrophin staining is uniformly severely diminished to completely absent. However, in a high proportion of DMD patients less than 1% of the fibers stain intensely with dystrophin, indicating revertant fibers in which a secondary somatic mutation has taken place. In BMD the amount of dystrophin staining is variable as are the clinical findings.

In suspected cases of BMD immunocytochemical staining for other sarcolemmal proteins including sarcoglycans, caveolin, and α-dystroglycan, or immunobiochemical analysis of dysferlin and calpain proteins are equally important, as the limb girdle muscle dystrophies might be very similar in clinical presentation especially in adolescence and early adulthood. Subsequently, DNA analysis should be performed guided by the results of protein analysis.

Treatment/management

By inducing specific exon skipping during messenger RNA splicing, antisense compounds given by intramuscular administration have been claimed to correct the open reading frame of the *DMD* gene and thus to restore dystrophin expression in patients with DMD. However, this finding warrants further studies.

Rehabilitation with the aim to contain optimal mobility is of paramount importance. Special attention should be given to the prevention of contractures when ambulation is ultimately lost. When contractures are present surgery can release the contractures, but it does not improve function. Scoliosis is often corrected in order to improve wheelchair comfort. Respiratory function improvement by spinal surgery has not been proven.

A systematic review addressing the use of corticosteroids in DMD based on randomized controlled trials (RCT) of prednisolone or deflazacort in DMD revealed that 0.75 mg prednisolone/kg/day showed improvement of muscle strength and function for 6 months to 2 years. The adverse effects of corticosteroid therapy have been of concern since the daily regime showed significantly more short-term adverse effects. However, as compared to placebo treatment they were usually not severe. There are no sufficient data on long-term side effects. Because of these adverse effects, pulsed or alternate regimes have been tried. In a small RCT a functional effect of a regimen of 10 days on and 20 days off 0.75 mg prednisolone/kg for 6 months was found. Notwithstanding, the adverse effects of cushingoid appearance, irritability, and hyperactivity were twice as common in the prednisolone group as in placebo. Although the use and the dosage are still under discussion, there is general consensus that after education prednisolone therapy should not be withheld from boys with DMD. In BMD no such studies have been performed.

In DMD the decrease in respiratory function determines the life expectancy. Since the introduction of non-invasive positive pressure ventilation (NIPPV) life expectancy has increased from around 19 to 26 years. Symptoms include excessive daytime somnolence, insomnia, nightmares, snoring, and early morning headache. Repeated pulmonary function tests should be done to time the initiation of NIPPV. NIPPV is usually indicated when nocturnal saturation falls below 80% for 5 minutes or more. When the saturation is lower than 92% during daytime, NIPPV should also be given during the day.

Ultimately all boys with DMD, a large proportion of BMD patients, and some female carriers develop a dilated cardiomyopathy, eventually leading to heart failure. To assess cardiac function it is advocated to monitor the cardiac function by ECG and echocardiography. This should be carried out every 2 years in DMD patients younger than 10 years and annually thereafter. In BMD patients and female carriers every 5 years seems appropriate provided cardiac function is not compromised. When the left ventricle is dilated patients or carriers should be initially treated with an angiotensin converting enzyme (ACE) inhibitor, which is said to delay further progression significantly. When progression is shown β-blockers are indicated.

Further reading

Brooke HM, Fenichel GM, Griggs RC, *et al*. Duchenne muscular dystrophy: patterns of clinical progression and effects of supportive therapy. *Neurology* 1989; 39: 475–81.

Eagle M, Baudouin SV, Chandler C, *et al*. Survival in Duchenne muscular dystrophy: improvements in life expectancy since 1967 and the impact of home nocturnal ventilation. *Neuromusc Dis* 2002; 12: 926–9.

Hoogerwaard EM, Bakker E, Ippel PF, *et al*. Signs and symptoms of Duchenne muscular dystrophy and Becker muscular dystrophy among carriers in the Netherlands: a cohort study. *Lancet* 1999; 353: 2116–9.

Manzur AY, Kunter T, Pike M, Swan A. Glucocorticoid corticosteroids for Duchenne muscular dystrophy. *Cochrane Database Syst Rev* 2004; 2: CD003725.

Muntoni F, Torelli S, Ferlini A. Dystrophin and mutations: one gene, several proteins, multiple phenotypes. *Lancet Neurol* 2003; 2: 731–40.

Nigro G, Comi LI, Politano L, Brain RJ. The incidence and evolution of cardiomyopathy in Duchenne muscular dystrophy. *Internat J Cardiol* 1990; 26: 271–7.

Tyler KL. Origins and early descriptions of "Duchenne muscular dystrophy." *Muscle Nerve* 2003; 28: 402–22.

Chapter 59
Facioscapulohumeral muscular dystrophy

George W. Padberg
Radboud University Nijmegen Medical Centre, Nijmegen, The Netherlands

Introduction

Facioscapulohumeral muscular dystrophy (FSHD) is an autosomal dominant myopathy with a high mutation rate (approximately 10% of all gene carriers, up to 40% of mitotic origin) and causally related to a deletion of an integral number of 3.3 kb repeats at the D4Z4 locus on chromosome 4q35.

Epidemiology

FSHD has a prevalence of 1:21 000 in the Caucasian population. Although asymptomatic cases (±30% of all gene carriers) have been taken into consideration, this number might be on the conservative side.

Mean onset of the disease is in the second decade of life, with a large variation from childhood to late adulthood.

Clinical features

FSHD most likely manifests itself first with – often asymmetrical (50%) – facial weakness, which frequently goes unrecognised. Initial complaints are usually due to shoulder muscle weakness (80%), while those caused by ankle dorsiflexor (10%), pelvic girdle (5%), and facial (5%) muscle weakness are less commonly mentioned. On clinical examination almost invariably shoulder girdle weakness is present, which is often asymmetrical. A proportion of gene carriers do not progress beyond this. At age 60 approximately two-thirds of all gene carriers have developed ankle dorsiflexor weakness and 50% pelvic girdle weakness. After this age 20% of patients are wheelchair-dependent outdoors. Females tend to have a milder course.

Dysphagia and dysarthria are rare features; lingual hypoplasia and facial immobility have been reported in severe cases. Respiratory function is related to the severity of the disease, but less than 1% of patients require ventilatory support. Cardiac muscle involvement has been debated for a long time; conduction defects occur slightly more frequently than in the normal population. Muscle pain (50–80%) and fatigue (35–60%) are neglected symptoms in the older literature. Contractures are rare, with the exception of ankle contractures. Pectus excavatum occurs more frequently (5%) than expected.

Subclinical high tone hearing loss (75%) and retinal vasculopathy with teleangiectasis (60%) only rarely lead to deafness or visual loss, except in the infantile form (onset before age 10). The latter represents the more severe end of the clinical spectrum with often marked facial weakness and early wheelchair dependency. In Japan this form appears to be associated with mental retardation and epilepsy; recently other studies have suggested the preclinical presence of central nervous system (CNS) involvement in FSHD of adolescent onset.

Pathophysiology

Initially all attempts to demonstrate a transcript from the D4Z4 repeat failed. Attention shifted to a position effect hypothesis. One author found distance, and deletion-size related upregulation of three genes proximally in 4q35. Each repeat contains two homeodomains and an open reading frame. D4Z4 was found to be evolutionarily conserved. Its putative gene, DUX4, was found recently to be expressed in FSHD myoblasts and appears to act as a pro-apoptotic protein. These results need to be confirmed and the various lines of pathophysiological evidence reconciled.

Investigations

Routine investigations including serum creatine kinase activity, electromyography, and muscle biopsy are not diagnostic.

Reduction of the D4Z4 repeat of chromosome 4q35 to 10 or less units causes FSHD with onset and severity roughly related to the residual number of repeats.

International Neurology: A Clinical Approach. Edited by Robert P. Lisak, Daniel D. Truong, William M. Carroll, and Roongroj Bhidayasiri. © 2009 Blackwell Publishing, ISBN: 978-1-4051-5738-4.

A complete deletion of D4Z4 does not lead to FSHD. The 4q telomere comes in two allelic variants, but only a deletion in the A variant leads to disease. DNA diagnostics is hampered by an almost identical repeat on chromosome 10q26 and the occurrence (10%) of repeat exchanges between chromosomes 4 and 10. A triple DNA analysis leads to the diagnosis in the majority of cases. FSHD patients show hypomethylation of the D4Z4 repeat. A more severe hypomethylation is found in the occasional patient with a classical FSH phenotype and no D4Z4 deletion.

Treatment

No causally related therapies are available. Prednisone, albuterol, and creatine appeared not to be beneficial. Calcium-entry blockers, folic acid and a myostatin inhibitor have been tested negatively in pilot studies. Aerobic training was found to have a moderate effect. Uncertainty about the duration of the effects warrants additional studies. Results on myostatin inhibitors are pending.

Further reading

Lemmers RJLF, de Kievit P, van Geel M, *et al*. Complete allele information in the diagnosis of facioscapulohumeral muscular dystrophy by triple DNA analysis. *Ann Neurol* 2001; 50: 816–19.

van Overveld PG, Lemmers RJ, Sandkuijl LA, *et al*. Hypomethylation of D4Z4 in 4q-linked and non-4q-linked facioscapulohumeral muscular dystrophy. *Nat Genet* 2003; 35: 315–17.

Chapter 60
Scapuloperoneal syndrome

Georges Serratrice
Timone Hospital, Marseille, France

Introduction

Scapuloperoneal syndrome is defined by localized weakness and atrophy of shoulder girdle muscles (especially the trapezius, serratus anterior, pectoralis, and rhomboids) in combination with peroneal muscles (especially extensor digitorum longus, extensor hallucis longus, tibialis anterior, peroneus longus and brevis, and extensor digitorum brevis). This definition is sometimes too stringent for several reasons: weakness of adjacent muscles (e.g., humeral muscles in Emery–Dreifuss muscular dystrophy), loss of characteristic scapuloperoneal features as the disease progresses, or other neuromuscular diseases ("secondary cases") sometimes presenting with a scapuloperoneal distribution of weakness (e.g., acid maltase deficiency) (Table 60.1).

The nosology of cases reported under this heading remains uncertain. They were initially thought to be a variety of Charcot–Marie–Tooth disease. Others used the designation scapuloperoneal "myopathy" and classified it as a muscular dystrophy or as a variant of facioscapulohumeral dystrophy (FSHD). Several cases were considered variants of spinal muscular atrophy.

In most cases the nature of the pathologic change is unclear, albeit that in a number of disease entities the molecular genetic cause is unravelled.

Clinical features

If the "secondary" cases are excluded (Table 60.1), two main groups can be distinguished using clinical, electrophysiological, pathological, and genetic data:
1 Scapuloperoneal muscular dystrophy (including scapuloperoneal myopathy)
2 Scapuloperoneal neuropathy

International Neurology: A Clinical Approach. Edited by Robert P. Lisak, Daniel D. Truong, William M. Carroll, and Roongroj Bhidayasiri. © 2009 Blackwell Publishing, ISBN: 978-1-4051-5738-4.

Table 60.1 Neuromuscular diseases sometimes presenting with a scapuloperoneal distribution of muscle weakness.

- Myotonic dystrophy
- Calpainopathy (LGMD 2A)
- Desminopathy
- Acid maltase deficiency
- Inclusion body myopathy associated with dementia and Paget's disease caused by mutations in the valosin-containing protein gene
- Adult-onset reducing body myopathy
- Phosphorylase deficiency
- Some distal myopathies
  - Nonaka type (rimmed vacuoles)
- Mitochondrial myopathy
- Congenital myopathies (centronuclear, myotubular)
- Polymyositis

Scapuloperoneal muscular dystrophy

There are two types of dominantly inherited scapuloperoneal muscular dystrophies (hyaline body myopathy) and also an autosomal recessive form (type 3). Type 1 is caused by mutations in the four-and-a-half-LIM protein 1 on chromosome Xq, no loci have been identified for type 2 and type 3 is localized on chromosome 3p22.

Onset ranges from the first to the fifth decade. In type 1, wasting and weakness usually start in the peroneal muscles, especially the anterior tibialis, but sometimes the shoulder girdle muscles are primarily affected. Asymmetric involvement of the peroneal musculature can lead to a misdiagnosis of peroneal nerve compression. Wasting of shoulder girdle muscles is characteristic with winging of scapulae. Humeral muscles are often spared, as are the deltoid muscles (Figure 60.1). In types 2 and 3 neck flexors may also be involved.

The extensor digitorum brevis may be hypertrophic. Ankle contractures do occur. Reflexes are present and there are no sensory disturbances.

Hearing loss and cardiac involvement may be present in a proportion of type 1 patients.

Serum CK activity is slightly to moderately elevated. Electromyography (EMG) shows a myopathic pattern. Histological changes are variable but share the presence of hyaline bodies mostly in type I fibers.

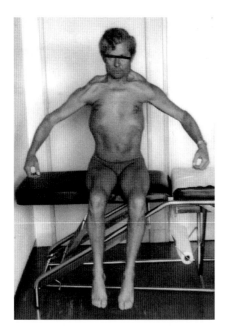

Figure 60.1 Scapuloperoneal myopathy. Normal aspect of the face, deltoids, upper arms, and forearms; winged scapulae, trapezius "hump," pectoralis atrophy, and bilateral peroneal atrophy.

The course is usually slow, with periods of stabilization, but may be more rapid in type 1 scapuloperoneal myopathy.

Another type of autosomal dominantly inherited hyaline body myopathy which can present with scapuloperoneal weakness is caused by mutations in the cardiac β heavy chain of the myosin gene (*MYH7*) on chromosome 14q11.2-q13 (myosin storage myopathy). This disorder is allelic to familial hypertrophic cardiomyopathy and Laing-type distal myopathy (see Chapter 64).

A small proportion of patients without facial involvement but otherwise "classical" features of facioscapuloperoneal muscular dystrophy show linkage to chromosome 4q35.

Emery–Dreifuss muscular dystrophy (see Chapter 63) initially shows rather a humeroperoneal distribution of muscle weakness associated with contractures and cardiac conduction disturbances. In due course there is scapular muscle involvement including winging of the scapulae.

Recently, in a family with an autosomal dominant scapuloperoneal syndrome described by Kaeser and considered to be neurogenic, mutations in the desmin gene were identified. Associated features included facial involvement, gynecomastia, dysphagia, and cardiomyopathy. Interestingly, a wide spectrum of findings ranging from near normal or non-specific pathology to typical myofibrillar changes with accumulation of desmin was found.

Scapuloperoneal neuropathy

Scapuloperoneal neuropathy, sometimes called Dawidenkow type, is a rare disease characterized by autosomal dominant inheritance, scapuloperoneal atrophy with glove and stocking sensory disturbances, pes cavus, areflexia, and slow nerve motor conduction velocities. In some patients chromosome 17p11.2 deletions were found rendering this entity a variant of hereditary neuropathy with liability to pressure palsies.

An equally rare autosomal dominantly inherited neurogenic scapuloperoneal syndrome with congenital absence of muscles and laryngeal palsy was mapped to chromosome 12q24.1-q24.31.

In conclusion, the clinician may easily be confused about the true nature of scapuloperoneal syndromes because in many patients EMG and pathology provide contradictory or non-specific data. In order to establish a precise diagnosis DNA analysis is required.

Treatment/management

There is no specific treatment. Referral to a rehabilitation physician in case of disabling weakness is useful. In diseases that can manifest with cardiac involvement close monitoring is needed.

Further reading

http://www.neuro.wustl.edu/neuromuscular/musdist/pe-eom. html#sp2.

Chapter 61
Myotonic dystrophy

Slobodan Apostolski and Vidosava Rakocevic-Stojanovic
School of Medicine, University of Belgrade, Belgrade, Serbia

Introduction

Myotonic dystrophy (DM, also known as dystrophia myotonica or Steinert's disease) is the most common form of muscular dystrophy in adults associated with myotonia and distinctive abnormalities of other organ systems. It is an inherited autosomal dominant disorder with genetic heterogeneity in which mutations in two unrelated genes cause similar disease phenotypes called DM1 and DM2, respectively. DM1 is characterized by variable penetrance and by an increase of disease severity in subsequent generations within a family (anticipation).

Epidemiology

The prevalence of DM1 is approximately 5 per 100 000 in most American and European populations. The highest prevalence was found in the Quebec province of Canada (189 per 100 000). The incidence of DM1 is approximately 1 per 8000 live births. DM1 is less common in Southeast Asia and rare in South and Central (sub-Saharan) Africans.

The majority of patients develop clinical symptoms and signs in early adult life.

Pathophysiology

Myotonic dystrophy type 1 (DM1) is caused by an aberrantly expanded CTG repeat in the 3'-untranslated region of the DM protein kinase (*DMPK*) gene on chromosome 19q13.3. Myotonic dystrophy type 2 (DM2) is caused by an expanded CCTG tetranucleotid repeat in the first intron of the zinc finger protein 9 (*ZNF9*) gene on chromosome 3q21.

The transcription of the expanded allele produces mutant RNA which contains unusually long tracts of CUG or CCUG repeats. The mutant RNA accumulates in nuclear foci, binds specific RNA binding proteins, muscleblind-like 1 (MBNL1) and CUG-binding protein 1 (CUG-BP1), and alters splicing of the insulin receptor, dystrophin, and muscle-specific chloride channel (ClC-1) transcripts. The loss of MBNL1 protein activity is a primary pathogenic event in the development of RNA missplicing and aberrant expression of embryonic isoforms with clinical presentation of myotonia, muscle wasting, and insulin resistance.

Clinical features

Myotonic dystrophy type 1 (DM1)
Patients with DM1 have a characteristic appearance with frontal baldness, eyelid ptosis, and wrinkled forehead, wasting of the masseter and temporal muscles, slender and malpositioned mandible, and thinness and slackness of other facial muscles with "inverted smile" (Figure 61.1).

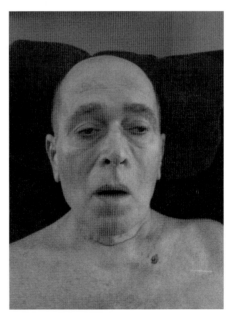

Figure 61.1 Myotonic dystrophy. The characteristic facial appearance with frontal baldness, ptosis, hollowing of the masseter and temporal muscles, and slackness of other facial muscles.

International Neurology: A Clinical Approach. Edited by Robert P. Lisak, Daniel D. Truong, William M. Carroll, and Roongroj Bhidayasiri. © 2009 Blackwell Publishing, ISBN: 978-1-4051-5738-4.

The atrophy and weakness of the sternomastoids and hyperlordosis of the neck ("swan neck") is almost invariably present. Nasal dysarthria, dysphagia, and weak and monotonous phonation are caused by weakness of the palatal, pharyngeal, and laryngeal muscles. The wasting and weakness of wrist extensors, finger extensors, and intrinsic hand muscles may be the earliest signs of the disease. In the lower extremities distal weakness and wasting involves mainly the anterior tibial and peroneal muscles, leading to foot drop. Disease progression is very slow, with gradual involvement of the proximal limb and truncal muscles. Walking disability may be very marked when a combination of weakness in knee extension and ankle dorsiflexion causes *genu recurvatum* ("back knee-ing"). The muscle stretch reflexes are lost or significantly reduced. The majority of patients are confined to a wheelchair within 25–30 years.

Myotonia expresses itself in the inability of muscle to relax after strong voluntary contraction ("action myotonia"). It commonly manifests as slowness in release of grip.

Spasm of the globe elevators can also be seen after forced eyelid closure with sudden lid release. Myotonia may also be seen as prolonged idiomuscular contraction following brief percussion ("percussion myotonia"). It can produce local depression in the thenar eminence by sustained contraction as well as dimpling of the tongue after percussion. Repeated contractions improve myotonia ("warm-up" phenomenon). Myotonia is increased by cold but is not as prominent a feature as in myotonia congenita. The myotonic phenomenon may not be elicited until after age 5. As the disease progresses, myotonia becomes difficult to detect because of muscle wasting. It may then only be demonstrated in the more proximal muscles.

The iridiscent posterior subcapsular cataracts (metachromatic or "Christmas tree") are found by slit-lamp examination in 90% of patients with DM1. At first dust-like, the cataract spreads slowly to involve other portions of the lens, interfering with vision. Cataract may be present even in completely asymptomatic adult patients. Slow saccades and decreased intraocular pressure may be additional ocular signs in DM1.

The heart is involved in the majority of patients with DM1 and approximately 90% of them show electrocardiographic (ECG) abnormalities. The most common are atrioventricular (AV) as well as intraventricular conduction defects. Sudden death caused by complete AV block is the worst cardiac complication in DM. The finding of QTc interval prolongation and late ventricular potentials correlates with the risk of malignant ventricular arrhythmia and sudden death. ECG changes do not correlate either with disease severity or with CTG repeat length. Cardiomyopathy and congestive heart failure occur far less frequently than conduction disturbances. The most prevalent echocardiographic changes are mitral valve prolapse and septal and myocardial fibrosis.

The prevalence of clinical diabetes mellitus is only slightly increased in DM despite the common findings of hyperinsulinemia, hyperglycemia, and insulin insensitivity. Testicular atrophy with hypotestosteronism, oligospermia, reduced libido or impotence, and sterility are frequent manifestations. Early male balding occurs commonly. Women may have a high rate of fetal loss and early menopause.

Diaphragmatic and intercostal muscle weakness may be the cause of impaired pulmonary vital capacity and impaired maximum expiratory pressure resulting in alveolar hypoventilation, chronic bronchitis, and bronchiectasis. Acute respiratory failure and pneumonia are the main causes of death in DM1. There is a greatly reduced life expectancy. In the adult phenotype the mean age of death is 55 years.

Gastrointestinal symptoms occur in as many as 80% of patients. Myotonia of the pharyngeal muscles may cause swallowing difficulties with a risk of aspiration. Dysphagia may be also caused by diminished esophageal motility and esophageal dilatation. Megacolon and fecal impaction are frequently seen due to a reduced colon activity.

Skull abnormalities include hyperostosis, enlargement of the paranasal sinuses, decrease in sella turcica size, and prognathism. Hypogammaglobulinemia caused by increased catabolism of IgG and IgM are immune system abnormalities in DM.

Central nervous system involvement includes a mild to moderate degree of mental retardation, dementia, paranoid personality changes, cerebral ventricular enlargement, and non-specific focal white matter lesions as well as diffuse gray matter atrophy. These symptoms lead slowly but progressively to intellectual and social deterioration. The large CTG expansion correlated with lower volumes of the cerebral frontal areas in adult patients with DM. Somnolence, a common problem, may be mistaken for narcolepsy and is associated with a disturbance of the night-time sleep pattern. Centrally mediated hypoventilation, a sleep-related breathing disorder, is characterized by an absence of the usual hyperpnea as a response to increased carbon dioxide concentration. This is associated with an abnormal sensitivity to barbiturates, morphine, and other drugs that depress the ventilatory drive.

Peripheral nerves may be also infrequently involved in DM and present as predominantly motor and axonal polyneuropathy.

Congenital myotonic dystrophy (CDM) occurs in 25% of offspring of mothers with DM1. The cause of CDM is the marked increase in the number of CTG repeats (more than 750) which occurs with maternal transmission.

It is characterized by profound hypotonia, facial diplegia, eyelid ptosis, a tented upper lip ("carp mouth"), jaw muscle weakness, but an absence of myotonia. Difficulties in sucking and swallowing and severe respiratory distress are common. Survivors may have delayed motor and speech development, mental retardation, arthrogryposis, and talipes.

Myotonic dystrophy type 2 (DM2)

DM2 is present in a large number of families of northern European ancestry. In Germany it has the same prevalence as DM1. In Europe, it has been called proximal myotonic myopathy (PROMM) or proximal myotonic dystrophy (PDM), while in the United States these patients have been described as having "DM with no CTG repeat expansion." The phenotype of DM2 resembles adult-onset DM1 with muscle weakness, myotonia, cataracts, diabetes, hypogonadism, hypogammaglobulinemia, and cardiac involvement. In comparison to DM1, the degree of muscle weakness and atrophy is typically mild until late in the course of the disease, affecting predominantly sternocleidomastoid muscles, elbow extensors, thumb and deep finger flexors, and hip girdle muscles. The patients have less symptomatic distal, facial, and bulbar weakness, and less pronounced clinical myotonia. Important differences also include the absence of a congenital form of DM2, an apparent lack of mental retardation in juvenile cases, and less evident central hypersomnia.

Investigations

Routine investigations of blood, urine, and cerebrospinal fluid (CSF) do not show significant abnormalities, except for a slightly raised serum creatine kinase (CK) activity in some adult cases, minimal γ-glutamyltransferase elevation, hypogammaglobulinemia, increased follicle-stimulating hormone in men with gonadal atrophy, and abnormal response to glucose loading in about 35% of patients. None of these tests is diagnostic.

Electromyogram (EMG) investigation reveals electrical myotonia, usually present in adult cases, random spontaneous activity at rest in some muscles, and myopathic, that is, low-amplitude, short-duration polyphasic motor unit potentials. Electric myotonia occurs during or after voluntary movement, after mechanical stimulation, or rarely spontaneously, and presents as bursts of repetitive potentials which wax and wane in both amplitude and frequency producing the sound of "dive bomber" or "motorcycle". DM2 has less elicitable waning-type electrical myotonia. Single-fiber EMG shows increased fiber density. Motor conduction velocities may be slightly slowed in patients with associated neuropathy.

Muscle biopsy may show large numbers of internal nuclei, increased variability in fiber size, ring fibers, and sarcoplasmic masses, as well as necrosis of muscle fibers and increased connective tissue. The rare eosinophilic cytoplasmic inclusions have been identified only in DM1.

DNA analysis is the definitive test for both types of DM. In DM1, an allele with expansion of the CTG trinucleotide repeat can be detected by polymerase chain reaction (PCR) and Southern blot analysis. The normal range for the DM1 allele is between 5 and 35 CTG repeats. Alleles ranging from 35 to 49 repeats are considered "premutation" alleles. In patients with 50–150 repeats the symptoms of the disease are mild, in those with 100–1000 repeats the disease is completely expressed, and congenital cases have usually more than 2000 repeats. The repeat length correlates with muscle strength, intelligence, and age of onset, but not with cardiac abnormalities, cataracts, diabetes, or hypogonadism. The size of CTG repeat expansion in DM1 usually increases upon intergeneration transmission, much more with maternal transmission. In contrast, the CCTG repeats in DM2 tend to be shorter in offspring after both maternal and paternal transmission. Prenatal diagnosis (chorionic villus sampling in the seventh to eighth week of pregnancy, or amniocentesis in the fourteenth to sixteenth week post conception) and genetic counseling are of great importance.

Treatment

There is no effective therapy for the progressive muscle weakness of myotonic dystrophy. The symptomatic therapy includes regular physiotherapy and lightweight orthoses which stabilize the ankle and knee joints. Cataract surgery is frequently required. Careful cardiac control for conduction disturbances is essential. Pacemaker insertion is strongly recommended for patients with advanced conduction system abnormalities as are home respirators for patients with respiratory insufficiency. Patients should be encouraged to lose weight. Hypersomnia may be treated with methylphenidate or modafinil and depression by imipramine or amitryptiline. Treatment of myotonia is indicated only if disability results from this symptom. Diphenylhydantoin has no side effects on cardiac conduction and is preferred over the anti-arrhythmic drugs (quinine, procainamide, mexiletine).

Further reading

Day JW, Ranum LPW. Myotonic dystrophies. In: Katirji B, Kaminski HJ, Preston DC, Ruff RL, Shapiro BE, editors. *Neuromuscular Disorders in Clinical Practice*. Boston: Butterworth Heinemann; 2002, pp. 1074–91.

Day JW, Ricker K, Jacobsen JF, *et al*. Myotonic dystrophy type 2. Molecular, diagnostic and clinical spectrum. *Neurology* 2003; 60: 657–64.

Harper PS, Rüdel R. Myotonic dystrophy. In: Engel AG, Franzini-Armstrong C, editors. *Basic and Clinical Myology*. New York: McGraw-Hill; 1994, pp. 1192–219.

International Myotonic Dystrophy Consortium (IDMC). New nomenclature and DNA testing guidelines for myotonic dystrophy type 1 (DM1). *Neurology* 2000; 54: 1218–21.

Lin X, Miller JW, Mankodi A, *et al*. Failure of MBNL1-dependent postnatal splicing transitions in myotonic dystrophy. *Hum Mol Genet* 2006; 15: 2087–97.

Chapter 62
Oculopharyngeal muscular dystrophy

Luis A. Chui[1,2] and Tahseen Mozaffar[1]
[1]University of California, Irvine, USA
[2]VA Long Beach Health Care System, Long Beach, California, USA

Introduction

Oculopharyngeal muscular dystrophy (OPMD) is a genetically determined adult-onset muscle disease that is associated with progressive weakness of the eyelid and extraocular muscles, manifesting as ptosis and ophthalmoplegia, and of the bulbar muscles, resulting in dysarthria and dysphagia. Inheritance is autosomal dominant, although rare recessive inheritance has been reported. It has unique myopathological features caused by short (GCG)n repeat expansions in the poly(A) binding protein nuclear 1 (*PABPN1*) gene. Even though a rare condition, the prevalence is disproportionately frequent in certain ethnic populations.

History

OPMD was originally included under the rubric of ocular myopathies; these disorders include ocular myopathies associated with mitochondrial DNA deletions, such as Kearns–Sayre syndrome (KSS). Even though the first reported case of progressive external ophthalmoparesis was described in 1868, it has been difficult in the literature to differentiate between different ocular myopathies. The first recognized case report of OPMD was from a French-Canadian family, described in 1915. This family had four members of the family affected by "progressive vagus-glossopharyngeal paralysis with ptosis," manifesting with late-onset ptosis and progressive dysphagia, resulting in death from starvation. Victor and colleagues termed this condition "oculopharyngeal muscular dystrophy" and reported 10 cases in three generations of a Jewish-American family of Eastern European origin. Tomé and Fardeau were the first to describe distinct tubular filaments within the muscle fiber nuclei in French patients with OPMD; these changes have now been confirmed in patients with OPMD of different ethnic origins.

International Neurology: A Clinical Approach. Edited by Robert P. Lisak, Daniel D. Truong, William M. Carroll, and Roongroj Bhidayasiri. © 2009 Blackwell Publishing, ISBN: 978-1-4051-5738-4.

Epidemiology

In North America, French-Canadians seem to be the most affected community, with prevalence of OPMD estimated to be around 1:1000. It is also particularly common in the Bukhara Jews living in Israel (prevalence estimated to be 1:600). Cases of OPMD have now been reported in 29 countries of the world so far. Cases of OPMD, though uncommon even in large Eastern and Midwestern neuromuscular clinics, are frequently seen in Southwestern USA, predominantly among Hispanic populations, in New Mexico, Arizona, and southern California. A recent report identified 216 patients seen at two hospitals that serve the entire population of New Mexico. Another cohort was reported in 1998 in California; these subjects were found to have similar mutations in the *PABPN1* gene as in the New Mexico cohort.

The origin of the OPMD mutation in New Mexico and California is not known. These cases may be from a new mutation(s) with geographical isolation (founder effect) at a "hot spot" in the genome that has a predilection for limited expansion. This mutation also may have been introduced by Spanish colonists who explored this region in the 1500s or by French-Canadian fur trappers in the 1800s. Many New Mexico patients trace their ancestry to colonial Spanish families that settled in New Mexico in the sixteenth and seventeenth centuries.

Pathophysiology

Autosomal dominant OPMD maps to chromosome 14q11.1 and is caused by short (GCG)n expansions in the first exon of the poly(A) binding protein nuclear 1 (*PABPN1*) gene. At the protein level this OPMD mutation causes the lengthening of a predicted N-terminus poly-alanine domain. *PABPN1* is an abundant, mostly nuclear protein involved in the polyadenylation of all messenger RNAs. The mutation causes a *proteinopathy*, a theme common to other repeat expansion disorders, with a resulting protein that is insoluble and resistant to proteosomal degradation. Gradual accumulation of these insoluble proteins gives rise to the intranuclear inclusions typical of OPMD. The expansion mutation in OPMD interferes with normal cellular trafficking of the *PABPN1* and its role in polyadenylation, thus interfering with crucial cellular processes.

Clinical features

Most patients become symptomatic in late adulthood, often presenting after the age of 50 years. There are two cardinal symptoms: eyelid ptosis and dysphagia, both of which are slowly progressive. In most cases ptosis is the first symptom, but in some cases dysphagia may manifest first. In families alert to OPMD, these manifestations may be noticed earlier, often by the middle of the third decade, but are often not bothersome until the fifth or sixth decade. Ptosis is always bilateral and can be quite severe. This often results in a compensatory contraction of the frontalis muscles and retrocollis, a pose referred to as Hutchinson's posture. External ophthalmoparesis is not an early feature of the disease. External ophthalmoparesis occurs late, but complete ophthalmoparesis is rare and diplopia is uncommon. Vision is not affected, but visual fields may be restricted because of ptosis. Dysphagia is initially to solids and progresses, with eventual inability to swallow liquids. Dysphagia can be severe, leading to malnutrition. Palatal hypomobility, pooling of secretions in the tracheobronchial tree, decrease in gag reflex, and palatal and laryngeal weakness with dysphonia are seen, usually in the later stages of the disease. Obstructive sleep apnea may be encountered frequently in these patients. Facial weakness can be seen as well. Though distal limb muscle weakness is most characteristic in Japanese OPMD patients (in which there are usually no *PABPN1* mutations), most patients outside Japan have predominant proximal muscle weakness. Weakness occurs symmetrically in the presence of atrophy. Tendon reflexes are diminished. Cardiac or significant respiratory involvement (external intercostal or diaphragmatic muscle involvement) is not a feature. The disease has a progressive course, with death occurring due to starvation or aspiration pneumonia. Aggressive medical and nutritional management considerably improves life expectancy in these patients.

Investigations

Serum creatine kinase (CK) activity is generally within normal limits, although CK can be raised up to two or three times in some patients, especially early in the disease.

Electromyographic studies show a myopathic pattern. Sensory and motor conduction velocities are usually normal.

Cine or manometric studies of the pharyngeal and laryngeal muscles show weak pharyngeal contractions but are normal in the upper esophageal sphincter; sphincter relaxation, however, is late and incomplete.

High serum levels of IgA and IgG were reported in French-Canadian patients and other ethnic groups.

Histopathologic changes in the muscle fibers are common to other muscular dystrophies, including loss of muscle fibers, increase in the number of nuclei, abnormal variation in muscle fiber size, increased interstitial fibrosis, and infiltration with adipose tissue. Autophagic rimmed vacuoles within muscle fibers are often found but may well be absent. These vacuoles are more frequent in type 1 than type 2 muscle fibers and seen more easily in limb than extraocular muscles. Electronmicroscopy shows characteristic intranuclear tubular filaments with an 8.5 nm outer diameter and 3 nm inner diameter.

Treatment/management

No treatment has been shown to slow down or reverse the steady progression typical of OPMD. Palliative measures improve the ptosis and dysphagia. These include use of glasses with props, blepharoplasty, with resection of the levator palpebrae muscles, and cricopharyngeal myotomy. The role of chemodenervation of the cricopharyngeal muscles with botulinum toxin to improve dysphagia is being explored.

Further reading

Becher MW, Morrison L, Davis LE, *et al*. Oculopharyngeal muscular dystrophy in Hispanic New Mexicans. *JAMA* 2001; 286: 2437–40.

Brais B. PABPN1 dysfunction in oculopharyngeal muscular dystrophy. In: Karpati G, editor. *Structural and Molecular Basis of Skeletal Muscle Diseases*. Basel: ISN Neuropath; 2002, pp. 115–8.

Brais B, Bouchard JP, Xie YG, *et al*. Short GCG expansions in the PABP2 gene cause oculopharyngeal muscular dystrophy. *Nat Genet* 1998; 18: 164–7.

Grewal RP, Karkera JD, Grewal RK, Detera-Wadleigh SD. Mutation analysis of oculopharyngeal muscular dystrophy in Hispanic American families. *Arch Neurol* 1999; 56: 1378–81.

Tomé FM, Fardeau M. Nuclear inclusions in oculopharyngeal dystrophy. *Acta Neuropathol* 1980; 49: 85–7.

Victor M, Hayes R, Adams RD. Oculopharyngeal muscular dystrophy. A familial disease of late life characterized by dysphagia and progressive ptosis of the eyelids. *N Engl J Med* 1962; 267: 1267–72.

Chapter 63
Emery–Dreifuss muscular dystrophy

Ronnie Karayan and Tahseen Mozaffar
University of California, Irvine, USA

Introduction

In 1961, Dreifuss and Hogan reported an X-linked muscular dystrophy initially believed to be a mild form of Duchenne muscular dystrophy in a kindred in which affected males ranged from 11 to 55 years of age. However, Emery and Dreifuss identified phenotypic differences, leading to the description of a novel disease in 1966. The name Emery–Dreifuss muscular dystrophy (EDMD) was coined 13 years later. An autosomal dominant form has since been identified.

Pathophysiology

X-Linked EDMD is caused by a mutation in the *EMD* gene, encoding a protein named emerin. The autosomal dominant form arises from *LMNA* mutations, encoding lamins A and C. *LMNA* mutations are associated with muscular dystrophies such as EDMD and limb girdle muscular dystrophy 1B, as well as lipodystrophy syndromes at times with developmental abnormalities and premature aging. Recently, phenotype clustering in patients with *LMNA* mutations showed that EDMD phenotypes were almost exclusively associated with missense mutations, in-frame deletions in childhood onset forms, whereas patients with adult onset mainly showed cardiac disorders or myopathy with limb girdle distribution, often associated with frameshift mutations.

Emerin and lamins A/C are localized to the nuclear membrane in tissues including skeletal and cardiac muscle.

The pathophysiology of EDMD has yet to be precisely defined, but these proteins are known to have a key role in modulating chromatin arrangement (an important component in gene expression) and in stabilizing the nuclear membrane during muscle contraction. A role in regulation of apoptosis has also been proposed.

Clinical features

EDMD most often presents in early childhood, though age of onset may range from the first year of life to the third decade. Disease progression and severity display considerable intra- and interfamilial variation, although this muscular dystrophy is typically considered relatively benign. EDMD is characterized by a clinical triad of (1) early contractures, (2) slowly progressive muscle weakness and atrophy in a humeroperoneal distribution in the early stages, and (3) cardiac conduction disturbances.

Contractures often occur prior to the occurrence of weakness, typically affecting the Achilles' tendons, elbows, and posterior cervical muscles. Limitation of forward flexion of the thoracic and lumbar spine occurs later. Muscle weakness initially affects the proximal arm and distal leg muscles, later involving the muscles of the scapula and pelvic girdle.

A distinctive feature of EDMD cardiomyopathy is the presence of atrioventricular conduction defects (even complete heart block), usually occurring after the second decade of life. Various rhythm disturbances and dilated cardiomyopathy are other manifestations. Occasional sudden death without preceding cardiac symptoms may occur, also in asymptomatic female carriers, warranting preventive pacemaker implantation.

Investigations

Diagnostic evaluation will show normal or moderately elevated serum creatine kinase activities, up to 20 times the upper limit of normal. Electromyography (EMG) will typically reveal a myopathic pattern.

Immunodetection of emerin in various tissues including muscle shows absence in 95% of individuals with X-linked EDMD. Immunodetection of lamins A/C is not as useful, as these proteins are defective, but not absent,

International Neurology: A Clinical Approach. Edited by Robert P. Lisak, Daniel D. Truong, William M. Carroll, and Roongroj Bhidayasiri. © 2009 Blackwell Publishing, ISBN: 978-1-4051-5738-4.

in patients with autosomal dominant disease. Definitive diagnosis rests with genetic testing.

Management

No specific treatment exists aside from standard evaluation and treatments applicable to most muscular dystrophies. Evaluation by a cardiologist is essential for both the patient and for asymptomatic female carriers.

Further reading

Benedetti S, Menditto I, Degano M, *et al*. Phenotypic clustering of lamin A/C mutations in neuromuscular patients. *Neurology* 2007; 69: 1285–92.

Bione S, Maestrini E, Rivella S, *et al*. Identification of a novel X-linked gene responsible for Emery–Dreifuss muscular dystrophy. *Nat Genet* 1994; 8: 323–7.

Bonne G, Di Barletta MR, Varnous S, *et al*. Mutations in the gene encoding lamin A/C cause autosomal dominant Emery–Dreifuss muscular dystrophy. *Nat Genet* 1999; 21: 285–8.

Dreifuss FE, Hogan GR. Survival in X-chromosomal muscular dystrophy. *Neurology* 1961; 11: 734–7.

Emery AE, Dreifuss FE. Unusual type of benign X-linked muscular dystrophy. *J Neurol Neurosurg Psychiatry* 1966; 29: 338–42.

Funakoshi M, Tsuchiya Y, Arahata K. Emerin and cardiomyopathy in Emery–Dreifuss muscular dystrophy. *Neuromuscul Disord* 1999; 9: 108–14.

Chapter 64
Distal myopathies

Nigel G. Laing[1] and Phillipa J. Lamont[2]
[1]University of Western Australia, Nedlands, Australia
[2]Royal Perth Hospital, Perth, Australia

Introduction

The distal myopathies are rare disorders predominantly affecting the strength of the distal limbs. Bjarne Udd in 2007 reviewed superbly the clinical phenotypes, pathological basis, and genetics of all known distal myopathies. Only certain points will be raised for further discussion.

Epidemiology

Distal myopathies are genetic disorders, dominantly or recessively inherited, or the result of new mutations not present in either parent. The incidence of distal myopathies in large parts of the world remains unknown. For some distal myopathies, particularly those such as Laing myopathy with relatively high new mutation rates, it is probable that the incidence is relatively uniform worldwide. However, some distal myopathies exhibit founder effects and less uniform prevalence around the world. Founder mutations in genetic isolates have led to higher incidences of Udd and Welander distal myopathies in Sweden and Finland, Nonaka myopathy in Japan, and hereditary inclusion body myopathy (hIBM) (which is allelic to Nonaka myopathy) amongst individuals of Middle Eastern descent. Some distal myopathies have to date only been described in single families (Table 64.1). According to Udd, the commonest distal myopathy in the world is likely to be Miyoshi myopathy.

Pathophysiology

Distal myopathy pathophysiology is beginning to be understood for those entities where the mutated gene has been identified. It is a mystery that mutations in proteins expressed in every muscle fiber in the body can cause myopathies with their effects restricted to distal muscles.

International Neurology: A Clinical Approach. Edited by Robert P. Lisak, Daniel D. Truong, William M. Carroll, and Roongroj Bhidayasiri.
© 2009 Blackwell Publishing, ISBN: 978-1-4051-5738-4.

Dysferlin is involved in muscle membrane repair and it has been hypothesized that damage gradually builds in susceptible muscles. Laing distal myopathy is caused by missense mutations to proline or deletion of amino acids within a restricted region of the tail of the myosin molecule, which should disrupt the ability of the coiled coil tail to form. How that leads to the distal myopathy is unknown.

Clinical features

These are outlined in Table 64.1. The earliest site of weakness is a valuable clue to diagnosis. Welander distal myopathy preferentially affects the hands, whereas all other distal myopathies initially affect the legs. Most affect the anterior compartment of the lower leg, but Miyoshi affects the posterior compartment. A "hanging big toe" is seen in both Laing and Udd distal myopathies. However, even with mutations in the same gene, the clinical phenotype can vary remarkably; for example, dysferlin mutations may produce the standard initial posterior lower leg Miyoshi distal myopathy, a limb-girdle muscular dystrophy phenotype (LGMD2B), or a distal myopathy with an anterior tibial compartment phenotype (DMAT). Caveolinopathy (caused by *Caveolin-3* gene mutations) which is also pleiotropic can manifest with foot drop or with a limb-girdle syndrome and is often associated with rippling of the muscle. A clinically significant cardiomyopathy is seen in several entities, such as myofibrillar myopathies.

Investigations

The combination of clinical phenotype, creatine kinase (CK), MRI/CT, and histopathological findings is the key to suspecting which distal myopathy a patient has.

Electromyography (EMG) is necessary to exclude neuropathy since distal myopathies may resemble motor-predominant peripheral neuropathies or distal anterior horn cell disease. MRI or CT are becoming increasingly useful as the suggestive pattern of muscle involvement for each

Table 64.1 Distal myopathies.

Distal myopathy	OMIM	Gene and/or location	Age of onset	Preferentially affected muscles	Pathology
Dominant					
Laing* (MPD1)	160500	Slow skeletal/beta cardiac myosin heavy chain (MYH7); 14q12	1–25, may delay walking	Anterior tibial, finger flexors, sternocleidomastoid, medial gastrocnemius	Type 1 fibers may be preferentially affected. Few rimmed vacuoles
Markesbery–Griggs	609452	ZASP; 10q22-q23	40s–50s	Distal legs and hands	Myofibrillar myopathy
Udd (tibial muscular dystrophy)	600334	Titin (TTN); 2q24	>35	Tibialis anterior, long toe extensors	Rimmed vacuoles
Welander	604454	2p13	>40	Hand function – thumb and index finger extension	Rimmed vacuoles
Distal myopathy 3 (MPD3)	610099	8p22-q11 or 12q13-q22	30–45	Hands and feet	Rimmed vacuoles, eosinophilic inclusions
Distal myopathy with vocal cord and pharyngeal dysfunction[†] (MPD2)	606070	5q	35–57	Feet and ankles, finger extensors, frequently vocal cord and pharyngeal weakness	Rimmed vacuoles
Vacuolar neuromyopathy[†]	601846	19p13.3	Late teens to early 50s	Lower leg	Rimmed vacuoles, filamentous bodies
Distal myopathy with early respiratory failure[†]	607569	Unknown	32–75	Tibialis anterior, respiratory muscles	Eosinophilic inclusions, rimmed vacuoles
Juvenile–adult onset[†] (Williams myopathy)		Unknown	Teens to 50s	Posterior leg anterior upper limb	Non-specific myopathy
Recessive					
Miyoshi myopathy	254130	Dysferlin (DYS); 2p13	15–48	Calf muscles, hand muscles but not intrinsic hand muscles	Dystrophy
Nonaka myopathy (distal myopathy with rimmed vacuoles) (DMRV, IBM2)	605820	GNE; 9p12-p11		Anterior tibial muscles, quadriceps is spared	Rimmed vacuoles, tubulofilamentous inclusions
Nebulin early onset		2q22	2–15	Anterior tibial muscles	Scattered and grouped atrophic fibers

OMIM: Online Mendelian Inheritance in Man.

* High new mutation rate.

† Described only in single families to date.

mutated gene is recognized. MRI/CT can also be used to guide which muscle is suitable for biopsy.

Muscle biopsy in the distal myopathies may show non-specific myopathic features such as variable fiber diameters, increased internal nuclei, and connective tissue, but many have more specific features such as rimmed vacuoles or the pathological changes of myofibrillar myopathy. The pathological features in genetically proven cases may, however, be highly variable. Genetic analysis is the gold standard in determining which distal myopathy the patient has. In time the classification of the distal myopathies may move to a genetic classification. However, there is currently both known and unresolved genetic heterogeneity in the distal myopathies.

Facioscapulohumeral muscular dystrophy (FSH) should be excluded in any patient presenting with a distal myopathy since FSH is common and pleiomorphic, including distal phenotypes without facial involvement. Similarly myotonic dystrophy should be excluded.

Treatment/management

There are to date no treatments for the distal myopathies. However, symptomatic management, such as ankle orthoses, can be extremely beneficial to patients.

Conclusions

New information about distal myopathies is accumulating rapidly, with gene discovery ongoing. Other research is aimed at understanding the pathobiology of the distal myopathies where the genes are known, and developing effective treatments. Interestingly, the genetic basis of Welander distal myopathy, the first major distal myopathy described, still has not been found, though it affects hundreds of patients in Sweden.

Further reading

Mercuri E, Jungbluth H, Muntoni F. Muscle imaging in clinical practice: diagnostic value of muscle magnetic resonance imaging in inherited neuromuscular disorders. *Curr Opin Neurol* 2005; 18: 526–37.

Udd B. Molecular biology of distal muscular dystrophies – sarcomeric proteins on top. *Biochim Biophys Acta* 2007; 1772: 145–58.

Chapter 65
Acute bacterial meningitis

Sudesh Prabhakar
Post Graduate Institute of Medical Education and Research, Chandigarh, India

Introduction

Acute bacterial meningitis (ABM) is a fulminant purulent infection of the meninges, characterized by fever, headache, and meningismus. The associated inflammatory reaction of the central nervous system (CNS) may result in altered sensorium, seizures, and raised intracranial pressure (ICP). The causative organisms vary in developing as compared to developed countries, depending upon the use of vaccination against *Hemophilus influenzae*. Despite the availability of potent newer antibiotics, the mortality rate in ABM remains significantly high (6–32%) in developing countries.

Epidemiology

The etiological agent for ABM depends upon the age of patients, their immunological status, and the country in which they reside. The epidemiology of bacterial meningitis has changed significantly in recent years, with almost complete elimination of *H. influenzae* type b in developed countries, due to vaccination against *H. influenzae*. *Streptococcus pneumoniae* and *Neisseria meningitidis* are the most common causative organisms of community-acquired bacterial meningitis in adults and are responsible for 80% of cases of meningitis.

Etiology

Bacterial meningitis due to *S. pneumoniae* is usually associated with pneumonia and sinusitis. The predisposing factors include head injury with basal skull fractures, and cerebrospinal fluid (CSF) rhinorrhoea, complement deficiency, diabetes, thalassemia major, and multiple myeloma.

Neisseria meningitidis, a common organism seen in the nasopharynx, is responsible for almost 25% of cases of meningitis in all age groups. The risk of invasive disease is mainly dependent upon the immune status of the individual and the virulence of the organism. In some cases the colonization leads to asymptomatic carrier state. Deficiency of any of the components of complement makes the individual highly susceptible to meningococcal infection.

The relative incidence of meningitis caused by *H. influenzae*, *S. pneumoniae*, and *N. meningitidis* is less in South East Asia compared to Western areas. Gram-negative bacilli such as *Klebsiella pneumoniae* and *Pseudomonas aeruginosa* are increasingly being recognized as important sources of community-acquired bacterial meningitis (CABM) as well as nosocomial meningitis. Most Indian studies report *S. pneumoniae* as the most common etiological agent of CABM. However, the commonly held view of *H. influenzae* being rare in Asia has been challenged in a study published by the World Health Organization (WHO), and large-scale vaccination for *H. influenzae* type b has been recommended for Asian countries as well.

Coagulase negative staphylococci and *Staphylococcus aureus* are common pathogens causing CSF shunt infections. Meningitis associated with other neurosurgical procedures is usually due to Gram-negative bacilli and staphylococci. Patients with defective cell-mediated immunity secondary to hematological malignancies, organ transplantation, cancer, and HIV infection develop *Listeria monocytogenes* meningitis. Patients with defective humoral immunity, on the other hand, are unable to control the infection due to polysaccharide-encapsulated bacteria such as *S. pneumoniae* and *N. meningitidis*. *Listeria monocytogenes* has become an increasingly important cause of meningitis in neonates, pregnant women, and the elderly. Food-borne human listeria infection has been reported from contaminated milk, soft cheese, and so on.

Recurrent meningitis usually occurs in association with head trauma, fracture of the base of the skull, and CSF rhinorrhea. It may also occur with meningomyelocele, parameningeal focus of infection, and post splenectomy cases.

International Neurology: A Clinical Approach. Edited by Robert P. Lisak, Daniel D. Truong, William M. Carroll, and Roongroj Bhidayasiri. © 2009 Blackwell Publishing, ISBN: 978-1-4051-5738-4.

Pathophysiology

Both *S. pneumoniae* and *N. meningitidis*, the common bacteria-producing meningitis, colonize in the naso-pharynx. They are transported across epithelial cells into the blood stream. Blood-borne bacteria reach the intraventricular choroid plexus, directly infecting the epithelial cells and CSF. The organisms, especially *S. pneumoniae*, migrate in between the epithelial cells to reach the CSF, where they multiply due to lack of host immune defense. The inflammatory reaction produced by the bacteria is mainly responsible for the neurological manifestations of bacterial meningitis.

The invasion of bacteria in the subarachnoid space (SAS) produces inflammation and release of tumor necrosis factor (TNF) and interleukins 1, 2, 6, and 8, causing significant reduction of cerebral blood flow. Later there is increased permeability of the blood–brain barrier, causing vasogenic edema. Microvascular thrombosis, vasculitis, and neuronal apoptosis produce cytotoxic edema. The edema leads to increased ICP.

Pathology

The meninges over the cerebral convexities in bacterial meningitis are usually yellowish-green in color. The exudates spread to basal cisterns and the posterior surface of the spinal cord. The exudate is very thick and localized to basal cisterns in *H. influenzae* infection, whereas in pneumococcal infection, the exudates are thinner and more extensive over convexities (Figure 65.1). In acute

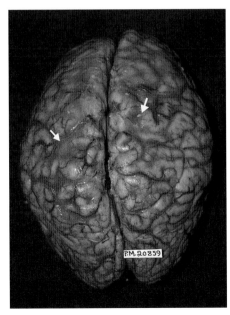

Figure 65.1 Gross photograph of brain showing exudates over the superolateral surface of bilateral cerebral hemispheres (arrows).

fulminant meningococcal meningitis, there may occasionally be no inflammatory exudate; however, there is significant interstitial edema. Microscopically, the exudates show neutrophils and bacteria in the early stage. In case of early treatment, these changes may vary. Within a week, the neutrophilic response may change to lymphocytic response. If the treatment is not adequate, it may produce a picture that mimics chronic meningitis such as tuberculous meningitis. The infection can also spread to veins leading to cortical venous thrombosis. As the exudates increase, the subarachnoid space is reduced and CSF flow may be compromised. Obstruction of foramina of Luschka and Magendie may result in communicating hydrocephalus.

Clinical presentation

The clinical presentation in a case of bacterial meningitis may be fulminant (overnight or within a few hours) or relatively subacute (over a few days). The presenting symptoms vary depending upon the age of the patient. Children usually present with fever, lethargy, altered sensorium, irritability, vomiting, respiratory symptoms, and headache whereas adults may have fever, headache, confusion, nausea, vomiting, photophobia, lethargy, or coma. Elderly persons may present with fever, progressing to confusion and coma. Nuchal rigidity, headache, and fever are seen in more than 90% of cases. Seizures as initial presentation or part of the illness may occur in 40% of cases. All adult patients, with the exception of the elderly and the majority of children, present with signs of meningeal irritation, that is, nuchal rigidity, Brudzinski's sign, and Kerning's signs. Presence of diffuse erythematous maculopapular rash suggests meningococcemia or enterovirus infection. In meningococcal meningitis, the rash becomes purpuric or petechial with the passage of time.

Diagnosis

ABM is an emergency. Once the diagnosis of ABM is suspected, blood culture is taken and empiric treatment started before CSF examination or CT scan reports are available. Antibiotics do not have major effects on cell count, Gram's stain, or polymerase chain reaction (PCR) examination.

Radiological investigations

CT scan prior to lumbar puncture is recommended in case of focal neurological deficit, new onset seizures, papilledema, unconsciousness, or immunocompromised state. MRI is preferred over CT scan as it delineates ischemia and edema in a better way. Contrast MRI shows evidence of meningeal enhancement, but it is not of specific diagnostic value.

Cerebrospinal fluid (CSF)

The CSF abnormalities characteristic of bacterial meningitis include an opening pressure of >180 mm of water, polymorphonuclear leucocytosis (>100 cells/µl), decreased glucose concentration (<40 mg/dl, CSF/serum glucose ratio of <0.4), and increased protein concentration (>45 mg/dl). CSF bacterial culture is positive in more than 80% of patients and Gram's stain in more than 60%. Latex agglutination (LA) test for detecting antigen of *N. meningitidis*, *S. pneumoniae*, *H. influenzae*, or *Streptococcus agalactiae* is very helpful in making a rapid diagnosis, especially in patients pretreated with antibiotics. PCR can detect a small number of viable and non-viable organisms in CSF and is a very helpful test in expert hands.

Differential diagnosis

Meningitis due to other causes

The differential diagnosis of a suspected case of ABM includes viral meningoencephalitis, particularly herpes simplex virus (HSV) encephalitis, fungal meningitis, tuberculous meningitis, carcinomatous/lymphomatous meningitis, meningitis associated with sarcoidosis, systemic lupus erthematosus (SLE), and lupus. The CSF findings, electroencephalogram (EEG) changes, and neuroimaging can distinguish ABM from HSV encephalitis. However, in 20–25% of patients with viral meningitis, CSF may show polymorphonuclear pleocytosis, which changes to lymphocytic reaction within 24 hours.

Fungal meningitis can present acutely in immunocompromised patients and CSF may show polymorphonuclear pleocytosis. The CSF should always be subjected to fungal smear and culture examination. Tubercular meningitis is usually a chronic infection with a history of a few weeks. Only occasionally in acute cases, initial polymorphonuclear leucocytosis may be there, which changes to lymphocytic response within a few days. Evidence of extracranial tuberculosis clinically or radiologically and CSF PCR examination are helpful in reaching diagnosis.

Subarachnoid hemorrhage (SAH)

SAH is a major differential diagnosis in an acute onset illness with headache, vomiting, and fever. Hemorrhagic CSF with leucocytosis clinches the diagnosis.

Subdural empyema

Subdural empyema and epidural abscess may mimic bacterial meningitis. The CSF shows normal sugar and mild mononuclear pleocytosis. Neuroimaging is diagnostic.

Table 65.1 Antibiotics used in empirical therapy for acute bacterial meningitis.

Indication	Antibiotics
Age of patient 3 months to 55 years	Ceftaxime or ceftriaxone + vancomycin
Age of patient less than 3 months to more than 55 years	Cefotaxime + ampicillin
All cases with chronic illness, organ transplant, pregnancy, malignancy, and immunosuppressive therapy	Ceftriaxone + vancomycin
Cases of hospital-acquired infections or meningitis following neurosurgical procedures	Ceftazidime + vancomycin + ampicillin

Treatment

Empirical antibiotic treatment

The treatment for ABM must start immediately after diagnosis is made. The emergence of penicillin- and cephalosporin-resistant *S. pneumoniae* has made these drugs useless for initial therapy. Ceftriaxone or cefotaxime provide good coverage for the *S. pneumoniae* group, group B streptococci, and *H. influenzae* and adequate coverage for *N. meningitidis*. Vancomycin is added in patients aged more than 3 months but less than 55 years, and those with hospital-acquired infections. Ampicillin should be added for coverage of *L. monocytogenes* in children less than 3 months and adults more than 55 years of age. In hospital-acquired meningitis, a combination of ceftazidime and vancomycin should be given to cover Gram-negative organisms and staphylococci. Ceftazidine is the only drug effective for CNS infections with *Pseudomonas aeruginosa* (Table 65.1).

Specific treatment

Penicillin G is the antibiotic of choice for susceptible strains of *N. meningitidis*. Hence, if the organism is sensitive or moderately sensitive, penicillin G should be substituted. A 7-day course of intravenous therapy is sufficient for a routine uncomplicated case of meningococcal meningitis. In resistant cases, the empirical treatment can be continued depending upon sensitivity. The same is the case for *S. pneumoniae*. Sensitivity should be tested for penicillin and cephalosporine. Usually CSF is sterile within 24–36 hours of therapy. Failure to sterilize suggests antibiotic resistance. The treatment should be continued for 10–14 days for meningitis due to *S. pneumoniae*, *H. influenzae*, and group B streptococci. Meningitis due to *L. microcytogenes* and enterobacteriaceae needs treatment for 3–4 weeks (Table 65.2).

Meropenem is the preferred drug for meningitis due to *P. aerugenosa*. Linezolid is a newer antibiotic with activity against *S. pneumoniae*, *S. aureus*, and *Enterococcus faecalis*.

Table 65.2 Antibiotic dose schedule in acute bacterial meningitis.

	Infants and children	Adults	Dosing interval
Penicillin G	0.3 mU/kg/day IV	24 mU/day	Every 4–6 hours
Ampicillin	300 mg/kg/day IV	12 g/day	Every 4 hours
Ceftriaxone	100 mg/kg/day IV	4 g/day	Every 12 hours
Cefotaxime	100–150 mg/kg/day IV	8–12 g/day	Every 4 hours
Nafcillin	200 mg/kg/day IV	9–12 g/day	Every 4 hours
Oxacillin	200 mg/kg/day IV	9–10 g/day	Every 4 hours
Cefepime	150 mg/kg/day IV	6 g/day	Every 8 hours
Meropenem	120 mg/kg/day IV	6 g/day	Every 8 hours
Vancomycin	60 mg/kg/day IV	2–3 g/day	Every 6 hours

However, some cases of resistance have been reported in *E. faecium* and *S. aureus*.

Role of steroids

Early use of dexamethasone has been shown to improve the outcome in adults with ABM. It reduces the unfavorable outcome as well as death. Treatment for a period of 4 days is sufficient and effective. Dexamethasone should be used in both pneumococcal and meningococcal meningitis at the initiation of therapy either before or along with the first dose. The mechanism of action is by inhibiting the synthesis of the inflammatory cytokines and by decreasing CSF outflow resistance.

Prevention

Hemophilus influenzae, type b conjugate vaccine has decreased the incidence of Hib meningitis in children in developed countries. Polyvalant vaccine containing a polysaccharide capsule of groups A, C, Y, and W135 is recommended for high-risk children over 2 years of age. Vaccinations are available against pneumococci and meningococci as well and are recommended in high-risk children. All those coming into intimate contact with patients with meningococcal meningitis should be given prophylactic rifampicin at a dosage of 10 mg/kg in children and 600 mg/day in adults for 2 days. In case of any contraindication for use of rifampicin, a single intramuscular injection of ceftriaxone may be given.

Prognosis

Bad prognostic signs in ABM include obtunded sensorium at admission, seizures within 24 hours of admission, signs of raised intracranial pressure, extremes of age, delay in start of treatment, and associated immune deficiency. Very low CSF sugar (40 mg%) and very high protein (>300 mg/dl) are observed in patients with poor outcome.

Third, sixth, seventh, and eighth cranial nerves may be involved in the course of ABM, but can recover. Deafness, however, may be permanent, especially in children.

Complications

The spread of infection can lead to focal cerebritis and subsequent abscess formation. Focal signs such as hemiparesis usually imply complications, for example, abscess, cerebritis, arteritis, or cerebral venous sinus thrombosis, and require urgent imaging. Subdural effusion and empyema are other important complications in *H. influenzae* and Gram-negative meningitis, particularly in children. These patients manifest with persistent fever, focal neurological deficit, and enlarging head circumference in the absence of hydrocephalus, and may require surgical management.

Hydrocephalus may be an important complication in ABM especially with *H. influenzae* infection because of thick basal exudates and may require drainage.

Further reading

Invasive Bacterial Infections Surveillance (IBIS) Group of the International Clinical Epidemiological Network. Are *H. influenzae* infections a significant problem in India? A prospective study and review. *Clin Infect Dis* 2002; 34: 949–57.

Mani R, Pradhan S, Nagarathna S, Wasiulla R, Chandermukhi A. Bacteriological profile of community acquired bacterial meningitis. A ten year retrospective study in a tertiary neuro care center in south India. *Indian J Med Microbiol* 2007; 25: 108–14.

Prasad K, Singh S, Gaekwad S, Sarkar C. Pyogenic infections of the central nervous system. In: Misra UK, Kalita K, Shakir RA, editors. *Tropical Neurology*. Texas: Landes Biosciences; 2003, pp. 50–74.

Roos KL. Acute bacterial meningitis. *Semin Neurol* 2000; 20: 293.

van de Beek D, de Gans J, Spanjaard L, Wersfert M, Reitsma JB, Vemeulen M. Clinical features and prognostic factors in adults with bacterial meningitis. *N Engl J Med* 2004; 351: 1849–59.

van de Beek D, de Gans J, Tunkel AR, Wijdicks EF. Community acquired bacterial meningitis in adults. *N Engl J Med* 2006; 354: 44–53.

Chapter 66
Brain abscess

Gagandeep Singh
Dayanand Medical College and Hospital, Ludhiana, India

Introduction

Brain abscess, a suppurative process involving the cerebral parenchyma, was recognized as early as 460 BC by Hippocrates. More recently, several pioneering neuro-surgeons, including Paul Broca, Victor Horsley, and William Macewen, optimized surgical approaches to brain abscess, which until the middle of the nineteenth century were the only options in the successful management of this condition. In the 1950s, the introduction of penicillin dramatically impacted its management and outcome. The next major advance was the introduction of computed tomography (CT), which led to early and straightforward diagnosis. Finally, recently, a shift in the microbiological spectrum of brain abscesses has been noted with increasing frequencies of fungal and tubercular etiologies owing to the emergence of acquired immune-deficiency syndrome and the widespread use of immunosuppressive drugs in cancer and transplant patients.

Brain abscesses are rare in developed countries; only about two to three cases may be seen among non-immunocompromised subjects in a year even in tertiary-care hospitals. In resource-poor countries, however, these may represent up to 8% of all intracranial space-occupying lesions.

Etio-pathogenesis

The brain abscess results from either contiguous spread from infected paranasal sinuses, middle ears, and mastoid bones or remote spread from dental abscesses, lungs, and infected heart valves or mechanical introduction by penetrating wounds and neurosurgical procedures. Over the years, a shift in the spectrum of the underlying conditions from otitic and sinus infections to abscesses resulting from trauma and neurosurgical procedures has been noted. The causative micro-organism(s) and hence

appropriate antibiotic treatment is largely determined by the underlying predisposing condition. *Streptococci* sp. and *Bacteroides fragilis* are the usual infecting organisms in abscesses arising from paranasal sinus, otitic, and dental infections and in patients with congenital cyanotic heart disease. When infection develops from the lungs, a mixed flora is usually encountered, but exotic organisms such as *Nocardia*, *Actinomycetes*, and *Mycobacterium* sp. may also be isolated. *Staphylococcus* sp. is the predominant organism isolated from abscesses complicating trauma and neurosurgical procedures. With stringent microbiological technique, pathogens can be isolated in up to 85% of cases; multiple pathogens are found in up to 20% of cases.

The location of the abscess is also determined by the source of infection: abscesses originating from sinus infections are frontal in location, otitic and mastoid infections seed in the temporal lobe or cerebellum, and hematogenous infections are distributed to various lobes in proportion to cerebral blood flow. From the pathogenic standpoint, a series of well-defined stages characterize the development of a parenchymal abscess: early cerebritis (days 1–5), late cerebritis (days 6–10), early capsule formation (days 11–15), and late capsule formation (more than 16 days). The pathological stages have bearing on the imaging diagnosis of the brain abscess. Throughout all stages, the abscess is hypointense on T1- and hyperintense on T2-weighted sequences and is surrounded by variable degrees of edema (Figure 66.1a). Ill-defined gadolinium enhancement characterizes the early cerebritis stage and transforms to irregular ring-like enhancement in the late cerebritis and smooth ring-like enhancement in the capsular stage (Figure 66.1b). In the capsular stage, the abscess wall forms a hypointense rim on T2 images (Figure 66.1a).

Clinical features

In keeping with the pathological evolution of brain abscess described above, the clinical course is often subacute. Symptoms comprise of fever, headache (due to increased intracranial tension), and focal neurological deficits. However, this symptom triad might be missing, with

International Neurology: A Clinical Approach. Edited by Robert P. Lisak, Daniel D. Truong, William M. Carroll, and Roongroj Bhidayasiri.
© 2009 Blackwell Publishing, ISBN: 978-1-4051-5738-4.

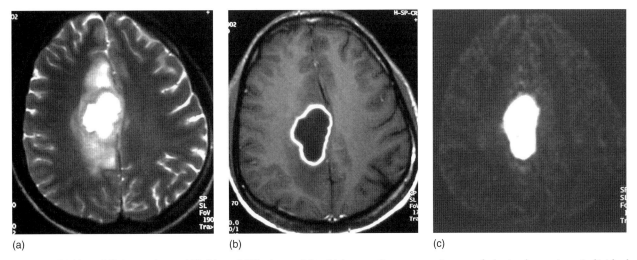

(a)   (b)   (c)

Figure 66.1 T2 (a), gadolinium-enhanced T1 (b), and diffusion-weighted (c) magnetic resonance images of a brain abscess in an individual with evidence of bronchiectasis.

headache and alternation in consciousness as the only presenting features. Other symptoms include seizures, malaise, photophobia, and neck stiffness. During bedside examination, attention should be directed towards detecting evidence of raised intracranial tension and the originating site of infection (e.g., lungs, heart, dental cavity).

Differential diagnosis

A common diagnostic dilemma is the differentiation of brain abscess from high grade glioma with a necrotic center. Diffusion weighted imaging (DWI) using echo planar spin echo sequences and *in vivo* proton magnetic resonance spectroscopy appear to hold promise in this differentiation. Pyogenic abscesses demonstrate hyperintensity on DWI (Figure 66.1c) as well as reduced apparent diffusion coefficients due to restricted water diffusion. Tumors do not exhibit these characteristics, though false positives can occur due to epidermoids, chordomas, and lymphomas.

Treatment and prognosis

The management of brain abscess depends upon the stage, location, number, and co-morbid factors (Table 66.1). During the early cerebritis stage, or in the presence of multiple abscesses without evidence of raised intracranial tension, medical management is indicated. When capsule formation and central necrosis ensues, surgical management, usually stereotactic aspiration of the abscess cavity, is the preferred initial management. A stereotactic approach is advantageous inasmuch as it allows histological distinction from neoplastic conditions, provides

Table 66.1 Treatment options in brain abscess.

Treatment options	Indications
Antibiotics alone	• Deep-seated (brainstem or basal ganglionic), small abscess • Single or multiple abscess(es), in which the microbial organism can be isolated from the primary site of infection (e.g., lungs) • Abscess in early cerebritis stage • Underlying immunocompromised state
Dexamethasone	• Transient use in event of raised intracranial tension • Profoundly altered sensorium
Anticonvulsants	• Usually administered except in deep-seated abscesses
Stereotactic aspiration	• To obtain material for microbial isolation • Biopsy to differentiate from tumors • Abscesses in eloquent areas
Open excision	• Abscesses that recur despite repeated aspiration • Multiloculated abscess(es) • Abscess associated with a sinus tract (usually complicating trauma)

material for microbiological identification and antibiotic sensitivity, and is considerably less damaging to neural tissue. Resort to open excision is undertaken in the case of an abscess that does not respond to multiple aspirations, multiloculated abscess(es), and the presence of a sinus tract that allows refilling of the abscess.

Antibiotic treatment is administered for several weeks irrespective of whether or not surgical treatment is undertaken. The choice of antibiotic regimen is dictated by the underlying predisposing condition and the suspected organism. Initial empirical treatment comprises of a third-generation cephalosporin (either cefotaxime, 6–9 g/day in divided doses, or ceftriaxone, 4 g/day in divided doses) and metronidazole (2 g/day in divided doses) but should also include either naficilin (12 g/day in divided doses) or vancomycin (2 g/day in divided doses) in the case of an abscess-complicating trauma and neurosurgical procedures.

Mortality due to brain abscess remains as high as 10–20% despite advances in diagnosis and treatment. In addition, long-term neurological sequelae such as epilepsy and persistent focal neurological deficits are encountered in as many as 60% of cases.

Further reading

Carpenter J, Stapleton S, Holliman R. Retrospective analysis of 49 cases of brain abscess and review of the literature. *Eur J Clin Microbiol Infect Dis* 2007; 26: 1–11.

Goodkin HP, Harper MB, Pomeroy SL. Intracerebral abscess in children: historical trends at Children's Hospital Boston. *Pediatrics* 2004; 113: 1765–70.

Habib AA, Mozaffar T. Brain abscess. *Arch Neurol* 2001; 58: 1302–4.

Reddy JS, Mishra AM, Behari S, *et al*. The role of diffusion-weighted imaging in the differential diagnosis of intracranial cystic mass lesions: a report of 147 lesions. *Surg Neurol* 2006; 66: 246–50.

Sharma BS, Gupta SK, Khosla VK. Current concepts in the management of pyogenic brain abscess. *Neurol India* 2000; 48: 105–11.

Chapter 67
Subdural empyema

Sandi Lam[1] and Tien T. Nguyen[2]
[1]University of California, Los Angeles, USA
[2]Fountain Valley Regional Hospital and Medical Center, Fountain Valley, USA

Introduction

Subdural empyema is a focal purulent infection between the dura and arachnoid mater, with few anatomic barriers to spread. More than 95% of subdural empyemas occur intracranially rather than in the spinal neuraxis. Subdural empyemas comprise 15–22% of focal intracranial infections, with historically high mortality prior to the widespread availability of antibiotics. Seventy to 80% of cases occur over the cerebral convexities, and also parafalcine, on the tentorium, and infratentorially.

Epidemiology/pathophysiology

The male:female ratio is 3:1. Most cases of subdural empyema occur as a result of direct extension of infection rather than by hematogenous spread. In contrast, most subdural empyemas in infants result from infection of subdural effusions from meningitis.

Local infection can spread into the intracranial compartment and subdural space from the frontal, sphenoid, or ethmoid sinuses from osteomyelitis or through retrograde thrombophlebitis of the valveless diploic veins. Most cases of complicated sinusitis occur in otherwise healthy men aged 20–40 suffering from chronic otitis media, mastoiditis, cranial traction devices, neurosurgical postoperative infections, compound skull fractures, or penetrating head trauma. Infections of pre-existing subdural fluid collections are also associated with subdural empyemas. Pulmonary or hematogenous etiologies are rare; tuberculous infections have also been reported.

International Neurology: A Clinical Approach. Edited by Robert P. Lisak, Daniel D. Truong, William M. Carroll, and Roongroj Bhidayasiri.
© 2009 Blackwell Publishing, ISBN: 978-1-4051-5738-4.

Clinical features

Patients present with neurologic symptoms due to mass effect, inflammation of the brain and meninges, and/or thrombophlebitis of cerebral venous drainage. Focal deficits or seizures develop with disease progression.

Common presenting features of subdural empyema include fever, headache, meningismus, altered mental status, hemiparesis, nausea/vomiting, sinus tenderness, local swelling/inflammation, seizures, speech difficulty, homonymous hemianopsia, and papilledema.

Cranial nerve palsies and visual changes are apparent on examination.

Investigations

While MRI is recognized to be more sensitive in showing morphologic detail, detecting intraparenchymal abnormalities, and delineating the extent of infection, CT is usually first carried out because of availability and the need for timely diagnosis. In cases associated with sinusitis, head CT may show sinus opacification, air-fluid levels, or bony erosion.

CT is most helpful when obtained with and without intravenous (IV) contrast, allowing differentiation from chronic subdural hematoma (SDH) or postoperative changes. CT findings (Figure 67.1) include a hypodense subdural lesion, enhancing especially along the medial border at the pial surface, inward displacement of the gray–white junction, and effacement of the ventricles, cortical sulci, and/or basal cisterns. Mass effect is often caused by edema rather than by the empyema itself. Edema is more prominent in cases of subdural empyema complicated by cortical venous thrombosis (with or without venous infarction), cerebritis, or associated cerebral abscess.

On MRI, subdural empyemas generally appear hypointense on T1-weighted images with rim enhancement following gadolinium administration, hyperintense on T2-weighted images, and with high signal on diffusion-weighted images (DWI).

Early in the disease course, imaging may be unrevealing. If the initial head CT is normal yet clinical suspicion

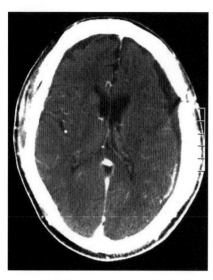

Figure 67.1 Head CT with contrast showing bilateral subdural empyemas in a patient who had previously undergone burr hole evacuation of bilateral subacute subdural hematomas.

Table 67.1 Common causative organisms in cases of subdural empyema.

Associated etiology	Common organisms
Paranasal sinusitis	Alpha-hemolytic streptococci Staphylococci Anaerobic/microaerophilic streptococci Aerobic Gram-negative bacilli *Bacteroides* species
Otitis media, mastoiditis	Alpha-hemolytic streptococci *Pseudomonas aeruginosa* *Bacteroides* species Staphylococci
Trauma or postsurgical infection	Staphylococci Aerobic Gram-negative bacilli
Meningitis (child)	*Streptococcus pneumoniae* *Hemophilus influenzae* *Neisseria meningitidis* *Escherichia coli*
Meningitis (neonate)	Group B streptococci Enterobacteriaceae *Listeria monocytogenes*

of subdural empyema persists, a repeat CT or MRI is warranted.

Laboratory studies

Complete blood count shows leukocytosis with predominance of polymorphonuclear neutrophils. Erythrocyte sedimentation rate and C-reactive protein are elevated, but generally less than 100 mm/h. Blood, urine, and sputum should be cultured to identify potential organisms. Additional preoperative workup should include screening for electrolyte abnormalities and metabolic dysfunction.

Lumbar puncture is not recommended given the potential risk of cerebral herniation. Cerebrospinal fluid (CSF) findings are typically non-specific, showing sterile pleocytosis with predominant polymorphonuclear neutrophils, elevated protein, and normal to low glucose levels. Gram stain and CSF cultures are negative in more than 85% of cases. Normal and sterile CSF samples do not rule out the diagnosis of subdural empyema.

Causative organisms vary with the source of primary infection (Table 67.1). Sterile intraoperative cultures are reported in up to half of cases, presumably as a result of preoperative administration of antibiotics.

Treatment/management

Broad spectrum antibiotic therapy should be started as soon as possible with coverage for aerobic and anaerobic organisms. Recommended empiric therapy for adult patients includes penicillin, a third-generation cephalosporin, and metronidazole. Antibiotics may be tailored according to Gram stain, culture, and sensitivity results. Duration of antibiotic therapy is recommended at 4–6 weeks, lengthened to 6–8 weeks with osteomyelitis. In subdural empyemas following neurosurgical procedures or trauma, penicillin should be substituted by vancomycin as part of the initial empiric antibiotics. For neonates and children, empiric antibiotic choices are the same as for meningitis treatment, which vary by local rates of microbial drug resistance. Anticonvulsants are administered prophylactically, and are necessary if seizure activity occurs.

Surgical management is indicated in almost all cases of subdural empyema. There is no consensus on the optimal surgical approach between burr hole drainage or craniotomy for debridement and drainage. The purulent material tends to be in a fluid state early in the disease process, and loculations develop over time. Repeat procedures may be required. Definitive surgical management of infected sinus disease should also be undertaken. A limited number of subdural empyema cases managed non-surgically have been reported, but this treatment strategy is not considered except in cases with very limited extension, no mass effect, no neurologic symptoms, and early favorable response to antibiotics.

Unfavorable prognostic indicators include age over 60 years, poor neurologic status at time of presentation, rapidity of disease progression, delay in starting antibiotics, and subdural empyema resulting from trauma or surgery. Mortality with treated cases of subdural empyema reaches 5–20%. Up to half of patients have neurologic deficits at the time of discharge from hospital, 15–35% with hemiparesis, and up to 30% with persistent seizures.

Further reading

Greenberg MS. *Handbook of Neurosurgery*, 5th ed. New York: Thieme; 2001.

Osborn MK, Steinberg JP. Subdural empyema and other suppurative complications of paranasal sinusitis. *Lancet Infect Dis* 2007; 7: 62–7.

Chapter 68
Epidural abscess

Sandi Lam[1] *and Tien T. Nguyen*[2]
[1]University of California, Los Angeles, USA
[2]Fountain Valley Regional Hospital and Medical Center, Fountain Valley, USA

Introduction

Epidural abscess develops between the skull and the dura mater. The adherence of the dura to the skull limits expansion of intracranial epidural abscesses; however, a parameningeal focus of infection involving the dural venous sinuses can cause a septic thrombophlebitis. Autopsy studies reveal evidence of associated subdural abscess formation in 80% of epidural abscesses.

Epidemiology/pathophysiology

Intracranial epidural abscesses arise from direct extension in association with sinusitis, cranial osteomyelitis, direct penetrating trauma, or postoperative infection.

In the spine, there is a relatively large space in the epidural compartment between the dura and the vertebral bodies, allowing extensive extension of spinal epidural abscesses. The pathophysiology of epidural abscess in the spine differs from that of intracranial epidural abscesses, and the etiology of these spinal infections can be hematogenous or from direct extension of a contiguous local infection. The focus of this chapter will be limited to intracranial epidural abscesses.

The incidence of intracranial epidural abscess is estimated to be at least nine times less than spinal epidural abscess. There is a male predominance, with the highest incidence in the second and third decades of life.

Clinical features

Patients with intracranial epidural abscess generally present with signs and symptoms of infection and an expanding intracranial mass lesion such as fever, headache, altered mental status, malaise, nausea, vomiting, focal neurologic deficits, seizures, sinus tenderness/local swelling, and evidence of wound infection in more than 90% of patients who had undergone craniotomy. The clinical presentation is generally described as more indolent when compared to subdural empyema, although cases may vary.

Investigations

Complete blood counts reveal leukocytosis with an elevated percentage of polymorphonuclear neutrophils and possibly band forms. Erythrocyte sedimentation rate is usually elevated, but represents a non-specific finding. Blood, urine, and sputum should be cultured to identify potential organisms and sources. Other tests should include electrolytes, blood urea nitrogen, creatinine, blood glucose, liver function tests, coagulation panel, chest X-ray, and electrocardiogram for pre-operative evaluation, for correction of electrolyte abnormalities, and to screen out underlying metabolic dysfunction while directing the choice of antibiotics for medical treatment.

Lumbar puncture is not recommended for intracranial epidural abscess since there is the potential risk of brain herniation due to increased intracranial pressure. It is known that cerebrospinal fluid (CSF) studies often show moderate pleocytosis with predominantly polymorphonuclear neutrophils, with moderately elevated protein, and normal to low glucose levels. Gram stain and CSF cultures are negative in more than 75% of cases. Normal and sterile CSF samples do not rule out the diagnosis of intracranial epidural abscess.

CT of the head is the most widely available and accessible imaging modality, and should be obtained with and without contrast (to help differentiate from chronic epidural hematoma and postoperative changes), and demonstrates a hypodense enhancing extra-axial lesion, often crescentic or lenticular in shape. MRI of the brain with and without gadolinium enhancement has higher sensitivity and may provide more detail in delineating the extent of infection. The signal of an intracranial epidural abscess on MRI is hyperintense on T2WI, variable on T1WI, and enhancing with gadolinium administration especially along the periphery of the lesion (Figure 68.1).

International Neurology: A Clinical Approach. Edited by Robert P. Lisak, Daniel D. Truong, William M. Carroll, and Roongroj Bhidayasiri. © 2009 Blackwell Publishing, ISBN: 978-1-4051-5738-4.

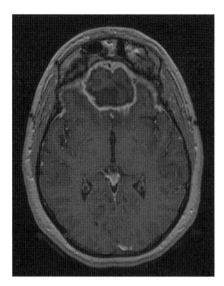

Figure 68.1 MRI T1-weighted image with gadolinium showing an extra-axial rim enhancing lesion of the frontal fossa in a patient who had previously undergone ethmoid sinus surgery.

Table 68.1 Common causative organisms in cases of intracranial epidural abscess.

Associated etiology	Common organisms
Paranasal sinusitis	Alpha-hemolytic streptococci Staphylococci Anaerobic/microaerophilic streptococci Aerobic Gram-negative bacilli *Bacteroides* species
Otitis media, mastoiditis	Aerobic and anaerobic streptococci *Pseudomonas aeruginosa* *Bacteroides* species Enterobacteriaceae Staphylococci
Penetrating trauma	Staphylococci Aerobic Gram-negative bacilli *Clostridium* species
Postoperative	Staphylococci Enterobacteriaceae *Pseudomonas aeruginosa* *Proprionibacterium* species

It is also expected to show restriction on diffusion-weighted image (DWI) sequences. This lesion may be contiguous to an area of skull osteomyelitis, sinusitis, skull fracture, or craniotomy defect.

Causative organisms vary with the primary etiology of infection (Table 68.1). Up to 50% of intraoperative Gram-stain cultures are sterile, presumably as a result of preoperative empiric antibiotic administration.

Treatment/management

Empiric broad spectrum antibiotics should be started as soon as possible, and may be subsequently tailored according to Gram stain, culture, and sensitivity results. Initial empiric therapy should provide coverage for Gram-positive cocci, Gram-negative bacilli, and anaerobes. The usual recommended empiric antimicrobial therapy includes a penicillin, metronidazole, and a third-generation cephalosporin. In the case of penetrating trauma or postoperative infection, the penicillin should be substituted with vancomycin. The course of antibiotic therapy is usually at least 6 weeks, and extended to 8 weeks or longer in the presence of osteomyelitis.

Prophylaxis for seizures is recommended, and anticonvulsants are mandatory if seizure activity occurs.

Burr holes or craniotomy for decompression, debridement, and drainage of epidural abscess is warranted in the majority of cases. Delay in surgical intervention has been associated with significant morbidity and mortality. Reoperation may be necessary in cases of persistent or recurrent suppurative infection.

The neurologic status at time of presentation is generally a good predictor of neurologic outcome. Delays in diagnosis or treatment are associated with increased morbidity and mortality. Mortality is estimated at 10–20% from treated intracranial epidural abscess.

Further reading

Hlavin ML, Kaminski HJ, Fenstermaker RA, *et al*. Intracranial suppuration: a modern decade of postoperative subdural empyema and pidural abscess. *Neurosurgery* 1994; 34: 974–81.

Krauss WE, McCormick PC. Infections of the dural spaces. *Neurosurg Clin N Am* 1992; 3: 412–33.

Tunkell AR. Subdural empyema, epidural abscess, and suppurative intracranial thrombophlebitis. In: Mandell GL, Bennet JE, Dolin R, editors. *Mandell, Douglas, and Bennett's Principles and Practices of Infectious Diseases*. Philadelphia: Elsevier Churchill Livingstone; 2005, pp. 1165–8.

Chapter 69
Intracranial septic thrombophlebitis

D. Nagaraja and D.K. Prashantha
National Institute of Mental Health and Neurosciences (NIMHANS), Bangalore, India

Introduction

Cerebral venous and sinus thrombosis (CVT) predominantly affects young adults, with a predilection for women. Its prevalence is 5×10^{-6} and it accounts for 0.5% of all strokes. The etiology of CVT is diverse and includes coagulation disorders, pregnancy and puerperium, dehydration, malignancy, head injury, and local, regional, or systemic infections. The infection-related CVT differs from aseptic CVT (Table 69.1) and can be categorized based on the sinuses or the veins that undergo thrombosis.

Septic cavernous sinus thrombosis

Cavernous sinus is the most frequently involved area in the septic CVT, accounting for 70% of cases. In patients reported between 1940 and 1960, 60% had infections involving the medial third of the face, nose, orbits, tonsil, and soft palate, whereas sphenoid and ethmoid sinuses were the more frequent sites during 1961–1984.

Bacteriology

The major organisms are *Staphylococcus aureus*, streptococci, and pneumococcal species. Other pathogens include Gram-negative and tubercular bacilli, bacteroids, *Aspergillus*, malaria, trichinosis, and viral infections like HIV and CMV.

Clinical presentation

Symptoms start in one eye and move to the other quickly. Most frequent symptoms are periorbital swelling and headache followed by drowsiness, diplopia, photophobia, and ptosis. Predisposing infection may be present in one-third, and over two-thirds of patients have fever, proptosis, chemosis, cranial nerve palsies (III, IV, VI), and papilledema. Approximately half of patients will have altered sensorium, neck rigidity, and abnormal ear, nose, and throat (ENT) examination. Decreased visual acuity,

International Neurology: A Clinical Approach. Edited by Robert P. Lisak, Daniel D. Truong, William M. Carroll, and Roongroj Bhidayasiri.
© 2009 Blackwell Publishing, ISBN: 978-1-4051-5738-4.

Table 69.1 Differences between septic and aseptic cerebral venous and sinus thrombosis (CVT).

	Septic CVT	Aseptic CVT
Incidence	Rare	5×10^{-6} per year
Gender predilection	No	Women
Common site(s)	Cavernous sinus	Superior sagittal and transverse sinus
Onset	Acute	Variable
Role of anticoagulation	Uncertain	Definite
Recurrence(s)	Exceptional	Variable (0–11.7%)
Neurological outcome	Variable, based on the sinus involved	Good in more than 80%
Mortality	Varied (12–78%)	4% in acute phase

abnormal pupils, hypo- or hyperesthesia of the face, and depressed corneal reflex are observed in a quarter, and seizures and hemiparesis in a minority. An infrequent finding may be an engorged, palpable frontal vein.

The thrombosis can extend to other dural sinuses and cortical veins resulting in hemorrhagic infarctions and abscess formation. Pituitary insufficiency and syndrome of inappropriate antidiuretic hormone secretion have also been reported.

Laboratory findings

The majority of patients reveal peripheral leucocytosis. Cerebrospinal (CSF) analysis shows evidence of paramenigeal infection or meningitis in nearly 80% of patients. Blood culture may be positive in patients with a rapidly progressive course and in those who have not received antibiotics previously.

Neuroimaging features

High resolution contrast CT scan and MRI (Figure 69.1) are helpful in documenting the thrombosis of cavernous and other sinuses, associated complications, and etiology. Contrast enhanced CT scan may show widening of the cavernous sinus, filling defects, enhancement of the walls, and dilated superior ophthalmic veins. In a series of eight patients with septic cavernous sinus thrombosis, evaluated by CT and MRI, six had bilateral cavernous sinus

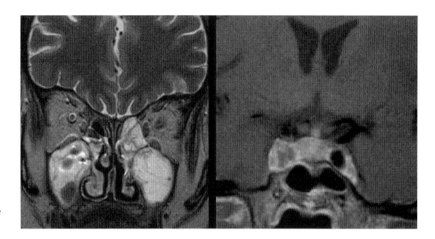

Figure 69.1 Post-contrast T1 coronal image showing bulging, enhancement, and filling defect in the right cavernous sinus. Note the non-visualization of the right carotid artery due to thrombosis.

thrombosis while others had variable affection of the posterior part of cavernous sinus, superior ophthalmic veins, carotid artery, and other dural sinuses. Orbital venogram, once considered as diagnostic, is rarely required.

Treatment and outcome

Therapeutic protocol includes antibiotics, anticoagulation, and antiedema measures. The antibiotic therapy should be based on culture and sensitivity pattern from the primary site of infection or CSF. The empirical antibiotic regimen consists of a third-generation cephalosporin (cefotaxime), metronidazole, and an antistaphylococcal agent such as nafcillin or vancomycin. The duration of antibiotic therapy depends on many factors and often exceeds 2 weeks. The evidence for the efficacy for anticoagulation is limited by its rarity but may be considered after excluding hemorrhagic infarct. The surgical drainage of the paranasal air sinuses can be considered when the aggressive medical management fails. Its mortality has reduced from nearly 100% to 30% and a full recovery can be expected in nearly 40% of cases.

Septic lateral sinus thrombosis

Lateral sinus is the second most commonly involved area in septic CVT, with the common primary site of infection being otitis media.

Clinical presentation

The most common symptoms in decreasing order of frequency are headache, ear ache, and vomiting. A history of ear infection is present in nearly half of patients.

Examinations often reveal posterior auricular swelling due to the obstruction of the emissary mastoid vein – the "Greisinger sign" – purulent discharge from the ruptured tympanic membrane, or an erythematous tympanic membrane. Other features include fever, papilledema, neck rigidity, and sixth cranial nerve palsy. Less frequent findings include altered sensorium, hemiparesis, decreased visual acuity, and nystagmus.

Laboratory findings

The common isolates include *Proteus* species, *Staphylococcus aureus*, *Escherichia coli*, *Pseudomonas*, bacteroides, and anaerobic streptococci. Peripheral leucocytosis is noted in more than two-thirds of patients. CSF pressure is elevated in 77% and features of parameningeal infection are noted in one-third of patients. CSF analysis may, however, be normal.

Neuroimaging findings

As the primary site of infection is the middle ear in most patients, imaging of the mastoid is essential. X-ray may exhibit increased density, loss of air trabeculae, and bony sclerosis of the mastoid(s) and lytic lesion in the temporal or parietal bones. Contrast enhanced CT scans may reveal a filling defect in the sinus and concomitant cerebritis, brain abscess, and hemorrhagic infarcts. Digital subtraction angiography can confirm the thrombosis.

Treatment and outcome

Awaiting the culture and sensitivity report, a combination of third-generation cephalosporin with activity against *Pseudomonas* (ceftazidime), an antistaphylococcal agent such as nafcillin or vancomycin, and metronidazole to cover the anaerobes may be started. Most patients require surgery for chronic otitis media. Other measures include antiedema agents and management of complications such as brain abscess and hydrocephalus. Anticoagulation is not recommended. Mortality is around 12% and about 13% of sufferers are left with chronic sequelae such as otitic hydrocephalus, facial palsy, hemiparesis, eighth nerve dysfunction, and decreased visual acuity.

Septic superior sagittal sinus thrombosis

Unlike in aseptic CVT, superior sagittal sinus is less frequently involved in septic CVT. The most common predisposing conditions are meningitis (48%) and sinusitis

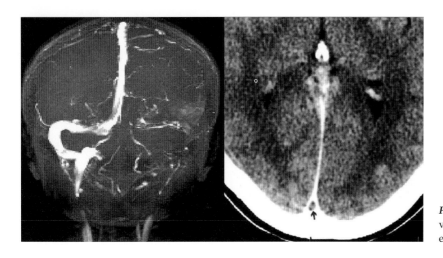

Figure 69.2 MR venography showing non-visualization of right transverse sinus. Contrast enhanced CT scan showing the empty delta sign.

(17%) involving the ethmoid and maxillary sinuses. It has also been described following frontal sinusitis, infection in tonsil, lungs, and pelvis, and lateral sinus thrombosis.

Clinical presentation

The most common symptoms are seizures, headache, and confusion. Nearly a third of patients have a history of predisposing factors. The most frequent findings on examination are fever and altered sensorium, while a few may have hemiparesis, neck rigidity, and papilledema.

Laboratory findings

The most frequent isolates are *Streptococcus pneumoniae*, β-hemolytic streptococci, and *Klebsiella*. Peripheral leucocytosis and elevated CSF pressure are common.

Neuroimaging observation

Contrast enhanced CT scan shows empty delta sign (Figure 69.2), gyral enhancement, and cerebral edema. The plain scan may show hemorrhagic infarcts when there is involvement of cortical veins. Angiography is the most definitive method, but with the advent of CT and MRI, it is rarely used as a diagnostic tool in an acutely ill patient.

Treatment and outcome

There has been little improvement in the mortality (a fall from 100% to 78%) despite development of many newer antibiotics. Optimal treatment includes intravenous antibiotics and antiedema measures. The empirical antibiotics are similar to those used in community-acquired bacterial meningitis. Anticoagulation is not recommended.

Septic cortical thrombophlebitis

Thrombosis of the cortical veins has been postulated as an important cause of seizures and focal deficits in a patient with bacterial meningitis. Out of the ten cases of isolated septic cortical vein thrombosis proven by autopsy, angiogram, or at surgery, nine patients had meningitis, two had subdural empyema, and four had otitis media. All but one had fever, seven had focal deficits, and five patients had seizures. All patients were in altered sensorium at admission. The most common organism was *Streptococcus pneumoniae*. Three of the five survivors had persistent focal neurological deficits.

The treatment includes antibiotics, surgical drainage of the foci of infection whenever possible, antiedema measures, and supportive care.

Conclusion

Septic CVT is an important cause of mortality and significant morbidity. Its early recognition and treatment with appropriate antibiotics and antiedema measures, and surgery whenever required, may improve the mortality and morbidity.

Further reading

Bousser MG, Ferro JM. Cerebral venous thrombosis: an update. *Lancet Neurol* 2007; 6: 162–70.

DiNubile MJ, Boom WH. Septic cortical thrombophlebitis. *J Infect Dis* 1990; 161: 1216–20.

Nagaraja D. Brain veins and their diseases. In: Toole JF, editor. *Cerebrovascular Disorders*, 5th ed. Philadelphia: Lippincott Williams & Wilkins; 1999, pp. 481–506.

Schuknecht B, Simmen D, Yuksel C, Valavanis A. Tributary venosinus occlusion and septic cavernous sinus thrombosis: CT and MRI findings. *Am J Neuroradiol* 1998; 19: 617–26.

Southwick FS, Richardson EP Jr, Swartz MN. Septic thrombosis of the dural venous sinuses. *Medicine (Baltimore)* 1986; 65(2): 82–106.

Chapter 70
Encephalitis due to bacterial infections

Karen L. Roos and Jennifer Durphy
Indiana University School of Medicine, Indianapolis, USA

Introduction

Encephalitis is a syndrome of fever and headache accompanied by an altered level of consciousness, a focal neurologic deficit, or seizure activity. Cerebrospinal fluid (CSF) analysis typically demonstrates an increased number of white blood cells and an increased protein concentration. Electroencephalography (EEG), fluid-attenuated inversion recovery (FLAIR), and diffusion-weighted MRI may demonstrate focal abnormalities. Encephalitis is distinguished from encephalopathy which is an altered or depressed level of consciousness with EEG evidence of diffuse slowing and an absence of a CSF inflammatory response. Although herpes viruses and arthropod-borne viruses are frequently the etiological agents of encephalitis, bacteria may also cause encephalitis.

Mycoplasma pneumoniae

Mycoplasma pneumoniae is the causative organism of 7–30% of cases of community-acquired pneumonia, but an uncommon cause of encephalitis. In a review of all published reports on patients with *M. pneumoniae* childhood encephalitis in the English language literature from 1972 to 2003, there were only 58 well-defined cases. *Mycoplasma pneumoniae* is more likely to cause a delayed or post-infectious immune-mediated neurological disorder than an acute encephalitis due to direct invasion of brain parenchyma by the pathogen. The clinical presentation of encephalitis includes fever, headache, vomiting, an altered level of consciousness, and seizure activity.

Diagnosis is made by a combination of a positive CSF culture or polymerase chain reaction (PCR) or both, with or without acute and convalescent serologic tests

demonstrating a fourfold increase in *M. pneumoniae* IgG, or by detection of *M. pneumoniae* in throat specimens by culture or PCR or both with confirmatory serologic tests. The diagnosis cannot rely exclusively on a single elevated IgM or IgG titer as there are many false-positive serologic results from serum. A history of preceding flu-like or respiratory symptoms prior to the onset of neurologic disease and chest radiograph evidence of a pulmonary infiltrate are supportive evidence of encephalitis due to this bacteria. Spinal fluid analysis demonstrates a lymphocytic pleocytosis in the majority of cases, but a pleocytosis of polymorphonuclear leukocytes has been reported as well. A CSF lymphocytic pleocytosis would be expected in an immune-mediated disorder, whereas a pleocytosis of polymorphonuclear leukocytes is more suggestive of acute bacterial infection of the CNS. Bickerstaff's brainstem encephalitis, which is a syndrome of progressive ophthalmoplegia and ataxia with disturbance of consciousness or hyperreflexia, has also been reported in association with *M. pneumoniae* infection. *Mycoplasma pneumoniae* was detected by PCR analysis of a throat swab and anti-GQ1b antibodies were detected in serum. Anti-GQ1b ganglioside antibodies have been detected in other immune-mediated neurologic syndromes following bacterial infections, including Miller–Fisher and Guillain–Barre syndromes.

Antimicrobial therapy should be initiated for the patient with signs and symptoms of encephalitis with a positive CSF culture or PCR for *M. pneumoniae* and/or a CSF pleocytosis of polymorphonuclear leukocytes. The recommended therapeutic agents are either a macrolide (erythromycin or azithromycin), tetracycline, chloramphenicol, or a fluoroquinolone. Patients with respiratory symptoms and chest radiograph evidence of a pulmonary infiltrate should also be treated with antimicrobial therapy. A delay between respiratory symptoms and the neurological disorder and evidence of a CSF lymphocytic pleocytosis are suggestive of an immune-mediated encephalitis, and treatment with high dose intravenous corticosteroid therapy, intravenous immunoglobulin, or plasma exchange is recommended. In these patients, *M. pneumoniae* is often detected by PCR in throat swabs, but not CSF specimens.

International Neurology: A Clinical Approach. Edited by Robert P. Lisak, Daniel D. Truong, William M. Carroll, and Roongroj Bhidayasiri.
© 2009 Blackwell Publishing, ISBN: 978-1-4051-5738-4.

Listeria monocytogenes

Listeria monocytogenes is a gram-positive bacillus that contaminates food and infection is acquired from coleslaw, hot dogs, Mexican-style cheese that contains unpasteurized milk, soft cheeses (Brie, Camembert), and delicatessen foods. Once in the gastrointestinal tract, the organism can directly invade the intestinal epithelium. *Listeria monocytogenes* is an intracellular parasite with a unique ability to infect neighboring cells without ever becoming extracellular. The organism uses host cell actin filaments to form filopodial projections which are engulfed by neighboring phagocytic cells. *Listeria* is then able to escape the lysosome of its new cell and repeat the process. Portal circulation carries the pathogen from the gut to the liver where *Listeria* becomes concentrated in the reticuloendothelial cells. A bacteremia then ensues. The central nervous system is infected during the bacteremia or by intra-axonal spread. *Listeria monocytogenes* can gain access to cranial nerves through the oral mucosa and via retrograde axonal spread infect cranial nerve nuclei in the brainstem.

The T-cell-mediated immune response of the host is important in determining the risk of the disease. Individuals with impaired cell-mediated immunity due to pregnancy, organ transplantation, AIDS, cancer, chemotherapy, or immunosuppressive therapy are at increased risk of disease. In addition to immune status, age (neonates and individuals over the age of 50), and underlying medical conditions (diabetes and alcoholism) increase the risk for listeriosis and central nervous system infection. Healthy individuals can develop *Listeria* infections as well.

Listeria monocytogenes may cause a meningoencephalitis characterized by fever and headache and an altered level of consiousness. Nuchal rigidity, focal neurologic signs, and seizures are less common. The organism may also cause a brainstem encephalitis, also referred to as a rhomboencephalitis. There may be a prodromal phase consisting of headache, nausea, vomiting, fever, and malaise. This is followed by the onset of cranial nerve palsies, cerebellar deficits, and long-tract motor or sensory deficits. A prodromal phase is not mandatory, as brainstem signs can develop without fever or headache.

Diagnosis is made by demonstrating the organism in blood cultures and examination of the CSF. The majority of patients with *L. monocytogenes* meningoencephalitis have a CSF pleocytosis with a predominance of polymorphonuclear leukocytes. Approximately 25% have a lymphocytic pleocytosis. The glucose concentration may be normal or decreased. In the majority of cases the organism can be cultured from CSF. In *Listeria* brainstem encephalitis, there is a high signal intensity lesion on T2-weighted, diffusion, and FLAIR MR. Spinal fluid analysis demonstrates a lymphocytic or monocytic pleocytosis. The absence of a CSF pleocytosis has also been reported.

There are a number of features particular to *L. monocytogenes* meningoencephalitis as compared with meningoencephalitis due to the other bacterial etiologies: (1) the presentation is typically acute but may be subacute, (2) nuchal rigidity is less common, (3) the presentation may be characterized by brainstem signs and symptoms, (4) blood cultures are often positive (75% of cases), (5) spinal fluid analysis may demonstrate a lymphocytic pleocytosis or be normal, and (6) the CSF glucose concentration may be normal.

Ampicillin is the recommended antimicrobial agent for the treatment of *L. monocytogenes* central nervous system (CNS) infections. The dose of ampicillin is 150 mg/kg/day for neonates (in an 8-hour dosing interval), 300–400 mg/kg/day for infants and children (in a 4- to 6-hour dosing interval), and 12–15 g/day for adults (in a 4- to 6-hour dosing interval). The duration of treatment is 2–3 weeks. Gentamicin is added to ampicillin in patients who are severely ill. Trimethoprim–sulfamethoxazole can be used in patients who are allergic to penicillin.

Whipple's disease

Whipple's disease is caused by the bacteria *Tropheryma whipplei* and was first described by George H. Whipple in 1907. Whipple's disease is characterized by two stages. There is a prodromal stage of chronic intermittent nonspecific symptoms, primarily migratory arthralgias, diarrhea, and fever. This is followed over the course of several years by a steady-state stage of weight loss, abdominal pain, fever of unknown origin, and diarrhea with symptoms of involvement of other organs, in addition to the gastrointestinal tract. The pathognomonic neurologic sign of Whipple's disease is oculomasticatory, or oculofacialsketetal, myorhythmia. Oculomasticatory myorhythmia consists of pendular horizontal convergent–divergent oscillations of both eyes synchronous with involuntary contractions of the jaw and tongue. Fifty percent of patients have a vertical gaze palsy at presentation. Myoclonus and cerebellar ataxia have also been reported. Cognitive changes are common, affecting 71% of patients with neurologic involvement, and take the form of dementia, delirium, memory loss, somnolence, apathy, depression, or anxiety. *Tropheryma whipplei* has a predilection for the hypothalamus and brainstem. Magnetic resonance imaging (MRI) may demonstrate atrophy of the hippocampus, or focal or multifocal ring-enhancing lesions with edema or multifocal white matter hyperintensities on T2-weighted imaging. Patients with supranuclear vertical gaze palsies may have rostral brainstem lesions or normal MRIs.

Whipple's disease may be diagnosed by periodic acid-Schiff (PAS) staining of small-bowel-biopsy specimens.

The organism may be identified by PCR in CSF or jejunal tissue obtained by biopsy. Spinal fluid analysis is usually normal, but a low-grade pleocytosis and a mild elevation of the protein concentration have been reported. The CSF PCR test to detect nucleic acid of *T. whipplei* is a useful test, although the sensitivity of this assay has not been determined.

The recommended treatment is 2 weeks of parenteral streptomycin (1 g/day) with penicillin G (1.2 million units/day) or ceftriaxone (2 g every 12 hours). This is followed by the oral administration of 160 mg of trimethoprim and 800 mg of sulfamethoxazole twice per day for 1–2 years. There have been reports of CNS relapse when tetracycline or penicillin were used alone.

Cat-scratch disease

Cat-scratch disease is caused by the gram-negative bacillus *Bartonella henselae*. The disease was first described in 1950. Its "typical" presentation is that of fever, an erythematous papule at the inoculation site, and a regional lymphadenopathy that develops 2 or 3 weeks after a cat scratch or bite. Cat-scratch disease is considered a benign, self-limiting disease in an immunocompetent individual and usually resolves in a few months. In approximately 10% of patients, there will be an "atypical" disease, such as encephalitis, neuroretinitis, endocarditis, or Parinaud oculoglandular syndrome.

The pathogenesis of cat-scratch disease encephalitis has not yet been defined. It is not clear if encephalitis is due to direct invasion of the brain by bacilli, as has been demonstrated in histopathological examination of brain tissue at autopsy, a vasculitis, or if this is a parainfectious immune-mediated process, such as an acute disseminated encephalomyelitis.

Cat-scratch encephalitis occurs from within a few days to up to 2 months following the presentation of "typical" cat-scratch disease. The most common symptoms of encephalitis are convulsions and status epilepticus. Other symptoms include persistent headache, lethargy, malaise or combative behavior, and ataxia. Aphasia, transient hemiplegia, and hearing loss may also occur.

The diagnosis of cat-scratch disease encephalitis is based on the detection of *B. henselae* antibodies in a single serum titer of more than 1:64, which has both sensitivity and specificity approaching 100%. Seroconversion may not occur until the third week of illness. PCR of lymph node tissue and culture are also used in diagnosis, but are less widely available. In approximately one-third of patients with cat-scratch disease encephalitis, there is a CSF pleocytosis with a lymphocytic predominance and an increased protein concentration. Fifty percent of patients have an elevated erythrocyte sedimentation rate and 25% an elevated peripheral leukocytosis.

Electroencephalography in the majority of patients will show diffuse background slow wave activity, indicative of encephalopathy. Findings on MRI and CT imaging studies are either negative or non-specific, demonstrating focal or diffuse white and gray matter abnormalities.

The preferred treatment for "typical" cat-scratch disease is supportive therapy only. A number of antibiotics have been shown to be efficacious, including rifampin, doxycycline, ciprofloxacin, trimethoprim–sulfamethoxazole, and azithromycin. Antimicrobial therapy with intravenous doxycycline 200 mg twice daily is recommended for patients with cat-scratch encephalitis. One study showed dramatic clinical improvement with the use of high-dose corticosteroids.

Prognosis is generally good, with full recovery in most patients within a month and the remainder within a year. There are, however, anecdotal reports of patients with persistent disability and partial seizures requiring long-term treatment.

Brucellosis

Infection with *Brucella* is acquired through the inhalation of infected aerosolized particles, through contact with animal parts, and through the consumption of unpasteurized dairy products. Four species of *Brucella* cause human disease: *B. melitensis*, *B. abortus*, *B. suis*, and *B. canis*. Brucellae are small, gram-negative coccobacilli. Consider this organism as the causative agent of encephalitis in veterinarians, farmers, abattoir workers, individuals who work in microbiology laboratories, and the household contacts of individuals with these occupations.

Brucella invades the mucosa, after which a bacteremia occurs. Initial symptoms are fever, headache, sweats, and malaise. A malodorous perspiration is pathognomonic. On physical examination, there may be evidence of lymphadenopathy, hepatomegaly, or splenomegaly. Central nervous system involvement in brucellosis can present as a meningitis, an encephalitis, a brain abscess, or demyelinating disease. Examination of the CSF demonstrates an increased number of white blood cells, an increased protein concentration, and a decreased glucose concentration. Diagnosis is made by isolation of the organism from blood culture, a positive indirect enzyme-linked immunosorbent assay (ELISA), isolation of the organism from CSF, evidence of *Brucella* agglutinating antibodies in CSF, or identification of bacterial nucleic acid by PCR. Treatment guidelines are based on the recommendations of the World Health Organization. Doxycycline 100 mg twice daily for 6 weeks is used in combination with either streptomycin or rifampin. Monotherapy is not recommended due to the risk of relapse with a single antibiotic.

Legionnaires' disease

Legionnaires' disease was first described in 1976 during an epidemic of pneumonia in Philadelphia that resulted in 34 deaths. The recognition of the disease was followed by a number of anecdotal reports and small case series in the 1980s of encephalopathy, cranial nerve palsies, cerebellar dysfunction, myelopathy, peripheral neuropathy, and myositis. Since then, only a rare case of legionnaires' disease with neurological complications has been reported, and few physicians today include *Legionella pneumophilia* in a differential diagnosis of bacterial etiologies of encephalitis.

Diagnosis depends on serology, isolation of the organism by culture, or evidence of *L. pneumophilia* by direct fluorescent antibody (DFA) test of a specimen obtained by bronchoalveolar lavage.

Historically treatment of encephalitis associated with *L. pneumophilia* pneumonia has been with rifampin and erythromycin or rifampin and azithromycin. Rifampin monotherapy is not recommended as resistance may develop.

Summary and recommendations

Encephalitis may be caused by a bacteria or occur as a parainfectious immune-mediated process following a bacterial infection. Every patient with encephalitis should have Gram's stain and blood cultures and examination of CSF. A PCR has recently become available to detect bacterial nucleic acid in serum. CSF should be sent for Gram's stain and bacterial culture, and broad range and meningeal-specific PCR to detect bacterial nucleic acid.

When *M. pneumoniae* is the suspected causative organism because of a history of preceding flu-like or respiratory symptoms prior to the onset of neurologic disease, obtain a chest X-ray, send CSF for culture and PCR for *M. pneumoniae*, and obtain acute and convalescent serology to demonstrate a fourfold increase in *M. pneumoniae* IgG. A delay between respiratory symptoms and the neurological disorder in association with evidence of a CSF lymphocytic pleocytosis is suggestive of an immune-mediated encephalitis. Send serum for anti-GQ1b ganglioside antibodies.

Whipple's disease causes a clinical presentation of a subacute encephalitis. The organism may be identified by PCR in CSF or jejunal tissue obtained by biopsy.

Inquire about a new kitten and a scratch or bite. Look for an inoculation site and examine the patient for lymphadenopathy. The diagnosis of cat-scratch disease encephalitis

is based on the detection of *B. henselae* antibodies in a single serum titer of more than 1:64. Seroconversion may not occur until the third week of illness.

Encephalitis due to a species of *Brucella* should be considered in the patient who has contact with animals or who has ingested unpasteurized dairy products. The diagnosis requires isolation of the organism from blood or CSF, a positive ELISA, evidence of *Brucella* agglutinating antibodies in CSF, or identification of bacterial nucleic acid by PCR.

Legionnaires' disease associated with acute encephalitis is rarely reported today. In a patient with pneumonia and encephalitis in whom the causative organisms cannot be identified by sputum, blood, and CSF culture, consideration can be given to bronchoalveolar lavage for a direct fluorescent antibody test for *L. pneumophilia*.

Further reading

Antal EA, Loberg EM, Bracht P, Melby KK, Maehlen J. Evidence for intraaxonal spread of *Listeria monocytognes* from the periphery to the central nervous system. *Brain Pathol* 1984; 11: 432–8.

Armstrong RW, Fung PC. Brainstem encephalitis (rhomboencephalitis) due to *Listeria monocytogenes*: case report and review. *Clin Infect Dis* 1992; 14: 815–21.

Bartt R. *Listeria* and atypical presentations of *Listeria* in the central nervous system. *Semin Neurol* 2000; 20(3): 361–73.

Carithers HA, Margileth AM. CSD. Acute encephalopathy and other neurologic manifestations. *Am J Dis Child* 1991; 145: 98–101.

Dalton MJ, Robinson LE, Cooper J, *et al.* Use of Bartonella antigens for serologic diagnosis of CSD at a national reference center. *Arch Intern Med* 1995; 155(15): 1670–6.

Daxboeck F, Blacky A, Seidl R, Krause R, Assadian O. Diagnosis, treatment and prognosis of *Mycoplasma pneumoniae* childhood encephalitis: systematic review of 58 cases. *J Child Neurol* 2004; 19: 865–71.

Fenollar F, Puechal X, Raoult D. Whipple's disease. *N Engl J Med* 2007; 356: 55–66.

Fraser DW, Tsai TR, Orenstein W, *et al.* Legionnaires' disease: description of an epidemic of pneumonia. *N Engl J Med* 1977; 297: 1189–97.

Kennedy DH, Bone I, Weir AI. Early diagnosis of legionnaires' disease: distinctive neurological findings. *Lancet* 1981; 1: 940–1.

Kimmel DW. Central nervous system Whipple's disease. In: Noseworthy JH, editor. *Fifty Neurologic Cases from Mayo Clinic.* New York: Oxford University Press; 2004, pp. 39–40.

Lorber B. Listeriosis. *Clin Infect Dis* 1997; 24: 1–11.

Margelith AM. Antibiotic therapy for CSD: clinical study of therapeutic outcome in 268 patients and a review of the literature. *Pediatr Infect Dis J* 1992; 11: 474–8.

Pappas G, Akritidis N, Bosilkovski M, Tsianos E. Brucellosis. *N Engl J Med* 2005; 352: 2325–36.

Sanger JM, Sanger JW, Southwick FS. Host cell actin assembly is necessary and likely to provide propulsive force for intracellular movement of *Listeria monocytogenes*. *Infect Immun* 1992; 60: 3609–19.

Solera J, Martinez-Alfaro E, Saez L. Meta-analysis of the efficacy of rifampicin and doxycycline in the treatment of human brucellosis. *Med Clin* 1994; 102: 731–8.

Steer AC, Starr M, Kornberg AJ. Bickerstaff brainstem encephalitis associated with *Mycoplasma pneumoniae* infection. *J Child Neurol* 2006; 21: 533–4.

Weston KD, Tran T, Kimmel KN, Maria BL. Possible role of high-dose corticosteroids in the treatment of CSD encephalopathy. *J Child Neurol* 2001; 16: 762–3.

Chapter 71
Mycobacterium tuberculosis

Einar P. Wilder-Smith
National University of Singapore, Singapore

Introduction

Tuberculosis (TB) re-emerged as a major health problem at the end of the 1980s due to the explosive emergence of HIV and the development of drug resistance of the *Mycobacterium*. Compounding this are the often reduced resources available to screen and investigate those at risk of TB. Prompt diagnosis and treatment is crucial to reduce the number of people dying from TB, which the World Health Organization (WHO) estimated at 1.6 million in 2005 alone.

Achieving a diagnosis can be challenging, particularly in view of the non-specificity of many of the clinical presentations and the constraints on investigative methods often encountered in countries with high incidence rates. This contributes to delayed onset of recognition and treatment, explaining at least in part the often poor clinical outcomes. Even though drug resistance to TB is increasing alarmingly, the majority of deaths from TB still occur in drug-sensitive disease, highlighting the importance of early disease recognition and treatment as well as preventive measures.

This chapter focuses on TB infection of the nervous system, which mainly affects the brain and the spinal cord. *Mycobacterium tuberculosis* is nearly always the infecting agent and other non-tuberculous mycobacteria are only very rarely pathological, apart from opportunistic infection in AIDS patients.

Epidemiology

As estimated by the WHO, 8.8 million new TB cases occurred in 2005. Of these, 7.4 million were in Asia and sub-Saharan Africa. A total of 1.6 million people died of TB, including 195 000 patients infected with HIV.

Although in 2005 the TB incidence rate was stable or in decline for the first time in many years, the total number of new TB cases was still rising slowly, because of a growing case load in African, eastern Mediterranean, and South-East Asian regions.

The majority (more than 85%) of new TB cases involve the lungs and only around 1% of all TB affects the nervous system, mainly in the form of meningitis and meningoencephalitis. The most important risk factor for TB of the nervous system disease is immunosuppression. This explains why a third of nervous system TB occurs in children and patients infected with HIV, the latter having a five-fold increased incidence.

As *M. tuberculosis* is ubiquitous, the majority of people are exposed to TB during their lifetime. The number of pathogens and an intact immune response determine whether disease will develop or not. Other important determinants of a successful immune response are age, nutrition status, diabetes, HIV, and immunosuppressive drug treatments such as steroids and chemotherapy.

Pathophysiology

All tuberculosis starts with the inhalation of TB bacilli and subsequent multiplication within the alveoli. From here there is spread to other organs via the bloodstream. Central nervous system (CNS) TB develops from "Rich foci" which are subependymal or subpial accumulations of bacilli, which within the brain are most commonly located in the Sylvian fissure. Here with growth they rupture into the subarachnoid or ventricular space to cause meningitis. Accumulation and subsequent growth of TB bacilli in other locations results in local disease such as tuberculomas or abscesses. Extracerebral sites that result in neurological disease are the spinal vertebrae where the hematogenously spread bacillus lodges preferentially in the anterior or inferior angle of the vertebral body. From here the disease spreads to the intervertebral disc which is typically destroyed and spreads to the adjacent vertebral body.

Tuberculous meningitis (TBM)
Typically, a thick exudate of the leptomeninges develops predominantly over the basal regions of the brain with

International Neurology: A Clinical Approach. Edited by Robert P. Lisak, Daniel D. Truong, William M. Carroll, and Roongroj Bhidayasiri.
© 2009 Blackwell Publishing, ISBN: 978-1-4051-5738-4.

involvement of the basal cisterns. This process predisposes to cerebrospinal fluid (CSF) obstruction and not infrequently results in communicating or obstructive hydrocephalus. As the disease progresses, ependymitis develops and spreads to other CNS sites. The exudate is composed of a network of mononuclear cells, red blood cells, neutrophils, lymphocytes, and varying numbers of tubercle bacilli. With disease progression, the predominant cell type is lymphocytic. One of the consequences of the exudate is irritation of the by-standing brain vessels which may occlude either through direct participation in the inflammatory process or through reactive vasoconstriction.

In childhood, TBM often manifests several weeks after the primary infection, explaining why the majority of cases of TBM show evidence of an active primary complex.

Tuberculoma and abscess

Tuberculomas consist of Langerhans' cells, epitheloid cells, and lymphocytes. Typically the center contains caseous material in which TB bacilli can be demonstrated. In children, tuberculomas of the brain are more frequent infratentorially, whereas in adults there is supratentorial preference. Liquefication of the caseous core of a tuberculoma results in the formation of abscesses which are often larger and multilobulated in immune-compromised individuals. Abscesses are made up of large numbers of neutrophils and numerous TB bacilli. Neurological deficits depend on the site of the tuberculomas and cause symptoms and signs as a result of arachnoiditis, vasculitis, and compression.

Clinical features

Co-infection with HIV does not alter the clinical presentation but increases the number of complications.

Tuberculous meningitis (TBM)

Fever, headache, and anorexia are the most frequent presenting symptoms of TBM. The most common clinical sign is meningism (40–80%) followed by coma (30–60%) and cranial nerve palsies (30–50%), of which sixth nerve palsy is by far the most common (30–40%). Seizures (generalized or partial) occur in 50% of children but only in 5% of adults. Hemiparesis is less common and noted in 10–20% of cases. Physicians should be aware that fever may be absent and that neurological signs can rapidly progress to coma.

In about 75% of cases of TBM and more frequently in children, extrameningeal TB – mostly seen over the lungs – is present. TBM is classified into three grades which with increasing severity predict increasing mortality. A fully oriented patient with no focal neurology is graded 1. Grade 2 is scored with a Glasgow Coma Scale of 10–14 with or without focal neurology and Grade 3 with a Glasgow Coma Scale of less than 10.

Tuberculomas

In the brain, tuberculomas produce signs through their irritative and space-occupying characteristics. India has a particularly high incidence of intracerebral tuberculomas which often present with seizures.

Tuberculosis of the spine (often termed Pott's disease) frequently results in a tender spine prominence or angulation (gibbus) with neurological deficit at the lower thoracic motor and sensory level. About half of those with spinal disease manifest paraparesis. In countries with high standards of living, those affected are usually elderly; in countries where TB is common, those affected are predominantly below 20 years of age. Pott's disease often occurs without evidence of other TB foci. Early manifestations are back pain and stiffness. In about half of cases, a paraspinal cold abscess develops that follows along ligamentous tracks, draining into distant regions such as the iliac crest, groin, or buttock. Spread along the spine is known to sometimes skip several spinal levels.

Investigations and diagnosis

Tuberculous meningitis

Diagnosis depends on a high index of suspicion. Examination of the CSF is essential and identification of acid-fast bacilli clinches the diagnosis. Meticulous microscopic technique and use of more than 5 ml of CSF results in detection in 60% of cases. Cultures take 6 weeks and are positive in approximately 70%. Characteristic is a lymphocyte-predominant CSF cell count of less than 1500 cells/mm^3, low glucose (less than 0.5 CSF to blood ratio), and moderately elevated protein levels. In early disease, cells may be predominantly polymorphonuclear. PCR does not better bacteriological diagnostic accuracy in untreated CSF samples but may be superior when treatment has already commenced. The typical neuroradiological triad accompanying TBM is basal meningeal enhancement (the most consistent), hydrocephalus, and (least common) supratentorial ischemia. These changes are, however, non-specific and can also be seen with other diseases such as viral meningoencephalitis, cryptococcal disease, metastasis, sarcoidosis, and lymphoma. Figure 71.1 shows leptomeningeal and ependymal enhancement in a patient with TBM.

Tuberculoma and abscess

Verification of tuberculomas and abscesses ultimately remains histological and should if possible be attempted prior to initiation of treatment mainly to exclude differential diagnoses.

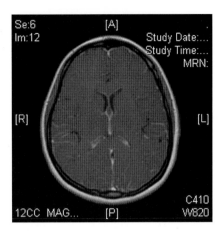

Figure 71.1 Gadolinium-enhanced axial MRI using T1-weighted sequence showing diffuse leptomeningeal enhancement with peri-ependymal enhancement of the lateral ventricles.

Treatment

Medication

Since delay of treatment can be fatal, treatment should be initiated when clinical and laboratory findings are compatible. Nine to 12 months of multiple drug therapy is recommended, although a recent review suggested 6 months may be sufficient in areas with low levels of bacterial resistance. The first 2 months of intensive treatment require quadruple therapy with isoniazid (10 mg/kg/day), rifampicin (10 mg/kg/day), and pyrazinamide (30 mg/kg/day), with the addition of one of the following: ethambutol, streptomycin, or ethionamide. Isoniazid – which shows excellent CSF penetration – should be given together with rifampicin for the continuation phase of treatment from months 3 to 9. Intolerance to one or more of the medicines during the intensive phase of treatment necessitates prolonged treatment. Pyridoxine therapy (100 mg/day) should be given with isoniazid therapy to prevent the development of peripheral neuropathy.

Adjunctive corticosteroids (prednisone 1–3 mg/kg/day or dexamethasone 0.3–0.5 mg/kg/day in a reducing dose regimen) significantly reduce mortality across all severity grades irrespective of co-infection with HIV. For this reason, steroids should be administered in all cases from day 1 of treatment in a tapering dose for the first 1–2 months.

Despite increasing resistance to antituberculous drugs worldwide, implications for treatment are not yet clear. Although bacilli resistant to isoniazid and rifampicin show worse clinical outcomes, the clinical implications of single drug resistance are as yet unclear. Currently, detection of resistance to isoniazid should result in prolonged treatment with a regimen that includes pyrazinamide. Identifying patients with multidrug resistance can be difficult, as many will be dead by the time bacteriological sensitivities arrive. Therefore when standard treatment fails to halt disease progression, drug resistance should be considered and at least three previously unused drugs should be prescribed, of which one should be a fluoroquinolone.

Neurosurgical

The best treatment for hydrocephalus remains unclear as there have been no trials comparing the treatment options. Serial lumbar punctures, ventriculoperitoneal, or atrial shunting have all been successfully used. As CSF circulation and reabsorption is often lastingly abnormal, permanent approaches of CSF drainage in the form of shunting are currently considered preferable.

Further reading

Bernaerts A, Vanhoenacker FM, Parizel PM, *et al.* Tuberculosis of the central nervous system: overview of neuroradiological findings. *Eur Radiol* 2003; 13: 1876–90.

Fitzgerald D, Haas DW. *Mycobacterium tuberculosis.* In: Mandall GL, Bennett JE, Dolin R, editors. *Principles and Practice of Infectious Diseases*, 6th ed. Philadelphia: Elsevier/Churchill Livingstone; 2005, Chapter 248, pp. 2852 ff.

Thwaites GE, Tran TH. Tuberculous meningitis: many questions, too few answers. *Lancet Neurol* 2005; 4: 160–70.

van Loenhout-Rooyackers JH, Keyser A, Laheij RJF, Verbeek ALM, van der Meer JWM. Tuberculous meningitis: is a 6-month treatment regimen sufficient? *Int J Tuberc Lung Dis* 2001; 5(11): 1028–35.

WHO. *Mycobacterium tuberculosis.* www.who.int/tb/publications/ global_report/2007/key_findings/en/index.html.

Chapter 72
Mycobacterium avium

Einar P. Wilder-Smith
National University of Singapore, Singapore

Mycobacterium avium (MA) only rarely infects the human nervous system and then only in severe immunosuppression syndromes, most commonly that accompany HIV infection. Central nervous system disease can result from the disseminated form of MA which may occur when CD4 counts drop below $100/mm^3$. Disseminated MA has been reported more frequently in developed countries (the United States and Europe) and is particularly rare in Africa.

The initial infection is via the gastrointestinal tract or the lung with subsequent hematogenous spread to the brain, where disease presents as a space-occupying lesion. Diagnosis can only be achieved by histological means. Surgical removal remains the most effective treatment, as antimycobacterial drugs are generally ineffective. Recently, treatment cocktails including macrolides (clarithromycin, azithromycin) have shown improved results in disseminated MA.

Further reading

Gordin FM, Horsburgh CR. *Mycobacterium avium* complex. In: Mandell GL, Bernett JW, Dolin R, editors. *Principles and Practice of Infectious Diseases*, 6th ed. Philadelphia: Elsevier/Churchill Livingstone; 2005, Chapter 250, pp. 2897–909.

International Neurology: A Clinical Approach. Edited by Robert P. Lisak, Daniel D. Truong, William M. Carroll, and Roongroj Bhidayasiri. © 2009 Blackwell Publishing, ISBN: 978-1-4051-5738-4.

Chapter 73
Leprosy

Minh Le[1,2]

[1]University Medical Center, Ho Chi Minh City, Vietnam
[2]The University of Medicine and Pharmacy, Ho Chi Minh City, Vietnam

Introduction

Leprosy (Hansen's disease) is a result of chronic infection by *Mycobacterium leprae*, affecting mainly the peripheral nerves, upper respiratory airways, anterior eye segments, and the testes.

Bacteriology and epidemiology

Mycobacterium leprae ($0.5 \times 4.0\,\mu m$) is an acid-fast bacillus (AFB) stained by the Ziehl–Neelsen method in smears and by the Fite–Faraco method in tissue sections. Staining properties of *M. leprae* in skin smears or biopsy specimens are important in the assessment of therapeutic efficacy of antileprotics: viable organisms stain solidly, whereas degenerate organisms stain irregularly and eventually become non-acid-fast. Non-viable organisms in tissues or in smears can be detected by silver staining methods. *Mycobacterium leprae* has a preference to infect cooler body areas, and is characterized by a long incubation period.

The prevalence of leprosy has recently decreased globally. According to the World Health Organization (WHO), there were 1.83 million people in the world affected by active leprosy in 1995. Prevalence rates vary geographically, with 75% of leprosy occurring in southern Asia, 12% in Africa, and 8% in the Americas. Leprosy today prevails in the poor tropical areas of the world.

The most important source of leprosy is infected humans, but armadillos, chimpanzees, and monkeys are other reservoirs.

Pathogenesis and immunity

Transmission through secretions from the nasal mucosa of untreated patients is thought to be the main route of infection. Direct skin-to-skin contact, mother's milk, and transplacental infection are other alternatives.

Bacteremia is present in up to 15% of paucibacillary patients and is common in multibacillary patients. *Mycobacterium leprae* invades peripheral nerves via the blood vessels of the perineurium, and causes infection of endothelial cells leading to ischemia of the nerves.

The characteristics of host cell-mediated immunity determine the clinical manifestation of the disease as described by the Ridley–Jopling classification. Lepromatous Hansen's disease is characterized by strong proliferation of AFB, anergy to lepromin, minimal inflammatory response, and disseminated nerve and skin lesions.

Tuberculoid Hansen's disease is characterized by intense cell-mediated immunity, delayed hypersensitivity response to lepromin, intense inflammatory lesions that cause local destruction of infected nerves, and rare AFB detected in skin and nerves.

Borderline forms share the characteristics of the two extremes.

Table 73.1 shows the clinical and histopathological classification of leprosy based on the Ridley–Jopling classification. The WHO Classification of Leprosy, which is based on the burden of AFB in tissues and the number of skin lesions, determines two main forms of leprosy: paucibacillary (PB) leprosy in which patients have skin smears negative for AFB, or five or fewer cutaneous lesions; multibacillary (MB) leprosy in which patients have positive skin smears for AFB, or more than five skin lesions. "Single-lesion" paucibacillary is the third category of the WHO classification. The WHO classification under PB would include indeterminate form (I), tuberculoid form (TT), and borderline tuberculoid (BT) of the Ridley–Jopling classification; MB would include midborderline (BB), borderline lepromatous (BL) and lepromatous form (LL). Single-lesion PB would include I and TT.

Clinical features

Skin lesions with associated sensory loss and enlarged peripheral nerves are the cardinal symptoms and signs of leprosy. Sensory disturbances are the outstanding

International Neurology: A Clinical Approach. Edited by Robert P. Lisak, Daniel D. Truong, William M. Carroll, and Roongroj Bhidayasiri. © 2009 Blackwell Publishing, ISBN: 978-1-4051-5738-4.

Table 73.1 Clinical and histopathological classification of leprosy.

Clinical features	Histopathologic features
Tuberculoid form	
Few well-defined anesthetic macules or plaques; neural involvement common	Granulomas with or without giant cells; rare bacilli; nerve damage; no subepidermal freezone
Borderline forms	
Borderline tuberculoid	
More lesions, borders less distinct; neural involvement common	Similar to TT but with occasional bacilli, usually in nerves; subepidermal freezone
Midborderline	
More lesions than BT, borders vague; neural involvement common	Epithelioid cells and histiocytes; focal lymphocytes; increased cellularity of nerves; bacilli readily found, mostly in nerves; subepidermal freezone
Borderline lepromatous	
Numerous lesions, borders vague; less neural damage than in BB	Histiocytes, few epithelioid cells, some foamy cells; bacilli plentiful in nerves and histiocytes; subepidermal freezone
Lepromatous form	
Multiple macules, nodules, or diffuse infiltrations; symmetrically neural lesions develop late	Foamy histiocytes with large numbers of bacilli; few lymphocytes; numerous bacilli in nerves; minimal intraneural cellular infiltration; subepidermal freezone
Indeterminate form	
Vaguely defined, hypopigmented, or erythematous macules	Small lymphocytic infiltrates around nerves and appendages; rare bacilli, usually in nerves

features of this disease, and include anesthesia or hypesthesia to pain and temperature, and sometimes paresthesias or dysesthesias. Often sensory abnormalities precede paralysis, with impaired temperature and touch often linked.

Tuberculoid

TT patients have single or few macules or indurated skin lesions which are hypopigmented, hypoesthetic, and anhydrotic. Cutaneous nerves and superficial peripheral nerve trunks are often enlarged in the region of lesions. The commonly involved nerves that present with hypertrophy are the great auricular, ulnar, radial, fibular, and sural nerves. Cold nerve abscesses due to intense response to bacilli within nerves can occur in larger nerve trunks of TT patients. Calcifications of nerves in long-standing cases of PB leprosy may be sufficiently intense to appear on X-ray. Acrodystrophy and autoamputation are the common late complications of neuropathy, in which loss of pain is predominant.

Lepromatous leprosy

LL is characterized by the infiltration of the skin with a predilection for the ears, central portion of the face, and extensor surfaces of the thighs and forearms. The scalp, palms, soles, and midline of the back are not usually involved. Skin lesions include macules, nodules, papules, ulcerations, and diffuse myxedema-like involvement.

Sensory loss is commonly first distributed to the ear helices, nose, malar regions, dorsal surface of the hands, forearms, feet, and dorsolateral surfaces of the lower legs. Other areas are the upper respiratory tract from the nasal mucosa to the larynx, the eye, lymph nodes, and testes. Commonly detected affected nerves are the ulnar, posterior tibial, common peroneal, and the median and facial nerves. The preservation of tendon reflexes is one particular aspect of the clinical findings of neuropathy associated with leprosy that should be mentioned as this can help differentiate from length-dependent neuropathies where tendon reflex loss is a hallmark.

Borderline leprosy

Borderline leprosy is the intermediate group in which patients' resistance to the micro-organism varies from weak to strong. This group includes three subgroups: BT, BB, and BL. This area of the spectrum is unstable, and such borderline patients can swing back and forth within the two extremes of TT and LL (Figure 73.1). The essential characteristics of these subgroups are shown in Table 73.1.

Indeterminate leprosy

Indeterminate leprosy usually presents as hypopigmented, or slightly erythematous, poorly defined macules. Texture, the amount of hair, sensation, and sweating in the affected area are, at the most, only slightly changed.

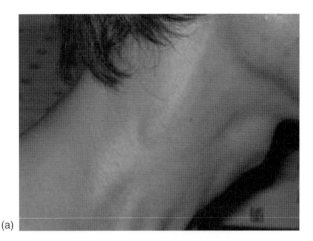

(a)

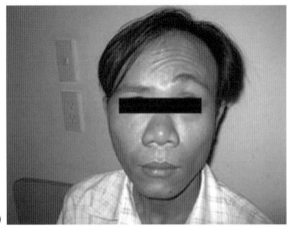

(b)

Figure 73.1 (a) Enlargement of the right great auricular nerve in borderline tuberculoid (BT) leprosy. (b). Same patient with facial paralysis on the right side, and hypoesthetic macular lesions of the upper and middle right hemiface.

Because of this vague and non-specific feature, indeterminate lesions can be diagnosed only with close cooperation between clinician and pathologist.

Lucio's leprosy

Lucio's leprosy is a particular form of the disease in which there is highly anergic and very diffuse infiltration of skin. Obstructive vasculitis causes massive dermal infarcts and ulcers can later supervene as this form of leprosy progresses. *Pure neural leprosy* affects peripheral nerves in the absence of skin lesions.

Leprosy reactions

Treating physicians need to be aware of inflammatory immune reactions that can occur during the progress and the treatment of leprosy because of their harmful effects on patients. Two main types of acute reactions can supervene during leprosy: type 1 reaction, or reversal reaction, and type 2 reaction, or erythema nodosum leprosum.

Reversal reactions occur in tuberculoid leprosy and in borderline leprosy, and represent an episodic upgrading of cell-mediated immunity. There is an exacerbation of previous lesions, with associated negative skin smears for AFB and a good response to anti-inflammatory therapy. Clinical findings include aggravation of previous skin lesions, new skin lesions, and neuritis, which usually appears during the first few months following initiation of chemotherapy. By way of repeated reversal reactions, borderline lesions may gradually change toward tuberculoid leprosy or tuberculoid lesions toward scar tissue. Permanent neurologic deficits may result unless anti-inflammatory treatment is quickly initiated.

Erythema nodosum leprosum (ENL) occurs in approximately half of lepromatous patients, though it may also occur in borderline lepromatous patients. These type 2 reactions often arise after several months of therapy, but may develop in untreated patients. The clinical findings of ENL include malaise, fever, painful indurated cutaneous nodules, painful peripheral nerve lesion, iridocyclitis, orchitis, and arthritis. Hepatomegaly and splenomegaly also rarely occur. ENL is the result of antigen–antibody complex deposition and results in complement fixation with subsequent cell lysis.

Diagnosis

The cardinal signs of leprosy are hypoesthetic lesions of the skin, enlarged peripheral nerves, and AFB in skin smears.

A careful physical examination of the entire skin surface and superficial peripheral nerves to look for skin lesions, sensory changes, peripheral nerve enlargement, and motor deficit (e.g., facial paresis, claw hand, foot drop) is necessary for the diagnosis. Sensory changes are the most important criterion for clinical diagnosis of leprosy. Leprosy is diagnosed clinically, but histopathological evaluation is useful to confirm the diagnosis, for classification, and the identification of pure neural leprosy.

Definitive diagnosis of leprosy is based upon the demonstration of AFB in skin scrapings, skin or nerve biopsies, or nasal secretions. Biopsy specimens should be taken from the edges of the lesions. Skin smears should be from multiple sites, and include the edges of macules or plaques, nodules, earlobes, or nasal mucosa.

The histopathological features of TT leprosy and LL leprosy differ. Destruction of the architecture of cutaneous nerves by granulomatous inflammation is the main histopathological finding in TT leprosy. Large numbers of AFB are detected in Schwann cells, macrophages, and axons of involved nerves in LL leprosy, together with a combination of Wallerian degeneration and segmental demyelination.

Other investigations

The lepromin test consists of the intradermal inoculation of 0.1 ml of lepromin (a suspension of heat-killed *M. leprae*) and is used to test the patient's immune response toward *M. leprae*. Evaluation of this response is based on the measurement of the diameter of induration at the injection site 3–4 weeks post-inoculation (Mitsuda reaction). This skin test is never used as a diagnostic test of leprosy, as many in the general population are reactive. A strong response to lepromin is seen in TT and BT (>5 mm), intermediate reactions in BL and BB (3–5 mm), and a weak or absent response in LL (0–2 mm).

The study of motor and sensory nerve conduction velocities can be helpful in demonstrating abnormality in the nerve trunks and branches and often predates clinical characteristics. It can also be useful to monitor nerve function.

Differential diagnosis

The differential diagnoses of leprosy are extensive and include sarcoidosis, syphilis, yaws, granuloma annulare, leishmaniasis, lupus erythematodus, superficial mycoses, onchocerciasis, streptocerciasis, lymphoma, psoriasis, pityriasis rosea, neurofibromatosis, syringomyelia, lead toxicity, diabetes mellitus, primary amyloidosis, sensory polyneuropathies, other mononeuropathies, and familial hypertrophic neuropathy.

Antileprotic treatment

Specific leprosy treatment, prevention of disease spread, and treatment of deformities are the main objectives for the management. Optimum management of this chronic disease should be comprehensive and requires the cooperation of internists, neurologists, orthopedic surgeons, ophthalmologists, and physical therapists.

Because of known drug-resistant strains of *M. leprae* toward dapsone, rifampicin and other antibiotics, monotherapy with any antileprotic is discouraged. The multidrug therapeutic (MDT) regimen recommended by WHO is based on the classification of leprosy into PB and MB. The paucibacillary regimen includes 600 mg rifampicin given once a month under supervision, plus 100 mg dapsone daily for 6 months. The minimum treatment for patients with single lesions consists of this regimen.

The multibacillary regimen includes 600 mg rifampicin and 300 mg clofazimine given once a month under supervision, plus 100 mg dapsone/day and 50 mg clofazimine/day for at least 12 months (WHO recommendation). In some countries, 24 months of treatment are still given.

Prothionamide, ethionamide, or minocycline may be used as a substitute for clofazimine when there is hyperpigmentation of the skin from clofazimine. Pefloxacin, ofloxacin, clarithromycin, and minocycline are currently used in clinical trials and may later be included in the MDT regimen.

Treatment of leprosy reactions

Reactions in leprosy are considered a medical emergency. Immobilization by splint, analgesics, and prednisone are the mainstay of the treatment of acute neuritis in reversal reaction. Prednisone up to 80 mg daily is given initially then tapered off over 2–3 months to a minimally effective level as long as neuritis persists. Long-term corticosteroid therapy may be given preferably in an alternated-day regimen. The efficacy of clofazimine in reversal reactions has not been established. Specific treatment of *M. leprae* by antileprotic agents is continued during management for reversal reactions.

Mild analgesics are required for milder forms of ENL. Severe forms of ENL require more vigorous treatment with steroids or thalidomide. Thalidomide is used at the initial dose of 100 mg three to four times daily then gradually tapered to the minimum effective level. Thalidomide is prescribed only for males and females without reproductive potential. Increasing the dosage of clofazimine up to 300 mg/day is another treatment alternative, but effect only takes place after 4–6 weeks. Prednisone is often used when thalidomide cannot be used. Iridocyclitis should be managed aggressively by combined systemic anti-inflammatory treatment and local corticosteroids. Sometimes surgical measures are needed to control increased intraoccular pressure.

Further reading

Meyers WM. Leprosy. In: Guerrant RL, Walker DH, Weller PF editors. *Tropical Infectious Diseases: Principles, Pathogens, and Practice*, 2nd ed, Vol. 1. Philadelphia: Elsevier-Churchill Livingstone; 2006, pp. 436–47.

Sabin TD, Swift TR, Jacobson RR. Neuropathy associated with infections – leprosy. In: Dyck PJ, Thomas PK, editors. *Peripheral Neuropathy*, 4th ed, Vol. 2. Philadelphia: Elsevier-Saunders; 2005, pp. 2081–108.

WHO Expert Committee on Leprosy. Seventh Report, WHO Tech Rep Ser No. 874. Geneva: WHO; 1998.

Chapter 74
Neurosyphilis

Jonathan Carr
University of Stellenbosch, South Africa

Introduction

The classical substrate for neurosyphilis was the overcrowded urban environment of the nineteenth century. Neurosyphilis was in decline well before the advent of the penicillin era, suggesting a substantial role for changing socio-economic conditions similar to tuberculosis, the incidence of which declined before the introduction of streptomycin.

In the early twenty-first century, neurosyphilis is seen predominantly in two major groups. In the developed world, the manifestations of neurological syphilis appear largely to be associated with ongoing localized epidemics amongst men who have sex with men (MSM). The developing world probably recapitulates the circumstances seen in the developed world over a century ago, with conditions of urban crowding and poor access to health care. To an extent, parts of the developing world represent a time capsule, in which the effects of the antibiotic era are not present, largely because medical care is limited. Overlapping these two extremes are the marginalized populations of the developed world, for whom access to health care providers is limited as a result of historical or social factors such as drug abuse.

The prevalence of syphilis and neurosyphilis mirrors that of HIV infection. Currently, the burden of syphilis is likely to be greatest in the developing world, and is causally related to a high frequency of unprotected sex with multiple partners. In the developed world unprotected sexual behavior is likely responsible for the high prevalence in MSM and other high risk populations.

Pathophysiology

The primary stage of syphilis is typically characterized by a chancre, although this may be absent or not visible to the patient. The secondary stage is characterized by a skin rash and lymphadenopathy but may additionally be complicated by uveitis and meningitis. Secondary syphilis is also the period in which invasion of the nervous system occurs, and abnormal cerebrospinal fluid (CSF) findings are common. The definition of tertiary syphilis varies widely but is typically assumed to include cardiovascular and neurological complications.

Neurosyphilis shares the major features of other chronic meningitides, including findings of a meningoencephalitis with a chronic inflammatory cell infiltrate of the leptomeninges and superficial cortex. Involvement of the leptomeninges is associated with changes in the vessels, with subintimal proliferation. The pathological features of neurosyphilis can be similar to those of tuberculous meningitis. However, there is a unique involvement of the parenchyma with loss of neurons and gliosis with neurosyphilis. The clinical correlates of the two major pathological processes of neurosyphilis, vascular occlusion and involvement of cortex and white matter, are varied. Classically, the syndromes have been described pathologically, and comprise acute syphilitic meningitis, meningovascular neurosyphilis, general paresis of the insane, and tabes dorsalis. The notion that these represent an orderly progression of events with a defined time course has given way to ideas of syndrome overlap of some of the early or late forms. Few reliable studies of the natural history of neurosyphilis exist, and all are hampered (including modern studies) by the great difficulty in establishing the latency from when syphilis was first contracted until the time that a particular neurosyphilitic presentation develops. Currently, the most common manifestations of neurosyphilis are acute syphilitic meningitis, stroke, and neuropsychiatric syphilis. Tabes dorsalis is an extremely rare entity, as are gummata.

Clinical features

Given that the clinician may be faced with weak data to support a clinical diagnosis of neurosyphilis, it is important to emphasize that atypical forms of neurosyphilis or formes frustes are controversial entities with little evidence to support their existence. Reports on atypical presentations of neurosyphilis have tended to be small series

International Neurology: A Clinical Approach. Edited by Robert P. Lisak, Daniel D. Truong, William M. Carroll, and Roongroj Bhidayasiri. © 2009 Blackwell Publishing, ISBN: 978-1-4051-5738-4.

in which the descriptions have in fact been compatible with standard forms of neurosyphilis, or else contaminated by inclusion criteria that were over-inclusive and hence included patients who did not have neurosyphilis. Although neurosyphilis may be rare in developed countries, the presentations are likely to be similar to those seen in developing countries.

The decision to investigate for neurosyphilis with lumbar puncture is usually made in the setting of positive serum serology associated with a clinical presentation compatible with neurosyphilis. However, the Centers for Disease Control and Prevention (CDC) recommend lumbar puncture for patients who are HIV-positive with late latent syphilis (i.e., asymptomatic syphilis acquired more than a year previously). Some authorities in the United States have recommended lumbar puncture for HIV-positive patients if the serum rapid plasma reagin (RPR) is greater than 1:32. Similarly, criteria for neurosyphilis in HIV-infected patients have been expanded to include patients with positive serum serology and a white cell count greater than $20/\mu l$ or a cell count greater than 5 associated with a positive CSF fluorescent treponemal antibody (FTA). Potential difficulties with this approach would include the presence of CSF abnormalities in many patients with secondary syphilis, who would not be expected to progress to neurosyphilis, and the presence of CSF pleocytosis in many HIV-positive patients.

Neurosyphilis presents in a restricted number of ways (despite its reputation as the great imitator). The following syndromes represent the majority of presentations.

Neuropsychiatric

This is usually a combination of delirium superimposed upon dementia, frequently associated with behavioral change that gradually worsens over months. Dementia is global and has a guarded prognosis for recovery. Although they occur, hallucinations and delusional behavior are not common. Physical examination usually reveals hyperreflexia, prominent facial reflexes, and tremor. Argyll Robertson pupils are an uncommon finding. This presentation is likely to correspond to that known traditionally as general paresis, a form of parenchymal neurosyphilis. The latency of onset of this condition is unlikely to be decades as is sometimes reported, and there is likely to be moderate overlap with meningovascular disease.

Stroke

Large and small vessel involvement may occur. Large vessel involvement may give rise to strokes in the middle cerebral artery territory, sometimes related to internal carotid disease. Strokes of varying ages in different vascular territories are also seen, as well as disease of the posterior circulation, the latter giving rise to small lacunar infarctions of the brainstem. Radiologically, there may be evidence of diffuse small vessel disease also.

Encephalopathy with seizures

This group overlaps with neuropsychiatric neurosyphilis. Patients may present with generalized tonic–clonic or complex partial seizures, and either may manifest initially with status epilepticus. A common electroencephalography (EEG) correlate is the presence of periodic lateralized epileptiform discharges. Patients are often noted subsequently to have a global cognitive impairment.

Spinal cord

A common presentation is acute stroke of the spinal cord, resulting in spinal shock. Gradually progressive spastic paraparesis is also seen, possibly on an ischemic basis, and a diffuse syphilitic myelitis has also been reported, of uncertain etiology.

Meningitis

Two forms of meningitis are seen. Acute meningitis associated with fever and neck stiffness is a manifestation of secondary syphilis and may be associated with a rash. A more chronic condition associated with cranial nerve palsies (sometimes multiple) also occurs, and is likely to represent a relatively pure form of meningovascular neurosyphilis.

Tabes dorsalis

Tabes has become extremely uncommon. Classically, tabes is associated with loss of reflexes, usually the ankle, sometimes with Argyll Robertson pupils and bladder dysfunction, and with loss of posterior column function. The latter results in Charcot joints, characterized by joint destruction and sclerosis, commonly in the knee.

HIV and neurosyphilis

Multiple reports were published in the late 1980s on the unexpectedly high frequency (and possibly novel) presentations of syphilis associated with HIV infection, proposing that neurosyphilis had become a more aggressive disease in the setting of immunosuppression. The major syndromes were those of acute meningitis, stroke, and uveitis. Many of the presentations were associated with secondary syphilis, and it is likely that the epidemic of syphilis which was taking place in the United States at the time was responsible for the increased number of cases seen. In many of the reported cases, CD4 counts were above 200, indicating relative sparing of the immune system. The descriptions of the manifestations of neurosyphilis in HIV-positive patients match those of well-described syndromes in the pre-HIV era, and the latency from infection to development of neurosyphilis is unlikely to have been reduced. It is appropriate to reiterate that reported aggressiveness of neurosyphilis associated with HIV infection is based on an assumption of predictable development of neurosyphilitic syndromes; however, the information in both the pre- and post-HIV era concerning latency from acquiring syphilis to the development of neurosyphilis is poor.

Ocular syphilis

The place of ocular syphilis in the classification of the complications of syphilitic infection is uncertain. Although classified by the CDC as neurosyphilis, it is unclear if ocular syphilis should receive the same treatment. However, there is unlikely to be clear evidence indicating what course the clinician should follow, and the most conservative course of assuming that ocular syphilis should be treated as neurosyphilis should probably be followed. Common manifestations include uveitis, interstitial keratitis, and optic neuritis.

Investigations

Treponema pallidum cannot be cultured without great difficulty, and serological testing together with neuroimaging represent strong surrogate markers. Polymerase chain reaction (PCR) is relatively insensitive and is not widely available. In a significant proportion of cases, neither the clinical presentation nor the special investigations allow the clinician to diagnose the presence of neurosyphilis with certainty.

In general, screening tests in the serum such as the RPR and Venereal Disease Research Laboratory (VDRL) are sensitive, and it is very likely that a negative FTA in serum excludes the possibility of neurosyphilis. In the CSF, a positive serological test to confirm the presence of neurosyphilis is important. In CSF, the VDRL is specific but lacks sensitivity (false negatives can occur), whereas the FTA is sensitive but is associated with false positives. Approximately, 20–33% of cases of neurosyphilis will have a negative VDRL in CSF. As in the serum, a negative FTA in CSF is highly likely to exclude neurosyphilis. Usually, features of disease activity such as elevated lymphocyte count, protein, and IgG index will be found in CSF. All tests of this nature are likely to have better predictive values when applied to populations where the prevalence of the disease is relatively high, whereas if the prevalence is low, the predictive values of the tests decline. The most frequent finding on MRI in cases with neuropsychiatric presentations is cerebral atrophy. Patients presenting with stroke will not uncommonly have evidence of previous events, and both large and small vessel disease may be seen.

Treatment/management

Treatment

The current CDC treatment regimen is aqueous crystalline penicillin G (benzyl penicillin) 18–24 mU/day,

administered intravenously (IV) as 3–4 mU every 4 hours or continuous infusion, for 10–14 days. Uveitis has been treated with benzathine penicillin alone. Penicillin-allergic patients may be treated with ceftriaxone 2 g daily for 10–14 days or doxycycline 200 mg twice daily for 28 days.

Treatment of HIV positive patient with neurosyphilis

HIV-positive patients should receive the same treatment as non-HIV-positive patients.

Follow-up

The principal issues in terms of follow-up are when repeat examination of the CSF should be obtained, and how to interpret the results. The available information is scanty and recommendations vary widely from follow-up at 6 months or less to follow-up at 1–2 years. Of the CSF parameters, cell count will respond most rapidly, and protein levels and IgG index more slowly. Although the cell count will tend to fall substantially by 6 months, it is unlikely that in all cases the cell count will be normal by that time. Regarding serology in CSF, the VDRL is insensitive, and typically has low titers, giving rise to a floor effect. There is potentially a 1:2 dilution margin of error in determination of VDRL titers, and the results of CSF serology are likely to have low utility in determining response to treatment. Given that changes in CSF will be slow to occur, early monitoring of CSF is unlikely to be beneficial, but the decision of when to monitor CSF is largely one of clinical judgment. Currently, CDC recommendations are that HIV-infected persons should be clinically evaluated and undergo serological testing at 3, 6, 9, 12, and 24 months after therapy. The CDC notes that "Although of unproven benefit, some specialists recommend a CSF examination 6 months after therapy."

Further reading

Adams RD. *Principles of Neurology*, 6th ed. New York: McGraw-Hill; 1997, pp. 722–8.

Goh BT, Voorst Vader PC. European guideline for the management of syphilis. *Int J STD AIDS* 2001; 12(Suppl 3): 14–26.

Golden MR, Marra CM, Holmes KH. Update on syphilis. Resurgence of an old problem. *JAMA* 2003; 290(11): 1510–14.

Timmermans M, Carr J. Neurosyphilis in the modern era. *J Neurol Neurosurg Psychiatry* 2004; 75: 1727–30.

Chapter 75
Lyme disease

Patricia K. Coyle
Stony Brook University Medical Center, Stony Brook, USA

Introduction

Lyme disease (borreliosis) is the clinical illness produced by infection with the bacterial spirochete *Borrelia burgdorferi*. Virtually all cases are from tick bites, with rare congenital transmissions. Blood-borne infection is possible, but no cases are documented.

Epidemiology

Lyme disease is the major tickborne infection in the United States (US) and Europe. It occurs in at least 50 nations in North America, Europe, and Asia, with limited cases from Russia, China, Japan, and possibly Mexico. The forested regions of central Europe and Sweden account for most European Lyme disease, while in the US the organism is endemic in over 15 states and reported from 49 states. The three major US foci are the northeast (Maine to Maryland), the Midwest (Wisconsin and Minnesota), and the West Coast (northern California and Oregon).

Demographics

Lyme disease affects all ages and both genders, but is most common in young boys aged 5–19 years and adults aged 30 years or older. Highest attack rates are associated with prolonged outdoor endemic area exposure. Infection can also occur with very brief exposure, backyard exposure, or one-time travel to an endemic region. In temperate climates there is a seasonal incidence, with most infections presenting in late spring and summer.

Tick vector

The vector for *B. burgdorferi* is the black-legged hard shell *Ixodes* tick. These ticks are very tiny (poppy-seed size).

They live for 2 years and feed three times, at each life stage (larva, nymph, adult).

In the Northeast and North Central United States, the black-legged hard shell deer tick (*Ixodes scapularis*) transmits *B. burgdorferi*. In the Pacific Coastal states it is the Western black-legged tick (*Ixodes pecificus*). In Europe the vectors are *Ixodes ricinis* and *Ixodes persulcatus*.

Organism

Borrelia burgdorferi is a Gram-negative organism 10–30 μm long and 0.2–0.25 μm wide. It consists of a protoplasmic cylinder, periplasm with flagella, and an outer membrane. The complete genome of the B31 strain has been sequenced, with a 950 kb linear chromosome and 9 linear and 12 circular plasmids.

Environmental triggers influence organism gene expression, which differs in the tick, the host, and the test tube. *Borrelia burgdorferi sensu lato* complex contains at least ten distinct genospecies, but only three are pathogenic. *Borrelia burgdorferi sensu stricto*, a fairly virulent strain, is responsible for all North American and some European cases. *Borrelia afzelii*, present in Europe and Asia, causes mild dermatologic disease, while *Borrelia garinii* in Europe and Asia causes neurologic disease.

Clinical expression

Target organs
Lyme disease targets the skin, musculoskeletal, cardiac, and nervous systems. Based on 119 965 US patients reported from 1992 to 2004, 68% had the characteristic skin rash, 33% had arthritis, 8% had facial palsy, 4% had radiculopathy, 1% had meningitis or encephalitis, and 1% had heart block.

Disease stages
Like all spirochetal infections, Lyme disease occurs in phases separated by quiescent periods. Patients can present in any stage. Early local infection occurs within 30 days of spirochete inoculation. It involves erythema migrans (EM), the pathognomonic rash at the tick bite site. Early

International Neurology: A Clinical Approach. Edited by Robert P. Lisak, Daniel D. Truong, William M. Carroll, and Roongroj Bhidayasiri. © 2009 Blackwell Publishing, ISBN: 978-1-4051-5738-4.

infection can also manifest as a flu-like illness during summertime, associated with seroconversion. Early disseminated infection occurs within 3 months of spirochete inoculation, and coincides with spirochete spread through dermal tissues, blood vessel invasion, and spirochetemia. In addition to multifocal EM, other recognized early dissemination syndromes involve the nervous, cardiac, and musculoskeletal systems. Late persistent infection refers to recrudescent disease more than 3 months after inoculation. It also involves suggestive skin, musculoskeletal, and nervous system syndromes.

Extraneural manifestations

EM is the most common manifestation of Lyme disease and occurs in up to 90% of cases. It is an expanding red macule/papule at the tick bite site, typically 7–10 (range 1–30) days after inoculation. Large numbers of spirochetes are present in the skin. Rashes that appear within 24 hours after tick bite, or that resolve within 48 hours without treatment, are not EM. EM is typically painless. It expands over several days to become quite large. It may show central clearing, a classic bull's-eye formation. However, there are many atypical forms. Any unusual rash during summertime in endemic regions should raise concerns about Lyme disease. EM can be accompanied by a multisymptom flu-like complex, with fatigue, myalgias, arthralgias, headache, fever, chills, stiff neck, and regional lymphadenopathy. Prominent respiratory or gastrointestinal complaints are rare.

Acrodermatitis chronica atrophicans, associated with *B. afzelii*, is a late/persistent infection of skin which occurs in Europe. Spirochetes have been cultured from skin lesions as late as a decade after initial infection. Elderly women are preferentially affected. The chronic skin lesion appears particularly on sun-exposed surfaces such as the lower leg.

Musculoskeletal involvement involves arthralgias and myalgias early on. Lyme arthritis with joint swelling is typically an oligoarticular large joint involvement. The knee is most commonly involved, with intermittent swelling and pain. It can be associated with a Baker cyst.

Cardiac involvement is now rarely seen. It is an early dissemination syndrome involving fluctuating atrioventricular block. Other reported manifestations include acute myopericarditis, mild left ventricular dysfunction, cardiomyopathy, pericarditis, and in Europe a chronic dilated cardiomyopathy.

Neurologic Lyme disease

Neurologic involvement can occur at all stages of Lyme disease, and involves both central (CNS) and peripheral nervous system (PNS) syndromes. Spirochetes may seed the CNS very early, coincident with or even before a detectable EM. More commonly neurologic involvement occurs coincident with the spirochetemia of early dissemination post-EM. Headache and stiff neck should always raise a concern about CNS seeding.

Early dissemination is associated with isolated cranial nerve palsy. This is largely facial nerve involvement, which can be bilateral in up to a third of patients. In the US, this is the most common neurologic syndrome. The facial nerve palsy is invariably accompanied by multisystem complaints (headache, palpitations, arthralgias/myalgias, stiff neck, fatigue, "foggy brain"). Much more unusual is involvement of other cranial nerves (such as III, IV, VI, VIII, V, or rarely II). Early dissemination is also associated with meningitis or encephalomyelitis. The meningitis mimics aseptic (viral) meningitis, but can be accompanied by facial nerve and radicular involvement. Acute cerebellar syndromes and transverse myelitis have also been associated with early dissemination. The most common neurologic syndrome in Europe is acute painful radiculoneuritis (referred to as Bannwarth syndrome), characterized by radicular and myotomal features. It often begins with severe intrascapular pain. Patients go on to focal deficits such as winging of the scapula, and may show simultaneous EM and facial nerve involvement. Despite floridly inflammatory cerebrospinal fluid (CSF), headache and meningismus are typically absent.

Late persistent infection neurologic syndromes involve chronic encephalopathy, axonal polyradiculoneuropathy, and encephalomyelitis. Late Lyme encephalopathy most often occurs in patients who received prior antibiotic therapy that was not optimal for a CNS-based infection. Patients show subtle cognitive disturbances in memory, attention, and processing speed. Cognitive deficits are rarely so marked as to produce true dementia. Late infection chronic polyneuropathy is very unlike the acute dissemination PNS syndrome. It is quite subtle, with occasional paresthesias or shock-like pains, and requires electrophysiologic testing to document peripheral involvement with a predominantly axonal component. This syndrome seems to be much rarer in recent years. Chronic encephalomyelitis is probably the rarest neurologic syndrome, seen particularly in Europe and associated with *B. garinii*. It can mimic brain tumor, multiple sclerosis, or movement disorders. Unusual neurologic syndromes associated with *B. burgdorferi* infection include myopathy, stroke-like, or vasculitic syndromes, multifocal encephalitis, and acute CNS inflammatory demyelinating disease (post-infectious encephalomyelitis).

Diagnosis

Diagnosis requires endemic area exposure. Time spent out of doors, especially in high risk areas, increases the likelihood of Lyme disease. Lyme disease also produces suggestive syndromes. The EM rash is so pathognomonic that it requires no supportive laboratory data and establishes the diagnosis. Multifocal EM documents dissemination. The other suggestive syndromes associated with early dissemination or late stage infection should be supported by laboratory data.

Unfortunately, there is no reliable direct infection assay. Culture is impractical: it requires specialized facilities and media, takes weeks for the organism to grow out, and provides high yield only in limited circumstances (punch biopsy of the EM site). Detection of spirochete nucleic acid using polymerase chain reaction (PCR) gives a reasonable yield in synovial fluid but a poor yield in CSF and serum/plasma. The spirochetes are tissue tropic and do not float free in body fluids. They are not detectable in blood except briefly during the dissemination period. Finally, no useful antigen test is available.

The most valuable diagnostic laboratory test remains serology. However, seropositivity indicates historic exposure rather than active infection. Currently, a two tier system is used. The first tier employs a rapid screening test, typically direct or indirect ELISA (enzyme-linked immunosorbent assay) (which is preferred to immunofluorescent assay (IFA)) using spirochetal sonicate preparations or less commonly recombinant proteins. Since spirochetes contain over one hundred organism-specific and non-specific antigens, legitimate false positives occur. Controls can show strong non-specific p41 flagellin or p58–60 heat shock protein responses, with resulting positive ELISA. Dental work can seed benign mouth spirochetes to result in a false positive first tier serology, as can high titers of autoantibodies with cross reactivity. Low positive or fluctuating positive ELISA should always raise concerns about a false positive. The second tier test is a more labor-intensive Western blot. In the US, Western blot has been partially standardized. Positive IgM Western blot must have two of three bands (23, 39, 41). Positive IgG Western blot must have 5 of 10 bands (18, 23, 28, 30, 39, 41, 45, 58, 66, 93). Recently a C6 peptide antibody assay has been offered, which purportedly boosts specificity. It uses the IR6 region (a unique 25 amino acid recombinant peptide sequence) of the surface protein VlsE. Unfortunately, as currently configured, it is not sufficiently sensitive or specific to serve as a single-tier test.

Seronegative cases of Lyme disease occur (probably less than 10%). Early antibiotics can abort the typical humoral response, and create such a seronegative.

CSF is generally abnormal in neurologic cases, and is more inflammatory early on. However, spirochetes have been isolated from normal CSF. In Europe inflammatory CSF is required for diagnosis, while in the US normal CSF is not felt to exclude neurologic involvement. The most valuable CSF test is intrathecal anti-*B. burgdorferi* antibody production, which requires paired CSF and serum samples. In Europe all neurologic cases show intrathecal antibody production, while in the US only 60% of Lyme meningitis cases show it. Mononuclear pleocytosis

(sometimes with a plasma cell component) and increased protein are suggestive but non-specific findings. CSF oligoclonal bands and elevated IgG index are present in all European cases but noted in less than 20% of US cases.

Other helpful diagnostic tests include electrophysiologic studies to document suggestive PNS involvement (polyradiculoneuropathy, median nerve entrapment, myopathic process). Magnetic resonance imaging (MRI) is typically normal, but may show lesions in up to 25% of cases. There is no characteristic pattern; the most frequently reported findings are of small, peripheral, vasculitic-like lesions. Brain single photon emission computed tomography (SPECT) shows abnormal blood flow pattern in late Lyme encephalopathy. Cognitive function testing can document objective abnormalities (but without a unique pattern). All the above objective abnormalities can improve post treatment.

Therapy

Lyme disease is a bacterial infection that responds to appropriate antibiotic therapy, started as soon as possible. Local infection and dissemination syndromes spontaneously clear, but will do so faster with treatment. Late syndromes do not spontaneously clear, but following treatment slowly improve over months.

EM is treated with oral antibiotics (doxycycline, amoxicillin, cefuroxime axetil). Doxycycline is used at 100 mg twice a day (pediatric dose: 2 mg/kg twice a day), amoxicillin at 500 mg three times daily (50 mg/kg/day in three divided doses), and cefuroxime axetil at 500 mg twice a day (30 mg/kg divided twice a day). EM is treated for 14–21 days. Doxycyline covers *Ehrlichia* infection (a tick co-pathogen) as well, so it is generally preferred. Doxycyline is not recommended in children under the age of 8 or in pregnant or lactating women, because of concerns about adverse dentition effects.

Neurologic Lyme disease is treated with intravenous ceftriaxone, a third-generation cephalosporin. The standard dose is 2 g daily for 14–30 days (pediatric dose: 50–75 mg/kg daily). It is a convenient outpatient therapy. A peripherally inserted central catheter (PICC) line or midline can be inserted and used for the duration of treatment. Acidophilus is taken daily to avoid pseudomembraneous colitis. For very severe late infections, treatment is sometimes extended up to 8 weeks.

Approximately 5–15% of those with penicillin allergy are allergic to cephalosporins. This can be assessed through formal testing. Desensitization protocols are available, or an alternative regimen can be used. Alternatives include cefotaxime at 2 g three times daily (pediatric dose: 100–200 mg/kg daily in three or four divided doses), doxycycline (typically 200 mg twice a day for better CNS penetration), or penicillin G at 18–24 mU daily divided every 4 hours (200 000–400 000 U/kg, divided every 4 hours).

Prevention

Preventive strategies include avoidance of tick-infested habitats, use of personal protective measures, reduction of tick populations, and daily tick checks, since the tick has to feed for longer than 24 hours to transmit infection. A single dose of 200 mg of doxycycline, if given within 72 hours of tick bite, shows 87% efficacy in preventing EM. EM developed in only 0.4% of cases (1:235) vs 3.2% (8:247) of those who received placebo. At the current time no human preventive vaccines are available.

Tick co-pathogens

Ticks are fairly dirty reservoirs. Ixodid ticks may contain multiple *B. burgdorferi* strains, other spirochetes, *Babesia microti*, the *Ehrlichia Anaplasma phagocytophilum*, viruses (tick-borne encephalitis virus in eastern Europe and Asia, Powassan deer tick virus in eastern South America), *Rickettsia* species, Bartonella, and other agents yet to be identified. It is possible to get dual infections, which may impact the severity of Lyme disease.

Pathogenesis

Pathology
The neuropathology of Lyme disease shows little overt destruction. Spirochetes are sparse and extracellular. CNS findings include mild meningeal and perivascular mononuclear inflammation, occasional spirochetes, microglial modules, mild spongiform changes, and rarely obliterative vasculopathy, demyelination, or granulomatous changes. PNS findings are consistent with axon damage, epineural, perineural, perivascular and vasa nervorum inflammation, and angiopathy. Muscle has shown focal myositis, interstitial inflammation, focal necrosis, and rare spirochetes. This lack of damage suggests that immunologic/inflammatory factors are important.

Pathophysiology
There are many different strains of *B. burgdorferi,* with different virulence and tissue tropism properties that factor into disease expression. *Borrelia burgdorferi* can persist for years undetected. Except during early infection, there are very small numbers of organisms within infected tissues. This implicates immune/inflammatory factors in pathogenesis. The bacterium produces inflammation out of proportion to spirochete numbers. Spirochetal lipoproteins activate the immune system. At least 132 genes encode putative lipoproteins, predominantly surface proteins, membrane proteins, and immunogens. *Borrelia burgdorferi* outer surface lipoproteins activate macrophages/monocytes, endothelial cells, neutrophils, and B cells, and induce cytokines including chemokines. Spirochetes are extracellular but tissue tropic. They bind to endothelium, platelets (via integrins), and most mammalian cells (via glycosaminoglycans). They are often associated with extracellular matrix collagen fibers. Spirochetes generate cross-reactive immunity to a number of autoantigens, which may also play a role in pathogenesis.

Chronic Lyme disease

Chronic Lyme disease (also called chronic Lyme or post Lyme syndrome) is a poorly understood syndrome which is a clinical issue in the United States. There are no consensus diagnostic criteria. The most logical definition involves patients who are treated for Lyme disease but experience persistent problems that date to their infection. This most often involves nonspecific and subjective pain (headache, arthralgias, myalgias), fatigue, paresthesias, and cognitive issues. Unfortunately, patients who have unexplained complaints without a history of Lyme disease are also diagnosed. They have been treated with unusual antibiotics, prolonged courses, or combination therapy. The etiology of chronic Lyme disease is not known, but probably encompasses several entities. First, it may reflect persistent infection not eradicated by prior antibiotics. This would seem most likely in patients who had a CNS infection but received only oral antibiotics. In a limited number of formal studies, most patients do not appear to show antibiotic responsiveness. Second, it could involve sequelae of infection by an unrecognized tick copathogen. Third, it could represent an immune-mediated syndrome. Chronic Lyme arthritis, which occurs in up to 10% of Lyme arthritis patients, is a non-antibiotic-responsive immune-mediated syndrome which is linked to certain HLA-DR4 alleles, and characterized by a strong systemic and synovial immune response against the OspA protein. In a single patient with persistent neurologic complaints, CSF studies showed a T-cell clone responsive to both spirochete and autoantigen epitopes. Other potential causes include reinfection with *B. burgdorferi*, fixed deficit, an alternative diagnosis (such as vascular headache), and hypochondriosis.

Further reading

Belman AL, Iyer M, Coyle PK, *et al*. Neurologic manifestations in children with North American Lyme disease. *Neurology* 1993; 43: 2609–14.

Feder HM, Johnson BJB, O'Connell S, *et al*. A critical appraisal of "Chronic Lyme disease". *N Engl J Med* 2008; 358: 428–31.

Halperin JJ, Shapiro ED, Logigian E, *et al*. Practice parameter: treatment of nervous system Lyme disease (an evidence-based review): report of the quality standards subcommittee of the American Academy of Neurology. *Neurology* 2007; 69(1): 91–102.

Logigian E, Kaplan R, Steere A. Chronic neurologic manifestations of Lyme disease. *N Engl J Med* 1990; 323: 1438–44.

Stanek G, Strie F. Lyme borreliosis. *Lancet* 2003; 362: 1639–47.

Steere AC. Lyme disease. *N Engl J Med* 2001; 345: 115–24.

Chapter 76
Fungal infections of the central nervous system

Thomas C. Cesario
University California, Irvine, USA

Introduction

Fungal infections of the central nervous system (CNS) are less common than bacterial infections but can be devastating and difficult to treat. They can exist in nature as primary pathogens; however, they often prey on compromised patients.

Candidiasis

Among the most commonly encountered fungi are members of the *Candida* genus, including agents such as *Candida albicans*, *Candida glabrata*, *Candida parapsilosis*, and *Candida tropicalis*. These organisms can be found on the normal host, especially after antibiotic therapy, or may exist in patients predisposed to colonization such as individuals with diabetes mellitus or AIDS, transplant patients, or chemotherapy patients. These fungi also may be encountered in neonates and individuals suffering from congenital immune deficiency diseases. *Candida* organisms exist worldwide.

In the largest reviews of *Candida* meningitis, headache and fever were common; sensorium was altered in some patients. Symptoms often existed for long periods prior to diagnosis – as long as 21 months. Cerebrospinal fluid (CSF) findings typically showed pleocytosis, but polymorphonuclear or lymphocytic cells also predominated. Cultures of the CSF grew *Candida* but with some difficulty, often requiring repeated taps and special efforts. Amphotericin plus flucytosine is the preferred treatment.

Candida meningitis also has been reported in neonates in association with disseminated infection, prematurity being a risk factor. The clinical features are similar to those of other systemic infections although CSF findings seem somewhat inconsistent. It has been reported in both children and adults with cancer, CSF shunts, and HIV. This infection may occur in adults as either an isolated CNS infection or as part of disseminated candidiasis. The disease has a relatively prolonged course and a 50% mortality rate. The best prognosis is in patients with CSF shunts when the device is removed and the patients treated. Diagnosis is often made by culture of CFS although more than one lumbar puncture may be needed. There may also be other inflammatory CNS changes. Patients should be treated at least initially with amphotericin and flucytosine, but newer antifungals such as micafungin and andalufungin may turn out to be equal or better alternatives.

Aspergillosis

Aspergillus species are ubiquitous in nature in soil, water, and organic materials. They typically do not pose a threat for the immunocompetent patient but may be cultured from the body particularly after broad spectrum antibiotic therapy. In contrast, they may induce disease in compromised individuals including patients with cancer, especially with hematologic malignancies, HIV, transplants, high dose steroid therapy, or other immunocompromised states. The organisms may produce either meningitis or a localized aspergilloma. In many cases *Aspergillus* tends to invade blood vessels and as such may induce vascular obstruction with downstream consequences. Typically patients have CNS disease resulting from infection in other organs, especially the lungs. Findings usually include those associated with mass lesions including focal neurological deficits and mental status changes. Meningitis occurs in a similar setting and may be manifest by fever, mental status changes, seizures, and focal deficits. Attempts to culture the organism can be difficult, but other organs besides the CNS can be cultured because the disease is usually disseminated. Where lesions are localized, surgical intervention plus antifungal therapy may be critical. Where the disease involves the meninges or is diffuse, antifungal therapy including either voriconizole, posoconazole, itraconazole, or caspofungin should be instituted immediately. Prognosis is guarded at best.

International Neurology: A Clinical Approach. Edited by Robert P. Lisak, Daniel D. Truong, William M. Carroll, and Roongroj Bhidayasiri. © 2009 Blackwell Publishing, ISBN: 978-1-4051-5738-4.

Cryptococcosis

Cryptococcus and related fungi are encapsulated yeast that can be detected in nature. There are three pathogenic varieties of *Cryptococcus*: neoformans, neoformans variant grubii, and neoformans variant gattii. The first two of these are found throughout the world in areas where bird droppings are common and when rotting vegetation is in the vicinity. The gattii variety is cultured from river red gum trees and forest red gum trees common to Australia but also in areas receiving exported red gum trees, including California.

CNS infection with cryptococci is a threat to immunocompromised patients. While infection of the lung can be seen in individuals without apparent underlying disease, this is usually not the case with infection in the nervous system. When the immune system, and particularly delayed hypersensitivity, is intact the organism tends to be confined to the lung where it is initially inhaled. Cryptococcal pneumonia, lung nodules, or lung abscesses may be seen in otherwise normal patients and may resolve on their own. On the other hand, when underlying disease such as hematological malignancies, AIDs, or severe pharmacological immune suppression is present, this organism may escape the lung and target other organs for metastatic infections. The preferred extrapulmonary site is the meninges and to a lesser extent the prostate, skin, and bones. Before effective AIDS treatment was available 5–10% of these patients in the United States and as many as 30% in Africa developed cryptococcal meningitis. Typically, 300–500 cases of non-AIDS-related cryptococcal meningitis are seen annually in the United States.

In AIDS patients, the manifestations of disease are slightly different but the signs and symptoms of CNS cryptococcal disease are similar. The most significant findings are those associated with chronic meningitis. The incubation period is often weeks and can be longer than a month. Generally, in the more immune-suppressed patients this period will be shorter. Disease onset is typically associated with headache and there may be altered consciousness, focal neurological signs and indications of increased intracranial pressure when obstruction to the flow of the CSF occurs. Fever and meningismus may or may not be present. Signs and symptoms of CNS cryptococcal infection may be gradually progressive over many months or years but invariably if untreated leads to death. Complications may occur including blindness and intracranial hypertension. Cryptococci in the brain also may produce mass lesions that typically present as other space-occupying masses.

Diagnosis of CNS infection is made by examination of the CSF using the cryptococcal latex agglutination test (LACT); serum LACT often supports diagnosis, and is positive in 70% of non-AIDS patients and over 90% of AIDS patients with CNS infection. The organism is also cultured on ordinary bacterial culture media, from the CSF, bone marrow, blood, or urine. The CSF, in cases of cryptococcal meningitis, will have 10–100 cells/ml usually, but not always, with lymphocytic predominance. Low CSF glucose and high CSF protein concentrations may be present and likely correlate with the disease duration and burden of the fungi. The LACT needs to be titered in the CSF as it is a therapeutic index and has significant prognostic implications. Culture of the CSF is important. If examination of the CSF is precluded by severe intracranial hypertension or mass effect, attempts to culture the organisms from other sites and serum LACT may be useful. Radiological examinations including computerized tomography (CT) and magnetic resonance imaging (MRI) show no diagnostic abnormality specific to cryptococcal disease but may show changes similar to those seen in other cases of chronic meningitis or mass lesions.

Therapy should be initiated with amphotericin (0.5–0.7 mg/kg/day) plus flucytosine (100–150 mg/kg/day in four divided doses) for the first 2 weeks and followed by oral fluconazole (400 mg/day) if the patient improves. If the patient fails to improve or has poor prognostic indicators, a repeat lumbar puncture is indicated. The amphotericin/flucytosine combination should be continued if the initial response to therapy is poor until cultures are negative. Antifungal treatment including fluconazole should be continued until the cultures are negative and the LACT titer falls to levels less than one to eight. Other CSF abnormalities are expected to return to normal during treatment. AIDS patients require continuous suppressive treatment with fluconazole at 200 mg/day when the patients have completed the course of therapy.

Patients need to be continuously monitored after treatment in case of relapse, including repeat lumbar puncture at periodic intervals until there has been no evidence of relapse for at least 1 year. The majority of patients will do well, but bad prognostic indicators include the severity of the underlying disease, very high CSF LACT titers, and failure to respond to treatment.

The course of treatment outlined above generally yields good results and has reduced the mortality rate to 5–20% dependent in part on the population being studied.

Coccidioidomycosis

Coccidioides immitis is a dimorphic fungus which grows in semi-arid regions of the world including the southwestern United States, northern Mexico, Guatemala, Nicaragua, Bolivia, Paraguay, Venezuela, Argentina, and Columbia. The organism grows in its saprobic state a few inches below the surface. It forms small regions on its filaments called arthroconidia which are prone to break free. During the dry season they are often aerosolized and can be carried long distances when it is windy. When inhaled, arthroconidia are converted within 2 days to the parasitic spherule. These enlarge and ultimately contain multiple endospores. Inhalation from the soil has been the predominant means by which humans acquire the fungus. The organism is quite infectious and individuals living in endemic areas have a skin test conversion rate of 3% per year.

When inhaled, *Coccidioides* initially becomes an asymptomatic or mildly symptomatic infection of the lung that does not precipitate a visit to a physician. The incubation period is 7–21 days. While up to half of patients may have some radiographic evidence of infection in the lung, only 5–10% develop pulmonary residuals including cavitary lesions. Erythema nodosum and erythema multiforme are also seen during the infection. Patients with intact cellular immune systems rarely develop complications from dissemination. However, certain ethnic groups are prone to developing disease from dissemination and these include Filipinos, Mexicans, and Blacks. Pregnant women, especially in the third trimester, patients receiving immunosuppressants, patients with diabetes, hematological malignancies, and AIDS may experience severe problems from dissemination.

Less than 1% of patients develop disseminated disease that requires attention. The usual sites where the presence of the fungus becomes evident include the meninges, bone, particularly the vertebrae, joints, skin, and components of the genitourinary system. The meninges, however, are among the most important and most frequent of these. Patients who develop coccidioidal meningitis have headache which is often one of the first signs. As the disease progresses, they will develop other signs and symptoms that may include gait disturbances, focal findings, altered consciousness, cranial nerve signs, and papilledema as evidence of basilar meningeal inflammation. Fever is common and meningismus may be seen in about half the cases. Left untreated the disease will inevitably progress to death within 2 years. Complications include hydrocephalus in 30–50% of patients and brain infarction.

The diagnosis of coccidioidal meningitis rests largely on the examination of the CSF. The cell count is usually between 100 and 1500 cells/ml^3, most of which will be lymphocytes. As the disease progress, the glucose level in the CSF will fall and the protein level will rise to concentrations in the range of 250 mg. Higher concentrations occur with obstruction to the flow of the CSF. The organism may be cultured from the CSF but only in about 15% of cases. The specific diagnosis is usually made by detection of antibodies in the CSF using the complement fixation method. Repeated examinations are sometimes necessary to find the antibody in spinal fluid, but it usually is detectable within 3 weeks after the onset of the symptoms.

Fluconazole in doses of 400–800 mg/day is recommended. Patients should begin to experience symptomatic relief after the onset of treatment, but if they continue to progress and show evidence of failing to respond, intrathecal amphotericin is instituted. This may be delivered intracisternally or through an Ommaya reservoir. Doses are adjusted, beginning with 0.01 mg and increasing as tolerated, with a maximum dose of 1.5 mg being given. The dosing interval may also be adjusted from daily to weekly as indicated. With this regimen it can be expected that 75–80% of patients will respond. Other agents may also be effective including itraconazole, posoconazole, and lipid encapsulated amphotericin. There is less experience with these other agents.

Mucormycosis (zygomycosis)

The Phycomycetes are an order of fungi that includes both the Mucorales and the Entomorphthorales, agents responsible for nasal diseases. The Mucorales include three species of filamentous agents which are largely responsible for the disease of mucormycosis. These agents are ubiquitous in the environment and frequently encountered through the aerosol route, but only compromised patients are at serious risk from these fungi. Patients with diabetes, especially when acidotic, those on steroids, with hematologic malignancies, transplant history, AIDS, renal or hepatic failure, who are malnourished, or have immune deficiencies face a significant threat from these agents. Rarely, people who have no underlying disease encounter problems from these organisms.

The most common form of nervous system infection with the Phycomycetes is rhinocerebral mucormycosis. This begins in the sinuses and nasal cavities and gradually erodes through tissues and in blood vessels to invade intracranial structures and cause infarction of cerebral tissue. Symptoms often include nasal stuffiness, purulent nasal discharge, sinus pain, and headache. Signs include fever, black eschars in the nose and sometimes on the hard palate, periorbital edema, proptosis, and eventually blindness. Signs and symptoms relate to the route by which the fungus spreads. Cavernous sinus thrombosis may occur. When the frontal lobes become involved, obtundation may develop. Less commonly, there are instances of isolated metastatic lesions to the brain, with development of symptoms related to mass effect and localisation.

Invasive fungal rhinosinusitis is a life-threatening infection. Diagnosis is established by demonstration of the fungal filaments in tissue sections. Current therapy includes amphotericin and extensive surgical debridement. Experimentally there is some evidence that posoconazole may be useful. With maximal therapy the mortality rate ranges from 25% to 75% depending in part on the underlying disease and the stage at which diagnosis is established and treatment undertaken.

Histoplasmosis

Histoplasma capsulatum is a dimorphic fungus whose physical state is related to the temperature of its environment. In nature it is in the mycelial state and in humans it is in the yeast phase. Moist, shady soil, fertilized with bird or bat droppings in moderate climates is the favored environment for the organism. *Histoplasma* has been found in the United States in the Mississippi and Ohio River valleys. It has also been found in Latin America and along the St Lawrence River. In addition, cases have been identified in Europe and Asia.

Man acquires *Histoplasma* by inhaling the infectious microconidia. The majority of infections are without symptoms and only about 5% will develop a self-limited flu-like illness. Most problematic cases evolve into subacute pulmonary infections with focal infiltrates and hilar or mediastinal nodes. Cavities may result. Nodular lung lesions may go on to calcify. Immunocompromised patients who fail to contain the organism and progress to dissemination can acquire serious disease with multiorgan involvement including mucous membranes, liver, spleen, and bone marrow. Of these cases, 5–25% will develop CNS disease, either solid intracerebral lesions or basilar meningitis. The solid lesions will present as mass lesions and the basilar meningitis may have the typical meningeal array of signs and symptoms including fever, meningismus, and abnormal CSF. Diagnosis is established by culture (25–50% positive) or detection of antigen or antibody in the CSF. Often it is necessary to culture the organism from other sites, particularly bone marrow, to detect antigen in urine or serum or antibody in serum. Treatment consists of amphotericin (1.0–1.5 g total dose given over 30–40 administrations) or lipid-encapsulated amphotericin (3–5 mg/kg/day to a total dose of 100–150 g) daily for 6–12 weeks, followed by suppression with itraconazole (200 mg twice or thrice daily) or fluconazole (600–800 mg/day). With this regimen there is a 20% failure rate but a relapse rate that can be as high as 40%. Lipid formulations of amphotericin B can be associated with less infusion-related toxicity and less nephrotoxicity.

Blastomycosis

Blastomyces dermatitidis is a dimorphic fungus from North and South America, Europe, Africa, and Asia. There is insufficient information about the environment in which it exists, but it appears to be a soil organism found along riverbeds particularly in areas with organic matter as part of the soil. The pathogenesis of the disease is very similar to histoplasmosis, with the organism entering the lung and primary disease being pulmonary in nature. Dissemination can occur, but it is primarily a disease of the immunocompetent person, affecting skin, bone, the genitourinary tract, and CNS. Approximately 10% of cases involve the CNS, causing either nodular lesions in the brain or a basilar meningitis. The CNS disease has the same features as histoplasmosis but is more difficult to diagnose as culture from the CSF appears harder and serologies are less reliable. Besides culturing multiple sites in the body, particularly bone marrow, involved tissue, and urine, serologies should be done and biopsies with histological examination for the organism carried out. The only treatment known so far is amphotericin.

Further reading

Casado JL, Quereda C, Corral I. Candidal meningitis in HIV infected patients. *AIDS Patient Care STDS* 1998; 12: 681–6.

Friedman JA, Wijdicks FM, Fulgham J, Wright AJ. Meningoencephalitis due to *Blastomyces dermatitidis*. *Mayo Clin Proc* 2000; 75: 403–8.

Gorbach S, Bartlett R, Blacklow N. *Infectious Diseases*. Philadelphia, PA: WB Saunders; 1998.

Kleinschmidt-Demasters BK. Central nervous system aspergillosis: a 20 year retrospective study. *Hum Pathol* 2002; 33: 116–24.

Pagano L, Ricci P, Tonso A, *et al.* Mucormycosis in patients with hematological malignancies: a retrospective study of 37 cases. *Br J Haematol* 1997; 99: 331–6.

Shih CC, Chen YC, Chang SC, Luh KT, Hsieh WC. Cryptococcal meningitis in non HIV infected patients. *Q J Med* 2000; 93: 245–51.

Sundaram C, Mahadevan A, Laxmi V, *et al.* Cerebral zygomycosis. *Mycoses* 2005; 48: 396–407.

Treseler C, Sugar A. Fungal meningitis. In: Scheld WM, Wispelwey B, editors. *Infectious Disease Clinics of North America*, Vol. 4. Philadelphia, PA: WB Saunders; 1990, pp. 789–808.

Voice RA, Bradley SF, Sangeorzan JA, Kauffman CA. Chronic candidal meningitis: an uncommon manifestation of candidiasis. *Clin Infect Dis* 1994; 19: 60–66.

Wheat LJ, Musial CE, Jenny-Avital E. Diagnosis and management of central nervous system histoplasmosis. *Clin Infect Dis* 2005; 40: 844–52.

Williams PL. Coccidioidal meningitis. *Ann N Y Acad Sci* 2007; 1111: 377–84.

Chapter 77
Introduction to protozoans of the central nervous system

Marylou V. Solbrig
University of Manitoba, Winnipeg, Canada

Apex predators try to kill and eat you immediately on the prairie or *veldt*, while parasites try to infect but keep you alive. Protozoans are obligate intracellular parasites. Generally, they cause mild or persistent subacute infections, and protozoan diseases are among the most common and successful parasitic diseases of man. However, when protozoans access an immunoprivileged site such as the brain or eye, or spread to an immunocompromised host, these organisms produce severe infections.

Protozoans pathogenic for man are found in both rich and poor countries, in both tropical and temperate climates. The number of infected hosts, plus the low success rates and high CNS toxicities of the best available treatments for some, render protozoan diseases significant contributors to the global burden of infectious diseases. The medical needs related to pathogens in this group, especially their neurologic complications, remain challenging and incompletely met.

Malaria is the most important parasitic disease of man. It affects over 1 billion people worldwide and causes 1–3 million deaths per year, many from cerebral malaria. Malaria, transmitted by the bite of infected *Anopheles* mosquitoes, poses a heavy burden in tropical communities, threatens non-endemic countries, and presents a danger to travelers. Drug resistance has evolved and, despite efforts, successful vaccines have not been developed.

The genus *Trypanosoma* contains many species of protozoans. *Trypanosoma cruzi*, the cause of Chagas' disease in the Americas, and the two trypanosome subspecies that cause human African trypanosomiasis, *Trypanosoma brucei gambiense* and *T. brucei rhodesiense*, are the only members of the genus that cause disease in humans.

In South America where an estimated 8% of the population is seropositive, *T. cruzi* is spread by an infected assassin bug bite, transfusion, transplant, or *in utero* exposure. American trypanosomiasis (Chagas' disease) is a significant cause of cardiovascular and thromboembolic

disease and there is no specific therapy to treat chronic disease.

Human African trypanosomiasis is associated with complex public health and epizootic problems, such that eradication has not been possible. The tsetse fly is the vector and infection reservoirs are present in cattle and other animals. In man, once nervous system treatment is required, therapy can be unsatisfactory due to poor tolerance and high toxicity of medications.

Amoebae species are global pathogens. *Entamoeba histolytica* occurs in fecally-contaminated water, food, or hands. Free-living amoebas of genera *Acanthamoeba*, *Naegleria*, and *Balamuthia* have been isolated from fresh and brackish water throughout the world. Any part of the body may be affected by *Entamoeba* via hematogenous dissemination from the colon or liver. Acanthamoeba cause corneal, systemic, or cerebral disease. *Naegleria* causes a meningoencephalitis that is usually fatal.

Toxoplasmosis is a worldwide pathogen, spread from contaminated hands, food, or water, or acquired *in utero* or via transplant. Seropositive populations are found in many temperate zones. Seropositive populations approaching 100% are reported in some moist tropical climates. A known cause of congenital infections and retinochoroiditis, toxoplasmosis had been a rare opportunistic infection of immunocompromised patients until the time of AIDS. Early in the AIDS epidemic, cerebral toxoplasmosis was the most frequent cause of focal cerebral lesions in HIV disease.

The protozoans of neurologic importance in man are presented in the chapters that follow. Their diagnosis is considered when evaluating neurologic illness in residents in endemic regions, in travelers to endemic areas, in individuals who are immunosuppressed due to medication or concurrent disease, in recent recipients of transfusions or transplants, in neonates who acquired infection *in utero*, or in others with pertinent exposures.

International Neurology: A Clinical Approach. Edited by Robert P. Lisak, Daniel D. Truong, William M. Carroll, and Roongroj Bhidayasiri. © 2009 Blackwell Publishing, ISBN: 978-1-4051-5738-4.

Chapter 78
Amoebic disease of the central nervous system

Melanie Walker
University of Washington School of Medicine, Seattle, USA

Introduction

Free-living amoebas *Acanthamoeba* species, *Balamuthia mandrillaris, Entamoeba histolytica,* and *Naegleria fowleri* cause extremely rare and sporadic central nervous system (CNS) infections. Typically, *N. fowleri* produces primary amoebic meningoencephalitis (PAM), which is clinically indistinguishable from acute bacterial meningitis. Infection by other amoebas causes granulomatous amoebic encephalitis (GAE), which is a more subacute or chronic infection. The presentation of GAE can mimic a brain abscess, aseptic or chronic meningitis, or CNS malignancy. While *Entamoeba* spp. are the least likely to invade the CNS, they deserve mention because they are the most common human amoebic pathogens.

Epidemiology

Although these one-celled protozoa are simple in form, amoebas are found abundantly in a variety of habitats all over the world. Amoebas thrive in aquatic environments – freshwater as well as ocean – and in the upper layers of the soil. Many have adapted parasitic lifestyles on the body surface of aquatic animals, as well as in the internal organs of both aquatic and terrestrial animals. Few animals escape invasion by some type of amoeba, and humans are no exception. Some are harmless, but others are pathogenic and can impart serious disease burden: amoebic dysentery affects hundreds of millions of people worldwide, causing mortality second only to malaria.

While amoebic CNS diseases are rare, cases have been reported worldwide, which reflects the ubiquity of the organisms. Warmer climates (and warmer seasons of the year) tend to harbor a higher number of *reported* cases. While most reports come from the United States, Australia,

and Europe, this is likely secondary to identification and/or reporting bias.

These infections are almost always fatal and it is likely that many cases go unrecognized. Only a handful of survivors of PAM have been reported. The high mortality rate is multifactorial: diagnosis is difficult and response to therapy is poor-to-marginal, and the contribution of immunosuppression in some patients also impacts outcome. In most individuals with PAM or GAE, a diagnosis is not made until after death. PAM has been reported in infants as young as 4 months, but it appears to be most common in the first three decades of life. Although persons of any age can be affected by GAE, infection appears more commonly in individuals at the extremes of age. Immunosuppression can contribute to CNS dissemination and also primary infection in GAE, but does not appear to play a role in PAM.

Pathophysiology

PAM secondary to *N. fowleri* is an exceptionally uncommon result of CNS invasion of a healthy host, following the very common exposure to the amoeba during routine activities of daily living. For unknown reasons, not all individuals who harbor the amoeba develop disease. Young children frequently carry the organism asymptomatically in their nasopharyngeal tract. Infection develops over a period of hours to 2 weeks after swimming, diving, bathing, or playing in warm, usually stagnant, freshwater. *Naegleria fowleri* is believed to migrate through the cribriform plate near the site of entry in the nasopharynx, along the fila olfactoria and blood vessels, and into the anterior cerebral fossa. Extensive inflammation, necrosis, and hemorrhage develop rapidly into meningoencephalitis.

In contrast, GAE appears to result from either acanthamoebic keratoconjunctivitis, which is the uncommon spread of the amoeba from the cornea into the CNS, or hematogenous spread of all of these ubiquitous organisms (e.g., *Acanthamoeba* or *Balamuthia* spp.) from primary inoculation sites in the lungs or skin into the CNS. Abscesses and focal granulomatous infections result, and, as such,

International Neurology: A Clinical Approach. Edited by Robert P. Lisak, Daniel D. Truong, William M. Carroll, and Roongroj Bhidayasiri.
© 2009 Blackwell Publishing, ISBN: 978-1-4051-5738-4.

it is not uncommon to see bilateral intracranial pathology. *Entamoeba histolytica* is the most common pathogen responsible for amoebic dysentery. The organism is transmitted in cyst form from feces-contaminated food or water by way of food handlers (usually asymptomatic carriers), flies, cockroaches, and from sexual contact. The infective cyst stage develops into a trophozoite in the small intestine. Trophozoites readily die outside the body, but while inside they release an enzyme that dissolves tissue which allows them to penetrate beyond the intestinal mucosa. If the disease disseminates beyond the gastrointestinal tract, abscesses may develop on the brain, in the lungs, heart, or other tissues, and death can result.

Clinical features

As with all neurologic disease, signs and symptoms are referable to the anatomic location more than the underlying disease mechanism. As such, it is difficult to make a definitive diagnosis based on clinical findings. Amoebic CNS disease presents a number of diagnostic challenges; however, there may be some clues for the astute health care provider. PAM presents with severe headache and other meningeal signs, such as, fever, vomiting, and focal neurologic deficits, and tends to evolve quickly (less than

10 days). Initial symptoms are typically not recognized as dangerous by many patients, since they may be vague. Rapid progression to coma and death is the most common clinical scenario with PAM. *Acanthamoeba* spp. cause mostly subacute or chronic GAE, with a clinical picture of headaches, altered mental status, and focal neurologic deficit, which generally progresses to death over several weeks. Additionally, *Acanthamoeba* spp. can cause granulomatous skin lesions, keratitis, and corneal ulcers following corneal trauma or in association with contact lens use – which may provide an early opportunity for treatment. Non-contact lens users and contact lens users with safe lens care practices can become infected. However, poor contact lens hygiene and exposure to contaminated water may increase the risk among contact lens users.

Investigations

While amoebic disease can be difficult to diagnose, laboratory evaluation offers the highest likelihood of pathogen identification. Light microscopy is accessible in almost every medical setting around the world. Neuroimaging with CT or MRI can be helpful in managing acute treatment; however, imaging alone will not provide a definitive diagnosis. Imaging and pathologic findings in amoebic CNS disease are discussed in Table 78.1.

Table 78.1 Imaging and pathologic findings in amoebic CNS disease.

	Laboratory diagnosis	CT scan	MRI scan
Granulomatous amoebic encephalitis (GAE)			
Acanthamoeba spp., *Balamuthia mandrillaris, Entamoeba histolytica*	Microscopic examination of stained smears of biopsy specimens (brain tissue, skin, and cornea) or of corneal scrapings may detect trophozoites and cysts. Confocal microscopy or cultivation of the causal organism, and its identification by direct immunofluorescent antibody, may also prove useful. An increasing number of PCR-based techniques (conventional and real-time PCR) have been described for detection and identification of free-living amoebic infections in the clinical samples listed above. Such techniques may be available in selected reference diagnostic laboratories. Because *Entamoeba* spp. disseminate from the intestinal tract to the brain, wet mounts and permanently stained preparations (e.g., trichrome) of fresh stool samples should be used for diagnosis	Multiple bilateral enhancing lesions involving the cerebral cortex and underlying white matter, with mild mass effect; hemorrhage commonly seen within the lesion(s). May also appear as solitary space-occupying lesions associated with mass effect	Multifocal lesions showing T2 hyperintensity and a heterogeneous or ring-like pattern of enhancement. Hemorrhage within the lesion can be confirmed with gradient echo imaging. May also present as a mass lesion with linear and superficial gyriform pattern of enhancement
Primary amoebic meningoencephalitis (PAM)			
Naegleria fowleri and other spp.	A wet mount of CSF may detect motile trophozoites, and a Giemsa-stained smear will show trophozoites with typical morphology	May be normal in early disease; later findings include evidence of generalized edema and basilar meningeal enhancement	Edema can be visualized on T2 sequence even early in the course of disease; obliteration of vessels secondary to edema can lead to infarction; basilar meningeal enhancement can be seen subacutely

Table 78.2 Treatment for amoebic disease of the CNS.

Infection	Drug	Adult dosage	Pediatric dosage
Acanthamoeba spp.		*In vitro* data only* for pentamidine, ketoconazole, and flucytosine	
Balamuthia mandrillaris		Data only as adjunct to surgical therapy[†]	
Entamoeba histolytica[‡]	Primary: metronidazole	750 mg TID × 7–10 days	35–50 mg/kg/day in 3 doses × 7–10 days
	Alternative: tinidazole[§]	2 g once daily × 5 days	50 mg/kg/day (maximum 2 g) × 5 days
Naegleria fowleri and other spp.	Amphotericin B[¶]	1.5 mg/kg/day in 2 doses × 3 days, then 1 mg/kg/day × 6 days	1.5 mg/kg/day in 2 doses × 3 days, then 1 mg/kg/day × 6 days

*In children, combination therapy with oral trimethoprim/sulfamethoxazole, rifampin, and ketoconazole may provide benefit.
[†]Case reports up to the time of publication suggest that flucytosine, pentamidine, fluconazole and sulfadiazine (plus either azithromycin or clarithromycin) may provide additional benefit. Prior to initiating non-standard therapy we recommend consulting with the CDC or reviewing current literature.
[‡]Treatment should be followed by a course of iodoquinol or paromomycin in the dosage used to treat asymptomatic amoebiasis.
[§]Ornidazole may also be used (outside the USA).
[¶]Adjunct therapy with either miconazole + rifampin or rifampin + ornidazole may also provide benefit.

Treatment/management

Rapid diagnosis is essential to the survival of patients with amoebic CNS disease. Identification of the organism allows more appropriate selection of medication, but there are other considerations. If the lesion(s) are discrete, surgical resection should be considered whenever possible. In the case of *Balamuthia* infection, prognosis is most favorable when surgery and antimicrobials are adjunct measures. In all cases of disease, the clinician must first provide supportive management. This often requires treatment of increased intracranial pressure using steroids, osmolar therapy, mechanical decompression, or even drainage in severe cases. Symptomatic and supportive care should be aggressive and with care to avoid neuroactive medications that might complicate evaluation of mental status, especially where neuroimaging is not readily available. Treatment for amoebic disease of the CNS is outlined in Table 78.2.

Further reading

CDC. DpDx: Laboratory Identification of Parasites of Public Health Concern (online). Available at http://www.dpd.cdc.gov/dpdx/default.htm.

Marciano-Cabral F, Cabral GA. *Acanthamoeba* spp. as agents of disease in humans. *Clin Microbiol Rev* 2003; 16(2): 273–307.

Singh P, Kochhar R, Vashishta RK, *et al.* Amoebic meningoencephalitis: spectrum of imaging findings. *Am J Neuroradiol* 2006; 27(6): 1217–21.

The Medical Letter. Drugs for Parasitic Infections (online). Available at http://www.themedicalletter.org/.

Walker MD, Zunt JR. Neuroparasitic infections: cestodes, trematodes, and protozoans. *Semin Neurol* 2005; 25(3): 262–77.

Chapter 79
Toxoplasmosis of the central nervous system

Marylou V. Solbrig
University of Manitoba, Winnipeg, Canada

Introduction

Toxoplasmosis is an infection caused by *Toxoplasma gondii*, a microscopic protozoan, so named because the organism was first identified in North African rodents called gondis.

Epidemiology

Toxoplasma gondii is an obligate intracellular protozoan infecting man, other mammals, and birds. Present in migratory birds, the parasite is worldwide, known on every continent but Antarctica.

Humans can be infected at any time during their lives. Almost all infections of man are acquired by mouth, by ingestion of oocysts or tissue cysts. The exceptions are infections acquired *in utero* and after tissue transplant.

Oocysts can be present in cat feces, and tissue cysts may be found in undercooked meat. The sexual part of the protozoa's life cycle occurs in the intestine of domestic cats and other felines, called definitive hosts. The infectious oocysts are then shed in their feces. Small vertebrates such as rodents and birds feeding on the ground become infected. *Toxoplasma* cysts form in muscle and brain, where the parasite remains, waiting to be eaten by cats to complete the life cycle. Other ground-feeding animals, such as cattle, pigs, sheep, and deer, can become infected and are sources of infection for man. Dogs, after rolling in cat excrement, can transmit oocysts on their fur to the hands of petting children. Unfiltered municipal drinking water and well water has been implicated in *Toxoplasma* transmission.

In utero, infection occurs when the fetus is infected via the bloodstream from a mother who developed primary infection during pregnancy. Primary infection may also be acquired from a *Toxoplasma*-infected tissue or organ donor. The risk is highest for heart and bone marrow transplantations, and less for lung and kidney.

In the normal host the risk of developing encephalitis during primary *Toxoplasma* infection is low. Ten percent to 50% of adults in North America and up to 80% in Central America have antibodies to *Toxoplasma* although no history of the disease. Roughly 20% of the populations studied in Europe and over 60% in tropical areas of Asia and Africa are seropositive. In moist tropical areas of South America, close to 100% of the population over the age of 40 may have antibodies. While the percentage of seropositive individuals is lowest in dry desert areas, oocytes may survive in areas of flooded or irrigated land and account for foci for acquiring the disease. Only approximately 10% of acutely infected individuals (normal hosts) have clinical signs and symptoms, which are usually mild.

The risk of intrauterine infection is highest if maternal infection is acquired shortly before delivery. Infants infected in the first half of gestation have the highest rates of encephalitis. In AIDS patients with *Toxoplasma* antibody, the risk of recrudescence of active toxoplasmosis is at the time that CD4 cell counts fall below $200/\text{mm}^3$. Sulfonamides and cotrimazole used for pneumocystis prophylaxis have anti-*Toxoplasma* activity and decrease the risk of recrudescence.

Toxoplasma accounts for 30–40% of retinochoroiditis in the United States.

Pathophysiology

Toxoplasma infections are common in man, and usually asymptomatic, because immunity is acquired quickly to tachyzoites multiplying in cells.

The exceptions to asymptomatic diseases are those in an immature fetus, immunocompromised patients, or when infection involves immunologically privileged or sequestered sites, such as the brain or eye. Delay in developing effective immunity leads to a higher burden of organisms. As immunity develops, encysted bradyzoites develop in tissue. Cysts then rupture, leaving necrotic tissue and foci

International Neurology: A Clinical Approach. Edited by Robert P. Lisak, Daniel D. Truong, William M. Carroll, and Roongroj Bhidayasiri. © 2009 Blackwell Publishing, ISBN: 978-1-4051-5738-4.

for hypersensitivity reactions. In immunocompromised patients, freed bradyzoites will transform into tachyzoites that multiply and injure tissue.

Clinical features

Signs of systemic infection include macular rash, fever, muscle pain, adenopathy, and headache. Central nervous system (CNS) toxoplasmosis occurs after acute generalized infection in children and adults, after intrauterine infection, in immunocompromised patients, and as reactivated encephalitis or retinochoroiditis years after primary infection.

Primary

Primary infection in children or adults can be a mononucleosis-like syndrome with encephalitis or ocular disease. The patients develop a febrile syndrome with lymphadenopathy, splenomegaly, macular rash, muscle pain, myocarditis, headache, and encephalitic syndrome characterized by seizures, tremors, varying degrees of impaired consciousness, and inflammatory spinal fluid. Diffuse encephalitis occurs in transplant patients with primary infection.

Congenital

Toxoplasmosis in the newborn varies from asymptomatic to a progressive, fatal illness. Rash, jaundice, and hepatosplenomegaly can occur in the neonatal period.

Neurologic signs include seizures, hydrocephalus, microcephaly, retinochoroiditis, small cerebral calcifications, increased cerebrospinal fluid (CSF) protein, and inflammatory cells. Aqueductal occlusion is a complication of protracted encephalitis. There is periventricular vasculitis and necrosis of the lateral and third ventricular walls consistent with antigen–antibody reaction. Mild cases may have isolated chorioretinal scars.

Immunocompromised patients

Although *Toxoplasma* infection is almost always followed by chronic infection, acquired immunity keeps the infection controlled. Breakdown of this immunity by corticosteroids, AIDS, malignancies such as Hodgkin's disease, or in cases of heritable immunodeficiencies such as X-linked hyperIgM syndrome causes dissemination of infection and encephalitis.

Toxoplasma encephalitis has been the most frequent cause of focal CNS infection in patients with AIDS. Cerebral abscesses are found in patients with HIV infection, with focal signs developing over several weeks. Lesions are commonly in basal ganglia or at the corticomedullary junction. In one study, all patients with AIDS and hemiballism or chorea have been shown to have cerebral toxoplasmosis.

AIDS patients may also develop a diffuse, subacute encephalitis with CSF mononuclear pleocytosis, elevated protein, and low or normal glucose. In this form of toxoplasmosis, usually limited to the brain, proliferating *Toxoplasma* kill their host cells, namely astrocytes and neurons, then migrate to the next viable cell, where the process repeats itself. Tissue necrosis and high parasite burdens spread and eventually involve vessel walls, which leads to hypertrophic arteritis, thrombosis, infarction, and retrograde hemorrhage.

Retinochoroiditis

Toxoplasmosis is the most common cause of posterior uveitis in immunocompetent subjects and is associated with congenital or acquired infection. Retinochoroiditis in immunocompetent adults is accompanied by serologic evidence of long-standing chronic, usually asymptomatic, infection.

Retinochoroiditis involves the *retina posteri* and secondarily spreads to choroid and vitreous. Patients have a painless blurred vision, usually in one eye. On ophthalmological examination, there is a yellowish necrotic retinal focus with indistinct margins. If acute, there is a vitreous haze, and whitish scars and peripheral hyperpigmentation if old. Often, multiple lesions at various stages of inflammation and healing are seen, as well as frosted branch angiitis. Progressive intraocular infection, panophthalmitis, and orbital cellulitis can occur.

Examples of ocular and cerebral toxoplasmosis are shown in Plate 79.1.

Investigations

Serologic tests for antibody are used to support a clinical diagnosis of toxoplasmosis, measuring antibody with the dye test, direct *Toxoplasma* agglutination test, indirect immunofluorescent antibody, or enzyme-linked immunosorbent assay (ELISA). Diagnosis of acute infection can be made by detection of both IgG and IgM antibodies to *Toxoplasma* in serum. IgM, IgA, and IgE measure a more recent antibody response than IgG, and are useful for diagnosing congenital toxoplasmosis when passively transferred IgG maternal antibody could obscure diagnosis in the neonate.

Antibody titers are usually high with active toxoplasmosis in the CNS and may be low with active chorioretinitis and in AIDS patients. In the latter cases, antibodies may be non-diagnostic, low, or may not reliably distinguish recent, remote, or inactive infection. As such, serologic tests may not be dependable in AIDS patients and a diagnosis of toxoplasmosis is based on identification of the agent, its antigens, DNA, or response to empiric antibiotic treatment within 2 weeks.

Treatment

The combination of sulfadiazine and pyrimethamine is the classic and probably best means of treating active disease. The addition of folinic acid avoids hematologic toxicity without interference with antibiotic efficacy.

Recommended drug therapies for cerebral toxoplasmosis are pyrimethamine + sulfadiazine + leucovorin or pyrimethamine + sulfadiazine + folinic acid followed by suppressive regimens with the same agents in AIDS patients. Atovaquone with or without pyrimethamine can also be considered. Individuals who have completed initial therapy for *Toxoplasma* encephalitis should continue treatment indefinitely unless immune reconstitution with a CD4+ T cell count greater than 200/μl occurs as a consequence of highly active antiretroviral therapy (HAART). Patients should be followed with periodic MRI scans or other neuroimaging modality. Clindamycin is an alternative in cases of sulfadiazine allergy. Although spiramycin has poor CNS penetration, it concentrates in the placenta and can treat toxoplasmosis during pregnancy. Congenital infection is treated with oral pyrethamine and sulfadiazine daily for 1 year. An alternative regimen of spiramycin plus prednisone has been shown to be efficacious.

Patients with ocular toxoplasmosis should be treated for 1 month with pyrimethamine plus either sulfadiazine or clindamycin. Primary prophylactic regimens use pyrimethamine–sulfadoxine (Fansidar) with folinic acid, dapsone–pryimethamine or trimethoprim–sulfamethoxazole (Cotrimoxazole, Bactrim).

Further reading

Frenkel JK. Toxoplasmosis. In: Connor DH, Chandler FW, Schwartz DA, Manz HJ, Lack EE, editors. *Pathology of Infectious Diseases*, Vol. 2. Stamford, CT: Appleton & Lange; 1997, pp. 1261–78.

Frenkel JK. Toxoplasmosis. In: Aminoff MJ, Daroff RB, editors. *Encyclopedia of the Neurological Sciences*, Vol. 4. San Diego: Academic, an imprint of Elsevier Inc; 2003, pp. 544–9.

Kaplan JE, Masur H, Holmes KK. Guidelines for preventing opportunistic infections among HIV-infected persons – 2002. Recommendations of the US Public Health Service and the Infectious Diseases Society of America. *MMWR Recomm Rep* 2002; 40: 4499–503.

Ramsey RG, Gean AD. Neuroimaging of AIDS. I. Central nervous system toxoplasmosis. *Neuroimaging Clin N Am* 1997; 7(2): 171–86.

Remington JS, McLeod R, Thulliez P, Desmonts G. Toxoplasmosis. In: Remington JS, Klein JO, Wilson CB, Baker CJ, editors. *Infectious Diseases of the Fetus and Newborn Infant*, 6th ed. Philadelphia: Elsevier Saunders; 2006, pp. 947–1091.

Chapter 80
Cerebral malaria

Polrat Wilairatana and Srivicha Krudsood
Mahidol University, Bangkok, Thailand

Introduction

Cerebral malaria may be defined strictly as unrousable coma (i.e., non-purposeful response or no response to a painful stimulus) during malaria infection. Although cerebral malaria is generally the result of infection by *Plasmodium falciparum*, it can rarely be caused by *Plasmodium vivax*.

Epidemiology

Malaria infects approximately 5% of the world's population. At the end of 2004, 107 countries and territories had areas at risk of malaria transmission, where some 3.2 billion people live. An estimated 350–500 million clinical malaria episodes occur annually; most of these are caused by *P. falciparum* and *P. vivax. Falciparum* malaria causes more than 1 million deaths each year. The vast majority of fatal cases occur in African children, many of whom succumb to cerebral malaria, which has a mortality rate of around 20%. In most developed countries, malaria is seen in migrants or people returning from traveling in malaria-endemic areas.

Pathology

The hallmark histopathological feature of cerebral malaria is engorgement of cerebral capillaries and venules with parasitized (PRBC) and non-parasitized (NPRBC) red blood cells. Sequestration of PRBCs in cerebral microvessels is significantly higher in the brains of cerebral malaria patients than those with non-cerebral malaria. Cerebral edema is not a major pathological process.

International Neurology: A Clinical Approach. Edited by Robert P. Lisak, Daniel D. Truong, William M. Carroll, and Roongroj Bhidayasiri.
© 2009 Blackwell Publishing, ISBN: 978-1-4051-5738-4.

Pathophysiology

Sequestration

Red blood cells containing mature forms of parasites sequestering in deep vascular beds of vital organs may be responsible for the major organ complications. In cerebral malaria, sequestration is maximal in the brain. The prognosis of severe malaria is thought to be related to sequestered parasite biomass.

Cytoadherence

Plasmodium falciparum is the only species of human malaria that induces cytoadherence of PRBCs to vascular endothelium. Cytoadherence causes sequestration of PRBCs in capillary and venules.

Cytokines

In severe malaria, blood concentrations of both pro-inflammatory cytokines and anti-inflammatory Th2 cytokines are elevated, but there is an imbalance in patients with fatal diseases. The cytokines promote cytoadherence of PRBCs and mechanical obstruction in the brain microcirculation. Nitric oxide (NO) production is increased via inducible NO synthase (iNOS) in severe malaria.

Other factors

Both PRBCs and NPRBCs have reduced deformability (RD) and are associated with poor outcome. Impaired RD promotes destruction of red blood cells and impairment of microcirculatory flow.

Pathogenesis of coma

Consciousness can be impaired by various interacting mechanisms. Inhomogeneous obstruction of cerebral microcirculation by sequestered PRBCs causes hypoxia and net lactate production in the brain, but without infarction of the brain tissue. Local overproduction of NO or other cytokines may impair neurotransmission. However, the relative contributions of these mechanisms may differ in adults and children. Seizures are an important cause of

	Children	Adults
Coma	Rapidly develops after convulsion	Gradually develops in 2–3 days or after generalized convulsion
Convulsions	More than 80% of cases with history of convulsions, 60% occur during admission; more than 50% of cases with recurrent focal motor, 34% with tonic–clonic, 14% with partial with secondary generalization, 15% with subtle or electrographic; status epilepticus is common	20% of cases, mostly generalized tonic–clonic; status epilepticus is rare
Neurological signs	More than 30% of cases have brain stem signs and are associated with increased intracranial pressure; retinal abnormalities in 60%; brain swelling identified by CT scan in 40%	Symmetrical upper motor-neuron signs are common; brain stem signs and retinal abnormalities are less common
Conscious recovery	Rapid, 1–2 days	Slower, 2–4 days
Mortality	19–75% of deaths occur within 24 hours of admission	20%; 50% occur within 24 hours
Neurological sequelae	11% of cases	Less than 5% of cases

Table 80.1 Clinical features of cerebral malaria in children and adults. (Adapted and reprinted from Idro R, Newton CRJC, *Lancet Neurol* 2005; 4: 828, with permission from Elsevier.)

impaired consciousness in children. Coma in malaria is not caused by increased intracranial pressure.

Cerebral malaria caused by *P. vivax*

Major organ dysfunction is rarely reported in *P. vivax* malaria. If a patient with *P. vivax* exhibits severe malaria (commonly associated with *P. falciparum*), the infection is presumed to be mixed. Although "pure" *P. vivax* could cause cerebral malaria, the pathogenesis of cerebral malaria in *vivax* malaria remains unknown.

Clinical features

Clinical manifestations of malaria differ considerably depending on the intensity of malaria transmission. In low transmission settings, symptomatic malaria occurs at all ages and cerebral malaria occurs both in adults and in children. Pregnant women are at greater risk of developing severe disease. In high transmission settings, severe malaria is confined to the first few years of life. Cerebral malaria is the major presentation of severe malaria in low and medium transmission settings, but when malaria transmission is very intense, it is less common, and occurs almost exclusively in infants and young children.

The clinical hallmark of malaria is fever. Cerebral malaria is a clinical syndrome characterized by coma at least 1 hour after termination of a seizure or correction of hypoglycemia, detection of asexual forms of *P. falciparum*

or *P. vivax* in blood smear, and exclusion of other encephalopathy causes. This definition is useful for comparisons of different studies. There are different clinical features of cerebral malaria in African children and Southeast Asian adults (Table 80.1). It remains unclear whether these differences are associated with age or immunity.

The common presentation of severe malaria in children is coma with convulsions, severe anemia, respiratory distress (acidosis), and hypoglycemia. The earliest symptom of cerebral malaria in children is usually fever. Depth of coma may be assessed by using the Glasgow Coma Scale for adults and the Blantyre Coma Scale for children. The scales can be used repeatedly to assess either improvement or deterioration. In Southeast Asia, where malaria transmission is much lower than in Africa and protective immunity is not acquired, all age groups can suffer from severe malaria, but young adults are the most affected group. The main complications of severe malaria in adults include cerebral malaria, renal failure, jaundice, and pulmonary edema. In both high and low transmission areas, pregnant women are vulnerable to hypoglycemia, pulmonary edema, and severe anemia.

In cerebral malaria, the onset of coma may be sudden, often following a generalized seizure, or gradual, with initial drowsiness, confusion, disorientation, delirium, or agitation, followed by unconsciousness. Extreme agitation is a poor prognostic sign. The length of prodromal history is usually several days in adults, but can be as short as 6–12 hours in children. A history of convulsions is common. Focal signs are relatively uncommon. The febrile patient has no signs of meningism, although passive resistance to neck flexion is not uncommon and hyperreflexion

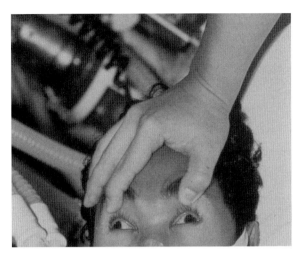

Figure 80.1 Dysconjugate gaze in a man with cerebral malaria; the optic axes are not parallel in the horizontal plane (© Polrat Wilairatana).

of the neck may occur in severely ill patients. Abnormal posturing including decorticate, decerebrate rigidity, and opisthotonos may be found; it is associated with intracranial pressure and recurrence of seizures.

In some children, extreme opisthotonos may lead to a mistaken diagnosis of tetanus or meningitis. The eyes may show a divergent gaze (Figure 80.1), with normal oculocephalic reflexes. Pupil and corneal reflexes are usually normal. However, in children with profound coma, corneal reflexes and "doll's eye" movements may be abnormal. Malarial retinopathy is better than any other clinical or laboratory feature in distinguishing malarial from nonmalarial coma (Plate 80.1a–c). Retinal hemorrhage can be seen in about 15% of cases. Patients with papilledema have increased risk of death. Cranial nerve involvement is rare. Muscle tone and tendon reflexes are often increased, but can also be normal or reduced. Abdominal reflexes are absent and the plantar reflexes are extensor in approximately half of cases.

Post-malaria neurological syndromes (PMNS)

Neurological sequelae occur in less than 5% of adults recovering from cerebral malaria. In children, residual neurological abnormalities are more common, with approximately 11% still having symptoms at the moment of discharge, including hemiplegia, cortical blindness, diffuse cortical damage, tremor, isolated cranial nerve palsies, and aphasia. In children, these are associated with profound and protracted coma, anemia, and prolonged convulsions. Symptoms completely resolve over 1–6 months in over half of the children, but a quarter will be left with major residual neurological deficits.

More subtle cognitive impairments in children as late neurological sequelae are common, particularly in comatose patients with concomitant multiple seizures, deep/ prolonged coma, hypoglycemia, and clinical features of intracranial hypertension. Other late neurological complications, including psychosis, encephalopathy, parkinsonian rigidity and tremor, fine tremor, and cerebellar dysfunction may occur following recovery from cerebral malaria.

There appears to be strong interaction between mefloquine and cerebral malaria, such that 5% of patients who receive mefloquine after severe malaria develop PMNS (a risk 10–50 times higher than following mefloquine treatment of uncomplicated malaria). Mefloquine should not be used following cerebral malaria.

Poor prognostic factors

In adults, depth of coma, agitation, oliguria, jaundice, and shock are important clinical predictors of poor outcome. Metabolic acidosis, raised plasma, or cerebrospinal fluid lactate are useful prognostic markers. Parasitemia with more than 4% parasitemia in nonimmune patients is associated with occurrence of complications or death.

Impaired consciousness or respiratory distress predicted 84% of deaths in African children. Other features associated with fatal outcome include hypoglycemia, increased plasma lactate or acidosis, increased cerebrospinal fluid lactate concentration, and mature parasites (more than 20% with visible malaria pigment).

Diagnosis

Cerebral malaria should be considered in comatose patients with a history of fever who have been in malaria-endemic areas or have been exposed to other risks of malaria infection (e.g., blood transfusion). The diagnosis should be confirmed by thick and thin blood films or rapid diagnostic tests, or dipstick detection of *P. falciparum* antigens *Pf*HRP2 and *p*LDH, which have a diagnostic sensitivity similar to that of microscopy, but do not require an experienced microscopist. Although *P. vivax* rarely impairs consciousness, patients with *P. vivax* malaria and conscious alteration should be considered as cases of cerebral malaria. Cerebral malaria should be considered in any patient with coma and malaria parasitemia, until proven otherwise.

Differential diagnosis of cerebral malaria includes hypoglycemia and bacterial or viral meningoencephalitis.

Sudden unexplained deterioration may result from hypoglycemia or sepsis. It is extremely unusual for a patient with *P. falciparum* cerebral malaria to have a negative blood smear. When it does happen, it is the result of previous antimalarial treatment, but in such cases *Pf*HRP2 tests are still positive. If the smear and *Pf*HRP2 tests are negative for *P. falciparum*, the patient has another cause of coma apart from *P. falciparum*.

Management

Resuscitation
Because most cerebral malaria patients die within 24 hours of admission, emergency or intensive care unit (ICU) care with attention to treatment of shock, severe metabolic acidosis, respiratory failure, and seizures is needed.

Antimalarial treatment
In cerebral malaria, an effective parenteral antimalarial drug should be given. Oral antimalarial drugs may have erratic absorption from the gastrointestinal tract during severe malaria. In general, chloroquine should not be used because most *P. falciparum* infections are resistant to chloroquine. Infusion can be given in normal saline or 5% or 10% dextrose. Oral treatment should be started as soon as the patient can swallow reliably enough to complete a full course of treatment.

Option 1: artesunate
Artemisinins are active at both early and late stages, whereas quinine takes effect during the later stages of parasite development. Intravenous artesunate is significantly superior to quinine in the treatment of severe malaria. The dose of intravenous or intramuscular artesunate is 2.4 mg/kg given over 3 min on admission, followed by the same dose after 12 and 24 hours, and then 2.4 mg/kg daily until the patient is able to take oral medication. Treatment should be completed with oral artesunate 2 mg/kg daily to complete 7 days of treatment *or* with a 3-day course of artemether–lumefantrine (Coartem®) *or* with atovaquone 20 mg/kg/day + proguanil 8 mg/kg/day for 3 days.

Option 2: artemether
A loading dose of artemether 3.2 mg/kg is given intramuscularly as a single dose on day 1. However, intramuscular artemether should not be given to patients in shock because absorption is unreliable. A maintenance dose is 1.6 mg/kg once a day starting on day 2 until the patient is able to tolerate oral medication. Treatment should be completed with oral artesuante 2 mg/kg daily to complete 7 days of treatment *or* with a 3-day course of artemether–lumefantrine (Coartem®) *or* with atovaquone 20 mg/kg/day + proguanil 8 mg/kg/day for 3 days.

Option 3: quinine/quinidine
Quinine
A loading dose of 20 mg salt/kg of quinine dihydrochloride over 4 hours should be given followed by 10 mg salt/kg every 8 hours (each given over 4 hours time). If there is a history of mefloquine or quinine administration within 24 hours before admission, the loading dose of quinine should not be given. A maintenance dose of 10 mg salt/kg is given by infusion over 4 hours every 8 hours. Doses should be reduced by 30–50% after the third day of treatment to avoid accumulation of the drugs in patients who remain seriously ill. However, a minimum of three doses of intravenous quinine should be given before changing to oral treatment. Intravenous quinine can cause hypoglycemia, and blood glucose should be monitored every 4 hours. Once the patient is able to tolerate oral medication, treatment should be completed with a full course of Coartem® for 3 days or oral quinine 10 mg salt/kg every 8 hours to complete the remainder of a total 7 days of quinine treatment. In areas of multidrug-resistant malaria, quinine should be combined with oral clindamycin 5 mg/kg 3 times a day for 7 days. If clindamycin in unavailable, use doxycycline 3 mg/kg once a day for 7 days, or oral tetracycline 4 mg/kg 4 times a day for 7 days. Doxycycline and tetracycline should not be given to children under 8 years old or to pregnant women. However, clindamycin can safely be given to these groups.

In settings where intravenous administration is not possible, quinine can be given intramuscularly. Intramuscular quinine is painful and sclerosant if given undiluted (300 mg/ml). It should be diluted in sterile water or normal saline at a ratio of 1:3 to 1:5 and injected into the anterior thigh, never the buttock, to avoid the risk of sciatic nerve damage. A minimum of three doses of quinine should be given before changing to oral treatment. Survival outcomes of patients treated with quinine or artemether are similar.

Quinidine
In settings where quinine is not available (e.g., the United States), quinidine may be given. Quinidine gluconate in normal saline 10 mg base/kg is intravenously administered over 1 hour, then 0.02 mg base/kg/min. Electrocardiographic monitoring is advisable.

Option 4: artesunate suppositories
In situations where it is not possible to give parenteral antimalarials, an artesunate suppository of 10 mg/kg is given and the dose repeated if the suppository is expelled within 1 hour. If it is not possible to refer the patient, repeat the dose after 24 hours.

Antimalarial treatment for asexual blood stages of "cerebral malaria" from *P. falciparum* and *P. vivax* malaria is similar. Although most *P. vivax* is chloroquine-sensitive,

Table 80.2 Non-recommended ancillary treatments for cerebral malaria.

Corticosteroids
Other anticerebral edema agents (mannitol, urea)
Oxypentifylline
Prostacyclin
Other anti-inflammatory agents
Iron chelating agents
Dichloroacetate
Low molecular weight dextran
Antitumor necrosis factor antibodies
Hyperimmune serum
Cyclosporin A
Adrenaline
Heparin
Hyperbaric oxygen

chloroquine is not recommended for treatment in this severe form of *vivax* malaria. Antimalarial drugs that kill asexual blood stages of *P. falciparum* can also kill asexual blood stages of *P. vivax*, but not any hypnozoites in the liver following *vivax* infection. Radical cure of *vivax* infection requires treatment with primaquine (0.25–0.5 mg base/kg daily together with food for 14 days; adult dose 15–30 mg) if pregnancy and G6PD deficiency have been excluded. In mild G6PD deficiency, intermittent therapy with a reduced dose of primaquine (0.6–0.8 mg base/kg for 6 weeks; adult dose 45 mg) to eradicate hypnozoites may be given.

Supportive treatment

Many cerebral malaria patients have multiple organ failure. If patients have renal failure, metabolic acidosis, or respiratory failure, hemofiltration/dialysis or ventilation,

respectively, is lifesaving and should be started early. Convulsions are very common in children with cerebral malaria; however, choice and dose of a seizure prophylactic drug have not been well established and this is currently not recommended. The treatment of convulsions in cerebral malaria with intravenous (or, if possible, rectal) benzodiazepines or intramuscular paraldehyde is similar to that for repeated seizures from any cause.

A number of ancillary treatments which, in the past, may have benefited select groups of patients, presently cannot be universally recommended. These are listed in Table 80.2.

Acknowledgments

We would like to acknowledge Elsevier for permission to use Table 80.1 and Dr Nicholas A.V. Beare and the *American Journal of Tropical Medicine and Hygiene* for permission to use Plate 80.1(a–c).

Further reading

Beare NAV, Taylor TE, Harding SP, Lewallen S, Molyneux ME. Malarial retinopathy: a newly established diagnostic sign in severe malaria. *Am J Trop Med Hyg* 2006; 75: 790–7.

Idro R, Newton CRJC. Pathogenesis, clinical features, and neurological outcome of cerebral malaria. *Lancet Neurol* 2005; 4: 827–40.

White NJ. Malaria. In: Cook GC, Zumla AI, editors. *Manson's Tropical Diseases*, 21st ed. London: WB Saunders; 2003, pp. 1205–95.

WHO. *Guidelines for Treatment of Malaria*. Geneva: WHO; 2006.

Wilairatana P, Looareesuwan S, Walsh DS. Chemotherapy of cerebral malaria. *CNS Drugs* 1997; 7: 366–80.

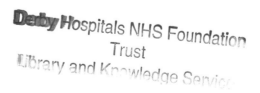

Chapter 81
Trypanosomiasis

Francisco Javier Carod-Artal
Sarah Network of Rehabilitation Hospitals, Brasilia DF, Brazil

American trypanosomiasis

Introduction

Trypanosome are parasitic protozoa that infect millions of poor people in tropical regions. American trypanosomiasis or Chagas' disease (CD) is an acute or chronic infection caused by the flagellate protozoan *Trypanosoma cruzi*.

Humans become involved when infected vectors infest cracks and holes of poor housing. Infection is acquired by the transmission of *T. cruzi* via the bite of the kissing bug of the family *Reduviidae*. The entry of trypanosomes through the wounded skin or mucous membrane is facilitated by the scratching of the bite by the sleeping victim.

Trypanosomes can also be transmitted through infected blood (transfusion, drug abusers), transplant donation, and rarely by oral ingestion. Congenital transmission affects 1–10% of babies born from infected mothers.

Epidemiology

Trypanosoma cruzi infection is widespread, from southern Chile, Argentina, and Brazil, throughout South and Central America. More than 20 million people have chronic infection, with approximately 50000 deaths each year. Up to 8% of the South American population is seropositive, but only 10–30% have symptomatic disease.

Population migrations from endemic countries towards developed nations have increased in recent decades, and CD has reached areas outside its traditional geographic boundaries. More than 100000 Latin American immigrants with *T. cruzi* infection are currently living in the United States. In Europe, 2% of Latino-American immigrants who live in Berlin are CD seropositive.

Clinical features

Acute infection occurs most often in childhood. It is usually asymptomatic, but can present with cutaneous lesions (chagoma; orbital edema or Romaña's sign), fever, lymphadenopathy, and hepatosplenomegaly. In untreated acute cases, myocarditis and meningoencephalitis can occur.

Most infected persons remain asymptomatic in a latent stage that may last years. Only positive antibodies for CD can be detected in this indeterminate form of the disease.

Cardiac and gastrointestinal involvement are the most frequent clinical features of chronic CD. Megaesophagus and megacolon provoke dysphagia and constipation. Chronic cardiomyopathy affects 30% of patients 10–30 years after initial infection. Chagasic cardiomyopathy is characterized by congestive heart failure, sudden cardiac death, arrhythmias, and thromboembolism.

Chagasic myocardiopathy is independently associated with ischemic stroke. Apical aneurysm, congestive heart failure, and cardiac arrhythmias are risk factors in chagasic stroke. Prevalence of apical aneurysm in CD stroke patients is around 37%. However, stroke may be the first manifestation of CD in patients with mild or undetected systolic dysfunction. Chagasic patients without associated vascular risk factors and no clinical evidence of heart failure are also at risk of stroke.

In Brazil, more than 40% of CD patients are diagnosed as having CD after their first stroke. Brain embolism should be suspected in cases of occlusion of the middle cerebral artery (MCA) or its branches (Figure 81.1). The MCA territory is the most common recipient site for cardioembolism, as observed in at least 70% of CD stroke patients.

Pathophysiology of chronic chagasic cardiomyopathy

Parasite persistence and autoimmune responses explain part of the spectrum of chronic CD. Myocardial fibrosis in the chronic disease results from several factors: (1) myocardial cell destruction due to direct tissue damage by *T. cruzi*; (2) inflammatory response responsible for progressive neuronal damage and microcirculation alterations; and (3) neuron involvement with selective parasite destruction of postganglionic parasympathetic neurons in the heart.

International Neurology: A Clinical Approach. Edited by Robert P. Lisak, Daniel D. Truong, William M. Carroll, and Roongroj Bhidayasiri.
© 2009 Blackwell Publishing, ISBN: 978-1-4051-5738-4.

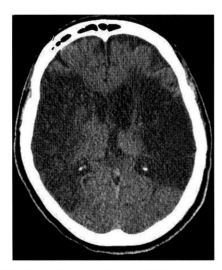

Figure 81.1 CT scan showing bilateral middle cerebral artery infarction in a Chagas' disease stroke patient.

Investigations

Trypanosoma cruzi may be observed by direct examination of fresh blood during the acute phase. Xenodiagnosis and hemocultures are used as indirect parasitological techniques. Serologic diagnosis of CD includes indirect fluorescent antibodies (immunofluorescence test), hemagglutination test, and enzyme-linked immunosorbent assay (ELISA). Parasite DNA can be detected by polymerase chain reaction (PCR) during the chronic stage.

Abnormalities in electrocardiogram (ECG), such as left anterior fascicular block, right bundle-branch block, and atrial fibrillation are common in the chronic cardiac form of CD. Arrhythmias may be detected in patients with normal ejection fraction. Frequently observed ECG features are decreased left ventricular dysfunction, diminished ventricular ejection fraction, systolic wall motion abnormalities, apical aneurysm, and left ventricular thrombosis.

Treatment/management

Treatment is available for acute disease (including congenital and transfusion transmission) and for reactivation of chronic infection. Trypanocide drugs are useful mainly against circulating trypomastigotes, and decrease parasitemia and mortality. Nifurtimox (8–10 mg/kg, for 30–120 days) and benznidazole (5–10 mg/kg, for 30–60 days) are drugs of choice. Side effects include nausea and vomiting, bone marrow hypoplasia, dermatitis, and toxic polyneuritis.

Although recent clinical trials have reported high rates of parasitologic cure in children with early chronic *T. cruzi* infection, there is still no specific effective therapy for the chronic stage of the disease.

Management of chronic chagasic cardiomyopathy involves use of anti-arrhythmic drugs and diuretics. Some patients may require a pacemaker due to severe atrioventricular conduction block. Secondary prevention with oral anticoagulation should be considered in CD patients with stroke and heart failure, atrial fibrillation, or apical aneurysm.

Prevention of the disease should be achieved by vector control and improvement in basic housing conditions in endemic areas.

Human African trypanosomiasis

Introduction

Human African trypanosomiasis (HAT), also called sleeping sickness, is caused by *Trypanosoma brucei*. This protozoan parasite is transmitted to humans by the bite of the tsetse fly (*Glossina* genus). East African HAT is caused by *Trypanosoma b. rhodesiense*, whereas the West African form is provoked by *T. b. gambiense*. Both HAT subtypes differ in their tempo of infection as a result of the greater adaptation of *T. b. gambiense* to the human host. *Trypanosoma b. gambiense* represents more than 90% of reported cases and causes a chronic infection.

Epidemiology

HAT occurs in no less than 36 African countries. Sixty million people who live mainly in rural parts of sub-Saharan Africa are at risk of contracting sleeping sickness. Annual incidence has been estimated at 300,000 cases. Poor surveillance, wars, and increasing parasite resistance are some of the reasons that may explain the re-emergence of HAT.

Pathophysiology

The tsetse fly bite erupts into a red sore and within 1–3 weeks the person can experience the first stages of the disease. This hemolymphatic phase is characterized by fever, headache, painful chancre, and aching muscles and joints. As the disease progresses, the trypanosomes multiply in subcutaneous tissues, blood, and lymph. This provokes specific organ dysfunction such as myocarditis, skin lesions, and hepatosplenic involvement. The late stage or encephalitic stage occurs when the parasites cross the blood–brain barrier to infect the central nervous system (CNS). This process can take years with *T. b. gambiense* whereas *T. b. rhodesiense* infection develops rapidly and invades the CNS after a few months or weeks.

Clinical features of encephalitic stage

Neurological symptoms can develop over many months or years and, if not treated, the disease is invariably fatal. The most common neurological features are (1) behavioral disturbances (changes in personality, irritability, violent behavior, agitation, confusion, delusions, hallucinations, delirium); (2) alteration of the circadian rhythm and sleep disturbances (daytime hypersomnolence, nocturnal insomnia, narcolepsy); (3) focal impairment (motor weakness, dystonia, paresthesias, abnormal movements, tremor, slurred speech, seizures); and (4) peripheral involvement (polyneuritis, muscle fasciculation).

Investigations

Screening of people at risk helps identify patients at an early stage. Diagnosis should be made as early as possible and before the advanced stage.

Persistent parasitemia is common in *T. b. rhodesiense*, and diagnosis can be made by identifying trypanosomes in peripheral blood or tissues (lymph node aspirate, bone marrow). *Trypanosoma b. gambiense* parasitemia is usually cyclical due to the greater adaptation to the host; serological tests (card agglutination trypanosomiasis test) can help in the diagnosis.

Cerebrospinal fluid (CSF) analysis is mandatory to rule out late-stage disease at which lymphocytic pleocytosis (>20 white blood cells (WBC)/μl), raised CSF protein (50–200 mg/ml), increased intrathecal IgM synthesis, and the presence of trypanosomes can be detected. However, there is not a universal consensus as to how late-stage disease should be diagnosed using CSF criteria in HAT.

Differential diagnosis includes malaria (both diseases may co-exist), leishmaniasis, typhoid fever, viral encephalitis, neuro-AIDS, and chronic tuberculosis meningitis.

Treatment/management

The main approach to controlling HAT is to reduce the reservoirs of infection and the presence of the tsetse fly.

Pentamidine is used to treat the first stage of *T. b. gambiense* infection, whereas intravenous suramine is the drug of choice for *T. b. rhodesiense*. Side effects include renal failure, anaphylaxis, and neurological complications for suramine, and hypo/hyperglycemia and hypotension for pentamidine.

The only effective drug for the late-stage disease in both types of HAT is the trivalent arsenical melarsoprol (Mel B). Mel B has many undesired effects, the most important of which is a severe post-treatment reactive encephalopathy (PTRE). PTRE occurs in about 10% of cases and may prove fatal in up to 50% of these. Accurate staging of the disease is essential because of the potentially fatal complications of melarsoprol treatment. The use of steroids in HAT remains controversial. In a large study, a combination of melarsoprol and prednisolone reduced the incidence of PTRE and fatalities in *gambiense* disease. A more recent alternative drug for late-stage *gambiense* disease may be eflornithine.

Further reading

Carod-Artal FJ, Vargas AP, Horan TA, Nunes LG. Chagasic cardiomyopathy is independently associated with ischemic stroke in Chagas' disease. *Stroke* 2005; 36: 965–70.

Schmid C, Richer M, Bilenge CM, *et al*. Effectiveness of a 10-day melarsoprol schedule for the treatment of late-stage human African trypanosomiasis: confirmation from a multinational study (IMPAMEL II). *J Infect Dis* 2005; 191: 1922–31.

Chapter 82
Rickettsial and parasitic infections

Oscar H. Del Brutto
Hospital-Clìnica Kennedy, Guayaquil, Ecuador

Introduction

Rickettsial and parasitic infections of the central nervous system (CNS) produce pleomorphic diseases. These infections cause a wide range of pathologic lesions and may be associated with a number of clinical syndromes, including acute, subacute, or chronic meningitis, acute or subacute encephalitis, stroke, space-occupying brain lesions, and myelopathy.

Epidemiology

Rickettsial diseases are mainly zoonoses affecting rodents and other mammals. Humans can acquire the diseases through the bite of an insect vector or, in the case of Q fever, by inhaling the causative agent. Most cases of CNS parasitosis occur when humans become accidental intermediate hosts of the parasite. Rickettsial and parasitic infections affect millions of people living in the developing world. In addition, massive emigration of people from endemic to non-endemic areas has contributed to the widespread diffusion of some formerly geographically restricted rickettsial and parasitic diseases.

Pathophysiology

Rickettsiae are obligate intracellular, Gram-negative, pleomorphic coccobacilli found in the alimentary tract of insects and arthropods. Rickettsial diseases can be classified into three groups based on clinical, epidemiologic,

and pathogenetic similarities: the typhus group, the spotted fever group, and a miscellaneous group that includes Q fever and ehrlichiosis. With the exception of Q fever, these diseases produce systemic angiitis characterized by microvascular injury of multiple organs, including the lungs, liver, kidneys, heart, and CNS. This angiitis is mainly related to the proliferation of rickettsiae within endothelial cells of small vessels, which causes endothelial swelling and necrosis, increased vascular permeability, recruitment of mononuclear inflammatory cells, liberation of procoagulant factors, and the formation of microthrombi with luminal occlusion. There is increasing evidence that a complex interaction between rickettsiae and the host's immune system may be responsible for the many types of pathologic lesions that these conditions cause in humans.

Parasites can be classified as protozoa and helminths (cestodes, nematodes, and trematodes). The former are unicellular microorganisms, whereas the latter are multicellular organisms with complex life cycles that usually require two or more hosts to complete them. Parasites are complex microorganisms that interact with the host's immune system in different ways. This interaction in which the host tries to drive out the infection while the parasite attempts to live in a hostile environment may be even more harmful to the host than the infection itself.

Most parasites known to infect humans have a special predilection to lodge in the CNS, where they cause significant morbidity and mortality. Parasites may enter the CNS by the hematogenous route or by ectopic migration of their larvae.

International Neurology: A Clinical Approach. Edited by Robert P. Lisak, Daniel D. Truong, William M. Carroll, and Roongroj Bhidayasiri. © 2009 Blackwell Publishing, ISBN: 978-1-4051-5738-4.

Chapter 83
Cestodes

Oscar H. Del Brutto
Hospital-Clìnica Kennedy, Guayaquil, Ecuador

Neurocysticercosis

Introduction

Neurocysticercosis (NCC) occurs when humans become intermediate hosts of *Taenia solium*. Humans are definitive hosts of this cestode and both humans and pigs can be intermediate hosts. Humans acquire cysticercosis mainly by ingesting food contaminated with *T. solium* eggs or via the fecal–oral route in individuals harboring the adult parasite in the intestine.

Epidemiology

NCC is endemic in Latin America, sub-Saharan Africa, and Asia, although mass immigration has increased its prevalence in the United States (US) and some European countries. NCC is a major cause of acquired epilepsy worldwide.

Pathophysiology

Cysticerci are vesicles containing an invaginated scolex similar to adult *T. solium*. Parasites can be located in brain parenchyma, the ventricular system, subarachnoid space, and spinal cord. Parenchymal cysts usually lodge in the cerebral cortex or basal ganglia. Ventricular cysticerci may attach to the choroid plexus or float in the ventricular cavities. Subarachnoid cysts manifest in the sylvian fissure or in cisterns at the base of the brain. Spinal cysticerci are found either at the cord parenchyma or in subarachnoid space.

After entering the central nervous system (CNS), cysticerci elicit few inflammatory changes in surrounding tissues and are in a vesicular stage. Parasites can remain in this stage for years or may enter, as a result of the host's immune attack, in a process of degeneration. The three stages of involution through which cysticerci pass are the colloidal, granular, and calcified stages.

Inflammatory reactions around cysticerci induce pathological changes in the CNS. Within brain parenchyma, such reactions are associated with edema and reactive gliosis. At the subarachnoid space, the leptomeninges thickens, with entrapment of cranial nerves and blood vessels. Luschka and Magendie's foramina are occluded by the thickened leptomeninges, with subsequent development of hydrocephalus. Ventricular cysticerci also elicit a local inflammatory reaction if attached to the choroid plexus or to the ventricular wall. In such cases, ependymal cells proliferate and may block cerebrospinal fluid (CSF) transit at the cerebral aqueduct or at Monro's foramina, causing obstructive hydrocephalus.

Clinical features

Seizures are the most common manifestation of NCC. Focal signs of subacute or acute onset have also been described. Others present with intracranial hypertension sometimes associated with seizures or dementia; hydrocephalus is the most common cause of this syndrome. Intracranial hypertension may also occur in patients with ventricular cysts, causing obstructive hydrocephalus, and in those with cysticercotic encephalitis. The latter is a severe form of NCC resulting from the host's immune response to a massive cysticercotic infection of brain parenchyma. Spinal cysticercosis causes root pain, weakness, and sensory deficits that vary according to the level of the lesion.

Investigations

Neuroimaging studies provide objective evidence about the location of cysticerci and the degree of host inflammatory response to parasites (Figure 83.1). Imaging findings include cystic lesions showing the scolex, parenchymal brain calcifications, and ring-enhancing lesions, and abnormal enhancement of the leptomeninges, hydrocephalus, and cerebral infarcts. In patients with subarachnoid or ventricular NCC, CSF analysis shows lymphocytic pleocytosis and increased protein contents with normal glucose levels. The most effective immune diagnostic test is serum immunoblot; however, false-positive results can occur in patients with cysticerci outside the CNS, and false-negative results are common in patients with a single cyst or with calcified lesions.

International Neurology: A Clinical Approach. Edited by Robert P. Lisak, Daniel D. Truong, William M. Carroll, and Roongroj Bhidayasiri. © 2009 Blackwell Publishing, ISBN: 978-1-4051-5738-4.

Treatment

Calcifications

Cysticidal drugs should not be used for calcifications. Antiepileptic drugs are advised for seizures. Seizure recurrence after antiepileptic drug withdrawal is high. Neuroimaging studies performed after seizure relapse have shown edema and abnormal contrast uptake around previously inert calcifications, suggesting that calcifications represent epileptogenic foci susceptible to reactivation when the inhibitory influence of antiepileptic drugs is withdrawn.

Cystic lesions

Praziquantel and albendazole provide clinical improvement and resolution of lesions in most patients with NCC. Praziquantel destroys more than 60% of lesions. Praziquantel dosages range from 10 to 100 mg/kg for 3–21 days. Albendazole, administered at daily doses of 15 mg/kg for 1 week, reduces the number of cysts by 86% (Figure 83.2). Patients with large subarachnoid cysts may require longer courses of albendazole. Corticosteroid administration is mandatory when treating these patients to ameliorate inflammatory reaction in the subarachnoid space, which can cause brain infarction.

A meta-analysis of randomized trials assessing the effect of cysticidal drugs found that such therapy results in better resolution of both colloidal and vesicular cysticerci and in lowered risk of seizure recurrence. Cysticidal drugs should not be used in patients with cysticercotic encephalitis; corticosteroids and osmotic diuretics are advised to reduce the inflammatory response associated with this condition. Most ventricular cysticerci should be removed by endoscopic aspiration to avoid adverse reactions related to the parasitic death.

Hydrocephalus

Patients with hydrocephalus due to NCC require a ventricular shunt. Continued administration of prednisone reduces the risk of shunt dysfunction, which is the greatest risk in these patients. Mortality is related to the number of surgical interventions to change dysfunctional shunts.

Echinococcosis

Introduction

Echinococcosis is caused by infection with larval *Echinococcus* spp. Canids are definitive hosts of these cestodes, and sheep, rodents, and humans can be intermediate hosts. Humans become infected by ingesting water or food contaminated with dog feces containing eggs of these tapeworms. After entering the body, eggs transform into cysts that grow in the CNS or other organs.

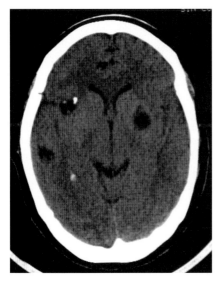

Figure 83.1 CT of the head showing cystic lesions and calcifications, highly suggestive of NCC.

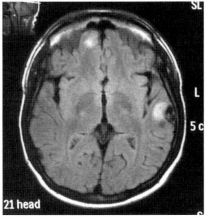 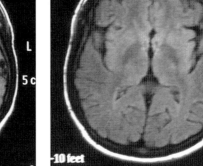

Figure 83.2 MRI of patient with cystic lesion located in left temporal lobe (a). After therapy, the lesion disappeared (b).

(a)　　　　(b)

Epidemiology

Echinococcus granulosus has been reported in Australia, Mediterranean countries, and North and South America. *Echinococcus multilocularis* is found in the Arctic, Canada, Europe, and countries of the former Soviet Union.

Pathophysiology

Cystic hydatid disease is caused by *E. granulosus*, and alveolar hydatid disease is caused by *E. multilocularis*. *Echinococcus granulosus* cysts are spherical and well demarcated from surrounding tissue. Cysts can be located in brain parenchyma, the ventricular system, subarachnoid space, epidural space, and the spinal canal. In contrast, *E. multilocularis* cysts are small, group in clusters, elicit a severe inflammatory reaction from the host, and tend to metastasize locally and distantly. These cysts are usually located within brain parenchyma.

Hydatid disease of the heart may cause a cerebral infarct. Hydatid cysts can grow within necrotic brain tissue, suggesting that embolic occlusion of an intracranial artery by fragments of a cyst broken within the heart may cause cerebral infarction.

Clinical features

Cystic hydatid disease of the brain is characterized by seizures or increased intracranial pressure. Focal neurological deficits result from strategically located cysts or from cerebral infarct caused by a cardiogenic brain embolism of cystic membranes. Cranial nerve palsies are common in patients with parasellar cysts due to involvement of the cavernous sinus. In alveolar hydatid disease, clinical manifestations include intracranial hypertension, seizures, and focal neurological deficits. Manifestations progress more rapidly and are more severe than those of cystic hydatid disease. Spinal cord involvement, associated with root pain and motor or sensory deficits, may be observed in both forms of hydatid disease.

Investigations

Cystic hydatid disease presents on neuroimaging studies as a single, large, non-enhancing lesion. Some lesions show calcifications. Cysts located in the subarachnoid space may be multiple and confluent. Epidural cysts have a bi-convex shape or multilocular appearance and may be associated with bone erosion. In alveolar hydatid disease, lesions are multiple, surrounded by edema, and show ring-like enhancement. CT best demonstrates bone erosion in vertebral bodies in patients with hydatidosis of the spinal canal. Immunologic diagnosis is not accurate due to cross-reactions with other parasitic diseases or false-negative results in patients with intact cystic hydatid lesions.

Treatment

Cystic hydatid disease of the brain requires surgery. Accidental rupture of the cyst may cause allergic reactions or recurrent hydatid disease due to spillage of the cyst's contents. Experience with albendazole for cerebral cystic hydatid disease is scarce. Albendazole can be given before surgery to prevent hazards of transoperative rupture of cysts or postoperatively to treat recurrent hydatid disease. Clinical deterioration may occur during therapy due to intense inflammatory reaction surrounding the dying cyst.

Treatment of patients with cystic hydatid disease of the spine includes decompressive laminectomy, removal of cysts, excision of involved bone, and stabilization of the spine. Albendazole is advised to reduce the risk of recurrent hydatid disease after surgery.

Surgical removal of alveolar cysts of the brain usually requires resection of adjacent tissue. Albendazole administration should follow or even precede the surgical procedure or may be used as primary therapy for patients with inoperable alveolar hydatid disease. With this approach, 90% of lesions regress or remain static.

Further reading

Del Brutto OH. Neurocysticercosis. *Semin Neurol* 2005; 25: 243–51.

Del Brutto OH, Roos KL, Coffey CS, Garcia HH. Meta-analysis: cysticidal drugs for neurocysticercosis. *Ann Intern Med* 2006; 145: 43–51.

García HH, Del Brutto OH. Neurocysticercosis: updated concepts about an old disease. *Lancet Neurol* 2005; 4: 653–61.

Schantz PM. Echinococcosis. In: Guerrant RL, Walker DH, Weller PF, editors. *Tropical Infectious Diseases. Principles, Pathogens & Practice.* Philadelphia: WB Saunders; 1999, pp. 1005–25.

Chapter 84
Trematodes: schistosomiasis

Sureshbabu Sachin and Manjari Tripathi
All India Institute of Medical Sciences, New Delhi, India

Introduction

Schistosomiasis, the second most common parasitic infection after malaria, is caused mainly by three species of *Schistosoma*, namely *S. haematobium, S. mansoni,* and *S. japonicum*. Eggs of the organism have been discovered in Egyptian and Chinese mummies. Today, schistosomiasis plagues the lives of millions of people in the developing world.

Epidemiology

According to the 2002 World Health Organization (WHO) Expert Committee report, 79 countries are endemic for *Schistosoma*. South America, sub-Saharan and southern Africa, and the Middle East are the main foci. Additional areas are added to the list every year as a result of international travel and migration of the infected population.

Pathogenesis

The eggs or parasite can reach the spinal cord retrogradely from portal venous systems through Batson's vertebral plexus (see Figure 84.1). Aberrant migration of parasites, dissemination of eggs via porto-systemic shunts, and emboli from the heart can bring the infection to the brain. Neuroschistosomiasis is produced by a predominantly cellular inflammatory response to antigenic products released by parasite eggs. The infection rate can be increased by co-infection with the HIV virus.

Clinical features

The early phase of infection is manifested by a hypersensitivity reaction to schistosomulae (also known as

Katayama fever), characterized by fever, fatigue, malaise, myalgia, right upper quadrant pain, bloody diarrhea, non-productive cough, eosinophilia, and pulmonary infiltrates. Rarely, aseptic meningitis can develop. In the chronic phase, presentation varies depending upon the location of the parasite.

Neurological complications can occur during all phases of schistosomiasis, the most common of which is transverse myelitis. In broad terms, neurological involvement can be classified into either cerebral or spinal schistosomiasis.

Cerebral schistosomiasis
Patients with the cerebral form of schistosomiasis may present with acute or subacute onset of headache, altered sensorium, seizures, and focal neurological deficits. Space-occupying lesions with significant mass effect, multiple focal lesions spanning the cerebral hemispheres, as well as non-specific granulomas with surrounding edema are the underlying pathology in most cases. Neurological deficits may be in the form of hemiparesis, visual impairment, dysphasia, or ataxia, depending on the location of these lesions.

Sometimes, the picture may resemble that of a malignant cerebral neoplasm with progressive evolution of symptoms and features of raised intracranial pressure. Multiple strokes can result from small vessel vasculitis or cardioembolism due to associated endomyocardial fibrosis. Partial motor seizures may be the sole manifestation in some cases. Heavy parasitic infection in undernourished children can lead to cognitive impairment. Asymptomatic infection of the brain is also prevalent in endemic regions.

Spinal schistosomiasis
The spinal form presents with progressive ascending weakness with bladder, bowel, and/or sexual dysfunction. Lumbar and radicular pain radiating down the legs precedes weakness in the majority of cases. Systemic features are usually lacking. Atypical presentations include cauda equina syndrome, progressive myelopathy resembling spinal cord tumor, and anterior spinal artery infarction. A large proportion of patients with myelopathy develop significant disability.

International Neurology: A Clinical Approach. Edited by Robert P. Lisak, Daniel D. Truong, William M. Carroll, and Roongroj Bhidayasiri. © 2009 Blackwell Publishing, ISBN: 978-1-4051-5738-4.

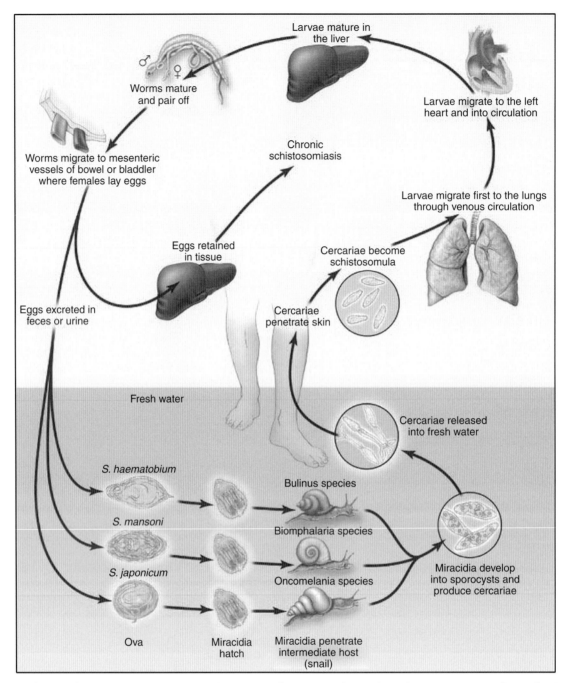

Figure 84.1 Life cycle of schistosoma. (Reproduced with permission from Ross *et al. N Engl J Med* 2002; 346: 1212–20. Copyright 2002 Massachusetts Medical Society. All rights reserved.)

Investigations

Histopathological examination with identification of larva is the gold-standard for diagnosis of neuroschistosomiasis. Short of this, diagnosis can be made on clinical grounds supported by imaging and laboratory data.

Cerebral lesions may be single or multiple, involving the cerebral hemispheres and, occasionally, the cerebellum. On imaging, lesions appear hyperintense on T2, with surrounding vasogenic edema. Cord lesions are usually isointense on T1 and hyperintense on T2 with cord expansion. Central linear enhancement, surrounded by multiple enhancing punctate nodules, is specific, but peripheral enhancement is equally common.

Several serological techniques including enzyme-linked immunosorbent assay (ELISA), indirect hemagglutination, and recently recombinant peptide antigen assay are used in the diagnosis of *Schistosoma* infection. A positive

Table 84.1 Etiology of eosinophilic meningitis.

Infectious	Non-infectious
Parasitic	Malignancy
Angiostrongylus cantonensis	Hodgkin's disease
Gnathostoma spinigerum	Non-Hodgkin's lymphoma
Baylisascaris procyonis	Esinophilic leukemia
Other helminths	Medications
Neurocysticercosis	Ciprofloxacin
Cerebral paragonimiasis	Ibuprofen
Neurotrichinosis	Intraventricular vancomycin
Cerebral toxocariasis	Intraventricular gentamicin
Cerebral/spinal schistosomiasis	Intraventricular iophendylate dye
Fungi	Ventriculoperitoneal shunts
Coccidioides immitis	Hypereosinophilic syndrome
Bacteria, rickettsiae, viruses	

test is indicative of only prior exposure and hence finds limited use in endemic zones. Other problems encountered with neuroschistosomiasis are delayed seroconversion and cross-reactivity with other helminthic antigens. CSF examination may reveal raised protein with mildly reduced glucose as well as lymphocytes and eosinophils on microscopy. Other specimens, such as urine and stool, rarely show ova with characteristic morphology.

Differential diagnosis (see Table 84.1) includes other causes of eosinophilic meningitis and space-occupying lesions, such as tuberculoma, toxoplasma, neoplasms, abscess, and cysticercosis. Spinal disease should be differentiated from transverse myelitis, spinal cord tumors, cysticercosis, tuberculosis, and angiostrongyliasis.

Biopsy of brain and spinal cord lesions reveals granuloma formation with extensive inflammation and vasogenic edema. Calcification, arteritis, and ova may be noted.

Treatment

Praziquintal is the drug of choice; a single dose of 40 or 60 mg/kg is effective in most cases. Side effects are mild and include nausea, vomiting, malaise, and abdominal pain. Resistance to praziquintal is an emerging problem in endemic countries, where the drug has been used for several years. Concurrent administration of albendazole may control co-existent helminths, but does not have any impact on the trematode. Corticosteroids (preferably dexamethasone) can be combined with antihelminthics in the spinal and the cerebral forms.

A ventriculoperitoneal shunt is required in cases of obstructive hydrocephalus, especially in those caused by posterior fossa lesions. In spinal schistosomiasis, decompressive laminectomy with surgical resection of the lesion and liberation of the roots is indicated in severe cases not responding to medical therapy.

Artemether, when given with praziquintal, controls the secondary infection rate. Artemether can also be used as a prophylactic agent for high-risk groups such as flood relief workers, tourists, and fishermen in endemic regions. Vaccines developed against the target antigen glutathione *S*-transferase are being investigated.

The importance of neurorehabilitative measures in paraplegic patients cannot be overemphasized. However, to avail these treatment options to underdeveloped and developing countries is a challenging public-health issue.

Further reading

Ferrari TC, Moreira PR, Cunha AS. Spinal cord schistosomiasis: a prospective study of 63 cases emphasizing clinical and therapeutic aspects. *J Clin Neurosci* 2004; 11: 246–53.

Gryseels B, Polman K, Clerinx J, Kestens L. Human schistosomiasis. *Lancet* 2006; 368(9541): 1106–18.

Ross AG, Bartley PB, Sleigh AC, *et al*. Schistosomiasis. *N Engl J Med* 2002; 346: 1212–20.

Chapter 85
Nematodes

Manjari Tripathi and Sureshbabu Sachin
All India Institute of Medical Sciences, New Delhi, India

Trichinosis

Trichinosis is a parasitic disease caused by infection with *Trichinella spiralis*.

Epidemiology
Humans are infected with trichinosis by consuming contaminated pork or wild game. The disease is common in Africa, Central and South America, Asia, and Eastern European countries. The life cycle of trichinosis is shown in Figure 85.1.

Clinical features
Severity ranges from asymptomatic to fatal. Initial symptoms may include nausea, diarrhea, fever, headache, maculopapular rash, periorbital and facial edema, chemosis, trismus, and dysphagia. Myalgia is common, particularly in the calf and forearm. Severe cases may include myocarditis.

In 10–20% of cases, central nervous system (CNS) involvement is seen; this is usually associated with heavy *Trichinella* infection. Such cases present with agitated behavior, delirium, and headache. Cranial nerve deficits, paresis, aphasia, convulsions, and cerebellar syndromes may occur. Venous infarction and intracerebral bleed are rare.

Investigations
Eosinophil count is often above 300/mm^3 and increases 10–12 days after infection. Absence of eosinophilia may indicate poor prognosis. Erythrocyte sedimentation rate (ESR) and creatine phosphokinase (CPK) may be raised. Electromyogram is myopathic, with muscle irritation presenting as fibrillation potentials. Muscle biopsy, which may be false-negative if performed in the first 2 weeks of infection, is necessary to confirm diagnosis. Microscopically, specimens reveal motile larvae coiled within a connective tissue pseudocyst.

Enzyme-linked immunosorbent assay (ELISA) is specific for excretory–secretory product of muscle larvae and for the tyvelose antigen. Cerebrospinal fluid (CSF) shows mildly elevated protein, occasional eosinophilia, and, rarely, larvae. Brain CT may show multiple small hypodense lesions in the cerebral cortex and white matter. Small intracerebral bleeds and infarcts have been reported on MRI. Myalgia with extraocular muscle involvement can be seen in thyrotoxic ophthalmopathy, pseudotumor oculi, or extraocular infiltration due to other causes.

Differential diagnosis of trichinosis infection includes myositis and a wide range of CNS syndromes and infections. Positive results from at least two screening tests are required to confirm diagnosis.

Treatment
Albendazole at 800 mg/kg in four divided doses for 7–14 days is the recommended treatment. Steroids may be needed in severe infection to prevent a Jarisch–Herxheimer-like reaction. Symptomatic treatment includes analgesics and antipyretics.

Gnathostomiasis

Gnathostomiasis is caused by several species of *Gnathostoma*, particularly *Gnathostoma spinigerum*.

Epidemiology
Humans are infected by eating raw or undercooked fish, poultry, or pork. Infection is most prevalent in Thailand, followed by Japan, Mexico, Myanmar, China, India, the Philippines, Malaysia, Sri Lanka, Indonesia, Australia, Laos, Cambodia, Vietnam, and Ecuador.

Clinical features
Eosinophilic myeloradiculitis and eosinophilic meningitis are the main neurological syndromes associated with gnathostomiasis.

Patients with eosinophilic myeloradiculitis present with severe radicular pains involving the limbs, trunk, and cervical and perianal regions, accompanied by motor, sensory, and autonomic dysfunction. Meningeal symptoms

International Neurology: A Clinical Approach. Edited by Robert P. Lisak, Daniel D. Truong, William M. Carroll, and Roongroj Bhidayasiri. © 2009 Blackwell Publishing, ISBN: 978-1-4051-5738-4.

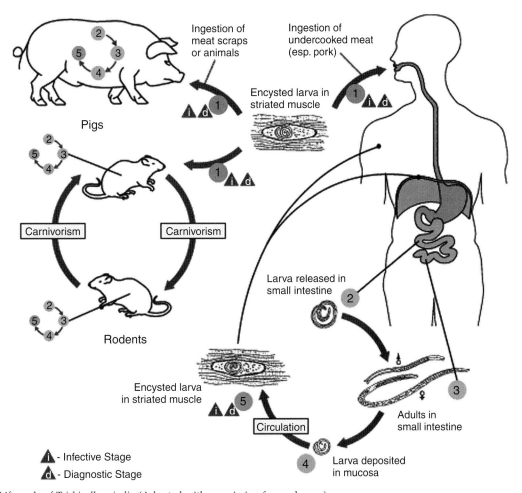

Figure 85.1 Life cycle of *Trichinella spiralis*. (Adapted with permission from cdc.gov.)

may be associated. Cranial nerve palsies, headache, visual impairment, and altered sensorium may be seen in high cervical cord lesions.

Patients with eosinophilic meningitis present with headache, vomiting, photophobia, and nuchal stiffness. Fever is uncommon. Seizures, altered sensorium, and cranial nerve palsies can occur. Neurological sequelae are common, and mortality due to intracerebral hemorrhage is seen in 7–25% of cases (see Table 85.1).

Investigations
In CSF, white blood cell count (WBC) greater than $500/\mu l$ and eosinophilia more than 10% with raised protein and normal or mildly reduced glucose, red blood cells (RBCs), and xanthochromia may be observed.

Fuzzy white matter hyperintensities, multiple intracerebral hemorrhages, basal ganglia hyperintensities, and nodular enhancement are noted on brain MRI. Hyperintense intramedullary lesions with cord expansion are seen on spine MRI. Immunoblot is specific.

Differential diagnoses for the cerebral form includes tuberculoma, toxoplasma, neoplasms, abscess, and cysticercosis; the spinal form includes other causes of transverse myelopathy.

Treatment
The role of antihelminthic treatment is not established in neurological disease. Corticosteroids can produce symptomatic relief.

Angiostrongyliasis

Angiostrongyliasis, caused by the parasite *Angiostrongylus cantonensis*, is the most common cause of eosinophilic meningitis.

Epidemiology
Humans become infected by ingestion of raw or undercooked terrestrial snails and slugs, or via transport hosts such as freshwater prawns, frogs, fish, and planarians and, rarely, contaminated lettuce. Major outbreaks have been reported in Thailand, Taiwan, Hawaii, Vietnam, Malaysia, Indonesia, the Philippines, Japan, Papua

Feature	Gnathostomiasis	Angiostrongyliasis
Root pain	Prominent	Rare
Illness	Severe	Less severe
Complications	Coma with respiratory failure	Coma without respiratory failure
CSF	Clear/xanthochromic, with RBCs	Clear/turbid, no RBCs
WBC	<500/µl	150–2000/µl
Eosinophilia	60% of cases	>95% of cases
MRI	Focal lesions and large hemorrhagic tracts	Small hemorrhagic tracts
Other	Intracerebral/subarachnoid hemorrhage and bleeding in brainstem	

Table 85.1 Differentiating features between gnathostomiasis and angiostrongyliasis.

New Guinea, and the United States. The disease is most common in young adults and children, with male predominance seen in some reports.

Clinical features

The typical neurological syndrome is eosinophilic meningitis. Patients present with headache, retro-orbital pain, nuchal stiffness, photophobia, and visual blurring. Systemic features include fatigue, malaise, myalgia, paresthesiae, abdominal pain, vomiting, and rash. Fever has been reported in some outbreaks. Cranial nerve palsies, behavioral disturbances, seizures, myeloradiculitis, and persistent cognitive impairment may also occur. The disease usually takes a benign course with neurological sequel. Coma and mortality are rare (see Table 85.1).

Investigations

CSF is clear or mildly turbid. WBC is 150–2000/µl. Eosinophils are greater than 10%. Protein is elevated. Glucose may be normal or reduced. Peripheral blood eosinophilia may be observed.

MRI shows multiple hyperintense signals in the cerebral hemispheres, white matter, and cerebellum. Enhancing lesions in the cisterns, stick-like pial enhancement, basal ganglia hyperintensities, prominent Virchow–Robin spaces, and linear tracks are also seen. Immunoblot ELISA confirms diagnosis.

Treatment

Albendazole administered for 2 weeks may reduce headache. Corticosteroids produce symptomatic relief.

Further reading

Lo Re V III, Gluckman SJ. Eosinophilic meningitis. *Am J Med* 2003; 114(3): 217–23.

Pozio E, Gomez Morales MA, Dupouy-Camet J. Clinical aspects, diagnosis and treatment of trichinellosis. *Expert Rev Anti-infect Ther* 2003; 1: 471–82.

Punyagupta S, Juttijudata P, Bunnag T. Eosinophilic meningitis in Thailand. Clinical studies of 484 typical cases probably caused by *Angiostronglus cantonensis. Am J Trop Med Hyg* 1975; 17: 551–61.

Chapter 86
Rickettsial disease

Clarisse Rovery and Didier Raoult
Université de la Méditerranée, Marseille, France

Introduction

The classification of the Rickettsiaceae family has undergone important changes over the past 20 years due to the generalization of the use of gene sequencing and genetic phylogeny. In this chapter, we focus on Rickettsiae. Rickettsiae are intracellular alpha proteobacteria associated with eucaryotic hosts (arthropods or helminths). Based on antigenic and genetic data, Rickettsiae are divided into three groups: (1) the spotted fever group (SFG) accounts for most of tick-borne rickettsioses, (2) the typhus group (TG), which includes *Rickettsia prowazekii*, the agent of epidemic typhus, transmitted by body louse, and *Rickettsia typhi*, the agent of murine typhus, transmitted by rat and cat fleas, and (3) *Orientia tsutsugamushi*, the agent of scrub typhus, transmitted by chiggers.

Until recently, the diagnosis of rickettsioses was confirmed almost exclusively by serologic methods. Serology does not allow discriminating rickettsiae belonging to the same group. The recognition of multiple distinct rickettsioses during the last 20 years has been greatly facilitated by broad use of cell culture systems and the development of molecular methods for the identification of rickettsiae. As a consequence, during 1984 through 2007, 11 additional rickettsial species or subspecies were identified as emerging rickettsioses. Another consequence is that there are more than one rickettsiose in one country. Description of the known rickettsioses could have included these new emerging rickettsioses, which could explain the variable clinical descriptions of the first described rickettsioses.

Symptomatic evidence of central nervous system (CNS) involvement is a frequent feature in rickettsial infections. Such involvement is a result of the systemic nature of these infections and their propensity for invasion of endothelial cells. The degree of insult to the CNS varies according to the various rickettsial infections.

Epidemiology

The geographic and temporal distribution of rickettsioses is mainly determined by their vectors (Table 86.1, Figure 86.1). Louse-transmitted diseases occur worldwide. Lice tend to parasitize individuals who live in crowded conditions and exhibit poor hygiene, preferentially in cold places and during wars. Common fleas such as dog, cat, and rat fleas are reported worldwide, as are their transmitted diseases – murine typhus and flea-borne spotted fever (caused by *Rickettsia felis*). Tick species are highly dependent on their environment; very few are found worldwide, with the exception of *Rhipicephalus sanguineus*, the dog tick, vector of *Rickettsia conorii* (in the Old World). Therefore, tick-transmitted diseases are usually restricted to parts of the world where they can be fed by the local fauna. Tick behavior may determine the targeted human population and the seasonality. It may also influence the clinical presentation. For example, *Amblyomma* ticks are aggressive hunting ticks. They frequently attack in groups. This behavior explains clustered cases and several inoculation eschars in African tick bite fever.

Pathophysiology

Rickettsiae are intracellular parasites of phagocytes that invade the CNS as part of a systemic infection. Rickettsiae can be divided into two categories according to their targets during natural infection: (1) organisms that parasitize vascular endothelial cells (*Rickettsia rickettsii, R. conorii*, TG Rickettsiae), and (2) organisms that parasitize both endothelial cells and phagocytes (*O. tsutsugamushi*). In terms of their intracellular niches, *O. tsutsugamushi* and the Rickettsiae lyse the phagosome and replicate predominantly in the cytoplasm of host cells. The central pathophysiological event of *Rickettsia* infection, including CNS infection, has been identified as parasitism of vascular endothelial bacteria by blood-borne bacteria. Histological studies have confirmed rickettsial invasion of vascular endothelial cells in the brains of humans and experimentally infected mice. Rickettsiae

Table 86.1 Main clinical and epidemiological features of Rickettsiae infection.

Group	Organism	Arthropod vector	Main clinical features	Prominent neurological features
Spotted fever group				
Rocky Mountain spotted fever	*Rickettsia rickettsii*	Tick	No eschar, rash often purpuric, 2–5% fatality rate	Encephalitis, meningitis, meningoencephalitis, deafness, central nerve palsies, Guillain–Barré polyneuropathy
Mediterranean spotted fever	*Rickettsia conorii conorii*	Tick	Single eschar, 2–5% fatality rate	Encephalitis, meningitis, meningoencephalitis, deafness, central nerve palsies, Guillain–Barré polyneuropathy
Israeli spotted fever	*Rickettsia conorii israelensis*	Tick	Eschar less frequent (10%) than in Mediterranean spotted fever	Encephalitis, meningitis, meningoencephalitis
Astrakhan fever	*Rickettsia conorii caspia*	Tick	Eschar (23%), maculopapular rash (100%)	Hearing loss (14%)
Indian tick typhus	*Rickettsia conorii indica*	Tick	Rash usually purpuric, eschar rarely found	
Siberian tick typhus	*Rickettsia sibirica sibirica*	Tick	Rash (100%), eschar (77%), and lymphadenopathy	Encephalitis, rare, usually mild
Lymphangitis associated rickettsioses	*Rickettsia sibirica mongolitimonae*	Tick	Eschar (75%) may be multiple, rash (63%), lymphangitis (25%), and adenopathy	Meningitis, cerebellitis (two unreported cases)
Japanese spotted fever	*Rickettsia japonica*	Tick	Eschar (91%), rash (100%), and lymphadenopathy less frequent than in scrub typhus	Meningoencephalitis
African tick bite fever	*Rickettsia africae*	Tick	Outbreaks and clustered cases common (74%), fever (88%), eschars (95%) which are often multiple (54%), maculopapular or vesicular rash (50%) and lymphadenopathy	Sub-acute neuropathy
Queensland tick typhus	*Rickettsia australis*	Tick	Rash (100%) sometimes vesicular, eschar (65%), and lymphadenopathy	Confusion, transient visual hallucinations, seizures, rare
Flinders Island spotted fever	*Rickettsia honei*	Tick	Rash (85%), eschar (25%), and lymphadenopathy (55%)	Not reported
Tick-borne lymphadenopathy	*Rickettsia slovaca*	Tick	Typical large eschar on the scalp with cervical lymphadenopathy, fever and rash rare	Meningoencephalitis, very rare
Far-eastern spotted fever	*Rickettsia heilongjiangensis*	Tick	Rash, eschar, and lymphadenopathy	Not reported
Rickettsial pox	*Rickettsia akari*	Mite	Eschar and rash often vesicular	Not reported
	Rickettsia felis	Flea	Rash	Not reported
Typhus				
Epidemic typhus	*Rickettsia prowazekii*	Human louse	Rash (40%)	Encephalitis, frequent
Murine typhus	*Rickettsia typhi*	Flea	Rash (20–40%)	Encephalitis, less frequent than in epidemic typhus (<5%), subacute meningitis or meningoencephalitis
Scrub typhus	*Orientia tsutsugamushi*	Chigger (thrombiculide mite)	Eschar, generalized lymphadenopathies, rash rare	Encephalitis, meningitis, deafness

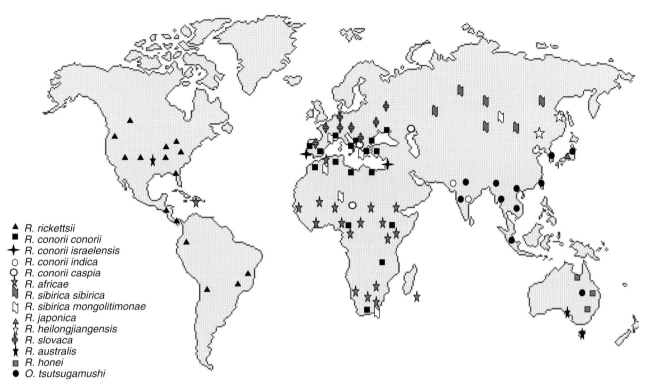

Figure 86.1 Geographic distribution of the spotted fever group rickettsioses and of scrub typhus.

▲ *R. rickettsii*
■ *R. conorii conorii*
✚ *R. conorii israelensis*
○ *R. conorii indica*
◐ *R. conorii caspia*
⬢ *R. africae*
▧ *R. sibirica sibirica*
⬗ *R. sibirica mongolitimonae*
△ *R. japonica*
⬠ *R. heilongjiangensis*
⬡ *R. slovaca*
✦ *R. australis*
▪ *R. honei*
● *O. tsutsugamushi*

invade and multiply at focal points in these small blood vessels, causing necrosis and proliferation of endothelial cells and development of platelet-fibrin thrombi at the site of damage, resulting in partial or even complete occlusion of the vascular lumen. These changes are associated with a perivascular inflammatory response, initially consisting of polymorphonuclear and monocytic cells, with the subsequent appearance of lymphocytes, macrophages, and plasma cells. This is the late phase of vascular damage, in which the immune response plays a major role. The classically described "typhus nodules" in the brain show similar pathology.

Clinical features

For many years, fever, rash, and headache were considered the diagnostic clue for rickettsial diseases. Indeed, this remains a major triad, but cases of spotless Rocky Mountain spotted fever (RMSF) have been reported, and many of the newly described rickettsial diseases have no rash. Major findings in rickettsioses include fever in a patient with exposure to a potential vector that may be associated with rash, inoculation eschar, or localized lymphadenopathy. Table 86.1 shows the major clinical symptoms with specificities according to the different species of Rickettsiae.

Spotted fever group rickettsioses
Rocky Mountain spotted fever

In the early phases of the disease, most patients have non-specific signs such as fever, headache, malaise, arthromyalgias, and nausea. Abdominal signs, especially in children, are often prominent, sometimes leading to erroneous diagnosis such as acute appendicitis. Only approximatively 60% of patients recall a tick bite. The rash appears late in the course of the disease (3–5 days) and may be absent in 10% of patients. In contrast with most other SFG rickettsioses, *R. rickettsii* does not generally elicit an eschar at the tick-bite site. So, when only non-specific symptoms dominate the clinical presentation, misdiagnosis and treatment delay can occur. The frequency and the severity of neurological signs depend on the severity of the illness. Headache is frequent (79–91%) and is one of the most consistent clinical findings in RMSF. Neurological complications are frequently the cause of death. Serious CNS complications include stupor, delirium, seizures, ataxia, papilledema, focal neurological deficits, and coma. Coma is more likely to occur in fatal than in non-fatal cases. Cranial and peripheral nerve palsies can occur, of which hearing loss is the most frequent. The incidence of meningeal signs is about 20% and among them about 60% had abnormalities of the cerebrospinal fluid (CSF). The white blood cell (WBC) count in the CSF is rarely more than $100/mm^3$. Polymorphonuclear leucocytes may predominate, but more commonly, lymphocytes predominate. Abnormalities in neuroimaging studies are not common in patients with RMSF, and when present they are often subtle. Since RMSF may present without rash, this illness must be considered in the differential diagnosis of every patient with encephalitic manifestations in endemic countries, especially if an appropriate epidemiological history is present. In general, the CNS manifestations resolve in parallel with the fever if adequate treatment is begun early in the course of illness. However, neurological sequelae are common following RMSF. They include learning disabilities, behavioral disturbance, depression, transverse myelitis, aphasia, and deafness.

Mediterranean spotted fever

After an asymptomatic incubation of 6 days (1–16 days), the onset of Mediterranean spotted fever (MSF) is abrupt and typical cases present with high fever (above 39°C), flu-like symptoms (headache, chills, arthromyalgias), and a black eschar (tache noire) at the tick bite site. Eschar is indolent and is usually localized on the trunk, legs, and arms. Usually the rash follows the fever within 2–3 days. In rare cases, fever may be absent (1–4% of cases) or is delayed until the fifth day. Gastrointestinal symptoms may be present in about 30% of patients and are more likely to be present in children. Headache is a common sign in MSF and is usually intense. Neurological complications occur in 10–15% of MSF cases. Hearing loss is the most frequent complication. Meningitis can occur but is less frequent than in RMSF. Serious CNS complications include stupor, delirium, seizures, ataxia, focal neurological deficits, and coma, and are usually associated with other organ failures representing the "malignant form" of MSF. This very severe form accounts for 5–6% of MSF cases and has a high mortality.

Other SFG rickettsioses

Table 86.1 lists the main clinical signs of other SFG rickettsioses and identifies which of them can manifest with neurological symptoms.

Typhus group rickettsioses
Epidemic typhus

The majority of patients with epidemic typhus experience the abrupt onset of fever and malaise. A severe headache is nearly invariably present in patients with typhus and has been used as a key clinical criterion for identifying suspected cases in epidemics, as well as severe leg myalgias. Infected patients may also complain of a number of other non-specific symptoms including cough, abdominal pain, nausea, and diarrhea. The rash of epidemic typhus classically begins several days after the onset of symptoms, appearing as a red macular or maculopapular eruption on the trunk that later spreads centrifugally to the extremities. Rash is rarely observed on dark skin. The majority of patients with epidemic typhus manifest one or more abnormalities in CNS function. Common neurological symptoms include confusion and drowsiness. Coma, seizures, and focal neurological signs may develop in a minority of patients. Delirium and coma are reported in 35% and 39% of fatal cases, respectively.

Murine typhus

Murine typhus is common in northern Africa, southern Europe, and South-East Asia. It is typically a mild illness. The onset of illness is usually abrupt with non-specific symptoms such as fever, headache, chills, and myalgias. Gastrointestinal symptoms are particularly common in children. Rash occurs in 20–54% of patients near the end of the first week of illness. It typically begins as a maculopapular eruption on the trunk and spreads peripherally. Symptoms of severe CNS disease such as seizures, stupor, and ataxia are infrequent, found in less than 5% of patients. However, cases of subacute aseptic meningitis or meningoencephalitis have been reported in patients with murine typhus without rash or other systemic findings. These cases suggest that neurological involvement in murine typhus is more common than previously described and that murine typhus should be included in the diagnosis of subacute meningitis, especially if an appropriate epidemiological history is present.

Scrub typhus

Scrub typhus is extremely common in Asia and specifically in South-East Asia. Scrub typhus may begin insidiously with headache, anorexia, and malaise, or start abruptly with chills and fever. Macular or maculopapular rash are frequently absent. More than 50% of patients have an eschar at the inoculation site. The eschar may develop before the onset of systemic symptoms, and can occur in multiple locations. Generalized lymphadenopathy occurs in the majority of patients. The neurological signs are similar in many respects to other rickettsial diseases in that headache is nearly always present. Meningismus or meningitis has been found in 5.7–13.5% of patients. However, in a series of 25 patients who underwent lumbar puncture in the absence of overt signs, 48% had a reactive spinal fluid showing a mild mononuclear pleiocytosis. Scrub typhus should be considered one of the causes of aseptic meningitis in areas of endemy. A small proportion of patients develop tremors, delirium, altered mental status, and coma. Acute hearing loss occurred in 6 out of 72 patients in Thailand.

Investigations

Culture remains extremely difficult for these organisms, and diagnosis mainly relies on serology and polymerase chain reaction (PCR). The reference technique for serology is immunofluorescence. Many cross-reactions are observed, and precise species determination of the infecting agent may be difficult. Testing of several antigens on the same slide to compare reactivity may help in discriminating among cross-reacting agents. Western blot may be more specific in early sera and cross-absorption may help to discriminate SFG rickettsiae.

PCR is an appropriate tool for the diagnosis of rickettsioses. Skin biopsy of the inoculation eschar is the best clinical sample for SFG rickettsiae, preferably before antibiotherapy. Molecular amplification with PCR, from eschar biopsy, ethylenediaminetetraacetic acid (EDTA), blood, or ticks, targets different genes (citrate synthase, *ompA*, *ompB*, "gene D") and allows the detection and identification of the causal agent with certitude. Biopsies can also be used for immunochemistry. Blood sample is the best clinical sample for scrub typhus for PCR.

Treatment

Early empirical antibiotic therapy should be prescribed in any suspected rickettsioses, before confirmation of the diagnosis. Early treatment may prevent many but not all cases in which CNS complications occur. Other variables such as age and glucose-6-phosphate dehydrogenase (G6PD) deficiency may be important factors in the risk of neurological complications. The most useful treatment in children and adults is doxycycline. In children, the risk of dental staining by doxycycline is negligible when a single, relatively short (5- to 10-day) course of treatment is administered. It can be prescribed in a short course (1 day for typhus, scrub typhus, and MSF). Chloramphenicol should not be prescribed because it is less active then doxycycline for RMSF.

Further reading

Drevets DA, Leenen PJ, Greenfield RA. Invasion of the central nervous system by intracellular bacteria. *Clin Microbiol Rev* 2004; 17(2): 323–46.

Marrie TJ, Raoult D. Rickettsial infections of the central nervous system. *Semin Neurol* 1992; 12(3): 213–24.

Parola P, Paddock C, Raoult D. Tick-borne rickettsioses around the world: emerging diseases challenging old concepts. *Clin Microbiol Rev* 2005; 18(4): 719–56.

Chapter 87
Acute, recurrent, and chronic viral meningitis

Larry E. Davis[1,2]
[1]New Mexico VA Health Care System, Albuquerque, USA
[2]University of New Mexico School of Medicine, Albuquerque, USA

Introduction

Viral meningitis is the most common infection of the central nervous system (CNS). The illness occurs worldwide, with the highest incidence in children and young adults. The term meningitis refers to inflammation of the meninges. Aseptic meningitis is a broad term that includes most meningeal mononuclear cell inflammatory processes not due to pyogenic bacteria, tuberculosis, or fungi. The Centers for Disease Control and Prevention define aseptic meningitis as a clinically compatible illness diagnosed by a physician, with no laboratory evidence of bacterial or fungal meningitis. The syndrome has multiple etiologies, but viruses cause the majority of cases. Recurrent meningitis refers to meningitis that recurs at definite intervals. Between the episodes, the patient is asymptomatic and usually has normal cerebrospinal fluid (CSF). Chronic meningitis refers to persistence of clinical meningitis symptoms and CSF inflammatory cells for more than 3–4 weeks. Meningoencephalitis is a term used when a virus infects both the meninges and brain parenchyma, with the patient developing signs of both meningitis and encephalitis.

Epidemiology

Viral meningitis is common around the world. Reports of aseptic meningitis regularly appear from Europe, Asia, Africa, Australia, and South America. When the viral cause is determined, the majority are enteroviruses. Often the same enterovirus serotypes simultaneously are circulating around the world.

The true incidence of viral meningitis is unknown. In the United States, aseptic meningitis is not a reportable disease, but estimates of the annual number of aseptic meningitis cases range from 75 000 to 150 000. Generally the incidence of adult viral meningitis ranges between 10 and 20 per 100 000 population per year . However, one report from Finland found the annual incidence of viral infections of the meninges and/or brain of children to be much higher – about 700 per 100 000.

The majority of cases are due to enteroviruses, mumps virus, herpes simplex virus, and arboviruses. Cases of meningitis from herpes simplex 2 meningitis and human immunodeficiency virus mainly develop in young sexually-active adults. Most cases of viral meningitis occur in summer in temperate climates at a time of prevailing of enteroviruses. Table 87.1 lists many of the viruses recognized as causing meningitis.

Pathophysiology

Viral meningitis begins with a primary focus of infection associated with the virus's route of entry – the gastrointestinal tract for enteroviruses, respiratory tract for mumps, subcutaneous tissue following mosquito or tick bite for arboviruses, and genital skin infection for herpes simplex virus type 2.

Spread to distant areas from the primary site occurs by viremia or infection of adjacent peripheral nerves such as in herpes simplex 2 virus infection. For most viruses, progeny virions spread from the initial body site into adjacent blood vessels or lymphatic channels. A viremia of varying duration then develops. For a viremia to cause meningitis, several important host barriers must be overcome. The reticuloendothelial system (RES) is an efficient filter of viruses circulating in the blood. However, some viruses overcome the RES by infecting vascular endothelial cells and constantly releasing viral particles into the blood. Other viruses circumvent the RES by infecting circulating blood cells.

Humoral and cellular immune responses also effectively terminate viremias. Because the primary infection triggered the host immune response days earlier, the incubation period is critical for enabling the host to produce neutralizing antibody, usually of the IgM class. Unfortunately the humoral immune response is not

International Neurology: A Clinical Approach. Edited by Robert P. Lisak, Daniel D. Truong, William M. Carroll, and Roongroj Bhidayasiri. © 2009 Blackwell Publishing, ISBN: 978-1-4051-5738-4.

Table 87.1 Causes of viral meningitis.

Common viruses	Comments
Enteroviruses	Account for over 50% of all cases in every country
Herpes simplex, types 2 and 1	Mainly in young sexually-active adults who acquire genital herpes
Arboviruses (West Nile, Western equine, Eastern equine, St Louis, California, Powassan, Japanese B, Jamestown Canyon, Toscana, tick-borne encephalitis, and many other viruses)	Incidence is seasonal when the vector is prevalent in the community
Mumps	Very common in children from countries that do not routinely administer childhood mumps vaccine, but sporadic cases occur from vaccination failures or waning immunity to mumps virus in developed countries
Less common causes	
Varicella-zoster virus	Can occur in immunocompetent and immunosuppressed patients with or without a rash
Lymphocytic choriomeningitis virus	Can occur from exposure to infected pet or wild rodents
Human immunodeficiency virus	Patients are symptomatic mainly during the primary infection, but CSF viral persistence occurs
Human T-cell lymphotropic virus, type 1	Low-grade lymphocytic meningitis with slowly progressive myelopathy
Poliovirus	Sporadic or clusters of cases occur in developing countries that lack strong poliovirus immunization programs. Meningitis without paralysis occurs in about 4% of primary infections
Live virus vaccines (mumps, measles, rubella, poliovirus)	Uncommon but recently has been associated with some strains of the mumps vaccine
Uncommon causes	
Parvovirus B19	Identified so far only in children or with immunosuppression
Adenovirus	Occurs rarely in immunosuppressed individuals
Reovirus	Mainly occurs in infants
Rhinovirus	Rare even in children
Cytomegalovirus	Mainly occurs in immunosuppressed individuals, especially AIDS
Human herpes virus 6	Rarely occurs in infants
Epstein–Barr virus	Mainly occurs in immunosuppressed individuals
Parainfluenza and influenza virus	Rare even in epidemics. Most patients with influenza and meningismus have normal CSF
Rubeola virus (measles)	Occurs mainly as a meningoencephalitis or post-viral encephalitis and occurs in countries without active childhood immunization programs
Rotavirus	Mainly seen in young children

always successful in terminating the viremia, particularly in immunosuppressed individuals.

The final hindrance for a virus to reach the CNS is the blood–brain barrier, which is usually highly effective in preventing all micro-organisms from reaching the meninges. These barriers successfully prevent viral entry into the CNS over 95% of the time.

Eradication of a viral infection within the meninges depends on the host's immune system as antiviral drugs are available for very few CNS viruses. Unfortunately, viral clearance of a CNS infection is less efficient than for infections elsewhere in the body since the brain and meninges have limited host defenses. Antibody titers in CSF are markedly lower than that of serum; few lymphocytes

are in normal CSF; and the brain lacks a lymphatic system. Nevertheless during active viral infection, immune monocytes invade the meninges, gamma interferon and other cytokines are released by the monocytes, and neutralizing antibody enters the CSF to normally destroy the virus.

Clinical features

Acute viral meningitis
Most cases of viral meningitis have a mild prodrome that begins a few days before the onset of headache. Enteroviral prodromes occur 1–3 days before onset of the

Table 87.2 Signs and symptoms of acute viral meningitis.

Common	Less common
Fever	Stupor
Headache	Seizures
Stiff neck	
Anorexia, nausea, vomiting	**Rare**
Photophobia	Focal neurologic signs
Irritability	Papilledema
Relative preservation of mental status	Babinski sign
	Coma

acute illness and range from gastrointestinal symptoms, pharyngitis, herpangina, and conjunctivitis, to rashes that may involve the hand, foot, and mouth. Patients with herpes simplex meningitis often have genital vesicles 1–7 days before the meningitis, but many recurrences lack genital vesicles. Arbovirus prodromes may include low-grade fever, myalgia, malaise, arthralgia, macular rashes, and gastrointestinal upset. Although parotitis is the classical sign of mumps developing several days before the meningitis, up to half the patients develop symptoms of the mumps meningitis either before the swelling of the parotid gland or without parotitis.

The onset of the meningitis is usually abrupt and explosive, becoming intense within a few hours. The classic triad for viral meningitis has been fever (which is seldom high), severe diffuse headache (which is often pounding), and stiff neck of varying severity. Table 87.2 lists the signs and symptoms of viral meningitis by their relative frequency. Patients with aseptic meningitis have a relative preservation of their mental status. Due to the headache, they seldom concentrate well or perform difficult mental tasks but are generally not disoriented, confused, or hallucinatory. If the mental status is markedly depressed, the diagnosis of meningoencephalitis should be considered. Although nuchal rigidity has been considered typical for viral meningitis, studies suggest that it is present only in about half of patients. The presence of papilledema, focal neurologic signs, or coma suggests that the patient may have another form of CNS infection.

Infants less than 2 years of age often present with non-specific signs such as fever, anorexia, lethargy, and irritability. Nuchal rigidity is noted in only one-fourth of cases. Signs of an upper respiratory or gastrointestinal infection and rash may also be present.

Recurrent viral meningitis

Recurrent viral meningitis is uncommon. A review of 46 reported cases of recurrent aseptic meningitis found that over 90% are due to herpes simplex virus (95% of cases from HSV-2 and 5% from HSV-1). Patients are young adults (mean age 37 years), with a slight female predominance, who experience benign recurring episodes of fever, severe headache, photophobia, and meningismus lasting 2–5 days followed by spontaneous recovery. Less

than half the patients recall experiencing genital herpetic lesions. The total number of episodes ranges from 3 to 9, with the time to recurrence varying from weeks to months or years. Over time the recurrences become less common. The syndrome, originally called Mollaret's meningitis, appears to be mainly due to recurrent HSV meningitis.

About 5% of patients with recurrent meningitis lack evidence of herpes simplex viral infection in the CSF. Rare cases have been associated with recurrent enterovirus infections, often of different serotypes. DeBiasi and Tyler review the many other causes that occasionally produce recurrent aseptic meningitis which include repeated exposures to drugs or biological products that trigger aseptic meningitis, intracranial and intraspinal tumors and cysts that periodically leak antigenic material into the CSF, and systemic connective tissue diseases.

Chronic viral meningitis

Persistence of viruses in the CNS is extremely rare in healthy individuals. When it happens, the viral persistence is mainly due to adaptation of the virus to evade the host immune response or the host immune response being deficient. HIV is the most common persistent meningeal virus and occurs by the virus evading and impairing the host immune response. Viral persistence develops early during the primary infection with viral invasion of the brain and meninges. From that point, the CSF contains HIV in varying viral titers usually accompanied by a low-grade lymphocytic pleocytosis. HIV may cause symptomatic meningitis during the primary infection but seldom causes chronic meningeal symptoms.

Viral and other infectious agents can be persistent in meninges when the host immune system is impaired, such as in AIDS or other immunosuppressive illnesses. Usually the infectious agent is one that does not persist in a healthy individual. Chronic viral infections of the meninges of immunosuppressed patients are recognized with several viruses including cytomegalovirus, enteroviruses, poliovirus, West Nile, Epstein–Barr, herpes simplex, and varicella-zoster.

Differential diagnosis

The differential diagnosis of acute aseptic meningitis is broad but mostly due to viruses (Table 87.1). There are other causes, including bacteria, Rickettsia, protozoa, helminths, parameningeal conditions, drugs, biological products, systemic or immunologically-mediated diseases, and neoplasms, as listed in Table 87.3.

The causes of chronic meningitis are broad and rarely include viruses. More common causes are other infectious agents (bacteria, fungi, parasites), vasculitis, connective tissue diseases, sarcoidosis, chronic administration of drugs producing idiosyncratic meningitis, chemical

Table 87.3 Non-viral causes of aseptic meningitis.

Other infectious agents

Bacteria

Borrelia burgdorferi (Lyme disease), *Treponema pallidum* (syphilis), *Leptospira* sp., *Brucella* sp., *Bartonella* sp. (cat scratch fever), agents of bacterial endocarditis, *Mycoplasma pneumonia*

Rickettsia

Rickettsia rickettsii (Rocky mountain spotted fever), *Rickettsia prowazekii* (typhus), *Rickettsia conorii*, *Orientia tsutsugamushi*, *Ehrlichia chaffeensis*, *Anaplasma* sp. (human granulocytic ehrlichiosis), *Babesia* sp.

Protozoa and helminths

Taenia solium (cysticercosis), *Toxoplasma gondii*, *Trichinella spiralis* (trichinosis), *Chlamydia trachomatis*, *Strongyloides stercoralis* (eosinophilic meningitis or hyperinfection syndrome), *Angiostrongylus cantonensis* and *Baylisacaris procyonis* (eosinophilic meningitis), *Naegleria fowleri* (amoebic meningitis)

Parameningeal conditions

Sinusitis, epidural or subdural empyema, mastoiditis, cranial osteomyelitis, infection or inflammation related to ventricular shunts, posterior fossa surgery, brain abscess, venous sinus thrombosis, subarachnoid hemorrhage

Drugs

Trimethoprim–sulfamethoxazole, ibuprofen, sulindac, tolmentin, naproxen, rofecoxib, diclofenac, ketoprofen, azathioprine, sulfasalazine, ciprofloxacin, amoxicillin, metronidazole, cephalosporins, pyrazinamide, isoniazid, carbamazepine, lamotrigine, ranitidine, phenazopyridine, chemical meningitis treated with drugs, air, or radiographic agents instilled into CSF, chymopapain injections into spinal area

Biologic products

Muromonab-CD3 murine monoclonal antibody OKT3, intravenous gammaglobulin (IVIg), influenza vaccine (killed virus)

Systemic or immunologically-mediated diseases

Sarcoidosis, systemic lupus erythematosus, rheumatoid arthritis, polyarteritis nodosa, granulomatous arteritis, mixed connective tissue disease, Sjögren's syndrome, lymphomatoid granulomatosis, Wegener's granulomatosis, sarcoidosis, Behçet's disease, Kawasaki disease, Vogt–Koyanagi–Harada syndrome, familial Mediterranean fever, status epilepticus, post-infectious syndromes

Neoplastic diseases

Leukemia, leptomeningeal carcinoma, lymphoma, craniopharyngioma, teratoma, astrocytoma, medulloblastoma, dermoid and epidermoid cysts

---

Table 87.4 Distinguishing CSF features between viral and bacterial meningitis.

CSF feature	Viral meningitis*	Bacterial meningitis*
White blood cells	Predominantly mononuclear	Predominantly neutrophils
Protein	Normal to mildly elevated	Elevated
Glucose	Normal to minimally depressed	Depressed
Lactate	Normal	Elevated
Gram stain of sediment	Negative	Positive
Bacterial culture	Negative	Positive

*These CSF features are usually present, but all the features will not necessarily be present in every patient.

meningitis from antigen leakage of CNS tumors into the CSF, and leptomeningeal cancer metastases, which have been extensively reviewed in Davis (2006).

Investigations

In the workup of a patient, the first step is to utilize the history and neurologic examination to establish a high suspicion of meningitis and to help distinguish meningitis from other CNS problems. The key to proving the patient has meningitis is to perform a lumbar puncture and examine the CSF. The opening CSF pressure should be obtained and from 10 to 20 ml of CSF is collected in several sterile tubes. Important tests to be ordered include CSF cell count with differential white cell count, glucose level, protein level, Gram stain of spun CSF sediment, and tests to determine the etiology, including bacterial culture, relevant CSF polymerase chain reaction (PCR) assays, and possibly viral culture. The presence of a CSF white blood cell pleocytosis establishes the diagnosis of meningitis.

Analysis of the CSF usually allows distinction between bacterial and aseptic meningitis. Table 87.4 lists CSF findings supportive of viral and bacterial meningitis. The CSF of most viral meningitides contains a predominance of mononuclear cells with a mean of 60–100 cells/mm^3 and a range of white blood cells from 10 to 600/mm^3. Occasionally if the CSF is examined in the first 12–24 hours of the viral meningitis, a transient predominance of neutrophils can be seen that converts to a lymphocytic predominance the following day.

A simultaneous serum glucose is helpful in determining whether the CSF glucose is depressed. CSF/serum glucose ratios below 50% are usually considered abnormal, as is a CSF glucose level below 40 mg/dl. Although viral meningitis usually has a normal glucose level, a few viruses (mumps, lymphocytic choriomeningitis) may produce a mildly depressed CSF glucose level typically from 30 to 40 mg/dl. In patients with CSF glucose levels less than 25 mg/dl, bacterial, fungal, or tuberculous meningitis should be considered. CSF protein levels are usually at the upper limit of normal, or elevated as high as 100 mg/dl, and CSF oligoclonal bands are unusual in the acute CSF sample.

In general, the fever in viral meningitis is low while it may be quite elevated in bacterial meningitis. Likewise, the peripheral white blood cell count in viral meningitis is often normal or slightly elevated, while it may be quite elevated in bacterial meningitis.

Once the CSF points to aseptic meningitis, the final diagnostic step is to identify the viral etiology. In general the yield of virus isolation from CSF is below 50% and rapidly declines to less than 10% over several days. Viruses that are most commonly isolated from CSF include enterovirus, mumps, and lymphocytic choriomeningitis. It is also possible to isolate the virus from other body sites, including throat, nasopharynx, stool, and skin lesions. Unfortunately, virus isolation from non-CNS sites does not automatically mean that that virus was the cause of the viral meningitis. This is particularly true for enteroviruses that often cause asymptomatic gastrointestinal infections in the summer or for herpes simplex virus that often produces a silent salivary viral reactivation with any acute febrile illness.

Because of the difficulty in isolating virus from CSF, polymerase chain reaction (PCR) assays have become popular. Viral PCR assays are rapid (often less than 1 day), less expensive than virus culture, have over 80–95% sensitivity and specificity depending on the virus, and can detect viral nucleic acid up to 1–2 weeks after disease onset. CSF PCR assays for enterovirus, herpes simplex, and HIV are now the standard for CSF diagnosis.

Recently "multiplex" CSF PCR assays have been developed that utilize multiple primers simultaneously in a single reaction mixture to amplify nucleic acid from a group of viruses. In one study of 787 CSF samples sent with a suspicion of a CNS infection, a "multiplex" PCR assay with eight different viral primers found 30% to be positive for viruses. However, clinical judgment must be used in interpreting the results of CSF PCR assays since occasionally dual viral infections are found and patients not suspected of a meningeal infection have had positive PCR assays.

A third method for establishing the etiology of viral meningitis is by demonstration of specific intrathecal antibody synthesis. Identification of specific IgM antibody in CSF is a common method to diagnosis West Nile virus neuroinvasive disease. CNS infection with varicella-zoster virus can also be diagnosed by demonstration of varicella-zoster antibody in CSF.

In patients with viral meningitis, cranial CT or MRI scan with gadolinium is generally normal. However, in chronic viral meningitis or meningoencephalitis, the MRI may show focal brain or spinal cord abnormalities depending on the virus. Electroencephalography is usually normal in aseptic meningitis but occasionally shows transient diffuse abnormalities that become normal by 1 week.

Treatment/management

Historically patients with aseptic meningitis are hospitalized, given antinausea medication, administered intravenous fluids for dehydration, and placed on age-appropriate medications for fever and headache. The majority of patients are given broad-spectrum antibiotics until the CSF bacterial cultures return and also may be given acyclovir for possible atypical herpes encephalitis until the CSF HSV PCR assay returns. The hospital duration ranges from 3 to 15 days.

Until recently, there has been little emphasis on establishing the specific etiology of the aseptic meningitis because seldom did a specific viral diagnosis affect treatment options. However, with the wider availability of enterovirus PCR assays, studies of children with aseptic meningitis have shown that early use of this CSF PCR test can significantly shorten the duration of the hospitalization by 1–3 days, reduce the need for neuroimaging and electroencephalography, and reduce hospital costs by up to $3000 per patient.

Under ideal circumstances, patients with enterovirus meningitis could be discharged after 24 hours assuming (1) early enterovirus PCR assay (possible because 6-hour commercial PCR kits are available), (2) patients have improved symptomatically at 24 hours, and (3) CSF bacterial cultures are negative at 24 hours since over 90% of patients with bacterial meningitis have positive CSF bacterial cultures by 24 hours.

Currently there is no Food and Drug Administration (FDA)-approved antiviral drug for treatment of enteroviral meningitis. However, a recent study of adults with enteroviral meningitis reported that pleconaril therapy (200 mg orally three times daily for 7 days) significantly reduced the duration of the intense headache and shortened the course of the illness.

Episodes of acute and recurrent herpes simplex meningitis are widely treated with antiHSV drugs, for example, acyclovir, famciclovir, and valaciclovir, with likely beneficial effects. However, there have been no controlled studies to demonstrate that these antiHSV drugs significantly shorten the duration of headache and stiff neck. For patients hospitalized with acute HSV meningitis, treatment is often with acyclovir (10 mg/kg intravenously every 8 hours for 5–7 days). For treatment of subsequent episodes of recurrent meningitis, the patient may be given a prescription for valaciclovir (1000 mg two times a day orally for 3–5 days) to begin at the first sign of a viral meningitis attack or the patient may take valaciclovir 1000 mg orally every day to prevent attacks. Currently there are no studies to demonstrate either approach is beneficial.

Recovery and prognosis

Over 95% of patients with viral meningitis make a complete recovery. In one study of adults, 43% were symptom free at hospital discharge, 50% were symptom free by 3 months, and 7% had persistent mild cognitive deficits, mainly in concentration, longer than 3 months. A few studies have examined the cognition of individuals 1–2 years after acute aseptic meningitis and found the majority of patients were normal. In very young infants, the viral meningitis may cause more long-lasting cognitive problems.

Recurrent herpes simplex meningitis usually lessens in frequency of attacks over several years and the overall prognosis is excellent with full recovery after each episode. For persistent viral meningitis the prognosis is poorer, although the type of complications depend on the specific virus and the immune status of the individual.

Further reading

Davis LE. Subacute and chronic meningitis. *Continuum* 2006; 12: 27–57.

Davies NWS, Brown LJ, Gonde J, *et al.* Factors influencing PCR detection of viruses in cerebrospinal fluid of patients with suspected viral infections. *J Neurol Neurosurg Psychiatry* 2005; 76: 82–7.

DeBiasi RL, Tyler KL. Recurrent aseptic meningitis. In: Davis LE, Kennedy PGE, editors. *Infectious Diseases of the Nervous System.* Oxford: Butterworth-Heinemann; 2000, pp. 445–79.

Desmond RA, Accortt NA, Talley L, Villano SA, Soong S-J, Whitley RJ. Enterovirus meningitis: natural history and outcome of pleconaril therapy. *Antimicrob Agents Chemother* 2006; 50: 2409–14.

Gilden DH, Mahalingam R, Cohrs R, Tyler KL. Herpesvirus infections of the nervous system. *Nat Clin Pract Neurol* 2007; 3: 82–94.

Nowak DA, Boehmer R, Fuchs H-H. A retrospective clinical, laboratory and outcome analysis in 43 cases of acute aseptic meningitis. *Eur J Neurol* 2003; 10: 271–80.

Sawyer MH, Holland D, Aintablian N, Connnor JD, Keyser EF, Waecker NJ. Diagnosis of enteroviral central nervous system infection by polymerase chain reaction during a large community outbreak. *Pediatr Infect Dis J* 1994; 13: 177–82.

Shaiabi M, Whiteley RJ. Recurrent benign lymphocytic meningitis. *Clin Infect Dis* 2006; 43: 1194–7.

Chapter 88
The syndrome of acute encephalitis

Heng Thay Chong and Chong Tin Tan
University of Malaya, Kuala Lumpur, Malaysia

Introduction

Encephalitis refers to inflammation of the brain parenchyma. Patients with encephalitis often exhibit concomitant involvement of the meninges. Meningo-encephalitis, a similar condition, refers to meningitis and inflammation of the brain parenchyma and can resemble both encephalitis and meningitis at presentation. The most common cause of encephalitis is infection, although it can also be caused by an autoimmune mechanism, such as in limbic encephalitis and Rasmussen's syndrome. Worldwide, the most common cause of acute encephalitis is viral infection.

Epidemiology and etiology

The overall incidence of viral encephalitis is estimated to be 1–7.4 per 10^5 persons per annum; however, among children younger than 2 years of age, the incidence is as high as 16.7 per 10^5 persons per annum. This is in contrast to bacterial meningitis, which has an incidence of 36.3 per 10^5 persons per annum.

There are many viral causes of encephalitis (see Table 88.1). The most important endemic agents across wide geographical areas are the herpes viruses and the arboviruses (arthropod-borne viruses). Among encephalitic patients with a microbiological diagnosis in developed countries in Western Europe, North America, and parts of Asia, herpes viruses are the most common infecting agents. Herpes simplex virus is usually responsible for sporadic encephalitis, while the varicella zoster virus accounts for 7.5–22% of pediatric encephalitis in these countries. However, it is estimated that even in developed nations, the larger, undiagnosed proportion of encephalitides is caused by the arboviruses.

Numerically, Japanese encephalitis is the most common encephalitis worldwide, while the West Nile virus is more widespread and is found in parts of Europe, Russia, Africa, the Middle East, India, Indonesia, and, recently, North America. In Eastern Europe, tick-borne encephalitis is the most common. Rabies virus, another causative agent of encephalitis, is endemic in Latin America, Asia, and Africa.

Pathology

With the exception of viral agents such as rabies and Nipah virus, the pathology of most viral encephalitides is non-specific. However, the presence of some pathological features is suggestive of certain infections, such as Cowdry type A inclusion bodies in herpes simplex encephalitis. Light microscopic examination often shows inflammation and perivascular lymphocytic and mononuclear cell infiltrate. This is often accompanied by arteritis, necrosis of neural tissue, and neuronophagia with glial cell hyperplasia. Gliosis can ensue if the patient survives.

Clinical and laboratory features

Patients with acute encephalitis present with rapid onset of fever, headache, nausea, vomiting, seizures, respiratory, and abdominal symptoms. On examination, there is impairment of the conscious state, confusion, and focal neurological deficits.

Laboratory examination findings are often non-specific. Complete blood count may show lymphocytosis. The clotting profile may be abnormal in viruses that cause hemorrhagic complications. Electroencephalogram (EEG) often shows non-specific slow waves, although periodic lateralized epileptiform discharges are seen in herpes simplex encephalitis and in severe Nipah encephalitis. Imaging studies are also non-specific, showing gray and sometimes white matter involvement; however, herpes simplex virus has a predilection to cause necrotic and hemorrhagic changes.

Cerebrospinal fluid (CSF) examination typically shows raised opening pressure, lymphocytosis, and raised protein

International Neurology: A Clinical Approach. Edited by Robert P. Lisak, Daniel D. Truong, William M. Carroll, and Roongroj Bhidayasiri.
© 2009 Blackwell Publishing, ISBN: 978-1-4051-5738-4.

Table 88.1 Viruses that affect the central nervous system. Adapted from Johnson RT. *Viral Infections of the Nervous System*, 2nd ed. Philadelphia, Lippincott-Raven; 1998.

Primary human viruses	
Herpes viruses	Herpes simplex types 1 and 2, varicella zoster, Epstein–Barr virus, cytomegalovirus, human herpes virus 6
Enteroviruses	Polioviruses 1–3, coxsackievirus A1–22, 24, B1–6, echoviruses 1–7, 9, 11–27, 29–33, enteroviruses 68–71
Other	Mumps, measles, rubella, human immunodeficiency virus, human T-cell lymphoma virus, adenovirus, parvovirus B19, JC virus
Zoonotic viruses	
Arenavirus	Lymphocytic choriomeningitis virus, Lassa virus, Junin virus, Machupo virus, Guanarito virus, Sabia virus
Filovirus	Marburg virus, Ebola virus
Paramyxovirus	Nipah virus, Hendra virus
Rhabdovirus	Rabies virus, Mokola virus, Lyssavirus
Herpes virus	B virus (Herpes simiae or Cercopithecine herpesvirus 1)
Arthropod viruses	
Flaviviridae	*Mosquito-borne complex*: St Louis encephalitis virus, Japanese encephalitis virus, Murray Valley encephalitis virus, Kunjin virus, West Nile virus, Ilheus virus, Rocio virus *Tick-borne complex*: Far Eastern, Siberian, and Western European tick-borne encephalitis viruses, Negishi virus, Louping ill virus, Langat virus, Powassan virus, Omsk hemorrhagic fever virus, Kyasanur forest disease virus, Kadam virus and Royal farm virus (which consists of three subtypes: Karshi virus, Gadgets Gulley virus, and Alkhurma virus)
Bunyaviridae	California encephalitis virus, LaCrosse encephalitis virus, Jamestown Canyon virus, Snowshoe hare virus, Tahnya virus, Inkoo virus, Rift Valley virus, Toscana virus
Togaviridae (alphaviruses)	Eastern equine virus, Western equine virus, Venezuelan equine virus
Reoviridae (orbivirus)	Colorado tick fever virus

levels; sugar levels are often normal, although initially there could be polymorph leucocytosis. Specific diagnosis is made by serological studies, viral culture, or polymerase chain reaction (PCR) to detect specific viral genomes in CSF, or, in selected cases, by brain biopsy (Table 88.2).

Differential diagnoses

Differential diagnoses of viral encephalitis include other central nervous system (CNS) infections, autoimmune diseases, and metabolic diseases (Table 88.3). In up to three-quarters of patients, specific viral studies such as serology, PCRs, and viral culture do not yield positive results. However, certain clinical and laboratory features suggest viral encephalitis, including fever, headache, focal neurological deficits, focal seizure, the absence of systemic illness, typical CSF findings, and gray matter involvement in brain MRI. Acute disseminated encephalomyelitis is particularly difficult to distinguish from viral encephalitis, especially among children. However, MRI in acute disseminated encephalomyelitis often shows thalamic and white matter changes with less prominent gray matter involvement. Geographical location, history of exposure, and clinical presentation are the most helpful features to elucidate the likely causative agent.

Geographical location

The main viruses that cause human encephalitides are primary human viruses, zoonotic viruses, and arboviruses. Primary human viruses have worldwide distribution, while most zoonotic viruses and arboviruses have limited geographical distribution (see Figure 88.1). Rabies, an exception to the generally limited zoonotic viruses, can be carried worldwide by dogs and other wildlife, while bat lyssavirus is found only in Australian bats.

History of exposure

Zoonotic viruses are primarily carried by rodents, primates, horses, bats, pigs, and dogs. Most arboviruses are carried by mosquitoes and ticks, with a wide range of animals serving as reservoirs and amplifying hosts, including birds and small mammals. Domesticated animals

Investigation	Differential diagnoses and complications
Blood tests	Serum electrolytes; sugar level; renal function; liver function; arterial blood gases; thyroid function; peripheral blood picture; creatinine kinase; autoimmune markers; thick and thin film for malaria parasite; blood culture; serology for bacterial, treponemal, and rickettsial infection
Chest X-ray	Pneumonia or pneumonitis (atypical pneumonia, Nipah encephalitis); orthostatic or aspiration pneumonia (complication); pulmonary tuberculosis; pulmonary aspergillosis; disseminated candidiasis or cryptococcomas
Brain CT scan	Brain abscess; subdural hematoma; vasculitic stroke
Brain MRI	Hyperintense signal in gray or white matter, diencephalon, brainstem, and cerebellum; tuberculoma; cryptococcomas; toxoplasma encephalitis; vasculitic stroke; venogram (for sagittal sinus thrombosis)
Lumbar puncture	Opening pressure, cell count and biochemical analysis; Gram stain and Ziehl–Nielsen stain; serology for bacterial, treponemal, and viral infection; cryptococcal antigen; bacterial and mycobacterial culture; PCR for tuberculosis, enterovirus, herpes simplex virus, cytomegalovirus, and other viruses; viral culture; quantification of herpes simplex viral; DNA copy for prognostication
Electroencephalogram	Non-convulsive status epilepticus; triphasic waves (hepatic and metabolic encephalopathy); periodic lateralized epileptiform discharges, and focal slow waves
Brain biopsy	Necrosis; hemorrhage; intraneuronal or intranuclear inclusion body; Negri body; vasculitic changes; fluorescent *in-situ* hybridization

Table 88.2 Laboratory investigations.

Infective causes

Bacterial	Abscess; actinomycoses; *Bartonella henselae*; *Borrelia burdgorferi*; brucella; legionella; leptospira; *Listeria monocytogenes*; *Mycobacterium tuberculosis*; *Mycoplasma pneumoniae*; nocardia; *Salmonella typhi*; *Treponema pallidum*; *Tropheryma whippeli* (Whipple's disease)
Rickettsial	Ehrlichiosis; Q fever; Rocky Mountain spotted fever typhus
Fungal	Aspergillosis; blastomycosis; candidiasis; coccidioidomycosis; cryptococcosis; histoplasmosis
Parasitic	Malaria; *Nagleria fowleri*; toxoplasmosis; trypanosomiasis; schistosomiasis

Non-infective causes

Autoimmune diseases	Acute disseminated encephalomyelitis; Bickerstaff encephalitis; vasculitides involving the CNS; limbic encephalitis; Rasmussen's syndrome; system lupus erythematosus
Metabolic diseases	Mitochondrial disease; thyrotoxic storm; neuroleptic malignant syndrome; thrombotic thrombocytopaenic purpura; severe systemic sepsis; hepatic encephalopathy; uraemia; diabetic complications (hypoglycemia, hyperglycemia, hyperosmolar syndrome, diabetic ketoacidosis); nutritional deficiency (e.g., Wernicke's encephalopathy)
Other systemic diseases	Hypoxic encephalopathy; malignant hypertension; non-convulsive status epilepticus; sagittal sinus thrombosis; poisoning

Table 88.3 Differential diagnoses of viral encephalitis. (Adapted and modified from Kennedy PGE. Viral encephalitis. *J Neurol*, 2005; 252: 268–72, and Chaudhuri A, Kennedy PGE. Diagnosis and treatment of viral encephalitis. *Postgrad Med J*, 2002; 78: 575–83.)

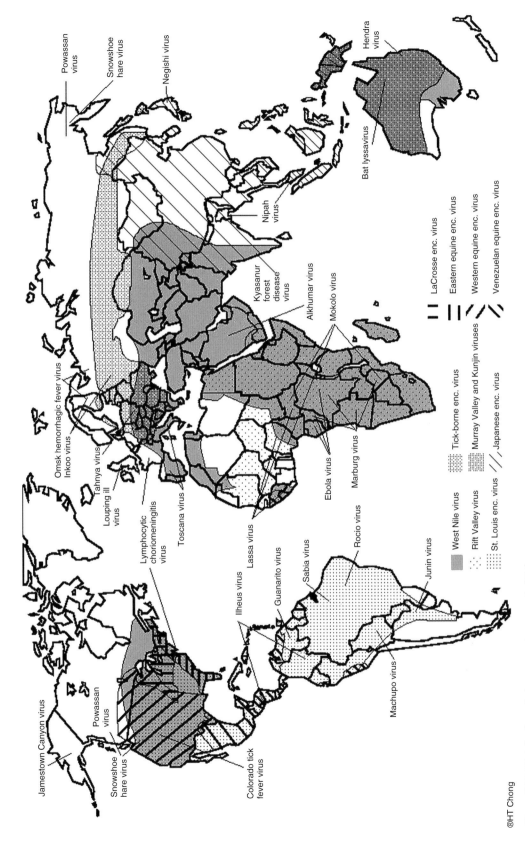

Figure 88.1 Distribution of viruses causing encephalitides.

©HT Chong

such as pigs, buffaloes, sheep, cattle, and camels can also serve as reservoirs.

Clinical presentation

Although most patients with encephalitis present with typical features as described above, certain viral agents such as rabies and Nipah virus can cause specific clinical features. Other viruses may have a predilection to infect children, the elderly, or the immunosuppressed. Specific viral symptoms and the patient profile can help in early diagnosis, especially when there are a limited number of viruses in the patient's geographical area. The specific clinical features of various viruses that cause encephalitis are listed in Table 88.4.

Management and prognosis

Treatment of viral encephalitis is broadly divided into supportive care, prevention and treatment of complications, specific antiviral therapy, and rehabilitation. At presentation, the patient's vital signs and conscious state should be closely monitored. Those who are ill should be managed in the intensive care unit. If there is significant impairment of the conscious state, as indicated by a low or rapidly deteriorating Glasgow Coma Scale score or if the patient is in status epilepticus, the patient should be intubated and mechanically ventilated for airway protection and prevention of aspiration pneumonia. Intravenous hydration and feeding through a nasogastric tube are also indicated, with meticulous attention paid to fluid, electrolyte, and acid base balance. Ripple mattress,

Table 88.4 Specific clinical features of viruses causing encephalitis.

Clinical features	Suggestive virus
Children	Japanese encephalitis virus; LaCrosse virus; enterovirus; adenovirus; poor outcome in Japanese encephalitis and Western and Eastern equine encephalitis
Elderly	West Nile virus; alphaviruses; worse outcome in St Louis, West Nile, Eastern equine, and Nipah encephalitis
Immunosuppressed host	Cytomegalovirus; JC virus (progressive multifocal leucoencephalopathy); measles virus (measles inclusion body encephalitis); recurrent enterovirus infection
Chronic or recurrent encephalitis	Measles virus (measles inclusion body encephalitis or subacute measles encephalitis and subacute sclerosing panencephalitis); Nipah virus; enterovirus in patients with immunoglobulin deficiency
Biphasic fever	Tick-borne encephalitis virus; Kyasanur Forest disease virus
Parkinsonism	Japanese encephalitis virus; West Nile virus; tick-borne encephalitis virus; Western equine virus
Cerebellar involvement	Varicella zoster virus; Junin virus
Brainstem involvement	West Nile virus; tick-borne encephalitis virus; St Louis virus
Spinal cord involvement	Japanese encephalitis virus; West Nile virus; rabies virus (paralytic rabies); tick-borne encephalitis virus; cytomegalovirus; human T-cell lymphoma virus type 1; human immunodeficiency virus
Autonomic involvement	Herpes simplex virus; Nipah virus; rabies virus (furious rabies)
Meningeal involvement	Enterovirus; Epstein–Barr virus; West Nile virus; parvovirus B9; lymphocytic choriomeningitis virus; Toscana virus; Colorado tick fever virus
Co-existing retinitis	Cytomegalovirus
Myoclonus, opsoclonus	Nipah virus; Japanese encephalitis virus; rabies virus; St Louis encephalitis virus
Urinary symptoms	St Louis encephalitis virus
Respiratory and/or abdominal involvement	LaCrosse virus; Nipah virus; Venezuelan equine virus; Guanarito virus
Bleeding diasthesis	Kyasanur Forest disease virus; arenavirus (Lassa, Junin, Machupo, Guanarito, and Sabia viruses); filovirus (Marburg and Ebola viruses)

Table 88.5 Specific treatment for viral infections of the central nervous system.

Virus	Therapy
Herpes simplex virus	Acyclovir 10 mg/kg, three times a day, IV, for 10–14 days; *or* valacyclovir *or* famciclovir
Cytomegalovirus	Ganciclovir 5 mg/kg, two times a day, IV, with/without foscarnet 60 mg/kg, three times a day, IV; valganciclovir; cidofovir
Herpes zoster virus	Acyclovir 800 mg, five times a day, IV, for 7–10 days; *or* famciclovir 500 mg, three times a day, for 7 days; *or* valacyclovir 1 g, three times a day, IV, for 7 days
Enterovirus	Pleconaril 5 mg/kg, three times a day, IV, for 10 days; *or* IV immunoglobulin for patients with immunoglobulin deficiency
Nipah virus	Day 1: ribavirin 2 g single dose; days 2–4: 1.2 g, three times a day Days 5–6: 1.2 g, twice a day Additional 1–4 days: 0.6 g, two times a day, orally
JC virus in HIV infection	Highly active antiretroviral agent therapy (HAART)
Rabies and bat lyssavirus	*Pre-exposure vaccination* Tissue culture vaccine in deltoid on days 0, 7, and 28; booster 1 year later; then every 2–5 years, depending on exposure *Minor wounds in patients with pre-exposure vaccination* Post-exposure vaccination with tissue culture vaccine • Five 1 ml deltoid IM injections on days 0, 3, 7, 14, and 30; *or* • Two 1 ml IM injections at two sites on day 0, followed by a single 1 ml injection on days 7 and 21; *or* • Eight 0.1 ml intradermal injections at eight sites (deltoid, suprascapular, abdominal, and anterolateral aspect of thighs) on day 0; four sites on day 7; single site on days 28 and 90 Double dose of vaccines at different sites on day 0 in immunosuppressed patients *Major or multiple wounds, or no pre-exposure vaccination* • Hyperimmune globulin at 40 IU/kg of hyperimmune equine antirabies serum; or 20 IU/kg of human rabies immunoglobulin; half infiltrate around the wounds (except digits), the other half IM (*not* in gluteal region); *and* • Post-exposure vaccination as above, double first dose of vaccine *Other management* • Clean wound with soap, iodine solution, or alcohol, then leave open without suturing for secondary healing • Remove foreign bodies and give tetanus toxoid and antibiotics for Gram negatives and anaerobes

coma nursing, regular positional change to prevent pressure sores, chest physiotherapy to prevent orthostatic pneumonia, and deep vein thrombosis prophylaxis are essential. Urinary catheter, if used, must be changed regularly with aseptic technique. Seizure must be rapidly controlled.

Specific antiviral therapy is only available in a few instances (Table 88.5). Because definitive diagnosis is often not available immediately and because of the prevalence and severity of herpes simplex encephalitis, most patients are empirically treated with acyclovir.

Overall, the outcome of viral encephalitis is relatively good, especially when compared to that of bacterial meningitis; actual mortality and morbidity depend on the etiologic agent and host factors. The overall mortality in children is only 4.5%, and only 8.1% develop neurological sequelae. However, the mortality rate remains high in herpes simplex encephalitis, Japanese encephalitis, Nipah encephalitis, and Eastern equine encephalitis.

Complications of viral encephalitis include cerebral salt-losing syndrome, syndrome of inappropriate antidiuretic hormone secretion, cerebral infarct, cerebral venous thrombosis, persistent neurological deficit, intellectual impairment, and epilepsy. Rehabilitation therapy,

therefore, is important in many patients recovering from viral encephalitis.

Specific viral encephalitides

Herpes simplex encephalitis
Epidemiology
Herpes simplex encephalitis is caused by herpes simplex virus type 1 in 90% of patients. In the other 10% of patients, often neonates or immunosuppressed individuals, it is caused by herpes simplex virus type 2. The incidence of herpes virus encephalitis is 0.1–0.84 cases per 10^5 per annum in developed nations, where it causes 16–24% of encephalitis with microbiologic diagnosis. Herpes simplex encephalitis occurs in all ages and at any time of year.

Pathogenesis
Herpes simplex infection is acquired when the virus, often carried by respiratory droplets, comes into contact with the mucosal surface of a susceptible individual. The virus replicates at the site of initial infection and, after being transported by retrograde axonal flow in the neuron to the

dorsal root ganglia, replicates again and establishes latent infection after being confined by host immune response. Occasionally, primary infection in neonates, pregnant women, or immunosuppressed hosts can occur and lead to systemic infection with multiorgan involvement.

Approximately two-thirds of encephalitis cases occur as a result of reactivation of latent infection; the other one-third is the result of primary infection. The route of access to the CNS is not totally understood, although evidence suggests that the virus gains access via the olfactory and trigeminal nerves, among others.

Pathology

Once the virus reaches the CNS, it infects neurons, causing ballooning of the cells, the appearance of chromatin, and degeneration of nuclei. The host immune response causes an influx of mononuclear cells, which leads to inflammation, necrosis, and, in severe cases, hemorrhage of the temporal and orbitofrontal lobes, as well as the cingulate and insular gyri in some cases. Microscopically, this is seen as vascular congestion, petechiae, perivascular cuffing, and necrosis. In approximately half of the patients, homogenous, eosinophilic, intranuclear inclusion bodies (Cowdry type A) are seen in the first week of infection. After 2 weeks, gliosis, glial nodules, and sattelitosis-neuronophagia appear, and it is at this time that widespread areas of hemorrhagic necrosis become prominent.

Clinical and laboratory features

Patients with herpes simplex encephalitis present abruptly with rapidly progressive fever, headache, vomiting, and autonomic dysfunction. Anosmia, personality changes, memory loss, and partial seizure are common, as are focal motor deficits, visual field defects, hemiparesis, ataxia, cranial nerve defects, and dysphasia. Complications of herpes simplex encephalitis include remote symptomatic epilepsy as well as persistent neurological deficits such as anosmia, dysphasia, motor deficits, poor memory, and even Klüver–Bucy syndrome. If left untreated, patients often progress rapidly to coma and death. Up to 20% of patients, however, develop a milder form of encephalitis without focal neurological deficits.

EEG shows unilateral or bilateral periodic lateralized epileptiform discharges. Brain CT scan shows hypodensity in the temporal lobe in up to 50% of patients. MRI of the brain shows hyperintensity in fluid-attenuated inversion recovery (FLAIR) and T2-weighted images in one or both of the temporal and orbitofrontal lobes, often extending up to the insular and cingulate gyri. In addition to the typical findings as stated above, CSF may also show xanthochromia, which indicates hemorrhage. Definitive diagnosis is made with PCR, which is over 90% sensitive and nearly 100% specific. False negatives may occur if the sample is taken after sufficient neutralizing antibodies are formed, if the sample is stored inappropriately for a prolonged period of time, or if the sample is stored in the presence of heme, which inhibits polymerase reaction. False-positive reaction may also occur due to carryover contamination.

Management and prognostic factors

The mortality rate is over 70% in untreated or inappropriately treated patients, and only 9% of survivors return to normal functions. Treatment with acyclovir reduces mortality by more than 70%, down to 20–30%. In immunocompromised patients, treatment with acyclovir may be necessary for 21 days due to possible resistance. In the general population, acyclovir-resistant herpes simplex virus occurs at a rate of 0.4%, but in the immunosuppressed, the rate is as high as 4–11%. A more favorable prognosis is seen in patients who are treated early, are younger than 30 years of age, have short duration of illness, a Glasgow Coma Scale score of more than 6, low viral load on CSF, and no hyperperfusion on single photon emission CT scan.

Rabies
Epidemiology

Rabies, a rhabdovirus, is spread by the bites of infected animals. Only 15% of victims bitten by rabid animals develop rabies. The likelihood of developing rabies after rabid animal bites depends on the species of animal, location, and severity of the bite, and whether the bite is through clothing that mechanically removes saliva from the teeth.

Rabies remains an important worldwide health problem with more than 35 000 reported human infections yearly; an estimated 25 000 of these occurring in India alone. Recently, rabies has reemerged in North America and a related virus, bat lyssavirus, was found in Australia. In the developing world infected dogs are the primary vectors in 90% of human infections, while in developed countries infection is caused by bats and small terrestrial mammals. The incidence of rabies is less than 0.1–1.0 cases per 10^5 persons in most countries, although it is as high as 3 cases per 10^5 persons in South Asia.

Pathogenesis

At the site of inoculation, the rabies virus infects muscle fibers and, by binding to the nicotinic acetylcholine receptor at the neuromuscular junction, gains entry into neurons. The virus then spreads retrogradely along the peripheral nerves to the CNS via fast axonal transport. After establishing infection in the CNS, the virus spreads along the parasympathetic nerves to various parts of the body, including the salivary glands in rabid animals.

Pathology

Rabies causes an acute non-suppurative meningoencephalomyelitis. Autopsy specimens often show perineural and perivascular mononuclear cell infiltrate, neuronophagia, ganglion cell degeneration, and glial nodules distributed widely in the brain, brainstem, spinal cord, and peripheral nerves. Intracytoplasmic inclusion bodies, or Negri bodies, contain viral ribonucleoprotein and are found in 80% of human patients, particularly in the pyramidal cells of Ammon's horn in the hippocampus, in Purkinje's cells in the cerebellum, and in the medulla.

Clinical features

Incubation usually lasts between 3 weeks and 2 months, although it can range from 5 days to 12 months. Facial inoculation, multiple severe bites, transmission by corneal transplantation, and accidental inoculation are associated with a shorter incubation period. Prodrome, which consists of fever, flu-like symptoms, mood changes, and, in a third of patients, localized pruritis, pain, or paraesthesiae at the site of bite, usually marks the first days of infection. Depending on whether the brain or spinal cord is predominantly involved, the patient could present with either furious (agitated) or paralytic (dumb) rabies.

Furious rabies, the more common presentation, involves the brainstem, the limbic system, the hypothalamus, and the autonomic center. It is characterized by hydrophobia, aerophobia, and episodic generalized arousal interrupted by periods of lucidity. Hydrophobia and aerophobia are caused by reflexive spasms induced by attempts to drink water or a draft of air on the skin. Initially, the spasm involves the diaphragm and other respiratory muscles, but later it involves other muscles and causes opisthotonos and generalized spasm. Episodic generalized arousal is associated with hyperesthesiae, hallucination, and agitated confusion. Between these episodes, however, the patient is alert, lucid, and rational. Other findings include rhisus sardonicus, meningism, cranial nerve palsy, upper motor neuron weakness, muscle fasciculations, and abnormal involuntary movement. Patients with furious rabies often progress to death within a week.

In patients with paralytic rabies, there is predominantly spinal cord involvement. Following the prodromal symptoms, the patient develops paralysis, paraesthesiae, pain, and muscle fasciculations, starting in the inoculated limb and gradually ascending to other parts of the body, causing quadriplegia, sphincteric disturbance, bulbar, and respiratory muscles palsy. Hydrophobia and aerophobia are usually absent, and the patient may survive for several weeks even without intensive treatment. Paralytic rabies is far less common than furious rabies and has been reported mainly in South and Central America in rabies transmitted by vampire bats.

Laboratory features

Brain MRI may be normal or show multiple T2-weighted images, hyperintensity in the medulla, pontine tegmentum, hypothalamus, basal ganglia, or thalamus, and minimal gadolinium enhancement. Confirmatory tests include serum neutralizing antibodies, nuchal skin biopsy, corneal impression smears, and brain biopsy. Recent advances in diagnostics include the use of PCR to detect the virus in saliva, skin biopsy, and in CSF.

Management

Pre-exposure vaccination and the treatment of rabid animal bites are outlined in Table 88.5. Modern tissue culture vaccine may cause mild local symptoms in approximately 15% of patients if given intramuscularly, or in 35% if given intradermally. Transient constitutional symptoms such as fever, headache, or flu-like symptoms may occur in approximately 7% of patients, and 10% may suffer from mild immune complex disease 3–13 days after booster injections. Older and less expensive nerve tissue-derived vaccines have variable potency and are associated with a high risk of autoimmune neurological diseases such as acute disseminated encephalomyelitis, mononeuritis multiplex, and Guillain–Barré syndrome.

Japanese encephalitis
Epidemiology

Japanese encephalitis virus, a flavivirus, is transmitted by the *Culex tritaeniorhynchus* mosquito between birds and pigs, both of which develop high viremia and are important in maintaining, amplifying, and transmitting the disease. Humans do not develop significant viremia and are thus a dead-end host, but they can become infected when living close to the enzootic cycle of the virus in rural areas. Japanese encephalitis has spread from East and South-East Asia to Russia, the Guam islands, India, and the northern tip of Australia. Today it is the most common cause of arboviral encephalitis, causing some 20 000–50 000 infections and 15 000 deaths annually, more than all other arboviruses combined. In endemic areas, it is a disease of children and young adults; however, when epidemics break out, non-immune adults, who are more likely to develop symptomatic infection, are also affected. In northern Asia, epidemics occur during the summer months, whereas in the south the disease is endemic, with outbreaks occurring in the monsoon months.

Pathogenesis and pathology

After the bite of an infected mosquito, the virus multiplies in the dermal tissue and lymph nodes, causing a transient viremia before invading further. The mechanism of entry into the CNS is unclear, but passive transfer through endothelial cells is thought to be important. In the brain, the virus causes diffuse encephalitis, seen macroscopically in autopsy specimen as focal petechiae or hemorrhage involving the gray matter. The thalamus, basal ganglia, and midbrain are severely affected. Microscopically, there is perivascular cuffing, mononuclear cell infiltration, and phagocytosis of dead cells. Immunologically, the patient mounts a rapid and effective IgM response within days, which limits viral replication and may facilitate lysis of infected cells. Cytotoxic T cells are believed to be important in the clearance of the virus as well. Patients who are not able to mount a humoral response are at risk of fatal outcome.

Clinical features

Only 1 in 25 to 1 in 1000 patients infected with Japanese encephalitis virus becomes symptomatic and naïve adults are more likely to be symptomatic than local populations in endemic areas. The reasons are not clear, but may be related to the age of patients when first exposed, different genetic susceptibility in different populations, partial protection from previous infections of other flaviviruses, or reporting bias. Symptoms range from mild, non-specific, flu-like illness to fatal meningoencephalitis. Severity depends on the route of viral entry, the size and virulence of the inoculum, and host factors, such as age, prior immunity, genetic factors, and general health.

In patients with encephalitis, fever, coryza, and diarrhea, followed by headache, vomiting, seizure, and an impaired conscious state develop after an incubation period of 5–15 days. Seizure is usually generalized and status epilepticus may occur, which carries a poorer prognosis. Older children and adults may present with abnormal behavior.

On examination, signs such as a mask-like face, tremor, generalized hypertonia, and cogwheel rigidity are seen in 70–80% of adults and 20–40% of children. Titubation, pill-rolling tremor, choreathetosis, orofacial dyskinesia, and upper motor facial nerve palsy are seen in approximately 10% of patients; these are believed to be due to the involvement of the thalamus and basal ganglia. Opisthotonus, opsoclonus, myoclonus, changes in respiratory pattern, decerebrate or decorticate posturing, and pupillary and vestibulo-ocular reflex abnormalities indicate brainstem involvement and may herald a poorer prognosis. Mortality is between 5% and 30%, particularly in younger children; and nearly a third of survivors have serious neurological sequelae. Some patients with Japanese encephalitis virus infection may present with flaccid paralysis of one or more limbs, probably due to anterior horn cell damage, and a third of these eventually develop encephalitis.

Laboratory features

Routine blood tests may show peripheral leucocytosis and hyponatremia due to the syndrome of inappropriate secretion of antidiuretic hormone (SIADH). EEG shows diffuse slowing, alpha-, theta-, or delta-coma, burst suppression, or epileptiform activities. Brain CT may show bilateral, non-enhancing hypodensity of the thalamus, basal ganglia, midbrain, pons, and medulla in half of patients. Brain MRI is more sensitive and shows more extensive involvement of the brainstem, thalamus, basal ganglia, cerebellum, and cerebral hemispheres on T2-weighted images. Single photon emission tomography shows hyperperfusion in the thalamus and the putamen.

Definitive diagnosis of Japanese encephalitis is made with IgM and IgG ELISAs, which have more than 95% sensitivity and specificity. PCR has been developed that is able to detect small amounts of the viral RNA, although its reliability is unknown.

Management

Prevention of Japanese encephalitis includes mosquito control programs and prevention of mosquito bites. Formalin-inactivated vaccines are given in three doses, on days 0, 7, and 30. Up to 20% of vaccine recipients report local side effects, which consist of swelling, tenderness, and redness, while 10% report mild systemic side effects of fever, chills, malaise, and headache. The risk of severe neurological side effects, such as encephalitis or encephalopathy, seizure, and peripheral neuropathy, is only 0.1–0.23 cases per 10^5 recipients. Recently, up to 1 case per 100 recipients in Europe, North America, and Australia reported a new pattern of side effects consisting of pruritis, urticaria, and facial angioedema. A live attenuated vaccine was produced in 1988 and proven to be effective in only two doses given at short intervals of 1–2.5 months.

There is no definitive antiviral agent for Japanese encephalitis infection, although various compounds, such as isoquinolone and α-interferon, have been used. Therefore, treatment is mainly supportive.

West Nile encephalitis
Epidemiology

Birds are natural reservoirs of West Nile virus, a flavivirus transmitted by the *Culex* mosquito from birds to humans and animals such as horses, domestic animals, and other mammals that are dead-end hosts. It is widely distributed across Africa, the Middle East, India, southern Europe, Russia, and North America. In the Nile Delta, approximately 40% of humans have antibodies against it. Although it is asymptomatic in endemic populations, outbreaks have occurred in South Africa, Europe, and Russia.

Pathology

Pathologically, West Nile virus causes encephalomyelitis and leptomeningitis. On histology section, microglial nodules with neuronal loss are seen in the gray and white matter of the cerebrum, hippocampus, thalamus, medulla, and, possibly, the anterior horn cells. There is also perivascular infiltration by mononuclear cells and focal inflammation of cranial nerves and the leptomeninges.

Immunohistochemical staining shows viral antigens in neuronal cytoplasm and processes associated with glial nodules.

Clinical features

In endemic areas, West Nile infection is often asymptomatic or self-limiting. In the Romanian outbreak in 1996, the ratio of clinical to subclinical infection was 1:140 to 1:320 and mortality was 4.3% in those with CNS involvement. Generally, symptomatic patients present 3–15 days after incubation with a flu-like illness, and half of the patients have a non-pruritic roseolar or maculopapular rash that usually lasts no more than a week. Less than 15% have CNS involvement, usually the elderly. This CNS involvement includes aseptic meningitis, encephalitis, myelitis, optic neuritis, and anterior horn cell involvement with flaccid paresis.

Severe neurological involvement is seen in non-endemic areas. In these patients, 30% develop meningitis and 60%, particularly those over 50 years of age, develop encephalitis. In those with encephalitis, common symptoms include fever, headache, nausea, vomiting, chills and rigors, myalgias, backache, and weakness. On examination, common signs are confusion, drowsiness, tremor, neck stiffness, myoclonus, ataxia, parkinsonism such as rigidity, bradykinesia, and postural instability, cranial nerve palsies such as dysphagia and absent corneal and gag reflexes, and brainstem dysfunctions such as nystagmus and apnoeic episodes. Some patients develop an asymmetric flaccid paralysis with areflexia and bladder dysfunction due to anterior horn cell involvement.

The overall mortality from West Nile infection in the recent North American outbreak was approximately 6%, although mortality was twice as high in those who were hospitalized. Patients over 68 years of age and those with flaccid paralysis fared the worst.

Laboratory features

In patients with encephalitis or meningitis, mild peripheral blood leucocytosis is common. CT scan of the brain is often normal, while MRI shows bilateral, focal T2 hyperintense lesions in the thalamus, basal ganglia, and pons in severely ill patients, and evidence of meningitis. EEG shows diffuse, irregular slow waves with sharp waves or seizure activities. Electromyography may show axonal neuropathy, probably reflecting anterior horn cell involvement, although in some patients, a demyelinating neuropathy is seen as well.

Infection is diagnosed with detection of IgM using ELISA or with a rising convalescent titer. West Nile cross-reacts with antibodies directed against other flaviviruses; therefore, the presence of specific IgM should be confirmed via plaque reduction assay to detect neutralizing antibodies. Viral isolation using the vero cell line is less sensitive but very specific. Other tests include virus gene sequencing or PCR; viral load can be quantified with real-time PCR.

Management

There is no specific treatment or human vaccine for West Nile encephalitis. Interferon-α, intravenous immunoglobulin, and ribavirin were used in the recent North American outbreak without definite success. Currently, management remains supportive.

Tick-borne encephalitis
Epidemiology

Tick-borne encephalitis is the most common encephalitis in Europe. There are three subtypes of the virus species: Far Eastern (previously Russian Spring and Summer), Siberian (previously West-Siberian), and Western European (previously Central European).

The viruses are transmitted by *Ixodes* and *Haemaphysalis* ticks. *Ixodes* ticks are found in Europe, the Baltic States, central Asia, and North Africa. Small mammals such as rodents and wolves act as the major reservoir and amplifying hosts for the viruses, and insectivores such as moles, hedgehogs, and shrews serve as additional reservoirs. Humans are dead-end hosts. Worldwide, 10 000–20 000 clinical cases are reported annually, particularly in Central and Eastern Europe, where it accounts for 29–54% of encephalitis with a diagnosis. The risk is highest among farmers, hunters, forest workers, and, in Russia, the unemployed. In more affluent countries, infection is contracted during outdoor leisure activities; men are therefore at higher risk of acquiring the disease. The incidence is as high as 80 cases per 10^5 persons per annum in parts of Finland, but generally ranges from 10 to 30 cases per 10^5 persons per annum. Seroprevalence varies from 1% (France) to 32.4% (Lithuania). The virus has been shown to be transmitted by goat milk in Slovakia. Tick-borne encephalitis is also found in the Jilin and Yunan provinces in China, and in Hokkaido, Japan.

Pathogenesis and pathology

Tick-borne encephalitis virus is found in tick saliva and is introduced into the skin through tick bites. The virus first infects the Langerhans cells, then invades the lymphoid and reticulo-endothelial system, where it spreads hematogenously to other organs, including the CNS. The route of entry into the CNS is not well delineated. Once inside the CNS, the virus causes widespread inflammation in the leptomeninges, cortical gray matter, brainstem, cerebellum, and spinal cord. Histologically, neuronal degeneration, necrosis, and neuronophagia are seen, with prominent perivascular inflammatory cell infiltration.

Clinical features

Serological surveys suggest that 70–95% of human infection is subclinical. In symptomatic patients, the virus causes a biphasic illness. After a median incubation period of 8 days (range 4–28 days), the patient complains of fever, myalgias, nausea, fatigue, and headache. This viremic phase usually lasts for 4–18 days. After an interval of 8–133 days 74–87% of patients present with CNS infection. Because the virus widely invades the CNS, tick-borne encephalitis can present in many clinical forms; approximately half (45–56%) of the patients have encephalitis, while others have meningitis, radiculitis, or myelitis ("poliomyelitic form"). Patients with encephalitis present with fever, headache, meningism, ataxia, confusion, cognitive impairment, altered consciousness, tremor, cranial nerve palsies, and, rarely, seizure. Eleven percent to 15% of patients have radiculitis or polyradiculoneuritis. Patients with myelitis present with lower motor neuron weakness of the neck and upper limbs, sparing the lower limbs.

Mortality is less than 1% in many European countries and is reportedly higher in Siberia (6–8%) and the Far East (20–40%). This could be due to either the more virulent strains of virus in these regions or bias in case ascertainment and hospitalization. Mortality is higher among adults than children. Up to 10% of patients suffer from permanent spinal paralysis; the proportion of patients with permanent disability was reported to be as high as 26–46%. Mortality is higher in older patients, patients with impaired consciousness, ataxia, abnormal MRI, pleocytosis of more than 300 cells/µl in CSF, and those with impairment of the blood–brain barrier.

Laboratory features

Thrombocytopenia and leukopenia are common in the viremic phase. In the meningoencephalitic phase, CSF analysis is similar to that of other viral encephalitides, although the serum and CSF albumin ratio often shows serious blood–brain barrier damage. CT scan is often normal, while MRI shows T2 hyperintensity in the thalamus, putamen, pallidum, and caudate nucleus. Because most patients present during the second phase of the illness when the antibody titer is high, viral isolation and PCR are not useful; ELISA of specific IgM is the main diagnostic method. However, antibodies to other flaviviruses cross-react with this assay, and neutralizing tests may be necessary in patients previously exposed to other flavivirus or to vaccination.

Management

There is no specific treatment for tick-borne encephalitis, and management is largely supportive. A vaccine with a protection rate of 95–98% is available and is given intramuscularly in three doses (the second dose in 2–12 weeks, the third dose in 9–12 months), with subsequent booster doses every 3–5 years, depending on exposure risk.

St Louis encephalitis
Epidemiology

St Louis encephalitis virus, a flavivirus, is the second most common cause of viral encephalitis in the United States. Although it occurs primarily in the Ohio–Mississippi Valley, human infection has been documented throughout the United States and the virus has been isolated from southern Canada to Argentina. It is carried by the *Culex* mosquito, and is amplified by passage between mosquitoes and birds. The virus spills out of the zoonotic cycle when there are a sufficient number of infected mosquitoes, causing waves of epidemic outbreaks in humans approximately every 10 years. Sentinel cases often occur in the elderly, due to the increased risk of clinical encephalitis and mortality.

Pathology

St Louis virus causes a meningoencephalitis with leptomeningeal infiltration by lymphocytes, macrophages, polymorphonuclear leukocytes, and plasma cells, particularly around the brainstem, the cerebellum, and in the Virchow–Robbin spaces. Neuronal death and neuronophagia occur in the brain parenchyma, where cellular nodules composed of monocytes, lymphocytes, and microglial cells are also seen. Gray matter, the substantia nigra of the midbrain, and thalamic nuclei are the most severely affected, although the cerebellum, pontine tegmentum, medulla, striatum, and spinal cord are variably affected as well.

Clinical features

There is a large range in the number of people infected by St Louis virus who actually develop clinical disease (1:800 to 1:100 000). While 40% of young adults and children who have clinically apparent illness suffer only from mild aseptic meningitis, 90% of the elderly with clinically apparent disease develop encephalitis. The onset of encephalitis can be abrupt or slow and is usually marked by fever, headache, dizziness, nausea, and malaise. Other clinical features include meningism, confusion, disorientation, tremor, unsteady gait, and apathy. Although the pathogenesis of involvement of the urinary tract is unknown, 25% of patients have urinary frequency, urgency, incontinence, or retention. Cranial nerve palsies are seen in 20% of patients. SIADH is occasionally seen. The disease progresses for up to a week before resolution, although in 30–50% of patients there is prolonged asthenia, irritability, tremor, insomnia, depression, poor memory, headache, and, in more severe cases, gait and speech disturbances, which can last up to 2 years. Mortality is approximately 5–20%, although in those over 75 years of age it is as high as 70%.

Investigation and management
Imaging studies are usually not helpful and diagnosis is made using serological tests. There is no specific antiviral agent; management, therefore, is largely supportive.

LaCrosse encephalitis
Epidemiology
The most common type of arboviral encephalitis in the United States is caused by the California serogroup of viruses, which are bunyaviruses. Out of the 15 viruses in this group, nearly all infection is caused by LaCrosse virus. The virus is transmitted by the *Aedes triseriatus* mosquito, with chipmunks and squirrels as the reservoirs and amplifying hosts. Like many other arboviruses, humans are incidental dead-end hosts. The incidence of LaCrosse encephalitis has been stable over the years, with approximately 70–100 cases per year, with a sharp peak in the summer months. More than 90% of cases occur in the central-eastern states of Minnesota, Wisconsin, Iowa, Illinois, Indiana, and Ohio, and more than 90% occur in those under 15 years of age. Males are twice as likely to contract the infection as females, probably reflecting differences in outdoor activity involvement. In endemic areas, 12.5–18% of residents are seropositive.

Pathology
Pathologically, LaCrosse virus causes an encephalitic process similar to that of other viral agents including neuronal and glial damage, perivascular cuffing around capillaries and venules, and, in fatal cases, cerebral edema. However, the virus has a predilection to affect the cortical gray matter of the frontal, temporal, and parietal lobes as well as the basal ganglia, midbrain, and pons.

Clinical features
The ratio of clinical to subclinical infection is not clearly known but can be as low as 1 case per 1000 persons. It usually affects children, and the median age of patients is 7 years. Fever is almost universal. Approximately 75% of patients have headache, and half have meningism; other features include seizure, altered conscious state, focal neurological deficits, abdominal pain, cough, and sore throat, and 12% progress to coma. The outcome is good, with a mortality rate of approximately 0.5% and an estimated 2% experiencing neurological sequelae, although 75% of children have abnormal EEG findings 3–4 years after infection. An estimated 6–20% of patients develop remote symptomatic epilepsy following infection with LaCrosse viral encephalitis.

Investigation and management
Diagnosis is made with ELISA of specific IgM or a four-fold rise in IgG in convalescent serum detected by complement fixation, hemagglutin inhibition, or immune fluorescence.

Serology is specific and sensitive. Treatment is supportive, as there is no specific antiviral agent. Because it affects mainly children, who are at risk of Reye's syndrome, salicylates should be avoided.

Alphaviruses
The alphaviruses belong to the Togaviridae family, three of which are of human significance – the Western, Venezuelan, and Eastern equine encephalitis viruses – which are all transmitted by mosquitoes and found in North and Central America.

Western equine virus
The Western equine virus is mainly transmitted by the *Culex tarsalis* mosquito. Birds are the main reservoirs; however, in late summer the mosquito switches its feeding pattern from birds to mammals, causing outbreaks in horses, mules, and humans. There have been fewer than five cases reported annually since the last outbreaks in the Red River Valley in 1975 and in Colorado in 1988.

Postmortem findings of the brain of a patient with Western equine encephalitis show edema and multiple necrotic foci, with or without cellular infiltrate, especially in the striatum, globus pallidus, substantia nigra, cerebral cortex, thalamus, pons, and, occasionally, spinal cord.

The ratio of clinical to subclinical infection ranges from 1 per 100 cases to 1 per 2000 cases, with an incubation period of 5–10 days. The virus causes a spectrum of clinical manifestations, from mild fever to aseptic meningitis to encephalitis. Infants are more susceptible to CNS disease and to developing neurological sequelae.

In those with encephalitis, the onset is sudden, heralded by fever, chills, headache, nausea, vomiting, and, uncommonly, respiratory symptoms. Within several days, the patient develops lethargy, drowsiness, meningism, photophobia, vertigo, impairment of conscious state, and, in severe cases, coma. In infants less than 1 year old, irritability, focal or generalized seizure, tremor, weakness (either upper or lower motor neuron lesion in origin), rigidity, and dyskinesia are common.

Recovery usually begins after 10 days; however, those who die often do so within 1 week. Mortality from Western equine encephalitis is only 3–5%, and adults often recover fully. However, 56% of infants less than 1 month, 16% of infants between 1 and 2 months, and 11% of infants between 2 and 3 months of age develop permanent and severe cognitive and motor impairment or seizures.

Venezuelan equine virus
Venezuelan equine virus consists of at least six subtypes, with types 1AB and 1C causing periodic but unpredictable outbreaks in Central and South America; the remaining serotypes are mainly enzootic and do not

cause human infection. Rodents are the main reservoir, equines the main secondary amplifying host, and *Culex* mosquitoes are the main vector. In epidemic outbreaks, *Ochlerotatus* and *Psorophora* species of mosquitoes are common vectors as well. Humans are infected when living in close settings with animals, such as in agricultural areas.

In human autopsy specimen, Venezuelan equine encephalitis virus causes meningoencephalitis with intense necrotizing vasculitis and cerebritis. Macroscopically, the brain appears congested and hemorrhagic. These changes are also observed in the gastrointestinal and respiratory tracts.

Venezuelan equine virus infection has an incubation period of 2–5 days, with most infections being clinically apparent. Clinical manifestation starts abruptly with fever, chills, occipital headache or retro-orbital pain, malaise, and myalgias in the back and thighs. Other symptoms include tachycardia, nausea, vomiting, and diarrhea. Neurological involvement is shown by photophobia, seizure, drowsiness, and confusion. In most patients, the illness subsides after 4–6 days, followed by a few weeks of asthenia. In some, however, the infection may be biphasic and recur 4–8 days after the initial onset. A small proportion of patients become comatose, although mortality is less than 1%.

Eastern equine virus

Eastern equine virus is the most lethal arboviral encephalitis in the United States. The chief vector is *Culiseta melanura*, a fastidious mosquito that is strictly ornithophilic and breeds only in a specific microenvironment of peat soil and dark, organic-rich water. Human infection only occurs when other, less fastidious, mosquitoes venture into this environment. The virus is found in the Atlantic and Gulf Coast regions of the United States, and in Wisconsin, Michigan, and Indiana. A different strain of Eastern equine virus is found in Central and South America, although human infection is very rare outside the United States.

Eastern equine virus causes either a systemic or a CNS infection. In the CNS, the virus causes an encephalomyelitis with neuronal death and vasculitic lesions in the frontal cortex, basal ganglia, and brainstem. Autonomic dysfunction may be severe and could lead to fatal heart failure and pulmonary edema.

Nearly all human infection by Eastern equine virus is symptomatic. Adults and older children may suffer only from systemic infection, although this can be followed by encephalitis. Young children are more susceptible to developing encephalitis and serious neurological sequelae. Systemic infection is characterized by abrupt onset of high fever, malaise, arthralgia, and myalgias, which usually last 1–2 weeks. In those who suffer from encephalitis, the onset is abrupt with high fever, headache, confusion, restlessness, drowsiness, nausea, vomiting, anorexia, diarrhea, seizure, and rapid progression to coma. Children may present with periorbital, facial, or generalized edema, tremor, muscle twitching, and meningism.

Mortality, which occurs 2–10 days after the onset of symptoms, is approximately 30%, although it can be as high as 80%, especially in the extremes of age. Serious neurological sequelae, which include severe intellectual impairment, personality changes, spastic paralysis, cranial nerve palsies, and epilepsy, occur in 70% of children. Long-term outcome is dismal, with only 10% of patients surviving beyond 9 years and a total of 3% having no neurological sequelae.

Laboratory features and management

Diagnosis of alphaviral infection is made serologically. For example, diagnosis of Venezuelan equine virus infection is made by ELISA, hemagglutination inhibition, neutralizing tests, or detection of viral antigen using indirect fluorescent antibody tests. There is no specific antiviral therapy and treatment is supportive. There are, however, effective equine vaccines against the alphaviruses.

Other encephalitides
Dengue virus

Dengue virus is a flavivirus transmitted by *Aedes* mosquitoes, which primarily infect humans and primates. It is endemic in the tropics and subtropics, especially in crowded, large metropolises. The virus causes an acute febrile illness with rash and severe myalgias and, in more severe cases, hemorrhages and hemorrhagic shock. CNS illness, characterized by headache, drowsiness, confusion, seizure, and focal neurological deficits, is seen in 1% of patients, particularly in those with severe illness. Whether dengue virus causes an encephalitis or an encephalopathy is still debated.

Nipah virus

The Nipah virus, which was first discovered in 1999 when it caused an outbreak of encephalitis in Malaysia, has since caused recurring sporadic outbreaks in Bangladesh and the neighboring state of West Bengal in India. Unlike other zoonotic viruses, it is a paramyxovirus originated from bats. The initial outbreak in Malaysia was believed to be transmitted to and amplified in pigs through bat excretion, then subsequently transmitted to humans. Human-to-human transmission was rare in the initial outbreak, though this was the dominant mode of transmission in some of the Bangladeshi outbreaks.

Pathologically, acute Nipah infection is characterized by systemic vasculitis with endothelial cell damage and necrosis as well as syncytial giant cell formation, which causes extensive thrombosis and parenchymal necrosis, particularly in the CNS and lungs. The virus then invades neurons, forming viral cytoplasmic and, less commonly, nuclear inclusion bodies, leading to diffuse encephalitis with focal neuronophagia, microglial nodule formation, and perivascular cuffing.

Following an incubation period of approximately 9 days (range 2–45 days), the patient presents with fever, headache, chills, myalgias, giddiness, drowsiness, seizures, confusion, and respiratory and abdominal symptoms. Severe hypertension, tachycardia, hyperthermia, segmental myoclonus, and focal neurological deficits are prominent features.

Mortality is approximately 40%. Poor prognostic factors include brainstem involvement, past history of diabetes mellitus, and presence of the virus in CSF. Ribavirin was shown in an open-label, historical control trial to reduce mortality by approximately 36%, although supportive management is equally important.

Enterovirus and EV71

The enteroviruses are the most common cause of aseptic meningitis worldwide, and 3% of these patients develop encephalitis. The enteroviruses are transmitted via a fecal–oral route, and humans are the only significant host. Among the many serotypes, certain serotypes predominate in a particular geographical locality; each serotype causes cyclical outbreaks when there are sufficient non-immunized individuals present, usually young children. Enteroviral infection of the CNS is usually mild and self-limiting, with the exception of enterovirus 71, which has been known to cause fatal outbreaks among young children in Bulgaria and in the Asia-Pacific region.

Enterovirus 71 infection manifests as the childhood exanthema known as hand–foot–mouth disease and is clinically indistinguishable from that caused by Coxsackie virus. In the CNS, the virus infects anterior horn cells, causing their death and leading to an acute flaccid paralysis; elsewhere in the CNS, the virus can cause meningitis, cerebellitis, and post-infectious neurological syndromes. The most severe form is brainstem encephalitis.

Patients with brainstem encephalitis, usually young children under the age of 5 years, present with fever, myoclonus, ataxia, nystagmus, and cranial nerve palsies. Although most patients recover, 10–20% develop neurological sequelae. Children with severe disease develop rapidly progressive neurogenic pulmonary edema, which has a mortality of over 80%. There is no proven treatment, although various agents, including pleconaril and intravenous immunoglobulin, have been tried. Treatment is therefore largely supportive.

Rift Valley encephalitis

Rift Valley virus is a Phlebovirus, from the family Bunyaviridae, a zoonotic virus first discovered in the 1930s in Kenya. The vector is the *Aedes* mosquito; buffaloes, cattle, sheep, and goats serve as reservoir and amplifying hosts. Rift Valley virus has caused major and recurring outbreaks of animal and human disease in Sub-Saharan Africa since the early 1900s, and has recently spread to northern Africa and the Sinai and Arabian peninsulas. The virus is transmitted by both mosquito bites and contact with infected animal carcasses and abortion and blood products.

In most patients, Rift Valley viral infection presents with fever, nausea, vomiting, and abdominal and respiratory symptoms. Less than 5% of patients develop meningoencephalitis, often late in the illness, with a clinical picture of confusion, meningism, hyperreflexia, and a depressed conscious state. Less than 8% of patients develop severe disease, characterized by hemorrhage, hepatitis, renal failure, retinitis, and encephalitis. Mortality is between 0.5% and 1.0% in most patients, but for those with severe disease, mortality is as high as 29–34%. Laboratory investigation shows elevated liver enzymes, hepatic and renal failure, and prolonged prothrombin and partial thromboplastin times. Treatment is supportive, as there is no specific antiviral agent.

Australian encephalitis – Murray Valley encephalitis and Kunjin encephalitis

Both Murray Valley encephalitis and Kunjin encephalitis viruses are closely related mosquito-borne flaviviruses endemic in Australia and Papua New Guinea. The primary vectors of both are *Culex* and *Aedes* mosquitoes. Water birds appear to be the major hosts. Murray Valley encephalitis can also be transmitted by *Anopheles* mosquitoes and, based on serological findings, other domestic and wild animals have been implicated as its hosts as well. Outbreaks may occur after periods of heavy rain and flooding.

CT scan of the brain in Murray Valley encephalitis shows hypodensity in the thalami, and brain MRI shows bilateral thalamic involvement that is hyperintense on T2- and hypointense on T1-weighted images.

Clinical Murray Valley encephalitis occurs in as few as 1 in 1000 infections, while Kunjin virus infection is milder and less common. Patients with Kunjin virus infection present with mild fever, headache, photophobia, rash, arthralgia, myalgias, lymphadenopathy, and, less commonly, encephalitis. Clinically, Murray Valley encephalitis and Kunjin encephalitis are indistinguishable. Patients with encephalitis often present with fever, drowsiness, cranial nerve palsies, dyskinesia, tremor, parkinsonism, and flaccid paralysis due to anterior horn cell involvement, and seizure may occur in children. Murray Valley encephalitis is more severe, with mortality between 20% and 30%, usually due to neurogenic respiratory failure, and severe neurological sequelae are seen in 20% of survivors.

Diagnoses of Murray Valley and Kunjin encephalitides are made by ELISA and treatment is supportive.

Further reading

Calisher CH. Medically important arboviruses of the United States and Canada. *Clin Microbiol Rev* 1994; 7(1): 89–116.

Chong HT, Tan CT. Central nervous system infections. In: Feigin VL, Bennett DA, editors. *Handbook of Clinical Neuroepidemiology.* Hauppauge, NY: Nova Science; 2007, pp. 339–89.

Haglund M, Günther G. Tick-borne encephalitis – pathogenesis, clinical course and long-term follow-up. *Vaccine* 2003; 21(Suppl 1): S11–18.

Solomon T. Exotic and emerging viral encephalitides. *Curr Opin Neurol* 2003; 16: 411–8.

Chapter 89
Post-viral cerebellitis

Heng Thay Chong and Chong Tin Tan
University of Malaya, Kuala Lumpur, Malaysia

Introduction

Post-viral cerebellitis is also known as acute cerebellitis and acute cerebellar ataxia. It is a syndrome characterized by rapid onset of cerebellar dysfunction often after an infection or vaccination.

Epidemiology

The actual incidence of post-viral cerebellitis is not known, though it is estimated to be $2/10^4$ to $1/10^5$ per annum. It is seen most commonly in children under 6 years of age, usually after a viral infection or vaccination. Infective agents associated with this condition are the varicella zoster virus, Epstein–Barr virus, and enterovirus, though case reports have implicated other agents such as parvovirus, mumps virus, hepatitis A virus, human herpes virus 6, herpes simplex virus, *Borrelia burdgorferi*, *Coxiella burnetti*, mycoplasma, legionella, *Neisseria meningitis*, typhoid fever, pertussis, scarlet fever, diphtheria, and malaria. It is also seen after vaccination for varicella zoster virus, hepatitis B, and rabies virus.

Pathogenesis

There is much debate on the pathogenesis of acute cerebellitis. Epidemiological, clinical, and laboratory features suggest that the illness is autoimmune in origin in most patients as (1) the disease occurs after recovery from the acute infection; (2) it is also seen in patients receiving vaccination; (3) case reports suggest that it responds to steroids; and(4) various autoantibodies have been found to be associated with it, such as antibodies against Purkinje cells, centrosomes, myelin-associated glycoprotein, and glutamate receptor (δ2 autoantibodies). In some patients, however, polymerase chain reaction has detected genomes of various infective agents in cerebrospinal fluid, such as varicella zoster virus, herpes simplex virus type 1, and mycoplasma, suggesting that, at least in these patients, the cerebellitis is a result of direct infection. The benign nature of this illness has precluded extensive pathologic study, although available studies suggest that it is closely related to acute disseminated encephalomyelitis and multiple sclerosis.

Clinical features

Clinically, the patients, usually children under 6 years of age, present with acute onset of limb or truncal ataxia, nystagmus, dysmetria, and dysarthria on average 9 (range 2–21) days after the prodromal infection or vaccination. Fever, headache, confusion, and meningism are rare, and prompted some to define these patients as having acute cerebellitis as distinguished from those who have only cerebellar signs. The former are said to have acute cerebellar ataxia. The illness is self-limiting in most patients, and most patients improve in 1–4 weeks. However, 10–30% of patients may have persistent ataxia or dysarthria. Poorer prognosis is associated with older age, Epstein–Barr infection, and perhaps the presence of lesions in MRI.

The differential diagnoses in children is broad and includes poisoning and drug side effects, acute disseminated encephalomyelitis, hydrocephalus, central nervous system infection, hyponatremia, hypocalcemia, posterior fossa tumor, neuroblastoma, cerebellar hemorrhage, acute labyrinthitis, and metabolic diseases such as Hartnup disease and maple syrup urine disease.

Investigations

The peripheral blood analysis is usually normal, though in some there is lymphocytosis. CT scan of the brain is usually normal as well. Electroencephalography shows slow waves in only 20% of patients. MRI of the brain often shows hyperintense lesions in the cerebellum in T2-weighted images. Cerebrospinal fluid analysis shows mild lymphocytic pleocytosis in 25–50% of patients, and

International Neurology: A Clinical Approach. Edited by Robert P. Lisak, Daniel D. Truong, William M. Carroll, and Roongroj Bhidayasiri. © 2009 Blackwell Publishing, ISBN: 978-1-4051-5738-4.

protein level is normal or slightly elevated during the later part of the illness. Viral identification techniques such as polymerase chain reaction may occasionally yield positive viral genome, though in most the associated infective agent is identified by serologic study. Varicella zoster virus is the most commonly identified agent, seen in about 25–35% of patients, and mumps virus in another 20%. Other agents such as mycoplasma and Epstein–Barr virus account for less than 5% each. In about 20% of patients the inciting agent is not found.

Management

No randomized controlled trials have been conducted on the treatment of post-viral cerebellitis, though steroid and intravenous immunoglobulin have been used in small series and case reports. Because of the association with varicella zoster virus and the uncertainty in the pathogenesis of this illness, acyclovir is often given as well, especially in immunosuppressed patients or in those with features suggestive of cerebellitis such as fever, confusion, and meningism. There is, however, no evidence of its efficacy in these situations. As patients with this illness have relatively good outcome and there is a lack of specific treatment, management should be focused on the prevention of falls and the identification and treatment of alternative diagnoses that carry worse prognoses.

Further reading

Davis DP, Marino A. Acute cerebellar ataxia in toddler: case report and literature review. *J Emerg Med* 2003; 24(3): 281–4.

Nussinovitch M, Prais D, Volovitz B, Shapiro R, Amir J. Post-infectious acute cerebellar ataxia in children. *Clin Pediatr* 2003; 42: 581–4.

Chapter 90
Subacute and chronic viral infections

Ellen Gelpi and Herbert Budka
Medical University of Vienna, Vienna, Austria

Introduction

Subacute and chronic viral infections of the central nervous system (CNS) encompass a group of viral diseases usually characterized by a progressive neurological disorder that resembles a neurodegenerative disease, usually leading to death. In contrast to acute viral infections, subacute and chronic viral infections show a considerably longer incubation period that lasts for many months or years, usually due to viral latency in the nervous system that exists for a long period before an inflammatory reaction occurs. In many of these infections, systemic symptoms are marginal when compared to the neurological disorder. In this chapter we describe chronic enteroviral encephalomyelitis, measles inclusion encephalitis, subacute sclerosing panencephalitis (SSPE), progressive rubella panencephalitis, and progressive multifocal leukoencephalopathy (PML). Retroviral infections are described in detail in other chapters of this book.

In addition to the identification of causative agents, it is important to understand the mechanisms by which the viruses escape general immune surveillance, reach, and persist in the CNS, and lead to a slowly progressing disease. The host reactions to the infections, special interactions between the viruses and target cells, as well as mutations of the virus genomes may account for their persistence in the CNS and the emergence of atypical disease forms.

Epidemiology

Chronic enteroviral encephalomyelitis is a rare condition that presents in patients with altered immunity. Depending on the underlying disease, age at presentation varies from 16 years in individuals with agammaglobulinemia to 39 years in those with combined variable immunodeficiency. There is no gender predilection.

Measles inclusion body encephalitis develops within several months after acute measles infection. It usually affects children with depression of cell-mediated immunity, most frequently in leukemia or lymphoma or related treatment. Males and females are equally affected.

SSPE occurs in patients without immunological impairment several years after an initial early infection by the measles virus. The age of manifestation ranges from 1 to 35 years of age, although most often it affects patients between 5 and 15 years of age. The interval from acute measles infection to SSPE onset also varies, from an average of 7 years to exceptionally long intervals of up to 22 years.

SSPE has been observed in many ethnic groups, with an annual incidence of approximately 1 case per million children per year or 1 per 100 000 cases of measles, although more recent data suggest an incidence of 1 per 10 000 after acute infection. The estimated risk varies between 0.4 and 9.7 cases per million patients with measles infection in Western countries. A decline in frequency has been noticed in most developed countries, whereas it continues to be high in developing countries, most likely due to inadequate vaccine coverage or circulation of atypical measles virus strains. For example, the prevalence in India and Pakistan was estimated to be 10 cases per million in the general population. SSPE affects more males than females at a 2:1 ratio. The risk is much greater in patients who contract measles in the first year of life, and is extremely reduced (10- to 20-fold reduction) by measles vaccination when administered before exposure to wild measles virus.

Progressive rubella panencephalitis is a very rare disease. It manifests usually between 8 and 20 years of age after congenital or, less frequently, childhood rubella.

PML is usually an opportunistic infection. It affects patients of any age with immunosuppression due to lymphoproliferative disease, as well as those with genetic deficiencies, chronic inflammatory and infectious diseases such as tuberculosis, sarcoidosis, and rheumatoid arthritis, and those with iatrogenic immunosupression for the treatment of autoimmune or neoplastic disorders or organ transplantation. Males and females are affected equally. More than 50% of young people and 75% of

International Neurology: A Clinical Approach. Edited by Robert P. Lisak, Daniel D. Truong, William M. Carroll, and Roongroj Bhidayasiri. © 2009 Blackwell Publishing, ISBN: 978-1-4051-5738-4.

adults have serological evidence of polyomavirus infection without disease manifestation. The incidence of PML had dramatically increased with the advent of the AIDS epidemic, but is progressively declining due to the restoration of immunity in HIV infection using highly active antiretroviral therapy (HAART).

Pathophysiology

These viruses do not have a selective affinity for neurons; they affect glial cells and induce tissue damage throughout the CNS. Once viruses have invaded the CNS after entrance by oral or respiratory routes, they interact with susceptible cells that carry a specific receptor site on the cytoplasmic membrane.

Chronic enteroviral encephalomyelitis is usually caused by Echoviruses and is associated with alteration of humoral immunity, such as agammaglobulinemia, or combined variable immunodeficiency.

The *measles* virus, which precedes *measles inclusion body encephalitis* and *SSPE*, is an RNA virus of the genus *Morbillivirus* that belongs to the family Paramyxoviridae. The virus has several important proteins in the nucleocapsid (NP), matrix (M), and envelope (hemagglutinin (H) and fusion (F) proteins). These proteins are involved in the process of binding to the cell-surface receptor (H protein), fusion of the envelope with the cell membrane (H and F proteins), entry into the cell, RNA transcription, assembly of nucleocapsids and envelope proteins, and budding of the virus through the membrane to form a mature virion. The measles virus genome continuously changes due to the accumulation of mutations in certain regions that may introduce new biological characteristics over time. The most variable regions are those encoding the M, H, and F proteins. It has been postulated that these changes could permit clonal expansion of the mutated virus within the brain and its spread via local cell fusion. This allows the virus to escape the immune system, which in SSPE induces a humoral hyperimmune response, producing high titers of antibodies to viral proteins other than the M protein. This strong humoral immune response provides a continuous selective pressure that favors clonal expansion of the mutated virus. The presence of circulating maternal antibodies to the measles virus during the first few months of life may similarly promote the emergence of mutant clones and contribute to the increased risk of SSPE that follows infection at a very early age.

Another mechanism observed in experimental studies that may explain atypical measles virus infection after immunization with formalin-inactivated vaccine is that certain surface-specific IgG antibodies to H proteins may enhance the entry of the measles virus into monocytes and macrophages and thus promote the spread of virus among Fc gamma receptor-expressing host cells.

Progressive rubella panencephalitis is caused by an RNA virus of the genus *Rubivirus*, which belongs to the Togaviridae family. The disease is still poorly understood. Patients usually have normal cell-mediated immunity and humoral immunity and show high levels of antibodies against the rubella virus in serum and in the CNS. Antibodies and T-cells directed against the rubella virus may alter the vasculature and react against autologous antigens such as myelin basic protein, proteolipid protein, and galactocerebrosides, thus inducing autoimmune-mediated brain damage through molecular mimicry between viral and host epitopes.

PML is caused by the JC virus (*polyomavirus hominis 2*), a papovavirus of the polyomavirus subfamily. The JC virus has double-stranded, circular DNA wound in a superhelix that is surrounded by a nucleocapsid. Several proteins of the nucleocapsid are needed to bind the virus to the cell receptor, allow the virus to enter the cell, transport the virus into the nucleus, initiate transcription of viral proteins, and, finally, for the virus to produce new virions that will be released from the cell within approximately 2 days of infection through cell lysis. Oligodendrocytes support productive JC infection, which leads to cell lysis and consequent demyelination. In contrast, astrocytes do not support productive infection, but a non-permissive infection of these cells may lead to their morphological transformation and resulting bizarre appearance.

In the general population, the JC virus probably establishes latent infection in extraneural tissues (in B lymphocytes and kidney), and possibly in the CNS. Immunodepression is associated with increased hematogeneous dissemination of the JC virus and its spread to the CNS. Another possibility of CNS infection is viral reactivation after latency within the CNS.

Clinical features

Chronic enteroviral encephalomyelitis
Clinical symptoms may include myelopathy with paraparesis, ascending sensory loss, and bladder dysfunction. Some patients suffer from an encephalopathic syndrome characterized by insidious headache, lethargy, intellectual decline, seizures, optic atrophy, pyramidal and extrapyramidal motor disturbances, or a combination of both myelopathic and encephalopathic signs and symptoms. In addition, many patients show systemic manifestations of the enteroviral infection. Neurological symptoms usually progress over years, with or without periods of clinical improvement.

Measles inclusion body encephalitis
Measles inclusion body encephalitis is characterizd by the onset of encephalitic symptoms including seizures (often

epilepsia partialis continua) or confusion as well as myo-clonus and a variety of neurological deficits 1–6 months after recovery from acute measles infection. The disease may progress to coma and in most cases to death within a few weeks of onset. A small percentage of patients have survived but with severe neurological dysfunction.

Subacute sclerosing panencephalitis (SSPE)

The clinical course of SSPE can be divided into four disease stages, although it may be variable. The first stage is characterized by insidious intellectual impairment and behavioral abnormalities. At least 50% of patients develop visual disturbances due to macular chorioretinitis, which may be the first manifestation of disease. The second stage develops 1–2 months later, with acceleration of intellectual decline, frequently associated with prominent repetitive symmetrical myoclonic jerks and characteristic electroencephalogram (EEG) changes. Focal or general-ized seizures might also appear. This stage may last for 2–3 months. In the third stage, which usually lasts for 1–4 months, patients become uncommunicative and develop various neurological symptoms combining ataxia, spasticity, choreoathetosis, and dystonia, with gradual disappearance of myoclonus. The fourth and final stage may last for months or years and is characterized by stupor, autonomic disturbances, and coma, eventually leading to death. Although the natural history of SSPE is often difficult to predict, the clinical course is generally steadily progressive, leading to death within 1–3 years. Nevertheless, long-term survival rates of more than 10 years and spontaneous stabilizations, remissions, and relapses in different disease stages have been described.

Progressive rubella pancenephalitis

Clinical symptoms progress slowly and intermittently and combine insidious intellectual deterioration and ataxia, often associated with seizures and progressive demen-tia. Spasticity, choreoathetosis, and myoclonus appear thereafter. A perimacular pigmentary retinopathy may develop. Although the neurological deficits associated with congenital rubella infection may be non-progressive, generally disease evolves over several years, until the patient becomes decerebrate and eventually dies.

Progressive multifocal leukoencephalopathy (PML)

PML usually presents insidiously, with diverse neurologi-cal deficits according to the site of brain damage. Initial symptoms may be personality changes and intellec-tual impairment over a period of several days to weeks. Neurological signs include paralysis, mental deterioration and confusional states, visual loss, sensory abnormalities, and ataxia. These signs take a progressive course, usually leading to coma and death in less than 1 year. Seizures are rare.

Investigations

To make a diagnosis of a subacute or chronic viral infec-tion, it is of utmost importance to obtain data on the history of vaccinations, infections in childhood, and con-genital infections. Cerebrospinal fluid (CSF) analysis may reveal signs of inflammation and protein increase, except in cases of PML, which usually has a normal cell count and protein level. Serological investigations are useful, and determination of IgM and IgG antibodies to viruses may be sufficient to make a diagnosis. In addition, deter-mination of antibody titers in CSF, isolation of the virus, and detection of viral nucleic acid using polymerase chain reaction (PCR) are possible for most of these infections and represent the core diagnostic tests. The occurrence of oligoclonal IgG in the CSF in SSPE and in progressive rubella panencephalitis with virus-specific antibodies suggests a local production of immunoglobulin within the CNS.

In SSPE, a marked increase in CSF IgG and high mea-sles virus antibody titers in both serum and CSF can be detected. Measles-specific IgG antibodies represent nearly 10–20% of total serum IgG and about 75% of total CSF IgG. Low titers of rubella-specific IgM in serum sam-ples may indicate virus persistency and an impairment of the shut-off mechanism of IgM synthesis.

Neuroimaging may be useful. In SSPE, CT scan may show white matter hypodensities involving the frontal, parietal, occipital, temporal, and periventricular regions, varying degrees of cerebral atrophy, and basal ganglia hypodensities. MRI may be normal or may show focal or diffuse white matter signal changes, signal alterations in basal ganglia, or brain atrophy. In addition, some studies have shown changes in neurometabolite concentrations according to clinical status and disease stage (increase of myoinositol until stage 3 and a reduction in stage 4) using magnetic resonance spectroscopy (MRS). In PML, radiological findings may simulate those of a brain tumor, although a mass effect is uncommon. MRI usually shows multiple small white matter hyperintense lesions. In SSPE, EEG may show a characteristic pattern composed of peri-odic complexes with high-voltage slow waves that are not suppressed by diazepam injection during EEG recording. In rare cases with unusual clinical or neuroradiological features, brain biopsy has facilitated diagnosis.

Neuropathological findings

Chronic enteroviral encephalomyelitis

Brain tissue shows an unspecific, patchy, non-necrotizing, chronic meningoencephalitis of variable severity and uneven distribution, affecting both gray and white mat-ter. In the subarachnoidal space, lymphocytic infiltrates and macrophages are observed. In the brain parenchyma, perivascular lymphocytic cuffs and microglial nodules are usually detected. Neuronal loss and gliosis are seen. Viral inclusion bodies are lacking, although some studies have detected viral antigens in neurons and astrocytes using immunohistochemistry.

Measles inclusion body encephalitis

Histological examination of brain tissue may show scattered inflammatory foci or normal-appearing brain parenchyma. Lesions may include reactive gliosis, perivascular accumulation of lymphocytes, microglial proliferation, and macrophages; some multinucleated cells have been found. Neurons and, less frequently, astrocytes and oligodendrocytes may contain prominent nuclear and/or cytoplasmic eosinophilic inclusion bodies (Plate 90.1a). Viral nucleocapsids can be demostrated using electronmicroscopy. Immunohistochemisty usually detects abundant viral antigen (Plate 90.1b).

Subacute sclerosing panencephalitis (SSPE)

The histological changes of SSPE are those of an encephalitis with lymphocytic infiltrates and macrophages in the meningeal space, brain parenchyma, and perivascular areas. Histological changes in the gray matter of gray matter (including the cerebral cortex, basal ganglia, thalamus, and brainstem) induces neuronal loss, reactive astrocytosis, marked microglial activation, and patchy inflammatory infiltrates. White matter can also be affected (panencephalitis), showing gliosis, eventual demyelination, and scattered lymphocytic infiltrates. Intranuclear viral inclusions are variably frequent on plain histology but may be detected in abundance via immunohistochemistry. In long-standing disease, destructive changes may be prominent and viral products may no longer be demonstrable by immunohistochemical or ultrastructural methods, but viral RNA can still be detected using *in situ* hybridization. The cerebellum and spinal cord may also be affected. In addition, in long-standing disease, neurofibrillary tangles may occur in similar distribution to those observed in Alzheimer's disease, affecting the hippocampus and cerebral cortex, the nucleus basalis of Meynert, the hypothalamus, and raphe nuclei. These tangles are composed of paired helical filaments and immunoreact with antibodies directed against phosphorylated tau protein. Oligodendroglial tangles have also been found in single SSPE cases.

Progressive rubella pancenephalitis

Only a few cases of progressive rubella pancenephalitis have been studied in detail in postmortem brain tissue. Histology reveals widespread neuronal loss and gliosis of gray matter with perivascular lymphocytic aggregates and microglial nodules. The white matter shows severe gliosis and characteristic amorphous and globular, PAS-positive, mineralized material within blood vessel walls. Viral inclusions are not seen.

Progressive multifocal leukoencephalopathy (PML)

PML causes a multifocal and progressive degeneration of mainly white matter with foci of patchy demyelination, giving the appearance of moth-eaten holes or of large demyelinated areas (Plate 90.1c). Lesions range in size from a few millimeters to extensive involvement of cerebral and cerebellar hemispheres. Parieto-occipital regions are more frequently involved. In rare cases, the spinal cord may be affected. Infected oligodendrocytes show enlarged, glassy, and homogeneous amphophilic nuclear inclusions (also known as PML cells) (Plate 90.1d). These cells are usually found at the borders of PML lesions. In addition, macrophages and large, bizarre astrocytes, which may be mistaken for tumorous astrocytes, as in glioblastoma, are observed (Plate 90.1d). Inflammatory infiltrates are rare. The JC virus is detectable in brain sections using immunohistochemistry (Plate 90.1d, inset), electron microscopy, and *in situ* hybridization, usually in oligodendroglial (PML) cells and, to a lesser extent, in astroglia. The JC virus can also be demonstrated in cells that do not show morphological changes.

Treatment/management

For most of these diseases there is no specific antiviral treatment. Management of the patient is based on supportive and symptomatic measures. It is pivotal to prevent the disease by vaccination if available. Recovery from the underlying immunosuppressive condition may improve neurological symptoms. Some patients affected by chronic enteroviral encephalomyelitis have responded to intravenous immunoglobulin therapy, but others have not. Even though not yet Food and Drug Administration (FDA)-approved, pleconaril has been made available for compassionate use on patients with chronic enteroviral encephalomyelitis. Some authors have reported successful use of the nucleoside analogue ribavirin to treat *subacute measles inclusion body encephalitis*. Disease-modifying agents, such as isoprinosine, intravenous immunoglobulins, oral prednisolone, levamisole, amantadine, and methylprednisolone, have been used for the treatment of SSPE, but with no obvious clinical effect. The immunomodulator inosiplex is one of the few drugs that has been partially effective in the treatment of SSPE. PML has had a fatal clinical course, with patients usually dying within 6 months of disease onset. While specific antiviral treatment has been unsuccessful, treatment of the underlying cause of immunosuppression and newer pharmacotherapies that reverse immunosuppression may induce remission of PML.

Further reading

Budka H. Viral infections. In: Garcia JH, Budka H, McKeever PE, Sarnat HB, Sima AAF, editors. *Neuropathology – The Diagnostic Approach*. Philadelphia: Mosby; 1997, pp. 353–91.

Frey TK. Neurological aspects of rubella virus infection. *Intervirology* 1997; 40(2–3): 167–75.

Johnson RT. *Viral Infections of the Nervous System*, 2nd ed. Philadelphia: Lippincott-Raven; 1998.

Love S, Wiley CA. Viral diseases. In: Graham DI, Lantos PL, editors. *Greenfield's Neuropathology*, 7th ed. London: Arnold; 2002, pp. 50–7.

Rima BK, Duprex WP. Molecular mechanisms of measles virus persistence. *Virus Res* 2005; 111(2): 132–47.

Steiner I, Budka H, Chaudhuri A, *et al*. Viral encephalitis: a review of diagnostic methods and guidelines for management. *Eur J Neurol* 2005; 12(5): 331–43.

Chapter 91
Prion diseases

Ellen Gelpi and Herbert Budka
Medical University of Vienna, Vienna, Austria

Introduction

Transmissible spongiform encephalopathies (TSE) or prion diseases represent an irreversible and fatal degeneration of the central nervous system leading invariably to death. The disease is considered to be caused by a conformational isomer of the host prion protein that is predominantly expressed in the brain but also in other tissues. Different types of human diseases have been described:

1 *Sporadic forms* (arising spontaneously, without obvious origin):
- sporadic Creutzfeldt–Jakob disease (sCJD)
- sporadic fatal insomnia (sFI).

2 *Genetic forms* (mutations or insertions in the prion protein gene on chromosome 20):
- genetic (familial) CJD (gCJD)
- fatal familial insomnia (FFI)
- Gerstmann–Sträussler–Scheinker disease (GSS).

3 *Acquired forms* (transmitted from contact with external prions):
- variant CJD (vCJD) (contact with BSE prions)
- iatrogenic CJD (iCJD) (inadvertent transmission by invasive medical procedures).

Animal TSEs comprise scrapie affecting sheep and goats, chronic wasting disease affecting North American cervids, transmissible mink encephalopathy, feline spongiform encephalopathy, and bovine spongiform encephalopathy affecting cattle. This chapter deals only with human disease forms.

Epidemiology

Creutzfeldt–Jakob disease is a rare disease, with a worldwide incidence of about 1–2 cases per million per year. *Sporadic CJD* is the most frequent form that occurs spontaneously, with an average age of onset between 60 and 70 years. Five to 15% of cases of CJD are *familial/genetic cases*, inherited in an autosomal dominant way. Nearly 400 cases of *iatrogenic CJD* have been reported. The most important sources of iatrogenic transmission have been human dura mater grafts and human growth hormone (hGH) obtained from cadaveric sources. The duration of hGH treatment ranges between 1 and 13 years (median 6.4 years) and the appearance of symptoms between 11 and 15 years. The long incubation period could be explained by low titers of infectivity present after dilutions, admixture from different donors, and the peripheral route of administration. Cadaveric human hormone preparations were used until the mid-1980s; synthetic recombinant hormones have been produced thereafter. Cases of iCJD after transplantation of lyophilized dura mater obtained from commercial dura mater grafts (produced before 1987) have most frequently been reported in Japan. The incubation period varies between 1.5 and 23 years. Single cases were reported after neurosurgery and corneal grafting.

Kuru was recognized in the late 1950s in the Fore tribe in Papua New Guinea to be due to ritualistic cannibalism. It affected mostly adult women and children over 4 years of age, as in the cannibalistic feasts, women and children ate the less desirable tissues, including CNS tissue.

In 1996, *variant CJD* was identified in the United Kingdom. A causal link between vCJD and bovine spongiform encephalopathy (BSE) in cattle was first hypothesized, and there is now overwhelming epidemiological and experimental evidence that prions causing BSE and vCJD are the same. The most plausible route of exposure is via BSE-contaminated food. Contamination of the human food chain most likely resulted from CNS tissue in mechanically recovered meat used in the manufacture of processed products. The incubation period seems to be 5–10 years, but a length of several decades cannot be excluded. vCJD mostly affects individuals under 40 years of age. As of February 2009, 212 patients with variant CJD have been reported, the majority in the UK (168) and France (23), and a few cases in Spain (5), the Republic of Ireland (4), the Netherlands (3), the USA (3), Portugal (2), Italy (1), Saudi Arabia (1), Canada (1), and Japan (1).

There is one important polymorphism at codon 129 of the *PRNP*, coding for either methionine (M) or valine (V).

International Neurology: A Clinical Approach. Edited by Robert P. Lisak, Daniel D. Truong, William M. Carroll, and Roongroj Bhidayasiri. © 2009 Blackwell Publishing, ISBN: 978-1-4051-5738-4.

It represents a risk factor for iatrogenic and variant CJD and influences the clinical and neuropathological phenotype of sporadic and genetic TSEs. In the normal population, MV heterozygotes represent 50%, MMs 39%, and VVs 11%, in contrast to sCJD cases where MM homozygotes represent around 70%. To date, all vCJD cases are MM homozygotes. Additionally, the phenotype of certain gTSEs is strongly influenced by codon 129 such as in the D178N mutation: when the mutated allele encodes methionine in codon 129, FFI is observed, whereas a CJD phenotype predominates when the mutated allele encodes valine.

The combination of this polymorphism with the prion protein type (type 1 and type 2; see "Pathophysiology") is the basis of the molecular and phenotypic classification of sCJD into six subtypes.

Pathophysiology

The name "prion" was created to designate a "proteinaceous infectious particle." The current *protein-only hypothesis* indicates that the infectious agent (prion) causing TSE represents a conformational change of a normal host-encoded protein called PrP^c (PrP = prion protein, c = cellular) present in all cells of the body, but predominantly expressed in the brain on the surface of neurons. The disease-associated, newly formed PrP^{sc} (sc derives from scrapie) is enriched in beta-sheets and may interact with PrP^c and cause the latter to adopt the beta-sheet conformation of PrP^{sc}, initiating a self-perpetuating process that results in increasing PrP^{sc} concentrations. PrP^{sc} cannot be degraded by common enzymatic activity and accumulates around neurons and axons. It is suggested that the loss of function of PrP^c combined with the accumulation of PrP^{sc} in the brain induces neurodegeneration. Some mutations and insertions in the *PRNP* gene apparently favor the spontaneous conversion of PrP^c to PrP^{sc}, which could account for the genetic forms of human prion diseases.

Western blot isoform patterns of PrP^{sc} are classified on the basis of electrophoretic mobility of the non-glycosylated protein band as type 1 (21 kDa) or type 2 (19 kDa) and by differences in the glycoform ratio.

Transmission of prions can occur within the same species or between species. Infection by the oral route, as in Kuru and vCJD, requires that prions enter the body by the digestive tract, where PrP^{sc} can be found in Peyer's patches and the enteric nervous system. It was suggested that myeloid dendritic cells mediate transport within the lymphoreticular system. Neuroinvasion is thought to occur through the peripheral nervous system via the autonomic splanchnic nerve that enters the spinal cord, or via the vagus nerve to the brain.

The infectivity of different tissues can be demonstrated by bioassays. Experimental data from Brown and colleagues in 1994 demonstrated highest transmission rates for iatrogenic CJD (100%), Kuru (95%), and sCJD (90%), and considerably lower ones for most familial forms of the disease (68%).

Clinical features

Sporadic CJD (sCJD)

The most frequent initial symptoms are cognitive decline, cerebellar symptoms, ataxia, behavioral change, dizziness, visual complaints (especially cortical blindness), and dementia. Later patients exhibit a combination of various neurological symptoms including movement disorders and pyramidal signs accompany the dementia, representing a rapidly progressive global encephalopathy. Myoclonus, and in the terminal phase akinetic mutism, are prominent features. The disease leads invariably to death, generally due to respiratory or systemic infection in the terminal stage, after less than 2 years, on average after about 6 months. The six molecular subtypes of sCJD show variability in age, clinical signs at onset, and duration of illness.

Genetic TSEs

Genetic or familial CJD is similar to sporadic forms in clinical parameters and laboratory variables, but might have earlier onset and longer duration of disease. In FFI, the onset age is younger, mainly 25–60 years, and the duration can be from 6 months to 3 years. Its main clinical manifestations are alterations of circadian rhythm and autonomic disturbances with insomnia and autonomic dysregulation, but myoclonus and dementia are also prominent. The principal clinical features of Gerstmann–Sträussler–Scheinker are cerebellar symptoms.

Iatrogenic CJD (iCJD)

The clinical presentation of iCJD seems to depend on the site of inoculation: after neurosurgery, dementia predominates, while after peripheral transmission (e.g., growth hormone), cerebellar symptoms predominate. In dural grafts, however, the location of the graft does not seem to influence the clinical manifestation of disease, which is mostly cerebellar and myoclonic.

Kuru

Kuru is characterized by intense tremor and instability in gait, bulbar signs such as dysarthria and dysphagia, and less prominent cognitive decline.

Variant CJD (vCJD)

vCJD differs from classical sCJD in that psychiatric and sensory symptoms are the most frequent initial clinical features. Because no neurological alterations at examination may be detected at early stages of the disease, patients are frequently referred to a psychiatrist. Duration of disease is also longer than in sCJD, with a median of 14 months (6–38 months). Later, dementia and myoclonus are frequent, but choreiform movements, pyramidal signs, cerebellar symptoms and rigidity, and vertical gaze weakness have also been described.

Investigations

There is no blood or serologic test to definitely diagnose a prion disease. Current clinical criteria (Table 91.1)

Table 91.1 Clinical diagnostic criteria for surveillance purposes according to the World Health Organization (WHO, 2003).

Sporadic CJD

Definite
- Neuropathological/immunohistochemical confirmation

Probable
- Rapidly progressive dementia and at least two of the following symptoms:
  ○ Myoclonus
  ○ Visual or cerebellar problems
  ○ Pyramidal or extrapyramidal features
  ○ Akinetic mutism
- And typical EEG and/or positive 14-3-3 (disease duration less than 2 years)

Possible
- Like probable, but disease duration less than 2 years and EEG and/or 14-3-3 negative or not performed.

Variant CJD

I (A) Progressive neuropsychiatric disorder
  (B) Duration of illness more than 6 months
  (C) Routine investigations do not suggest an alternative diagnosis
  (D) No history of potential iatrogenic exposure
  (E) No evidence of a familial form of TSE
II (A) Early psychiatric symptoms*
  (B) Persistent painful sensory symptoms†
  (C) Ataxia
  (D) Myoclonus or chorea or dystonia
  (E) Dementia
III (A) EEG does not show the typical appearance of sporadic CJD‡ (or no EEG performed)
  (B) Bilateral pulvinar high signal on MRI scan
IV (A) Positive tonsil biopsy§

Definite: IA *and* neuropathological confirmation of vCJD¶

Probable: I *and* 4/5 of II *and* III A *and* III B, or I *and* IV A

*Depression, anxiety, apathy, withdrawal, delusions.
†This includes both frank pain and/or dysesthesia.
‡Generalized triphasic periodic complexes at approximately 1/s.
§Tonsil biopsy is not recommended routinely, nor in cases with EEG appearances typical of sCJD, but may be useful in suspect cases in which the clinical features are compatible with vCJD and MRI does not show bilateral pulvinar high signal.
¶Spongiform change and extensive PrP deposition with florid plaques, throughout the cerebrum and cerebellum.

cover suspected cases with high sensitivity (97%) and moderate specificity (65%). Additional techniques such as electroencephalogram (EEG) findings, determination of 14-3-3 protein in cerebrospinal fluid (CSF), and MR neuroimaging improve the accuracy of diagnosis. Nevertheless, several differential diagnoses must be taken into account: Alzheimer's disease, diffuse Lewy body disease, vascular dementia, inflammatory encephalopathies in younger people, Hashimoto encephalopathy, and paraneoplastic syndromes can present with symptoms fulfilling the surveillance criteria for possible or probable CJD.

Electrophysiological studies

In sCJD, the EEG shows a typical morphology with periodic sharp-wave complexes (PSWC), some with triphasic morphology, with a duration of 100–600 ms and an intercomplex interval of 500–2000 ms. It is important to remark that other disorders such as hepatic encephalopathy, hypoglycemia, SIADH (syndrome of inappropriate ADH secretion), brain abscesses, and drugs (lithium, baclophen) may cause similar EEG alterations. According to this, EEG has a sensitivity of 66% and a specificity of 74%, and can be observed during progression of disease, but may disappear at the terminal stages of disease. In vCJD, PSWC have been only observed in single cases at late disease stage.

Cerebrospinal fluid

The detection of 14-3-3, a neuronal protein that increases in the CSF after tissue damage, has the highest sensitivity (94%) and specificity (84%) for the clinical diagnosis of sCJD. Nevertheless, it is not diagnostic for CJD as it may be present in conditions with neuronal destruction such as stroke, encephalitis, or tumor. Some false negative results have been reported, especially at the onset of clinical symptoms and, in some cases, it turned positive with the progression of disease. In genetic forms and in vCJD it is not a useful marker. Other proteins that have been studied are tau, beta-amyloid, neuron-specific enolase, and S100 protein, which, however, have lower sensitivity and specificity and are not first choice, even if tau shows a multifold increase in patients with sCJD beyond the range seen in Alzheimer's disease or other dementing disorders.

Neuroimaging

Brain MRI may demonstrate bilateral areas of increased signal intensity in the caudate nuclei and putamina on long repetition time images in sCJD, and a bilateral pulvinar high signal in vCJD. In fluid-attenuated inversion recovery (FLAIR) images and diffusion-weighted MRI, ribbon-like high signal intensity changes in the cerebral cortex can be observed.

Genetic analysis

Genetic analysis is recommended in all suspected cases when possible, as an aberration is suggested by a family history in only half of genetic cases. Furthermore, knowledge of the codon 129 polymorphism is important to predict the clinical course and to rate the result of additional investigations such as EEG and 14-3-3.

Brain biopsy

Brain biopsy has a role in suspected CJD only when treatable alternative diagnoses are under consideration. Because of local variability in the distribution of typical histological changes and PrP^{sc} deposits, the chance of false negative results of a brain biopsy must be considered. In addition to central nervous system (CNS) tissue, the thymus, lymph nodes, tonsil, spleen, liver, adrenal gland, and rectum may contain PrP^{sc} in vCJD. Tonsillar biopsy has been advocated as a potentially relevant examination in the diagnosis of vCJD and is currently included in clinical diagnostic criteria of vCJD (Table 91.1).

Postmortem investigations

Every suspected case of any form of CJD should be confirmed by neuropathology after death of the patient whenever possible. In order to use adequate safety precautions for the postmortem examination, the pathology laboratory should be notified of the suspected diagnosis. Classical histopathological features include spongiform change, neuronal loss, and astrogliosis. Amyloid plaques are rarely seen in sCJD, in contrast to vCJD which shows abundant amyloid plaques, many of them surrounded by vacuoles (called "florid plaques") as hallmarks. In GSS, multicentric amyloid plaques are the defining criterion, while FFI is characterized by severe gliosis of the thalamus and olivary nuclei without prominent spongiform change. Immunohistochemistry or Western blot for the detection of PrP^{sc} is needed for definitive neuropathological diagnosis in cases with non-classical histopathology.

Therapeutic approaches to prion diseases

To date, no effective treatment of prion diseases is available. Experimental approaches in cell culture, cell-free systems, and animal models have used diverse compounds to block prion conversion and accumulation by targeting the substrate PrP^c or directly the PrP^{sc} (e.g., polyanionic and polycationic compounds, tetrapyrrolic compounds, polyene antibiotics, tri- and tetracyclic compounds, beta sheet breakers, immunomodulatory agents, statins, and inhibitors of intracellular signalling pathways) and have shown somewhat promising results, but there is little evidence that these drugs are efficient against prion diseases *in vivo*.

The difficulty of treatment resides in the following: (1) most of these compounds would only be effective if administered before the onset of clinical disease, (2) some drugs do not effectively cross the blood–brain barrier (e.g., pentosan), and (3) there is no blood or serologic test to definitely diagnose prion diseases. One of the most important needs in prion investigation is a diagnostic tool to detect carriers in the infective stage, before cerebral damage manifests itself, followed by treatment before disease becomes evident.

Preventive measures

One important characteristic of prions is their extreme resistance to conventional sterilizing procedures such as heat, irradiation (UV and ionic), and chemicals (alcohol, formaldehyde, ethylenoxid, etc.). To avoid and prevent transmission to other persons, (neuro-)surgical instruments must undergo special decontamination procedures or be disposed of after potential contact with prions. The proven efficacious inactivating methods are treatment with sodium hydroxide and subsequent autoclaving at 134°C. Conventional care of patients in hospital or at home is not associated with a transmission risk.

Additionally, blood might be a vehicle of prions in variant CJD (not sporadic CJD), and four cases of transfusion-associated vCJD have been reported to date. As the incubation period of variant CJD might last for several years, asymptomatic carriers might be blood donors, with implications for transfusion services and blood products.

Further reading

Brown P, Gibbs CJ Jr, Rodgers Johnson P, *et al.* Human spongiform encephalopathy: the National Institutes of Health series of 300 cases of experimentally transmitted disease. *Ann Neurol* 1994; 35: 513–29.

Budka H. Neuropathology of prion diseases. *Br Med Bull* 2003; 66: 121–30.

Parchi P, Giese A, Capellari S, *et al.* Classification of sporadic Creutzfeldt–Jakob disease based on molecular and phenotypic analysis of 300 subjects. *Ann Neurol* 1999; 46(2): 224–33.

Trevitt CR, Collinge J. A systematic review of prion therapeutics in experimental models. *Brain* 2006; 129(Pt 9): 2241–65.

WHO. WHO manual for surveillance of human transmissible spongiform encephalopathies including variant Creutzfeldt–Jakob disease. *WHO Communicable Disease Surveillance and Response.* Geneva: WHO; 2003.

Will RG, Ironside JW, Zeidler M, *et al.* A new variant of Creutzfeldt–Jakob disease in the UK. *Lancet* 1996; 347(9006): 921–5.

Zerr I, Pocchiari M, Collins S, *et al.* Analysis of EEG and CSF 14-3-3 proteins as aids to the diagnosis of Creutzfeldt–Jakob disease. *Neurology* 2000; 55(6): 811–5.

Chapter 92
HIV and the acquired immunodeficiency syndrome: an overview of neurological complications

Bruce J. Brew
St Vincent's Hospital, Sydney, Australia

Introduction

HIV-related neurological complications are important to distinguish and recognize because they are common, treatable, and easily mistaken for other, more "classical," neurological disorders. A method of classifying these complications is discussed in this chapter as are certain principles that are important to the clinician. Finally, a clinical approach to these disorders is advanced.

Epidemiology

At least one-third of patients with advanced HIV disease will present with a neurological complication, sometimes in the absence of known HIV infection. With advancements in the treatment of HIV and the correlating number of individuals living with HIV infection, an even greater number of patients living with less advanced infection will experience one or more neurological complications. At autopsy, more than 80% of HIV patients have cerebral pathology, ranging from evidence of HIV encephalitis to opportunistic infections and lymphoma. At least half will have some evidence of a peripheral neuropathy. Given the current world burden of HIV disease, the neurological complications of HIV are now far more common than multiple sclerosis, motor neuron disease, and other neuropathologies that have traditionally been the focus of the medical community. Indeed, HIV-associated dementia is now the most common cause of dementia in young to middle-aged persons.

Pathophysiology/clinical features

Perhaps more than any other disease, HIV can mimic many diseases, some of which are untreatable. Neurologists

International Neurology: A Clinical Approach. Edited by Robert P. Lisak, Daniel D. Truong, William M. Carroll, and Roongroj Bhidayasiri. © 2009 Blackwell Publishing, ISBN: 978-1-4051-5738-4.

unaware of existing HIV infection may mistakenly diagnose the patient with disorders such as Huntington's chorea, multisystem atrophy, and Guillain–Barré syndrome, to name only a few.

Determining the degree of HIV infection at the time of neurological involvement, or "time-locking," is the first principle for the clinician, as neurological complications are directly related to the degree of advancement of HIV disease. Indeed, because the stage of HIV infection can help determine both the severity and pathology of neurological disease, time-locking should be determined *before* further assessing any present neuropathology.

The next principle important to the clinician is that of parallel tracking, as certain complications can and often do involve several parts of the nervous system at the same time. This may change the "classical" presentation of some disorders and may complicate the interpretation of test results: CSF abnormalities such as a mononuclear pleocytosis frequently occur as "background" phenomena without any direct clinical correlation.

The third principle is that of layering. Complications can and often do involve one part of the nervous system and layer upon one another at different points of time in the course of HIV disease. The fourth and final principle is that of unmasking, wherein previously compensated deficits may be "unmasked" by the occurrence of an additional insult.

Opportunistic infections common to HIV patients such as cryptococcosis and cytomegalovirus infection (CMV) can have neurological complications, even in the presence of adequate systemic response to therapy. Other disorders such as *Mycobacterium avium* complex infection (MAC) and Kaposi's sarcoma (KS) rarely involve the CNS. In approaching the patient with neurological complications related to HIV, it is important to employ the latter-mentioned principles in conjunction with an appreciation of the importance of co-existing and past disease as well as therapies.

Investigations

While several classification schemes have been promulgated in the literature, the most clinically useful is that which groups complications according to the stage of HIV disease at presentation of the complication. Stages of HIV are usually determined by CD4 cell count: CD4 > 500 (early), CD4 < 500 but >200 (moderately advanced), and CD4 < 200 (advanced). The latter is often known already or can be broadly gained from careful clinical assessment focusing on systemic features such as weight loss, oral candidiasis, and retinal cotton wool spots. Moreover, simple routine laboratory tests may reveal such indicators as lymphopenia, raised erythrocyte sedimentation rate, and elevated serum protein.

Treatment/management

Most neurological complications of HIV disease are treatable. Indeed, HIV-associated dementia is the only viral dementia that can be treated, often leading to significant improvement if not full recovery. Cryptococcal meningitis and cerebral toxoplasmosis can similarly be successfully treated.

Pharmaceutically, the antiretroviral drug zidovudine may lead to a myopathy, while didanosine and stavudine can cause peripheral neuropathy. On the other hand, certain medications may decrease the likelihood of neurological complications. Cotrimoxazole lessens the risk of developing not only pneumocystis carinii pneumonia but also toxoplasmosis, and fluconazole decreases the risk of cryptococcal meningitis. Highly active antiretroviral therapy (HAART) is the only treatment for progressive multifocal leukoencephalopathy.

Further reading

Brew BJ. *HIV Neurology*. New York: Oxford University Press; 2001, Chapters 3–4, pp. 32–42.

Chapter 93
Human immunodeficiency virus: biology and general overview of seroconversion and early infection

Alexandros C. Tselis

Wayne State University School of Medicine, Detroit, USA

Introduction

Human immunodeficiency virus (HIV) disease has prominent neurological manifestations and is probably the most common cause of viral encephalitis and other brain infections around the world. In this chapter, we discuss the biology of the virus and clinical aspects of initial infection. While there are two groups of HIV, HIV-1 and HIV-2, because HIV-1 is the dominant type, both in number and severity, we will deal exclusively with this virus, and refer to it as HIV.

Epidemiology

There are three overall groups of HIV, the M (or Main) group, the O (Outlier) group, and the N (non-M and -O) group. The M group consists of nine subgroups, or clades: A, B, C, D, F, G, H, J, and K. Each clade differs from the others by >20% in the ENV region of the genome (see below) and by >15% in the GAG region. The O and N groups appear to affect only a minority of patients. There is a geographic distribution of local clade prevalence; for instance, clade B is found in North America and Europe, while clades A, C, D, and H are found in Africa, and clades J and K in Zaire and Cameroon, respectively. Some viral isolates have sequences from different clades in different parts of their genomes. These arose as recombinants from simultaneous infection of one individual by viruses from two or more clades, and are now known as circulating recombinant forms (CRFs).

Antigens for most commercially available enzyme-linked immunosorbent assay (ELISA) tests are based on clade B viruses from North America and Europe, which have received the bulk of research and clinical trials. These tests may lose sensitivity for viruses of other clades

or even groups. Further, viruses of other clades may respond to commonly used antiretroviral drugs in a different manner. HIV-1 group O and HIV-2 viruses tend to be resistant to non-nucleotide reverse transcriptase inhibitors (NNRTIs), and HIV-1 clade G may be less susceptible *in vitro* to protease inhibitor drugs.

Pathophysiology

The HIV virion consists of two identical (diploid) single-strand 9 kb RNA molecules enclosed within a capsid surrounded by a lipid envelope. The virus transcribes its RNA into DNA by reverse transcriptase (RT) and inserts the resultant DNA into the genome of the infected cell by an integrase (IN).

The viral genome consists of the typical retroviral LTR-GAG-POL-ENV-LTR structure, incorporating the regulatory long terminal repeat (LTR) and genes for structural (GAG, or group-specific antigen), polymerase (POL), and envelope (ENV) proteins, along with accessory genes (tat, vpr, vpu, nef), as shown in Figure 93.1. The viral genome is translated as a polyprotein, which is then cleaved into functional component proteins by the viral-encoded protease (PR) segment of the polyprotein. GAG encodes for the structural proteins present in the virion, which include the matrix protein (MA), capsid protein (CA), p7, and nucleocapsid protein (NC). POL encodes for three

International Neurology: A Clinical Approach. Edited by Robert P. Lisak, Daniel D. Truong, William M. Carroll, and Roongroj Bhidayasiri. © 2009 Blackwell Publishing, ISBN: 978-1-4051-5738-4.

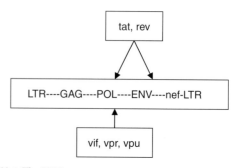

Figure 93.1 The HIV genome.

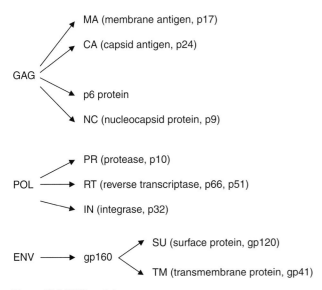

MA (membrane antigen, p17)

CA (capsid antigen, p24)

GAG

p6 protein

NC (nucleocapsid protein, p9)

PR (protease, p10)

POL ——→ RT (reverse transcriptase, p66, p51)

IN (integrase, p32)

SU (surface protein, gp120)

ENV ——→ gp160

TM (transmembrane protein, gp41)

Figure 93.2 HIV proteins.

proteins: a PR, an RT, and an IN. Finally, ENV codes for the envelope glycoprotein gp160, which is cleaved into two viral surface proteins, gp120 and gp41. gp120 attaches the virus to the cell, and gp41 induces fusion between the viral envelope and cell membrane. The proteins are shown in Figure 93.2.

HIV infects a spectrum of cells, but CD4+ T lymphocytes and macrophages are most prominently involved. To achieve infection, the HIV envelope gp120 protein attaches to a CD4 molecule as well as to one of two possible "coreceptors," CXCR4 or CCR5. The CD4 molecule, expressed on lymphocytes and macrophages, is considered the "main" viral receptor. CXCR4 coreceptors, expressed on T lymphocytes, select for infection by so-called X4 viruses, while CCR5 coreceptors are expressed on macrophages and select for R5 viruses. The precise tropism of the virus is in part dictated by sequences in the gp120 protein that bind to either CXCR4, resulting in a T-lymphotropic (or T-tropic) virus, or CCR5, resulting in a macrophage-tropic (M-tropic) virus. T-tropic strains replicate to high titer in cells of the MT-2 cell line, cause the cells to fuse in a syncytium (syncytium-inducing or SI), and have cytopathic effects in cell culture. M-tropic strains replicate to low titer in MT-2 cells, are non-syncytium-inducing (NSI), and have low pathogenicity.

Once the virus penetrates the cell, subsequent events depend on the viral strain and type of cell infected. HIV RNA, bound to viral proteins including RT, is released into the cell cytoplasm. If the cell is permissive, RT reverse transcribes the viral RNA into a complementary DNA copy, cDNA, which is then converted into double-stranded DNA (ds cDNA). The ds cDNA, along with viral proteins MA, vpr, and IN, forms the so-called "preintegration complex", which is directed into the nucleus of the cell, where the ds cDNA is inserted into the host cell's

genomic DNA. At that point, infection may become latent or it can be productive, transcribing incorporated cDNA into viral RNA and producing virions.

Clinical features

HIV infection is classified into several stages depending on viral load, clinical characteristics, and CD4 count. Acute retroviral syndrome is defined as the first few weeks of HIV infection, before the development of anti-HIV antibodies. Primary or early HIV infection is defined as the first few months following development of anti-HIV antibodies. This is followed by a clinically latent state, in which there are no clinical signs or symptoms of disease. Advanced HIV infection or AIDS is defined by several criteria, including a low CD4 count (below 200 cells/μl), the presence of any one of several particular opportunistic infections, and certain HIV-specific syndromes such as HIV dementia, HIV-associated sensory neuropathy, and HIV-associated vacuolar myelopathy.

Acute HIV infection may be entirely asymptomatic, but often is characterized by acute illness, with fever, sore throat, fatigue, weight loss, maculopapular rash, and myalgia. Some findings on physical examination include oral ulceration, exudative pharyngitis, thrush, genital or rectal ulceration, and adenopathy. Acute retroviral syndrome can resemble other acute systemic infectious diseases such as infectious mononucleosis, secondary syphilis, hepatitis A or B, measles, and toxoplasmosis and may be accompanied by aseptic meningitis.

In acute infection, blood-borne dissemination results in viral deposition in various organs and can manifest as organ-specific syndromes. These may be the result of cytopathic effects or immunopathology. HIV can be isolated from CSF very early in the course of infection. Occasionally, acute retroviral syndrome can involve the nervous system most prominently. HIV syndromes in the central nervous system (CNS) include encephalitis and acute myelopathy. In the peripheral nervous system (PNS), Bell's palsy, acute brachial plexopathy, and inflammatory demyelinating polyneuropathy can occur. Sensory ganglionitis, cranial nerve palsies, progressive myopathy, and acute rhabdomyolysis have also been reported. Pathogenesis of these syndromes is unclear and may not involve direct infection of neural cells, but may reflect the effects of generalized immune activation. The outcome of these illnesses is unpredictable, but often quite good.

Investigations

Upon initial infection, particularly with M-tropic strains, only part of the viral inoculum replicates to a high initial titer. The inoculum breaches the mucosal barrier and encounters Langerhans' cells, which express both CD4 and CCR5 molecules, thus possibly selecting the M-tropic part of the inoculum. The Langerhans' cells migrate to local draining lymph nodes, become activated dendritic cells, and infect CD4+ lymphocytes. Virus becomes detectable in the local lymph nodes within a few days. This is followed by a burst of viremia with systemic dissemination. The blood viral load is initially high, but as cell-mediated immunity is activated, drops to a steady level, or "set point." A high set point is predictive of a more rapid progression to AIDS. Initially, the number of CD4+ T cells drops, while the number of CD8+ cells increases, so that the CD4:CD8 ratio is inverted. As the set point is approached, the CD4 count recovers. In the untreated host, the CD4 count then decreases very slowly and symptomatic AIDS occurs in about 10 years.

After the set point is achieved and antiretroviral medication is initiated, measurements of viral load reveal the dynamics of viral generation. Cells productively infected with virus have an average lifetime of approximately 2 days. Plasma viral load has a half-life of about 6 hours; decay of plasma virus is slightly faster than that of peripheral blood mononuclear cell-associated virus. The viral generation time, from release of a virion to release of "daughter" virions after infection of a new cell, is approximately 2.6 days. It is estimated that 10 billion virions are produced every 24 hours.

In the original burst of viremia, HIV is deposited in various tissue compartments and establishes infection in each of them, particularly in the CNS. Usually, the initial virus is of R5 M-tropic phenotype. The compartments are relatively isolated, and the virus evolves in each compartment independently from the others. Thus, early on, HIV isolates from blood and cerebrospinal fluid (CSF) may have the same phenotype, but late in the course of the infection the phenotypes can differ.

Treatment/management

In acute inflammatory demyelinating polyneuropathy, standard treatment of intravenous immunoglobulin or plasmapheresis may be used. For rare syndromes, such as acute encephalitis, there is no treatment established. Treatment with antiretroviral drugs strongly suppresses viral load and may penetrate the blood–brain barrier; however, since the natural history of this syndrome is unknown, the benefit of this regimen is unclear.

Further reading

Cornblath D, McArthur J, Kennedy P, Witte A, Griffin J. Inflammatory demyelinating neuropathies associated with human T-cell lymphotropic virus type III infection. *Ann Neurol* 1987; 21: 32–40.

Davis L, Hjelle B, Miller V, *et al.* Early viral brain invasion in iatrogenic human immunodeficiency virus infection. *Neurology* 1992; 42: 1736–9.

Douek D, Picker L, Koup R. T cell dynamics in HIV-1 infection. *Annu Rev Immunol* 2003; 21: 265–304.

Haseltine W. Molecular biology of the human immunodeficiency virus type 1. *FASEB J* 1991; 5: 2349–60.

Hollander H, Levy J. Neurologic abnormalities and recovery of human immunodeficiency virus from cerebrospinal fluid. *Ann Intern Med* 1987; 106: 692–5.

Kassutto S, Rosenberg E. Primary HIV type I infection. *Clin Infect Dis* 2004; 38: 1447–53.

Parry G. Peripheral neuropathies associated with human immunodeficiency virus infection. *Ann Neurol* 1988; 23: S49–S53.

Peeters M, Toure-Kane C, Nkengasong J. Genetic diversity of HIV in Africa: impact on diagnosis, treatment, vaccine development and trials. *AIDS* 2003; 17: 2547–60.

Schacker T, Collier A, Hughes J, Shea T, Corey L. Clinical and epidemiologic features of primary HIV infection. *Ann Intern Med* 1996; 125: 257–64.

Simpson D, Bender A. Human immunodeficiency virus-associated myopathy: analysis of 11 patients. *Ann Neurol* 1988; 24: 79–84.

Chapter 94
HIV-related CNS disorders

Girish Modi, Kapila Hari, and Andre Mochan
University of the Witwatersrand, Johannesburg, South Africa

Aseptic meningitis

Introduction

Aseptic meningitis is a clinicopathological syndrome, the cardinal symptoms of which are headache, fever, and meningism. Defining cerebrospinal fluid (CSF) findings includes a mononuclear pleocytosis, normal or mildly raised protein, and normal glucose levels. The causes are mainly viral infections and it is usually a self-limiting illness.

Aseptic meningitis in HIV may be caused by HIV itself or by an opportunistic infection (OI), by non-infectious inflammatory processes, or by central nervous system (CNS) neoplasia. In terms of direct infection, HIV has been identified throughout the course of infection in CSF by polymerase chain reaction (PCR) or viral culture techniques. HIV-associated aseptic meningitis occurs in several different settings: at the time of seroconversion, during the course of the disease, and with the use of highly active antiretroviral treatment (HAART). Aseptic meningitis in these HIV-related settings presents as an acute, self-limiting illness (often with a cranial neuropathy, e.g., facial nerve palsy), as acute symptomatic meningitis, or as chronic asymptomatic meningitis.

Epidemiology

Aseptic meningitis is the second most common type of meningitis in HIV-positive patients, the most common being cryptococcal meningitis. The incidence or prevalence of aseptic meningitis in HIV cannot be accurately determined because it is most often asymptomatic. Frequencies of 0.5–1.0% have been reported. No gender, ethnic, geographical, or clade-related differences have been described.

Pathophysiology

Meningeal inflammation occurs as a result of HIV breaching the meningeal blood–CSF barrier or due to autoimmune processes that cause non-infectious inflammation. Meningeal invasion can occur either via the hematogenous route or by neurotropic spread. Meningeal irritation elicits the protective reflex of neck stiffness and can cause headache and cranial nerve palsies.

Clinical features

The illness is typically biphasic, initially producing non-specific constitutional symptoms followed by the classical features of headache, malaise, fever, neck stiffness, rigors, photophobia, nausea, and vomiting. A characteristic skin rash such as that of varicella zoster (VZV) may precede or occur in conjunction with the syndrome. Rare features include cranial neuropathies, confusion, somnolence, seizures, and personality changes.

Investigations

The typical CSF profile in aseptic meningitis is that of a lymphocytic pleocytosis of less than 500 cells/mm, normal or mildly elevated protein, normal glucose, and negative bacterial antigen tests. Early CSF analysis may reveal a neutrophil predominance. CT or MRI may help exclude suspected structural disease such as parameningeal infectious foci but are generally not necessary.

Treatment/management

Management is symptomatic. If bacterial or partially-treated bacterial meningitis is suspected, empiric antibiotics should be commenced. HSV-1, HSV-2, severe Epstein–Barr virus and VZV infections can be treated with acyclovir, and antiretrovirals can be considered for HIV as well. Corticosteroids are not recommended due to inhibitory effects on immune responses.

Prognosis

Outcome is generally excellent, with full recovery in 5–14 days after symptom onset. Headaches, light-headedness, and fatigue may persist in some patients. Natural history is determined by the natural history of the HIV infection and its effects on immunity.

International Neurology: A Clinical Approach. Edited by Robert P. Lisak, Daniel D. Truong, William M. Carroll, and Roongroj Bhidayasiri. © 2009 Blackwell Publishing, ISBN: 978-1-4051-5738-4.

HIV-associated cognitive impairment

Introduction

Cognitive impairment in HIV is caused either by the virus itself or by opportunistic disease. The latter occurs from progressive immunosuppression and includes systemic and CNS infections (cryptococcal meningitis, toxoplasma encephalitis, progressive multifocal leukoencephalopathy, or PML) and neoplasia (lymphoma).

HIV neurocognitive illness comprises a spectrum ranging from mild (neuropsychologically impaired, NPI), to moderate (minor cognitive motor disorder, MCMD), to severe (HIV-associated dementia, HAD).

Epidemiology

The HIV epidemic can be described in three phases. The first of these is the illness prior to the introduction of antiretrovirals, followed by the era of monotherapy with zidovudine (AZT), and now, more recently, the era of HAART.

Primary HIV-related neurocognitive illness is now the most common preventable and treatable neurocognitive illness in people under the age of 50. Prior to the introduction of antiretrovirals, dementia was a common manifestation of late disease, occurring in over 50% of AIDS patients. With AZT, dementia rates and overall mortality decreased, leading to an increase in patients with MCMD and NPI. This has been further influenced by HAART, particularly in developed regions of North America and Europe, dominated by the clade B strain of HIV-1, where HAART is standard management.

The clade C virus is linked to an estimated 50% of infections globally and is associated with the rapidly growing epidemics in sub-Saharan Africa and parts of Asia, including India and China. Until recently, there has been little data published on HIV-related neurocognitive impairment from non-clade B regions. HIV dementia was believed to be a minor problem in these developing regions when compared to the overwhelming burden of OIs. The low prevalence was thought to be due to underdiagnosis, underreporting, and short life expectancy. Subsequent frequencies were found to be higher, with reported figures of 38% in South Africa (clade C), up to 35% in India (clade C), and 31% in Uganda (clades A and D). The influence of clade subtype on the spectrum of cognitive dysfunction is minimal, if any.

Pathophysiology

Once within the brain, HIV segregates selectively, with the highest levels found in the basal ganglia, subcortical (especially frontal) white matter regions, and frontal cortex. This peculiar regional distribution is unexplained, but may be related to viral entry via CSF, to patterns of monocyte trafficking within the brain, or to relative differences in the selective vulnerability of particular neuronal populations or brain regions.

Neuropathological features include white matter pallor, microglial nodules, multinucleated giant cells, and gliosis, a constellation termed HIV encephalitis (HIVE). Damage to synaptic and dendritic structures dominates over neuronal loss. The extent of histopathological involvement and severity of clinical dementia correlate poorly, indicating that biochemical and immunological factors determined by host–virus interactions rather than structural damage are responsible for neuropathogenesis.

Neurotoxicity occurs directly from viral proteins (gp120, gp41, tat, nef) or indirectly from macrophage factors (quinolinic acid, prostaglandins, leucotrienes), cytokines, and chemokines (TNF-α, IL-1, IL-6, IL-10, interferons). Blood–brain barrier disruption may additionally promote access of neurotoxins from the systemic infection to the extracellular CNS compartment. Excitotoxicity via activation of *N*-methyl-*D*-aspartate (NMDA) receptors may be the final common pathway.

Clinical features

HIV-associated cognitive impairment manifests over a period of weeks to months, with the triad of cognitive decline, behavioral abnormalities, and motor dysfunction.

Cognitive domains initially affected include verbal and visual memory (retrieval rather than recognition), complex sequencing, mental flexibility, and visual construction. This presents clinically with impaired short-term memory, poor concentration and attention, and executive dysfunction with mental slowing and impaired judgement. Patients complain of increasing forgetfulness and losing track of events, items, or even occurrences; complex daily tasks take longer to complete.

Behavioral abnormalities include apathy, inertia, loss of libido, irritability, blunting of emotional responses, and waning interest in work and hobbies, ultimately leading to social withdrawal. Early symptoms are subtle and may be misdiagnosed as depression. Delirium, mania, and psychosis can be the presenting feature in up to 10% of cases.

Early motor symptoms are mild and consist of psychomotor retardation that leads to difficulties with fine finger movements and balance problems. Patients report deterioration of handwriting and a tendency to drop things. Gait difficulties are present from early stages and resemble impaired postural reflexes seen in patients with extrapyramidal disease. Early in the illness, neurological examination is normal except for mild slowing of repetitive movements (e.g., finger tapping), subtle saccadic and smooth pursuit eye movement abnormalities, and increased deep tendon reflexes. With progression of the disease, process spasticity (especially of lower limbs), clonus, frontal release signs, tremor, and incontinence develop.

Seizures and myoclonus can occur in late disease. In advanced dementia, signs of co-occurring myelopathy and/or peripheral neuropathy may contribute to abnormal motor findings. Focal neurological signs such as hemiplegia, hemianopia, and hemisensory impairment, and focal cortical signs such as apraxia, agnosia, or aphasia are absent and their presence is suggestive of other pathologies. In late- or end-stage disease, dementia becomes global, with mutism, abulia, and incontinence.

NPI, MCMD, and HAD form part of a continuum in which activities of daily living are unaffected in NPI and MCMD. NPI can only be diagnosed by formal neuropsychological testing, whereas MCMD shows clinical impairment in complex tasks of daily living.

Investigations

Laboratory tests or parameters cannot reliably establish the diagnosis of HIV-associated cognitive impairment. Differential diagnoses include delirium secondary to drugs and metabolic derangements, encephalopathies due to substance abuse or head injury, CNS opportunistic disease (meningitis and focal brain lesions), and primary psychiatric conditions.

CSF in HAD is usually normal or non-specifically abnormal, with a lymphocytic pleocytosis, mildly elevated protein, and detectable viral RNA (aseptic meningitis syndrome). CSF analysis excludes other etiologies, in particular cryptococcal and tuberculous meningitis, neurosyphilis, cytomegalovirus (CMV) encephalitis, and PML. Since the introduction of HAART and resultant viral suppression attained by most patients, CSF viral load is no longer useful as a potential marker of CNS infection.

Structural imaging with CT or MRI is integral to diagnostic evaluation. Age-inappropriate cerebral atrophy with corresponding ventricular enlargement is a typical finding. Increasing ventricular size consistent with subcortical tissue loss has been shown to mirror progressive clinical deterioration. On T2-weighted MRI sequences, especially with fluid attenuated inversion recovery, this appears as patchy confluent high-intensity white matter signal changes sparing subcortical U fibers.

Neuropsychological testing can be used for screening purposes in high-risk asymptomatic or early symptomatic patients and for follow-up evaluation in patients with established cognitive impairment. Appropriate normative standards are not available for large parts of the developing world.

Treatment/management

HAART has led to a decreased frequency of HIV dementia and improved cognitive performance in some patients with established deficits and may delay or prevent the onset of symptoms in others. Despite this, there are no specific consensus treatment guidelines on when to initiate antiretrovirals and which drug combination to use. Current evidence supports commencement of HAART at the earliest stage of neurocognitive impairment irrespective of immunological suppression because the severity of impairment at initiation appears to be the strongest predictor of persistent neuropsychological deficits. CNS penetration of antiretrovirals is a controversial issue in relation to choice of drug. Symptomatic treatment of depression, anxiety, psychosis, or mania in patients with HIV neurocognitive impairment remains an integral part of management.

HIV-associated disorders in children

Introduction

AIDS is now a leading cause of childhood morbidity and mortality. Pediatric HIV is mainly acquired through vertical mother-to-child transmission. Other routes of infection include horizontal transmission through sexual abuse or transfusion of contaminated blood products. Adolescent HIV infection follows the same modes of transmission as that seen in adults, that is, sexual exposure and intravenous drug use.

The predominant neurological manifestation of HIV in children is a progressive HIV encephalopathy (PHE) caused by direct infection. OIs and malignancies do not contribute significantly to HIV-associated CNS disorders in childhood except in developing regions.

Epidemiology

An estimated 2.3 million children worldwide are living with HIV/AIDS, with nearly 2000 new infections and 1500 deaths occurring daily. This refers mainly to the developing world, and in particular sub-Saharan Africa, where less than 10% of HIV-positive pregnant women have access to appropriate measures to prevent mother-to-child transmission. In the developed world, pediatric HIV has ceased to be a significant problem as a result of effective use and delivery of antiretrovirals during pregnancy, elective cesarean section, and infant formula feeding.

In the United States and Europe, HAART has reduced the frequency of PHE from 9% to 35% early in the HIV epidemic, to 0–2% currently. The few available studies from sub-Saharan Africa report cognitive and motor developmental delay affecting 15–40% of HIV-infected children. There are no published data on the effects of HAART in this population. PHE in Latin America occurs in 32–36% of HIV-positive children. CNS OIs are relatively frequent, at 34% in a Brazilian hospital-based study and 12% in Argentina. The latter study documented a remarkable reduction of severity and frequency of PHE after the introduction of HAART. Data from Asia are inadequate.

Pathophysiology

The interaction between fetal astrocytes and endothelial cells is crucial to the development of the integrity of the blood–brain barrier (BBB). This occurs during early gestation. HIV directly compromises BBB development by restricted or non-productive CD4 receptor-independent infection of astrocytes. In the immature brain, this is pivotal to the development of PHE. The restricted infection of astrocytes causes neuronal dysfunction via loss of supporting growth factors and impaired neurotransmitter reuptake with resultant excitotoxicity. Macrophages, microglia, and multinucleated giant cells harbor productive HIV infection. Infected macrophages initiate an inflammatory cascade, which is compounded by their interactions with astrocytes, leading to the amplification of neurotoxic cytokine production. Neuronal loss in PHE is thought to be secondary to these processes and therefore an indirect result of HIV infection. Active infection of neurons or neuronal progenitor cells remains controversial, but low levels may occur in children.

Clinical features

PHE presents with a well-defined triad of: (1) acquired microcephaly due to impaired brain growth, (2) progressive motor dysfunction, and (3) loss, plateau, or delay of neurodevelopmental milestones.

Acquired microcephaly is diagnosed by the demonstration of stagnating or decreasing serial measurements of head circumference in children under 2 years of age. In older children with closed skull sutures, impaired brain growth is seen as progressive parenchymal atrophy on serial neuroimaging.

Progressive motor dysfunction results from pyramidal tract abnormalities and presents with impaired fine motor function and, ultimately, loss of gross motor skills. Tone is often spastic. Motor milestones either are not achieved or can be lost. Extrapyramidal dysfunction with parkinsonian features of rigidity, drooling, and hypomimic facies may occur; cerebellar involvement is rare. Advanced disease leads to a spastic, bedridden state. The motor syndrome evolves symmetrically. Focal deficits should alert to possible underlying structural brain disease such as a mass lesion or infarct.

Neurodevelopmental delay typically presents with a global cognitive deficit involving language and visiospatial integration skills, attention, concentration, and executive function. Poor language development, especially of expressive language, often precedes other cognitive and motor impairments. Behavioral problems such as social withdrawal, apathy, mood disorders, and impulsiveness are other symptoms. These abnormalities may be a primary manifestation of the encephalopathy or secondary to other psychosocial or biological factors.

The clinical disease pattern of PHE varies widely with respect to age of onset, rate of progression, and domain(s) of functional impairment. Onset of PHE is most common in the first year of life, with incidence rates of 9.9% in the first year, 4.2% in the second year, and less than 1% thereafter. Rates of progression vary widely, with rapid decline over a few months or a gradual deterioration. Early disease onset, especially when accompanied by advanced immune suppression, predicts a more rapid and aggressive course and high mortality. Timing of vertical and horizontal infection has also been found to be a prognostic indicator.

Static encephalopathies, presenting either as a non-progressive deficit or with neurodevelopmental delay, are also described. In contrast to PHE, there is no regression and there may be spontaneous improvement. These encephalopathies may be directly due to HIV infection or secondary to other neurological insults such as premature birth, prenatal exposure to toxins or infectious agents, genetic factors, or head injury.

The frequency of OIs is low in children compared to that of adults. Commonly reported OIs are CMV encephalitis, *Candida albicans* meningitis, and micro-abscesses secondary to septicemia. The spectrum of OIs in developing countries is poorly documented. Endemic infections such as tuberculosis may play a larger role than in developed countries. Co-infection of HIV and malaria may aggravate the neurodevelopmental delay in affected children; in malaria-endemic areas, severe falciparum malaria alone results in neurocognitive impairments in up to 24% of children.

Strokes, both cerebral infarction and intracranial hemorrhage, have been described in HIV-infected children. The frequency is lower than that seen in adults. Hemorrhage can occur due to a tumor or thrombocytopenia. Cerebral infarction can be caused by vasculitis resulting from meningitis, or cardioembolic disease secondary to cardiomyopathy. A rare but characteristic intracranial aneurysmal vasculopathy, characterized by fusiform aneurysms affecting the arteries around the circle of Willis, has been reported in pediatric AIDS cases.

Seizures occur more commonly in HIV-infected children than the age-equivalent HIV-negative population. Primary CNS lymphoma and metastatic lymphoma to the CNS have been described. Myelopathies are rare in children and are due to reactivated infections such as CMV. Vacuolar myelopathy is distinctly uncommon in children.

Investigations

CSF analysis is often normal, even in patients with florid PHE. Non-specific findings are common and include a slightly raised protein and lymphocytic pleocytosis. Intrathecal antibody production, oligoclonal bands, and markers of immune-activation can be detected in children with PHE, but also in neurologically normal subjects. HIV viral RNA is usually present in the CSF and may loosely correlate with PHE severity. Suppression of CSF viral load is utilized as a marker of response to treatment. CSF findings can be helpful in establishing the diagnosis of certain OIs and neoplasms.

CT scans reveal varying degrees of cerebral atrophy, with corresponding ventriculomegaly, white matter hypodensities, and bilateral symmetrical calcifications of the basal ganglia. MRI is more sensitive to detect atrophy and white matter changes, but less sensitive for calcifications. Serial imaging studies are useful to document neuropathological progression, but quantitative and volumetric studies have not yet been standardized as useful surrogate markers for early diagnosis or disease progression in clinical practice.

Standard neuropsychological and neurobehavioral assessment tools are useful to document neurodevelopmental deficits and progression. Test results require careful interpretation, as a child's performance may be influenced by a multitude of biological and psychosocial factors other than the encephalopathy. In addition, HIV-positive children are more likely to be exposed to poor socioeconomic circumstances and low levels of maternal education, and are more likely to suffer from compounding illnesses such as birth asphyxia, anemia, and malnutrition.

Psychometric testing is unavailable to children in most developing countries due to lack of human resources and skills. Standard assessment tools still need to be validated in regions outside the United States and Europe.

Treatment/management

Effective prevention of mother-to-child transmission can eradicate pediatric HIV altogether. HAART should be initiated at the onset of PHE. However, the ideal timing of commencement and choice of regimen are yet to be determined.

HIV-associated myelopathies

Introduction

Myelopathies in HIV/AIDS are less frequent than encephalopathies and occur mainly with advanced disease. Myelopathy etiologies in HIV include infections, neoplasms, vascular disease, and metabolic derangements. Infectious myelopathies caused directly by HIV are vacuolar myelopathy (VM), acute transient myelopathy, and relapsing and remitting myelitis. Other infectious etiologies include CMV, HSV-1 and 2, VZV, HTLV-1, measles, JC virus, tuberculosis (TB), *Pseudomonas*, syphilis, *Nocardia*, *Cryptococcus*, *Aspergillus*, and *Toxoplasma gondii*. Neoplastic causes are primary CNS lymphoma (PCNSL), metastatic lymphoma, astrocytoma, and plasmacytoma. Necrotising vasculitis and disseminated intravascular coagulation (DIC) are some of the described vascular causes.

Epidemiology

Myelopathy frequencies in HIV/AIDS range from 5% to 10%, compared with HAD frequencies of 15–30% and distal sensory polyneuropathy (DSP) frequencies of 15–50%. In the United States, myelopathy occurs with frequencies of 5–10% in HIV/AIDS. In the South African black population, myelopathy frequency is 3%. Data from other regions are not widely available.

The most prominently reported spinal cord disease in HIV/AIDS is vacuolar myelopathy, accounting for 5–10% of HIV-related neurological disease (or 20–55% of HIV myelopathy) in the United States. It is less common in clade C regions or in areas where infections dominate. VM accounts for 4% of HIV neurological disease in Japan (clade B), 1% in Brazil (clade B), and 2% in South Africa (clade C). In South Africa, TB is the most common cause of myelopathy in HIV (18–50%).

Pathophysiology

The pathological feature of VM is patchy vacuolization, occurring mainly in the thoracic region and predominantly affecting the lateral and dorsal columns. Axonal damage is a secondary phenomenon. There is no significant inflammatory infiltrate.

The exact pathogenesis of VM is unknown. HIV-infected macrophages, microglia, and astrocytes secrete immunoactive substances that are myelin-toxic. These include TNF-α, IL-1, and IL-6. TNF-α mediates oligodendrocyte and myelin injury through the generation of reactive oxygen species. Oxidative damage to oligodendrocyte membranes causes increased consumption of antioxidants (e.g., glutathione) and methyl groups, which are essential in myelin maintenance.

S-adenosylmethionine (SAM), the universal methyl group donor, is deficient in HIV patients with neurological disease and in vitamin B_{12} deficiency, accounting for the striking pathological similarities (i.e., the vacuolar change). It is likely that cytokines released by HIV-infected macrophages lead, via SAM depletion, to a metabolic disorder that causes white matter vacuolization in VM. Co-occurrence of SAM depletion and macrophage activation in immune-suppressed HIV-negative individuals (e.g., those with hematological malignancies or organ transplantation) can produce a clinically and pathologically identical myelopathy.

Clinical features

VM presents as a slowly progressive, spastic paraparesis with lower limb weakness, hyperreflexia, and extensor plantar responses. Sensory findings are less prominent, with sensory ataxia (20%) and a co-existent distal sensory neuropathy (53%). A sensory level is rare (13%). Bladder disturbance occurs uncommonly. VM has been observed to co-occur with HAD and DSP as a possible distinctive syndrome.

TB causes transverse myelitis, spinal meningitis/arachnoiditis, and Pott's disease of the spine, leading to cord compression. Back pain, spinal tenderness, and fever are characteristic features. Patients present with varying degrees of paraplegia or tetraplegia. TB myelopathy can occur at any stage of HIV infection and is common in endemic areas.

HSV-1 and 2 cause acute transverse myelitis at any stage of HIV. CMV causes lumbosacral radiculomyelitis in severe immune suppression. VZV also presents as a transverse myelitis. Co-infection of HIV and HTLV-1 has been reported in HTLV-1 endemic regions. Syphilitic meningomyelitis in HIV is rarely described. *Toxoplasma gondii* uncommonly causes myelitis in isolation or in conjunction with focal cerebral lesions.

Investigations

CSF in VM is non-specific (raised protein with lymphocytic pleocytosis). MRI is usually normal, but there may be atrophy of the thoracic cord and non-specific increased signal intensities on T2 images. Increased T2 cord signal and meningeal and nerve root enhancement have been described in viral and post-viral myelitides, in particular with CMV. In TB of the spine, vertebral body and intervertebral disc involvement appear as low signal on T1- and as high signal on T2-weighted images; irregular endplates and enhancing paraspinal collections have been documented. Lymphoma shows focal areas of low signal on T1- and high signal on T2-weighted images, with patchy contrast enhancement.

Treatment

There is no specific therapy for VM. Neither HAART nor vitamin B_{12} supplementation have shown consistent improvement or delayed progression of VM. CMV spinal cord disease can improve with the use of ganciclovir alone or in combination with cidofovir. Herpes simplex infections respond to acyclovir. HTLV-1 associated myelopathy responds temporarily to intravenous corticosteroids. TB disease of the spine responds well to standard treatment. Syphillitic myelitis responds very well to high-dose intravenous penicillin therapy. Early diagnosis of a *Toxoplasma gondii* myelitis and therapy with sulfadiazine and pyrimathamine produces a good response. Primary CNS lymphoma responds to appropriate chemotherapy.

Further reading

Ances BM, Ellis RJ. Dementia and neurocognitive disorders due to HIV-1 infection. *Semin Neurol* 2007; 27: 86–92.

Berger JR, Levy RM. *AIDS and the Nervous System.* Philadelphia: Lippincott Williams & Wilkins; 1997.

Gendelman HE, Lipton SA, Epstein L, Swindells S. *The Neurology of AIDS.* New York: Chapman and Hall; 1998.

Modi G, Hari K, Modi M, Mochan A. The frequency and profile of neurology in black South African HIV infected (clade C) patients – a hospital-based prospective audit. *J Neurol Sci* 2007; 254: 60–4.

Tan SV, Guiloff RJ. Hypothesis on the pathogenesis of vacuolar myelopathy, dementia and peripheral neuropathy in AIDS. *J Neurol Neurosurg Psychiatry* 1998; 65: 23–8.

Van Rie A, Harrington PR, Dow A, Robertson K. Neurologic and neurodevelopmental manifestations of pediatric HIV/AIDS: a global perspective. *Eur J Paediatr Neurol* 2007; 11: 1–9.

Victor M, Ropper AH. *Adams and Victor's Principles of Neurology.* New York: McGraw-Hill; 2001.

Chapter 95
HIV neuropathy

Giorgia Melli[1] and Ahmet Höke[2]
[1]National Neurological Institute "Carlo Besta", Milan, Italy
[2]Johns Hopkins University, Baltimore, USA

Introduction

There are many types of peripheral neuropathies associated with HIV infection, but few are specific to HIV. From the earliest reports, it appeared that there was a link between the type of neuropathy and the stage of HIV infection, and that certain non-HIV-specific neuropathies may have been over-represented in the HIV-infected population. Many of these disorders are indistinguishable from those that occur in association with other viral diseases.

Since the introduction of highly active antiretroviral therapy (HAART) in 1996, central nervous system (CNS) complications of HIV infection have declined dramatically. The incidence and prevalence of peripheral nervous system (PNS) complications of HIV, however, remain high and may be increasing. Most prospective studies find the prevalence of peripheral neuropathy to be 30–40%, and advanced HIV disease is the main risk factor.

HIV-associated sensory polyneuropathies

Introduction

There are two main forms of HIV-associated predominantly sensory polyneuropathies. The first is distal symmetric polyneuropathy (DSP), associated with advanced HIV-1 infection, and the second, most commonly called antiretroviral toxic neuropathy (ATN), is due to antiretroviral neurotoxicity. While clinically and physiologically similar, these disorders are different in etiopathogenesis.

Epidemiology

The incidence of HIV-associated sensory neuropathies is as high as 40% and represents the most common peripheral neuropathy in HIV-infected individuals. Increases in the incidence of glucose intolerance in patients treated with protease inhibitors may contribute to the development of sensory neuropathy, affecting predominantly small, unmyelinated fibers.

Clinical features

In both DSP and ATN, initial symptoms are distal painful burning dysesthesias and allodynia that start in the toes and slowly progress up the legs. As the disease progresses, dysesthesias may reach the knees, but rarely involve the hands. At later stages, patients complain of numbness; examination confirms the distal loss of sensory function. Sensory thresholds are raised to all modalities, especially those that test small fiber functions. Ankle reflexes are almost universally lost. Deep tendon reflexes at the knees are often normal but may be brisk. In such instances, concomitant myelopathy should be considered. Although patients may complain of weakness, it is rarely found on examination. The only clinical feature that may differentiate DSP from ATN is a recent history of neurotoxic antiretroviral drug use, which is indicative of ATN. Even if the offending drug is discontinued, most patients experience worsening of symptoms for 1–2 months due to a phenomenon termed "coasting." Later, most patients will see an improvement in symptoms, but often they never return to a completely asymptomatic state.

Investigations

Laboratory investigations in DSP and ATN patients are relatively unrevealing. General screening tests for other etiologies of neuropathy are often negative. Cerebrospinal fluid (CSF) analysis may show slightly elevated protein in a small number of patients. Cell counts are usually normal and, in fact, CSF pleocytosis should raise the possibility of concurrent opportunistic infection. In earlier stages, electrophysiological studies may be normal and diagnosis may require use of skin biopsies to evaluate the intra-epidermal nerve fiber density. In advanced DSP, nerve conduction studies reveal a length-dependent axonal polyneuropathy.

Treatment/management

Treatment of DSP and ATN is similar to many other neuropathies that have predominantly painful sensory involvement. Painful neuropathic symptoms can be

International Neurology: A Clinical Approach. Edited by Robert P. Lisak, Daniel D. Truong, William M. Carroll, and Roongroj Bhidayasiri. © 2009 Blackwell Publishing, ISBN: 978-1-4051-5738-4.

controlled by oral agents such as tricyclic antidepressants, antiepileptics, and opioid drugs or by topical capsaicin or anesthetics such as lidocaine formulations. There is no proven therapy for the underlying disease.

Inflammatory demyelinating polyneuropathies (IDPs)

Pathophysiology
Both acute and chronic forms of IDPs can occur at the time of seroconversion. Because of the similarities to HIV-1-seronegative IDPs, it is likely that HIV-1-seropositive IDP occurs on an immunopathogenic basis.

Clinical features
Clinical features of HIV-1-infected individuals with IDP are not different from those patients without HIV-1. Presentation may be acute, with progression in less than 4 weeks, or chronic, with disease onset occurring over several months. In the majority of cases, motor symptoms dominate. Cranial nerves may be involved, and respiratory paralysis occurs in acute cases.

Investigations
Several features distinguish HIV-1-seronegative individuals from HIV-1-seropositive individuals with IDP. First, Guillain–Barré syndrome may occur during HIV-1 seroconversion so that serial testing is required. Second, circulating CD4/CD8 T-cell ratios are inverted in HIV-1 cases. Third, in contrast to the usual absence of cellular response in CSF in HIV-1-seronegative IDP, patients with HIV-1 IDP frequently have CSF pleocytosis. Fourth, many patients have polyclonal elevations of serum immunoglobulins that can range up to several grams per deciliter. This may not be specific to IDP, but may be an indication of chronic antigenic stimulation and immunoglobulin production in HIV-1-infected individuals.

Treatment/management
Immunomodulatory treatments used in HIV-1-seronegative patients are often effective in HIV-1-seropositive patients as well. Intravenous immunoglobulins and plasma exchange can be safely used, but corticosteroids need to be administered carefully, especially if there is risk of opportunistic infection.

Opportunistic infections of the PNS

Opportunistic infections in HIV-positive patients have declined dramatically in developed countries with access to antiretroviral therapy, but remain a major problem in the developing world. Most opportunistic infections affect the CNS, but some have unique presentations in the PNS.

Cytomegalovirus (CMV)
Introduction
CMV is an opportunistic viral infection that results in polyradiculoneuropathy. In almost all reported cases, this syndrome occurs in those with AIDS.

Clinical features
Over a short time period, a neurologically well individual develops a cauda equina syndrome that is asymmetrical and predominantly motor. Lower back pain with radiation into one leg may be the earliest symptom, followed by urinary incontinence. Asymmetrical leg weakness and saddle sensory disturbance develop. The syndrome rapidly advances to a flaccid paraplegia with bowel and bladder disturbance. In most cases, the disease remains at this stage for some period of time. The disease may ascend with arm weakness or cranial nerve involvement.

Investigations
CSF analysis reveals polymorphonuclear pleocytosis, hypoglycorrhachia, and elevated protein. Frequently, CSF viral cultures reveal CMV. Polymerase chain reaction (PCR) for CMV DNA is frequently detectable in a shorter period of time. Evidence of CMV is usually found in retina, blood, and urine. Electrodiagnostic studies reveal evidence of axon loss in lumbosacral roots with fibrillations and positive sharp waves in leg muscles. There is little or no evidence of demyelination.

In AIDS patients, polyradiculopathy may have causes other than CMV, such as lymphomatous meningitis or syphilis; CSF studies are most helpful in distinguishing these syndromes. Sural nerve biopsies in this syndrome have been relatively unrevealing.

Treatment/management
Ganciclovir is the first choice of treatment and can result in stabilization or improvement, although ganciclovir-resistant cases have been reported. In such cases, foscarnet can be used.

Herpes zoster
Introduction
Herpes zoster infections of peripheral nerves and the spinal cord are well-known complications of HIV-1. These may involve any cranial or spinal peripheral nerves and may also involve the brain or spinal cord in severely immunocompromised patients.

Clinical features
Clinically, the disorders are indistinguishable from those occurring in HIV-seronegative individuals, although in individuals with AIDS the disease may be more aggressive.

Investigations

Herpes zoster infection is uncommon in young, healthy individuals; HIV-1 testing should be performed in an otherwise asymptomatic young individual with appropriate risk factors.

Mononeuropathy multiplex

Epidemiology

Multiple mononeuropathies due to vasculitis that occurs in symptomatic HIV-1 infection have been reported. These cases have occurred primarily in individuals with advanced HIV-1 infection.

Clinical features

Data suggest that clinical presentations in HIV patients are similar to those of other series of patients with vasculitic neuropathy.

Investigations

Nerve biopsies show all features previously described in patients with vasculitic neuropathy, including cellular infiltrates, perineurial infarcts, inter- and intrafascicular variability in the degree of nerve injury, and active axonal degeneration. The hallmark is necrotizing vasculitis.

Treatment/management

Firm conclusions about the role of therapy cannot be made due to limited data. Intense immunotherapy may worsen a compromised immune system and lead to opportunistic infections, but intravenous immunoglobulin seems to be relatively safe.

Neuropathy in diffuse infiltrative lymphocytosis syndrome (DILS)

Pathophysiology

DILS is characterized by CD8 hyperlymphomatosis and visceral organ infiltration, which can involve peripheral nerves.

Clinical features

Most patients have a sicca syndrome and multivisceral involvement without overt lymphoma. DILS is often symmetric, acute or subacute in onset, and almost always painful.

Investigations

Electrophysiology suggests an axonal process and biopsies reveal axonal neuropathy with diffuse CD8 cell infiltrates.

Treatment/management

Most patients respond to either antiretroviral treatment or steroid therapy.

Further reading

Cornblath DR, Hoke A. Recent advances in HIV neuropathy. *Curr Opin Neurol* 2006; 19: 446–50.

Hoke A, Keswani SC, McArthur JC. Current therapy for HIV sensory neuropathy. *Curr Treat Op Infect Dis* 2003; 5: 467–75.

Polydefkis M, Yiannoutsos CT, Cohen BA, *et al.* Reduced intraepidermal nerve fiber density in HIV-associated sensory neuropathy. *Neurology* 2002; 58: 115–19.

Sacktor N. The epidemiology of human immunodeficiency virus-associated neurological disease in the era of highly active antiretroviral therapy. *J Neurovirol* 2002; 8(Suppl 2): 115–21.

So YT, Olney RK. Acute lumbosacral polyradiculopathy in acquired immunodeficiency syndrome: experience in 23 patients. *Ann Neurol* 1994; 35: 53–8.

Chapter 96
Myopathies in HIV infection

Mirela E. Toma,[1] Alejandra Gonzalez-Duarte,[2] and David M. Simpson[1]
[1]Bronx Lebanon Hospital, New York, USA
[2]Instituto Nacional de Ciencias Medicas y Nutricion Salvador Zubiran, Mexico DF, Mexico

Introduction

Skeletal muscle involvement can occur at any stage of HIV infection and can be secondary to multiple causes (Table 96.1). Most neuromuscular complications occurring in HIV patients are HIV related, secondary to the toxic effects of antiretrovirals (ARVs) or, less frequently, to opportunistic infections. The most common ARV associated with myopathy is zidovudine (AZT), which has affinity for mitochondrial DNA polymerase-gamma, the enzyme required for mitochondrial DNA replication. Other nucleoside reverse transcriptase inhibitors (NRTIs), particularly the so-called d-drugs ("ddC" or zalcitabine, "ddI" or didanosine, "d4T" or stavudine), may also induce mitochondrial dysfunction or toxicity, but these are less commonly associated with myopathy.

A relatively rare form of myopathy that resembles Guillain–Barré syndrome, referred to as HIV-associated neuromuscular weakness (HANWS), presents in association with hyperlactemia and NRTI exposure. Metabolic manifestations range from asymptomatic hyperlactemia to acute severe lactic acidosis syndrome.

Epidemiology

HIV myopathy is uncommon; the incidence of myopathy in the era of ARVs varies between 1% and 28.7%. The most common risk factors are AZT exposure and the presence of a pre-existing myopathy. The incidence of NRTI myopathy has declined as the use of AZT is less frequent; however, it is still a concern in some developing countries.

Pathophysiology

The pathogenesis of HIV myopathy is likely immunological. The presence of CD8-positive lymphocytes,

together with diffuse expression of major histocompatibility complex (MHC) class I antigens on myofibers, suggests that HIV myopathy is a T-cell-mediated and an MHC class I-restricted cytotoxic process. HIV myopathy has been reported during immune reconstitution with highly active antiretroviral treatment (HAART), occurring in the context of a rapid restoration of T-cell subsets. Clinical improvement with corticosteroids and intravenous immunoglobulins (IVIGs) supports an autoimmune etiology.

NRTI myopathy is thought to be mediated by mitochondrial dysfunction. Toxicity is produced by inhibition of DNA polymerase-gamma, the enzyme required for mitochondrial DNA replication.

Clinical Features

The main clinical manifestation of HIV myopathy and NRTI myopathy is progressive, symmetrical weakness of limb-girdle muscles and neck flexors. Patients report difficulty in climbing stairs and performing tasks requiring proximal arm function. Myalgia, especially in the thighs, is present in only half of the patients. Functional testing often demonstrates difficulty in rising from a seated position or from a squatted position. Deep tendon reflexes are often preserved unless there is coexisting peripheral neuropathy. The development of myopathy following initiation of AZT or other NRTIs, as well as improvement of myopathy after subsequent withdrawal of the offending drug, distinguishes NRTI myopathy.

Investigations

Elevation of the serum skeletal muscle enzyme creatine kinase (CK) is helpful in diagnosis, although not a specific marker. Usually, serum CK levels are elevated approximately two to four times the normal values, but sometimes levels are normal or exceed 1000 IU/l. The CK level correlates with the degree of myonecrosis but not with the degree of muscle weakness.

Electromyography (EMG) is a sensitive diagnostic test, with up to 94% diagnostic yield. EMG shows short, brief,

International Neurology: A Clinical Approach. Edited by Robert P. Lisak, Daniel D. Truong, William M. Carroll, and Roongroj Bhidayasiri. © 2009 Blackwell Publishing, ISBN: 978-1-4051-5738-4.

Table 96.1 Myopathies and their causes in patients with HIV.

HIV-associated myopathy	Complications of ARVs*	Miscellaneous
• Polymyositis • Inclusion body myositis • Nemaline rod myopathy • Diffuse infiltrative lymphocytosis syndrome (DILS) • HIV-wasting syndrome • Vasculitic processes	• AZT[†] toxicity • Toxicity related to other NRTIs[‡] • HANWS[§] • HIV-associated lipodystrophy syndrome • IRIS[¶]	• Opportunistic infections • Rhabdomyolysis

*ARVs: antiretrovirals; [†]AZT: zidovudine; [‡]NRTIs: nucleoside-analog reverse transcriptase inhibitors; [§]HANWS: HIV-associated neuromuscular weakness syndrome; [¶]IRIS: immune restoration syndrome.

polyphasic motor unit action potentials that recruit with early and full interference patterns, with or without associated irritative activity.

Muscle biopsy confirms diagnosis. Histopathological features of HIV myopathy are similar to those of polymyositis in seronegative individuals, including scattered necrotic and basophilic fibers, multiple foci of mononuclear inflammatory cells within fascicles, and focal invasion of non-necrotic muscle fibers by inflammatory cells. Immunohistological features show endomyseal infiltrates with CD8-positive cells, macrophages, and CD4-positive cells. Muscle biopsy of patients with AZT myopathy have been reported to show ragged red fibers (RRF) on modified trichrome staining, which is considered a hallmark of mitochondrial dysfunction. The percentage of RRF correlates with the severity of clinical myopathy. However, the specificity of mitochondrial changes in AZT myopathy have been questioned, given their presence in myopathy unassociated with AZT. Other histological changes of AZT myopathy include myofibrillar alterations, degeneration, necrotic fibers, and inflammatory infiltrates.

Treatment/management

Given the likely immune-mediated pathogenesis of HIV myopathy, the primary treatment strategy for HIV-associated myopathy is immunotherapy. However, there have been no controlled therapeutic trials. When a patient has only mild immunosuppression, corticosteroids might be considered, as in HIV-negative polymyositis. A dose of 1 mg/kg of prednisone or 60–80 mg/day is administered and tapered according to clinical response, predominantly based on improvement in strength. For patients with moderate to advanced HIV disease, the risk of further immunosuppression associated with corticosteroids makes long-term use inadvisable. In this setting, IVIG (2 g/kg divided over 2–5 days monthly) may be given. In our experience, if no response is noted after a trial of 2–3 months of treatment, IVIG may be suspended. In patients with myopathy receiving AZT or another NRTI with potential mitochondrial toxicity, withdrawal of the agent may be tried.

Further reading

The German Neuro-AIDS Task Group. Peripheral nerve diseases and myopathies associated with HIV infection. *Nervenarzt* 2000; 71: 442–50.

Authier FJ, Chariot P, Gherardi RK. Skeletal muscle involvement in human immunodeficiency virus (HIV)-infected patients in the era of highly active antiretroviral therapy (HAART). *Muscle Nerve* 2005; 32: 247–60.

Authier FJ, Gherardi RK. Muscular complications of human immunodeficiency virus (HIV) infection in the era of effective antiretroviral therapy. *Rev Neurol (Paris)* 2006; 162: 71–81.

Brew BJ, Tisch S, Law M. Lactate concentrations distinguish between nucleoside neuropathy and HIV neuropathy. *AIDS* 2003; 17: 1094–6.

Nakagawa M, Maruyama Y, Sugita H, Osame M. Nationwide survey of neurologic manifestations of acquired immunodeficiency syndrome in Japan. *Intern Med* 1997; 36: 175–8.

Chapter 97
HIV-associated cerebral opportunistic infections

Bruce J. Brew
St Vincent's Hospital, Sydney, Australia

Introduction

Opportunistic infections (OIs), the result of reactivation of previously latent infection, occur in advanced HIV disease with low CD4 cell counts, usually below 200 cells/μl. Sometimes OIs occur when the CD4 cell count is rising and HIV viral load is dropping, namely with the use of highly active antiretroviral therapy (HAART), due to the immune reconstitution syndrome. Several infections may occur at the same time. The best clinical approach is to determine whether the clinical picture is *dominantly* diffuse or focal.

Diffuse complications

Cryptococcal meningitis
Introduction
Cryptococcal meningitis, a treatable and curable condition, is a frequent complication of advanced HIV disease. Clinical vigilance is paramount, as patients may present only with headache.

Epidemiology
Cryptococcal meningitis has a variable prevalence depending on geography (2% in northern Europe to 20–30% in Africa and South East Asia), and whether fluconazole and HAART are already being taken.

Pathophysiology
Most cases are related to *Cryptococcus neoformans* var. *neoformans*.

Clinical features
Headache and fever are the dominant manifestations. Drowsiness occurs in 20% of cases. Less common are cranial neuropathies, incoordination, seizures, and transient, ischemic-like episodes.

International Neurology: A Clinical Approach. Edited by Robert P. Lisak, Daniel D. Truong, William M. Carroll, and Roongroj Bhidayasiri. © 2009 Blackwell Publishing, ISBN: 978-1-4051-5738-4.

Investigations
Virtually all patients have a positive cryptococcal antigen in blood. Evaluation with the CT or MRI followed by cerebrospinal (CSF) analysis should be performed. Imaging reveals associated mass lesions compatible with cryptococcomas and gives a baseline evaluation of ventricle size.

In 75% of cases, the CSF shows a mononuclear pleocytosis (usually ≤20 cells/mm^3), elevated protein and, less frequently, depressed glucose. CSF cryptococcal antigen is usually positive. Fungal cultures performed on CSF determine sensitivities to antifungal agents.

The most important prognostic factor is the CSF open pressure ≥250 mm H$_2$O. The other factors include depressed consciousness, hyponatremia, depressed CSF glucose, CSF white cell count (WCC) below 20/mm^3, and CSF cryptococcal antigen titer ≥1024.

Treatment/management
Antifungal therapy, consisting of either fluconazole or amphotericin B, should start when diagnosis is confirmed. Increasing data point to the superiority of amphotericin B, particularly if the patient is obtunded. Some clinicians advise 2 weeks of amphotericin B followed by fluconazole. Fluconazole should be administered as a loading dose intravenously followed by at least 400 mg/day.

Acute treatment should continue for 10–12 weeks, after which time a repeat CSF study should be performed. If the patient is doing well, a maintenance dose of 200 mg/day of fluconazole should be instituted. Raised intracranial pressure should be treated aggressively with acetazolamide, frequent lumbar punctures, possibly mannitol, and, in difficult patients, by lumbar drain or ventriculostomy. To prevent immune restoration exacerbation of cryptococcal disease, HAART is commenced 1 month after antifungal therapy. If the patient is on HAART, it should be continued. Maintenance therapy can be discontinued if HIV viral load becomes undetectable and CD4 cell counts are above 200/μl for several months.

Tuberculous meningitis (TBM)
Introduction
Tuberculous meningitis (TBM), particularly in Africa and parts of Asia, is a significant cause of a non-focal deficit.

Epidemiology

In general, HIV-related TBM is associated with a higher burden of TB than TBM in non-HIV patients. TBM occurs in up to 10% of HIV-infected patients, especially in developing countries and among intravenous (IV) drug users.

Clinical features

Fever (83–89%), headache (59–83%), and altered mental status (43–71%) are common symptoms, while cough with sputum production occurs in approximately 20% of patients. Meningeal signs occur in 65% and focal deficits in 19% of patients. Half have no preceding TB-related symptomatology.

Investigations

Imaging often reveals meningeal enhancement, hydrocephalus, and, sometimes, focal brain lesions. CSF reveals lymphocytic pleocytosis of approximately 200 cells/μl. However, up to 16% of patients have acellular CSF, 43% normal protein, and 14% normal glucose. Elevated CSF concentrations of adenosine deaminase are non-specific. Direct smears of CSF are positive for TB in 25% of patients, while polymerase chain reaction (PCR) approaches 80%. Half have a chest X-ray showing pulmonary infiltrates and cavitating lesions. The CD4 cell count is usually below 200 and certainly below 400 cells/μl.

Treatment/management

Combination therapy, initially with corticosteroids, is required. There is a higher rate of adverse drug reactions, particularly with rifampin; the dose should be halved when used in combination with protease inhibitors. Isoniazid (with pyridoxine 50–100 mg/day) and pyrazinamide are bactericidal and cross into the CSF. Rifampin is preferred over ethambutol because it is bactericidal. Three drugs should be given for at least 2 months, followed by two drugs for 4 months. After initiation of therapy, hydrocephalus, hyperimmune response, or infarcts related to an arteritis may occur. Response should be assessed at 2 months with repeat CSF analysis. Therapy for at least 9 months may be necessary. TBM is treatable and curable with early diagnosis.

Cytomegalovirus (CMV) encephalitis
Introduction

CMV encephalitis is an uncommon, treatable complication of advanced HIV disease.

Epidemiology

CMV encephalitis occurs in at least 6% of patients with advanced HIV disease not on HAART; the incidence is much lower in HAART-treated patients. The mean CD4 cell count is 13 cells/μl, and almost all have a count of less than 50 cells/μl.

Pathophysiology

CMV is the consequence of reactivation of previously latent herpes infection.

Clinical features

Patients present with confusion (70–90%), apathy (60%), headache (30–50%), fever (16%), incoordination (10%), and, sometimes, seizures developing over 3.5 weeks. One-quarter have brainstem involvement with vertical or horizontal gaze-evoked nystagmus, internuclear ophthalmoplegia, and cranial neuropathies. CMV infection is often present elsewhere, usually the retina.

Investigations

Brain imaging often shows periventricular ependymal or meningeal enhancement. CSF shows polymorphonuclear pleocytosis (in 25% of patients), depressed glucose (in 33%), and raised protein (in 83%). CSF PCR for CMV DNA is positive in more than 90% of patients, sensitivity and specificity values are 80%, and positive and negative predictive values are 86–92% and 95–98% respectively.

Treatment/management

Ganciclovir and foscarnet are administered for approximately 3 weeks, followed by half the dose as maintenance until there is a sustained CD4 cell count above 100 cells/μl. Approximately half the patients improve and the other half stabilize or deteriorate. HAART should be commenced 1 month after anti-CMV treatment. Without treatment, the mean time to death is 8.5 weeks.

Focal complications

Cerebral toxoplasmosis
Introduction

Cerebral toxoplasmosis is one of the most common causes of a focal brain lesion in patients not on HAART, even in the developing world. All focal brain lesions in patients with advanced HIV disease are considered cerebral toxoplasmosis until proven otherwise.

Epidemiology

Seroprevalence of past toxoplasmosis infection varies from 80% in Europe to 30% in North America. Eating contaminated red meat or food contaminated by cat feces containing oocysts increases the risk of contracting toxoplasmosis.

Pathophysiology

Toxoplasma gondii is an intracellular parasite that exists in three forms: the tachyzoite, the bradyzoite, and the oocyst.

Clinical features

Headache (60%), a focal deficit with fever (70%), confusion (40%), and seizures (25%) occur. Less common are movement disorders and brainstem deficits. Systemic manifestations are uncommon.

Investigations

Seropositivity to toxoplasma establishes possible cerebral toxoplasmosis, but up to 16% may be seronegative. Brain imaging, especially MRI, is useful: a single lesion or periventricular lesions favor cerebral lymphoma, while lesions of deeper parts of the brain favor toxoplasmosis. Thallium brain single photon emission computed tomography (SPECT) scanning can differentiate toxoplasmosis from cerebral lymphoma. CSF PCR for *Toxoplasma gondii* is positive in 60% of patients. Most patients with toxoplasmosis have a CD4 count of less than 100 cells/μl.

Treatment/management

Pyrimethamine (75–100 mg/day), folinic acid (10–15 mg/day), and sulfadiazine (6–8 g/day) are recommended; clindamycin is useful (2400–4800 mg/day) in sulfa-allergic patients. Where sulfadiazine is not available, cotrimoxazole may be effective. Approximately 30% of patients require alternative therapy (azithromycin, clarithromycin, atovaquone, doxycycline, or dapsone).

Patients may deteriorate in the first days because of hemorrhage or edema. Edema can be treated in the short term with mannitol; corticosteroids should be avoided due to the confounding effect if the diagnosis is lymphoma. Clinical and radiological response occurs after 10 days, and by 6 weeks 30% of patients have complete resolution. Persistent lesion enhancement on imaging indicates continued treatment. Maintenance therapy can be instituted when there is no lesion enhancement. HAART should commence 1 month after antitoxoplasmosis therapy.

Tuberculosis (TB)
Introduction

Tuberculosis (TB) with central nervous system (CNS) involvement occurs at an earlier stage of HIV disease than do other infections.

Clinical features

The two forms of focal tuberculous brain involvement, tuberculoma (tuberculous granuloma) and tuberculous abscess, have concurrent clinical features of headache, focal deficits, and seizures. Tuberculous abscess often presents with fever, while tuberculomas are often multiple, sometimes with tuberculous meningitis co-existing. Half the patients have respiratory disease.

Investigations

A positive Mantoux test can be helpful, but negative results occur in up to 66% of those with a CD4 cell count less than 200 cells/μl; assessing cutaneous anergy may help interpret negative tests. Chest X-rays, sputum smears, blood cultures, and PCR for TB from blood can help. Tuberculomas on CT are solid-enhancing or ring-enhancing, possibly with calcification and mild-to-minimal mass effect. MRI shows nodular rim-enhancing lesions that are hypointense, isodense, or hyperintense on T2-weighted images. Tuberculous abscesses on CT are hypodense lesions with significant mass effect and peripheral enhancement, while MRI shows lesions with central hyperintensity on T2.

Treatment
See Chapter 71.

Progressive multifocal leukencephalopathy (PML)
Introduction

PML, a common complication of HIV, is a subacute demyelinating disease of the CNS, resulting from infection of oligodendrocytes and astrocytes by the JC virus (JVC). HAART can stabilize and improve PML.

Epidemiology

Up to 4% of patients with advanced HIV develop PML; this figure has not significantly changed with HAART.

Pathophysiology

JCV is a double-stranded DNA virus encapsulated in an icosahedral protein. It remains latent in cells of the reticuloendothelial system until reactivated, usually due to immunodeficiency. Clinicians believe JCV is transported into the brain by infected blood cells. JCV may infect oligodendrocytes and B cells, but probably not monocytic cells.

Clinical features

Hemiparesis, speech disturbances, cognitive dysfunction, headache, and ataxia are the presenting symptoms, usually developing over several weeks. In 60% of patients, there is a single clinical localization.

Investigations

Seropositivity in normal adults is at least 80%, thereby invalidating diagnostic utility. PCR amplification of JCV DNA and RNA in peripheral blood mononuclear cells, plasma, and urine is not helpful, as asymptomatic viremia occurs in normals. CT is normal or reveals hypodensity without mass effect that rarely enhances. Cranial MRI reveals single or multiple areas of T2 high-signal intensity in white matter. Mild contrast enhancement may occur in 15% of patients. CSF cell count and glucose are usually normal, but CSF protein is mildly to moderately elevated in 50% of cases. The mean CD4 cell count ranges from 30 to 104 cells/μl. One-third of patients have plasma HIV viral loads below detection.

CSF PCR for JCV DNA has a sensitivity of 65% and a specificity of 92%. The most definitive test is brain biopsy.

Treatment/management

HAART increases median survival from 11 weeks to 46.4 weeks. Some patients worsen during the first weeks of HAART, probably due to immune restoration disorder. Cytarabine has a limited role. Cidofovir, α-interferon, and topotecan are ineffective. Patients with a CD4 cell count of more than 50 cells/μl have a better prognosis, as do patients under 45 years old. Approximately 10% of patients experience spontaneous remission and survive beyond 1 year, while 5% live beyond 1 year, with a mean survival of 42 months. Untreated, the average survival is 3–4 months.

Further reading

Bertschy S, Opravil M, Cavassini M, *et al*. Discontinuation of maintenance therapy against toxoplasma encephalitis in AIDS patients with sustained response to anti-retroviral therapy. *Clin Microbiol Infect* 2006; 12(7): 666–71.

Brew BJ. *HIV Neurology*. New York: Oxford University Press; 2001, Chapters 7–11, pp. 91–123.

Chayakulkeeree M, Perfect JR. Cryptococcosis. *Infect Dis Clin North Am* 2006; 20(3): 507–44.

Dedicoat M, Livesley N. Management of toxoplasmic encephalitis in HIV-infected adults (with an emphasis on resource-poor settings). *Cochrane Database Syst Rev* 2006; (19)3: CD005420.

Offiah CE, Turnbull IW. The imaging appearances of intracranial CNS infections in adult HIV and AIDS patients. *Clin Radiol* 2006; 61(5): 393–401.

Thwaites GE, Duc Bang N, Huy Dung N, *et al*. The influence of HIV infection on clinical presentation, response to treatment, and outcome in adults with tuberculous meningitis. *J Infect Dis* 2005; 192(12): 2134–41.

Chapter 98
HIV-associated lymphoma: neurologic complications

Bruce J. Brew
St Vincent's Hospital, Sydney, Australia

Introduction

HIV-associated lymphoma may involve the nervous system either as primary central nervous system lymphoma (PCNSL) or as systemic lymphoma with neurological metastases. These conditions are different in terms of epidemiology, pathophysiology, clinical features, and treatment.

Primary central nervous system lymphoma (PCNSL)

Epidemiology

Highly active antiretroviral therapy (HAART) has reduced the occurrence of PCNSL in advanced-disease HIV patients by 50%. In HAART-naïve patients not taking cotrimoxazole, PCNSL is the second most common cause of a mass lesion after toxoplasmosis; in patients taking HAART this is likely no longer true, though rigorous data are lacking. The median CD4 cell count of HIV patients who develop PCNSL is generally below 50/µl, although occasionally cases occur in the normal range. HAART has improved the median survival rate of patients who develop PCNSL from 32 days to 48 days and the 12-month survival rate from 4% to 12%.

Pathophysiology

PCNSL is a diffuse non-Hodgkin's lymphoma arising in the CNS that is almost always secondary to unchecked reactivation of Epstein–Barr virus (EBV) brought on by immune deficiency which then promotes B-cell proliferation, leading to gene arrangement and PCNSL.

Clinical features

Usually patients present with confusion (51%), focal deficits (30–60%), headache (30–40%), seizures (22%), and fever. Ocular involvement is uncommon.

Investigations

Brain imaging with CT or MRI often shows a single enhancing lesion with edema, usually in the frontal lobe, periventricular region, and, less often, the basal ganglia. Posterior fossa involvement is found in less than 10% of patients. Magnetic resonance spectroscopy may show changes in phosphorylethanolamine consistent with the diagnosis. Thallium single photon emission computed tomography (SPECT) imaging has some diagnostic utility; patients with lesions >2 cm in dimension have increased thallium uptake.

Polymerase chain reaction (PCR) for EBV has a sensitivity of 83–100% and specificity of 94–100%. However, there is concern that these figures are less favorable in patients who develop PCNSL while taking HAART. Cerebrospinal fluid (CSF) cytology may be positive in up to 30% of cases.

When other diagnostic methods fail, brain biopsy can be useful. However, false-negative results, which may reflect the lympholytic effect of previous corticosteroid treatment, may occur (5–33%), morbidity is as high as 11%, and death occurs in up to 8% of patients.

Treatment/management

Treatment for PCNSL can be considered when the definitive diagnosis has been made by one of the previously mentioned techniques or when there has been failure to respond to a trial of antitoxoplasmosis therapy. While there is no curative therapy, treatment can increase the patient's life span and quality (see Table 98.1).

Radiotherapy, corticosteroids, and HAART should be administered when possible. Because PCNSL is multicentric, there is no value in surgical removal of any identifiable tumor. HAART-related improvement in immune function decreases the risk of death from an opportunistic infection and possibly curtails PCNSL progression.

Table 98.1 Factors associated with increased survival in patients with PCNSL.

1. Completion of radiotherapy (especially at least 30 Gy)
2. Highly active antiretroviral therapy (HAART)
3. Few or no previous AIDS-defining illnesses
4. Absence of non-focal neurological symptoms, such as confusion

International Neurology: A Clinical Approach. Edited by Robert P. Lisak, Daniel D. Truong, William M. Carroll, and Roongroj Bhidayasiri. © 2009 Blackwell Publishing, ISBN: 978-1-4051-5738-4.

While chemotherapy is generally not recommended, there may be a role in some otherwise well patients.

Systemic lymphoma

Epidemiology

Systemic lymphoma occurs in 5–10% of advanced-disease HIV patients. This figure may change as patients live longer on HAART, as evidence suggests that the risk of developing lymphoma is related in part to the duration of HIV disease. Data thus far have shown that HAART has not led to a decrease in the incidence, contrary to its effects on PCNSL incidence.

The CNS is involved in approximately 20% of patients with systemic lymphoma and usually takes the form of leptomeningeal disease. Median CD4 cell count for systemic non-Hodgkin's lymphoma is just under 200 cells/μl.

Pathophysiology

Systemic lymphoma with CNS metastases is almost always of non-Hodgkin's type. It is related to EBV infection in only half the patients.

Clinical features

Brain metastases lead to confusion, focal deficits, and, sometimes, seizures. Leptomeningeal involvement occurs in up to 10% of cases, causing a compressive spinal cord syndrome or multilevel deficits with the characteristic finding of scattered absent deep tendon reflexes.

Investigations

In patients with brain metastases, brain imaging with CT or MRI shows multiple enhancing lesions. In cases with leptomeningeal disease, CSF cytology is frequently positive.

Treatment/management

Intrathecal chemotherapy, usually with methotrexate or cytarabine, should be given in addition to systemic chemotherapy. While there is some controversy as to whether HAART should be given concurrently due to concerns regarding additive myelotoxicity, most physicians do recommend contemporaneous HAART. Caution should be used regarding: (1) the additive myelotoxicty when zidovudine is a component of HAART, (2) the additive risk of neuropathy when stavudine or didanosine are components of HAART and vinca alkaloids are part of chemotherapy, and (3) protease inhibitors as part of HAART due to effects on the cytochrome P450 system.

Radiotherapy combined with chemotherapy has some efficacy for localized disease. Chemotherapy regimens often include the use of granulocyte-macrophage colony-stimulating factor (GM-CSF) for chemotherapy-induced neutropenia. Leptomeningeal disease is treated with intrathecal methotrexate.

Further reading

Cingolani A, Fratino L, Scoppettuolo G, Antinori A. Changing pattern of primary cerebral lymphoma in the highly active antiretroviral therapy era. *J Neurovirol* 2005; 11(Suppl 3): 38–44.

Gerstner E, Batchelor T. Primary CNS lymphoma. *Expert Rev Anticancer Ther* 2007; 7(5): 689–700.

Palmieri C, Treibel T, Large O, Bower M. AIDS-related non-Hodgkin's lymphoma in the first decade of highly active antiretroviral therapy. *QJM* 2006; 99: 811–26.

Parekh S, Ratech H, Sparano JA. Human immunodeficiency virus – associated lymphoma. *Clin Adv Haem Oncol* 2003; 1(5): 295–301.

Quinn D, Newell M, De Graaff B, *et al*. Human immunodeficiency virus related primary central nervous system lymphoma: factors influencing survival in 111 cases. *Cancer* 2004; 100(12): 2627–36.

Chapter 99
Peripheral nervous system complications of HTLV-1 myelopathy: HAM/TSP and related syndromes

Abelardo Araújo,[1,2,3] *Marco A. Lima,*[1] *and Marcus Tulius T. Silva*[1]

[1]Evandro Chagas Clinical Research Institute, Rio de Janeiro, Brazil
[2]The Federal University of Rio de Janeiro, Rio de Janeiro, Brazil
[3]University College, Dublin, Ireland

Introduction

Many infective agents can affect peripheral nerves and muscles. Peripheral neuropathies (PN) and myopathies can be associated with human T-lymphotrophic virus type 1 (HTLV-1), although less commonly than with HIV infection. HTLV-1 is the etiologic agent of a group of neurologic syndromes known as the HTLV-1 neurologic complex, the most common of which is HTLV-1-associated myelopathy/tropical spastic paraparesis (HAM/TSP), a chronic myelopathy. Rarely, a related retrovirus, HTLV-2, can induce a syndrome similar to HAM/TSP.

Epidemiology

Ten to 20 million individuals carry HTLV-1. Endemic foci of HTLV-1 are found in southern Japan, the Caribbean, sub-Saharan Africa, the Middle East, South America, the Pacific Melanesian Islands, and Papua New Guinea. In the United States and Europe, HTLV-1 has been identified among intravenous drug users (IDU), female sex workers, recipients of multiple blood transfusions, and immigrants from endemic areas. HTLV-2 is more prevalent in some Native American groups and in IDU worldwide, sometimes associated with HIV or hepatitis C. HTLVs can also be transmitted from mother to child through perinatal exposure or breastfeeding.

Pathophysiology

HTLVs are single-stranded RNA retroviruses with reverse transcriptase activity that leads to DNA transcription of the virus and random integration into the host genome.

Once integrated, such proviruses can persist latently, escaping immune surveillance. HTLV-1 has a unique region, called *pX*, that encodes two crucial proteins for activation of host genes and virus replication: *tax* and *rex*. CD8+ cytotoxic T-lymphocytic response to *tax* plays a decisive role in the pathogenesis of HAM/TSP. HTLV-1 infects mostly CD4+ T lymphocytes; approximately 10% of these become infected with HAM/TSP. The hallmark of HTLV-1-infected T cells is the expression of activation markers, resulting in proliferation of peripheral blood mononuclear cells *in vitro*. These cells produce and induce secretion of a variety of cytokines. In contrast to HTLV-1, HTLV-2 preferentially infects CD8+ T cells.

Only 2–3% of individuals infected with HTLV-1 develop HAM/TSP. Factors associated with HAM/TSP development include a high anti-HTLV-1 antibody titer, high proviral load, and female gender. Pathological features of HAM/TSP include degeneration and demyelination of pyramidal, spinocerebellar, and spinothalamic tracts. These lesions are associated with hyaline thickening of blood vessels both in the spinal cord and, to a lesser extent, in the brain, sometimes with perivascular infiltrates, astrocytic gliosis, and foamy macrophages.

The mechanism by which HTLV-1 induces neurological diseases is unknown. The most accepted theory of how HTLV-1 infection leads to nervous system damage is the bystander damage hypothesis, which holds that specific CD8+ cytotoxic T lymphocytes sensitized against viral antigens interact with HTLV-1-infected CD4+ cells inside the central nervous system (CNS), secreting myelinotoxic cytokines and stimulating microglia to secrete cytokines such as TNF-α, which are also myelinotoxic.

The blood–peripheral nerve barrier limits entry of many substances and biological agents into the peripheral nerve microenvironment. However, the barrier is absent at the dorsal root ganglia and in the terminal branches of sensory and motor nerves; these sites may allow entrance and retrograde transport of neurotoxic or inflammatory substances and could explain the occurrence of PN even in the absence of HAM/TSP.

International Neurology: A Clinical Approach. Edited by Robert P. Lisak, Daniel D. Truong, William M. Carroll, and Roongroj Bhidayasiri. © 2009 Blackwell Publishing, ISBN: 978-1-4051-5738-4.

Polymyositis (PM) and inclusion body myositis (IBM) have been found in HTLV-1-infected individuals. Muscle damage is not related to direct invasion of muscle fibers by the virus, but to an immune-mediated process. In PM, the cell-mediated T-cell response appears to be driven against antigens of the HTLV-1 *tax* protein. With IBM, the process seems to be mediated by a clonally-driven sub-population of activated T cells that attack MHC-class I-expressing muscle fibers.

Clinical features

HAM/TSP

Patients present with symptoms of myelopathy and serological evidence of HTLV-1 infection. (See Table 99.1 for a summary of the World Health Organization (WHO) diagnostic criteria for HAM/TSP.) Differential diagnoses of HAM/TSP include the spinal form of multiple sclerosis, vacuolar myelopathy of HIV infection, familial spastic paraparesis, primary lateral sclerosis, spinal cord compression, vitamin B_{12} deficiency, lathyrism, Konzo, neuroschistosomiasis, Lyme disease, syphilis, and HTLV-1-negative TSP.

HAM/TSP has a slow onset and chronic, steady progression, although it can exhibit rapid deterioration. Progression occurs mainly during the first or second year of disease, then stabilizes. Approximately 60% of patients have weakness of the lower limbs as the first symptom. Bladder dysfunction, as well as impotence in males, ensues. Other symptoms include back pain, paresthesiae of lower limbs, xerosis, xerophthalmia, and xerostomia. Neurological examination reveals a spastic gait, spastic paraparesis, hyperreflexia, and extensor plantar responses. A Romberg sign and abnormal deep or superficial sensory signs may be observed. Neurological manifestations such as amyotrophic lateral sclerosis-like syndrome, PN, cognitive dysfunction, and myopathy have been described. Multiple mononeuropathy has been described and carpal tunnel syndrome is relatively common.

Peripheral neuropathy (PN)

The reported frequency of HTLV-1 PN has varied from negligible to 32%. In a recent clinical, electrophysiological, and anatomopathological study, PN was identified in HTLV-1-infected individuals without HAM/TSP: 21 out of 335 patients (6.3%) had clinical and/or electrophysiological abnormalities suggestive of a polyneuropathy. A higher prevalence of PN in HIV/HTLV-2 coinfection was reported, suggesting that HTLV-2 could be a predisposing cofactor for development of PN in HIV-infected patients. This could also apply to HTLV-1 infection, given that it shares many biological similarities with HTLV-2.

Table 99.1 WHO guidelines for diagnosis of HAM/TSP.

Clinical	
Age and sex	Sporadic and adult; female predominant
Onset	Usually insidious
Main neurological manifestations	Chronic spastic paraparesis, slow progression, sometimes static after initial progression
	Weakness of lower limbs, especially proximally
	Bladder disturbance is an early feature; constipation occurs later; impotence and decreased libido
	Sensory symptoms more prominent than objective physical signs
	Impaired vibration sense
	Low lumbar pain with radiation to legs
	Hyperreflexia of lower limbs, often with clonus and Babinski's sign; hyperreflexia of upper limbs with positive Hoffmann's and Trömner's signs; exaggerated jaw jerk
Less frequent neurological findings	Cerebellar signs, optic atrophy, deafness, nystagmus, cranial nerve deficits, hand tremor, absent or depressed ankle jerk
Other neurological manifestations	Muscular atrophy, fasciculation, polymyositis, peripheral neuropathy, polyradiculopathy, cranial neuropathy, meningitis, encephalopathy
Systemic non-neurological manifestations	Pulmonary alveolitis, uveitis, Sjögren's syndrome, arthropathy, vasculitis, ichthyosis, cryoglobulinemia, monoclonal gammopathy, adult T-cell leukemia/lymphoma
Laboratory	
Blood	HTLV-1 antibodies or antigens
	Lobulated lymphocytes
	Viral isolation when possible
CSF	HTLV-1 antibodies or antigens
	Lobulated lymphocytes
	Mild to moderate increase of protein
	Viral isolation when possible

PN associated with HTLV-1 is characterized by paresthesiae, burning sensations, and abnormal superficial sensation distally in a stocking and-glove distribution, coupled with abolished ankle jerks. A comprehensive history and neurological examination should lead to precise diagnosis. Dysautonomia is frequent but underdiagnosed in most HAM/TSP patients. Dizziness, orthostatic hypotension, discomfort in the neck or shoulders, dry skin with excessive sweating, and sexual impotence are associated with specific electrophysiological abnormalities.

Cases of acute or chronic polyradiculoneuropathy and chronic sensory neuropathy presenting as severe impairment of propioceptive and kinesthetic sensation associated with HTLV-1 have been described, but there is uncertainty about the role of the infection.

Myopathy

Clinical presentation of HTLV-1-related PM is similar to that of idiopathic PM, including symmetrical and proximal weakness and varying degrees of myalgia. Bulbar muscles are clinically affected in one-third of cases. Deep tendon reflexes are diminished or abolished but look normal or even increased in patients with HAM/TSP. Rheumatologic, cardiac, and respiratory manifestations are present in HTLV-1-seronegative PM, but less common in HTLV-1-related PM.

IBM occurs predominantly in males over 50 years of age. Onset is insidious and slowly progressive, which can delay diagnosis. Proximal and distal muscles are affected in an asymmetrical manner. Quadriceps, volar, and ankle dorsiflexor muscles are affected early; extraocular muscles are spared; one-third of patients have mild sensory neuropathy.

Investigations

Enzyme-linked immunosorbent assay (ELISA) or particle agglutination assays are the most common screening tests for HTLV-1. Western Blot assay confirms diagnosis. Polymerase chain reaction (PCR) can distinguish HTLV-1 from HTLV-2 and detect DNA in tissue or other biological specimens.

Systemic laboratory abnormalities typical of HAM/TSP include the presence of atypical lymphocytes in peripheral blood smears ("flower-cells"), hypergammaglobulinemia, increased β-2-microglobulin, increased proportion of CD4+ cells, and false-positive Veneral Disease Research Laboratory (VDRL) test. CSF findings include moderate pleocytosis and raised protein content. These are typical of the first few years of disease and tend to decline. Oligoclonal bands and increased intrathecal antibody synthesis specific for HTLV-1 antigens have been described. Cerebral white-matter lesions can be seen in

patients with HAM/TSP on MRI, and spinal cord edema and atrophy can be detected in acute and chronic phases of disease, respectively.

Electrophysiological studies identify polyneuropathy in approximately 50% of HAM/TSP patients and show predominantly sensory-motor polyneuropathy with axonal or mixed components. Specific electrophysiological studies for dysautonomia reveal mainly dysfunction of the sympathetic nervous system, with impairment of cardiovascular and sweat control. Data suggest that spinal nerve roots are involved in the inflammatory response observed in the spinal cord of some HAM/TSP patients. Perineural and perivascular infiltrates, decreased number of myelinated fibers, mixed axonal degeneration and segmental demyelination, the presence of myelin globules and ovoids, and perineural fibrosis have also been found (Figure 99.1). Inflammatory infiltrates initially contain CD8+ and CD4+ T cells and foamy macrophages; later, CD8+ T cells predominate.

Diagnosis of HTLV-1-related myopathies via clinical findings is corroborated by muscle enzyme measurements, electromyography, and tissue biopsy. Creatine kinase is elevated 5- to 50-fold in patients with PM but is normal or mildly elevated (up to 10-fold) in patients with IBM. Anti-Jo-1 antibody is the most common myositis-specific autoantibody; sensitivity of this test in the HTLV-1-infected PM population may be lower than that of the general population. Electromyography is usually abnormal in both conditions and shows features consistent with inflammatory myopathy, including

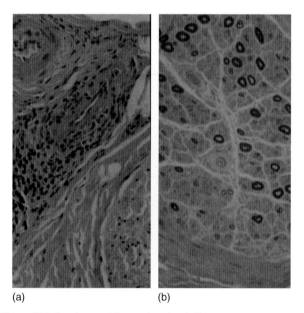

(a)   (b)

Figure 99.1 Sural nerve biopsy showing inflammatory mononuclear cell infiltrates in the epineura close to blood vessel wall (a – H&E 40×) and loss of large and small myelinated fibers (b – toluidin blue 40×).

increased insertional activity, small polyphasic motor unit action potentials, and early recruitment. Muscle biopsy in HTLV-1-related PM demonstrates endomysial and perivascular mononuclear infiltrates, variability in fiber size, and scattered necrotic and regenerating fibers; there is no apparent direct muscle invasion. In IBM, characteristic findings include a mononuclear inflammatory infiltrate predominantly in endomysial and muscle fibers with one or more rimmed vacuoles that arise singly or in multiples. Electron microscopy shows 15–21 nm cytoplasmatic and intranuclear tubulofilaments.

Treatment/management

There is no effective treatment for HAM/TSP. Various studies have shown that optimal results are obtained with administration of steroids and α-interferon; azathioprine, pentoxifylline, and high-dose vitamin C are less effective. Immunomodulatory therapies, including anti-inflammatory drugs, may have beneficial effects in HAM/TSP patients with peripheral nerve dysfunction, particularly when started early. HTLV-1 neurological syndromes can be treated with high doses of oral prednisone or intravenous methylprednisolone. Pain or burning sensations associated with PN can be treated with amitryptiline, gabapentin, or carbamazepine.

Data support the use of immunosuppressive and immunomodulatory drugs in HTLV-1-seronegative PM as well. Satisfactory clinical response in 50% of patients treated with prednisone at doses of 1 mg/kg with or without azathioprine (2–3 mg/kg) has been observed. Methotrexate, cyclophosphamide, and intravenous immunoglobulin can be used in refractory cases or when steroids are contraindicated. No treatment has been proven effective for IBM.

Further reading

Araujo A, Silva MT. The HTLV-1 neurological complex. *Lancet Neurol* 2006; 5(12): 1068–76.

Gilbert DT, Morgan O, Smikle MF, Simeon D, Barton EN. HTLV-1 associated polymyositis in Jamaica. *Acta Neurol Scand* 2001; 104(2): 101–4.

Grindstaff P, Gruener G. The peripheral nervous system complications of HTLV-1 myelopathy (HAM/TSP) syndromes. *Semin Neurol* 2005; 25(3): 315–27.

Osame M. Pathological mechanisms of human T-cell lymphotropic virus type I-associated myelopathy (HAM/TSP). *J Neurovirol* 2002; 8(5): 359–64.

Silva MT, Harab RC, Leite AC, Schor D, Araujo A, Andrada-Serpa MJ. HTLV-1 proviral load in asymptomatic carriers, HTLV-1-associated myelopathy/tropical spastic paraparesis, and other neurological abnormalities associated with HTLV-1 infection. *Clin Infect Dis* 2007; 44(5): 689–92.

Chapter 100
Multiple sclerosis

Robert P. Lisak[1] and Jun-Ichi Kira[2]
[1]Wayne State University School of Medicine, Detroit, USA
[2]Kysuhu University, Fukuoka, Japan

Introduction

Multiple sclerosis (MS) is the most common cause of neurologic disability among young adults in the temperate regions of the western hemisphere, Europe, and Australia/New Zealand. There has been an increase in our understanding of the pathogenesis of MS although the etiology is unknown. Even more remarkable has been the emergence of disease modifying treatments (DMT), treatments that have been shown to have a positive effect on the course of the disease. Imaging studies have been critical in allowing earlier diagnosis as well as to understand the evolution of the disease from its earliest presentation.

Epidemiology

MS is not evenly distributed geographically but increases, in general, as one moves north or south from the equator. In countries with long north/south dimensions, such as the United States, the same pattern is observed, though Japan is an exception to this; here the incidence and prevalence are much lower than other highly industrialized countries at the same latitude. Prevalence worldwide varies, with highs of 30–150/100 000, a mid-range of 5–30/100 000, lows of less than 30/100 000, Japan with 1.4/100 000, to virtually no disease. Migration studies support the concept that with regard to MS it is important where one is born and raised for the first 10–15 years of life. Generally the increased risk of developing MS by being born and raised in regions of high prevalence accompanies the migrant to low prevalence regions and vice versa. Among Ashkenazi Jews, however, who have a high prevalence, their offspring who are born in Israel, a region where Sephardic Jews and Arabs have a relatively low prevalence, retain the high risk even though they were predicted to acquire the low prevalence. Studies

have suggested that some of these geographic differences are becoming less striking, particularly for certain populations such as white females in the United States, and are non-existent for other populations such as black men. Reports suggest that the incidence of MS is increasing, and that this increase cannot be solely attributed to better and more widely available diagnostic techniques or diagnostic criteria.

There are clearly racial/ethnic differences throughout the world that likely represent genetic factors rather than being solely related to environmental factors. In Japan the prevalence is much lower than in Western countries and as described later frequently has a different clinical presentation. Among the many potential environmental factors postulated to contribute to the higher incidence and prevalence of MS in certain geographic regions are the previously mentioned genetic/ethnic differences, amount of sunlight, infectious agents, particularly viral infections, products of industry in the environment, and dietary differences. In the case of viruses, infection with common viruses at a later age, perhaps because of better hygiene, has long been a popular theory, as has infection with a particular virus in a susceptible population. Differences in the immune system in individuals living in temperate climates where the predominant intracellular infectious agents are viruses requiring a Th1-weighted response as opposed to tropical climates where parasitic diseases elicit Th2-weighted responses have been suggested to be involved in the geographic distribution of MS. This theory is in part based on the current evidence that the focal inflammatory/demyelinating lesions in the white matter are in large part initiated by Th1 lymphocytes.

In countries with highly heterogeneous ethnic/racial populations such as the United States, the disease is seen more frequently in Caucasians when compared with African-Americans, although it is much more common than previously believed in that population. MS is virtually unknown in black Africans in Africa and rare in individuals of Oriental origin in both countries of origin and living in countries such as the United States. The relapsing–remitting presentation of the disease (relapsing–remitting MS; RRMS) is more common in women than men (approximately 2:1), with evidence that

International Neurology: A Clinical Approach. Edited by Robert P. Lisak, Daniel D. Truong, William M. Carroll, and Roongroj Bhidayasiri. © 2009 Blackwell Publishing, ISBN: 978-1-4051-5738-4.

it is or is becoming even higher, particularly in childhood onset. Patients who present with progressive disease without remissions from the onset (primary progressive MS; PPMS) seem to be equally represented (1:1). The age of onset is most frequently between 20 and 40 years of age, although there is increasing recognition of onset in teenage and prepubertal children as well as patients in their 40s and 50s. PPMS patients tend to be older at the age of onset.

There is an increased familial incidence of MS, with 1–5% incidence in first-degree relatives. In different studies, concordance in siblings is 1–2%, dizygotic twins 2–5%, and monozygotic twins about 30–40%. Thus MS is not an inherited disease in the sense of a mutation in a single gene (Mendelian inheritance). It is more likely the effect of changes in multiple genes and their protein products that are not pathogenic on their own, or interactions with one another and with environmental factors. In addition there is evidence that there are genes involved in resistance to MS and others that may determine severity/ course of the disease.

Pathology, pathogenesis, and etiology

Pathology

MS has been viewed as a multifocal inflammatory disease of central nervous system (CNS) myelin with later secondary axonal damage. Modern immunopathologic techniques, pathologic specimens from cases of shorter duration, and rediscovery of pathological findings in the earliest studies of MS have expanded our understanding of the pathology and pathogenesis. Neuroimaging has also been instructive to understanding the pathology and clinical course. It is suggested that there are two distinct processes to MS, inflammation and degeneration. This is an oversimplification and is partly dependent on a definition of inflammation as being the presence of gadolinium-enhancing lesions on MRI. Nevertheless the relative emphasis of each mirrors the clinical features of relapsing and progressive clinical phases.

The hallmark lesions in the white matter of patients with MS are the perivascular (perivenular) inflammatory lesions consisting of T and B lymphocytes, monocytes/macrophages, and plasma cells. Demyelination, often in a vesicular pattern with myelin phagocytosis by macrophages, is characteristic. Microglial activation and reactive astrocytes are seen. These are classified as acute lesions and are thought to evolve into chronic active lesions where the inflammatory cells are at the edge of the lesion. Further evolution results in areas of demyelination with minor amounts of infiltrating inflammatory cells, known as chronic inactive lesions. These various lesions constitute the plaques, which are frequently confluent and often macroscopic (Plate 100.1). Some acute lesions resemble delayed hypersensitivity reactions (type I). In studies of biopsy and early autopsy material, the most common lesions (type II) are similar to the type I lesions but with deposition of activated complement. They likely represent a combination of delayed hypersensitivity and antibody-mediated immune reaction. Increase in IgG is found in the CNS in patients with MS. Studies have shown that some of this IgG is specific for several myelin antigens. Type I and II lesions contain oligodendrocytes and oligodendrocyte precursors. There is some remyelination, eventually insuffcient and/or repeated attacks, or other factors eventually block effective remyelination. Lesions with significant remyelination are termed shadow plaques.

Two less common types of acute lesions have been identified. Type III is characterized by oligodendrocyte death probably by apoptosis, with characteristics suggestive of a dying-back oligodendrogliopathy and uneven demyelination with some similarities to Balo's concentric sclerosis but on a microscopic scale. There are similarities to hypoxic lesions of myelin. Type IV lesions show even demyelination, but oligodendrocytes appear as if they are undergoing cytotoxic death, perhaps via toxin or infection. Modest numbers of inflammatory cells are found in type III and IV lesions. It has been proposed that all acute lesions in individual patients are of one type throughout the relapsing course of their disease. Others posit that individual patients may have different types of lesions in different sites and at different times in their disease course, and further that one type of lesion may evolve into another. Additionally immunohistologic and proton magnetic resonance spectroscopic (MRS) studies of so-called normal-appearing white matter (NAWM) reveal abnormalities that apparently precede the classic pathologic changes described above and before focal abnormalities can be seen on standard diagnostic MRI. Clusters of apoptotic oligodendrocytes have been reported in NAWM with activated microglia in the absence of other inflammatory changes, suggesting that the inflammatory lesions in white matter are a consequence of primary changes in oligodendrocytes in patients with the appropriate genetic make-up. The rediscovery of axonal pathology in early inflammatory lesions as well as changes in *N*-acetyl aspartate (NAA) by MRS in lesions has been responsible for a change in paradigm, with MS being viewed as a neurodegenerative disease. While inflammation in the white matter likely leads to dysfunction and damage to axons and neurons upstream early in the disease, much of the permanent disability in MS is due to loss of axons and neurons which may represent more direct damage to these cells. In patients with SPMS and PPMS, conventionally viewed as non-inflammatory on the basis of a lack of gadolinium enhancement of focal lesions, though gadolinium enhancement is not equivalent to inflammation or cellular infiltration, there is diffuse inflammation in the brain (SPMS and PPMS) and germinal follicle-like lesions in the meninges (SPMS) as well as within the brain.

There is a view that of the one-third of Japanese MS patients who clinically have predominantly optic nerve and spinal cord clinical manifestations (optic spinal MS; OSMS), virtually all actually have neuromyelitis optica (NMO) with antibodies to aquaporin 4 (AQP4). Yet a substantial number of Japanese appear to have MS by the usual clinical and imaging criteria. In OSMS, MS lesions severely affect both the optic nerve and the spinal cord and are frequently necrotic (see also Chapter 101). Tissue destruction is most prominent at the optic chiasma and from the lower cervical to the thoracic spinal cord. Microscopically, not only demyelination but also axonal degeneration, cavity formation, and in some cases microhemorrhage are seen in the lesions. Vessel wall thickening and capillary proliferation are also commonly observed in these lesions. Usually, many lipid-laden macrophages are present; however, the degree of perivascular inflammatory cell cuffing is variable. Thus there is pronounced infiltration of lymphocytes together with neutrophils in some and virtually no inflammatory cells in others. It remains to be elucidated whether the wide range of variability in inflammatory cell infiltrates reflects distinctions of immune mechanisms operative for lesion development. Recently the deposition of IgM and complement components as well as the preferential loss of AQP4 in astrocytes in excess of myelin basic protein loss in myelin in perivascular lesions has been described in autopsied Japanese OSMS cases. This supports the predominant involvement of humoral immunity in such cases.

Pathogenesis and etiology

MS is widely viewed as an autoimmune disease and in most forms of MS the immune system is involved in the disease pathogenesis, but the evidence for true autoimmunity is indirect. The current concept of the pathogenesis of RRMS is that CD4+ Th1-cells capable of recognizing a component of CNS myelin become activated, perhaps in response to an infectious agent by molecular mimicry and through sequential/orchestrated cytokines and chemokines affecting adhesion molecules and their ligands enter the CNS through an altered blood–brain barrier. On recognizing their cognate antigen presented by antigen presenting cells (APC), likely microglia, additional cytokines and chemokines recruit additional inflammatory cells. These include additional CD4 cells, CD8 cells, monocytes/macrophages, dendritic cells, B-cells, and plasma cells and further contribute to lesion formation. Plasma cells seen in lesions might be maturational products of B-cells. B-cells, monocytes/macrophages, and dendrite cells, as well as microglia, are APC, can interact with T-cells and further contribute to the lesion formation. These cells and their products, such as tumor necrosis factor-α and lymphotoxin, directly and indirectly, by generating toxic products such as nitric oxide, peroxynitrite, and free radicals, mediate damage to myelin, presumably to oligodendrocytes,

and also to axons. In the type II lesions antibodies directed at one or more components of myelin bind to myelin and cause damage by deposition and activation of complement cascade. Th17 cells producing IL-17 are also likely to be important in lesion formation. CD8+ T-cells may cause damage to axons, and excitatory neurotransmitters may also damage oligodendrocytes, axons, and neurons. Cytokines and chemokines may alter the function of oligodendrocytes, astrocytes, and neurons/axons. Demyelinated axons upregulate sodium channel numbers which then spread along the bare internode and in the short run may allow demyelinated axons to regain function. Continued excess activation of channels may eventually lead to axonal damage. Downregulatory cytokines are also likely to be important in limiting lesion activity. Astrocyte hypertrophy and hyperplasia (gliosis) leads to scarring which among other factors may combine to eventually limit remyelination, restoration of impulse transmission and functional recovery. The pathogenic mechanisms mediated by the inflammatory cells and activated microglial nodules in SPMS and PPMS are not known but are likely to contribute to slow continuing axonal loss. End-stage changes in neurons may represent failure of mitochondria, but the mechanisms leading to these changes are not understood.

Clinical presentation

Symptoms, signs, and course

The symptoms and signs of MS involve dissemination in space in the CNS, and in the RRMS presentation dissemination in time. The symptoms and signs can be quite variable although there are some that are more common, particularly early in the course of the disease (Table 100.1). Many patients present with subacute, occasionally acute, onset of a single symptom representing a single lesion (monosymptomatic); others have polysymptomatic onset. Subtle signs of other lesions may be apparent in monosymptomatic-onset patients. Clinically isolated syndrome (CIS) is a commonly used if imperfect term for the presentation of a first attack (relapse) of symptoms of MS occurring in a patient of appropriate age, with other possible etiologies being excluded. The chances of a patient going on to a diagnosis of MS is often predictable from the MRI and cerebrospinal fluid (CSF) findings with this first episode. The most common symptoms at onset are paresthesias and/or decreased sensation, weakness, abnormal gait and/or limb ataxia, decreased vision (optic neuritis), and diplopia. Vertigo and bladder/bowel dysfunction can be experienced early in the disease, and sphincter and sexual dysfunction are very common as the disease relapses and progressive disability accumulates. Fatigue is a common symptom, causing major difficulties in work and daily living. Cognitive problems are common and can be detected with neuropsychologic testing in up to

Table 100.1 Symptoms in MS.

Blurred or loss of vision*
Diplopia*
Loss of balance and/or clumsiness of limbs*
Weakness of limbs*
Paresthesias with/without decreased sensation*
Lhermitte's sign*
Band-like sensation around chest or abdomen
Fatigue
Bladder dysfunction*
Bowel dysfunction
Sexual dysfunction
Pain of various types including trigeminal neuralgia
Stiffness/spasms
Vertigo*
Dysarthria*
Dysphagia
Cognitive complaints
Depression
Seizures
Pseudobulbar behavior
Paroxysmal episodes

* Patients with marked segmental sensory deficits, lower motor neuron weakness, or marked increase in tone may manifest hypo- or even arreflexia in some regions.

Table 100.2 Common neurological signs in MS.

Abnormal reflexes (absent superficial reflexes, hyperreflexia, Babinski, hyporeflexia*)
Weakness
Spasticity
Impairment of vibratory sensibility
Decrease in proprioception/position sense
Impairment of sense of pain, light, touch, and/or temperature
Ataxia of gait and/or trunk
Limb dysmetria with/without tremor
Abnormalities of eye movement including internuclear ophthalmoplegia, nystagmus
Decrease in visual acuity, visual fields, color vision
Pallor of the optic disc
Afferent pupillary defect
Dysarthria (cerebellar, pseudobulbar, and/or bulbar)
Decrease in facial sensation
Facial weakness
Abnormalities of mood (signs of depression)
Cognitive dysfunction

* Patients with marked segmental sensory deficits, lower motor neuron weakness, or marked increase in tone may manifest hypo- or even arreflexia in some regions.

30–50% of patients, but severe dementia is rare. Disorders in mood including depression are frequent and inappropriate euphoria and uncontrolled crying and/or laughter (pseudobulbar behavior) are also seen. Seizures occur, usually later in the course, but are uncommon. Signs on neurological examination confirm the multifocal and diffuse nature of the disease, especially over time (Table 100.2).

In Japanese patients with OSMS selective and severe involvement of the optic nerves and spinal cord is characteristic (see also Chapter 101). Compared with patients with the conventional form of MS (CMS), which shows multiple involvement of the CNS including the cerebrum and cerebellum, OSMS patients show a significantly higher age at onset, female preponderance, greater disability (higher expanded disability status scale; EDSS), higher frequency of bilateral and severe optic neuritis and acute transverse myelitis, and a lesser frequency of secondary progression. On MRI, OSMS patients also show a higher frequency of longitudinally extensive spinal cord lesions (LESCLs) extending over three or more vertebral segments than CMS patients (Figure 100.1). In Western MS patients, less than 3% have such LESCLs. By contrast, in Asians, LESCLs are seen in more than half of OSMS patients, while about one-quarter of CMS patients also have these lesions. LESCLs in OSMS patients are present from the lower cervical to thoracic cord whereas they are preferentially found in the cervical cord in CMS patients. Not unexpectedly given their definitions, cranial MRI shows a significantly lower frequency of brain lesions fulfilling Barkhof criteria in OSMS than in CMS patients.

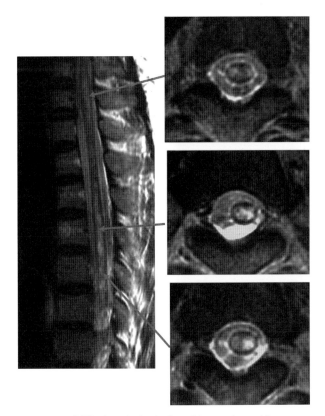

Figure 100.1 MRI of cervical spinal cord in a patient with Japanese ocular spinal MS (OSMS); T2-weighted image.

Patients with MS have a modest decrease in life expectancy, and somewhere between 50% and 80% of patients in the era preceding the introduction of disease modifying therapies (DMT) developed a progressive course and significant disability. It is still not clear whether DMT prevent or even slow the onset of SSPMS. We do not know if the percentage of treated patients with RRMS going on to develop SPMS will be less than in the past or if there will be a delay in the development of SPMS. Although some series report 10–30% of patients have benign disease at 10 and 20 years of disease, the percentage at 30 or more years is likely to be no more than 5–10%.

Diagnosis

The diagnosis of MS is still based on dissemination of lesions in the CNS in time and space with no alternative diagnosis by a physician experienced in the diagnosis of MS. The current criteria employ MRI (Figure 100.2), CSF analysis, and visual evoked responses (VEP) added to the clinical history and neurological examination to allow for an earlier diagnosis. Other laboratory tests and imaging studies help eliminate other diagnostic possibilities.

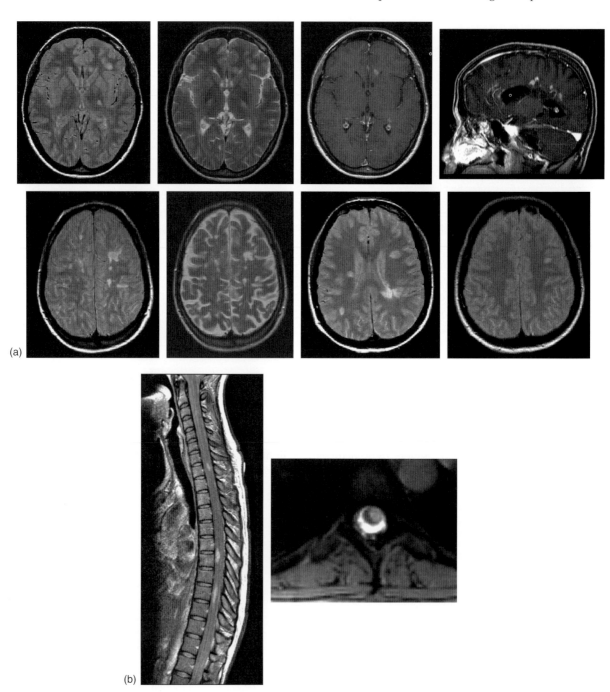

Figure 100.2 MRI in a patient with MS. (a) MRI of brain T2, proton density, fluid-attenuated inversion recovery (FLAIR), and T1 images demonstrating classic lesions including gadolinium enhancement on T1 sequences. (b) MRI of cervical and thoracic spine demonstrating three separate lesions on sagittal sequences and one of the lesions in axial sequence. (Courtesy of Dr Omar Khan.)

The diagnosis is not difficult when there are clearcut relapses of typical symptoms with objective evidence of dissemination of lesions limited in and limited to the CNS by neurological examination, such as visual loss, dyschromatopsia, disc pallor and an afferent pupillary defect, internuclear ophthalmoplegia and other brain stem findings, paraparesis with or without spasticity, ataxia of gait and/or limbs, and sensory deficits. PPMS and PRMS can still pose problems in diagnosis, as can atypical presentations of RRMS. The differential diagnosis varies with the clinical presentation depending on the part of the nervous system implicated as well as whether the onset and course is acute, subacute, or progressive. With an acute onset the differential includes vascular diseases, certain infectious processes and immunologically mediated diseases, including vasculitides, subacute onset from tumors, certain subacute infections, other immunologically mediated diseases, as well as combined systems degeneration and paraneoplastic syndromes, and a progressive pattern from tumors, inherited disorders, spinal cord compression, and HTLV-1 associated myelopathy. Imaging, CSF, and laboratory testing should be rational, based on the symptoms, signs, and onset/course of the disease.

In CSF oligoclonal bands and an increase in the IgG index are found significantly less frequently in OSMS than CMS or Western MS patients (about 25% versus 60% respectively in Japan and 80–90% in MS in Western countries, depending in part on the technique employed), while marked pleocytosis (50 cells/μl) and neutrophila are encountered significantly more commonly in OSMS than CMS or Western MS patients. Anti-AQP4 antibodies or NMO-IgG are found in 50–60% of patients having OSMS with LESCLs (in Japanese patients, 30% of OSMS with and without LESCLs, and about 15% of all Japanese MS). In Japan both anti-AQP4 antibody-positive MS and anti-AQP4 antibody-negative OSMS patients with LESCLs demonstrate higher frequencies of severe optic neuritis and acute transverse myelitis than anti-AQP4 antibody-negative CMS patients. With spinal cord MRI, LESCLs in anti-AQP4 antibody-positive MS patients predominantly involve the central gray matter of the thoracic cord, while those in anti-AQP4 antibody-negative OSMS patients extend from the cervical through the thoracic spinal cord and show a pattern of entire cord involvement. However, even in anti-AQP4 antibody-positive MS patients, ovoid lesions in the periventricular white matter of the cerebrum and short lesions in the peripheral white matter of the spinal cord frequently coexist with LESCLs. Thus, there is overlap and transition among anti-AQP4 antibody-positive MS patients who fulfill the definite NMO criteria, anti-AQP4 antibody-negative OSMS patients, and anti-AQP4 antibody-negative CMS patients. Anti-AQP4 antibodies occur in up to 75% of patients with classic NMO (see Chapter 101).

Treatment

Treatment of MS encompasses four areas: (1) maintenance of general health measures, as MS has only a modest effect on life expectancy; (2) symptomatic therapy; (3) treatment of relapses; and (4) disease modifying therapy (at this time treatments are immunomodulatory and/or immunosuppressive).

Treatment of symptoms

Therapy involves the use of medications as well as non-pharmacologic physical treatments that are generally related to the nature of the symptom and the lesions responsible for those symptoms, with some modification based on the disease. Not all symptoms need to be treated. It is important to remember to balance therapeutic effects with side effects and tolerability. Close communication between physicians and other health professionals with patients and families in helping patients deal with this chronic disorder is important.

Spasticity is best treated by a combination of physical therapy and medication. Occupational therapy is often helpful for problems with hands. Some degree of spasticity is often useful for patients in helping with ambulation; in some it is critical for the ability to transfer. Baclofen is a useful and generally well-tolerated and safe agent. Doses are best titrated and can range from 5 mg bid-tid to 160–200 mg/day, the higher doses generally reserved for non-ambulatory or limited ambulatory patients, when intrathecal infusions may be required. Limiting side effects include an increase in weakness, sleepiness, and fatigue. Other medications include tinazidine, as a solitary agent or in combination with baclofen, the drugs acting on different channels/receptors within the CNS. It is necessary to build this agent up very gradually since sleepiness, fatigue, lightheaded sensation, and hypotension are not uncommon. Benzodiazepines can be helpful, particularly as a nighttime dose, but sleepiness can limit use. Dantrolene may prove effective, but weakness and significant hepatic damage can occur in chronic use. Paroxysmal hypertonia, including "spasms," can sometimes be effectively treated with anticonvulsant drugs. Repeated local injections of botulinum toxin can provide help for months but eventually need to be repeated. Casting by physiatrists and other combined treatments may be required for deforming spasticity. A major advance in the treatment of spasticity is the intrathecal baclofen pump.

Fatigue is an frequent and often disabling symptom in MS. Patients experience several types, including fatigue due to effort (work- and exercise-induced worsening which recovers upon rest), fatigue due to depression (often present early in the day, even upon waking), fatigue due to difficulties with sleep (nocturia, sleep apnea, etc.), and the classical sense of fatigue that is often overwhelming and triggered by very little if any effort. Treatment includes energy conservation and naps or other periods of rest. Amantadine (100 mg qd-bid) and modafinil (100–400 mg/day) can be helpful.

Bladder dysfunction is common, interfering with daily activities, and can lead to complications including urinary tract infections, skin infections and breakdown, nephrolithiasis, and rarely renal failure. There are three basic patterns of dysfunction, and urodynamics may be needed to plan therapy in some instances. Some patients have difficulty in retaining urine, with urgency, frequency, incontinence, and at times nocturia. Other patients have difficulty voiding, with hesitancy, double voiding, and at times overflow incontinence. Most have a combination of problems because of detrussor sphincter dysynergy. Urinary retention (>100–150 ml post-voiding residual) is to be avoided and requires intervention. If there is no significant retention, anticholinergic drugs, including long-acting and skin patch formulations, or tricyclic antidepressants can prove useful if there is not excessive urinary retention. The latter can readily be determined by measuring post-voiding residual. If there is significant retention with recurrent infections or ureteral reflux, intermittent catheterization is preferable to indwelling urethral or suprapubic catheters. In some, ileal conduits, electrical stimulation, or intravesical botulinum toxin will be useful. Bowel dysfunction likewise can result in mixed symptoms, such as urgency, constipation, obstipation, and/or incontinence. The latter is hardest to manage. A bowel training program and working with patients on both bladder and bowel management permit patients to better manage their lives.

Sexual dysfunction is common, generally under-appreciated, and affects women as well as men. Treatment with phosphodiesterase type 5 inhibitors, intrapenile suppositories, or injections of prostaglandin alone or in combination with other drugs is helpful for some men. Counseling of couples is very important.

Pain is common in patients with MS and treatment depends on the type of pain. Those with abnormal gait or posture may have accentuated musculoskeletal pain including degenerative spine disease. Advanced spasticity including spasms can be painful and treatment should be directed at the spasticity/spasms. Neuralgia and neurogenic pain accompanying paroxysmal tonic spasms, segmental puritis, and band-like sensations may require a combined approach. If simple analgesics do not suffice anticonvulsant drugs such as gabapentin, pregablin, carbamazepine, phenytoin, and topiramate can help control pain. Trigeminal neuralgia can also be treated in the same manner. There is seldom any reason to treat Lhermitte's phenomenon.

Depression can usually be satisfactorily treated with antidepressant medications and counseling. Mood swings, pseudobulbar behavior, and inappropriate euphoria are harder to treat and there are as yet no proven treatments. Off-label uses of other psychoactive drugs alone or in combination may be partially effective. Cognitive problems are difficult to treat and there is little evidence that inhibitors of CNS acetylcholinesterase or CNS excitotoxicity are particularly effective in most individuals. Tremor and ataxia are difficult to treat and agents used for essential tremor have limited efficacy. Rarely patients may benefit from deep brain stimulation.

Treatment of relapses

All relapses need not be treated. Preventing relapses in RRMS is an important goal, but there is little evidence that treating relapses affects long-term prognosis. Relapses that cause a significant adverse effect on a patient's activities of daily living or ability to work are treated with corticosteroids (CS), generally intravenous methylprednisolone (MP) at a total of 1 g/day for 2–5 days. Oral CS may be equally effective, but additional studies testing very high dose oral CS need to be performed to show equal efficacy without an increase in side effects and/or tolerability. While various post-IVMP oral CS tapering schedules are widely employed with some theoretical basis, there are no large controlled prospective randomized studies indicating that they have any effect on degree of recovery from the relapse or the onset of the next relapse. Plasma exchange may be useful for CS refractory relapses.

Disease modifying therapies (DMT)

The development of agents that modify the course of MS, at least for several years, has changed the face of management of MS. In many countries there are currently three types of available therapies for RRMS: the interferon (IFN)-βs, glatiramer acetate, and natalizumab. There are currently two formulations of IFN-β1a and in some countries two formulations of IFN-β1b of recombinant IFN-β: IFN-β1b (non-glycosylated and differing in two amino acids from human IFN-β1a), administered subcutaneously (SC) every other day, and IFN-β1a (glycosylated) given either SC three times a week or intramuscularly once a week. Evidence suggests dose and particularly frequency of administration matter; the only two head-to-head studies favored the high dose/high frequency regimes, and although controversy continues, early treatment seems as important. In addition, neutralizing antibodies (NAbs) occur commonly in patients treated with the subcutaneous IFN-β medications and persistent high titers of NAbs reduce the therapeutic effect. Weekly intramuscular IFN-β1a is clearly less immunogenic. Controversy exists over the best way to measure NAbs and availability and cost of testing in some countries limit the widespread routine use of NAbs. Patients receiving IFN-β1 therapy require monitoring of blood counts and liver function tests (LFTs). Significant long-term adverse effects have not been seen in patients receiving these medications who are properly monitored. There are significant side effects involving tolerability, but these can generally be managed.

Glatiramer acetate (GA) is a preparation of random polymers of four basic amino acids which inhibits development of experimental autoimmune encephalomyelitis (EAE), a model of MS. Not an interferon, it seems to have several mechanisms of action that differ from the interferons. Administered SC daily, there do not seem to be any NAbs. GA does not affect either bone marrow elements or LFTs and it is very well tolerated. Some patients develop occasional self-limited immediate post-injection reactions and others chronic lipoatrophy. The recently completed large, randomized, prospective, double blind, head-to-head studies comparing GA with interferons in RRMS show GA to be as effective.

Natalizumab is a partially humanized monoclonal antibody directed against the α4 integrin peptide of VLA4, a ligand for vascular adhesion molecule (VCAM). EAE can be prevented and treated by antibodies to α4 integrin since the interaction of VLA4 and VCAM is required for the entry of pro-inflammatory CD4 T-cells into the CNS through the altered blood–brain barrier. Natalizumab administered intravenously every 28 days markedly reduces both relapse rate and gadolinium enhancement on MRI compared to placebo. The comparative efficacy of IFN-β or GA and natalizumab for the treatment of RRMS is uncertain since no head-to-head study has been performed. Side effects including a slight increase in serious infections compared to placebo were acceptable, and at the time of writing the risk of progressive multifocal leukoencephalopathy (PML) was estimated to be 1 per 1000. PML was reported in two patients who received IFN-β plus natalizumab and a patient with Crohn's disease treated with natalizumab and immunosuppressant therapy. Recently it has been reported in several patients only receiving natalizumab. For this reason it is used as a solitary agent and usually for those with DMT refractory RRMS. A program of very close monitoring for patients treated with natalizumab is required.

RRMS patients who are rapidly progressing with frequent relapses may be considered for immunosuppressant medications such as cyclophosphamide or mitoxantrone to induce remission, followed by GA or IFN-β1, but there are no large randomized studies to support this approach routinely. In the future it is likely that a number of other medications will be available for this situation. Mitoxantrone is also used for treatment of SPMS.

Treatment of clinically isolated syndrome (CIS)

Several studies indicate that treatment of patients with CIS with IFN-β1 delays the onset of the defining second relapse and/or MRI defining lesion to meet the criteria of MS as does a study of glatiramer acetate. Although useful to have proven, it is not surprising; CIS with defined MRI criteria and other disorders ruled out usually is the first clinical episode of MS. From these studies combined with evidence from the MS pivotal trials and non-placebo controlled extensions of them, early treatment seems to be beneficial, but whether this should include all such patients in the absence of a helpful biomarker remains controversial. Severity of deficit from the first attack, lesion load or volume, evidence of atrophy or non-gadolinium-enhancing T1 hypointensities on initial or repeat MRI in 3–6 months have all been suggested as guidelines to treat CIS patients with DMT.

Treatment of SPMS, PPMS, and PRMS

SPMS treatment remains a major challenge. Although IFN-β1b is an approved treatment for SPMS, it seems clear that this should be reserved for patients with superimposed relapses or gadolinium-enhancing lesions. It is not clear yet if there is a subset of mitoxantrone-responsive SPMS patients and it has significant side effects (cardiac, increased susceptibility to infection, and leukemia) and tolerability issues. Cyclophosphamide should be reserved for patients with very rapid progression. There is little to recommend methotrexate or azathioprine and there are no large controlled studies of other agents or autologous stem cell transplantation. No treatments have been proven to significantly slow progression in PPMS, although there is post-hoc analysis suggesting that males might benefit from GA. Patients with progressive onset but with one or more clearcut relapses (PRMS) are often treated as SPMS since there are no studies on patients with this relatively uncommon pattern of disease.

Further reading

Boissy A, Fox RJ. Current treatment options in multiple sclerosis. *Curr Treat Options Neurol* 2007; 9: 176–86.

Boster A, Eden G, Frohman E, *et al.* Intense immunosuppression in patients with rapidly worsening multiple sclerosis: treatment guidelines for the clinician. *Lancet Neurol* 2008; 7: 173–83.

Compston A, Coles A. Multiple sclerosis. *Lancet* 2002; 359(9313): 1221–31.

Frohman EM, Racke MK , Raine CS. Multiple sclerosis – the plaque and its pathogenesis. *N Engl J Med* 2006; 354(9): 942–55.

Kira J. Multiple sclerosis in the Japanese population. *Lancet Neurol* 2003; 2: 117–27.

Lisak RP, Hohlfeld R. Repair and retention of neuronal structures in multiple sclerosis: identifying markers, metrics and correlates of treatment success. *Neurology* 2007; 68(Suppl 3): S1–S96.

Lucchinetti C, Bruck W, Parisi J, Scheithauer B, Rodriguez M, Lassmann H. Heterogeneity of multiple sclerosis lesions: implications for the pathogenesis of demyelination (see comments). *Ann Neurol* 2000; 47(6): 707–17.

Matsuoka T, Matsushita T, Kawano Y, *et al.* Heterogeneity of aquaporin-4 autoimmunity and spinal cord lesions in multiple sclerosis in Japanese. *Brain* 2007; 130: 1206–23.

Misu T, Fujihara K, Kakita A, *et al.* Loss of aquaporin 4 in lesions of neuromyelitis optica: distinction from multiple sclerosis. *Brain* 2007; 130: 1224–34.

Chapter 101
Neuromyelitis optica (NMO) or Devic's disease

William M. Carroll
Sir Charles Gairdner Hospital, Nedlands, Australia

Introduction

Cases conforming to neuromyelitis optica (NMO) and what became eponymously known as Devic's disease after the publications of Eugene Devic (1894) and François Gault (1895) were first recognised by Albutt (1870) and Aoyama (1891). On the experience of a relatively small number of cases, they described a syndrome of transverse myelitis (MY) associated with simultaneous or sequential optic neuritis (ON), which often proved fatal. Nowadays less severe forms, often relapsing, are also recognised and in turn considered part of the spectrum of inflammatory demyelinating diseases (IDD).

Clinical and laboratory features and diagnostic criteria

Typically the ON and MY are severe and temporally associated, especially in monophasic cases, but involvement at these two sites of predilection can be widely separated in time. The ON can result in blindness or significant visual impairment, and the MY in paraplegia, sphincter dysfunction, and respiratory failure. However, the clinical spectrum has been broadened by increasing recognition of this syndrome. Not only can the ON and MY be separated by a variable period of time, even years in some instances, but also involvement at these sites can be recurrent, vary in severity, or be restricted to optic nerve and/or spinal cord. Relapsing NMO (RNMO) has a female:male ratio of up to 7:1, whereas monophasic NMO with closely associated MY and ON has a more equal gender ratio, and commonly commences in the fourth and fifth decades. Familial NMO occurs rarely. Features that help predict RNMO are the older age of onset, female gender, and short interval between the first two relapses. The selective emphasis of spinal cord and optic nerve involvement and the severity of the attacks

usually mean that up to half the patients with NMO will be severely disabled within 5 years.

The clinical phenotype differs from most cases of multiple sclerosis (MS) and so do the laboratory investigations. MRI in the early stages uncommonly shows intracranial lesions, and typically spinal cord lesions are located centrally rather than peripherally and extend longitudinally for three or more vertebral segments (see Chapter 100, Figure 100.1). Intracranial lesions, if they occur early in the disease, can involve the central regions of the brain stem and diencephalon or periventricular areas (Figure 101.1) and infrequently present as atypical large hemisphere lesions. Later in the course of RNMO lesions more typical of MS may develop. In the cerebrospinal fluid (CSF) a pleocytosis of more than 50 leucocytes/mm^3 is common, sometimes with neutrophils, the CSF protein is frequently elevated, and oligoclonal bands (OCB) are infrequently demonstrated.

The clinical phenotype of NMO may be associated with other autoimmune diseases, such as systemic lupus erythematosus (SLE), vasculitides, Sjögren's syndrome, autoimmune thyroid disease, myasthenia gravis, and infections such as pulmonary tuberculosis and neurosyphilis. Even in the absence of clinical features of these diseases, cases of NMO may carry the serological markers, such as ANF.

Diagnostic criteria were proposed in 1999 (Table 101.1) in order to distinguish RNMO from conventional MS (CMS). Modification of these criteria (2006) on the basis of MRI and Aquaporin-4 (AQP-4) serological positivity remain contentious, though are likely to prove useful in segregating this condition.

Pathology and pathogenesis

Studies of both Caucasian and Japanese cases have been remarkably similar and reflect both the severity of the insult and the proposed antibody-mediated pathogenesis. Macroscopically there are large areas of demyelination of white matter tracts and central gray matter, often associated with cavitation. Microscopically there is necrosis and axonal injury, marked loss of

International Neurology: A Clinical Approach. Edited by Robert P. Lisak, Daniel D. Truong, William M. Carroll, and Roongroj Bhidayasiri. © 2009 Blackwell Publishing, ISBN: 978-1-4051-5738-4.

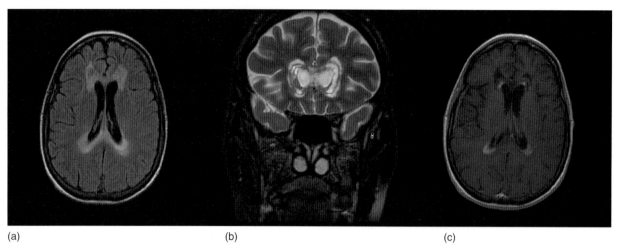

Figure 101.1 T2 axial (a), coronal fluid-attenuated inversion recovery (FLAIR) (b), and T1 post-gadolinium (c) MRI sections from a sero AQP-4 positive NMO patient showing enhancing symmetrical periventricular and callosal lesions. (Courtesy of Dr BG Weinshenker.)

Table 101.1 NMO diagnostic criteria.

(a) Criteria for the diagnosis of NMO* (Wingerchuk DM *et al. Neurology* 1999; 53: 1107–14)	(b) Proposed diagnostic criteria for NMO (Wingerchuk DM *et al. Neurology* 2006; 66: 1485–9)
Absolute criteria	**Definite NMO**
Optic neuritis	Optic neuritis
Acute myelitis	Acute myelitis
No evidence of clinical disease outside of the optic nerve or spinal cord	At least two of three supportive criteria
	1. Contiguous spinal cord MRI lesion extending over atleast three vertebral segments
Supportive criteria	2. Brain MRI not meeting diagnostic criteria for MS
Major	3. NMO-IgG seropositive status
Negative brain MRI at onset (does not meet Paty criteria)	
Spinal cord MRI abnormality extending over atleast three vertebral segments	
CSF pleocytosis of >50 leucocytes/mm^3 or >5 neutrophils/mm^3	
Minor	
Bilateral optic neuritis	
Severe optic neuritis with fixed visual acuity <20/200 in at least one eye	
Severe, fixed, attack-related weakness (MRC grade ≤2) in one or more limbs	

*Diagnosis requires all absolute criteria and one (major) or two (minor) supportive criteria.

oligodendrocytes, and demyelination. In recent lesions there is a prominent cellular infiltrate of macrophages, granulocytes, eosinophils, and some T lymphocytes in a perivascular distribution, while hyalinized blood vessels and fibrosis are present in early and late lesions. Perivascular staining patterns of immunoglobulin (mainly IgM) and congruent complement C9$_{neo}$ are also characteristic features of early lesions. Together, these findings suggest a prominent role for humoral auto-immune mechanisms.

The finding of a serum IgG antibody in 73% of Caucasian cases of RNMO and 58% of the equivalent Japanese optico-spinal MS (OSMS) cases, subsequently shown to target the AQP-4 water channel, supported this proposition. Although the anti-AQP-4 antibody is not IgM and is yet to be demonstrated to be pathogenic, the distribution of lesions in RNMO is characteristically in regions where this water channel is found in high concentration. Recent studies have demonstrated that AQP-4 staining is lost in spinal cord lesions of NMO, together with the depletion of astrocytes, suggesting that AQP-4 or astrocytes may be intimately involved in the pathogenesis of this condition. Finally, the anecdotal observations by clinicians that plasma exchange and the therapeutic targeting of B cells may be more effective treatments (see below) than conventional disease modifying therapies currently available for CMS further supports the antibody-mediated hypothesis.

Epidemiology and immunogenetics

The overall population prevalence of RNMO is unknown, but the prevalence relative to MS varies according to ethnic and genetic backgrounds. It is relatively more common than MS among pigmented non-Caucasian populations of Asia, Africa, North America, Australasia, and some minority groups such as Romany gypsies. While the prevalence in the overall population has not been established, given that its relative prevalence in the IDD is approximately 3–4% in Caucasians and up to 30% in Japanese, where the overall prevalence of MS is approximately one-tenth, it is likely that prevalence of RNMO is of a similar order in both Caucasian and non-Caucasian populations. Arguments have been presented that the relatively higher prevalence in pigmented non-Caucasians represents a prototypic form of demyelinating disease, from which CMS evolved in Caucasian populations. Further, the situation is changing with a decreasing proportion of RNMO (or OSMS) Japanese patients; a change attributed to the effects of immunogenetic selection consequent upon increasing industrialization. Japanese with RNMO/OSMS have a higher degree of association with the HLA haplotype DPB1*0501, which is also present in 60% of the wider Japanese population, whereas Japanese with CMS share the same HLA haplotype of DRB1*1501 with Caucasian populations.

Relationship to other inflammatory demyelinating diseases and treatment

NMO, both monophasic and relapsing forms, can be differentiated from other inflammatory demyelinating diseases including MS on the basis of clinical phenotype, MRI and CSF findings, pathology, therapeutic response, and the serological biomarker of anti-AQP-4 antibody. Whether it is distinctly separable or represents one pole of the spectrum of demyelinating disease with CMS at the other is not yet absolutely clear. The remaining intermediate cases of demyelinating disease with an optico-spinal phenotype who may be AQP-4 antibody negative or differ in MRI appearances is where the situation remains unclear and may pose a therapeutic dilemma. On the other hand, recurrent forms of ON or MY, with typical longitudinally extensive MRI lesions, particularly if they are AQP-4 antibody positive, will be categorized as NMO and indeed have been referred to as NMO spectrum disorder. In such cases, even when the AQP-4 antibody is unavailable, it seems reasonable to assume that they form part of the NMO spectrum.

On the basis of anecdotal experience, the pathology of RNMO, the associated AQP-4 antibody, and the absence of evidence of clear efficacy with currently available demyelinating disease modifying treatments such as Interferon Beta and Glatirimer Acetate, treatments targeting humoral mechanisms are to be preferred. For acute treatment these include high-dose steroids (usually intravenous) with regimes of plasma exchange or intravenous immunoglobulin, and for longer-term prophylaxis, immunosuppression with agents including cyclophosphamide (1 mg/kg/day po), methotrexate (5–10 mg po once a week), the anti-B-cell monoclonal antibody Rituximab, or even the anti-B-cell proliferative monoclonal antibody Belimumab should be considered. Given the severity of the attacks in NMO, consideration should be given to their introduction after the first attack of ON or MY if other features such as ethnic background, MRI and CSF findings, and particularly the anti-AQP-4 antibody are present.

Conclusion

The position and relevance of NMO among IDD has changed dramatically since its original descriptions. From an uncommon condition considered a variant of MS, NMO has moved to center stage as the pathology, pathogenesis, epidemiology, clinical and imaging characteristics, and potential biomarking serology have provided a rational basis for its treatment and an opening from which to progress the understanding of more common forms of IDD.

Further reading

Kira J. Multiple sclerosis in the Japanese population. *Lancet Neurol* 2003; 2: 117–27.

Lennon VA, Kryzer TJ, Pittock SJ, Verkman AS, Hinson SR. IgG marker of optic-spinal multiple sclerosis binds to the aquaporin-4 water channel. *J Exp Med* 2005; 202: 473–7.

Lucchinetti CF, Mandler RN, McGavern D, *et al*. A role for humoral mechanisms in the pathogenesis of Devic's neuromyelitis optica. *Brain* 2002; 125: 1450–61.

Pittock SJ, Lennon VA, Krecke K, Wingerchuk DM, Lucchinetti CF, Weinshenker BG. Brain abnormalities in neuromyelitis optica. *Arch Neurol* 2006; 63: 390–6.

Chapter 102
Isolated inflammatory demyelinating syndromes (IIDS)

Ernest W. Willoughby
Auckland City Hospital, Auckland, New Zealand

Introduction

This chapter describes disorders characterized by focal non-infective areas of inflammation of the central nervous system (CNS), defined by the site affected: that is, the optic nerve (optic neuritis), spinal cord (myelitis), brainstem, or cerebral hemisphere. Usually only one area is affected clinically, but isolated inflammatory demyelinating syndromes (IIDS) may be multifocal, and a unifocal clinical syndrome may be accompanied by other asymptomatic focal lesions on MR scan. An alternative, less precise term is "clinically isolated syndrome" (CIS).

Of particular significance is the likelihood that these syndromes may be the first clinical manifestation of a chronic relapsing inflammatory disease of the CNS, especially multiple sclerosis or neuromyelitis optica (NMO), also known as Devic's disease. The focal inflammation may follow vaccination or a systemic viral infection, but IIDS does not include acute disseminated encephalomyelitis (ADEM), where there are widespread inflammatory CNS lesions with more diffuse clinical features.

Features common to all of the syndromes

Epidemiology

IDSS occur in all parts of the world and affect all racial groups, but there is considerable variation in the frequency of the syndromes in different parts of the world. The typical syndromes are most common in Western Europe and North America and in other temperate areas where the population is of predominantly European origin and where the prevalence of multiple sclerosis (MS) is high. This reflects the fact that the single most common cause of IDSS is a first clinical attack of MS. In Asia, Africa, and the Middle East where the prevalence of MS is much lower, IDSS are less frequent and often represent the first clinical

attack of NMO, which is more common in populations of Asian origin and probably also in Polynesians.

In general, optic neuritis and myelitis are substantially more common in all areas than syndromes affecting the brainstem or cerebral hemisphere, and are virtually the only syndromes seen as a manifestation of NMO. Women are affected about twice as often as men, with a peak age of onset of 20–35.

Clinical features

• Symptoms may appear relatively suddenly and characteristically worsen over several days or 2–3 weeks, reaching a plateau. Even without treatment, there is then gradual improvement over several weeks or months. Resolution may be complete or there may be residual neurologic deficit.
• Clinical manifestations are due primarily to involvement of major white matter tracts in the affected area. The severity varies considerably both in terms of the peak symptoms and the amount of residual disability. The degree of recovery relates in large measure to the extent of initial axonal damage.
• Pain may be a prominent symptom. It is related mainly to involvement of sensory pathways in the affected area.
• Except for general fatigue, there is usually no associated systemic upset such as fever, unless this is a manifestation of a preceding viral infection that may trigger IIDS.

Diagnosis

• MR scanning of the appropriate area is the key diagnostic investigation in distinguishing IIDS from other pathological processes producing similar symptoms. In addition, by demonstrating white matter scars resulting from previous, asymptomatic patches of CNS inflammation in other areas, particularly in the brain, MR has a role in determining the likelihood of further attacks, that is, if the IIDS is the first clinical manifestation of an already established chronic relapsing process, or potentially an isolated event.
• Cerebrospinal fluid (CSF) may show a mild lymphocytic pleocytosis, and the presence on electrophoresis

International Neurology: A Clinical Approach. Edited by Robert P. Lisak, Daniel D. Truong, William M. Carroll, and Roongroj Bhidayasiri. © 2009 Blackwell Publishing, ISBN: 978-1-4051-5738-4.

of oligoclonal IgG bands substantially increases the chances of further attacks in the future, indicating MS. Serum autoantibodies may show an underlying systemic connective tissue disorder.

Pathophysiology

• The inflammatory pathology has been studied mainly in large cerebral lesions. It is probably much the same at different sites with infiltration of lymphocytes and macrophages with myelin breakdown and variable amounts of axonal damage. There is controversy about the extent of oligodendrocyte loss as an early feature. Subsequent healing is characterized by remyelination with gliosis. In some cases, especially in NMO-type inflammation, there is more involvement of small vessels with necrosis and relatively little selective demyelination.

Treatment

• The main consideration is the use of high-dose corticosteroids, typically methylprednisolone 0.5–1.0 g daily, intravenously (IV) or orally, for 3–5 days, perhaps followed by a tapering course of oral steroids for 2–3 weeks. There is no established consensus on the most appropriate regimen. Steroids relieve acute symptoms, especially pain, and produce more rapid improvement, but evidence is lacking that the treatment reduces the amount of long-term residual disability. For severe attacks with limited improvement on steroids, plasmapheresis has been shown to be of benefit and intravenous immunoglobulin (IVIG) may possibly have a place.

• After recovery from an IDSS, if there is evidence that the episode represents the first manifestation of MS or NMO, another issue is consideration of ongoing immunomodulatory or immunosuppressive treatment to reduce the chance of future attacks. That is a complex decision, dependent on availability of costly treatments such as beta-interferon or glatiramer acetate and the likely nature of the underlying disease process.

Optic neuritis

Clinical features

This usually affects one eye but may be bilateral. Impairment of vision is most marked centrally with early reduction of color vision and worsening typically over several days. Pain in the eye is usual and aggravated by eye movement. Severity of visual impairment is very variable. A common and characteristic feature is temporary aggravation of visual impairment by exercise or exposure to heat (Uhthoff's phenomenon). Swelling of the optic disc is seen in only about one-third of cases, that is, the inflammatory process does not extend anteriorly to the optic nerve head (retrobulbar neuritis). Characteristically,

even when visual impairment is mild there is reduced papillary constriction to light, demonstrated most sensitively by alternately shining the light in each eye (relative afferent pupil defect). After several weeks, even with good return of vision, pallor of the optic disc (optic atrophy) commonly develops.

Differential diagnosis

This includes other disorders affecting the optic nerve, especially anterior ischemic optic neuropathy (usually painless and more abrupt in onset, often with altitudinal visual field defects), Leber's hereditary optic neuropathy (painless and progressive over weeks or months), and orbital idiopathic granulomatous disease or tumors. Chronic raised intracranial pressure or severe hypertension with papilloedema may present with acute impairment of vision in one eye as may disease of the eye itself, especially neuroretinitis (most commonly due to cat scratch disease), other retinal disorders, anterior uveitis, ocular larva migrans, and acute glaucoma. In the tropics onchocerciasis also needs consideration.

(Transverse) myelitis

Clinical features

Depending on the site of the main inflammatory focus (cervical or thoracic) there is paraparesis or quadriparesis of variable degree, often asymmetrical, with sensory impairment below the level of the lesion, plus bladder and bowel dysfunction. The term transverse myelitis relates to that clinical pattern with discrete demarcation of sensory change at a particular segmental level. Relatively mild disease with involvement of only part of the cord cross section is particularly likely to be a feature of a first MS attack. Pain in the spine may be marked and the distal sensory impairment may also be painful. If weakness is severe and develops rapidly, tone may be flaccid and tendon reflexes absent in the early stages. The extent of recovery is very variable.

Differential diagnosis

The first step is to distinguish myelitis from other causes of acute weakness, especially polyneuropathy. MR scanning usually will distinguish myelitis from other cord lesions such as tumors, abscesses, and vascular malformations and CSF will also help distinguish infections of the cord, especially with herpes and West Nile viruses and TB and, in tropical areas, schistosomiasis. The inflammation in IDSS may be localized as in MS, or more patchy, extending over several spinal segments with diffuse cord swelling and areas of enhancement with gadolinium, as in NMO.

Brainstem inflammatory lesions

Clinical features
Motor and sensory dysfunction in the limbs may be similar to that seen in cervical myelitis, with the additional features of cranial nerve lesions and/or cerebellar dysfunction.

Differential diagnosis
Tumors, vascular malformations, and infective processes are usually distinguishable by MR scan and CSF.

Cerebral hemisphere inflammatory lesions

Clinical features
Usually hemiparesis, hemisensory symptoms, or homonymous visual field defects are the clinical features. Headache is not consistently present and seizures may occur.

Differential diagnosis
Symptomatic lesions are usually large, characteristically with incomplete peripheral ring enhancement with contrast on CT or MR scan. A feature that helps distinguish this type of inflammation from tumors and abscesses on MR scan is a relative lack of mass effect for the size of the lesion. Progressive multifocal leukoencephalopathy usually has no or little enhancement.

Further reading

Balcer L. Optic neuritis. *N Eng J Med* 2006; 354: 1273–80.

Miller D, Barkhof F, Montalban X, Thompson A, Filippi M. Clinically isolated syndromes suggestive of multiple sclerosis. Part 1: Natural history, pathogenesis, diagnosis and prognosis. *Lancet Neurol* 2005; 4: 281–8.

Miller D, Barkhof F, Montalban X, Thompson A, Filippi M. Clinically isolated syndromes suggestive of multiple sclerosis. Part 2: Non-conventional MRI, recovery processes and management. *Lancet Neurol* 2005; 4: 341–8.

Pittock S, Lucchinetti L. Inflammatory transverse myelitis: evolving concepts. *Curr Opin Neurol* 2006; 19: 362–8.

Wasay M, Khatri I, Khealani B, Sheerani M. MS in Asian countries. *Int MS J* 2006; 13: 58–65.

Chapter 103
Acute disseminated encephalomyelitis

Brenda L. Banwell
University of Toronto, Toronto, Canada

Overview

Acute disseminated encephalomyelitis (ADEM) is considered to be a monophasic fulminant inflammatory demyelinating syndrome, more common in children, manifesting with encephalopathy and polyfocal neurological deficits. ADEM is hypothesized to occur as a consequence of mistaken immunological targeting of central nervous system (CNS) antigens following infectious or vaccine-mediated exposures. ADEM occurs in approximately 1/1000 children following acute infection with measles, which remains a major health issue in countries that do not have universal vaccination programs. Post-vaccinial ADEM is most clearly associated with exposure to vaccines that utilize neural tissue cultures as part of their production. Declining use of such vaccines has resulted in fewer vaccine-associated ADEM cases.

Current therapeutic strategies for ADEM include corticosteroids (CS), immune globulin (IVIg), and plasma exchange (PE), with the choice of therapy dictated by the clinical severity of the presentation. As many as 18–25% of children and 40% of adults with ADEM will experience recurrent disease, and most patients with recurrent disease will ultimately be diagnosed with multiple sclerosis (MS). Currently, there are no clinical, laboratory, or MRI features that reliably predict MS risk at the time of acute ADEM presentation.

Clinical features

Table 103.1 summarizes the key features reported in children and adults with ADEM. Most patients present with acute polysymptomatic neurological dysfunction accompanied by encephalopathy, and variably with seizures, meningism, or fever; 50–70% report a preceding infectious illness. Polyfocal features may include visual loss due to

unilateral or bilateral optic neuritis; limb weakness and sensory loss due to spinal cord involvement (transverse myelitis) or due to cerebral lesions; ataxia, dysarthria, tremor, and nystagmus due to involvement of the cerebellum; or oculomotor, motor, or sensory symptoms, and possibly respiratory depression resulting from involvement of the brainstem.

These presentations are characteristic of "classic" ADEM, but some diagnose ADEM in patients with any acute monofocal or polyfocal demyelinating presentation, provided that the MRI demonstrates multifocal white matter or deep gray nuclei lesions. Others permit inclusion of patients with acute, typically post-viral, neurological symptoms even in the absence of white matter lesions on MRI. Some, but not all, require alteration in sensorium (encephalopathy).

The International Pediatric Multiple Sclerosis Working Group has published consensus clinical definitions for ADEM, MS, and other acquired demyelinating syndromes (Table 103.2). While these definitions were created based on features of ADEM seen in children, the clinical features of ADEM in the adult population do not appear to vary significantly from those in childhood.

Laboratory findings in ADEM

Cerebrospinal fluid (CSF) pleocytosis (cell count >10/µl) and/or elevated CSF protein occurs in approximately 50% of children and 80% of adults with ADEM. CSF oligoclonal bands (OCBs) occur in 3–58% of patients with ADEM. OCBs may be transient in some patients, although few patients undergo repeated testing. OCBs were detected in 17% of children with ADEM who were ultimately diagnosed with MS, as compared to 92% of children for whom the first demyelinating event was typical of MS. Methodology is critical, and thus a large single laboratory study of patients with ADEM and MS is required to truly define the relative frequency of CSF OCBs. Serial CSF examinations are required to determine whether development of OCBs occurs later in the MS disease process in patients with an ADEM-like first MS attack.

International Neurology: A Clinical Approach. Edited by Robert P. Lisak, Daniel D. Truong, William M. Carroll, and Roongroj Bhidayasiri. © 2009 Blackwell Publishing, ISBN: 978-1-4051-5738-4.

Table 103.1 Summary of the key features of ADEM in children and adults.

	Preceding features	CSF oligoclonal bands	Sequelae	MS diagnosis
Pediatric ADEM	• Infection or fever (76%) • Systemic findings (42%)	0–29%	• 20% residual disability (mild) • Less than 5% mortality • Some mild cognitive impairment in some patients	18–26%
Adult ADEM	• Infection or fever in 33%	13–65%	• 50% residual deficits • Rare mortality • Some mild cognitive impairment in some patients	35%

ADEM: acute disseminated encephalomyelitis; CSF: cerebrospinal fluid; MS: multiple sclerosis.

Magnetic resonance imaging features of ADEM

MRI features of ADEM most commonly include multifocal, bilateral, asymmetric, hyperintense lesions of T2-weighted images scattered diffusely in the CNS white matter, often associated with increased signal in the deep gray nuclei. Spinal cord lesions may also be present, and tend to extend longitudinally to encompass multiple spinal cord segments. Although ADEM is a fulminant and acute process, gadolinium-enhancing lesions were detected in only 17–37% of well-characterized pediatric cohorts. In a single study of 40 adults with ADEM, 95% showed enhancement of at least one lesion, raising the possibility that gadolinium enhancement may be more commonly seen in adult-onset ADEM. Rarely, the emergence of white matter lesions may be delayed, with the development of lesions evident on MRI performed 5–7 days after clinical onset.

Figure 103.1 contrasts the typical MRI features of ADEM and MS. MRI features at presentation cannot be used to distinguish ADEM from the first attack of MS, as MRI features typical of ADEM can occur at the time of a first demyelinating attack in children and adults, and evolve over time into a pattern more consistent with MS. Accrual of clinically silent new lesions over time likely distinguishes MS from monophasic ADEM.

Differential diagnoses

The differential diagnosis of acute neurological illness in a previously well child or adult is broad. The key disorders that require exclusion include: (1) active, viral, or bacterial infection; (2) systemic or isolated CNS inflammatory disorders including vasculitis and sarcoidosis; (3) disseminated CNS malignancy (such as lymphoma, leukemia, or metastatic disease); (4) macrophage activation syndromes (seen almost exclusively in children); and (5) in all patients one must consider whether the acute demyelinating event is the first manifestation of MS. The key clinical features and specific investigations appropriate for the exclusion of these disorders are listed in Table 103.3.

Treatment

Treatment of acute ADEM typically consists of high-dose intravenous (IV) corticosteroids (CS) with the additional use of IVIg in CS-resistant or life-threatening cases. Although evidence-based treatment guidelines are lacking, proposed treatment protocols typically include IV CS (20–30 mg/kg/day for 3–5 days). Oral prednisone is typically then administered (initial dose of 1 mg/kg/day), and tapered over 3–4 weeks. Case series-level evidence exists for the use of IVIg (2 g/kg divided over 2–5 days) for patients who do not respond to CS therapy, and level I evidence exists for the use of PE (seven treatments over 14 days) in acute, life-threatening demyelination.

Outcome of ADEM

The outcome of ADEM is generally favorable, and over 85% of patients will recover with little or no sequelae. Children may recover more quickly than adults. Of patients with residual sequelae, motor impairment and minor cognitive deficits are the most notable.

Although ADEM is typically considered a monophasic illness, some patients experience a re-emergence of their initial clinical and radiographic features (recurrent ADEM), or may experience new episodes of meeting the criteria for ADEM with clinical and radiographic evidence of new disease (multiphasic ADEM) (Table 103.2). Recurrent and multiphasic ADEM are exceptionally rare in adults.

ADEM can also represent the first attack of MS. Among 296 children with acute demyelination, 29% initially diagnosed with ADEM were ultimately diagnosed with MS.

Table 103.2 Summary of the proposed definitions for acquired demyelinating disorders.

Diagnosis	Definition	Key clinical features	Key MRI features	Specific exclusions
Monophasic ADEM	• A first clinical attack with a presumed inflammatory or demyelinating cause, with acute or subacute onset that affects multifocal areas of the CNS • Symptoms may evolve over a period of 3 months	• Polyfocal features • Encephalopathy[*]	• Multifocal hyperintense *or* a single large T2 lesion(s) • Lesions in white matter and/ or deep gray nuclei • No evidence of chronic "black holes"[†]	• Prior events consistent with demyelination • Acute CNS infection • Alternative diagnosis[‡]
Recurrent ADEM	• New attack of ADEM with a recurrence of the initial symptoms and signs, three or more months after the first ADEM attack, without involvement of new clinical areas either by history, examination, or neuroimaging • Attack does not occur while on steroids, and occurs at least 1 month after completing therapy	• Polyfocal features • Encephalopathy[*]	• MRI shows no new lesions; original lesions may have enlarged	• Clinical or MRI evidence of new areas of demyelination • Attack occurs within 3 months of first ADEM episode (considered to then be part of initial ADEM illness)
Multiphasic ADEM	• ADEM followed by a new clinical attack also meeting criteria for ADEM, but involving new anatomic areas of the CNS • Attack does not occur while on steroids, and occurs at least 3 months after initial ADEM episode	• Polyfocal features • Encephalopathy[*]	• MRI shows new lesions; original lesions may have enlarged or resolved	• Attack occurs within 3 months of first ADEM episode (considered to then be part of initial ADEM illness) • Evidence of accrual of clinically silent new MRI lesions[§]
Multiple sclerosis	• Clinical or radiographic evidence of lesion dissemination in both space and time (as defined in Krupp *et al.*, 2007)	• Relapsing disease course • Monofocal or polyfocal features	• New lesions on repeat imaging (as described in Krupp *et al.*, 2007)	• Children with a first demyelinating event consistent with ADEM, must have two non-ADEM events to qualify for MS diagnosis
Neuromyelitis optica	• Must have ON and TM • Spinal cord lesion extending over three cord segments or NMO IgG positive	• Monophasic (i.e., single ON and TM episodes) • Relapsing NMO (recurrent ON and TM episodes)	• Longitudinally extensive spinal lesions • Increased T2 signal, swelling, or Gd enhancement of optic nerves • Brain lesions tend to be in hypothalamic region, midbrain, or in a pattern not otherwise consistent with MS	• Clinical features more consistent with MS

ADEM: acute disseminated encephalomyelitis; CNS: central nervous system; Gd: gadolinium; IgG: immunoglobulin; MRI: magnetic resonance imaging; MS: multiple sclerosis; NMO: neuromyelitis optica; ON: optic neuritis; TM: transverse myelitis.

[*]Encephalopathy is defined by (1) behavioral change (confusion, excessive irritability) or (2) alteration in consciousness (lethargy, coma).
[†]Chronic black holes are defined as areas of hypodensity on T1-weighted images that do not enhance with gadolinium, are bright on T2-weighted images, and persist on serial imaging.
[‡]A structured approach to disorders considered in the differential diagnosis of acute demyelination is available in recently published reviews (Hahn *et al.*, 2007).
[§]MRI evidence of new lesion formation occurring without clinical signs should not occur in patients with multiphasic ADEM, and would be more in keeping with MS.

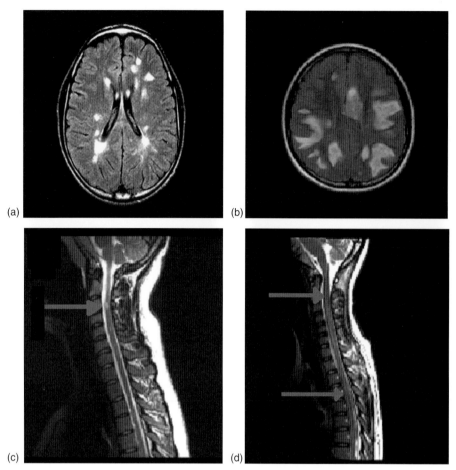

Figure 103.1 Typical MRI features of multiple sclerosis and ADEM. The figure contrasts the typical MRI features of MS and ADEM. (a) Axial fluid-attenuated inversion recovery (FLAIR) image: the typical MRI appearance of MS is characterized by multifocal, ovoid bright lesions with a predilection for the periventricular white matter. (b) Axial FLAIR image: MRI lesions in ADEM tend to be large, with ill-defined borders. Cortical involvement is commonly seen, as is involvement of the deep gray nuclei (not shown). (c) Sagittal T2 image: spinal MRI image demonstrates multiple, small spinal lesions in a patient with MS. (d) Sagittal T2 image: spinal MRI in a patient with ADEM with a single lesion extending longitudinally over multiple spinal cord segments.

In a prospective study, 132 children with ADEM were followed to determine factors predictive of MS. A first presentation that included optic neuritis, a family history of demyelination, MRI features meeting the criteria for lesion dissemination in space were associated with risk of a second demyelinating event. A longitudinal study of 84 children with ADEM followed for a mean of 6.6 years found multiphasic ADEM in 10%, none of whom met the criteria for MS. In a study of adults with ADEM, 38% were ultimately diagnosed with MS – no clinical, MRI, or CSF finding distinguished these patients from those with monophasic disease.

Pathobiology

Pathological studies of ADEM are restricted to biopsies of tumefactive lesions and autopsy studies of extremely fulminant disease. Pathological features that appear to distinguish ADEM from typical MS include: (1) all lesions appear to be of similar age; (2) inflammatory cells in ADEM tend to congregate in a sleeve-like pattern around CNS venules; and (3) inflammatory cells may invade vessel walls. Acute hemorrhagic leukoencephalitis (AHLE), a severe form of ADEM, is characterized by necrotizing angiitis of the venules and capillaries with ball and ring hemorrhage, myelin edema, and demyelination.

There are many similarities between ADEM and a model of acquired demyelination, experimental autoimmune encephalomyelitis (EAE). In EAE, myelin-reactive T cells lead to inflammatory demyelination. The frequency of myelin-reactive T cells is 10-fold higher in patients with ADEM relative to controls. T cells from patients recovering from ADEM secrete the Th2 cytokine interleukin 4.

In summary, prototypical ADEM is an acute, transient demyelinating illness of the CNS. Biomarkers that reliably distinguish ADEM from an ADEM-like first MS attack would be of enormous clinical importance.

Table 103.3 Diagnostic considerations in a patient with ADEM.

Disorder	Key clinical clues	Investigations
CNS infection	• Persistent fever • Systemic evidence of infection • Predominantly gray matter involvement • Exposure to infected contacts, or endemic exposures	• Blood and CSF cell counts and cultures, and PCR testing for infection • TB testing • Fungal cultures
Vasculitis, vasculopathy, and sarcoidosis	• Persistent and prominent headache • Systemic evidence of vasculitis (arthritis, carditis, rash) • *Note*: clinical, laboratory, and radiographic evidence of systemic disease may be absent in isolated CNS vasculitis	• ESR, CRP, ANA, dsDNA • ACE level • Antiphospholipid and anticardiolipin antibodies • CXR • MRA • Cerebral angiography • Brain biopsy
Malignancy	• History of prior malignancy	• Blood smear • CSF cytology • Brain biopsy
Macrophage activation syndromes	• Young age (typically less than 2 years) • History of similarly affected sibling or consanguineous parentage • Systemic signs of liver, skin, renal, or bone marrow involvement • Persistent fever	• Serum ferritin and triglycerides • Blood and bone marrow analysis for hemophagocytosis • Perforin expression in lymphocytes
Multiple sclerosis	• History of prior transient neurological deficits • Fatigue • Recurrent disease • Family history of MS	• CSF OCBs • Serial MRI scans • Rigorous and longitudinal observation

ACE: angiotensin converting enzyme; ADEM: acute disseminated encephalomyelitis; ANA: antinuclear antibodies; CNS: central nervous system; CRP: C-reactive protein; CSF: cerebrospinal fluid; CXR: chest X-ray; dsDNA: double-stranded DNA; ESR: erythrocyte sedimentation rate; MRA: magnetic resonance angiography; MRI: magnetic resonance imaging; MS: multiple sclerosis; OCBs: oligoclonal bands; PCR: polymerase chain reaction; TB: tuberculosis.

Further reading

Brass SD, Caramanos Z, Santos C, Dilenge ME, Lapierre Y, Rosenblatt B. Multiple sclerosis vs acute disseminated encephalomyelitis in childhood. *Pediatr Neurol* 2003; 29(3): 227–31.

Dale RC, de Sousa C, Chong WK, Cox TC, Harding B, Neville BG. Acute disseminated encephalomyelitis, multiphasic disseminated encephalomyelitis and multiple sclerosis in children. *Brain* 2000; 123(Pt 12): 2407–22.

Hahn J, Pohl D, Rensel M, Rao S, for the International Pediatric MS Study Group. Differential diagnosis and evaluation in pediatric multiple sclerosis. *Neurology* 2007; 68: S13–22.

Hollinger P, Sturzenegger M, Mathis J, Schroth G, Hess CW. Acute disseminated encephalomyelitis in adults: a reappraisal of clinical, CSF, EEG, and MRI findings. *J Neurol* 2002; 249(3): 320–9.

Hynson JL, Kornberg AJ, Coleman LT, Shield L, Harvey AS, Kean MJ. Clinical and neuroradiologic features of acute disseminated encephalomyelitis in children. *Neurology* 2001; 56(10): 1308–12.

Krupp L, Banwell B, Tenembaum S, for the International Pediatric MS Study Group. Consensus definitions proposed for pediatric multiple sclerosis. *Neurology* 2007; 68: S7–12.

Leake JA, Albani S, Kao AS, *et al.* Acute disseminated encephalomyelitis in childhood: epidemiologic, clinical and laboratory features. *Pediatr Infect Dis J* 2004; 23(8): 756–64.

Mikaeloff Y, Caridade G, Husson B, Suissa S, Tardieu M. Acute disseminated encephalomyelitis cohort study: prognostic factors for relapse. *Eur J Paediatr Neurol* 2007; 11(2): 90–5.

Murthy JM, Yangala R, Meena AK, Jaganmohan RJ. Acute disseminated encephalomyelitis: clinical and MRI study from South India. *J Neurol Sci* 1999; 165(2): 133–8.

Murthy SN, Faden HS, Cohen ME, Bakshi R. Acute disseminated encephalomyelitis in children. *Pediatrics* 2002; 110(2 Pt 1): e21.

Schwarz S, Mohr A, Knauth M, Wildemann B, Storch-Hagenlocher B. Acute disseminated encephalomyelitis: a follow-up study of 40 adult patients. *Neurology* 2001; 56(10): 1313–18.

Tenembaum S, Chamoles N, Fejerman N. Acute disseminated encephalomyelitis: a long-term follow-up study of 84 pediatric patients. *Neurology* 2002; 59(8): 1224–31.

Chapter 104
Osmotic demyelination syndromes

Ovidiu Bajenaru
University Hospital of Emergency, Bucharest, Romania

Introduction

Osmotic demyelination syndrome (ODS) is a clinicopathologic entity first described by Adams *et al.* in 1959 in chronic alcoholic patients as central pontine myelinolysis and defined pathologically as a symmetric area of myelin disruption in the center of the basis pontis. During the following years, patients have been described with similar lesions preferentially in the basis pontis but also with extrapontine myelinolysis or only in other brain areas without pons injury. The most often identified cause of this condition is the rapid medical correction of chronic hyponatremia.

Epidemiology

ODS is not a common medical condition. There are no epidemiological data concerning its prevalence or incidence. Initial descriptions of ODS were based on autopsy findings, so it has been considered as a medical entity with a high mortality. As imaging techniques have improved diagnosis and supportive care has also advanced, two types of consequences emerged: the number of survivors with or without neurologic sequelae reported is greater than initially expected, but also new difficulties in differentiating ODS from other pathologic entities have appeared.

Pathophysiology

ODS most often seems to be a consequence of a hyperosmotically-induced demyelination process, resulting from rapid intracellular/extracellular to intravascular water shifts producing relative glial dehydration and myelin degradation and/or oligodendroglial apoptosis. When chronic hyponatremia is rapidly corrected, reaccumulation of brain organic osmolytes is delayed and

brain cell shrinkage occurs, finally leading to ODS. To date, experimental models demonstrate brain demyelination only when sodium is rapidly corrected and not with gradual correction. However, these models do not take into account the underlying disorders that may be present in patients. Therefore, the nature and degree of insult required to trigger osmotic injury remains unclear, as long as normonatremic patients (alcoholic cirrhosis and intravenous fluid resuscitation, therapy with alpha-interferon) and those with hypernatremia (hyperosmolar diabetic coma, hypernatremia after peritoneal lavage with saline solution) have also been reported to develop ODS. Histologic characteristics of ODS include symmetric, midline demyelinating lesions in the pons and/or extrapontine areas (mostly in the bundles of myelinated fibers in the gray matter and in the white matter surrounded by massive gray matter, including the cerebellar and neocortical white/gray matter junctional areas, thalamus, and striatum, and even hippocampus), loss of oligodendrocytes, reactive gliosis, and relative preservation of axons. Proposed hypotheses concerning the mechanism of development of ODS include osmotic injury to the endothelium resulting in myelinotoxic factors or vasogenic edema and brain dehydration resulting in separation of the axon from its myelin sheath with resultant injury of oligodendrocytes, particularly at the interfaces of gray and white matter. Recent studies imply other mechanisms including (1) a decreased concentration of Na, K-ATPase in endothelial cell membrane in hyponatremia complicated by hypokalaemia; (2) particular vulnerability of oligodendrocytes to apoptosis; (3) a detrimental role of microglia with massive accumulation in demyelinating lesions which expressed the pro-inflammatory cytokines; and (4) complement activation following blood–brain barrier disruption.

Clinical features

As chronic hyponatremia is the most frequent condition associated with ODS, the first step in the diagnosis is the recognition of the predisposing risk factors for this electrolyte derangement. As mentioned, the first described patients with ODS were chronic alcoholic patients. The

International Neurology: A Clinical Approach. Edited by Robert P. Lisak, Daniel D. Truong, William M. Carroll, and Roongroj Bhidayasiri.
© 2009 Blackwell Publishing, ISBN: 978-1-4051-5738-4.

association with alcoholism continues to be particularly frequent (in up to 40% of cases), probably because alcohol itself interferes with sodium/water regulation by supression of antidiuretic hormone and also because these patients usually have inadequate nutrition. Other reported risk factors associated with ODS are liver disease and liver transplantation, sepsis, acute pancreatitis (particularly the necroticohemorrhagic form), adrenal insufficiency, the syndrome of inappropriate secretion of antidiuretic hormone (and the etiological conditions generating this syndrome), amyotrophic lateral sclerosis, use of antineoplastic agents such as cyclophosphamide, and use of drugs such as angiotensin converting enzyme inhibitors and thiazide diuretics. Anorexia nervosa represents a particular condition in which serum electrolyte abnormalities are attribuable to malnutrition, excessive water intake, or laxative and/or diuretic misuse follwed by rapid correction. Though hemodialysis has been reported as a risk factor for ODS, the frequency of this association is much less than one would expect, probably because urea is acting in renal failure as an "ineffective solute" that contributes to measured osmolarity but does not contribute to hypertonicity because it easily crosses cell membranes, thus protecting from the rapid shifts in sodium content. In some cases of neurological disturbances suspected to be due to ODS associated with first hemodialysis, the MRI apparent diffusion coefficient (ADC) map shows changes suggestive of interstitial brain edema (increased ADC). Similarly, ODS is very rare in diabetes mellitus despite the frequent electrolyte derangements and pronounced shifts in osmolarity.

It is important to mention that the clinical manifestations of ODS usually develop after a delay of some days (on average 4–6 days) after changes in sodium levels.

The classical presentation of ODS is related to its most frequent topographic location of lesions in the CNS: the central pons. The most suggestive clinical manifestations are dysphagia, dysarthria, ophthalmoplegia, and focal or generalized weakness progressing to quadriplegia. Less frequently, the central pons involvement generates a clinical picture of the "locked-in" syndrome. Extrapontine demyelinating lesions (usually but not always associated with central pontine involvement) have been described as having clinical manifestations in only 10% of cases. These include ataxia, parkinsonism, athetosis, dystonia, confusion, behavioral or personality changes, hallucinations, seizures, catatonia, and akinetic mutism, depending on the areas of the brain involved. However, extrapyramidal symptoms are less frequent because often they are masked by effects of pyramidal tract lesions and brainstem dysfunction. Symptoms may progress over days, and in severe cases may lead to coma or death or survival in a prolonged vegetative state, sometimes accompanied by myoclonus.

Differing from the classical view concerning the prognosis of ODS, modern imaging techniques have shown that some patients have a favorable prognosis, with clinical improvement during the following months after the acute stage of the disease. In many cases the improvement is associated with resolution of the lesions detected by MRI. There are more cases reported with movement disorders as sequelae of ODS, as parkinsonism, dystonia, or myoclonus associated or not with cognitive disorders. Of particular interest is the observation that the parkinsonism after ODS is usually dopa-responsive.

Investigations

Modern non-invasive imaging techniques, in particular MRI, have superseded auditory evoked potentials and CT scan. Today, brain MRI is the imaging technique of choice because it is superior to CT for the demonstration of lesions in central pons but especially of the extrapontine osmotic demyelinating lesions. These are hyperintense on T2- and hypointense on T1-weighted images. It is important to note that the MRI lesions can be significantly delayed in appearance, so in some instances it is necessary to repeat the MRI after 10–14 days. Bilateral changes in MRI signals may be seen in other conditions as well, including perinatal hypoxic-ischemic injury, carbon monoxide poisoning, and metabolic disorders. Patchy multifocal signal change may be seen also in acute disseminated encephalomyelitis, and other encephalitides such as Creutzfeldt–Jakob disease, small vessel disease, inflammatory microangiopathies, and mitochondrial diseases. Diffusion weighted imaging (DWI) has the capability of detecting lesions not detected on T2. In some cases DWI could help differentiate among demyelinating lesions and vasogenic edema. In other conditions, such as the posterior reversible encephalopathy syndrome, DWI cannot reliably differentiate from ODS but only in correlation with the clinical etiopathological context.

Treatment

As ODS frequently develops after the aggressive treatment of hyponatremia by any method, including water restriction, prevention of ODS by extremely cautious treatment of hyponatremia is required especially if hyponatremia has been present longer than 48 hours. There is no consensus about the optimal treatment of symptomatic hyponatremia, but a 5% increase in serum sodium concentration, not exceeding 12 mmol/l/day, is recommended as a reasonable target.

There are no clinical trials for treatment of established ODS. Supportive treatment is recommended. There are small case series reporting different therapies including corticosteroids, intravenous immunoglobulins, and thyrotropin-releasing factor, but results are difficult to interpret. Controlled clinical trials now underway will help to elucidate the role of arginine–vasopressin receptor antagonism in the treatment of hyponatremia.

Further reading

Adrogue HJ, Madias NE. Hyponatremia. *N Engl J Med* 2000; 342(21): 1581–9.

Chen CL, Lai PH, Chou KJ, Lee PT, Chung HM, Fang HC. A preliminary report of brain edema in patients with uremia at first hemodialysis: evaluation by diffusion-weighted MR imaging. *Am J Neuroradiol* 2007; 28(1): 68–71.

Martin RJ. Central pontine and extrapontine myelinolysis: the osmotic demyelination syndromes. *J Neurol Neurosurg Psychiatry* 2004; 75(Suppl 3): iii22–iii28.

Tomita I, Satoh H, Satoh A, Seto M, Tsujihata M, Yoshimura T. Extrapontine myelinolysis presenting with parkinsonism as a sequel of rapid correction of hyponatremia. *J Neurol Neurosurg Psychiatry* 1997; 62(4): 422–3.

Chapter 105
Concentric sclerosis (Baló's disease)

Takeshi Tabira

Graduate School of Juntendo University, Tokyo, Japan

Introduction

Concentric sclerosis is a demyelinating disease of the central nervous system (CNS), which is characterized by the annual ring-like alternate pattern of demyelinating and myelin preserved regions. The first case showing such lesions was reported by Otto Marburg in 1906 as "akute multiple sclerosis." Twenty years later, a similar case was reported by Joseph Baló as "encephalitis periaxialis concentrica." Because of the pathological characteristics, it is now widely accepted as "concentric sclerosis or Baló's concentric sclerosis (disease)." Although it is a rare condition worldwide, increased prevalence has been observed in the Philippines.

Pathology

Seventeen autopsy cases were collected in the Philippines from 1981 to 1999. All cases showed the typical concentric pattern of demyelination (Figure 105.1). Histologic studies demonstrate both demyelination and some axonal damage. Perivascular cuffs are seen in active demyelinating areas in one study and inflammatory cells include CD4, CD8, T-cells, and macropaghes. It has been suggested by some that there are aspects of the type III lesions described in relapsing–remitting MS (RRMS) that show similarities, on a smaller scale, to Balo's concentric sclerosis.

Epidemiology

In the pathologically verified cases the age of onset was 19–49 years (mean = 32.5) and the male to female ratio was 1:1.8. The Philippines is located in the tropical zone with high temperatures of over 30°C all year around; it is relatively cooler in October–January and is extremely hot in April–June. There was no seasonal preference in

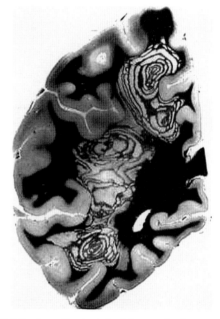

Figure 105.1 Section of brain stained for myelin demonstrating the typical pattern of demyelination in Balo's concentric sclerosis.

the disease appearance. The Philippines is composed of thousands of islands on 5–20°N. Main islands are Luzon, Mindanao, Negros, Panay, Samar, Mindoro, Cebu, and Leyte. The cases were collected in Luzon and Cebu because of the presence of autopsy facilities, but patients were seen in all areas of the Philippines. There was no particular overrepresented occupation or evidence to indicate it was contagious. Since the late 1990s the disease abruptly disappeared in the Philippines.

Clinical

Prodromal symptoms and signs such as fever and headache were present in 8 of 14 patients 4–30 days prior to onset of the disease. Reticence (muteness), urinary incontinence, and pyramidal signs were present in all patients. Generalized seizure was observed in 4 out of 16 cases. All cases except for one showed acute onset of the disease and died during the acute stage. One case showed a relapse

International Neurology: A Clinical Approach. Edited by Robert P. Lisak, Daniel D. Truong, William M. Carroll, and Roongroj Bhidayasiri.
© 2009 Blackwell Publishing, ISBN: 978-1-4051-5738-4.

4 years after the first attack, and died on the 28th day of the second attack. Ten patients died of secondary infection such as pneumonia and sepsis. It is interesting to note that four cases died of brain herniation. Duration of the illness was 5 days to 8 months (mean = 2.38 months) except for one which showed a relapse. There are some atypical presentations, but the clinical course, although not the pathology, is similar to what is now often called Marburg's variant of MS, a rapidly progressive "acute MS." The relationship between Baló's disease, particularly as described from the Phillipines, Marburg's acute MS, and Baló-like lesions in more typical MS is not clear.

Laboratory findings

Cerebrospinal fluid (CSF) findings were subtle. White blood cells (WBCs) were increased in 5 out of 15 cases, and the highest count was $59/mm^3$. Total protein was also mildly elevated (44–100 mg/dl) in 5 of the 15 cases.

WBCs in the peripheral blood were elevated in 10 of the 15 cases, but this was thought due to be secondary to infections.

Imaging

MRI scan can be suggestive of concentric sclerosis with large lesions which enhance in layers and are inhomogeneous on T2. Although such lesions are highly suggestive of this disease, other conditions such as infections or tumors must be ruled out.

Treatment

There have been no large series and no controlled clinical trials. Treatment with corticosteroids has been reported to have some effect in case reports/small series.

Further reading

Baló J. Encephalitis periaxialis concentrica. *Arch Neurol Psychiat* 1928; 19: 242–64.

Kuroiwa Y. Concentric sclerosis. In: Koetsier JC, editor. *Demyelinating Diseases*. Amsterdam: Elsevier; 1985, pp. 409–17.

Marburg O. Die sogenannte "akute multiple sklerose" (encephalomyelitis periaxialis scleroticans). *J Psychiatr Neurol* 1906; 27: 217–312.

Tselis AC, Lisak RP. Other deymyelinating diseases. In: Freedman MS, editor. *Multiple Sclerosis and Demyelinating Diseases. Advances in Neurology*, Vol. 98. Philadelphia: Lippincott Williams & Wilkins; 2006, pp. 335–49.

Chapter 106
Neurotoxicology

Nai-Shin Chu[1,2] *and Chin-Chang Huang*[1,2]
[1]Chang Gung University College of Medicine, Taipei, Taiwan
[2]Chang Gung Memorial Hospital, Taipei, Taiwan

Introduction

Neurotoxicity deals with the adverse effects on the structure and/or function of the nervous system that are caused by exposure to chemical, biological, or physical agents. These neurotoxic effects are manifest at many levels of the neuronal organization, leading to a disorder or disease.

Hundreds of agents are recognized as having neurotoxic potential in humans. These agents may have direct or indirect effects on the nervous system. The nervous system is particularly vulnerable because it has complex structure and function, it has a prolonged period of development, and even after maturation it is very active and has a high metabolic demand. Therefore, the nervous system's vulnerability to toxic agents depends heavily on its developmental state and the post-developmental functional specialization.

According to Schaumburg there are five well-recognized sources of postnatal human neurotoxic disorders: (1) pharmaceutical agents; (2) biological neurotoxic agents; (3) environmental chemical exposure; (4) occupational chemical exposure; and (5) self-administration of harmful agents. Therefore, many disorders are not necessarily caused by occupational or environmental exposure, but are patient initiated. Clinicians should be aware of these possibilities when dealing with neurotoxic diseases.

The chapter is divided into eight sections: (1) heavy metal intoxication, (2) pesticides, (3) food poisoning, (4) industrial intoxication, (5) household accident, (6) bacterial toxins, (7) plant toxins, and (8) regionally specific toxicities.

Heavy metal intoxication

Arsenic

Exposure to potentially toxic levels of arsenic may occur from drinking contaminated groundwater, working in mining and ore-smelting plants, accidental ingestion of pesticides, and, infamously, intentional homicidal ingestions. Most cases of acute arsenic poisoning are due to accidental ingestion of pesticides or insecticides, or by inhalation in occupational settings.

Both neuropathy and encephalopathy are common manifestations of acute arsenic exposure. Clinical features may include nausea, vomiting, bloody diarrhea, dizziness, diffuse muscle weakness, numbness, and paresthesia of the distal extremities. Respiratory symptoms can be seen in cases of inhalation exposure. Hypotension, cardiac arrhythmias, myoglobulinuria, and acute renal failure are not infrequent. In severe cases, seizures, coma, and death may follow.

Chronic encephalopathy is more common after exposure to organic arsenic than inorganic arsenic. The symptoms may include confusion, irritability, paranoid delusions, and auditory or visual hallucinations.

The neuropathy is a painful, axonal, length-dependent, sensory, peripheral axonopathy affecting all extremities. Symptoms usually begin 2–3 weeks after initial exposure and start with pain in the distal lower extremities, eventually involving the distal upper extremities.

Systemic abnormalities that may provide important clues to the diagnosis include weight loss, severe alopecia, and white horizontal lines on the nails (Mees' lines). Diagnosis can be confirmed by detecting elevated arsenic levels in the blood, urine, hair, or nail clippings.

Standard treatment consists of elimination of continued arsenic exposure and removal of arsenic by use of sulfur chelators, including dimercaptosuccinic acid or *D*-penicillamine.

Lead
Due to its extensive commercial use, lead has historically been one of the most common sources of heavy metal intoxication. Lead toxicity may occur from occupational exposure, that is, metal soldering, ore smelting, battery manufacturing, or industrial painting, or from non-occupational exposure, that is, accidental ingestion of lead paint by children, or exposure to contaminated water and foods. Children are at particular risk from oral ingestion of paint chips or contaminated soil.

International Neurology: A Clinical Approach. Edited by Robert P. Lisak, Daniel D. Truong, William M. Carroll, and Roongroj Bhidayasiri.
© 2009 Blackwell Publishing, ISBN: 978-1-4051-5738-4.

Characteristic systemic features of lead poisoning are abdominal pain, constipation, and a microcytic, hypochromic anemia. In general, peripheral neuropathy is commonly seen in adults, whereas acute lead encephalopathy is most common in children.

The peripheral neuropathy of lead toxicity is a pure motor neuropathy affecting the upper limbs more than the lower limbs, presenting as a symmetric or asymmetric wrist drop. The weakness may also involve other muscle groups of the distal upper extremities. Involvement of lower extremities, including isolated foot drop, also may occur.

Electrophysiologic studies reveal a wide range of abnormalities, from mild motor conduction slowing to denervation, indicating axonal involvement. Nerve biopsy reveals increased paranodal demyelination and internodal remyelination in mild-to-moderate neuropathies, and axonal degeneration in advanced neuropathies.

Symptoms of acute lead encephalopathy include lethargy, irritability, confusion, ataxia, and impaired motor functions. Chronic low-level lead exposure also causes encephalopathy. The symptoms are similar to those of acute lead toxicity, but the onset is insidious. The long-term effects of chronic low-level lead exposure have especially devastating effects on the still-developing nervous system of young children.

Laboratory diagnostic indicators of lead toxicity include elevated blood lead level, decreased blood delta-aminolevulinic acid (ALA-D), and basophilic stippling on blood smear.

Treatment requires eliminating continued exposure and initiating therapy to enhance excretion with chelating agents, such as ethylenediaminetetraacetic acid (EDTA), penicillamine, and British antilewisite.

Manganese

Manganese was initially used by the Egyptians and Romans in the manufacture of glass and ceramic. Today, it is widely employed in industry, primarily in the manufacture of steel and alloys. Several hundred cases of manganese poisoning have been reported, not only from mining regions of Chile, Egypt, Cuba, Morocco, India, and China, but also from industrial countries processing this metal for metal alloys, dry-cell batteries, paints, varnish, enamel, colored glass, and an antiknock agent in lead-free gasoline. Rarely, central nervous system (CNS) manganism occurs in agricultural workers who have chronic exposure to fungicide containing manganese.

The history of manganese neurotoxicity dates back to 1837, when Couper of Glasgow first reported a peculiar neurological syndrome somewhat similar to Parkinson's disease in five men working in a manganese ore-crushing plant in France. This report of "manganese crusher's disease" appeared only 20 years after Parkinson's essay on the shaking palsy in 1817.

Chronic manganese toxicity causes an extrapyramidal syndrome with features resembling those found in Parkinson's disease, Wilson's disease, and postencephalitic parkinsonism.

The clinical course of manganism can be divided into three phases: an initial phase of subjective symptoms, with or without a psychotic episode, lasting for a few months; an intermediate phase of evolving neurological symptoms, again for a few months; and an established phase with persisting neurological deficits. The onset is usually insidious and progressive. In general, miners have more severe neurological deficits than victims of other types of exposure.

The initial symptoms are usually subjective and non-specific, and may include fatigue, restlessness, headache, poor memory, reduced concentration, apathy, insomnia, diminished libido, somnolence, lumbago, muscle aches and cramps, and a generalized slowing of movement. Usually seen in miners, an episode of psychomotor excitement can be among the presenting symptoms, which include nervousness, irritability, nightmare, emotional lability, aggressive and destructive behavior, and bizarre compulsive acts. It has been referred to as *locura manganica* or "manganese madness."

In the intermediate phase, speech becomes monotonous, low in volume, halting, and sometimes stuttering; the face is expressionless with dazed appearance and intermittent grimace; handwriting can become tremulous, micrographic, and cramped; movements are generally slow and clumsy; gait is often impaired, body turn tends to be "en bloc," and walking backward is particularly difficult.

In the established phase, there is aggravation of neurological deficits and walking difficulty becomes more pronounced. A peculiar wide-based slapping gait and dystonic posturing of the foot with sustained plantar flexion may be seen and is termed "cock-walk" (Figure 106.1). Inability to walk backward because of severe retropulsion

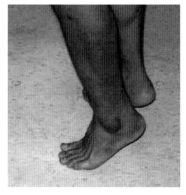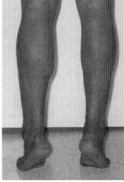

Figure 106.1 "Cock walk" posture and foot dystonia. Note that the patient walks on the metatarsopharyngeal joints.

is generally the most striking feature. Tremor is not a common finding, but when it does occur, it is usually postural rather than resting, and of low amplitude. Dystonic features are common, and tend to involve the face and foot.

Neurological deficits tend to become established 1–2 years after onset of the disease. Thereafter, neurological deficits may remain stable or improve following cessation of exposure, or continue to progress, even after elimination of the source of exposure. In our long-term, 20-year follow-up study, neurological symptoms continued to progress in the first 10 years and then stabilized in the second 10 years.

Neuropathological studies, although few, have consistently shown that the hallmark is the degeneration of the basal ganglia, principally confined to the medial segment of the globus pallidus and the pars reticulata of the substantia nigra. The putamen and the caudate nuclei are often affected, but to a lesser degree.

Our positron emission tomography (PET) studies, employing 6-fluorodopa to investigate the integrity of the dopaminergic nigrostraital pathways and D2 receptor ligand raclopride to investigate the dopaminergic postsynaptic function, are found to be generally normal. Our recent study on dopamine transporter binding using ^{99m}Tc-TRODAT-1 single photon emission computed tomography (SPECT) also reveals only a slight decrease in the uptake in the putamen in patients with manganism when compared to normal subjects, indicating that presynaptic dopaminergic terminals are not the main target of chronic manganese intoxication.

Although *L*-dopa has been shown to be effective in some reports, others have failed to detect a meaningful improvement.

Mercury

Neurological damage may occur in adults and children after poisoning with mercury compounds due to occupational exposure to fungicides containing organic mercury, ingestion of grain treated with these fungicides, or consumption of fish and shellfish contaminated by industrial wastes containing organic mercury (Minamata disease). Rarely, poisoning may result from inhalation of elementary mercury vapor in factories reprocessing mercury batteries or in glass blowers.

Mercury exists in elemental, organic, and inorganic forms. It is the only metal that is in a liquid state in its elemental form. The inorganic form may be classified in accordance with the oxidative state of the metal, whereas the organic form may covalently bind to an organic (carbon-containing) moiety, either as arylmercury or alkylmercury. The arylmercury is readily degraded into inorganic mercury ions in the biological system, whereas the alkylmercury is relatively stable and resists biodegradation.

Various forms of mercury are found in household items, manufacturing products, and water supplies. Among them, elementary mercury vapor and alkylmercury compounds are considered to be most neurotoxic.

Elemental mercury

Metallic mercury vaporizes readily even at room temperature. When inhaled, mercury vapor is efficiently absorbed through the alveolar membrane and has high affinity for the CNS, especially gray matters of the occipital cortex, the cerebellum, and various nuclei of the brainstem.

Prolonged exposure to mercury vapor, generally the result of occupational exposure, produces "battery refiner's disease" in workers reprocessing mercury batteries. The syndrome consists of a fairly well-defined set of neurologic and psychiatric features including fatigue, tremor, poor memory, cognitive impairment, social withdrawal, excitability, personality change, and emotional lability. In more severe cases, a fine trembling tremor appears in the fingers, tongue, eyelids, and lips. In addition, there is a progressive and incapacitating movement disorder consisting of titubation, truncal ataxia, generalized tremor, and multifocal myoclonus. Visual field may be constricted. The combination of increased excitability, tremor, and gingivitis has been thought as the classic triad of chronic mercury exposure.

Inorganic mercury salts

Human mercurous mercury poisoning is mainly due to the use of calomel in children's teething powder in the early twentieth century. Because of the redness of the hands and feet, it is referred to as "pink disease." Symptoms include acrodynia, photophobia, profuse sweating, anorexia, and insomnia. However, the primary target for mercuric salts is the kidney.

Neurotoxicity from mercury salts is usually not prominent, although prolonged exposure to mercuric oxide and mercuric nitrate may result in "mad hatter syndrome," which historically affected workers in the felt hat industry. This syndrome is similar to that observed in mercury vapor poisoning.

Organomercury compounds

The most neurotoxic compounds are methylmercury and ethylmercury, and the most notorious poisoning was the massive outbreak of methylmercury intoxication in Japan in the 1950s. It is called "Minamata disease" because it occurred in Minamata Bay, Kumamoto, due to industrial dumping of mercury-containing waste into the water supply. After entering the water, mercury was methylated by microorganisms and in turn ingested by aquatic species, that is, fish and shellfish, that were finally consumed by humans.

Neurological manifestations of methylmercury toxicity are paresthesia, tremor, ataxia, spasticity, visual and hearing loss, and encephalopathy. Prominent features are ataxia, chorea, athetosis, ballismus-like movements, and coarse tremor. Cognitive and memory deficits may be present. In severe cases, coma and death may occur.

The pathological hallmark of mercury poisoning is severe damage affecting the visual cortex and the granule cell layer of the cerebellum. In the cerebral cortex, degeneration and loss of neurons with gliosis are found. Damage to the basal ganglia, especially the putamen, is frequent and usually moderate to severe, but may be minimal.

Thallium

Thallium salts have been used for the treatment of many diseases, including tuberculosis, gonorrhea, syphilis, and scalp fungal infection. Recently, thallium has been utilized in the manufacturing of optical lenses, semiconductors, scintillation counters, imitation jewelry, and chemical catalysts.

Thallium toxicity generally occurs after ingestion of thallium-containing chemicals, rat poison, or contaminated foods. An outbreak of thallium poisoning was reported in California in 1932 and attributed to the use of a rodenticide for control of a ground squirrel infestation. Thallium poisoning has become rare after thallium was banned from use in pesticides in the 1970s. Currently, thallium toxicity is seen only in unintentional ingestion, usually linked to attempted homicides.

The clinical manifestations of acute thallium poisoning consist of the characteristic dermatological findings of alopecia, hyperkeratosis, and Mees' lines on the nails, as well as neurological symptoms including dysesthesia, painful neuropathy, muscle weakness, cranial nerve palsies, ataxia, tremor, convulsions, coma, and death.

Painful neuropathy is usually severe and excruciating, and is often the most prominent symptom of thallium poisoning. A debilitating encephalopathy may also occur and its symptoms may include hallucinations, paranoia, and cognitive impairment. The term "encephalopathia thallica" implies a variety of conditions, from giddiness, lack of drive, and memory impairment to a decline in intelligence and irreversible dementia. It should be pointed out that neuropathic and systemic symptoms of thallium toxicity are strikingly similar to those of arsenic poisoning.

Electrodiagnostic and nerve biopsy findings are consistent with an axonal degeneration primarily of the distal nerves involving both large and small myelinated fibers, and even unmyelinated fibers, particularly in the lower extremities.

There is no specific therapy for neuropathy and encephalopathy, but gastric lavage, activated charcoal, hemodialysis, and Prussian blue may assist in blocking further absorption and facilitating elimination.

Pesticides

Organophosphates

Organophosphates have been used in several major industries including pesticides, helminthicides, petroleum additives, modifiers of plastics, and chemical warfare. Organophosphates can be easily absorbed through pulmonary alveoli, skin, eyes, and the gastrointestinal tract following intentional (suicidal) ingestion, accidental exposure, or homicidal attempts. Most organophosphates can cause an acute cholinergic crisis via inhibition of acetylcholinesterase and then an intermediate syndrome because of neuromuscular junction block. Occasionally a delayed peripheral neuropathy may occur 2–3 weeks after exposure.

Acute effects of organophosphates are caused by slowly reversible or irreversible binding to acetylcholinesterase, leading to increased bronchial secretion, sweating, abdominal pain, and diarrhea. CNS effects include convulsions, confusion, irritability, and anxiety. Overactivity of nicotinic function may produce fasciculation and muscle weakness.

The intermediate syndrome usually develops within 24–96 hours after poisoning and affects the bulbar and ocular muscles, neck flexors, proximal limb muscles, and respiratory muscles. Electromyographic studies show fade on titanic stimulation, absence of fade on low-frequency stimulation, and absence of post-titanic facilitation, indicating a postsynaptic defect. The neuromuscular function defect has been the predominant cause of the paralytic symptoms. Atropine therapy has no effect on the intermediate syndrome.

Some organophosphates can produce delayed axonopathy with muscle cramps, muscle weakness, paresthesias, and decreased or absent tendon reflexes following single exposure. The pathogenetic mechanisms are inhibition and aging of the enzyme-neuropathy target esterase. The delayed neuropathy involves motor and sensory function and even myelopathy. Recovery is sometimes incomplete with residual muscle weakness and spasticity.

Triorthocresyl phosphate (TOCP) is a lipid-soluble, oily substance and its intoxication has been found in axonal neuropathy epidemics after drinking the adulterated Jamaica ginger extract known as "Jake." Severe damage to the peripheral nervous system (PNS) and spinal cord has resulted in permanent "Jake leg paralysis" in the United States.

Electrophysiological studies vary during the course of exposure in the acute, intermediate, and delayed syndromes. In acute intoxication and the intermediate syndrome, an atypical decremental response to repetitive nerve stimulation can be observed. In the delayed neuropathy, nerve conduction studies show reduced sensory and motor responses with signs of denervation.

The drug of choice in the treatment of acute muscarinic effects is atropine. Phosphorylated cholinesterase can be treated with oxime compounds such as pyrine-2-aldoxime methylchloride (2-PAM pralidoxime).

Food poisoning

Mushroom poisoning

Exposure to poisonous mushrooms usually occurs by accidental ingestion or in the setting of intended recreational use. Mushrooms that predominantly affect the nervous system produce an immediate response. Poisonous mushrooms belong to the genus *Amanita*, including *A. muscaria*, *A. regalis*, and *A. panthirina*, and the genus *Psilocybe*.

The CNS toxicity of *A. muscaria* is due to ibotenic acid and its derivative, muscimol. Ibotenic acid has structural and functional similarities to the excitatory neurotransmitter glutamate. It is estimated to be approximately eight times more active than glutamate and equipotent to *N*-methyl-*D*-aspartate (NMDA) in provoking the activity of cat spinal interneurons and Renshaw cells. In human experiments, both *Amanita* and muscimol poisonings produce ataxia, myoclonic jerks, somnolence, and euphoria. The effects of muscimol cannot be distinguished from those of ibotenic acid.

The CNS symptoms often include alterations in mental status, visual changes, hallucinations, agitation, and ataxia. In severe cases, seizures and psychosis may occur. Muscle fasciculations and anticholinergic symptoms such as flushing, mydriasis, and urinary retention are commonly seen.

Psilocybe mushrooms contain psilocybin and its more potent metabolite psilocin. These indolealkylamines are structurally similar to serotonin and interact with CNS receptors to produce a lysergic acid diethylamide (LSD)-like syndrome, including visual illusions, vivid hallucinations, euphoria, and reckless behavior. Anxiety, drowsiness, and dysphonia are common. Flushing, hypertension, tachycardia, and hyperthermia also occur frequently.

The acute neurotoxicity of mushrooms typically resolves completely and without chronic sequelae.

Industrial intoxication

Acrylamide

Acrylamide, a water-soluble, vinyl monomer, is an important industrial compound and has been widely used in chemical industries, including polyacrylamides such as flocculants for waste-water treatment, cosmetics, soil stabilization, adhesives, and grouts, and polyacrylamide gels in molecular laboratories.

Acrylamide monomer can be absorbed via inhalation, ingestion, and skin exposures, and is toxic to the PNS and CNS, while the acrylamide polymer is not. Numbness, muscle weakness in the distal limbs, and diffuse hyporeflexia or areflexia are experienced in the initial stage of acute intoxication. Action or intention tremor and a wide-based gait are common early signs. Excessive sweating, peeling skin, and contact dermatitis are frequently found.

The motor nerve conduction studies are characterized by mild abnormalities with reduced motor conduction velocities, while sensory nerve conduction studies are almost abnormal, particularly in the sensory nerve action potentials. The reduction of amplitudes is the most common early abnormality. Recent quantitative electrophysiological field studies indicate that significant differences in the vibratory thresholds of index fingers and great toes are noted between acrylamide-exposed workers and healthy controls.

Previously, distal axonopathy has been considered in acrylamide intoxication based on the observation that there is distal swelling and degeneration of large myelinated axons in both PNS and CNS. The fundamental axonal change is an accumulation of 10 nm neurofilaments. In recent animal studies, acrylamide intoxicated rats showed ataxia, hindlimb weakness, foot splay, and autonomic dysfunction. In the peripheral nerves, axonal degeneration is an epiphenomenon, related to long-term low-dose intoxication. With exposure to a higher dose of acrylamide for a shorter duration, nerve terminal dysfunction and degeneration are noted in electrophysiological, neurochemical, and morphological studies. However, recent animal studies have shown that nerve terminals are the primary site of intoxication in both the CNS and PNS, and that acrylamide produces a terminal neuropathy, not an axonopathy. In immunohistochemical studies of human skin biopsies, acrylamide also induces degeneration of small-diameter sensory nerves with epidermal nerve swelling in the early stage and a progressive loss of epidermal nerves in the late stage.

In addition, acrylamide disrupts presynaptic function via decreased release of neurotransmitters. Evidence also suggests that acrylamide may cause changes in thiol groups of proteins that are critically involved in the synaptic vesicle-membrane fusion and recycling.

Carbon disulfide (CS₂)

CS_2 is a colorless liquid organic solvent at room temperature and is used in the production of viscose rayon fibers and cellophane films. Acute exposure to large amount of CS_2 may cause narcosis, psychosis with delirium, seizure, mental impairment, and even death. In chronic exposure or repeated low dosage exposure to CS_2, there may be polyneuropathy, parkinsonism, intention tremor, and neuropsychological symptoms, such as sleep disturbance, depression, decreased concentration, and impotence.

Peripheral neuropathy induced by CS_2 includes distal muscle weakness, paresthesia, a glove- and stocking-like sensory impairment, and decreased or absent tendon reflexes. Electrophysiological studies show a reduction of compound muscle action potentials, prolonged distal latencies, and slowed nerve conduction velocities. The pathological studies on sural nerve biopsy reveal a decrease of fiber density, relative loss of large myelinated fibers, and degeneration of both axon and myelin. In animal studies, multiple axonal swelling with secondary demyelination develops in the node of Ranvier region. Electronmicroscopic examination reveals an accumulation of neurofilaments which is very similar to that with n-hexane or acrylamide intoxication.

After exposure to CS_2 for a few months, symptoms of manic-depressive psychosis, hallucination, and suicidal attempt may appear. Subsequently depressive mood is accompanied by tremor, incoordination, ataxia, and memory impairment. Following long-term exposure, there may be pyramidal tract symptoms and parkinsonism, with cogwheel rigidity, bradykinesia, and loss of balance.

Long-term exposure to CS_2 may lead to an increase in mortality due to coronary artery diseases, bradycardia, tachycardia, and/or other arrhythmias. Laboratory studies reveal an increase in β-lipoprotein, total cholesterol, triglyceride, and low density β-lipoprotein cholesterol. In addition, cerebral vascular diseases with multiple infarctions and reduced regional blood flow in the brain are observed (Plate 106.1).

The carbamide 2-mercapto-2-thiazolinone-5,2-thiothiazolidine-4-carboxylic acid (TTCA) is the most important metabolite in CS_2 intoxication. TTCA in the urine has been generally used as a biomarker. The level of urinary TTCA can reflect previous day's exposure.

The natural course of patients with CS_2 exposure has been rarely studied. In a few long-term follow-up studies, persistent damage to the peripheral nerves was noted even after CS_2 exposure had ceased for 3 years. In addition, the CS_2-induced parkinsonism and cerebellar damage cannot be recovered even with *L*-dopa treatment.

n-Hexane

n-Hexane is an aliphatic hexacarbon and an organic solvent. It has been widely used in many industrial processes, particularly in the production of glues, paints, adhesives, coating products, laminating plastics, press proofing, cleaning agents, shoes, leather, furniture, and vulcanizing procedures.

Exposure to *n*-hexane may cause a subacute onset and progressive course of axonal polyneuropathy in humans, involving both motor and sensory fibers in the distal extremities. *n*-Hexane is also present in certain glues and cements. Therefore *n*-hexane-induced polyneuropathy also has been found in those who sniff glue for recreation. Common symptoms include distal numbness, muscle weakness, and muscle wasting in the intrinsic muscles of the hand and foot. A loss of pin-prick, temperature, touch, vibratory, and position sensations is usually accompanied by diminished ankle jerks. In severely intoxicated patients, weight loss, anorexia, abdominal pain, and muscle cramps are also found. Some glue sniffers with high and prolonged exposure may develop dysarthria, swallowing difficulty, blurred vision, and autonomic disturbances. Hyperhidrosis or anhidrosis, blue discoloration, impotence, and reduced temperature of the distal limbs have been reported in patients with moderate or severe glue sniffing.

In patients with severe *n*-hexane intoxication, nerve action potentials usually cannot be elicited, particularly in the distal peroneal nerves. In other nerves, there are prolonged distal latencies, reduced amplitudes of compound muscle action potentials and sensory nerve action potentials, and profound slowing of nerve conduction velocities. Focal conduction block with temporal dispersion may occur in some cases, indicating a demyelinating nature. There are frequent fibrillation potentials and positive sharp waves with reduced recruitment pattern. Somatosensory, brainstem auditory, and pattern-reversal visual-evoked potentials also demonstrate abnormalities in the central pathways as well as the PNS.

Nerve biopsies and postmortem pathological studies reveal giant axons with segmental demyelination in the paranodal region. In giant axons, 10 nm neurofilaments accumulate in the distal nerve fibers and spinal cord. The histograms of the sural nerve biopsy confirm a predominant loss of large myelinated fibers. In experimental studies, degeneration of myelinated fibers may also occur in the spinal cord, medulla, inferior cerebellar peduncles, and cerebellar vermis.

The neurotoxic property of *n*-hexane and the related substance methyl *n*-butyl ketone is attributable to the common gamma-diketone metabolite 2,5-hexanedione (2,5-HD). This is a potent neurotoxin. However, other gamma-diketones including 3,6-octanedione can also cause neuropathy. In addition, detection of 2,5-hexanedione in the urine has been proved to be a biological marker.

A continuous progression of the neurological features is noted one to a few months after cessation of the toxic exposure. Prognosis is generally favorable if exposure to *n*-hexane ceases. Patients with mild or moderate polyneuropathy usually recover completely within 1–2 years. Severely affected patients also improve but sometimes have neurological sequelae, such as mild weakness, leg spasticity, and hyperreflexia 2–3 years later.

Toluene

Toluene is a major component of glue vapor. The acute CNS effects of toluene intoxication include headache, nausea, vomiting, confusion, euphoria, hallucination, ataxia, and conscious disturbance. Chronic exposure to toluene may also induce mainly CNS manifestations such as permanent encephalopathy with cognitive disturbance, cerebellar dysfunction, optic neuropathy, and neurosensory-type hearing loss. Cerebellar dysfunction is characterized by nystagmus, unsteady gait, ataxia, and intention tremor in both hands. Behavioral toxicology study reveals that toluene can induce hyperactivity, ataxia, addiction, insomnia, and memory impairments.

In addition to the CNS manifestation, chronic progressive polyneuropathy is also common in glue sniffers. Patients may develop muscle wasting, distal numbness, and hyporeflexia or areflexia. Although polyneuropathy resulting from glue sniffing is well recognized, the glue may contain other substances such as *n*-hexane, methyl-*n*-butyl ketone, benzene, and acetone. In a few reports, toluene was reported as the sole agent to induce peripheral neuropathy.

Brain MRI shows diffuse cerebral, cerebellar, and brainstem atrophy, loss of differentiation between the gray and white matters, and increased periventriular white matter lesions. Among the persistent neurological deficits attributed to toluene, cerebellar dysfunction is the commonest. Toluene appears to have only a low toxicity to the peripheral nerves.

Household accident

CO intoxication

Carbon monoxide (CO) is a worldwide environmental toxin and a leading cause of deliberate or accidental poisoning. Acute CO intoxication may induce hypoxic encephalopathy with variable degrees of brain damage, ranging from confusion to deep coma. Although approximately one-third of patients succumb during the acute intoxication, most of the remaining patients can recover completely from the first episode. However, 0.2–40% of the survivors develop delayed encephalopathy within 2–6 weeks after pseudorecovery.

The common clinical features include cognitive changes, sphincter incontinence, akinetic mutism, parkinsonism, and dystonia. Most patients have a prominent improvement particularly in sphincter incontinence and akinetic mutism, although some sequelae such as dystonia and cognitive impairment persist. The common neuroimaging changes are hyperintensity lesions in the basal ganglion, particularly in the globus pallidus and subcortical white matter (Figure 106.2). A steady improvement is also noted in the basal ganglion and subcortical white matter in serial brain MR images.

The neuropathologic changes in acute CO intoxication include necrosis, ischemia, and demyelination in the globus pallidus and cerebral white matter, spongy changes in the cerebral cortex, and necrosis in the hippocampus. In delayed encephalopathy, the characteristic findings are small necrotic foci and demyelinating changes in the cerebral white matter and globus pallidus. Demyelination with relative preservation of axons is prominent in the frontal lobes. The pathogenesis of the predominant involvement of the globus pallidus remains unclear, but ischemic changes may precede irreversible changes in some patients with CO intoxication.

Recovery from acute CO intoxication usually depends on the CO concentration, duration of hypoxia, and individual variation, while the prognosis of delayed CO encephalopathy is relatively good.

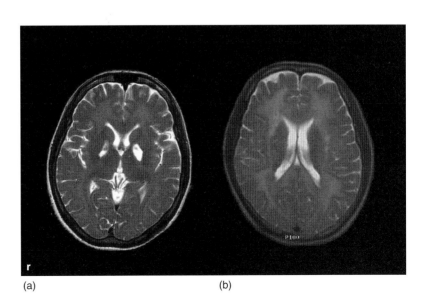

Figure 106.2 Brain MRI T2-weighted images in two patients with carbon monoxide intoxication showing high signal intensity lesions in the basal ganglia (a) and subcortical white matter of the frontal and occipital areas (b).

(a)　　　(b)

Bacterial toxins

Tetanus

Tetanus (lock jaw) still remains a considerable health problem in many parts of the world. It is an infection with *Clostridium tetani* that causes localized or generalized spasm of muscles due to the toxin produced by the causative organism. The organism is present in the excreta of humans and most animals, and in putrefying liquids and dirt. It is especially prevalent in fertilized or contaminated soil. The organism gains entrance to the human body through puncture wounds, compound fractures, or cut wounds.

Tetanus toxin blocks the inhibitory interneurons that synapse with motor neurons and also blocks the inhibition by the intermediolateral cells in the spinal cord.

The incubation period is usually between 5 and 10 days. Symptoms may be localized or generalized. Localized tetanus develops when the toxin spreads through the nerve. The symptoms are muscular spasms and contractions that are confined to the wounded limb or region. However, localized tetanus is relatively rare.

Generalized tetanus is usually ushered in by stiffness of the jaw (trismus) which is followed by stiffness of the neck, irritability, and restlessness. As the disease progresses, muscle stiffness and rigidity become generalized. The spasm of the back muscles may become so severe that the patient assumes the posture of opisthotonus. Rigidity of the facial muscles may give a characteristic facial expression of the so-called risus sandonicus. In addition, there are paroxysmal tonic muscle spasms, or generalized convulsions that may occur spontaneously, or may be precipitated by an external stimulus, such as a sudden noise or a touch. Spasm of the pharyngeal muscles may cause dysphasia, and spasm of glottis or respiratory muscles may produce cyanosis and asphyxia.

Basic management consists of tetanus toxoid (500–3000 u), human tetanus immune globulin, sedation, and debridement of the wound. Penicillin G is the most effective antibiotic for inhibiting further growth of the organism. Sedatives, muscular relaxants, and anticonvulsants are given to combat generalized spasms and convulsions. Intrathecal baclofen or intravenous dantrolene may be tried. Artificial ventilation may be required.

Plant toxins

Datura poisoning

The plants of *Datura* or jimson weed, including *Datura stramorium*, *Datura alba*, and *Datura suaveolens*, grow in the wild throughout the world, particularly tropical and subtropical areas.

Datura stramorium is comprised of several kinds of alkaloids, including atropine, hyoscyamine (daturine), and scopolamine. Scopolamine and atropine, which are structurally similar to the neurotransmitter acetylcholine, may interfere with the transmission of nerve impulses in the parasympathetic nervous system. Hyoscyamine has atropine-like effects more potent than natural atropine.

Ingestion of *D. stramonium* can cause acute anticholinergic syndrome, with dryness of the mouth, pupillary dilatation, blurred vision, facial flushing, palpitation, hypertension, disorientation, and even coma. This poisoning is usually caused by medication in releasing asthma, hallucinogens, or ingestion of contaminated grains. The onset of symptoms usually develops within 30 minutes to 2 hours after ingestion of *Datura*.

The severity of *Datura* poisoning appears to be related to the dosages of atropine and scopolamine and the pattern of onset. In cases of severe intoxication, patients may progress to convulsions, respiratory depression, stupor, coma, or even death. Recently, the incidence of this poisoning seems to have increased in oriental countries because the plants have been used for loss of vitality or in herbal drugs used as a remedy. Most of the abnormalities are reversible. The treatment of acute *Datura* poisoning includes gastric lavage and administration of activated charcoal. In severely intoxicated patients with seizures, uncontrolled hypertension, hallucinations, arrhythmia, or coma, physostigmine salicylate is indicated.

Regionally specific toxicities

Puffer fish poisoning

Puffer fish or fugu in Japanese has become well known in tales of fatal poisoning after ingestion of improperly prepared fugu, which is an expensive Japanese delicacy. There are 100–200 cases of puffer fish poisoning each year in Japan. The poisoning comes from tetrodotoxin, which is highly concentrated in the viscera (particularly the liver and ovaries) of the tetrodontiform fishes, including puffer fish (*Fugu poecilonotus*) and porcupine fish (*Diodon hystrix*).

Tetrodotoxin is an exceptionally potent voltage-gated sodium channel blocker, and the organs that contain sodium channels are affected. They include the brain, peripheral nerves, and skeletal muscle. Cardiac muscle and its sodium channels are less sensitive to tetrodotoxin than those of nerves.

Tetrodotoxin poisoning causes a rapidly progressive sensorimotor polyneuropathy that may affect bulbar and respiratory muscles. Numbness of the tongue and lips develops within minutes after ingestion. Limb weakness develops soon after and may result in flaccid quadriparesis. Symptoms of the autonomic nervous system are frequent, including vomiting, profuse salivation, excessive sweating, hypotension, bradycardia, and hypothermia.

Tetrodotoxin intoxication can be divided into four stages based on clinical signs: (1) numbness of the tongue and lips, and often of fingers occurs; (2) numbness progresses rapidly and limb paralysis occurs; (3) motor incoordination and paralysis develop; and (4) consciousness may progressively deteriorate and respiratory paralysis may cause death.

Sodium channel blockade underlies the pathophysiology of tetrodotoxin poisoning, which impairs the propagation of the nerve action potentials. Electrophysiological studies reveal reduced amplitudes of compound muscle action potentials and sensory nerve action potentials, slowing of sensorimotor conduction velocity without conduction block or temporal dispersion, and prolongation of distal and proximal (F-wave) motor latencies. Wave forms of compound muscle and sensory nerve action potentials appear normal. These abnormalities can be explained by the fact that, in mammalian myelinated fibers, most of the sodium channels are located at the node of Ranvier, with few in the internodal anoxal membrane. The nerve conduction abnormalities may rapidly improve in parallel with clinical recovery and a decrease in the urinary excretion of tetrodotoxin.

Treatment of puffer fish poisoning is supportive. No chemical antidotes are known and patients must be ventilated until the tetrodotoxin level is sufficiently reduced. Recovery may be dramatic.

Podophyllotoxin (Bajiaolian)

Podophyllum, or a herbal medicine referred to as Bajiaolian in Chinese, is the dried resin from the roots and rhizomes of *Podophyllum pelatum*. It has been applied as a cathartic, helmintic ointment for a variety of tumors and anogenital condylomata. Podophyllotoxin is thought to be the major ingredient of podophyllum. The toxin may affect the nervous system, bone marrow, liver, kidneys, and gastrointestinal system. The clinical features of podophyllotoxin poisoning include diarrhea, nausea, vomiting, tachycardia, oliguria, paralytic ileus, and nervous system symptoms. The CNS toxicity includes acute confusional state: hallucination, convulsion, coma, and even death. The PNS toxicity consists of autonomic and sensorimotor polyneuropathy. In most patients, sensory ataxia with a prominent loss of vibration and position sensations is noted.

The mechanism of cytotoxicity induced by podophyllotoxin is similar to that of colchicine: arrest of cellular mitosis in metaphase through the inhibition of microtubule formation and increased assembly of neurofilaments. Experimental animal studies reveal a disturbance of axonal transport with extensive disintegration of Nissl bodies in the ganglion neurons. Human sural nerve pathology shows a decrease in the number of large myelinated fibers, axonal degeneration, and disruption of myelin. On ultrastructural examination, atrophic axons with disorganized neurofilaments are very similar to those of vincristine-induced axonal-type polyneuropathy. There is improvement in motor weakness in 1 year follow-up; however, impairment of position and vibration sensations may still be present in the legs, consistent with the changes in nerve conduction studies.

Polychlorinated biphenyls (PCBs)

PCBs and the products of polychlorinated dibenzofurans (PCDFs) are toxic chemicals that have been widely used in the past. They contain approximately 209 congeners in active ingredients with variable toxicity to humans, most through contaminated food or environmental exposure. PCBs have been used as capacity insulators, in adhesion, and in electronics since the 1950s. Because thousands of tons of PCBs have been dispersed into the environment, leading to a serious contamination and slow breakdown, the use of these chemicals was abandoned in the United States in 1977.

There have been two notorious outbreaks of PCB intoxication: "Yusho" in Japan in 1968 and "Yu-Cheng" in Taiwan in 1979. The victims who consumed the contaminated rice oil developed chloracne, arthritis, headache, and general fatigue. In addition, hypothyroidism, menstrual abnormalities, reproductive disorders, and even slow cognitive development in the patients' descendants have been noted.

In about half the patients, there are neurological manifestations such as headache, dizziness, memory impairment, mental dullness, paresthesia or pain in the extremities, and hearing difficulty. Sensory symptoms are more prominent than motor symptoms. Nerve conduction velocity (NCV) tests show abnormalities of sensory or motor nerves in about half the patients. In CNS, acute PCB poisoning may induce irreversible neurobehavioral changes and persistent depression in adults, while chronic exposure of PCBs may produce sequential memory and learning deficits.

In long-term follow-up studies, sensory disturbance is usually more prominent than motor disturbance in PCB-intoxicated victims. However, the PNS abnormalities are not well correlated with the concentrations of PCBs/PCDFs in the blood.

In experimental studies, PCBs are profoundly neurotoxic to the dopaminergic system, causing neurobehavioral abnormalities and movement disorders in rats.

Conclusions

Neurotoxicity due to occupational or environmental exposure is not only an individual illness but also a public health matter. It is therefore important for clinicians to understand these neurotoxic diseases. Furthermore, many neurotoxic diseases are preventable.

In dealing with neurotoxic diseases, it is important to employ a multidisciplinary approach that may include neurobiological, neurophysiological, neuropathological, neurobehavioral, neuroimaging, neurogenetic, and public health specialities. Through such an approach, a better understanding of the neurotoxic disease may be achieved, and hopefully a better treatment may be realized.

Further reading

Chang LW, Dyer RS, editors. *Handbook of Neurotoxicology.* New York: Marcel Dekker; 1995.

Chen RC, Tang SY, Miyata H, *et al.* Polychlorinated biphenyl poisoning: correlation of sensory and motor nerve conduction, neurologic symptoms, and blood levels of polychlorinated biphenyls, quaterphenyls, and dibenzofurans. *Environ Res* 1985; 37: 340–8.

Chu NS, Huang CC, Calne DB. Manganese. In: Spencer PS, Schaumburg HH, Ludolph AC, editors. *Experimental and Clinical Neurotoxicology,* 2nd ed. New York: Oxford University Press; 2000, pp. 752–5.

Huang CC, Chu NS, Lu CS, *et al.* The natural history of neurological manganism over 18 years. *Parkinsonism Relat Disord* 2007; 13: 143–5.

Huang CC, Chu NS, Shih TS, *et al.* Occupational neurotoxic diseases in Taiwan: a review of the outbreaks and clinical features. *Chang Gung Med J* 1997; 20: 71–8.

Kuo HC, Huang CC, Tsai TH, *et al.* Acute painful neuropathy in thallium poisoning. *Neurology* 2005; 65: 302–4.

Kutsuma M, editor. *Minamata Disease.* Study Group of Minamata Disease. Japan: Kumamoto University; 1968.

Oda K, Araki K, Totoki T, *et al.* Nerve conduction study of human tetrodotoxication. *Neurology* 1989; 39: 743–5.

Schaumburg HH. Human neurotoxic disease. In: Spencer PS, Schaumburg HH, Ludolph AC, editors. *Experimental and Clinical Neurotoxicology.* New York: Oxford University Press; 2000, pp. 55–82.

Senenayake N, Karalliedde L. Neurotoxic effects of organophosphorus insecticides. An intermediate syndrome. *N Engl J Med* 1987; 316: 761–3.

Shih RD. Mushroom poisoning. In: Viccellio P, editor. *Emergency Toxicology,* 2nd ed. Philadelphia: Lippincott-Raven; 1998, pp. 1081–6.

Spencer PS, Schaumburgh HH, Ludolph AC, editors. *Experimental and Clinical Neurotoxicology,* 2nd ed. New York: Oxford University Press; 2000.

Chapter 107
Vitamin deficiency

Jacques Serratrice
Timone Hospital, Marseille, France

Introduction

These vital trace substances are generally associated with vitamin deficiency syndromes, but because health enthusiasm has reached passionate proportions for many individuals, physicians are encountering neurotoxic syndromes from overdosage.

The first recognized toxicity of vitamins was related to the fat-soluble vitamins (ADEK), but water-soluble vitamins (the others) have been found to be harmful at times when they are ingested in large quantities. Vitamin deficiencies, or overload, affect the central and peripheral nervous systems in several ways. Formerly, the knowledge of beri-beri was responsible for the discovery of thiamine and for the concept of vitamin B_1 deficiency. Even now there is still a significant incidence of beri-beri in underdeveloped countries. Moreover in these countries, alcoholism is a major factor in nutritional disorders as well as avitaminosis. At least some drugs utilized in the treatment of tuberculosis or hypertension are able to interfere with the enzymatic function of vitamin B_6.

In this chapter, after a brief recap on physiology, we discuss the most relevant neurological manifestations of deficiency or overload of the main vitamins.

Group B vitamins

The most important nutrients for the nervous system are vitamins and more specifically members of the B group.

Thiamine (B_1), its active form thiamine pyrophosphate (TPP), is critical in the intermediary metabolism of carbohydrate. TPP is involved in three enzyme systems: pyruvate dehydrogenase, which converts pyruvate to acetyl coenzyme A, α-ketoglutarate dehydrogenase, which catalyzes the conversion of α-ketoglutarate to succinate in the Krebs cycle, and transketolase, which catalyzes the pentose monophosphate shunt. A deficiency of TPP leads to elevated levels of serum pyruvate and occasionally lactate, reduced red blood cell (RBC) transketolase activity, and a corresponding increase in transketolase activity in response to added TPP (TPP effect). It is not understood how TPP deficiency leads to the hallmark pathology. Thiamine is most abundant in yeast, pork, legumes, cereal grains, and rice, and the recommended daily allowance of this vitamin is 0.5 mg/1000 kcal. The total body store is 30–100 mg, and it is present in the heart, skeletal muscle, liver, kidneys, and brain. Because there is a limited quantity stored, the supply must be constantly replenished. The half-life of thiamine is approximately 2 weeks, and patients may suffer severe neurological complications and even death after 6 weeks of total thiamine depletion. Patients at high risk of deficiency include adults who derive most of their carbohydrate from milled rice, alcoholics, and infants breast fed by malnourished mothers. Other potentially thiamine-deficient states include anorexia nervosa, post -gastric or -jejunoileal bypass, intractable vomiting following gastric stapling for morbid obesity, prolonged total parenteral nutrition, hyperemesis gravidarum, and severe malabsorption. Thiamine deficiency is also found in those who are prisoners of war or those who engage in a hunger strike. Thiamine deficiency has also been reported after long-standing peritoneal dialysis and hemodialysis.

Nicotinic acid or niacin deficiency: its name was changed to niacin in order to prevent confusion with the tobacco derivative nicotine. Niacin includes both nicotinic acid and nicotinamide, which form metabolically active nicotinamide adenine dinucleotide (NAD) and NAD phosphate (NADP), an end-product of tryptophan metabolism. More than 200 enzymes are dependent on NAD and NADP to carry out oxidation and reduction reactions, and these enzymes are involved in the synthesis and breakdown of all carbohydrates, lipids, and amino acids. Although niacin is endogenously produced in humans, exogenous intake is required in order to prevent deficiency. Niacin is found in meat, liver, fish, legumes, peanuts, enriched bread, coffee, and tea.

Pyridoxal phosphate is the active biochemical form of pyridoxine (B_6). It is a coenzyme of amino acid metabolism, particularly tryptophan and methionine. By inhibiting

International Neurology: A Clinical Approach. Edited by Robert P. Lisak, Daniel D. Truong, William M. Carroll, and Roongroj Bhidayasiri. © 2009 Blackwell Publishing, ISBN: 978-1-4051-5738-4.

methionine metabolism, excessive *S*-adenosylmethionine accumulates, which inhibits nerve lipid and myelin synthesis. Because tryptophan is required in the production of niacin, pyridoxine deficiency can produce a secondary niacin deficiency indistinguishable from primary pellagra. Pyridoxine is also involved in lipid and neurotransmitter synthesis. Dopamine, serotonin, epinephrine, norepinephrine, and gamma-aminobutyric acid (GABA) all require pyridoxine for their production.

The recommended daily allowance of pyridoxine is 2 mg. It is found most abundantly in enriched breads, cereals and grains, chicken, orange and tomato juice, bananas, and avocados. Patients at risk of pyridoxine deficiency include those with general malnutrition, prisoners of war, refugees, alcoholics, infants of vitamin B_6-deficient mothers, and patients using isoniazid and hydralazine. Pyridoxine is unique in that both the deficiency and toxic states result in a peripheral neuropathy.

Methylcobalamin is a cofactor of methionine synthase, a cytosolic enzyme that catalyzes the conversion of homocysteine and methyltetrahydrofolate to produce methionine and tetrahydrofolate. Methionine is further metabolized to *S*-adenosylmethionine, which is necessary for methylation of myelin sheath phospholipids and proteins. Tetrahydrofolate is the required precursor for purine and pyrimidine synthesis. In the mitochondria, adenosyl-cobalamin catalyzes the conversion of *L*-methylmalonyl-CoA to succinyl-CoA. Vitamin B_{12} (cobalamin) deficiency affects the neurological and hematological systems by impairing the function of these two enzyme systems. The total body store of cobalamin is 2000–5000 μg, half of which is stored in the liver. The recommended daily allowance is 6 μg/day, and the average diet provides 20 μg/day. Because the vitamin is tightly conserved through enterohepatic circulation, 2–5 years elapse before a subject develops cobalamin deficiency from malabsorption, and as long as 10–20 years are needed to induce a dietary deficiency from a strict vegetarian diet.

Pantothenic acid (B_5) is part of coenzyme A, an essential element of carbohydrate and fatty acid synthesis and degradation. Because of its ubiquity, no single neurological syndrome is known to be caused by pantothenate deficiency, with the exception of generalized malaise.

Vitamin B_1 deficiency
Gayet–Wernicke encephalopathy
Gayet–Wernicke encephalopathy is a polioencephalitis hemorrhage with pathological changes primarily affecting the gray matter around the third and fourth ventricles and aqueduct of Sylvius, as well as mammillary bodies, with punctate hemorrhages, gliosis, and vascular proliferation. These lesions are due to vitamin B_1 deficiency related either to deprivation or mainly to alcoholism. The onset is usually abrupt, with mental status changes that may include a global confusional state, memory loss,

and agitation. Rarely, patients develop stupor and coma. Ocular abnormalities include nystagmus, lateral rectus palsies, conjugate gaze palsy, ptosis, retinal hemorrhages, pupillary abnormalities, and scotomas. Ataxia may be severe, preventing an affected patient from standing without assistance. Finger-to-nose and heel-to-shin tests are often normal when the patient is tested in the bed. Truncal ataxia often becomes obvious only on standing or sitting, reflecting the midline degeneration of the superior division of the vermis. Polyneuropathy is present in over 80% of patients with Gayet–Wernicke encephalopathy. It presents with slowly progressive muscular weakness, sensory impairment, and hyporeflexia, accompanied by burning feet and lancinating pains. Calf tenderness is a prominent feature. Bilateral foot drop and even wrist drop may occur. Patients may also develop an autonomic neuropathy with orthostatic hypotension. Pyruvic acid is elevated. Thiamine therapy (1 g/24 hours intramuscularly) is very effective in preventing the development of Korsakoff's syndrome. The frequency of Gayet–Wernicke encephalopathy from autopsy series ranges from 0.8% to 2.8%. The disorder is probably underdiagnosed during life. Gayet–Wernicke encephalopathy is most common in alcoholics because patients are particularly susceptible to thiamine deficiency due to a combination of poor diet, inadequate intake and impaired absorption of vitamins, and overdependence on alcohol as a source of calories. Certain individuals may also have a genetic predisposition toward the development of Gayet–Wernicke encephalopathy owing to an abnormality of thiamine-dependent enzymes. Patients with thiamine deficiency may become acutely symptomatic when challenged with large doses of carbohydrate.

Korsakoff's syndrome
This amnesic syndrome is linked to thiamine deficiency in a chronic alcoholic either spontaneously or after a Gayet–Wernicke encephalopathy.

The salient features include anterograde amnesia (impaired ability to acquire new information) and retrograde amnesia (impaired ability to recall events that have been well established before the onset of the syndrome). Immediate memory (digit repetition) and remote memory (early life events) are relatively unaffected. Confabulation (momentary and fantastic rememory) is not constant and often associated with false recognition. Pathologically, there are symmetric lesions in both mammillary bodies (with necrosis, neuronal loss, hemorrhages) and bilateral medial thalami.

Unfortunately, complete recovery occurs only in 20% of patients.

Polyneuropathy (neuropathic beri-beri)
In polyneuropathy the main pathologic change is axonal degeneration with destruction of both axon and myelin

sheath. The most pronounced changes are observed in the distal part of the largest myelinated fibers. The nerve roots can be affected. Anterior horn and dorsal root ganglion cells undergo chromatolysis indicating axonal damage.

The peripheral neuropathy is characterized by symmetric sensorimotor impairment and hyporeflexia, most marked in the distal segments of the limbs. Pain is common in the initial period. Dysesthesia is prominent with a dull, constant ache in the feet and legs, or lightning pains. Cramps, band-like feelings, coldness of the feet, or burning in the soles are also common, worsened by contact with bedclothes or the ground (burning feet). The signs are those of sensory-motor neuropathy, initially with distal weakness and predominant cutaneous sensory loss. Nerve conduction study and electromyography generally reveal a moderate decrease of motor and sensory motor nerve velocity. Sensory action potentials are markedly reduced.

In some patients, severe leg edema, heart murmur, accentuated secondary pulmonary sound, and cardiac enlargement are present, together with a severe neuropathy, predominantly affecting distal motor function. The majority of patients cannot stand or walk. Serum level and urinary excretion of thiamine is reduced, while lactate in serum is increased. Good recovery is obtained by thiamine treatment.

Cerebellar degeneration

Thiamine deficiency probably plays a part in cerebellar degeneration, particularly in alcoholics. More frequent in men, this disorder is characterized by gait instability and ataxia. The full clinical spectrum of cerebellar syndrome gradually evolves. MRI shows cortical cerebellar atrophy. The pathological changes consist of degeneration of the cerebellar cortex, particularly of the Purkinje's cells. The syndrome is caused by nutritional deficiency rather than toxic effects of alcohol. Cerebellar ataxia improves with thiamine therapy.

Central pontine myelinolysis

Central pontine myelinolysis is related to profound electrolytic disturbances (severe hyponatremia) associated with hypoxia and vitamin B_1 deficiency. The nature of lesions is essentially demyelination involving the basis pontis. Clinical features are variable. Most patients who develop this syndrome usually have chronic medical illnesses. The patients may present with quadriparesis, pseudobulbar palsy, and locked-in-like syndrome over a period of several days. CT and MRI of the brain show a central pontine hypodensity. The treatment involves gradual correction of hyponatremia and vitamin B_1 supplementation.

Other syndromes related to thiamine deficiency

Henry Strachan, a British medical officer stationed in Jamaica, described in 1888 a syndrome of distal paresthesias, painful peripheral neuropathy, numbness associated with gait ataxia, muscle wasting and weakness, areflexia, amblyopia, hearing impairment, stomatitis, and orogenital dermatitis. Denny Brown and others found similar ailments among Allied troops liberated from prisoner-of-war camps after World War II. In these patients, other symptoms included sensorineural deafness, dizziness, confusion, spastic paraparesis, foot drop, Wernicke's encephalopathy, and rare cases of neck extensor weakness and myasthenic bulbar weakness. Poor nutrition, hard physical labor, and concurrent infection were thought to be exacerbating factors. In Fisher's autopsy series of Canadian prisoners of war, the most prominent pathological finding was demyelination of the posterior columns of the thoracic and cervical spinal cord. This demyelination accounted for the loss of vibration and joint position sense and sensory ataxia. Pathologically, the optic and auditory nerves showed moderate to severe demyelination.

The disease progresses to irreversible optic atrophy. Nutrition and vitamin supplementation may improve the vision. It is related to vitamin B_1 deficiency (also B_2, B_6, and B_{12}) and tobacco.

Nicotinic acid deficiency
Pellagra

Pellagra continues to occur in parts of Africa and Asia, especially in populations dependent on corn as the principal source of carbohydrate. In developed countries niacin deficiency is seen in alcoholics and patients taking isoniazid. There is a single case report of a patient developing nicotinic acid deficiency after valproic acid therapy. Pregnant women are protected from niacin deficiency owing to their enhanced ability to convert tryptophan to niacin endogenously, particularly in the third trimester.

Pellagra, or rough skin, affects the skin, the gastrointestinal system, and the central nervous system, hence the classic triad of the "three Ds" – dermatitis, diarrhea, and dementia. In industrialized countries, particularly among alcoholics, niacin deficiency may present only with encephalopathy. Patients may have altered sensorium, diffuse rigidity of the limbs, grasping, and sucking reflexes. Dementia and confusion are the most common findings, followed by diarrhea (50%) and dermatitis (about 30%). The initial symptoms can be insomnia, fatigue, nervousness, irritability, and depression. Detailed neurological examination may disclose psychomotor slowing, apathy, and memory impairment. Sometimes, an acute confusional psychosis dominates the clinical picture. Spinal cord and peripheral nerve defects have also been reported. Peripheral neuropathy is frequent and may be indistinguishable from neuropathic beri-beri. Spinal cord involvement is different from spinal spastic syndrome (frequent in prisoner-of-war camps) or from tropical spastic paraparesis (caused by human T-cell leukemia (HTLV) infection, or a toxic effect of cassava ingestion).

The cerebral pathology of pellagra is most marked in the large cells of the motor cortex, Betz's cells, although similar changes can be observed to a lesser extent in the pyramidal cells of the cortex, the large cells of the basal ganglia, the cells of the cranial motor and dentate nuclei, and the anterior horn cells of the spinal cord. The affected cells appear swollen and rounded, with eccentric nuclei. Co-existing deficiencies of thiamine and pyridoxine are common, especially in alcoholics.

Hartnup's disease, an autosomal recessive defect in tryptophan absorption of the gastrointestinal system and kidney, can give a clinical picture identical to pellagra that is also responsive to niacin administration.

Carcinoid syndrome can produce niacin deficiency. Because all tryptophan is diverted to the production of serotonin in this disorder, none is available for the production of nicotinic acid, thereby predisposing to deficiency in the absence of supplementation.

Supraphysiologic doses of niacin (1.5–3.0 g daily) have been used successfully in the treatment of hypercholesterolemia, further reducing the mortality caused by coronary artery disease. Side effects of high-dose niacin include flushing, hyperuricemia, hyperglycemia, and elevations in liver enzymes.

In the evaluation of potential niacin deficiency, nicotinic acid metabolites can be identified in the urine. The administration of 40–250 mg of niacin daily is usually adequate to reverse most of the symptoms and signs of niacin deficiency. With proper therapy, the prognosis for the resolution of neurological symptoms is excellent.

Nicotinic acid deficiency encephalopathy in alcoholic patients

In 1940, Jolliffe *et al.* described a syndrome characterized by clouding of consciousness, cogwheel rigidity, and grasping reflexes. Patients were treated with nicotinic acid and recovered rapidly. The status of the syndrome and its relation to pellagra remain uncertain.

Chronic niacin deficiency

Chronic niacin deficiency is a dramatic example of how nutritional deficiency could affect mental function in childhood.

Vitamin B$_{12}$ deficiency

The most common cause of vitamin B$_{12}$ deficiency is pernicious anemia or autoimmune parietal cell dysfunction. The mean age of diagnosis is 60 years, with a female-to-male ratio of approximately 1.5:1. In white populations, the incidence of the disease increases with age, peaking after age 65. In Hispanic and African populations, there is an overall younger age distribution, especially among women. When using radioassay-derived serum cobalamin levels below 200 pg/ml or elevated levels of homocysteine and methylmalonic acid as diagnostic criteria,

the prevalence of vitamin B$_{12}$ deficiency from all causes ranges from 7% to 16%.

The brain, spinal cord, optic nerves, and peripheral nerves may also be involved in pernicious anemia. The spinal cord is usually affected first and often exclusively. The term *subacute combined degeneration* is used to designate the spinal cord lesion in pernicious anemia and to distinguish it from other forms of so-called combined system disease, in which the posterior and lateral columns are affected. Symptoms of nervous system disease occur in the majority of patients with pernicious anemia. The initial symptoms are usually generalized weakness and paresthesias described as tingling, pins and needles, or other vague sensations. They are localized to the distal parts of all four limbs in a symmetrical pattern; occasionally the lower extremities are involved before the upper ones. As the illness progresses, the gait becomes unsteady. Then, the legs become weak and spastic. If the disease remains untreated, an ataxic paraplegia with variable degrees of spasticity and contracture may develop.

When only paresthesias are present, there may be no objective signs. The examination may disclose the impairment of the posterior and lateral columns of the spinal cord, predominantly of the former. Loss of vibration sense is by far the most consistent sign; it is more pronounced in the legs than in the arms, and frequently it extends over the trunk. Position sense is usually impaired as well. The motor signs include weakness, spasticity, changes in tendon reflexes, and clonus, associated with extensor plantar responses. These signs are usually limited to the legs. The patellar and Achilles' reflexes can be diminished, increased, or even absent. With treatment, the reflexes may return to normal or become hyperactive. The gait at first is predominantly ataxic, later ataxic and spastic.

Sensory disturbances are of spinal or peripheral distribution.

Psychiatric disturbances are frequent, ranging from irritability, apathy, somnolence, paranoia, and emotional lability to a marked confusional, depressive psychosis, or intellectual deterioration.

Visual impairment may be the sole manifestation in pernicious anemia; examination discloses symmetrical centrocecal scotoma and optic atrophy in the most advanced cases.

The cerebrospinal fluid (CSF) is usually normal.

Pathology shows diffuse degeneration of white matter, brain, and spinal cord with vacuolated aspect and gliosis.

The paresthesia and ataxia are due to lesions in the posterior columns, and this may also account for the loss of tendon reflexes. Weakness, spasticity, increased reflexes, and Babinski signs depend on involvement of corticospinal tracts. The spinothalamic tract explains the finding of a sensory level on the trunk. The distal and symmetrical impairment of superficial sensation and the loss of tendon reflexes that occur in some cases are due to involvement of peripheral nerves.

Nerve conduction velocity is reduced. Reduction of sensory action potentials is usual.

The pathophysiology of nervous alteration is not known.

Diagnosis is based on assay of cobalamine serum concentration, Schilling test, megaloblastic and macrocytic anemia, and antibodies to intrinsic factor, parietal cells, and IgG.

Treatment is aimed at the underlying disorder: restoring dietary imbalance, supplementing of pancreatic enzymes, administering of antibiotics, taenicids, corticosteroids, intestinal motility-decreasing drugs, and bile salt sequestering agents, as well as cobalamine (parenteral) substitution therapy with cobalamine 2000 µg intramuscularly per day during the first 2 weeks and 100 µg intramuscularly every month thereafter. In some cases, oral supplementation is effective.

Pyridoxine (vitamin B₆)

Antagonists of pyridoxine are used in tuberculosis and hypertension. Hydrazines and isoniazid (INH) produce pyridoxal-hydrazones, biologically inactive compounds which are excreted, suggesting a carbonyl-trapping effect, which also includes other compounds such as furadantine. Excretion of xanthurenic acid is increased in these conditions. Deficiency affects the blood, skin, and nervous system. The skin changes are indistinguishable from pellagra, probably due to the close interaction of niacin and pyridoxine. Pyridoxine improves the microcytic anemia of alcoholics as well as the anemia associated with pyridoxine-responsive seizures in infants. Pyridoxine-deficiency neuropathy in man was produced in long-term experiments with the antagonist desoxypyridoxine; it also appears during concomitant treatment with antagonist drugs. The characteristic peripheral nerve involvement usually affects distal symmetric sensory nerves with "burning feet" sensations. Pain can be so severe that it interferes with sleep. Weakness generally occurs later, with initial motor disturbances usually consisting of moderate weakness of the toe and foot.

The nerve lesions are primarily axonal. The pathogenesis of hydralazine neuropathy and clinical manifestations are similar to those of INH neuropathy. Favorable response to vitamin B₆ administration is observed.

CNS involvement is manifested by dizziness, drowsiness, lethargy, anorexia, vomiting, or psychotic episodes, occasionally similar to Korsakoff's syndrome.

In children, hyperexcitability is common, generally culminating in seizures. Pyridoxine dependency is a rare disease, inherited as an autosomal recessive trait. It is characterized by the early onset seizures, sometimes even in utero, failure to thrive, hypertonia-hyperkinesia, irritability, tremulous movements ("jitter-baby"),

exaggerated auditory startle (hyperacusis), and later, if untreated, psychomotor retardation. Excretion of pyridoxine and its catabolic end-product 4-pyridoxic is decreased. The specific laboratory abnormality is an increased excretion of xanthurenic acid in response to a tryptophan load. Neuropathologically, brain weight is below normal as there is a decreased amount of central white matter in the cerebral hemispheres and a depletion of neurons in the thalamic nuclei and cerebellum, with gliosis. The administration of 50–100 mg of vitamin B₆ ablates the seizure, and daily doses of 40 mg permit normal development.

Excess pyridoxine also results in a peripheral neuropathy. Megadoses of pyridoxine produce a sensory neuropathy, generally in excess of 2 g/day, but have been reported in long-standing use of as little as 200 mg/day. Symptoms of paresthesia, ataxia, and burning feet occur 1 month to 3 years after starting pyridoxine. Sural nerve biopsies show reduced myelin fiber density and myelin debris, suggesting axonal degeneration. After stopping pyridoxine, all patients improve, but the condition resolves entirely in only a few.

Pantothenic acid deficiency (vitamin B₅)

Deficiency may possibly induce a sensory polyneuropathy, characterized by numbness and tingling of the hands and feet. However, there is no firm evidence that lesions of peripheral nerves may be caused by pantothenic acid deficiency alone. Administration of this vitamin may reverse the painful dysesthesiae of the "burning feet" syndrome. Experimentally, neuropathy with degeneration of large-diameter fibers in nerves and dorsal roots is produced.

Other vitamins

Alpha-tocopherol is the most active form of vitamin E present in humans. Tocopherol is absorbed and incorporated into chylomicrons in the small intestine. It is carried in portal blood to the liver, and alpha-tocopherol transfer protein (α-TTP) binds and recycles vitamin E in the liver for incorporation into low-density lipoproteins and very low-density lipoproteins. Once it is delivered to the cells, alpha-tocopherol serves as an antioxidant, preventing free radical peroxidation and injury to cell membranes. It is stored in adipose tissue, liver, and muscle. Deficiency can occur at any stage of tocopherol metabolism, resulting in reduced food intake, fat malabsorption, inhibition of enterohepatic circulation, mutation of α-TPP, and abetalipoproteinemia. Vitamin E is a fat-soluble vitamin found in abundance in vegetable oils and wheat germ. The recommended daily allowance is 10 mg for men and 8 mg for women. Patients at risk of the development of vitamin E deficiency include those who have hypobetalipoproteinemia or abetalipoproteinemia (Bassen–Kornzweig syndrome), other disorders of the pancreas and liver, such as cystic fibrosis and primary biliary atresia, familial vitamin E deficiency due to a defect in α-TTP, and other malabsorptive states that result in cholestasis such as Crohn's disease, ulcerative colitis, and celiac disease. Pregnancy increases vitamin E serum concentrations, but premature infants often have low levels of vitamin E due to a lack of adipose tissue as well as difficulty in transplacental migration of the vitamin. The majority of patients who have vitamin E deficiency are those with severe malabsorptive states present since birth or rare familial vitamin E deficiency due to transfer protein abnormalities. Vitamin E deficiency leads to axonal membrane injury, with resultant axonal degeneration of peripheral nerves, dorsal root ganglia, and posterior columns.

Vitamin C (ascorbic and dehydroascorbic acid) readily oxidizes to dehydroascorbic acid in aqueous solution. Because the latter can be reduced *in vivo*, it possesses vitamin C activity. Therefore, total vitamin C is measured as the sum of ascorbic and dehydroascorbic acid concentrations. Because of its antioxidant properties, it serves primarily as a biologic antioxidant in aqueous environments. Biosyntheses of collagen, carnitine, bile acids, and norepinephrine, as well as proper functioning of the hepatic mixed-function oxygenase system, depend on this property. Vitamin C in foodstuffs increases the intestinal absorption of non-heme iron. Overt deficiency is uncommon in developed countries. Tobacco smoking lowers plasma and leukocyte vitamin C levels.

Vitamin A, derived from β-carotene, is necessary for normal vision and reproduction. Deficiency leads to night blindness and corneal ulceration. Hypervitaminosis in pregnant mothers may lead to birth defects and learning disabilities.

Vitamin D is necessary for calcium absorption in the gut. Deficiency leads to osteomalacia, hypocalcemia, and hypophosphatemia, contributing to muscle weakness.

Other neuroavitaminosis
Vitamin E deficiency
Vitamin E deficiency could explain some ataxia, loss of tendon reflexes, ophthalmoparesis, and proximal muscle weakness with a high level of creatine kinase. However, the main characteristic syndrome is ataxia with vitamin E deficiency (AVED), which differs from Freidreich's ataxia. Mutation 744 del A of the αTTP gene is present. Three principal differences from Friedreich's ataxia are the frequency of head titubation, decreased visual acuity, and retinitis pigmentosa.

Another rare autosomal recessive disorder is Bassen–Kornzweig syndrome related to malabsorption of vitamin E and carrier lipoprotein not being synthesized in the liver. It is characterized by near absence of β-lipoprotein and a low level of cholesterol in the serum, retinal degeneration, and acanthocytosis (a thorny appearance of the red cells, with a chronic, progressive deficit, usually beginning in childhood, steatorrhea and retarded growth). The first neurological sign is hyporeflexia or absence of tendon reflexes in the second year of life. Later, a loss of position sense is found in the legs. Cerebellar ataxia of gait, trunk, and extremities, titubation, dysarthria, muscle weakness, ophthalmoparesis, Babinski's sign, and loss of pain and temperature sensations and other neurologic abnormalities. Mental backwardness is another feature; progression occurs over a few years and many patients are no longer able to stand and walk by the time of adolescence. Retinitis pigmentosa is observed.

Neuropathologic findings consist of demyelination of peripheral nerves and degeneration of nerve cells in the spinal gray matter and cerebellar cortex. Diagnosis is confirmed by the finding of acanthocytes, low serum cholesterol, and β (low-density)-lipoproteins.

Vitamin A deficiency
Vitamin A deficiency is very uncommon except in underdeveloped countries in childhood, where xerophthalmia induces blindness. Avitaminosis of vitamin A is the main cause of blindness in the world. Electroretinogram and electonystagmogram are useful tests. Vitamin A deficiency is sometimes induced by antiepileptic drugs (dihydantoin). Hypervitaminosis may also cause neurological symptoms, for example, pseudotumor cerebri (increased intracranial pressure and visual disturbances with normal brain imaging), ataxia, and bone and muscle pain. Chronic toxicity may occur with habitual daily intake of more than 10 000 µg.

Vitamin C deficiency
The classic symptom of vitamin C deficiency is scurvy, characterized by fatigue, depression, and widespread abnormalities in connective tissues, such as inflamed gingiva, petechiae, perifollicular hemorrhages, impaired wound healing, coiled hairs, hyperkeratosis, and bleeding into body cavities. In infants, defects in ossification and bone growth may occur. In some adults living on tinned foods (thermolability of vitamin C), asthenia, myalgias, and hemorrhages could appear. Ascorbic acid level is low in leucocytes and in plasma.

Vitamin D deficiency
This deficiency gives few neurological signs that generally occur in childhood, including muscle hypotonia and skull deformation. Adult patients often complain of pronounced fatigue with bone pain. The reason why muscle weakness occurs in such patients is unclear, and the phenomenon is explained only in part by low serum calcium.

Further reading

Bier JG, Corash L, Hubbard VS. Medical uses of vitamin E. *N Engl J Med* 1983; 308: 1063–71.

Carmel R. Cobalamin, the stomach, and aging. *Am J Clin Nutr* 1997; 66: 750–9.

Clayton PT. B$_6$-responsive disorders: a model of vitamin dependency. *J Inherit Metab Dis* 2006; 29: 317–26.

Green R, Kinsella LJ. Current concepts in the diagnosis of cobalamin deficiency. *Neurology* 1995; 45: 1435–40.

Harding AE, Matthews S, Jones S, *et al*. Spinocerebellar degeneration associated with a selective defect of vitamin E absorption. *N Engl J Med* 1985; 313: 32–5.

Ishii N, Nishihara Y. Pellagra among chronic alcoholics: clinical and pathologic study of 20 necropsy cases. *J Neurol Neurosurg Psychiatry* 1981; 44: 209–15.

Jollife N, Bowman KN, Rosenblum LA, Fein HD. Nicotinic acid deficiency encephalopathy. *JAMA* 1940; 114: 307–12.

Kril JJ. Neuropathology of thiamine deficiency disorders. *Metab Brain Dis* 1996; 11: 9–17.

Kumar N. Nutritional neuropathies. *Neurol Clin* 2007; 25: 209–55.

Lindenbaum J, Healton ES, Savage DG, *et al*. Neuropsychiatric disorders caused by cobalamin deficiency in the absence of anemia or macrocytosis. *N Engl J Med* 1988; 318: 1720–8.

Marcus R, Coulston AM. Water soluble vitamin, the vitamin B-complex and ascorbic acid. In: Shils ME, Olson JA, Shike M, editors. *Modern Nutrition in Health and Disease*, 8th ed. Philadelphia: Lea & Febiger; 1994, pp. 1547–90.

McCombe PA, McLeod JC. The peripheral neuropathy of vitamin B$_{12}$ deficiency. *J Neurol Sci* 1984; 66: 117–26.

Rueler JB, Girard DE, Cooney TG. Wernicke's encephalopathy. *N Engl J Med* 1985; 312: 1035–9.

Chapter 108
Starvation, Strachan's syndrome, and postgastroplasty polyneuropathy

Le Quang Cuong
Hanoi Medical University of Viet Nam, Ha Noi, Viet Nam

Starvation

Starvation is the most extreme form of malnutrition due to a severe reduction of vitamin, nutrient, and energy intake. According to the Food and Agriculture Organization of the United Nations, more than 25 000 people die of starvation every day, and more than 800 million people are chronically undernourished. On average, a child dies every 5 seconds from starvation.

Adequate nutrition has two components: necessary nutrients and energy, in the form of calories. It is not only the overall lack of nutrients and energy that results in susceptibility to disease, but also the ingestion of enough calories without a well-balanced selection of individual nutrients produces abnormalities. For example, children getting enough calories but not enough protein may suffer from kwashiorkor, but those who seemingly get adequate amounts of food without getting the minimum requirement of energy may suffer from maramus.

Starvation is caused by a number of factors including: anorexia nervosa, fasting, coma, stroke, famine, and severe gastrointestinal disease. The body combats malnutrition by breaking down its own fat and eventually its own tissue; therefore the body's structure and its functions are affected.

Characteristic symptoms of starvation include shrinkage of vital organs, such as the lungs, heart, ovaries, or testes, and because of this their functions diminish. This results in chronic diarrhea, anemia, reduction in muscle mass, weakness, low body temperature, decreased ability to digest food because of lack of digestive acid production, irritability, immune deficiency, edema (swelling from fluid under the skin), and decreased sex drive. In adults, anemia is the first sign of malnutrition followed by edema of extremities due to decreased albuminocemia, then loss of resistance to infection. Then the specific symptoms of nutrient deficiencies may appear. However, for children, chronic malnutrition is marked by growth retardation.

Treatment

An adequate and well-balanced diet is the key treatment. In cases of severe malnutrition, carefully prepared elemental diets, or even intravenous feeding, are necessary. Gradually solid foods should be introduced.

Strachan's syndrome

A syndrome of painful peripheral neuropathy, ataxia, optic neuropathy, and stomatitis among sugar cane workers was described by Henry Strachan in 1988. Other symptoms were found in allied troops liberated from prison camps following World War II, including neurosensorial deafness, dizziness, confusion, spastic leg weakness, and myasthenic bulbar weakness. In a series of autopsies of Canadian prisoners of war carried out by Fisher, the most prominent pathological finding was demyelination of the posterior columns of the thoracic and cervical spinal cord. In 1992–1993, a similar syndrome appeared in Cuba, with about 50 000 people developing an isolated or combined optic neuropathy, painful sensory neuropathy, dorsolateral myelopathy, neurosensorial deafness, spastic paraparesis, dysphonia, and dysautonomia. Proposed mechanisms included vitamin B complex and thiamine deficiency, cyanide intoxication, viral infection, and mitochondrial deletion. Infections appeared to precipitate or exacerbate symptoms. Evidence for peripheral nerve lesion has been mixed. Axonal degeneration of large myelinated fibers, observed in nerve biopsy, and slow nerve conduction velocity were reported. Almost all patients responded to early supplementation with vitamin B complex. Extensive studies in Cuba and in Africa revealed smoking, weight loss, and excessive alcohol intake as risk factors, and pregnant women are most vulnerable.

Due to the variation in clinical signs, this syndrome must be differentiated from other pathologies such as beri-beri, vitamin B_{12} deficiency, pellagra, tropical spastic paraparesis, tropical ataxic neuropathy of Africa, Leber's optic neuropathy, and nutritional amblyopia.

International Neurology: A Clinical Approach. Edited by Robert P. Lisak, Daniel D. Truong, William M. Carroll, and Roongroj Bhidayasiri. © 2009 Blackwell Publishing, ISBN: 978-1-4051-5738-4.

Treatment

Treatment consists of re-establishing a balanced diet with vitamin B complex and vitamin A supplementation.

Postgastroplasty polyneuropathy

After undergoing bariatric or weight reduction surgery, some cases develop a syndrome of acute or subacute sensory loss, weakness, and tendon areflexia that follows a period of dramatic weight loss and repeated bouts of protracted vomiting. Following a period of recurrent vomiting and precipitous weight loss, patients develop numbness and tingling in the soles of lower extremities. Distal or proximal weakness may develop. Patients have difficulty arising from a chair or climbing stairs. Pain is not a predominant feature, unlike the exquisitely tender calves often seen in thiamin-deficient neuropathy. Symmetrical loss of sensory feeling is often found in the extremities, as is weakness and areflexia, predominantly in the legs. Patients may develop quadriparesis and permanent disability. Some have been mistakenly diagnosed early in their course as having a conversion disorder. Some developed Wernicke's encephalopathy which occurs most commonly 2–8 months after surgery, mainly in individuals with weight loss greater than 7 kg/month. Changes in mental status, ocular abnormalities, and motor problems such as gait incardination and ataxia are the main clinical features of this disorder.

Nerve conduction studies show severe reduction of sensory and motor action potentials, variable slowing, and absent or prolonged late responses in this disorder. Electromyogram (EMG) shows diffuse denervation with consistent fibrillations. Pathological studies have shown lipid-laden neurons and Schwann cells surrounding demyelinating and degenerating axons. All these manifestations reveal an axonal and demyelinating sensorimotor polineuropathy.

Differential diagnosis

Guillain–Barré syndrome, cobalamin myeloneuropathy, other types of polyneuropathy, beri-beri, Strachan's syndrome, hypocalcemia, hypomagnesemia, and other disturbances of the peripheral nervous system should be considered.

Treatment

Although thiamine deficiency has been thought to be a cause, reports documenting low thiamine activity are lacking. Furthermore, on the one hand, the pathology is unlike any known nutritional neuropathy, and, on the other hand, some patients have developed the neuropathy despite adequate nutritional supplementation. The physiopathology of this disorder is unknown, but acute catabolism of lipid after bypass surgery is suggested. All patients following bariatric surgery should adhere to a strict dietary regimen with addition vitamins. If vomiting develops, parenteral nutrition plus thiamin and other vitamins should be administered. Most patients fully recover; however, some may have residual weakness and sensory loss, depending on the duration and severity of symptoms before treatment.

Further reading

Feit H, Glasberg M, Ireton C, Rosenberg RN, Thal E. Peripheral neuropathy and starvation after gastric partitioning for morbid obesity. *Ann Intern Med* 1982; 96: 453–5.

Fisher M. Residual neuropathological changes in Canadians held prisoner of war by the Japanese (Strachan's disease). *Can Serv Med J* 1955; 11: 157–99.

Food and Agriculture Organization of the United Nations. *The State of Food Insecurity in the World*. Rome: Food and Agriculture Organization of the United Nations; 2000.

McCathy M. Cuban neuropathy. *Lancet* 1994; 343: 884.

Sechi G, Serra A. Wernicke encephalopathy: new clinical settings and recent advances in diagnosis and management. *Lancet Neurol* 2007; 6: 442–55.

World Health Organization. *Management of Severe Malnutrition: A Manual for Physicians and Other Senior Health Workers*. Geneva: World Health Organization; 1999 (http://www.who.int/nut).

Chapter 109
Alcohol-related neurological disorders

Yuri Alekseenko
Vitebsk State Medical University, Vitebsk, Republic of Belarus

Pharmacological aspects

Alcohol can influence various structures of the nervous system and cause some potentially dangerous conditions. Development of alcohol-related disorders of the nervous system depends on the extent and the duration of alcohol abuse, nutrition, metabolic activity, and a variety of individual factors. Alcohol appears to be toxic to the central and peripheral nervous systems in a dose-dependent manner. Metabolism of ethanol is carried out in the liver by several enzymes, including alcohol dehydrogenase, aldehyde dehydrogenase, microsomal ethanol-oxidizing system, and peroxisomal catalase. Non-habituated patients metabolize ethanol at 13–25 mg/dl/hour. In alcoholic persons, this rate increases to 30–50 mg/dl/hour. Metabolism rates vary greatly between individuals. Clinical presentation of alcohol intoxication depends on blood concentrations and tolerance to ethanol. Acetaldehyde is a highly toxic metabolite of ethanol and, probably the major factor in alcohol-related damage of the nervous system. Chronic alcohol consumption is usually accompanied by malnutrition and vitamin deficiency, particularly of thiamine. On the other hand, it may be itself one of the most important causes of malnutrition, vitamin deficiency, and metabolic and electrolyte disorders. Alcohol affects several neurotransmitter systems within the brain: the glutamate, gamma-aminobutyric acid (GABA), dopamine, serotonin, and opioid systems. Alcohol produces opioid-related analgesic, pleasure, and stress-reducing effects. At the same time alcohol increases dopamine neurotransmission which mediates the pleasurable effects of alcohol via the mesolimbic dopamine system. Serotonin may also be linked to the pleasurable effects of alcohol, so different brain serotonin levels may provide for anxious and aggressive behavior in alcohol misusers. The interaction between alcohol and the GABA-benzodiazepine receptors is probably the major pathogenic mechanism responsible for the alcohol dependency and withdrawal syndrome. Alcohol may interact with neurologic and psychiatric medications with some undesirable effects and life-threatening complications.

Acute alcohol intoxication

Acute alcohol intoxication is a transient exogenous condition resulting from acute intake of sufficiently large amounts of alcohol. The clinical manifestations of acute alcohol intoxication depend on its amount but do not directly reflect the blood alcohol concentration. The general physical shape of the subject, individual metabolic rate, pre-existing somatic and neurologic disorders, and some additional intrinsic and environmental factors contribute to the clinical effects of ethanol intoxication.

There are three stages of acute alcohol intoxication which may be acceptable for different practical purposes:
1 Mild alcohol intoxication (blood alcohol concentration 0.5–1.5‰) is usually characterized by reduction of psychomotor capacities, loss of inhibitions, increased sociability and volubility, increased thirst for action, reduced control, and positional nystagmus.
2 Moderate alcohol intoxication (blood alcohol concentration 1.5–2.5‰) is typically manifested by euphoria or aggressive irritability, reduced self-criticism, daze, behavior strongly dependent on external cues, primitive explosive reactions.
3 Severe alcohol intoxication (blood alcohol concentration greater than 2.5‰) is usually associated with disturbance of consciousness, disorientation, anxiety, and agitation. Ataxia, dizziness, dysarthria, and nystagmus develop as a result of alcohol-induced dysfunction of the vestibulocerebellar system. At high concentrations, alcohol can cause severe autonomic dysfunction, coma, and death from respiratory depression and cardiovascular collapse. Concomitant traumatic brain injury, intoxication with psychotropic drugs, and metabolic coma should be excluded in patients with severe alcohol intoxication and progressive disorders of consciousness.

Pathological intoxication may be observed in some special circumstances in predisposed subjects, for instance,

International Neurology: A Clinical Approach. Edited by Robert P. Lisak, Daniel D. Truong, William M. Carroll, and Roongroj Bhidayasiri. © 2009 Blackwell Publishing, ISBN: 978-1-4051-5738-4.

in patients with brain injury and other neurological disorders. In such cases even a small amount of alcohol may cause a state of agitation or drowsiness with disorientation with respect to people and places, illusions, anxiety, fury, and violent behavior with complete amnesia for these events.

The treatment of severe alcohol intoxication should be provided according to standard protocols which are suitable for intoxications of other origin. In some cases haloperidol may be effective in the treatment of agitation with a low risk of cardiovascular side effects. Special therapy for patients with mild or moderate alcohol intoxication is usually not necessary.

Alcohol withdrawal

Patients who stop drinking demonstrate a spectrum of different symptoms ranging from mild sleep disturbance to alcoholic delirium. The severity of this withdrawal syndrome relates to a number of factors, but most importantly to the abruptness of withdrawal, level of alcohol intake, and the contribution of residual effects of previous drinking. Alcohol withdrawal usually starts 8–12 hours after the cessation or sufficient reduction of chronic alcohol consumption. The main symptom of all varieties of alcohol withdrawal is a 6–8 Hz tremor of the hands, which may also extend to the tongue and the eyelids. Alcohol withdrawal may cause insomnia, anxiety, hyperkinesias, nausea, vomiting, and signs of vegetative hyperactivity such as tachycardia, hypertension, hyperhydrosis, and mild hyperpyrexia. Some patients may complain of dryness of the mouth and headache. Alcoholic delirium develops in more serious cases and is clearly differentiated from uncomplicated alcohol withdrawal by disturbed orientation and clouded consciousness with agitation. These patients experience frightening visual or auditory hallucinations which last usually 5 or 6 days. Visual hallucinations typically consist of scenes with small moving animals or objects. Seizures may occur; they are usually brief, generalized, tonic–clonic in nature, and without an aura. They occur in a cluster of one to three seizures with a short postictal period. Partial seizures are not uncommon. In 30–50% of patients, the seizures progress to alcoholic delirium. Most seizures terminate spontaneously or are easily controlled with benzodiazepines. The peak incidence for seizures is around 36 hours (usually occurring between 12 and 48 hours) and for delirium around 72 hours. The alcoholic delirium is a self-limited disorder, which resolves spontaneously. At the same time it is always a life-threatening condition because of severe autonomic dysregulation (hyperthermia, respiratory disturbances, cardiac arrhythmias) and uncontrolled seizures. Medical treatment of alcoholic delirium consists of the administration of benzodiazepines (diazepam or chlordiazepoxide) or chlomethiazole to reduce agitation and the incidence of seizures. Alternatively gamma-hydroxy-butyric acid may be used. Beta-blockers (such as atenolol) reduce tremor and autonomic dysfunction. Neuroleptic drugs may be useful as an adjunctive therapy but may provoke seizures. In addition, parenteral thiamine is recommended. Any associated infection, dehydration, hypoglycaemia, or electrolyte disturbances should be treated.

Alcoholic dementia

Alcohol may have a direct neurotoxic effect on cortical neurons. Chronic alcohol consumption causes cerebral atrophy, particularly of the frontal lobes, with the involvement of both white and gray matter, and ventricular dilatation, which are confirmed by the computed tomography (CT) of the brain. Neuropathological studies show reduced numbers of neurons within the superior frontal cortex in alcoholic patients with dementia. Neuropsychological investigations demonstrate that alcoholic dementia involves generalized cognitive abnormalities and predominantly affects problem-solving abilities, whereas Wernicke–Korsakoff syndrome is distinguished by selective amnesia. At the same time diffuse brain damage, predominantly subcortical in alcoholic patients, may be caused by concomitant thiamine deficiency leading to Wernicke–Korsakoff syndrome. In general, cognitive impairment is quite common in alcoholics. So in fact it usually reflects varying combinations of acute and chronic brain damage including alcohol intoxication, vitamin deficiency, metabolic disorders, cerebrovascular diseases, and previous traumatic brain injuries. One should bear in mind that sometimes the cognitive impairment in alcoholic patients without any history of apparent head injury may be due to subdural hematoma. Some investigations have demonstrated that the neuroradiological signs of cerebral atrophy are at least partially reversible after the cessation of alcohol consumption. The reduction of cerebral atrophy seems to be accompanied by an improvement in cognitive function and takes some weeks to months. However, the extent of this improvement as well as its underlying mechanisms are still a matter of discussion.

Alcoholic cerebellar degeneration

Mild clinical signs of cerebellar dysfunction may be found in about a third of all chronic alcoholics. This alcohol-related cerebellar degeneration affects men more often than women and peaks in the fifth decade of life. The structural substrate of the disease is a degeneration of the anterior and middle parts of the cerebellum vermis.

Purkinje's cells of cerebellar cortex are more affected than other cerebellar neurons. Cerebellar degeneration not only seems to result from the direct toxic effects of alcohol or its metabolites, but also reflects some other factors, such as thiamine deficiency in Wernicke's encephalopathy. The clinical picture is characterized by a severe ataxia of stance and gait. Coordination of hands is only mildly disturbed. Dysarthria and oculomotor abnormalities are unusual. In many patients peripheral neuropathy of alcoholic or thiamine deficiency origin usually contributes to the ataxia. Although generally of gradual onset, alcoholic cerebellar degeneration may evolve to become relatively acute over the course of several weeks. The incidence of cerebellar ataxia does not quite correlate with the extent of lifetime alcohol consumption or the degree of cerebellar atrophy on computed tomography of the brain. It remains unclear why thiamine deficiency may cause Wernicke's encephalopathy in some patients but selective lesions of separate cerebellum parts in others. Cessation of alcohol consumption, thiamine, and other B vitamins should be recommended to all patients. If alcohol consumption is ceased, a further progression of the disease can be avoided, and in some cases certain improvement may be observed.

Marchiafava–Bignami disease

Marchiafava–Bignami disease is characterized by symmetrical demyelination and necrosis of the central parts of the corpus callosum and occasionally of the anterior and posterior commissures. It is usually observed in alcoholic patients after an excessive and long-term (greater than 20 years) consumption of alcohol. The disorder was originally associated with red wine consumption but is now known for other groups of alcoholic beverages and factors. The exact mechanisms of this disease remain poorly understood. The onset of the disease is usually acute. Disturbances of consciousness, seizures, gait apraxia, spasticity, signs of pyramidal tract involvement, dysarthria, and dementia are the most typical clinical features. Clinical presentation of this disorder is quite variable. The damage of the corpus callosum and adjacent cerebral white matter can be detected by MRI or high-resolution CT scanning. Modern imaging techniques (MRI, CT scan) allow the differentiation of various alcohol-related conditions, including central pontine myelinolysis and Wernicke's encephalopathy, during the patient's life. The disease is usually progressive and in most cases patients die after only a few days to a few months, or survive for many years with severe dementia. No specific treatment measures are known that reliably influence the outcome of the disease. However, high-dose intravenous corticosteroid treatment may be considered as an option in rapidly progressive cases.

Alcoholic amblyopia

Alcoholic amblyopia (tobacco–alcohol amblyopia) is a selective optic neuropathy which may be observed in some alcoholic patients. Alcoholic optic neuropathy seems to be associated with any deficiency of the B vitamins, as well as with exposure to cyanides, methanol, or combinations of these factors. The substrate of this optic neuropathy is symmetrical, bilateral, papillomacular demyelination, which starts in the retrobulbar region and develops retinofugally. Blurred vision or loss of vision is the main complaint of patients. These symptoms appear gradually within several days or weeks. Examination usually reveals symmetrical central scotomas and pallor of the temporal parts of the optic disk. Without appropriate treatment, alcoholic optic neuropathy can lead to irreversible optic nerve atrophy. Therapy includes the administration of B vitamins and a well-balanced diet and should be started as soon as possible. If the symptoms persist for more than a couple of weeks after the beginning of the therapy, the prognosis with regard to a full functional recovery remains doubtful.

Alcoholic myopathy

There are three different types of acute and chronic alcohol-related damage of muscles which may be observed in patients with alcohol abuse: rhabdomyolysis, hypokalemic alcohol myopathy, and chronic alcohol myopathy. Alcohol is probably the most frequent cause of acute rhabdomyolysis of non-traumatic origin. Seizures, vascular occlusion, physical exercise, prolonged muscle compression, drugs, toxins, infections, and extremes of temperature are less frequent but can also be responsible. Episodes of acute muscle weakness due to rhabdomyolysis usually follow bouts of excessive alcohol consumption and are associated with myoglobinuria. At the same time such an apparently slight muscle injury is often asymptomatic with only elevation of muscle enzymes in the serum. The most typical clinical manifestations are pain, swelling, weakness of affected muscles, and dark urine. The muscle lesion can lead to hyperkalemia and increased serum myoglobin and creatine kinase levels. Renal failure is a common complication of acute rhabdomyolysis. The possibility of rhabdomyolysis should be considered in any intoxicated patient with muscle tenderness and acute muscle paralysis. There is no specific therapy, but common measures of intensive therapy usually include water and electrolyte balance correction, enforced diuresis, and hemodialysis.

Hypokalemic myopathy in alcoholic patients usually develops because of frequent vomiting and increased loss of potassium through the gastrointestinal tract, whereas renal excretion of potassium is not changed. Painless muscle weakness, mainly affecting the proximal parts of the limbs, and decreased serum potassium level are the most typical clinical features. Significant increases in serum level of liver and muscle enzymes may be found. The therapy consists mainly of slow intravenous infusion of potassium chloride or potassium lactate. Monitoring of the electrocardiogram is necessary. The muscle weakness usually improves within 7–14 days.

Chronic alcoholic myopathy is probably one of the most prevalent skeletal muscle disorders in the western hemisphere and occurs in approximately 50–70% of alcohol misusers. This myopathy occurs independently of peripheral neuropathy, malnutrition, and secondary liver disease. Chronic alcoholic myopathy is characterized by selective atrophy of type II muscle fibers and the entire muscle mass may be reduced by up to 30%. Alcohol and acetaldehyde are potent inhibitors of muscle protein synthesis, and both contractile and non-contractile proteins are usually affected by acute and chronic alcohol exposure. Some possible mechanisms include free radical effects, and calcium and immunologic disturbances may play a role. The extent of the myopathy significantly correlates with the overall amount of the patient's alcohol consumption during his or her lifetime. Malnutrition or electrolyte disturbances are not thought to be important contributing factors. The main clinical features are painless atrophy and paresis of the proximal limb muscles. The pelvic girdle musculature is usually affected much more than the shoulder girdle. An associated cardiomyopathy is common. Besides, alcoholic myopathy may be accompanied by alcoholic polyneuropathy, which usually involves the more distal parts of the limbs. The serum creatine phosphokinase level may be elevated in one-third of patients. Electromyography and histological examination show non-specific myopathic features, which may be demonstrated in a significant number of all alcohol misusers with minimal or even absent clinical symptoms. Abstention from alcohol is considered to be the most important treatment measure. A well-balanced diet and physiotherapy should be recommended in addition. In general, alcoholic myopathy has a more favorable prognosis in comparison with alcoholic polyneuropathy.

Alcoholic polyneuropathy

The clinical presentation of alcohol-related polyneuropathy was described more than 200 years ago. Meanwhile the precise mechanisms of pathogenesis of alcoholic neuropathy remain unclear. Polyneuropathy may be found in 10–50% of alcoholic patients according to different diagnostic criteria and patient selection. Alcohol appears to exert a toxic effect on the peripheral nervous system in a time- and dose-dependent manner, so polyneuropathy is usually associated with frequent, heavy, and continuous alcohol consumption. Taking into account electrodiagnostic criteria, polyneuropathy may be detected in up to 90% of patients. A high incidence of alcoholic polyneuropathy is observed in women.

Direct neurotoxic effects of ethanol or its metabolites can cause alcoholic polyneuropathy. Acetaldehyde is one possible mediator of these effects among the ethanol metabolites. At the same time, nutritional and vitamin deficiencies including thiamine, other B-complex vitamins, and folic acid are quite often found in alcoholic patients with polyneuropathy. However, it is always difficult to separate alcohol effects from nutritional and vitamin deficiencies, especially thiamine. Although clinicopathologic features of the pure form of alcoholic polyneuropathy are uniform, they show extensive variations when thiamine deficiency is present. Hereditary polymorphism of aldehyde dehydrogenase-2 can explain the association of acetaldehyde accumulation due to the enzyme inactivity with alcoholic polyneuropathy in some selected patients. It is suggested that a minimal intake of 100 ml ethyl alcohol/day for 3 years precipitates the polyneuropathy.

Alcoholic polyneuropathy is predominantly axonal with the involvement of both afferent and efferent fibers. Clinical manifestations of alcoholic polyneuropathy can be summarized as slowly progressive (over months) abnormalities in sensory, motor, and autonomic functions. In general, symptoms are not quite specific and often indistinguishable from those in other forms of sensorimotor axonal neuropathy. The legs are usually affected earlier than the arms and more severely; so are the distal parts of the extremities in contrast to the proximal ones. Sensory symptoms include early numbness of the soles, hyperalgesia, paresthesias, and dysesthesia of the feet and legs, especially at night. Paresthesias might become unpleasant, even painful. The character of the pain may be variable: dull and constant or sharp and lancinating. Pain and paresthesias, which are commonly reported, usually worsen with even a light touch or any contact. Sometimes patients complain of cramping sensations in the muscles of the feet and calves, as well as a sensation of heat and burning. When the symptoms extend above the ankle level, the fingertips often become similarly involved, giving rise to the well-known stocking-and-glove pattern of sensory disturbances. When the proprioception fibers become involved, sensory ataxia occurs, contributing to gait difficulty, independent of possible concomitant alcoholic cerebellar ataxia. Motor manifestations usually include distal weakness and muscle wasting. Frequent falls and gait unsteadiness are common. These are secondary and mainly due to ataxia that is caused by cerebellar degeneration, sensory ataxia, or distal muscle weakness. Cranial nerve involvement is not common and is usually confined to the oculomotor and low cranial nerves. Symptoms such as dysphagia and dysphonia may appear secondary due to degeneration of the vagus nerve.

Autonomic disturbances are quite relevant clinical features. Excessive sweating of the soles and palmar surfaces of the feet, palms, and fingers is a common manifestation of alcoholic polyneuropathy. There are some signs of parasympathetic dysfunction including depressed heart rate responses, abnormal pupillary reactions, erectile dysfunction, and sleep apnea. Sympathetic dysfunction is quite rare, but it can lead to orthostatic hypotension and hypothermia. There are some visible trophic abnormalities such as thinning of the skin and alteration of nails, but trophic ulcers occur rarely.

Examination usually reveals distal sensory abnormalities, pain in muscles and superficial nerves, loss of tendon reflexes in the legs and less frequently in the arms, distal weakness, muscle atrophy, sweating of the feet and palms, sometimes ataxia, and gait disorders. Occasionally subjective complaints predominate over the mild sensory and motor disturbances.

Some details in regard to clinicopathologic heterogeneity of polyneuropathy should be mentioned. Clinical features of alcoholic polyneuropathy without thiamine deficiency are characterized by slowly progressive, sensory-dominant symptoms. Superficial sensation is predominantly impaired and painful symptoms are the major complaint. Pathologic features are characterized by small-fiber-predominant axonal degeneration. In contrast, the clinicopathologic features of alcoholic polyneuropathy with concomitant thiamine deficiency are variable, constituting a spectrum ranging from a picture of a pure form of alcoholic polyneuropathy to a presentation of non-alcoholic thiamine-deficiency polyneuropathy.

The natural course of alcoholic polyneuropathy is quite variable. Manifestations of polyneuropathy may not be apparent clinically, in spite of continued alcohol consumption. In most cases, well-known clinical symptoms steadily increase over the course of several weeks or months. Alcoholic patients often ignore early symptoms and seek help only when severe neurological disorders develop. Sometimes alcoholic polyneuropathy may present as acute- or subacute-onset sensorimotor polyneuropathy, clinically mimicking Guillain–Barré syndrome. Alcoholics with generalized axonal polyneuropathy are prone to pressure palsies at multiple sites. The prognosis of alcoholic polyneuropathy is generally good in the case of complete abstention from alcohol. Patients with mild to moderate polyneuropathy can significantly improve, but the improvement is usually incomplete in those with severe disorders. The recovery is presumed to be due to regeneration and collateral sprouting of damaged axons. The prognosis does not depend on age. At the same time, some findings suggest that the evidence of vagal neuropathy in long-term alcoholics is associated with a significantly higher mortality rate than in the general population. Deaths due to cardiovascular disease are a major factor.

The diagnosis is based on an accurate history of prolonged and excessive alcohol intake, clinical signs and symptoms, and electrophysiologic testing. Electromyography examination of the distal muscles of the lower extremities shows active denervation as well as chronic changes in the form of re-innervation patterns. Nerve conduction tests may be abnormal even before the emergence of clinical symptoms. Sural nerve biopsy often shows evidence of generalized distal axonal loss affecting both large and small fibers, with secondary segmental demyelination but without distinctive pathologic features. Thiamine levels are not consistently reduced, but the thiamine-mediated enzyme transketolase is often abnormal. In all alcoholic patients with sensorimotor polyneuropathy other causes of neuropathy (e.g., malignancy, diabetes, and nerve trauma) should be routinely excluded. In cases of acute or subacute manifestation of alcohol-related polyneuropathy, Guillain–Barré syndrome may be considered, although biopsy and electro-diagnostic studies usually reveal an axonal neuropathy, with normal cerebrospinal fluid (CSF) parameters. Patients have an increased risk of compression neuropathy and the interpretation of electro-diagnostic findings can be confusing because of superimposed mononeuropathies.

The treatment strategy is directed against further damage of the peripheral nerves supporting the restoration of functioning. It can be achieved by alcohol abstinence, a nutritionally balanced diet supplemented by all the B vitamins, physical therapy, and rehabilitation. Benfotiamine 320 mg/day for 4 weeks followed by 120 mg/day for at least 4 more weeks may be recommended. However, in the setting of ongoing alcohol consumption, vitamin supplementation alone is not sufficient for improvement in most patients.

Fetal alcohol syndrome

Maternal alcohol consumption during pregnancy can cause serious birth defects, of which fetal alcohol syndrome is the most devastating. Recognized by characteristic craniofacial abnormalities (smooth philtrum, thin vermillion, and small palpebral fissures) and growth retardation (intrauterine growth restriction and failure to have catch-up growth), this condition produces severe alcohol-induced damage in the developing brain and leads to cognitive impairment, learning disabilities, and behavioral abnormalities.

Ethanol and its metabolite acetaldehyde can alter fetal development by disrupting cellular differentiation and growth, disrupting DNA and protein synthesis, and inhibiting cell migration. Both ethanol and acetaldehyde modify the intermediary metabolism of carbohydrates, proteins, and fats. They also decrease the transfer of amino acids, glucose, folic acid, zinc, and other nutrients across the placental barrier, indirectly affecting fetal growth due to intrauterine nutrient deprivation.

The principal structural and functional neurological features of children with fetal alcohol syndrome include microcephaly, delayed or deficient myelination, agenesis or hypoplasia of the corpus callosum, intellectual impairment (mild to moderate mental retardation), cognitive impairment, developmental delay, irritability in infancy, hyperactivity in childhood or attention deficit/hyperactivity disorder, ataxia, and seizures.

Neuro-imaging studies reveal that in addition to the overall reduction of brain size, prominent brain shape abnormalities with narrowing in the parietal region and reduced brain growth in portions of the frontal lobe are present. Volumetric and tissue density findings demonstrate disproportionate reductions in the parietal lobe, cerebellar vermis, corpus callosum, and the caudate nucleus, suggesting that certain areas of the brain may be especially vulnerable to prenatal alcohol exposure.

In the absence of sensitive and specific biomarkers of exposure and given the common reluctance or inability of women to accurately disclose the quantity and frequency of their alcohol consumption, validating maternal reports of alcohol use is usually difficult. The risk of alcohol-related effects increases according to maternal alcohol consumption in a dose-dependent fashion. Furthermore, heavy episodic or binge drinking is the riskiest pattern of consumption. No level of alcohol consumption in pregnancy is known to be safe. So far as alcohol primarily affects brain development, drinking in all three trimesters poses a risk. As a consequence, pregnant women can reduce their risk of alcohol-related birth outcomes by reducing the dose or by discontinuing the consumption of alcohol as soon as possible or better before the pregnancy.

Further reading

Koike H, Sobue G. Alcoholic neuropathy. *Curr Opin Neurol* 2006; 19: 481–6.

McIntosh C, Chick J. Alcohol and the nervous system. *J Neurol Neurosurg Psychiatry* 2004; 75; 16–21.

Thier P. Acute and chronic alcohol-related disorders. In: Brandt T, Caplan L, Dichgans J, Diener HC, Kennard C, editors. *Neurological Disorders: Course and Treatment*, 2nd ed. San Diego: Elsevier Science; 2003, pp. 971–90.

Chapter 110
Peripheral neuropathies: overview

Friedhelm Sandbrink[1,2]
[1]Veterans Affairs Medical Center, Washington, USA
[2]Georgetown University, Washington, USA

Polyneuropathy affects numerous peripheral nerves simultaneously. *Mononeuropathy* indicates involvement of a single nerve, usually due to trauma, compression, vasculitis, or tumor infiltration. *Mononeuropathy multiplex* signifies simultaneous or sequential damage to multiple non-contiguous nerves, often due to vasculitis. In the advanced stage, deficits may become confluent and resemble polyneuropathy. *Neuronopathies* are diseases of nerve cell bodies including motor neuron diseases such as spinal muscular atrophies and sensory ganglionopathies.

Polyneuropathies are among the most common neurological disorders. Population-based estimates indicate a prevalence of 2–7%, more common in the elderly, and an annual incidence of 25–200/100000. In Western countries, the most common causes are diabetes mellitus and alcoholism. In other countries, infectious etiologies are prominent, especially leprosy. Table 110.1 shows some of the many causes of polyneuropathy. Even after diagnostic workup, the etiology remains unknown in one-third of patients (Table 110.1).

Most polyneuropathies fit the typical pattern of symmetric sensory predominant symptoms with distal onset, consistent with "length-dependent" or "dying-back" axonal polyneuropathy. The primary insult to neuron or axon causes degeneration in the distal parts of the nerve, most removed from the trophic influence of the nerve cell body. Failure of axonal transport results in wallerian degeneration distally with centripetal progression. Clinically, numbness or paresthesiae begin in the toes and feet. When the sensory symptoms reach to just below the knee level, the hands become affected and a stocking-and-glove sensory deficit pattern is said to be present and weakness and atrophy of distal muscles may follow.

In a patient with this typical pattern and a history or laboratory documentation of diabetes, alcohol abuse, vitamin B_{12} deficiency, uremia, or preceding exposure to a known neurotoxin or drug, further diagnostic workup is unlikely to change the diagnosis. Patients without an obvious cause may have "cryptogenic" polyneuropathy, but should undergo further testing including neurophysiology.

Table 110.1 Causes of polyneuropathy.

Hereditary
- Hereditary motor and sensory neuropathies
- Hereditary sensory and autonomic neuropathies
- Refsum's disease
- Familial amyloidosis
- Friedreich's ataxia
- Metachromatic leukodystrophy
- Krabbe's disease
- Abetalipoproteinemia
- Tangier disease
- Fabry's disease
- Porphyrias

Acquired
- Immune-mediated
  - Guillain–Barré syndrome
  - Chronic inflammatory demyelinating polyneuropathy
  - Multifocal motor neuropathy
  - Vasculitis
- Neoplastic and paraproteinemic
  - Paraproteinemias
  - Amyloidosis
  - Paraneoplastic
  - Tumor infiltration/compression
- Metabolic
  - Diabetes
  - Vitamin B_1, B_6, and B_{12} deficiency
  - Hypothyroidism
  - Uremia
  - Liver disease
- Infective and granulomatous
  - HIV-related
  - Leprosy
  - Lyme
  - Diphtheria
  - Sarcoidosis
  - Sepsis/multiorgan failure
- Drug-induced and toxic
  - Alcohol
  - Drugs
  - Toxins

Any atypical presentation, including predominant weakness, asymmetrical or anatomically restricted pattern, and an acute or relapsing course, indicates a shorter list of diagnostic possibilities (Figure 110.1). These patients

International Neurology: A Clinical Approach. Edited by Robert P. Lisak, Daniel D. Truong, William M. Carroll, and Roongroj Bhidayasiri. © 2009 Blackwell Publishing, ISBN: 978-1-4051-5738-4.

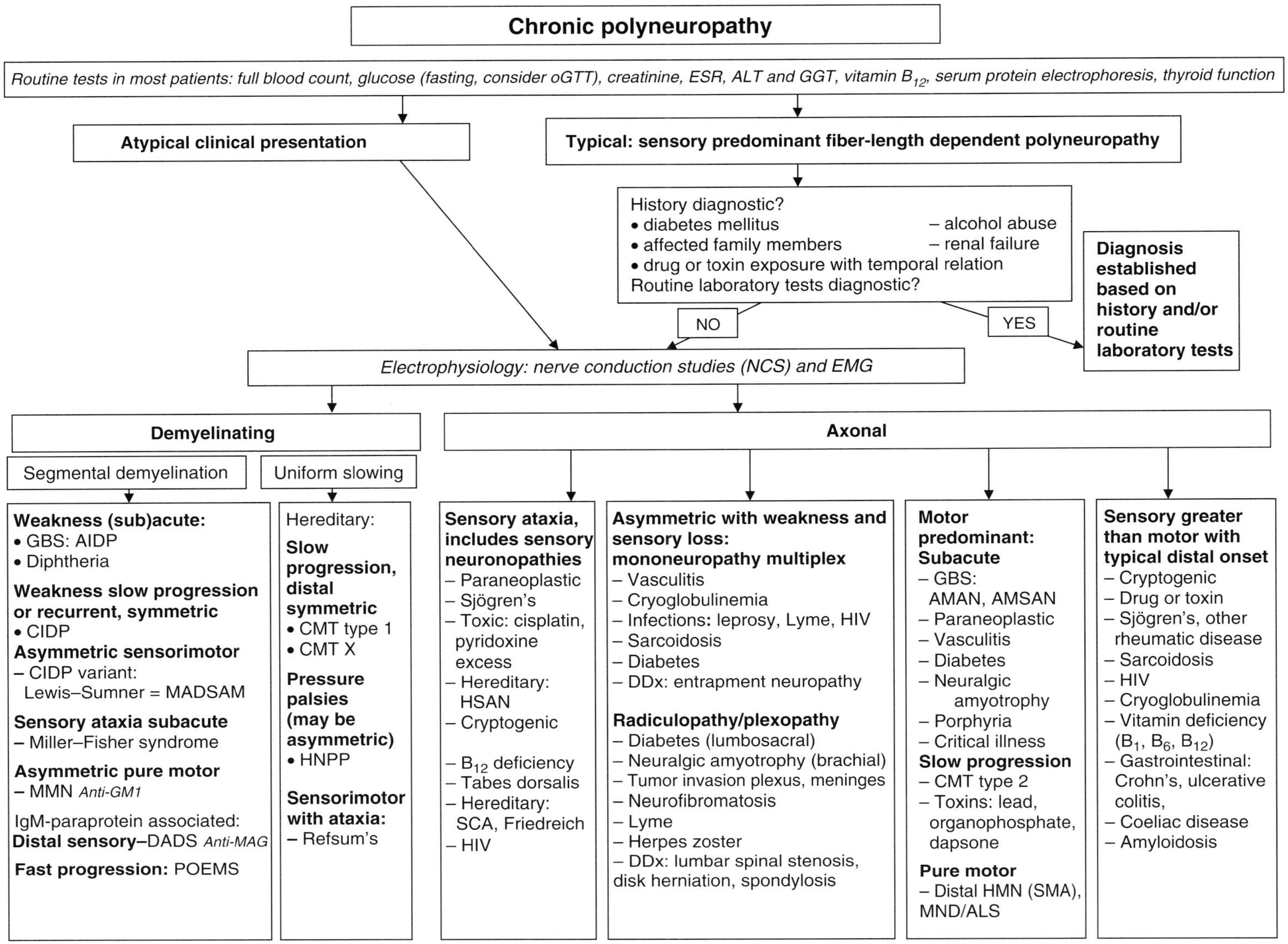

Chronic polyneuropathy

Routine tests in most patients: full blood count, glucose (fasting, consider oGTT), creatinine, ESR, ALT and GGT, vitamin B$_{12}$, serum protein electrophoresis, thyroid function

Typical: sensory predominant fiber-length dependent polyneuropathy

Atypical clinical presentation

History diagnostic?
• diabetes mellitus
• affected family members
• drug or toxin exposure with temporal relation
Routine laboratory tests diagnostic?

– alcohol abuse
– renal failure

YES → **Diagnosis established based on history and/or routine laboratory tests**

NO

Electrophysiology: nerve conduction studies (NCS) and EMG

Demyelinating

Segmental demyelination

Weakness (sub)acute:
• GBS: AIDP
• Diphtheria
Weakness slow progression or recurrent, symmetric
• CIDP
Asymmetric sensorimotor
– CIDP variant:
  Lewis–Sumner = MADSAM
Sensory ataxia subacute
– Miller–Fisher syndrome
Asymmetric pure motor
– MMN *Anti-GM1*
IgM-paraprotein associated:
Distal sensory–DADS *Anti-MAG*
Fast progression: POEMS

Uniform slowing

Hereditary:
Slow progression, distal symmetric
• CMT type 1
• CMT X
Pressure palsies (may be asymmetric)
• HNPP
Sensorimotor with ataxia:
– Refsum's

Axonal

Sensory ataxia, includes sensory neuronopathies
– Paraneoplastic
– Sjögren's
– Toxic: cisplatin, pyridoxine excess
– Hereditary: HSAN
– Cryptogenic
– B$_{12}$ deficiency
– Tabes dorsalis
– Hereditary: SCA, Friedreich
– HIV

Asymmetric with weakness and sensory loss: mononeuropathy multiplex
– Vasculitis
– Cryoglobulinemia
– Infections: leprosy, Lyme, HIV
– Sarcoidosis
– Diabetes
– DDx: entrapment neuropathy
Radiculopathy/plexopathy
– Diabetes (lumbosacral)
– Neuralgic amyotrophy (brachial)
– Tumor invasion plexus, meninges
– Neurofibromatosis
– Lyme
– Herpes zoster
– DDx: lumbar spinal stenosis, disk herniation, spondylosis

Motor predominant:
Subacute
– GBS:
  AMAN, AMSAN
– Paraneoplastic
– Vasculitis
– Diabetes
– Neuralgic amyotrophy
– Porphyria
– Critical illness
Slow progression
– CMT type 2
– Toxins: lead, organophosphate, dapsone
Pure motor
– Distal HMN (SMA), MND/ALS

Sensory greater than motor with typical distal onset
– Cryptogenic
– Drug or toxin
– Sjögren's, other rheumatic disease
– Sarcoidosis
– HIV
– Cryoglobulinemia
– Vitamin deficiency (B$_1$, B$_6$, B$_{12}$)
– Gastrointestinal: Crohn's, ulcerative colitis,
– Coeliac disease
– Amyloidosis

Figure 110.1 Diagnostic considerations in patients with polyneuropathy depending on clinical and electrophysiological pattern.

Abbreviations: oGTT: oral glucose tolerance test; ESR: erythrocyte sedimentation rate; ALT: alanin transaminase; GGT: gamma glutamyl transferase; EMG: electromyogram; GBS: Guillain–Barré syndrome; AIDP: acute inflammatory demyelinating polyneuropathy; CIDP: chronic inflammatory demyelinating polyneuropathy; MADSAM: multifocal acquired demyelinating sensory and motor neuropathy; MMN: multifocal motor neuropathy; DADS: distal acquired demyelinating sensory neuropathy; POEMS: peripheral neuropathy, organomegaly, endocrinopathy, M-component, and skin changes; CMT: Charcot–Marie–Tooth; HNPP: hereditary neuropathy with liability to pressure palsies; HSAN: hereditary sensory and autonomic neuropathy; SCA: spinocerebellar ataxia; HIV: human immunodeficiency virus; DDx: differential diagnosis; AMAN: acute motor axonal neuropathy; AMSAN: acute motor sensory axonal neuropathy; HMN: hereditary motor neuropathy; SMA: spinal muscular atrophy; MND/ALS: motorneuron disorder/amyotrophic lateral sclerosis.

(Modified from Mygland, *Acta Neurol Scand* 2007; 115(Suppl 187): 15–21 and Vrancken *et al.*, *J Neurol Neurosurg Psychiatry* 2006; 77: 397–401.)

should undergo neurophysiological testing to delineate the pathology.

The typical *axonal neuropathy* is characterized by reduced amplitudes of nerve action potentials with normal or only minor slowing of conduction velocities, affecting sensory more than motor fibers, in legs more than arms. Electromyography documents acute and/ or chronic denervation. Less commonly, axonopathies present as wallerian degeneration distal to single or multiple injury sites related to focal axonal interruption from trauma or vasculitis.

Myelinopathies with *uniform slowing of conduction velocity* are usually hereditary. *Segmental demyelination* is typical for acquired immune-mediated myelinopathies. Neurophysiological testing demonstrates marked slowing of conduction velocity (less than 70% of lower normal limit), severely prolonged distal latencies, and in particular conduction block or temporal dispersion. Conduction block is responsible for weakness and sensory loss. The clinical features of myelinopathies include early loss of reflexes, disproportionately mild muscle atrophy despite marked weakness, proximal muscle involvement, tremor, and enlarged nerves.

Small-fiber involvement is usually not detected by routine electrophysiology. It occurs in amyloidosis, diabetes, HIV, leprosy, hereditary sensory and autonomic neuropathies, Fabry's, and Tangier disease. Patients have impairment of pain and temperature modalities and autonomic dysfunction, including postural hypotension and syncope, heat intolerance due to impaired sweating, and cold extremities. Bladder or bowel dysfunction is common and erectile dysfunction occurs early in men. Autonomic deficits are also common in uremia and paraneoplastic neuropathies.

The differential diagnosis of painful neuropathies includes the small-fiber neuropathies, and also vasculitis, alcohol, porphyria, neuralgic amyotrophy, Guillain–Barré syndrome, entrapment neuropathies, and radiculopathies.

Laboratory testing in patients with undiagnosed polyneuropathy routinely includes full blood count, glucose (fasting, oral glucose tolerance test), creatinine, sedimentation rate, liver function tests, vitamin B_{12}, serum protein and immune electrophoresis, and thyroid function. Further testing is based on the clinical and electrophysiological presentation.

Cerebrospinal fluid (*CSF*) in acquired demyelinating polyneuropathies typically shows markedly increased protein in the setting of normal or only mildly increased cell count. CSF protein to a lesser degree is also elevated in diabetes and some of the inherited demyelinating neuropathies. CSF pleocytosis occurs in HIV or Lyme disease. Paraneoplastic neuropathies may result in increased CSF protein and cell count. Abnormal cytology is noted in meningeal carcinomatosis or lymphomatosis.

A *nerve biopsy* is most useful in patients with suspected vasculitis and amyloidosis, and may be needed in sarcoid, leprosy, or neoplastic infiltration. It may be helpful in acquired or hereditary demyelinating disorders, but is usually not required for diagnosis except polyglycosan body neuropathy. A trend nowadays has seen intradermal nerve histology replacing the traditional sural nerve biopsy.

Medical treatment of neuropathic pain is difficult. Simple analgesics including acetaminophen (paracetamol) and non-steroidal anti-inflammatory drugs (NSAIDs) are not effective. Opioid treatment is controversial and usually requires higher dosages than for nociceptive pain. Treatment with adjuvant pain medication includes antidepressants and anticonvulsants. Tricyclic antidepressants relieve burning and dysesthesiae and improve sleep. Nortriptyline, amitriptyline, or desipramine are used with initial doses of 10–25 mg at bedtime and gradually increased as tolerated. Side effects including sedation are frequently dose limiting and caution is advised in elderly patients and patients with cardiac arrhythmias. Serotonin-norepinephrine reuptake inhibitors (duloxetine, venlafaxine) may be helpful. Anticonvulsants include gabapentin, pregabalin, carbamazepine, and other sodium channel blocking agents. The topical agents capsaicin cream and lidocaine patches may also be helpful.

Further reading

Mygland A. Approach to the patient with chronic polyneuropathy. *Acta Neurol Scand* 2007; 115(Suppl 187): 15–21.

Vrancken AF, Kalmijn S, Buskens E, *et al*. Feasibility and cost efficiency of a diagnostic guideline for chronic polyneuropathy: a prospective implementation study. *J Neurol Neurosurg Psychiatry* 2006; 77: 397–401.

Chapter 111
Hereditary neuropathy

Liying Cui and Mingsheng Liu
Peking Union Medical College Hospital, Beijing, China

Introduction

The classification of hereditary neuropathies has been a source of confusion, as both clinical and genetic schemes are used. Based on clinical patterns, hereditary neuropathies are subdivided into three categories, reflecting the selective or predominant involvement of the motor or sensory peripheral nervous system. The most common group is *hereditary motor and sensory neuropathy (HMSN)*, also called Charcot–Marie–Tooth disease as it was first described by Charcot and Marie in France and Tooth in England in 1886, in which both motor and sensory nerves are affected. The second group is *hereditary sensory and autonomic neuropathy (HSAN)*, in which sensory dysfunction prevails and the autonomic nervous system is involved to a varying degree. The third group are the *distal hereditary motor neuropathies* that only affect the peripheral motor nervous system, and are also termed spinal muscular atrophies.

Hereditary motor and sensory neuropathy (HMSN)

HMSN or Charcot–Marie–Tooth (CMT) neuropathy refers to inherited peripheral neuropathies that affect motor and sensory nerves. It is a heterogenous group of disorders, and since 1991 more than 24 distinct genetic causes have been identified. Table 111.1 provides a framework for HMSN based on clinical and genetic information

Clinically, HMSN with autosomal dominant inheritance is subdivided on the basis of nerve conduction velocity into two types: HMSN I or CMT1 with slow conduction velocities (demyelinating) and HMSN II or CMT2 with normal or near normal conduction velocities (axonal). HMSN III is the clinical category for hypertrophic neuropathy with onset in infancy, termed Dejerine–Sottas disease (CMT3). CMT X is X-linked and has intermediately slowed nerve conduction velocity.

International Neurology: A Clinical Approach. Edited by Robert P. Lisak, Daniel D. Truong, William M. Carroll, and Roongroj Bhidayasiri.
© 2009 Blackwell Publishing, ISBN: 978-1-4051-5738-4.

Epidemiology

HMSN is the most common inherited peripheral neuropathy and one of the most common inherited neurological diseases. The exact prevalence is uncertain because of its clinical heterogeneity, but it is usually quoted as 40/100 000 of the population.

Pathophysiology

Inheritance of HMSN is most often autosomal dominant, with almost complete penetrance; less often it is autosomal recessive and rarely X-linked dominant or X-linked recessive. Seventy percent of cases of CMT1 result from duplication of the gene for a peripheral myelin protein (PMP22) on chromosome 17p11 (CMT1A), and 20% are caused by a point mutation in the gene for the myelin protein P0 (*MPZ gene*) on chromosome 1q22 (CMT1B). Other studies of the *PMP22* and *P0* gene expression in CMT1 and CMT3 (Dejerine–Sottas disease) have yielded discordant results. The disease termed hereditary liability to pressure palsies (HNPP) displays an aberration on chromosome 17 within the same gene as CMT1A, but in the form of a deletion rather than duplication of the *PMP22* gene. The identification of many new genes associated with CMT demonstrates the role of axonal transport and abnormal protein trafficking. Axonal signaling and the molecular architecture of both Schwann cells and neurons are of considerable importance in the pathogenesis of CMT.

Nerve biopsy in CMT1 demonstrates reduced numbers of myelinated nerve fibers; myelinated fiber histograms demonstrate a unimodal distribution with a broad middle peak and deficiency of both large and small myelinated fibers. Striking Schwann cell proliferation forming "onion bulbs" is a typical feature (Plate 111.1). The fascicular area is expanded because of endoneurial fibrosis. Teased nerve fibers show paranodal segmental demyelination and internodal remyelination.

In CMT2, the pathology demonstrates a decreased number of large-diameter myelinated nerve fibers; the loss is greater at distal sites. In plastic-embedded sections, features include loss of myelinated nerve fibers, axonal atrophy as demonstrated by an increase in the axon-caliber myelin thickness ratio, and small clusters of thinly

419

Table 111.1 Hereditary motor sensory neuropathies.

Disorder	Locus/gene	Inheritance	Protein	Mutation (frequency)
CMT1A	17p11.2/*PMP22*	AD	PMP22	Duplication (98%)
HNPP	17p11.2/*PMP22*	AD	PMP22	Deletion (80%)
CMT1B	1q22/*MPZ*	AD	MP0	Point mutation
CMT1C	16P13.1-P12.3/*LITAF*	AD	SIMPLE	Point mutation
CMT1D	10q21.1-q22.1/*EGR2*	AD	Early growth response protein 2	Point mutation
CMT2A	1p36/*KIF1B*	AD	Kinesin-like protein KIF1B	Point mutation
CMT2B	3q21/*RAB7*	AD	Ras-related protein Rab-7	Point mutation
CMT2C	12q23-24/unknown	AD	Unknown	
CMT2D	7p15/*GARS*	AD	Glycyl-tRNA synthetase	Point mutation
CMT2E	8p21/*NEFL*	AD	Neurofilament triplet L protein	Point mutation
CMT2F	7q11-21/*HSP27*	AD	Small heatshock protein 27, also called HSPB1	Point mutation
CMT4A	8q13-q21.1/*GDAP1*	AR	Ganglioside-induced differentiation protein-1	Point mutation
CMT4B1	11qww/*MTMR2*	AR	Myotubularin-related protein 2	Point mutation
CMT4B2	11p15/*CMT4B2*	AR	SET binding factor 2	
CMT4C	5Q32/*KIAA1985*	AR	Unknown	
CMT4D	8q24.3/*NDRG1*	AR	NDRG1 protein	
CMT4E	10q21.1-q22.1/*EGR2*	AR	Early growth response protein 2	
CMT4F	19q13.1-q13.2/*PRX*	AR	Periaxin	
CTMX	Xq13.1-q13.2/*PRX*	X-linked	Gap junction beta-1 protein (connexin 32)	

AD: autosomal dominant; AR: autosomal recessive.

myelinated, regenerating axons. Occasional onion-bulbs may also be encountered. Teased nerve fibers shows nerve wrinkling, myelin wrinkling, Wallerian-like degeneration, and remyelination. Remyelination can be distinguished from primary demyelination by the increased number of consecutive short internodal segments.

In CMT3 (Dejerine–Sottas disease), nerve biopsy shows a marked reduction of myelinated nerve fibers. Thinly myelinated fibers are prominent. Onion-bulb formation is usually more severe than in CMT1. Teased nerve fiber preparations demonstrate segmental demyelination or uniform, thinly myelinated fibers giving the appearance of hypomyelination. The unmyelinated fiber population remains relatively spared.

In HNPP, the number of myelinated nerve fibers is variable. In many cases, there is only a slight reduction, while others show an obvious loss. The diagnostic finding on nerve biopsy is the presence of sausage-shaped structures comprising redundant loops of myelin folded over and back on themselves. In plasticized sections, nerve fibers may appear hypermyelinated when the redundant loops adhere to the contour of the axon. In teased nerve fiber preparation, the thickened or swollen areas appear globular or sausage-like and in longitudinal section the thickened areas appear as focal enlargements. Electronmicroscopy of the large thickened fibers shows increased numbers of myelin lamellae and some demyelinated fibers, but the axons and Schwann's cells are normal (Figure 111.1).

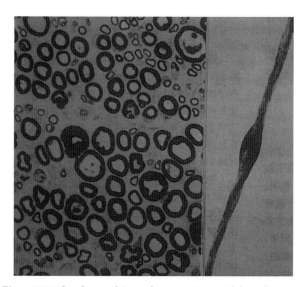

Figure 111.1 Sural nerve biopsy from a patient with hereditary neuropathy with liability to pressure palsies shows focal abnormally thickened myelin (tomacula). Many fibers have abnormally thin myelin. Teased nerve fiber preparations show regions of myelin thickening (tomaculi) that appears sausage-like. (Reproduced with permission from Chen Lin, *et al.*, *Zhonghua Shen Jing Ke Za Zhi* 1997; 30: 142–6.)

Clinical features
CMT1

CMT1 is the most common subtype of HMSN. It is autosomal dominant with onset in the first or second decade. About 20% of cases have no family history and represent new mutations. There are four genetic variants: 70% have CMT1A, 20% CMT1B, and 10% CMT1C or CMT1D. These variants cannot be distinguished by clinical or electrophysiological studies, although some evidence suggests that CMT1B may be slightly more severe.

The clinical presentation of CMT1 includes complete symmetry and slow progression over decades. Difficulty running, frequent ankle sprains, or stumbling and slapping of the feet are noted by the parents of young children. Adult patients have difficulty dating the onset of symptoms. Milder forms may not even be aware of neuropathy, and examination of family members may identify patients without symptoms. Distal muscle weakness and atrophy begins in the feet and legs and later involves the hands. The majority of patients have pes cavus and hammer toes. Sometimes it is these skeletal abnormalities that bring the patient to medical attention. In severe cases, clawing of the fingers may be seen. An early age of onset of motor impairment is predictive of a more severe course. Most patients do not complain of sensory impairment, but vibratory sensation is usually diminished with preserved joint position sense. Muscle stretch reflexes are absent, especially in lower limbs. The feet may become cold, swollen, and blue, secondary to muscle inactivity. There is usually no autonomic dysfunction.

CMT2
CMT2 is less common than CMT1. Genetic linkage has been established for six types of CMT2, all autosomal dominant. Clinically, CMT2A shows a striking resemblance to CMT1. The onset is often slightly later than in CMT1, sometimes in the second decade or even later. Families with CMT2B have been reported to have mutilating neuropathic ulcers. CMT2C may have vocal cord paralysis and respiratory muscle weakness. In severe cases, symptoms begin in infancy; the majority of patients have a more insidious onset. CMT2D more severely affects the upper limbs than the legs. The distinguishing feature is onset with hand weakness and atrophy, and there is preferential loss of muscle stretch reflexes and sensory loss in the upper extremities.

X-linked CMT neuropathy (CMTX)
CMTX is caused by genetic defects on the proximal long arm of the X chromosome (Xq13.1), the locus of the gene encoding the connexin 32 (Cx32) protein, which is expressed by myelinating Schwann cells and is necessary for the formation of gap junctions. More than 150 different mutations of the *Cx32* gene have been identified. With genetic testing, CMTX is nowadays more commonly diagnosed and represents the second most common form of CMT with at least 10–15% of all HMSN. Clinical findings are similar to CMT1. Peripheral nerves are often not palpably enlarged. The disease has an expanded clinical spectrum including demyelinating, intermediate, and axonal neuropathies, transient central nervous system dysfunction, mental retardation, and hearing loss. Females carrying the *Cx32* mutation may be asymptomatic or only mildly affected.

Dejerine–Sottas disease (CMT3)
The clinical classification of Dejerine–Sottas disease or HMSN III refers to a severe demyelinating form of HMSN with onset in early childhood and autosomal recessive inheritance. In recent classifications, Dejerine–Sottas disease as CMT3 identifies all the severe sensory and motor neuropathies with early onset, including autosomal recessive or dominant forms. The genes known to cause CMT3 include *PM22*, *P0*, and *EGR2*. Clinical onset is at birth or early childhood. Pain and paresthesiae in the feet occur early, followed by symmetrical weakness and wasting distally. Delayed motor milestones lead to inability to walk. Talipes equinovarus postures with claw feet and later claw hands are common. All sensory modalities are impaired distally, and tendon reflexes are absent. Miotic, unreactive pupils, nystagmus, and kyphoscoliosis have been observed. The enlarged nerves are not tender.

Hereditary neuropathy with pressure palsies (HNPP)

HNPP (also termed tomaculous neuropathy) is autosomal dominant, with onset in the second or third decade typically as multiple mononeuropathy. It is caused by a deletion of the *PMP22* gene, the same gene involved in CMT1A. In CMT1A, the gene is duplicated on one chromosome, and the total PMP22 protein is therefore increased. By contrast, in HNPP the gene is deleted from one chromosome, so that the PMP22 protein is predicted to be at half-normal levels. Patients usually present with episodic recurrent motor and sensory neuropathies caused by traction or compression. Weakness and sensory loss occur in an anatomic distribution of a specific peripheral nerve. The focal neuropathies and plexopathies are generally not painful. Focal nerve lesions are often provoked by slight or brief compression. Most commonly affected are the ulnar nerve (elbow), peroneal nerve (fibula head), median nerve (wrist), and radial nerve (spiral groove). In addition to recurrent focal neuropathies, most individuals with HNPP have a mild, slowly progressive, demyelinating sensorimotor neuropathy.

Investigations
The contribution of electrophysiology to our understanding and diagnosis of inherited neuropathy cannot be overemphasized. In both CMT1 and CMT2, the compound muscle action potentials (CMAPs) and

sensory nerve action potentials (SNAPs) are reduced in amplitude. Severe sensory nerve conduction abnormalities may be asymptomatic. In CMT1, there is severe and uniform slowing of nerve conduction velocity without conduction block, with lower limbs more affected than arms. Most patients have conduction velocities between 15 and 30 m/s. In CMT2, motor nerve conduction velocities are normal or mildly slow, and CMAP amplitudes are greatly reduced. SNAPs are also significantly reduced or absent, more severely in lower limbs. CMAP and SNAP amplitudes are more severely reduced in CMT2 than in CMT1, but temporal dispersion is more severe in CMT1. Conventional electromyogram (EMG) studies show neurogenic changes, including increased duration and amplitude of motor unit potentials and decreased recruitment patterns, most severe in distal lower limb muscles.

The cerebrospinal fluid (CSF) in CMT1 and CMT2 is usually normal. Some patients have mildly elevated CSF protein up to 80 mg/dl, rarely higher in CMT1.

Genetic tests for the most common types (CMT1A, CMT1B, CMT2 and CMTX) are available, and it is now possible to identify many more cases including sporadic ones. It is seldom necessary to resort to nerve biopsy for diagnosis; occasionally biopsy is necessary for patients with negative genetic testing to exclude chronic inflammatory demyelinating polyneuropathy .

In CMT3, unlike other forms of CMT, the CSF protein is usually elevated, in all likelihood because the spinal roots are enlarged. Nerve conduction velocities are markedly reduced, even when there is little or no functional impairment.

In HNPP, electrophysiological studies show focal slowing of conduction velocities and a loss of amplitude at the sites of entrapment affecting motor and sensory nerves. HNPP patients have some slowing of conduction velocities of distal motor and sensory nerves favoring a more generalized demyelinating neuropathy. CSF protein may be elevated. Nerve biopsies document localized nerve sheath thickening with duplication of the myelin lamellae.

Hereditary sensory and autonomic neuropathy (HSAN)

The HSAN is a clinically and genetically heterogenous group with five different clinical subtypes. With the exception of the autosomal dominant HSAN1, the other four types are autosomal recessive. Molecular genetic research has shown that at least eight loci and six genes are associated with HSAN.

Clinical features
HSAN I
HSAN I, the most common form, is linked to chromosome 9q22. Onset of this autosomal dominant neuropathy occurs between the second and fourth decade as a slowly progressive but marked sensory impairment with variable motor and minimal autonomic involvement. Patients come to clinical attention for foot ulcers or spontaneous pain. Impaired sensation in the lower limbs causes foot deformities and ulcerations, and some patients have Charcot joints. The sensory deficit is symmetrical and more severely affects the distal lower limbs. Sensory loss for pain and temperature predominates. Some patients show hyperhidrosis and anhidrosis at different stages, caused by denervation to the sweat glands. Muscle stretch reflexes are depressed or absent at the ankle and preserved at other joints. Distal muscle weakness is not prominent.

HSAN II
HSAN II is a rare autosomal recessive form. Patients present in early childhood with distal glove-and-stocking numbness in the upper and lower limbs. Later, the sensory loss affects all modalities with impairment of pain, temperature, and touch, including the trunk. Patients usually have digital ulcers and recurrent fractures. In most cases, the neurologic deficits are not or only slowly progressive.

HSAN III
HSAN III (also called Riley–Day syndrome or infantile dysautonomia) is autosomal recessive. It affects the development and survival of sensory and autonomic neurons, and is a catastrophic illness starting at birth. Patients demonstrate swallowing problems, episodes of vomiting, and intermittent unexplained fever. Absent lacrimation, profuse sweating, and labile blood pressure are common. On physical examination, the absence of fungiform papillae of the tongue is particularly important. Muscle stretch reflexes are usually absent. Muscle strength is normal. There is decreased nociception and temperature sensation over the entire body, whereas touch, vibration, and position sensation are retained. Many die in early childhood from recurrent pneumonia.

HSAN IV
HSAN IV represents a congenital variant of autosomal recessive HSAN. Autonomic disturbances are a predominant feature. Sweating is markedly decreased or absent, leading to episodic fever. Absent pain sensation promotes repeated traumatic and thermal injuries and severe mutilations of the hands and feet. Hyperactivity and emotional lability are common, and children often show mild mental retardation. On examination, there is widespread anhidrosis, decreased pinprick, deep pain and temperature sensation, with normal touch, vibration, and proprioception. Muscle strength and deep tendon reflexes are preserved. Patients may die from hyperpyrexia within the first years of life.

HSAN V

HSAN V, the least common HSAN, begins in infancy. Impaired nociception and temperature sensation leads to acral ulcers, painless fractures, and neurogenic arthropathies. Other sensory modalities are preserved, and autonomic function is normal except for decreased sweating in some patients. Muscle strength and tendon reflexes are normal. There is no mental retardation.

Investigations

Motor conduction velocity is normal or only mildly reduced in HSANs. EMG may reveal large motor unit potentials in distal muscles. SNAPs are reduced in amplitude or absent in HSAN I, HSAN II, and HSAN III, and normal in HSAN IV and HSAN V. The sympathetic skin response is absent.

Distal hereditary motor neuropathy (distal HMN)

The distal HMNs are often included in the inherited neuropathies and comprise about 10% of all inherited motor neuropathies. They are neuronopathies and usually termed spinal muscular atrophies (SMAs). A separate chapter is devoted to their discussion (Chapter 55). Patients usually present with weakness and atrophy in distal muscles. Sensory abnormalities are absent, although older patients may have a mild decrease in vibratory sensation. Distal HMNs have been tentatively classified into seven subtypes on the basis of clinical phenotype, age at onset, and mode of inheritance. Four subtypes are autosomal dominant: type I is juvenile, type II adult onset, type V affects the upper extremities preferentially, and type VII has vocal cord paralysis. The autosomal recessive forms are types III, IV, and VI, more severe and with earlier onset than the dominant forms. Electrodiagnostic examination of the SMAs reveals normal or near-normal SNAPs. Motor conduction velocities are normal or minimally slow, despite clinical evidence of weakness and atrophy and EMG evidence of denervation-reinnervation. Fasciculations may be encountered but are not nearly as prominent as in amyotrophic lateral sclerosis.

Other hereditary neuropathies

Refsum's disease (sometimes termed HMSN IV) is an autosomal recessive disorder (chromosome 10) resulting in accumulation of phytanic acid. Peripheral neuropathy is usually present by age 20. Other features include retinitis pigmentosa (night blindness), ichthyosis, and cerebellar ataxia. Muscle weakness and atrophy begins in the legs distally and later becomes generalized, accompanied by areflexia and large-fiber sensory impairment. Pes cavus and overriding toes (due to short fourth metatarsals) are diagnostic clues. CSF protein is elevated. Motor conduction velocities are markedly slowed, with either uniform or non-uniform changes. SNAPs are decreased or absent. Refsum's disease is treated by elimination of phytanic acid from the diet, and plasmapheresis may be helpful to reduce body stores of phytanic acid.

Familial amyloid polyneuropathy (FAP) often presents as small-fiber neuropathy, but large fiber function and motor fibers are usually affected in advanced disease. Decreased pain and temperature sensation is accompanied by stabbing, lancinating pains in the feet and autonomic dysfunction (impaired sweating, postural hypotension, constipation or diarrhea, etc.). Nerve entrapment (carpal tunnel syndrome) may occur from amyloid deposition. Several subtypes have been described, with types I and II linked to the transthyretin (TTR) gene on chromosome 18q11.

Friedreich's ataxia (see Chapter 48) manifests as childhood-onset ataxia and sensory greater than motor polyneuropathy. The disorder is autosomal recessive and is caused by triplet repeat expansion in a non-coding region of the frataxin gene on chromosome 9q. Features include ataxic gait, clumsiness, and other features of cerebellar ataxia, reduced or absent deep tendon reflexes, distal weakness and atrophy, scoliosis, and electrocardiogram (ECG) abnormalities.

In hereditary disorders of lipid metabolism, dysmyelination usually affects central and peripheral myelin, and central manifestations often overshadow the peripheral neuropathy. Polyneuropathy occurs in children with *metachromatic leukodystrophy* and *Krabbe's disease* (globoid cell leukodystrophy), both autosomal recessive. *Adrenoleukodystrophy or adrenomyeloneuropathy* is X-linked dominant; *abetalipoproteinemia* and *Tangier disease* are autosomal recessive.

Fabry's disease (see Chapter 157) is caused by X-linked deficiency of alpha-galactosidase. Affected boys or young men complain of burning or stabbing pain in hands and feet, especially with heat exposure or fever. Angiokeratomas (reddish purple skin lesions) are typical. Premature arteriosclerosis causes renal disease and early strokes. Routine nerve conduction studies are normal in this small-fiber neuropathy. Enzyme replacement therapy is available.

The *porphyrias* (see Chapter 163) are inherited disorders of defective heme synthesis. Three autosomal dominant forms cause peripheral neuropathy. Most common is acute intermittent porphyria, the others are variegate porphyria and hereditary coproporphyria. Drugs or hormonal changes precipitate attacks. Typically, acute abdominal pain is followed 48–72 hours later by sudden onset of proximal or distal weakness (resembling Guillain–Barré syndrome), with sensory findings less prominent. Tendon reflexes are diminished, but ankle jerks are often retained.

Respiratory insufficiency may occur, and autonomic abnormalities are frequent. Pain may present early in the legs or back. Agitation or psychosis is common. Some patients recover rapidly, others have slow improvement of weakness over many months. Acute intermittent porphyria is caused by abnormal porphobilinogen deaminase, and urinary levels of porphobilinogen and aminolevulinic acid are increased.

Treatment

No specific treatment is known for hereditary neuropathy, with the exception of some of the inherited metabolic disorders. Stabilizing the ankles by arthrodeses is indicated if foot drop is severe. Regular exercise, but avoiding excessive weight training, is important. Home-based, moderate-intensity resistance training can improve muscle function. In mild and early cases, fitting the legs with light braces and the shoes with springs to overcome foot drop can be helpful. Referral for occupational therapy service is strongly advised to address a variety of activities.

For patients with HSAN, the most important aspect of management is attending to acral ulcers to prevent sepsis and osteomyelitis. For patients with lancinating pain, a similar approach to other painful neuropathies is appropriate. In some patients immobilization of injured limbs and surgical correction of established deformities must be considered. Precautions should be taken to avoid direct exposure to the sun or activities resulting in overheating, because temperature regulation and sweating are impaired. Defective lacrimation requires special attention to dry eyes. Close observation for bone fractures and progressive scoliosis should be integrated into the care of these patients.

In addition to traditional approaches such as rehabilitation medicine, ambulation aids, and pain management, identification of the genes causing CMT has led to improved genetic counseling and assistance in family planning. Delineation of common molecular pathways in multiple forms of CMT may be exploited in future molecular therapies. Scientifically based clinical trials for CMT are currently being implemented. Techniques of gene therapy may become feasible options in the future.

Further reading

Chance PF. Inherited focal, episodic neuropathies: hereditary neuropathy with liability to pressure palsies and hereditary neuralgic amyotrophy. *Neuromol Med* 2006; 8(1–2): 159–74.

Chen L, Guo Y, Huan Y, *et al.* Clinical manifestations and pathology of tomaculous neuropathy. *Zhonghua Shen Jing Ke Za Zhi* 1997; 30: 142–6.

Cui L, Tang X, Li B. Clinical electrophysiological studies of peroneal muscular atrophy: report of 32 cases. *Zhongguo Yi Xue Ke Xue Yuan Xue Bao* 1989; 11: 175–9.

Emery AE. Population frequencies of inherited neuromuscular disease: a world survey. *Neuromuscul Disord* 1991; 1: 19–29.

Houlden H, King R, Blake J, *et al.* Clinical, pathological and genetic characterization of hereditary sensory and autonomic neuropathy type I. *Brain* 2006; 129: 411–25.

Nicholson G, Nash J. Intermediate nerve conduction velocities define X-linked Charcot–Marie–Tooth neuropathy families. *Neurology* 1993; 43: 2558–64.

Shy ME. Charcot–Marie–Tooth disease: an update. *Curr Opin Neurol* 2004; 17: 579–85.

Song S, Zhang Y, Chen B, *et al.* Mutation frequency for Charcot–Marie–Tooth disease type 1 in the Chinese population is similar to that in the global ethnic patients. *Genet Med* 2006; 8: 532–5.

Verhoeven K, Timmerman V, Mauko B, *et al.* Recent advances in hereditary sensory and autonomic neuropathies. *Curr Opin Neurol* 2006; 19: 474–80.

Chapter 112
Acquired neuropathies

Friedhelm Sandbrink[1,2]
[1]Veterans Affairs Medical Center, Washington, USA
[2]Georgetown University, Washington, USA

Immune-mediated neuropathies

Guillain–Barré syndrome (GBS)
Introduction
GBS is the most common cause of acute flaccid paralysis in Western countries and *acute inflammatory demyelinating polyneuropathy (AIDP)* is the most common subtype. The axonal variant of *acute motor sensory axonal neuropathy (AMSAN)* involves both motor and sensory fibers and is often more severe. Most common in China is *acute motor axonal neuropathy (AMAN)*. It lacks any sensory disturbance and is common in children. *Miller–Fisher syndrome* is characterized by areflexia, gait ataxia, and ophthalmoparesis. *Acute dysautonomia* is a rare variant with sympathetic and parasympathetic dysfunction. General features of all forms include a rapidly evolving neurological deficit (usually weakness) often with antecedent infection, areflexia, and elevated cerebrospinal fluid (CSF) protein.

Epidemiology
The annual incidence of GBS in Western countries is 1.2–1.9 per 100000, and the syndrome is slightly more common in men. In Europe and North America, the incidence ranges from less than 1 per 100000 in people younger than 30 years to 4 per 100000 in those older than 70 years. In Western countries, 90% of patients have AIDP and only 5% axonal subtypes. In contrast, in China GBS is less common in adults, with an incidence of 0.66 per 100000 for all ages. In northern China, 60–80% are AMAN; typically as summer epidemics in children and young adults. In Japan, AIDP is about as frequent as AMAN. AMSAN and Miller–Fisher syndrome are less common.

Most cases worldwide are sporadic, but summer epidemics of AMAN occur in China, and small clusters associated with bacterial enteritis caused by contaminated water are seen in tropical countries.

Pathophysiology
In two-thirds of patients, the disease follows within weeks of a preceding upper respiratory or gastrointestinal tract infection or, rarely, surgery, vaccination, or drug exposure. *Campylobacter jejuni* is a major cause of bacterial gastroenteritis throughout the world. It is found serologically in one-third of GBS patients in Western countries and more commonly in China. Other patients have serological evidence for preceding infection with *Mycoplasma pneumoniae*, Epstein–Barr virus, cytomegalovirus (CMV), viral hepatitis, or human immunodeficiency virus (HIV). Slightly increased risk of GBS was noted after influenza vaccination in 1976, with a steady decline since then. The only vaccine with significant risk for GBS is rabies vaccine containing brain material (risk 1:1000).

The antecedent infection presumably triggers an autoimmune response to peripheral nerve antigens by "molecular mimicry." In axonal GBS, a primarily antibody-mediated mechanism is likely as *C. jejuni* lipopolysaccharide and human gangliosides expressed on the motor axolemna of peripheral nerves share homologous epitopes. Serum antibodies against gangliosides GM1, GM1b, GD1a, or GalNAc-GD1a are found in axonal GBS. Autopsy studies in AMAN reveal axonal degeneration of motor fibers without demyelination.

In contrast, in AIDP, cell-mediated and humoral mechanisms are part of the autoimmune attack on peripheral nerve myelin. Lymphocytic infiltration and macrophage invasion of myelin sheath and Schwann's cells are seen. Experimental allergic neuritis, a rat model for AIDP, involves T-cell-mediated activation of lymphocytes against peripheral nerve myelin components. Antiganglioside antibodies and their target epitopes in AIDP are unknown. Epitopes implicated in Miller–Fisher syndrome are GQ1b and GT1a.

Clinical features
Patients typically present with symmetric weakness beginning in the legs and worsening quickly. Paresthesiae may be the initial symptom in AIDP and AMSAN. The leg weakness may be more pronounced distally or proximally, and typically ascends to the trunk

International Neurology: A Clinical Approach. Edited by Robert P. Lisak, Daniel D. Truong, William M. Carroll, and Roongroj Bhidayasiri.
© 2009 Blackwell Publishing, ISBN: 978-1-4051-5738-4.

and arms. Disease severity and progression vary greatly. Some patients have rapidly ascending weakness resulting in quadriplegia and life-threatening compromise of respiration and swallowing within hours. Other patients have only minimal weakness or slow progression over weeks. Most patients are maximally weak within 7–10 days and less in axonal variants. Facial weakness is common. Weakness of neck flexor muscles resulting in inability to lift the head against gravity indicates impending respiratory failure. Tendon reflexes may be normal or hypoactive for the first few days, but then are invariably lost. Sensory impairment is minimal in AIDP; distally decreased vibration sense may be found. In AMSAN, glove-and-stocking sensory deficit accompanies the weakness. Autonomic dysfunction occurs frequently including tachycardia, blood pressure fluctuations, sphincter dysfunction, paralytic ileus, and disturbed sweating. Cardiac arrhythmia, hypotension, or pulmonary failure may be life threatening.

Miller–Fisher syndrome begins with diplopia, evolving within days to rather complete ophthalmoplegia and followed by limb and gait ataxia. Pupillary reflexes are preserved. Mild distal paresthesiae and muscle weakness may be present.

Investigations

The typical CSF finding is protein elevation in the setting of normal cell count, frequently above 300 mg/dl. During the first few days after onset, protein elevation may not be present, and repeat CSF testing should be performed. About 10% of patients, however, lack protein elevation even on serial CSF testing. Transiently elevated IgG or positive oligoclonal bands are common. The cell count is usually normal or less than 10 cells/µl but rarely as high as 50–100 cells/µl. Pleocytosis in a patient with otherwise typical GBS suggests HIV and CMV infection.

Electrophysiological abnormalities may be minor at the onset of weakness, but eventually are found in 90% of patients. In AIDP, marked slowing of motor conduction velocities and conduction block document the demyelination. Prolonged or absent F-waves and increased distal motor latencies are typical early findings. Sensory nerve action potentials (SNAPs) may show a "normal sural-abnormal median pattern." Evidence of denervation and axonal loss is more pronounced in axonal variants. MRI may demonstrate gadolinium enhancement of lumbar nerve roots.

Serological testing has limited value. Elevated serum antibodies and positive stool culture for *C. jejuni* and serological testing (acute and convalescent samples) for Epstein–Barr virus (EBV), CMV, and *M. pneumoniae* are recommended. Antiganglioside antibodies may be present. HIV-serology may be indicated by the clinical context or CSF pleocytosis.

Diagnosis

GBS needs to be distinguished from other conditions with subacute motor weakness. *Diphtheric polyneuropathy* has a long latent period between the respiratory infection and subsequent weakness, slower evolution, and frequent paralysis of ocular accommodation. *Acute anterior poliomyelitis* is distinguished by meningeal irritation, fever, asymmetry of paralysis, and CSF pleocytosis. In *acute porphyria*, the neuropathy is preceded by abdominal pain, associated cognitive symptoms are common, and CSF is normal. *Toxic* (*N*-hexane inhalation, acrylamide, organophosphorus compounds, thallium or arsenic intoxication, heavy metals, biological toxins), *vasculitic*, and *critical illness neuropathies* may also begin acutely. CSF pleocytosis (more than 50 cells/µl) suggests *Lyme disease* or *HIV-associated polyradiculopathy* with superimposed CMV infection. *Tick paralysis* is an ascending motor paralysis developing 5–6 days after the tick has attached itself to a cutaneous site. Cranial nerve palsies and respiratory paralysis occur. CSF is normal. Symptoms promptly reverse with removal of the tick. Muscle disorders to consider include *acute rhabdomyolysis, periodic paralysis, inflammatory myopathy,* or severe *metabolic disturbances* (hypophosphatemia, hypokalemia). Neuromuscular junction disorders may present as subacute weakness. *Botulism* affects the ocular muscles and pupillary reflexes, and is separated by electrophysiology. *Lesions of the CNS,* such as acute basilar artery stenosis, spinal cord compression, or transverse myelitis, or *hysterical weakness* may occasionally present diagnostic difficulties.

Treatment

GBS is best managed in the intensive care setting, as good supportive care is essential. Forced vital capacity should be monitored; reduction below 1 l (15–20 ml/kg), shortness of breath, and retention of carbon dioxide are indications for elective intubation and assisted ventilation. Treatment of cardiac arrhythmia or marked blood pressure fluctuation is often necessary. Leg stockings and subcutaneous heparin reduce the risk of deep vein thrombosis. Skin breakdown and exposure keratitis in patients with facial weakness must be prevented. Even with complete quadriplegia, patients remain cognitively intact, and means of communication should be explored. Treatment of back pain or dysesthesiae may require opioid analgesics.

Immunotherapy is recommended in all GBS subtypes, especially for patients unable to walk. Randomized studies document equal efficacy of plasmapheresis and intravenous immunoglobulin (IVIg). Treatment is best instituted early; it reduces time to recovery and residual neurological deficit. There is no additional benefit of combining both therapies. Plasmapheresis involves removal of 200–250 ml/kg of plasma over 7–10 days and requires catheter placement for venous access. IVIg (0.4 g/kg/day for 5 days) is usually preferred, especially in adults with cardiovascular instability and in children. Corticosteroids are not beneficial.

Prognosis is generally good, with improvement over weeks to months being the rule. About 20% of patients are left with neurological disability, more common in AMSAN. Older age, early progression to maximal deficit (less than 7 days), severity at nadir, need for ventilatory support, and marked reduction in compound muscle action potential (CMAP) amplitudes indicate poor prognosis. Preceding *C. jejuni* and CMV infections are unfavorable, whereas EBV is associated with milder forms. Even with optimal treatment, mortality is 2–10% owing to complications such as respiratory failure and cardiac arrhythmia, which are more likely in AMSAN than AIDP. Most AMAN patients make a good recovery.

Chronic inflammatory demyelinating polyneuropathy (CIDP)

Introduction
CIDP is clinically similar to GBS but with a more protracted or relapsing course. CIDP is arbitrarily defined by progression of weakness over at least 8 weeks (or 2 months), whereas progression over 4–8 weeks indicates subacute inflammatory demyelinating polyneuropathy. About half of all CIDP patients have an atypical, often multifocal presentation.

Epidemiology
The prevalence is reported as 2.0–7.7 per 100 000, but it is likely underdiagnosed due to its clinical heterogeneity and stringent diagnostic criteria. It occurs in all ages, with peak in the fifth or sixth decade. CIDP is a fairly frequent diagnosis (about 20%) in patients with chronic polyneuropathy referred to neuromuscular centers.

Pathophysiology
A preceding infection is unusual and found in less than 10% of cases. Pregnancy may be a triggering factor. Immune-mediated mechanisms resulting in peripheral nerve demyelination are postulated, supported by the benefit of immunotherapy and the finding of lymphocytic infiltration and segmental demyelination in nerve biopsies. There are, however, no established target epitopes or serologic markers in typical CIDP.

Clinical features
CIDP begins insidiously or subacutely, and follows a steady or stepwise progressive (two-thirds of patients) or relapsing–remitting course (one-third, younger patients). Classically, CIDP is characterized by motor-predominant symptoms, with symmetrical weakness of distal and proximal muscles (strongly suggestive) in upper and lower extremities. Deep tendon reflexes are reduced or absent. Sensory involvement tends to affect vibration

and position sense more than pain or temperature. Initial sensory symptoms affecting the upper limbs are typical. A distal to proximal sensory gradient is noted, with fingers as frequently affected as the feet, resulting in numbness or tingling in glove-and-stocking distribution. Cranial nerve involvement is not common, but if present suggests CIDP. Constipation and urinary retention occur late.

About half of CIDP patients have an atypical presentation. A multifocal or asymmetric CIDP variant is called *multifocal acquired demyelinating sensory and motor neuropathy (MADSAM)* or *Lewis–Sumner syndrome (LSS)*. Pain, paresthesiae, and weakness suggest mononeuritis multiplex. Tinel's sign is commonly present. Electrophysiology documents a demyelinating disorder with persistent multifocal conduction block in sensory and motor nerves.

CIDP may also present with *sensory predominant* symptoms, including paresthesiae, dysesthesiae, and proprioceptive ataxia. Patients have usually subclinical motor involvement on electrophysiology. This CIDP variant resembles distal acquired demyelinating sensory neuropathy (DADS), but the latter is considered a separate entity because of IgM paraproteinemia and different treatment response.

Other CIDP variants are *pure motor* or *minimal symptoms* with only fatigability and minor paresthesia.

Investigation
CSF protein is usually increased with normal CSF cell count, but consistently less than in GBS.

Nerve conduction studies indicate a demyelinating neuropathy with superimposed axonal degeneration. Demyelinative criteria include marked slowing of nerve conduction velocities (below 70% of lower normal limit in nerves with reduced CMAP amplitudes), marked prolongation of F-waves, and prolonged distal latencies. Conduction block and temporal dispersion document segmental demyelination. CIDP should also be suspected if the CMAP amplitude is normal in a clinically weak muscle, or if SNAPs are normal despite marked sensory complaints.

The MRI findings of enhancement or hypertrophy of plexus or nerve roots including cauda equina may help confirm the diagnosis.

A nerve biopsy is usually not needed, but may be used when other studies are not diagnostic.

Diagnosis
Diagnostic criteria as published by the American Academy of Neurology in 1991 for research purposes include primarily patients with classical CIDP and are not sensitive enough for clinical use. More recent guidelines (2005) by the European Federation of Neurological Societies/Peripheral Nerve Society define CIDP as typical or atypical. Definite CIDP requires clear-cut demyelinating electrodiagnostic changes in two nerves or

probable demyelinating features in two nerves plus at least one supportive feature (CSF, biopsy, MRI, treatment response).

Chronic polyneuropathies resembling CIDP occur in chronic active hepatitis (B or C), HIV, lymphoma, diabetes, collagen vascular disorders, thyrotoxicosis, after organ and bone marrow transplants, nephrotic syndrome, and inflammatory bowel disease. The differentiation may be particularly difficult in diabetes patients who frequently exhibit more severe slowing of conduction velocities than other axonal polyneuropathies.

Treatment

Corticosteroids are considered beneficial in classical CIDP and its variants, based on a single non-blinded controlled trial and case reports. Plasmapheresis and IVIg were effective in double-blind trials. Comparitive studies indicate similar response rates to these three treatment modalities. Two-thirds of patients will respond to one of these therapies. Steroids may more likely induce a lasting clinical remission. Dosage recommendations range from 60 to 120 mg prednisolone daily to pulse methylprednisolone. A typical regimen is prednisolone 100 mg/day for 2–4 weeks, gradually tapered by 5 mg/week. Clinical response is expected at around 1.9 months. The dosage is reduced to the lowest maintenance dose that prevents relapse. IVIg is first-line therapy due to safety and effectiveness. It is given at 2 g/kg body weight (0.4 g/kg/day for 5 days or 1 g/kg/day for 2 days) and shows clinical benefit as early as 7 days. It may be repeated with 1 g/kg at 3 weeks. More than 80% of patients require maintenance infusions every few weeks (0.5–1.0 g/kg), with some patients requiring higher dosages, others less frequent infusions. IVIg may occasionally be stopped after years. Plasmapheresis is used if IVIg or corticosteroids are ineffective or contraindicated. Immunosuppressants are used in patients who fail standard therapies and include cyclophosphamide, cyclosporin A or tacrolimus, mycophenolate mofetil, the monoclonal antibodies rituximab and alemtuzumab, etanercept and interferons.

Multifocal motor neuropathy (MMN)

MMN is a rare disease (1 in 100 000) that mimics motor neuron disorder but responds to treatment. It is more common in men, with onset between age 20 and 50 years. The polyneuropathy presents as slowly progressive, predominantly distal, and asymmetric weakness, associated with muscle atrophy and fasciculations. It begins typically in the upper extremities, in the anatomical distribution of individual motor nerves. Muscle cramps are common. The disorder is purely motor; any sensory involvement is controversial. Many patients (35–50%) have IgM antibodies against GM1 and occasionally against other glycolipids (asialo-GM1, GD1a, or GM2). Electophysiological testing should be performed on multiple nerves including

proximal segments, in order to identify focal conduction block limited to motor nerves, and at sites usually not affected by entrapment. The electrophysiological findings in motor nerves are similar to Lewis–Sumner syndrome, but sensory involvement does not occur in MMN.

Some patients have the typical clinical presentation of MMN, but electrophysiological findings are axonal. These patients are diagnosed with an axonal variant, called *multifocal acquired motor axonopathy* (MAMA).

The primary treatment for MMN and MAMA is IVIg. Some patients seem to lose responsiveness to maintenance IVIg treatment over years. Corticosteroids and plasmapheresis are not effective.

Neuropathies with monoclonal gammopathies

Paraprotein-associated neuropathies comprise about 10% of neuropathies with otherwise unknown etiology, with neuropathy often the first symptom of the gammopathy. About 10% of neuropathy patients with gammopathy have an underlying hematological malignancy, including Waldenström's macroglobulinemia, multiple myeloma, solitary plasmacytoma, and primary amyloidosis.

In patients with *monoclonal gammopathy of unknown significance* (MGUS) who have neuropathy, the paraprotein is usually IgM and the electrophysiology suggests segmental demyelination. In contrast, in MGUS without neuropathy IgG is more common. About 5% of people over 70 years of age have MGUS, and the yearly risk of progression to malignancy is estimated at 2.7%.

Distal acquired demyelinating sensory (DADS) neuropathy is a slowly progressive symmetric polyneuropathy associated with IgM gammopathy. Antineural antibodies are commonly found in IgM neuropathy, and half of DADS patients have antibodies against the Schwann cell-based myelin-associated glycoprotein (anti-MAG). The polyneuropathy begins with distal paresthesiae and numbness. Weakness is minor, if at all present. After years, patients may develop ataxia, walking difficulty, and tremor. The electrophysiology is demyelinating, with more severe slowing of conduction velocity in distal nerves. Increased CSF protein is common. The prognosis is relatively good due to slow progression of sensory predominant symptoms. Treatment response to steroids is poor, but IVIg or rituximab may be beneficial.

Waldenström's macroglobulinemia is a lymphoplasmocytic lymphoma that produces IgM and may result in demyelinative neuropathy.

The polyneuropathy in *POEMS syndrome* (peripheral neuropathy, organomegaly, endocrinopathy, M-component, and skin changes) is rapidly progressive, with prominent motor involvement and severe disability within 1 year. The gammopathy is frequently IgG or IgA, with low levels of lambda light chain, and an osteosclerotic (myeloma) lesion or Castleman's syndrome is frequently present. Electrophysiological testing shows demyelinating features without conduction block, and severe axonal loss in the legs. POEMS does not respond to typical CIDP treatments.

In *amyloidosis*, light-chain deposition in nerves and other tissues results in a length-dependent sensory predominant polyneuropathy. The axonal neuropathy affects small fiber modalities, causing pain and autonomic dysfunction.

Polyneuropathy in mixed *cryoglobulinemia* associated with hepatitis C is sensory or sensorimotor, occasionally multifocal, and electrophysiologically is axonal in character .

Vasculitic neuropathies

Systemic vasculitides in collagen vascular disease often involve the peripheral nervous system. The typical clinical presentation is subacute *mononeuropathy multiplex*, less commonly distal *asymmetric or symmetric polyneuropathy*.

Neuropathy occurs in 50% of patients with systemic necrotizing vasculitis, including *polyarteritis nodosa* and *Churg–Strauss disease*. Mononeuropathy multiplex or polyneuropathy is present in 30% of *Wegener's granulomatosis*. Neuropathy is less common in *systemic lupus erythematosis* and *Sjögren's syndrome*. Vasculitic neuropathy in rheumatoid arthritis is rare, but entrapment neuropathies are often present. *Isolated vasculitic neuropathy* occurs occasionally without systemic vasculitis.

Necrotizing vasculitis results in inflammation and necrosis of blood vessel walls leading to nerve infarction and wallerian degeneration. The result is an acute or subacute step-wise progressive neuropathy.

Clinically, acute pain involving a cranial or peripheral nerve is followed by motor and sensory deficit in the distribution of the affected nerve. Within days or weeks, additional nerves are affected resulting in progressive mononeuropathy multiplex. With progression, the picture of distal asymmetric or symmetric polyneuropathy develops. Less commonly, vasculitic neuropathy presents primarily as symmetric polyneuropathy. Systemic symptoms include weight loss, fever, and anorexia.

Laboratory findings of systemic vasculitis include elevated sedimentation rate and other markers of inflammation or collagen vascular disease. Evidence of end-organ involvement may be present. Antineutrophilic cytoplasmic antigen (ANCA) antibodies are present in Wegener's granulomatosis. Electrophysiology reveals acute axonal nerve lesions, but may mimic conduction block on initial testing. If vasculitic neuropathy is suspected, nerve and muscle biopsy should be performed expeditiously. Perivascular and transmural mononuclear cell infiltrates with necrosis of the blood vessel walls and occlusion of epineural blood vessels are pathognomic.

Immunotherapy should be initiated as soon as the diagnosis is made. It typically includes steroids (prednisolone

Table 112.1 Neuropathies associated with diabetes.

Symmetric
(Distal) sensory or sensorimotor polyneuropathy
Autonomic neuropathy
Acute painful diabetic neuropathy

Focal/asymmetric
Polyradiculoplexopathies
• plexopathy: lumbosacral > brachial
• truncal radiculopathy: thoracic > abdominal
Limb mononeuropathy from nerve infarction
Limb mononeuropathies from nerve entrapment
Mononeuropathy multiplex
Cranial mononeuropathies: III > VI, IV > VII

60–100 mg daily, or pulse methylprednisolone), IVIg, or cyclophosphamide.

Metabolic neuropathies

Diabetic neuropathy

Neuropathy in diabetes may affect any part of the peripheral nervous system. Most common is diabetic polyneuropathy, followed by mononeuropathy, usually nerve entrapment such as carpal tunnel syndrome (Table 112.1).

Epidemiology

Careful history and examination may reveal evidence of diabetic neuropathy at the time of diagnosis of diabetes in 7.5% of cases and after 25 years in 50%. Mean time interval from onset of diabetes to symptoms of neuropathy is 8 years, shorter in diabetes type II than type I.

Pathophysiology

Diabetic polyneuropathy is more common in patients with prolonged hyperglycemia, and tight glucose control reduces the risk. According to the metabolic hypothesis, hyperglycemia leads to shunting of glucose into the polyol pathway, resulting in accumulation of sorbitol and fructose in nerve cells. Hyperglycemia causes non-enzymatic glycosylation of structural nerve proteins. The microvascular hypothesis postulates endoneurial hypoxia from capillary damage and increased vascular resistance. An autoimmune neuropathy may emerge from immunogenic alteration of endothelial cells.

Clinical features

The most common manifestation (70%) is distal *sensory or sensorimotor polyneuropathy*, often with autonomic features. It is a typical length-dependent axonopathy with large- and small-fiber sensory manifestations. A combination of negative (numbness) and positive (pain, paresthesiae) sensory symptoms is common. Asymptomatic patients often have ankle areflexia and diminished vibration sense distally. In severe cases, sensory ataxia occurs in combination with distal weakness, diabetic dysautonomia, Charcot's joints, and foot ulcers.

Diabetic neuropathy may manifest itself predominantly as *autonomic neuropathy*. Occasionally, an *acute painful polyneuropathy* occurs in type I shortly after diagnosis and is preceded by weight loss. It improves over months with glucose control and weight gain.

Diabetic polyradiculoplexopathy (diabetic amyotrophy) is a proximal diabetic neuropathy of presumably inflammatory vascular etiology. It usually affects the lumbosacral plexus (especially femoral and obturator nerves). Asymmetric pain (thigh, hip, or buttock) is followed days or weeks later by weakness and wasting of proximal leg muscles, with only minor sensory loss. Recovery takes up to 24 months, and often mild to moderate weakness persists. Diabetic truncal neuropathy results from ischemic radiculopathy, typically affecting a thoracic dermatome with sensory loss and severely painful dysesthesiae.

Mononeuropathies of sudden onset may affect a single nerve (femoral, sciatic, median, or ulnar) or multiple nerves in combination. The most common *cranial neuropathy* is oculomotor palsy with sparing of the pupillary reflex, with recovery in weeks to months. *Entrapment neuropathies* (median, ulnar, and peroneal) are common.

Investigations and diagnosis

All patients with unexplained neuropathy are checked for diabetes. Fasting glucose and HgbA1c are often used for screening, but oral glucose tolerance test is more sensitive and may identify patients with impaired glucose tolerance and neuropathy. Nerve conduction studies often reveal diminished amplitudes and slowing of conduction velocities that tends to be more pronounced than in other axonal polyneuropathies. CSF, if tested, shows mild to moderately increased protein. Typical polyneuropathy features in the context of longstanding diabetes are usually diagnostic, but 5–10% of patients may have a different cause. Painless proximal neuropathy is unusual and suggests CIDP.

Treatment

Tight control of diabetes is partially effective in preventing diabetic neuropathy. Patients with entrapment neuropathy may benefit from decompressive surgery. IVIg or steroids may be beneficial in subcategories of diabetic neuropathy, including diabetic amytrophy, neuropathy similar to CIDP, or mononeuritis multiplex.

Neuropathy from vitamin B$_{12}$ deficiency

Vitamin B$_{12}$ (cobalamin) deficiency affects the spinal cord as subacute combined degeneration and the peripheral nervous system as symmetric polyneuropathy. It is especially common in the elderly. Strict vegetarian diet is rarely the cause. In most cases, it results from impaired B$_{12}$ absorption in the gastrointestinal tract, due to inadequate gastric production of intrinsic factor (pernicious anemia, gastrectomy) or from disorders of the terminal ileum (coeliac disease, intestinal resection). Pernicious anemia is caused by autoantibody production against gastric parietal cells. Treatment with antacids and gastric proton pump inhibitors may be contributory. A rare cause is infection with fish tapeworm. Exposure to nitric oxide may precipitate symptom onset by inactivation of cobalamin.

The disease begins gradually with distal paresthesiae and weakness. Involvement of the spinal cord results in pyramidal tract signs (spastic paraparesis) and posterior column dysfunction (loss of vibration and position sense, sensory ataxia). Deep tendon reflexes may be decreased or increased. Isolated polyneuropathy without any myelopathy is unusual.

In untreated patients, B$_{12}$ levels are low. Patients with low normal B$_{12}$ levels (below 300 pg/ml) may become symptomatic. An increase in methylmalonic acid or homocysteine is confirmatory. Macrocytic anemia is common. Schilling test documents B$_{12}$ malabsorption.

Treatment with vitamin B$_{12}$ should be given parenterally in severe cases. A simple regimen is 1000 µg daily for a week, weekly for a month, and then monthly. After restoration of body stores, oral B$_{12}$ administration may be sufficient for maintenance. Treatment with folic acid only treats the macrocytic anemia, not the neuropathy, and may worsen the neurological deficits.

Other metabolic and endocrine neuropathies

In *chronic renal failure*, a typical sensory predominant axonal polyneuropathy is common. The prevalence is 10–80% depending on duration and severity of the uremia. Most bothersome are dysesthesiae in the feet, resulting in "burning feet" and resembling restless leg syndrome. Muscle cramps are common. In advanced uremia, distal weakness and autonomic dysfunction occurs. Electrophysiology is axonal, with more slowing of conduction velocity in patients with creatinine clearance below 10% of normal. Dialysis may prevent or improve the condition. Renal transplantation usually improves even severe uremic neuropathy.

In *hepatic insufficiency*, symptomatic neuropathy is uncommon and mild, with more common abnormalities on nerve conduction testing.

Hypothyroidism may cause mild axonal polyneuropathy with distal sensory manifestations.

Infectious neuropathies

Detailed descriptions of the most important infectious neuropathies are provided elsewhere, including designated chapters for leprosy, neurosyphilis, Lyme disease, and HIV neuropathy.

Neuropathy from nutritional causes and alcoholism

Neurological manifestations of malnutrition and alcoholism are discussed in detail in separate chapters. *Alcoholic polyneuropathy* is outlined here due to its relative frequency. Population studies from inner-city hospitals suggest that 10–15% of chronic alcoholics develop a neuropathy. It occurs alone or in combination with other alcohol-related disorders, such as alcohol-related seizures, Wernicke's encephalopathy, or Korsakoff's amnestic syndrome. It is subject to controversy whether the neuropathy associated with chronic alcoholism is the result of a direct "toxic" effect of alcohol or is due to associated nutritional deficiencies (thiamine) or chronic liver disease.

The polyneuropathy is typically symmetric and distal in glove-and-stocking distribution. In the legs, decreased sensation to light touch and vibration is usually present, and ankle jerks are depressed or absent. Painful paresthesiae are common. Weakness if present tends to be distal, but proximal weakness and atrophy may occur, and rapidly progressing weakness has been described. Gait disturbance is common, particularly in patients with superimposed alcoholic cerebellar degeneration or Wernicke–Korsakoff's disease.

Cessation of alcohol consumption and nutritional support are essential. Vitamins and minerals should be replaced, especially thiamine 100 mg daily, initially parenterally.

Further reading

Ashbury AK, Cornblath DR. Assessment of current diagnostic criteria for Guillain–Barré syndrome. *Ann Neurol* 1990; 27(Suppl): S21–4.

Boulton AJM. Diabetic neuropathy: classification, measurement and treatment. *Curr Opin Endocrinol Diabetes* 2007; 14: 141–5.

Cornblath DR, Feasby TE, Hahn AF, *et al.* Research criteria for diagnosis of chronic inflammatory demyelinating polyneuropathy (CIDP). *Neurology* 1991; 41: 617–18.

French CIDP Study Group. Recommendations on diagnostic strategies for chronic inflammatory demyelinating polyradiculoneuropathy. *J Neurol Neurosurg Psychiatry* 2008; 79: 115–8.

Hughes RA, Cornblath DR. Guillain–Barré syndrome. *Lancet* 2005; 366: 1653–66.

Joint Task Force of the EFNS and PNS. European Federation of Neurological Societies/Peripheral Nerve Society guideline on management of chronic inflammatory demyelinating polyradiculoneuropathy. *J Periph Nerv Syst* 2005; 10: 220–8.

Kuwabara S. Guillain–Barré syndrome. *Curr Neurol Neurosci Rep* 2007; 7: 57–62.

Léger JM, Behin A. Multifocal motor neuropathy. *Curr Opin Neurol* 2005; 18: 567–73.

Lewis RA. Chronic inflammatory demyelinating polyneuropathy. *Neurol Clin* 2007; 25: 71–87.

Lozeron P, Adams D. Monoclonal gammopathy and neuropathy. *Curr Opin Neurol* 2007; 20: 536–41.

Sandbrink F, Klion AD, Floeter MK. "Pseudo-conduction block" in a patient with vasculitic neuropathy. *Electromyogr Clin Neurophysiol* 2001; 41: 195–202.

Toothaker TB, Brannagan TH. Chronic inflammatory demyelinating polyneuropathies: current treatment strategies. *Curr Neurol Neurosci Rep* 2007; 7: 63–70.

Chapter 113
Plexopathies and mononeuropathies

Friedhelm Sandbrink[1,2]
[1]Veterans Affairs Medical Center, Washington, USA
[2]Georgetown University, Washington, USA

Plexopathies

The neural plexus is a network of nerve fibers that are formed by the spinal nerve roots, specifically the anterior primary rami of the mixed spinal nerves, and which reorganize into peripheral nerves distally.

The *cervical plexus* is formed in the lateral neck by the C1–C4 spinal nerves and has communication with the lower cranial nerves X–XII. The phrenic nerve (C4) is the most important nerve derived from the cervical plexus. Cervical plexopathies are rarely diagnosed. Injury occurs during radical neck dissection and from closed violent trauma such as motorcycle accidents, usually in combination with upper brachial plexus lesions. Neoplastic infiltration of the cervical plexus often presents with unrelenting pain in the neck, throat, or shoulder region that worsens with neck movement or swallowing. Clinical examination often does not reveal the mass lesion, but rather neck tenderness and palpable lymph nodes.

The *brachial plexus* receives input from the C5–T1 nerve roots that come together to form three trunks. The upper (C5–C6 root supply), middle (C7), and lower trunk (C8–T1) represent the supraclavicular portion of the brachial plexus. The nerve fibers reorganize into three anterior and three posterior divisions that are situated behind the clavicle. The infraclavicular portion of the brachial plexus includes the cords named in relation to the axillary artery as lateral, posterior, and medial (Figure 113.1). Most terminal nerves derived from the plexus originate from the cords within the axilla.

Brachial plexopathies are the most common plexus lesions, more commonly supraclavicular than infraclavicular. The supraclavicular plexopathies are divided into upper, middle, and lower plexus lesions, indicating involvement of the upper, middle, and lower trunk fibers, respectively. It is often clinically difficult to distinguish supraclavicular plexopathies affecting the trunks from disorders of the corresponding nerve roots or mixed spinal nerves.

Trauma is the most common cause of brachial plexopathies. The usual mechanism is traction of the supraclavicular plexus nerve fibers. It tends to damage the upper plexus (trunk) in particular. The *burner syndrome* occurs in athletes (especially young men in contact sports) who are subjected to forceful depression of the shoulder. It consists of a sudden, intense burning dysesthesia and anesthesia in the entire arm, often associated with weakness, and usually resolves quickly. *Rucksack (pack) palsy* is a transient weakness caused by direct compression of the upper trunk or long thoracic nerve by a heavy back pack. More severe injury occurs with excessive separation of the head and shoulder, as in motorcycle accidents, that results in traction of the upper trunk, all trunks, and/or the corresponding nerve roots. A *humerus fracture or dislocation* may injure the infraclavicular plexus or terminal nerves, especially the axillary nerve. *Postmedian sternotomy* (open-heart surgery) results in C8 nerve root or lower trunk brachial plexopathy, with weakness, paresthesiae, and pain in an "ulnar" distribution.

The nerve roots, particularly the ventral (motor) roots, are more vulnerable to traction injury than the plexus or peripheral nerves because of lesser amounts of collagen and lack of supporting epineurial and perineurial sheaths. *Traumatic nerve root avulsion* of C5 and C6 roots or upper trunk lesion result in *Erb–Duchenne palsy*. It may occur during delivery as a result of excessive lateral traction on the fetal head when delivering the shoulder. Motorcycle accidents frequently cause avulsion of upper brachial nerve roots (often combined with middle and lower levels) and result in severe disability from permanent motor and sensory deficits and root avulsion pain. Traumatic avulsion of C8–T1 nerve roots or the lower plexus is less common, resulting in *Dejerine–Klumpke palsy*. It is caused by traction on the abducted arm or by a fall where the outstretched arm grasps a fixed object to arrest the fall.

Neuralgic amyotrophy, also called *idiopathic brachial plexus neuropathy*, brachial plexitis, and Parsonage–Turner syndrome, is considered the second most common cause of brachial plexopathy (after trauma). Idiopathic neuralgic amyotrophy has an annual incidence of 2–3/100 000 persons and is twice as common in men as in women. It may occur at any age including childhood, but is most

International Neurology: A Clinical Approach. Edited by Robert P. Lisak, Daniel D. Truong, William M. Carroll, and Roongroj Bhidayasiri. © 2009 Blackwell Publishing, ISBN: 978-1-4051-5738-4.

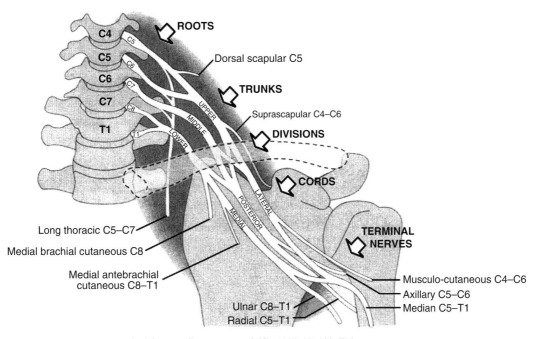

Figure 113.1 The brachial plexus. (Modified from Wilbourn, *Neurol Clin* 2007; 25: 139–71.)

common in the fourth and fifth decades. The attacks are assumed to be autoimmune in origin, and antecedent events are noted in half the patients, such as viral illness, vaccination, trauma, or surgery. The disorder affects the plexus and/or several individual peripheral nerves and tends to be patchy. Damage in the upper part of the brachial plexus combined with the long thoracic nerve and/or suprascapular nerve is the most common pattern (71% in a study by Van Alfen and van Engelen), but almost any nerve in the plexus may be affected. The disorder is bilateral in one-third of cases. The attacks typically begin with a severe, continuous pain in the shoulder or neck region that may radiate to the arm. Onset of pain is usually sudden, often overnight, but may be stuttering. Severe weakness in the shoulder girdle muscles typically develops a few days later, with range from less than 24 hours to several weeks. Occasionally, the weakness occurs without preceding pain. Fasciculations may be noted. Hypesthesia or paresthesia over the lateral shoulder or upper arm region occur frequently but can be quite subtle. Vasomotor dysfunction includes skin changes, edema, and increased sweating. Most patients improve at least partially over months to years. The continuous initial pain lasts for days to weeks, and is frequently followed by stabbing or shooting pains elicited by movements or prolonged posturing of the arm. On follow-up of 3 years and longer, chronic pain persists in almost half the patients. After 2–3 years, 10–20% of patients have moderate to severe residual paresis. Recurrent attacks years later are not uncommon.

Hereditary neuralgic amyotrophy (HNA) or familial brachial neuritis is an autosomal dominant disorder linked to mutations in the SEPT9 gene (a member of the cytoskeleton-related septin family) on chromosome 17q25. Some pedigrees have characteristic facial features, including hypotelorism. Attacks are similar to idiopathic neuralgic amyotrophy. The age at onset is earlier, with first attack in childhood or young adulthood. Nerves outside the brachial plexus are more commonly affected, such as the lumbosacral plexus, phrenic nerve, intercostal nerves, and recurrent laryngeal nerves (resulting in bilateral vocal cord paresis). Functional outcome is worse, with more severe maximum weakness and greater residual paresis. Repeated attacks are typical, triggered by factors such as stress, infections, or puerperium.

Most *malignant tumors* involving the brachial plexus are metastatic lung or breast carcinomas invading the lower plexus, especially the lower trunk and medial cord. Severe, persistent pain is the cardinal symptom, usually located in the shoulder and axilla, or radiating along the medial (ulnar) aspect of the forearm and hand. Progressive weakness of lower plexus (C8–T1) innervated muscles usually appears later, whereas parathesia is relatively uncommon. Horner's syndrome indicates invasion of the cervical sympathetic by paravertebral tumor near the first thoracic vertebra, for example, caused by "Pancoast" tumor at the apex of the lung.

Radiation-induced brachial plexopathy may follow months to years after radiation treatment, with a median of 1.5 years in breast cancer patients. The overall frequency is cited as 1.8–4.9% of treated patients, and is likely to be higher if total dose is more than 50 Gy, if fewer and higher doses are used (hypofractionation), or if combined with simultaneous chemotherapy. Radiation plexopathy tends to affect the upper plexus or whole plexus. Initial presentation is usually sensory with paresthesia and numbness in lateral cord (median nerve) innervated fingers, followed soon by weakness and loss of tendon reflexes. Edema of the affected extremity and chronic skin changes in the radiation field are typical. In contrast to neoplastic plexopathy, pain is inconstant and develops late.

Many patients with pain in the shoulder, arm, or hand are labeled with "thoracic outlet syndrome," but do not have a brachial plexus compression. *True neurogenic thoracic outlet syndrome* is also called *cervical rib and band syndrome*. It is a rare condition caused by a developmental anomaly. A taut fibrous band extends from the tip of a rudimentary cervical rib or from an elongated C7 transverse process to the first true thoracic rib. Sometimes, the cervical rib articulates directly with the first thoracic rib. Stretching of the distal T1 root or lower trunk fibers results in a predominantly motor syndrome. Typical presentation is unilateral weakness and wasting of hand muscles in a young to middle-aged woman, affecting the thenar eminence in particular. Intermittent, mild aching pain and sensory complaints in the ulnar aspect of the forearm and hand may be present, but pain is usually not severe. The entire arm and hand are sometimes developmentally smaller on the affected side. Vascular compression of the subclavian artery is rarely apparent clinically, and Adson's test (decrease in radial pulse with head turning to the affected side and deep inhalation) is often falsely positive. The congenital bony changes may be noted on X-ray, but the presence of a cervical rib does not prove the condition, and the band is usually radiolucent. MRI may document the band in some patients or demonstrate distortion of the brachial plexus. Surgical resection or sectioning of the offending band, not the first thoracic rib, is curative. The *droopy shoulder syndrome* occurs in young women who have low-hanging shoulders and long necks, resulting in chronic stretch of the brachial plexus. Horizontal or down-sloping clavicles on inspection and visualization of upper thoracic vertebrae on lateral cervical spine films support the diagnosis. Tapping over the plexus causes pain and paresthesia. Symptoms are worse with pulling the arms down and are relieved by pushing them up. The neurological examination and nerve conduction tests are normal. Treatment consists of exercises to strengthen the shoulder muscles. Surgical resection of the first thoracic rib or the anterior or middle scalene muscles is not indicated in these patients or other patients with arm pain who lack any objective neurological deficit, sometimes labeled as "disputed thoracic outlet syndrome."

The *lumbosacral plexus* is anatomically divided into the lumbar plexus (L1–L4) and the sacral plexus that is formed by the lumbosacral trunk (L4–L5) and S1–S3 roots. Anterior divisions of the lumbar plexus give rise to the obturator nerve and posterior divisions to the femoral nerve (Figure 113.2). The sciatic nerve is the main nerve of the sacral plexus, with the tibial nerve portion derived

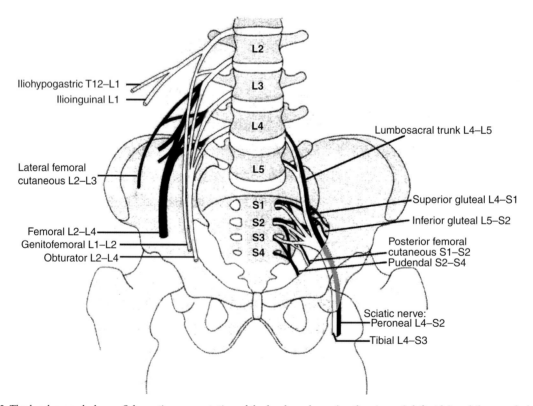

Figure 113.2 The lumbosacral plexus. Schematic representation of the lumbar plexus (on the viewer's left side) and the sacral plexus (right side). *Black portions* signify the nerves derived from the posterior divisions of the ventral primary rami, and *white portions* are derived from either the ventral primary rami or their anterior branches. (Modified from Wilbourn, *Neurol Clin* 2007; 25: 139–71.)

from the anterior divisions and the common peroneal nerve from the posterior divisions.

Traumatic injuries of the lumbosacral plexus are rare and usually associated with bony fractures of the pelvic ring or dislocations of the sacroiliac joint. A severe stretching force causes intradural nerve root avulsion and tearing of the arachnoid nerve root covering, and is detected on MRI or myelography as a pseudomeningocele or diverticulum-like outpouching.

Malignancy is the most common cause of lumbosacral plexopathy, usually by direct extension from the colorectum or cervix uteri, or from lymphomas and retroperitoneal sarcomas. The sacral plexus is more commonly affected than the lumbar plexus. Metastases cause 25% of malignant plexopathies and are often bilateral. Pain is usually the first symptom in malignant plexopathy. It is dull, aching, and constant, with worsening in the supine position. There is often superimposed sharp radicular pain in the lower back, hip, and thigh with lumbar plexopathy, and in the posterolateral thigh, calf, and foot in sacral plexopathy. Paresthesiae and weakness follow a few weeks later. During examination, the Valsalva maneuver or straight-leg raising may worsen the symptoms. Leg edema may be present, and involvement of sympathetic plexus fibers may cause a "hot-dry foot."

Radiation injury to the lumbosacral plexus is infrequent. It results from treatment of testicular and prostate cancer, cervix carcinoma, or lymphomas, with a latency of a few months to decades. As in the upper extremities, it presents initially without much pain, with weakness and paresthesiae predominating, sometimes bilateral but asymmetric. Bowel and bladder dysfunction is uncommon. Post-radiation malignant schwannoma of the plexus can develop up to 20 years later.

Diabetic lumbosacral radiculoplexopathy typically occurs in elderly patients with longstanding type 2 diabetes, often superimposed on diabetic polyneuropathy. Rather sudden onset of unilateral, sometimes asymmetric bilateral, aching pain in the thigh, hip, or buttock regions is followed days or weeks later by weakness and wasting of anterior and lateral thigh muscles. The femoral and obturator nerves seem to be affected predominantly. Minor sensory loss over the anterior thigh is often present. The knee jerk is usually absent on the affected side. The syndrome probably is caused by ischemic nerve injury secondary to microvasculitis. A similar syndrome also occurs rarely in non-diabetic patients. Recovery takes up to 24 months and in many cases mild to moderate weakness persists.

Lumbosacral plexopathy is occasionally caused by *retroperitoneal hemorrhage* into the iliacus muscle affecting femoral nerve fibers predominantly, or into the psoas muscle where a large amount of blood may be lost and cause a compartment syndrome.

Diagnosis

The most important studies in plexopathies are imaging and electrophysiology. MRI is more sensitive than CT in documenting brachial or lumbosacral plexus lesions. Tumors are more likely than radiation injury to show root or plexus enhancement on MRI, and positron emission tomography (PET) scanning is frequently positive. In neuralgic amyotrophy, MRI frequently detects signal abnormalities in the affected muscles of the shoulder girdle, and MR neurography documents a thickened and hyperintense plexus.

Electrophysiological studies are more helpful in the evaluation of brachial than lumbosacral plexopathies. In the legs, routine sensory studies only assess the sacral plexus and become unreliable in the elderly. Most plexopathies are axonal in nature and result in decreased sensory and motor nerve potential amplitudes. When present for several weeks, pathological spontaneous activity may be noted on electromyogram (EMG). In *neuralgic amyotrophy*, sensory abnormalities are often limited on nerve testing, due to patchy and predominantly proximal motor nerve involvement. In the arms, stimulation at the supraclavicular Erb point may document conduction slowing or conduction block located distal to the mid-trunk level. In a *trauma* patient with complete sensory loss of the arm, the presence of sensory nerve action potentials indicates a supraganglionic lesion, and thus root avulsion rather than plexopathy. Myokymic EMG discharges are typical of *radiation plexopathy*.

Treatment

Treatment is directed at the underlying pathology if possible. In neuralgic amyotrophy, high-dose steroids and immunoglobulin treatments are of uncertain value. In lumbosacral diabetic polyradiculoplexopathy, steroids are usually contraindicated, but immunoglobulins may be tried. In most instances, treatment of plexopathies is symptomatic, including management of neuropathic pain. Intractable pain in patients suffering from nerve root avulsion may be treated by dorsal root entry zone (DREZ) surgery or cervical cord spinal stimulation.

Mononeuropathies (entrapment neuropathies)

Entrapment neuropathy indicates dysfunction of a peripheral nerve that is compressed, stretched, or angulated by surrounding anatomic structures (Figure 113.3). Only the most common entrapment syndromes are discussed. In most instances, initial complaints are intermittent or gradually progressive numbness or paresthesiae. The pathophysiology is segmental demyelination resulting in slowing of nerve conduction velocity across the affected nerve segment or, if severe, conduction block. Axonal

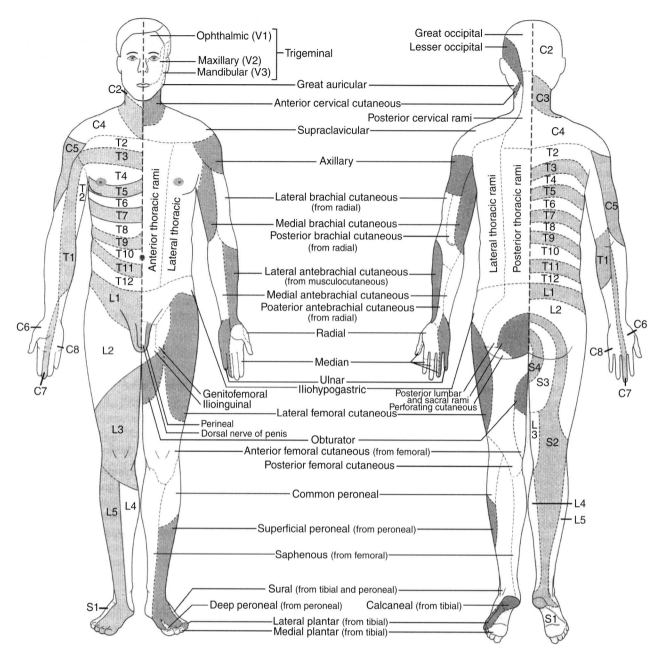

Figure 113.3 Cutaneous innervation. Schematic representation of the dermatomal (radicular) and peripheral nerve innervation from the anterior (left figure) and posterior aspect. Dermatomes are shown on the right side of the body (outer hemibodies) and the peripheral nerve distribution on the left side of the body (inner hemibodies). (Modified from Aminoff MJ, Greenberg DA, Simon RP, *Clinical Neurology*, 6th ed. Lange: McGraw-Hill; 2005, and Haymaker W, Woodhall B. *Peripheral Nerve Injuries*, 1st ed. Philadelphia: Saunders; 1945.)

degeneration is usually a secondary event indicating more severe nerve damage.

Entrapment neuropathies may be triggered by underlying systemic disease or hormonal changes, such as diabetes, hypothyroidism, acromegaly, pregnancy, rheumatological diseases resulting in inflammatory or degenerative arthritis (wrist), and previous trauma (elbow).

Early symptoms of a *focal median neuropathy* at the wrist (*carpal tunnel syndrome*) are pain and paresthesiae in the median nerve distribution (first three digits, lateral half

of digit 4, and thenar eminence). Painful paresthesiae in the hand and arm, sometimes including the upper arm and shoulder region, occur at night and are relieved by shaking the hand or arm. In advanced carpal tunnel syndrome, weakness and atrophy of thenar muscles develops. Examination reveals paralysis of the abductor pollicis brevis and opponens pollicis muscles. Sensory deficit is in the median territory of the hand, but not proximal to the wrist. Tinel's sign is positive, when percussion of the median nerve at the wrist causes paresthesiae in the nerve's distribution. Phalen maneuver is positive, when flexion of the wrist for 30–60 s reproduces or exacerbates the symptoms. The differential diagnosis includes proximal median nerve lesions, brachial plexopathy, and C6–7 radiculopathy.

Ulnar neuropathy at the elbow is the second most common entrapment following carpal tunnel syndrome. Numbness and paresthesia affect digit 5, the medial half of digit 4, and the ulnar aspect of the hand, but not the forearm to any significant extent. The elbow region may be painful and sensitive to touch. Repeated elbow flexion or pressure on the ulnar nerve (such as when leaning on the elbow) exacerbates the symptoms. Weakness, if present, affects intrinsic hand muscles including hypothenar muscles, interossei, and lumbricals. Ulnar innervated forearm muscles (M. flexor carpi ulnaris and M. flexor digitorum profundus) are typically less affected but may be atrophic in advanced disease. Claw hand (flexion of digits 4 and 5) occurs in severe ulnar neuropathy. Ulnar neuropathy at the elbow occurs at two different entrapment sites that are clinically similar but may be separated by electrophysiology. Compression at the sulcus ulnaris (retroepicondylar groove) is more common than entrapment of the ulnar nerve within the cubital tunnel (humeroulnar arcade).

In lesions affecting the ulnar nerve at the wrist or palm of the hand, sensory or motor changes in the hand may occur in isolation or in combination, depending on the specific lesion site within Guyon's canal. Such lesions may be differentiated from ulnar neuropathy at the elbow by intact sensation over the dorsal hand on clinical examination and by electrophysiological testing (dorsal ulnar cutaneous branch is not affected). Sensory deficits in the forearm imply a more proximal lesion, such as lower trunk or medial cord plexopathy and C8–T1 radiculopathy.

The *radial nerve* may be compressed in the axilla by crutches. Injury in the upper arm is caused by prolonged pressure, as seen in those who have slept heavily (often after inebriation) with an arm resting on a hard surface or in humerus fractures. Weakness of the finger and hand extensors with sparing of the triceps muscle is characteristic, with often only minor associated sensory symptoms affecting the area of the hand between the thumb and index finger.

Peroneal neuropathy is the most common entrapment of the lower extremity, usually at the fibular head, secondary to trauma or pressure (sitting with one leg resting over the opposite knee). Weakness affects toe and foot dorsiflexion (anterior tibial muscle) and foot eversion (peroneal muscles), with impaired sensation over the dorsum of the foot and distal leg.

The *tarsal tunnel syndrome* results from *tibial nerve* entrapment at the ankle inferior and posterior to the medial malleolus. Burning pain over the plantar surface of the foot, especially at night, is typical and weakness of intrinsic foot muscles may be noted.

In *meralgia paresthetica*, the lateral femoral cutaneous nerve is compressed in the lateral groin (inguinal ligament) resulting in burning pain, paresthesiae, and numbness in the anterolateral thigh region. There is no motor involvement. Predisposing factors are pregnancy and sudden weight gain or weight loss.

Diagnosis

Nerve conduction studies are usually diagnostic by documenting focal slowing at the entrapment site. Denervation on EMG documents axonal degeneration and therefore more severe entrapment.

Prevention and treatment

Avoidance of triggering factors (excessive repetitive wrist flexion and extension often with weight loading in carpal tunnel syndrome, leaning on elbows and repetitive elbow flexion in ulnar neuropathy, crossing of legs in peroneal neuropathy) is sometimes sufficient to allow recovery of nerve function. Additional measures include nocturnal wrist splints in carpal tunnel syndrome and elbow pads in ulnar neuropathy. Pharmacological treatment with a short course of anti-inflammatory agents is often helpful in carpal tunnel syndrome. Steroid injections into the wrist often provide temporary benefit but may be harmful. If deficits are severe or refractory despite conservative treatment, surgical division of the carpal tunnel ligament or ulnar nerve transposition may be indicated.

Further reading

Chance PF. Inherited focal, episodic neuropathies: hereditary neuropathy with liability to pressure palsies and hereditary neuralgic amyotrophy. *Neuromol Med* 2006; 8: 159–74.

Jaeckle KA. Neurological manifestations of neoplastic and radiation-induced plexopathies. *Semin Neurol* 2004; 24: 385–93.

Jillapalli D, Shefner JM. Electrodiagnosis in common mononeuropathies and plexopathies. *Semin Neurol* 2005; 25: 196–203.

Moghekar AR, Moghekar AR, Karli N, Chaudry V. Brachial plexopathies: etiology, frequency, and electrodiagnostic localization. *J Clin Neuromusc Dis* 2007; 9: 243–7.

Van Alfen N, van Engelen BGM. The clinical spectrum of neuralgic amyotrophy in 246 cases. *Brain* 2006; 129: 438–50.

Wilbourn AJ. Plexopathies. *Neurol Clin* 2007; 25: 139–71.

Chapter 114
Myasthenia gravis

Richard A. Lewis
Wayne State University School of Medicine, Detroit, USA

Introduction

Myasthenia gravis (MG) is an autoimmune disorder in which there is a failure of neuromuscular transmission due to binding of antibodies to proteins at the postsynaptic neuromuscular junction (NMJ). It is the quintessential autoimmune disease in that it has been demonstrated that antibodies have been shown to be present at the site of pathology and removal of the antibody is effective therapy. In addition, the disease can be transferred to animals by both passive transfer of immunoglobulin from myasthenic patients and immunization of animals with acetylcholine receptor (AChR).

Epidemiology

MG is relatively rare, with an annual incidence of 2–4 per million and a prevalence of about 100 per million. Like many other autoimmune disorders, there are two incidence peaks, one between 20 and 40 years of age with predominantly women affected (F:M = 4:1) and the other between 60 and 80 years of age without gender dominance. As many as 15% of cases may present before age 20. A transient neonatal MG due to passive placental transfer of maternal AChR antibody occurs in 10% of babies born to myasthenic mothers. This tends to last for 3–4 weeks and does not lead to future development of the disease.

The disease occurs worldwide without specific clustering. There is a strong correlation of young adult MG with HLA genotypes. These have been studied in Japanese, Chinese, Scandinavian, and other Caucasians. There is an increased incidence of MG and other autoimmune disorders in family members of MG patients, but there is no direct Mendelian inheritance. Twin studies have shown disease in both twins in only a minority of twins investigated.

International Neurology: A Clinical Approach. Edited by Robert P. Lisak, Daniel D. Truong, William M. Carroll, and Roongroj Bhidayasiri. © 2009 Blackwell Publishing, ISBN: 978-1-4051-5738-4.

Pathophysiology

Neuromuscular junction transmission and the acetylcholine receptor

Acetylcholine (ACh) is the transmitter at the neuromuscular junction. It is synthesized and stored in vesicles in the distal motor nerve terminal, with each vesicle containing approximately 10 000 ACh molecules, called a quantum. There is spontaneous release of quanta, but depolarization of the nerve terminal produces an inward flux of calcium which causes a large release of ACh quanta. The ACh binds to receptors on the postsynaptic muscle membrane. The AChR is a glycoprotein made up of five subunits which are arranged to form a channel. The two alpha subunits have binding sites for ACh and are the locations for AChR antibody binding.

Acetylcholine receptor antibody and the autoimmune disorder

The initial event in MG is unclear but is related to an autoimmune reaction, predominantly to the main immunogenic region (MIR) on the alpha subunit of the AChR. This initial event, particularly in patients with thymoma, may begin in the thymus. There is evidence that both T and B lymphocytes are important in the development of MG. The IgG AChR antibodies initiate a complement-mediated lysis of the postsynaptic muscle membrane. The resulting reduction in functional AChR causes a reduced effect of ACh on the muscle. Normally, the number of active receptors is more than enough to depolarize the muscle membrane, but with the loss of functional receptors in MG, this safety factor for transmission is lost and some muscle fibers will fail to depolarize during sustained muscular effort.

The role of the thymus

The association of thymoma and MG has been known for over 70 years. Most patients with thymoma and MG have AChR antibodies. The relationship of thymoma to anti-MuSK-related MG is not known (see the section 'Investigations' below). Thymoma is present in approximately 15% of MG patients, with a peak incidence at age 50 in both men and women. The presence of thymoma does not portend a worse prognosis or more severe disease and most patients will have persistent MG after surgical removal of the thymic tumor. CT or MRI of the chest will identify a mediastinal mass, but small thymomatous nodules may be identified histologically in radiologically unremarkable mediastinums. Malignant thymomas comprise a small fraction of thymic tumors. In the younger population, the thymus usually shows hyperplasia with increased germinal centers. Older patients who do not have thymoma usually have atrophic thymuses. There is fairly good evidence that in thymomas the humoral immune disorder develops within the thymus, but the evidence for this in hyperplastic thymuses is less clear. The thymus contains myoid cells with MIR epitope as well as titin and RyR epitopes.

Clinical manifestations

Symptoms and signs
The majority of patients present with diplopia and/or ptosis with or without other muscle involvement. Some may only have ocular symptoms, but over 85% develop other symptoms. Those who remain purely ocular for more than 2 years rarely generalize after that. Other manifestations include facial and jaw weakness, speech and swallowing problems, and proximal and/or distal limb muscle weakness. Most concerning is the involvement of respiratory muscles. A clue to the diagnosis is the diurnal fluctuation of the symptoms. Frequently the symptoms become worse with exercise. Respiratory insufficiency and inability to protect the airway are the major life-threatening symptoms. Fortunately, modern intensive care management and immunotherapy have improved the prognosis of MG to over 80% 5-year survival and at least 70% 10-year survival. Most patients respond to medications, but full remission in which the patient requires no medications occurs in less than 20% of cases.

The examination of the patient with suspected MG should include careful observation for variability of signs. For instance, ptosis may not be manifest initially but be evident intermittently during the examination. Speech may become more nasal as the patient is talking. Repetitive or sustained effort may bring out signs. Sustaining upgaze for 30 seconds may induce ptosis or having the patient raise his or her arms up may induce weakness of shoulder abduction. Neck flexion and extension may be particularly weak and jaw closure may be difficult. Some patients with anti-MuSK antibodies have particular problems with bulbar function and neck extension, sometimes with prominent muscle atrophy.

Associated disorders
Patients with MG have an increased incidence of other autoimmune diseases such as rheumatoid arthritis, systemic lupus erythematosus, pernicious anemia, and autoimmune thyroiditis. Some patients present with both MG and hyperthyroidism and it can be difficult to determine which disorder is causing the extraocular muscle problems.

Investigations

Antibody detection
Antibodies (Ab) directed against the AChR are found in 85% of patients with generalized MG and up to 70% in ocular MG. These predominantly IgG polyclonal antibodies are specific for MG, but binding antibody titer does not correlate with clinical severity. Of the 15% of patients who are AChR antibody negative, 40% have antibodies directed against Muscle Specific Kinase (MuSK). It is unclear whether MuSK antibodies are pathogenic and the incidence of MuSK Ab positivity in the Scandinavian population appears particularly low. Antistriational antibodies are seen in 30% of MG patients and high titers are seen more commonly in patients with thymoma or who have late onset. At least two antigens related to the striational antibodies have been described, titin and the ryanodine receptor.

Electrophysiologic studies
The physiologic effect of AChR antibodies is to reduce the muscle fiber response to acetylcholine release from the distal nerve terminal. The consequence of this is that there is a reduction in the safety factor of transmission. This is manifest in electrodiagnostic studies by a decrement in the compound motor action potential amplitude with repetitive stimulation at low rates of stimulation (2–5 Hz). This decrement worsens 1–4 minutes after exercise and has been a useful diagnostic test. However, it is not specific for MG, being seen in other neuromuscular junction disorders, and to a lesser extent in motor neuron disease and peripheral nerve disorders. Abnormal decrement is seen in approximately two out of three patients with generalized MG but less than 50% of patients with ocular MG.

The other consequence of the reduction in the safety factor of transmission is seen in the jitter and blocking that is found on single fiber electromyography (SFEMG). This technique looks at pairs of muscle fibers from the same motor unit. Normally, they will consistently fire in a time-locked fashion. With impaired neuromuscular transmission this firing is inconsistent and the interdischarge interval varies or "jitters" and fibers can fail to fire. These abnormalities occur in over 95% of patients with generalized MG but are also non-specific.

Diagnostic approach
A patient who has ptosis and diplopia with or without bulbar, neck, or limb weakness should be suspected of

having MG. Weakness that fluctuates or increases with activity should also raise suspicion. There are still regions in the world where one cannot test for AChR antibodies, and in those situations the diagnosis is dependent on demonstrating the electrophysiologic abnormality and/or finding a transient reversal of weakness after intravenous edrophonium (Tensilon®), a short-acting acetylcholinesterase inhibitor. This allows for ACh to remain at the muscle endplate, potentially overcoming the reduced safety factor of transmission. This Tensilon® test remains a useful examination tool but is used less frequently with the availability of laboratory testing for AChR antibodies. AChR antibodies are specific for MG and when detected are pathognomonic for the disease. If these are not detected, anti-MuSK antibodies can be looked for and repetitive stimulation and/or SFEMG can be performed.

Other diagnostic studies that are appropriate include laboratory testing for thyroid disease and autoimmune disorders. Creatinine kinase (CK) and antistriational antibody assays are of interest. A chest CT or MRI scan looking for a thymoma is important for patients identified as having MG.

Treatment/management

Physiologic therapy

Acetylcholinesterase inhibitors (AChEI) such as pyridostigmine, directed against AChE at nicotinic receptors, can substantially improve symptoms and in some instances provide complete reversal of symptoms as long as the medication is taken. This, however, does not treat the underlying immunologic disorder. Side effects are primarily related to cholinergic muscarinic effects on the gastrointestinal and cardiopulmonary systems. These can be controlled with atropine or similar medications. Excessive amounts of pyridostigmine can cause fasciculations and increased weakness, sometimes leading to cholinergic crisis. Pyridostigmine's effect tends to last for 3–4 hours. There is a slow release form of pyridostigmine which may be useful overnight but is not recommended for use during waking hours.

Immunosuppressive and immunomodulatory therapy

If AChEIs are not symptomatically effective then immunosuppressive agents are utilized. There have been very few large, double-blind, placebo controlled studies and recommendations are based on the clinical experiences described in the literature.

Corticosteroids have been used for over 40 years and are generally accepted as being effective. The clinical effects are usually apparent within 4–8 weeks and occur in over two out of three patients. There is a potential for clinical deterioration within 5–14 days of initiating high doses and

it is usually recommended to gradually increase the dose over a period of 7–14 days unless the situation is urgent and the patient hospitalized. Some patients may go into remission, but most require continued therapy. The usual side effects of corticosteroids are common but can be mitigated by alternate day dosing, the use of biphosphonates, and careful follow-up. Patients with purely ocular MG who do not respond to pyridostigmine may respond to low doses of corticosteroids, avoiding the complications of higher doses.

Azathioprine at doses of 2–3 mg/kg has been shown to be an effective steroid-sparing medication. It takes a minimum of 6 months and as much as 18 months before the full immunosuppressive effect is evident. Usually well tolerated with minimal long-term risk of malignancy, the patient must be carefully monitored for hepatic and bone marrow toxicity. These are sometimes seen with initiation but can also be dose related. The effectiveness of azathioprine as a single agent is less clear and has not been adequately studied.

Other immunosuppressives generally accepted as being effective in a significant number of patients include cyclosporine and cyclophosphamide. Both have significant side effects and potential toxicities. Two recent controlled trials with mycophenolate mofetil failed to find efficacy. Other immunosuppressives that have been considered, but with less documented experience, include methotrexate, tacrolimus, and rituximab.

Plasmapheresis, by removing circulating antibodies, can have a profound effect within days of initiation, and is therefore a highly effective agent to prevent or reverse myasthenic crisis. Its clinical effect is temporary, usually dissipating in 2–4 weeks, and it has a limited role in long-term management. The major problems with pheresis are venous access and complications of indwelling venous catheters as well as potential cardiopulmonary effects of fluid and metabolic shifts. Intravenous immunoglobulin (IVIg) has also been shown to be effective with a slightly lower complication rate but does not work quite as fast as plasmapheresis. It has the same temporary effectiveness but is more easily given intermittently over months to years.

Thymectomy is indicated for patients with CT or MRI evidence of a thymoma. The role of thymectomy in MG without radiologic suggestion of thymoma is less clear although it is commonly utilized. The literature suggests a greater benefit in younger patients with generalized MG who are AChR antibody positive. Patients over 45 years old with anti-titin or RyR antibodies appear to have the least benefit.

Drugs that can worsen MG

A number of drugs can exacerbate MG. The major ones include aminoglycosides, quinidine, procainamide, and magnesium products, but other medications including antibiotics and anti-arrhythmics have been implicated. The most striking drug relationship to MG is with D-penicillamine which, when given for other disorders such as rheumatoid arthritis, scleroderma, or Wilson's disease, can cause MG with AChR and striational antibodies, but the disease can remit with withdrawal of the drug.

Emergency care of myasthenic patients

Patients with swallowing or breathing problems and those with marked neck weakness and speech problems should be considered to be at risk for respiratory failure or aspiration pneumonia. They should be hospitalized and monitored closely, preferably in an intensive care setting. Respiratory status must be followed closely with parameters that assess respiratory muscle function, usually forced vital capacity, and negative inspiratory force. Oxygen saturation is insensitive to respiratory muscle weakness and is an inadequate guide to respiratory failure. Patients with good swallowing and who do not need airway protection may benefit from non-invasive ventilatory support. Plasmapheresis or IVIg should be initiated on an urgent basis if one is hoping to prevent intubation or to facilitate early extubation.

Further reading

Benatar M. A systematic review of diagnostic studies in myasthenia gravis. *Neuromuscul Disord* 2006; 16(7): 459–67.

Benatar M, Kaminski H. Medical and surgical treatment for ocular myasthenia. *Cochrane Database Syst Rev* 2006; (2): CD005081.

Conti-Fine BM, Milani M, Kaminski HJ. Myasthenia gravis: past, present, and future. *J Clin Invest* 2006; 116(11): 2843–54.

Gajdos P, Chevret S, Toyka K. Intravenous immunoglobulin for myasthenia gravis. *Cochrane Database Syst Rev* 2006; (2): CD002277.

Hart IK, Sathasivam S, Sharshar T. Immunosuppressive agents for myasthenia gravis. *Cochrane Database Syst Rev* 2007; (4): CD005224.

Jani-Acsadi A, Lisak RP. Myasthenic crisis: guidelines for prevention and treatment. *J Neurol Sci* 2007; 261(1–2): 127–33.

Parr JR, Jayawant S. Childhood myasthenia: clinical subtypes and practical management. *Dev Med Child Neurol* 2007; 49(8): 629–35.

Chapter 115
Lambert–Eaton syndrome

Johan A. Aarli
Haukeland University Hospital, Bergen, Norway

Introduction

In 1966, Lee Eaton, Edward Lambert, and E.D. Rooke reported that some patients with bronchial carcinoma develop muscular weakness in the shoulder and hip muscles, often with bilateral ptosis. They named it "myasthenic syndrome" because of its clinical similarities with myasthenia gravis. Eaton and Lambert later described the neurophysiological characteristics and the differences from myasthenia gravis (MG). In 1980, John Newsom-Davis and co-workers found that the condition may also be seen in patients who have no malignancies and that it may improve after plasma exchange. Today, the condition is named Lambert–Eaton myasthenic syndrome, often abbreviated to LEMS.

Epidemiology

LEMS can occur at any age, but is mainly seen in the middle-aged and in elderly persons. It used to be more common in men, but more recent reports now show almost equal incidence, probably because of an increasing occurrence of bronchial carcinoma in women.

LEMS is not especially prevalent in any part of the world. Although few studies of its epidemiology have been reported, there is nothing to indicate geographic variations, except that it will be less common in countries with a high percentage of children and young people.

The incidence of LEMS is less than 0.5 per million. The prevalence is much lower than it is for MG because of the poorer survival of LEMS patients with bronchial carcinoma. A prospective study found two cases of LEMS among 150 patients with small-cell lung carcinoma. In the province of South Holland, The Netherlands, LEMS was found to be 46 times less prevalent (2.32×10^{-6}) than MG (106.1×10^{-6}), whereas the annual incidence rate of

LEMS was 14 times lower (0.48×10^{-6}) than that of MG (6.48×10^{-6}), reflecting the poor survival of LEMS patients with small-cell lung carcinoma (SCLC). LEMS patients who do not have lung carcinoma carry a much better prognosis than the paraneoplastic cases.

Pathophysiology

LEMS is a presynaptic neuromuscular disorder. Patients with this disease have circulating antibodies against presynaptic voltage-gated calcium channels (VGCC). There are at least five types of such channels, N, L, T, P and Q. P and Q have the same α1 subunit and are usually referred to as P/Q-type. The antibodies found in sera of LEMS patients bind to the P/Q-type of VGCC and are found in more than 85% of patients. Antibodies against N type VGCC are also found, but are not specific for LEMS. VGCC are also present in the cell membranes of SCLC. The immune response found in paraneoplastic LEMS may therefore be primarily directed against the tumor.

Binding of these antibodies leads to downregulation in the presynaptic part of the endplate because of the effect of the specific IgG antibodies. Influx of Ca^{2+} is therefore reduced, which leads to decreased evoked quantal release of acetylcholine (ACh) and disruption of the presynaptic active zones, resulting in weakness of the involved muscles. The antibodies are also responsible for the autonomic dysfunction found in patients with LEMS.

Newsom-Davis and collaborators showed that the electrophysiological characteristics of LEMS could be reproduced in mice after infusion of LEMS plasma or IgG from LEMS patients.

The role of the VGCC antibodies has not been defined. They do not block the VGCC function directly, but may cross-link and thereby internalize them, leading to loss of VGCC. Interestingly, when the presence of P/Q-type calcium channel antibodies in patients with SCLC was studied, it was found that patients with LEMS had a better prognosis and a longer survival, while the presence of such antibodies in patients who did not have LEMS did not lead to a better prognosis.

International Neurology: A Clinical Approach. Edited by Robert P. Lisak, Daniel D. Truong, William M. Carroll, and Roongroj Bhidayasiri. © 2009 Blackwell Publishing, ISBN: 978-1-4051-5738-4.

Clinical features

The main symptoms of LEMS are muscle weakness and fatigue, especially of the legs. The weakness does not show diurnal variation and is not as pronounced as in MG. Diplopia is uncommon, but some patients may have a moderate bilateral ptosis. Cranial nerve symptoms are infrequent in LEMS. There is no clear fatiguability of skeletal muscles, as seen in MG. Instead, some patients report an initial increase of the muscle power after voluntary contractions, a phenomenon termed facilitation. The deep reflexes are usually weak or absent, but may become apparent after voluntary muscular contractions.

In addition, most LEMS patients have symptoms of autonomic dysfunction. Such symptoms are not seen in MG. LEMS patients may complain of dry mouth, absent sweating, constipation, bladder dysfunction, and impotence.

LEMS was first described in patients with malignant tumors, especially SCLC, which is present in about 50% of patients. In some patients, a bronchial carcinoma of the lung has already been detected when the weakness is noticed, but in 40% of patients, the myasthenic weakness is the first symptom to be detected. In most cases the cancer is found within 2 years after the onset of LEMS.

Around 50% of patients with LEMS have no detectable malignancies. The paraneoplastic and the non-tumor cases of LEMS are clinically indistinguishable, but patients with SCLC are usually older and have a history of smoking. Many non-tumor patients have associated autoimmune diseases, such as thyroiditis, pernicious anemia, celiac disease, juvenile onset diabetes mellitus, or Sjögren's syndrome. There is a high association with the MHC antigen HLA-B8, but also with HLA-DQ2 and HLA-DR3 in the non-tumor cases. HLA-B6 positivity correlates with a decreased risk of SCLC even among smokers. LEMS has also been described together with thymoma.

Investigations

The two most important investigations for the diagnosis of LEMS are (1) electrodiagnostic studies and (2) the detection of serum antibodies to the VGCC. Such antibodies have been reported in 75–100% of patients with LEMS and underlying cancer and in 90% of patients without. They may also be detected in a few MG patients and in patients with other autoimmune disorders. Some LEMS patients may have antibodies to the nicotinic acetylcholine receptor in low titers.

The electrodiagnosis of LEMS is based upon the characteristic electromyographic (EMG) pattern. The classical finding is small compound muscle action potential on supramaximal stimulation of the abductor digiti minimi muscle (down to 10% of normal) with rapid increase during rapid rates of stimulation (10–200/second). The incremental response may last for up to half a minute. It has been suggested that a 60% increment is a criterion that may be critical for the diagnosis of LEMS and this may differ in seropositive and seronegative LEMS, with a higher increment in the seropositive cases. In MG, supramaximal stimulation of a motor nerve leads to a decrement of the evoked muscle action potentials.

It is important to have CT or MRI of the chest to exclude chest malignancy. Bronchoscopy may be necessary if imaging studies are normal, but, in the presence of the characteristic EMG pattern, the probability of SCLC is high. LEMS has also been associated with lymphosarcoma, malignant thymoma, and carcinoma of the breast, stomach, colon, prostate, bladder, kidney, and gallbladder. Clinical signs usually precede cancer identification.

An HLA-B8 negative LEMS patient with a history of smoking should be suspected of an SCLC and has a worse prognosis than an HLA-B8 positive non-tumor case.

Treatment/management

When a diagnosis of LEMS is made, an extensive search for any underlying cancer is important, and the initial therapy should be aimed at treating the neoplasm. Removal of the tumor may lead to an objective improvement of the muscular weakness.

Plasma exchange has an effect upon the motor weakness, but not as marked as can be seen in patients with MG. As in MG, the effect is transitory and disappears after 4–5 weeks. Intravenous immunoglobulin can also improve muscle strength in a similar way. 3,4-diaminopyridine (a potassium channel antagonist) has an effect upon the symptoms of LEMS. Some patients with LEMS respond to prednisolone, and immunotherapy can be used in some cases. Acetylcholine inhibitors, standard treatment of MG, may also give some benefit in LEMS.

Further reading

Eaton L, Lambert EH. Electromyography and electric stimulation of nerves in diseases of motor unit: observations on myasthenic syndrome associated with malignant tumors. *JAMA* 1957; 163: 1117–24.

Lang B, Newsom-Davis J, Wray D, Vincent A. Autoimmune etiology for myasthenic (Eaton–Lambert) syndrome. *Lancet* 1981, ii: 224–6.

Oh SJ, Kurokawa Y, Claussen GC, Ryan HF Jr. Electrophysiological diagnosis criteria of Lambert–Eaton myasthenic syndrome. *Muscle Nerve* 2005; 32: 515–20.

Wirtz PW, Lang B, Graus F, *et al*. P/Q-type calcium channel antibodies, Lambert–Eaton myasthenic syndrome and survival in small cell lung cancer. *J Neuroimmunol* 2005; 164: 161–5.

Wirtz PW, Nijnuis MG, Sotodeh M, *et al*. Dutch Myasthenia Study Group. The epidemiology of myasthenia gravis, Lambert–Eaton myasthenic syndrome and their associated tumours in the northern part of the province of South Holland. *J Neurol* 2003; 250: 698–701.

Chapter 116
Neuromuscular transmission disorders caused by toxins and drugs

Zohar Argov

Hadassah-Hebrew University Medical Center, Jerusalem, Israel

Botulism

Botulism is a synaptic disorder caused by a neurotoxin that inhibits acetylcholine (ACh) discharge from motor and autonomic nerve endings by cleaving specific proteins essential for ACh vesicle docking. The toxin is excreted by the Gram-positive, spore-forming, anaerobic bacillus *Clostridium botulinum*. There are five types of this toxin and the three that are relevant for human diseases are A, B, and E. The spores, prevalent in soils worldwide, are heat-resistant, surviving food preparation methods that do not use temperatures of 120°C for long enough periods. Typically these are home-made, canned food like fish, vegetables, and potatoes.

There are four forms of botulism: "classical" food botulism, wound botulism, infant botulism, and occult (adult) botulism. A rare form is the complication after medical usage of the toxin in low quantities to overcome muscle overactivity. The potential use of botulinum toxin as a biological weapon (especially for terrorist attacks) should not be overlooked.

The clinical syndrome varies by the mode of toxin access into the body. In food-borne cases there is ingestion of the toxin from ill-prepared food. In wound-related cases (either traumatic or introduced by contaminated needles in drug abusers) the spores inhabit the oxygen-free environment of the tissue and the bacilli produce the toxin more slowly. In infant botulism the spores reside in the intestines and this is thought to be the case in the adult-onset "occult" botulism.

Once disseminated, the toxin produces a rather similar clinical picture of rapidly (hours to 1 day) progressive paralysis with autonomic failure. Symptoms and signs appear first in the cranial musculature, leading to ptosis, ophthalmoparesis, and speech and swallowing difficulties (the "4Ds": diplopia, dysarthria, dysphagia, and dysphonia). Generalized motor paralysis develops rapidly in a descending pattern, affecting the upper limbs first. Respiratory paralysis may then appear. Autonomic failure manifests commonly as dry mouth, constipation, pupilary abnormalities, and often also urinary retention and systemic hypotension. The fatality rate has markedly decreased in places with modern respiratory support facilities but is still as high as 10%. Where no critical medical care is present the death rate can reach 50%.

The diagnosis may be missed if the clinical pattern is not recognized, as the only confirmatory tests include isolation of the bacilli and especially identification of the toxin in body fluids and tissues. Rarely the bacilli are grown from tissue cultures and in many instances no biological confirmation can be established, especially if the samples are taken more than 48 hours after disease onset. The main sources are serum, stool, and, when relevant, wound samples. The mode of stool collection (especially in infants) and storage of samples should be known to prevent failure of diagnosis. The toxin is identified and typed in a biological test (a mouse model used in very specialized laboratories only). The main findings in the clinical electrodiagnostic laboratory are: small compound muscle action potential and increased jitter on single fiber electromyography (SFEMG). Decremental responses to low rate repetitive nerve stimulation and spontaneous activity on EMG of paralyzed muscles can sometimes be found.

Infant botulism usually occurs before age 6 months and starts mostly with constipation. Feeding difficulties, weak cry, and bulbar weakness with rapidly ensuing limb paralysis should alert the physician to the possible diagnosis. Honey consumption is considered a source of *Clostridium* spores (mainly type B) in 15% of infantile cases and its administration should be avoided before age 1. Adult intestines are resistant to bacilli growth, but prior abnormalities such as surgery, inflammatory bowel disease, and massive antibiotic treatment can reduce it.

The main mode of treatment is intensive care with good respiratory support systems until recovery, which may be as long as a few months, but usually is 2–8 weeks. Antitoxin administration remains controversial because this equine-borne treatment is associated with high

International Neurology: A Clinical Approach. Edited by Robert P. Lisak, Daniel D. Truong, William M. Carroll, and Roongroj Bhidayasiri. © 2009 Blackwell Publishing, ISBN: 978-1-4051-5738-4.

rate of serious allergic reactions. When given early, it reduces the respiratory failure period and fatality rate. The source of contamination should be rapidly identified in food-borne cases to prevent small epidemics. Other medications such as guanidine and aminopyridines have not been sufficiently studied to merit usage. In general, antibiotic use to treat the *Clostridium* infection is considered unnecessary.

Organophosphates (OP) intoxication

OP block the activity of acetylcholine esterase (AChE) and thus impair neuromuscular junction transmission as well as other cholinergic synapses. The main use of OP is as pesticides, and intoxication can occur not only on farms but also at work places, manufacturing sites, and at home (by accidental or suicidal consumption). Their development as a "nerve gas" for war and terror usage mandate the recognition of the clinical picture and the therapy of intoxication.

The clinical signs and symptoms of OP acute intoxication result from ACh accumulation in nicotinic, muscarinic, and central synapses. The neuromuscular signs include flaccid weakness and fasciculations and are associated with increased gland secretion, autonomic and smooth muscle overactivity, and central nervous system (CNS) features. Less recognized is the intermediate syndrome that occurs a few days after the acute intoxication (usually not a severe one) and results in proximal muscle weakness which may lead to respiratory failure and mimic other conditions. OP myopathic side effects in experimental animals have been reported, but their existence in humans is controversial.

Recognition of the clinical picture is the main step in the diagnosis; confirmation can be obtained by measuring AChE activity in erythrocytes.

Treatment includes removal of the patient from the contaminated environment (if necessary) and administration of three types of medications: (1) atropine that blocks muscarinic synapses in increasing doses until an effect is observed (doses may be extremely high); (2) oximes to reactivate the enzyme; and (3) diazepam to reduce CNS irritability. Supportive therapy is essential, especially mechanical respiration, as patients may recover after prolonged periods when new enzyme is regenerated.

Delayed neuropathy has been described after acute intoxication, but its potential development after low-grade chronic exposure has not been confirmed. Likewise the prolonged neuropsychological syndrome after exposure (acute or chronic) is controversial.

Neuromuscular junction (NMJ) disorders induced by medications

There is a growing list of drugs implicated in aggravating or inducing myasthenic syndromes. The clinical presentations include:

1 The appearance of myasthenia after short exposure to a medication. This condition is attributed to the various drugs' NMJ-blocking properties and is considered to appear in susceptible patients (i.e., those having subclinical myasthenia). This complication usually resolves when the offending medication is withdrawn, but in some cases the full picture of myasthenia gravis (MG) continues then to evolve.

2 The aggravation of a pre-existing NMJ disorder (usually MG but also Lambert–Eaton myasthenic syndrome (LEMS)). The most common situation is the administration of antibiotics to a myasthenic patient with infection. Other drugs have been implicated, usually those with a local anesthetic-like action.

3 Acute weakness or prolonged respiratory depression after uneventful anesthesia. This occurs when a drug with NMJ-blocking properties is given to the patient when the NMJ has not fully recovered from the anesthetic medications. Overuse of magnesium in the treatment of eclampsia can also lead to such an acute event.

4 The development of a chronic immune-mediated myasthenic syndrome after long-term exposure to a medication. This has mainly been described with penicillamine used for rheumatoid arthritis and is attributed to its effects on immune control. Recently statin-aggravated seropositive myasthenia has been identified.

Recognition and withdrawal of a potentially offending medication is the main therapeutic approach, but specific therapies that counter the blocking activity may be necessary.

Further reading

Argov Z, Kaminski HJ, Al-Mudallal A, Ruff RL. Toxic and iatrogenic myopathies and neuromuscular transmission disorders. In: Karpati G, Hilton-Jones D, Griggs RC, editors: *Disorders of Voluntary Muscle*. Cambridge, UK: Cambridge University Press; 2001, pp. 676–88.

Cherington M. Clinical spectrum of botulism. *Muscle Nerve* 1998; 21: 701–10.

Costa LG. Current issues in organophosphate toxicology. *Clin Chim Acta* 2006; 366: 1–13.

Midura TF. Update: infant botulism. *Clin Microbiol Rev* 1996; 9: 119–25.

Robinson RF, Nahata MC. Management of botulism. *Ann Pharmacother* 2003; 37: 127–31.

Chapter 117
Critical illness myopathy

Muhammad Al-Lozi and Alan Pestronk
Washington University in Saint Louis, St Louis, USA

Introduction

Critical illness myopathy (CIM) is characterized by weakness with inexcitable membranes and loss of myosin and thick filaments in muscle fibers. CIM was first described in patients with severe asthma who were treated with neuromuscular junction blockade and high doses of corticosteroids. The many different terms used to describe this entity include thick filament (myosin) loss, acute quadriplegic myopathy, acute necrotizing myopathy, and rapidly evolving myopathy with myosin loss. Some early authors noted numerous angular muscle fibers in muscle biopsies, ascribed the weakness to acute axonal damage, and described the syndrome as a critical illness polyneuropathy. Most investigators now agree that a myopathy is the primary cause of weakness. An axonal sensory neuropathy may occur along with the myopathy in some patients with CIM syndromes.

Epidemiology

Estimates of the incidence of CIM in patients in intensive care units vary widely depending on the definition of the syndrome. Mild to moderate proximal weakness with electrophysiology suggesting a myopathy may occur frequently in 20–76% of intensive care unit patients. A severe syndrome with rapidly progressive weakness and respiratory failure occurs in a small minority of patients. CIM is most prevalent in patients with severe critical illnesses who are treated with steroids, neuromuscular blocking agents, or aminoglycosides, and have a prolonged stay in an intensive care unit. CIM is mostly a disease of adults, but the syndrome also occurs in children.

Clinical features

CIM most commonly develops in patients in the intensive care unit with acute medical illnesses such as asthma, chronic obstructive pulmonary disease, sepsis, and respiratory distress syndrome, or surgical conditions, including severe trauma and organ transplantation. A similar myosin-loss myopathy syndrome occurs occasionally in ambulatory patients with myasthenia gravis who have been treated with high doses of corticosteroids. Weakness probably develops over a period of days to weeks. The exact evolution of the syndrome in individual patients may be difficult to define because of impaired sensorium due to sedation or encephalopathy. Weakness is often first appreciated during difficulties weaning patients off assisted ventilation. The pattern of weakness is symmetric and diffuse with more prominent involvement of proximal muscles. Facial weakness may occur, but ophthalmoplegia is rare. Tendon reflexes are either diminished or absent. Distal sensory loss occurs in some patients. The course is typically monophasic. The prognosis of CIM is largely determined by the underlying medical condition. If patients survive their medical illness, they usually have substantial improvement in strength and function over weeks to months.

Investigations

Serum creatine kinase (CK) level is high in some patients during the first 2 weeks and is usually normal after that time. Electrodiagnostic studies are important for the diagnosis. Compound muscle action potentials (CMAPs) are typically small, and contrast with normal nerve conduction velocities and distal latencies. Sensory nerve action potential (SNAP) amplitudes are relatively preserved but may be diminished or absent if there is an associated sensory neuropathy. Direct muscle stimulation can show decreased muscle excitability. Needle electromyography may show fibrillations/positive sharp waves, especially early in the disease course, and early recruitment of brief and small potentials, mainly proximally.

International Neurology: A Clinical Approach. Edited by Robert P. Lisak, Daniel D. Truong, William M. Carroll, and Roongroj Bhidayasiri. © 2009 Blackwell Publishing, ISBN: 978-1-4051-5738-4.

Table 117.1 Neurological disorders associated with respiratory failure and ventilator dependence.

Muscle	Neuromuscular junction	Nerve	Anterior horn cell	Central disorders
Critical illness myopathy	Myasthenic disorders	Guillain–Barré syndrome	Amyotrophic lateral sclerosis	Cervical myelopathy
Acid maltase deficiency	Botulism		Poliomyelitis	Brainstem encephalopathy
			West Nile infection	Central hypoventilation

Pathology

Muscle biopsy confirms the diagnosis and is useful in ruling out other potentially treatable causes of weakness. Muscle pathology (Plate 117.1) shows scattered small, angular, often basophilic, muscle fibers with enlarged nuclei. Reduced myosin ATPase stain at all pH levels in scattered muscle fibers is the hallmark of CIM. The myosin ATPase loss in individual muscle fibers may be diffuse or focal within the muscle fiber. Muscle fiber necrosis may occur early in the disease course. No inflammation or storage material is present. Immunocytochemistry shows selective loss of myosin with relative preservation of actin. Ultrastructural studies show loss of thick filaments and disorganization of sarcomeres.

Pathophysiology

The major pathophysiological changes in CIM are the selective loss of a major contractile protein (myosin) and the inexcitability of muscle membrane. The events that trigger these changes are not well defined. Some degree of weakness occurs in 20–50% of patients with systemic inflammatory response syndrome (SIRS) and mechanical ventilation for more than 1 week. It is postulated that SIRS may trigger a cascade of events that result in impairment of the microcirculation and delivery of oxygen and nutrients. Evidence of protein degeneration is supported by the increased calpain expression in atrophic muscle fibers. Muscle membrane inexcitability is associated with sodium channel inactivation.

Differential diagnosis

CIM should be differentiated from central nervous system and neuromuscular disorders that produce rapidly progressive generalized weakness, especially with prominent respiratory failure (Table 117.1). A central disorder may be especially entertained in patients with trauma and sepsis. Among the central causes, high cervical myelopathy or bilateral brainstem lesions may produce quadriparesis and respiratory muscle weakness. Early in the course of central lesions, diminished tendon

reflexes may simulate a peripheral disorder. The presence of an extensor plantar response is not a feature of CIM and suggests an alternative diagnosis. Neuromuscular conditions that may produce generalized weakness include disorders of muscle, neuromuscular junction, nerve, or anterior horn cells. Rhabdomyolysis is characterized by very high CK and myoglobinuria. Neuromuscular junction transmission may be affected in myasthenia gravis, botulism, hypermagnesemia, use of aminoglycoside, and neuromuscular blocking agents. Guillain–Barré syndrome and toxic neuropathies may produce an acute neuropathy that may mimic CIM. In patients with cancer, carcinomatous meningitis should be considered as a possible cause of generalized weakness.

Treatment

There is no specific treatment for CIM. Prophylactic treatment may play a role in preventing or minimizing the severity of the disease. Aggressive treatment of sepsis may help in reducing SIRS and the duration of intubation. Careful use of medications such as steroids, neuromuscular blocking agents, and aminoglycosides may minimize the risk. Recent data suggest that strict control of blood sugar may decrease the incidence of the disease, and supplementation with essential amino acids may minimize the catabolic effects of hypercortisolemia and bed rest.

Further reading

Al-Lozi MT, Pestronk A, Yee WC, Flaris N, Cooper J. Rapidly evolving myopathy with myosin-deficient muscle fibers. *Ann Neurol* 1994; 35: 273–9.

Bolton CF. Neuromuscular manifestations of critical illness. *Muscle Nerve* 2005; 32: 140–63.

Latronico N, Peli E, Botteri M. Critical illness myopathy and neuropathy. *Curr Opin Crit Care* 2005; 11: 126–32.

Pestronk A. *Critical Illness Myopathy/Neuropathy.* Neuromuscular Disease Center at Washington University in Saint Louis; 2008 www.neuro.wustl.edu/neuromuscular/msys/resp.html.

Stevens RD, Dowdy DW, Michaels RK, Mendez-Tellez PA, Pronovost PJ, Needham DM. Neuromuscular dysfunction acquired in critical illness: a systematic review. *Intensive Care Med* 2007; 33: 1876–91.

Chapter 118
Progressive muscle dystrophies

Stephan Zierz
University Halle-Wittenberg, Halle/Saale, Germany

Introduction

Progressive muscle dystrophies are a clinically and etiologically heterogeneous group of myopathies. Historically, the term muscle dystrophy was first introduced by Wilhelm Erb in 1891 for a progressive neuromuscular disorder ("dystrophia muscularis progressiva"). The term dystrophy was intended to describe the clinical and histological coexistence of features of muscle atrophy and hypertrophy. Various myopathological changes described in this disease constituted morphological criteria that are still valid. The expanding identification of numerous etiologically different inherited myopathies makes it now often difficult to define a progressive degenerative myopathy either as a muscular dystrophy or as a myopathy.

Thus, it seems somewhat arbitrary to classify, for example, the various forms of distal myopathies not as progressive dystrophies. Conversely, oculopharyngeal muscular dystrophy usually does not show dystrophic histopathological features. However, progressive muscle dystrophies are clearly differentiated from congenital muscular dystrophies (CMD and also recently MCD). This etiologically heterogeneous group of autosomal recessive disorders usually start at birth and lead to severe progressive disability. Many forms of MCD are not restricted to skeletal muscle but also involve the central nervous system (CNS) and the eye. Examples of MCD are Fukuyama MCD, muscle–eye–brain disease, Walker–Warburg syndrome, and MCD type Ulllrich.

A number of the more common causes of progressive muscle dystrophy are described in Chapters 57–64.

Dystrophinopathies

Dystrophinopathies are hereditary muscular dystrophies with different phenotypes caused by different mutations

Table 118.1 Clinical phenotypes of dystrophinopathies.

Asymptomatic elevation of serum creatine kinase (CK)
Exercise intolerance associated with myalgia and muscle cramps
Exercise-induced myoglobinuria
Slight limb girdle weakness
Quadriceps myopathy
Cardiomyopathy associated with mild muscle weakness
Cardiomyopathy without weakness of skeletal muscle
Becker type muscle dystrophy (BMD)
Duchenne type muscle dystrophy (DMD)

---

of the dystrophin gene in skeletal muscle. Dystrophin is a subsarcolemmal cytoskeletal protein encoded by a large gene on Xp21.

Dystrophinopathies are transmitted by X-linked recessive inheritance. The two major phenotypes of dystrophinopathy are Duchenne type (Duchenne muscle dystrophy, DMD) and Becker type (Becker muscle dystrophy, BMD). Dystrophin is usually absent or markedly reduced in DMD and is a lethal disorder by adolescence. BMD is a milder variant of dystrophinopathy and dystrophin is accordingly less reduced than in DMD. Increased knowledge of dystrophin pathology has identified a broad range of phenotypes (summarized in Table 118.1). The dystrophinopathies are dealt with in detail in Chapter 58.

Duchenne type (DMD)

The incidence of DMD is 1 in 3500–4000 male births. The very severe course of the disease is characterized by early manifestations of developmental delay, difficulty in running and climbing stairs, and frequent falls. During the first 3 years of life the calf muscles begin to enlarge. Between 3 and 6 years of age the gait becomes lordotic, Gowers' sign appears, and in the advanced stage involvement of the shoulder muscles (scapular winging), facial muscles, and neck flexors appears. Tendon reflexes diminish and are lost further in the disease course. Contractures develop at between 6 and 10 years of age. Loss of ambulation occurs by 10 years after onset. Kyphoscoliosis and significant weakness of respiratory muscles begins around 8 or 9 years and worsens steadily. The heart is commonly involved with degenerative

International Neurology: A Clinical Approach. Edited by Robert P. Lisak, Daniel D. Truong, William M. Carroll, and Roongroj Bhidayasiri. © 2009 Blackwell Publishing, ISBN: 978-1-4051-5738-4.

cardiomyopathy or conduction abnormalities. The mean age of death is 18 years mainly from respiratory failure and/or cardiac failure.

Becker type (BMD)

The incidence of BMD is 1 in 14 000 male births. Age at onset is usually about 12 years (range 1–70 years). BMD is characterized by a limb girdle weakness (pelvic girdle more than shoulder girdle) and calf hypertrophy. Loss of ambulation is in the fourth but may vary from 10 to 78 years (mean 35 years). Cardiac involvement in BMD is unrelated to the severity of the myopathy and cardiomyopathy and conduction abnormalities are common.

Dystrophinopathy in females

Because of the X-linked inheritance, nearly all patients are male. Nevertheless, mild manifestation of the disease in females ranges from calf hypertrophy and elevated CK to more marked limb girdle weakness in the following situations: failure of inactivation of the maternal X chromosome (manifesting carriers), Turner syndrome (X0), Turner mosaic (X/XX or X/XX/XXX), structurally abnormal X chromosome, and X-autosomal translocation.

Diagnosis and therapy

For this see Chapter 58.

Limb-girdle muscle dystrophies (LGMD)

This topic is considered in detail in Chapter 57. LGMD are autosomal recessive and dominant muscular dystrophies presenting with a progressive weakness predominantly affecting the proximal muscles (pelvic and shoulder girdle) resulting in the so-called limb-girdle syndrome. In later stages distal muscle weakness develops. As a phenotypic group LGMD has a highly variable genotype.

A genetic classification of LGMD divides it into LGMD1 with autosomal dominant inheritance and LGMD2 with autosomal recessive inheritance. Up to seven forms of LGMD1 and 13 forms of LGMD2 have been identified (Table 118.2) and are subdivided in chronological order of their identification using letters in alphabetical order. Interestingly, defects in some genes can cause either LGMD or other myopathies such as distal myopathy.

Epidemiology, diagnosis, and therapy

The incidence of LGMD is estimated to be at least 0.8 per 100 000, but is higher in inbred populations due to its mainly recessive inheritance (only 10% autosomal dominant inheritance). The most common forms are LGMD2A, 2B, 2I, and 2C–2F.

Clinically, it is usually not possible to distinguish between the different forms of LGMDs. Disease onset

Table 118.2 Classification of limb girdle muscle dystrophies (LGMD).

Inheritance	Gene/locus	Gene product
Autosomal dominant		
LGMD 1A	*TTID*	Myotilin
LGMD 1B	*LNMA*	Lamin A/C
LGMD 1C	*CAV3*	Caveolin-3
LGMD 1D	6q23	Unknown
LGMD 1E	7q	Unknown
LGMD 1F	7q32	Unknown
LGMD 1G	4p21	Unknown
Autosomal recessive		
LGMD 2A	*CAPN3*	Calpain-3
LGMD 2B	*DYSF*	Dysferlin
LGMD 2C	*SGCG*	γ-Sarcoglykan
LGMD 2D	*SGCA*	α-Sarcoglykan
LGMD 2E	*SGCB*	β-Sarcoglykan
LGMD 2F	*SGCC*	δ-Sarcoglykan
LGMD 2G	*TCAP*	Telethonin
LGMD 2H	*TRIM32*	E3-ubiquitin ligase
LGMD 2I	*FKRP*	Fukutin-related-protein
LGMD 2J	*TTN*	Titin
LGMD 2K	*POMT1*	Protein *O*-mannosyltransferase-1
LGMD 2L	*FCMD*	Fukutin
LGMD 2M	11p13-p12	Unknown

is variable, ranging from early childhood even to late adulthood. However, there are some features typical for certain forms, such as sudden onset in the teens and early difficulties in standing on tiptoe in LGMD2B. Pseudohypertrophy especially of the calves is typically seen in LGMD1C, 2C–F, and 2I. Cardiac involvement is frequently observed in LGMD 1B and 2I, together with early contractures in LGMD1B.

CK is elevated in most forms. Very high levels (20–150 times normal) are observed in LGMD 2B and 2C–F. Electromyography frequently shows a myopathic pattern but is otherwise non-specific.

Diagnosis requires muscle biopsy not only to exclude other myopathies presenting as a limb-girdle syndrome, but also for the detection of the defective protein either by Western blot or by immunohistochemistry. Histology reveals typical signs of muscular dystrophy. However, there are oligosymptomatic patients who show only slight histological changes and some LGMD show secondary inflammatory features, most prominent in LGM2B, which can cause difficultiy distinguishing myositis from LGMD.

Cardiac assessment requires electrocardiogram (ECG), echocardiography, and Holter-ECG.

There is no *specific* treatment at present. Some forms of LGMD (e.g., LGMD2L) or those patients with inflammation in muscle biopsy might respond to steroids. Cardiac treatment can include angiotensin converting enzyme (ACE) inhibitors, pacemaker, or implantable defibrillator.

Facioscapulohumeral muscular dystrophy (FSHD)

See also Chapter 59.

Prevalence of FSHD ranges from 1 per 20 000 to 1 per 455 000, depending on the geographical region. The historical description of Landouzy and Dejerine (1884) forms the basis of the current diagnostic criteria: (1) onset of the disease in facial or shoulder girdle muscles, and sparing of the extraocular, pharyngeal, and lingual muscles and the myocardium; (2) facial weakness in more than 50% of affected family members; (3) autosomal dominant inheritance in familial cases; (4) evidence of myopathy on electromyocardiogram (EMG) and muscle biopsy in at least one affected family member without biopsy features of alternative diagnoses.

FSHD is linked in 95% of cases to chromosome 4q35. A deletion of multiple copies of a tandem repeat consisting of 3.3-kb units (*D4Z4*) is associated with the disease (see also Chapter 59). Restriction enzyme cleavage with *Eco*RI/*Bln*I allows the distinction of the 4q35 locus from a homologous locus on chromosome 10q26 in most individuals. *Eco*RI/*Bln*I fragments in the range of 10–35 kb on chromosome 4q35 are assumed to be disease associated and can be detected by probe p13E-11 with a test sensitivity of 95% and a specificity approaching 100% at the 34-kb level. Sporadic cases occur, presumably the result of new mutations.

Symptomatic onset varies from infancy to middle age and the degree of involvement ranges from minimal facial weakness to severe generalized paresis. Usually, initial manifestations are difficulty elevating arms above the head, progressive winging of the scapulae, or an inability to close the eyes firmly, to purse the lips, and to whistle. Lips have a tendency to protrude. The lower parts of the trapezius muscle and the sternal parts of the pectorals are almost invariably affected, but, by contrast, the deltoids may seem to be large and strong. Wasting of the biceps muscle is usually less than the triceps muscle, and the brachioradialis seems spared so that the upper arm may be thinner than the forearm. Pelvic muscles are involved later and to milder degree and the pretibial muscles weaken, so that foot drop adds to the waddling (Trendellenberg) gait. Early disease may show asymmetric weakness and atrophy. FSHD progresses slowly; approximately 20% of patients eventually become wheelchair-dependent.

The clinical presentation of patients with FSHD-associated short fragments on chromosome 4q35 varies greatly and includes facial-sparing SHD, LGMD syndrome, distal myopathy, asymmetric brachial weakness, and FSHD with additional symptoms of chronic progressive external ophthalmoplegia (CPEO). Due to the extreme clinical phenotypic variability in patients with an FSHD genotype, atypical FSHD should be considered in patients with obscure and unclassified myopathies.

Although the genetic diagnosis of clinical FSHD is crucial, patients with unequivocal clinical features of classical Landouzy–Dejerine FSHD and without typical short *Eco*RI/*Bln*I fragments have been reported, suggesting that the FSHD phenotype might result from a number of different molecular mechanisms.

Oculopharyngeal muscular dystrophy (OPMD)

OPMD is an autosomal dominant disorder with onset in late life characterized by progressive ptosis of the eyelids, dysphagia, and proximal limb weakness. This topic is discussed in detail in Chapter 62.

Epidemiology
OPMD is a rare disease with an estimated prevalence of 1 per 100 000 in Western Europe. Large clusters of OPMD were found in Quebec (prevalence 1 per 1000), in Bukhara Jews (prevalence 1 per 600), Uruguayans, Spanish Americans living in New Mexico, and California. Nevertheless cases with OPMD have been reported worldwide.

Pathophysiology
OPMD is caused by a small expansion of a short polyalanine tract in the nuclear poly (A) binding protein 1 (PABPN1). Short GCG nucleotide expansions in the first exon of the *PABPN1* gene were first demonstrated to cause OPMD. The six wildtype GCG repeats were expanded to 7–13 GCG repeats. $(GCG)_7$ is associated with recessive OPMD and $(GCG)_{8-13}$ with dominant OPMD. Along with the $(GCG)_{7-13}$ nucleotide expansions, different combinations of GCA and GCG trinucleotides were also reported, all resulting in additional alanines in the N-terminal domain of PABPN1. The mechanism by which the polyalanine expansions in PABPN1 cause the disease is unclear. Wildtype PABPN1 stimulates the poly(A) RNA polymerase, rendering polyadenylation processive, and control of the length of poly(A) tails. It was shown that mutant PABPN1 aggregates contain mRNA and various proteins.

Clinical features
OPMD is a probable diagnosis in patients with familial occurrence of late-onset ptosis and swallowing difficulties. External ophthalmoplegia only evolves at very late stage of the disease. Additional symptoms include changes in voice and proximal atrophic limb weakness occurring almost regularly later in the course of disease. Dysphagia becomes so prominent that food intake is limited. Life expectancy is almost normal.

Investigations
Muscle biopsy reveals mild myopathic changes. Rimmed vacuoles are rather characteristic but not specific.

Neuropathic changes such as angulated fibers or fiber-type grouping have been described, but these changes may be age-related. The distinct ultrastructural hallmark of OPMD is the presence of tubulofilamentous intranuclear inclusions in skeletal muscle fibers of about 8.5 nm outer diameter. These inclusions contain mutated and aggregated PABPN1. To confirm the diagnosis in clinically suspected patients, molecular genetic testing is recommended.

Treatment

Ptosis can be treated with gathering of the eyelid; this method is reversible in contrast to the resection of the eyelid muscle. Dysphagia can be ameliorated by cricopharyngeal myotomy or by paralyzing these muscle with botulinum toxin. Finally, pharyngeal dilatation to widen the esophageal opening can be helpful. In advanced cases, alimentation might require gastrostomy.

Myotonic dystrophies

This topic is discussed in detail in Chapter 61. There are two clinically and genetically different myotonic dystrophies (DM), that is, DM1 (Curschmann–Steinert myotonic dystrophy) and DM2 (proximal myotonic myopathy, PROMM). In contrast to other myotonias, DM1 and DM2 show a progressive course of muscle weakness. Usually, muscle weakness is by far more disabling than myotonic symptoms. Sometimes myotonia might only be seen in EMG. DM1 and DM2 are both multisystemic diseases (Table 118.3). The diagnosis is mainly based on the typical clinical symptoms, on the characteristic myotonic changes in the EMG, and finally on the molecular findings of a CTG repeat expansion on chromosome 19q13.3 for DM1 and of a CCTG tetranucleotid repeat expansion

Table 118.3 Clinical features of myotonic dystrophy Curschmann–Steinert (DM1) and of PROMM (DM2).

Symptom/sign	DM1	DM2
Myotonia	+	+
Cataract	+	+
Paresis		
Facial	+	(–)
Distal	+	(–)
Proximal	(–)	+
Atrophy	+	–
Myalgia	–	+
Cardiac arrhythmia	+	(+)
Cognitive impairment	+	–
Endocrine abnormalities (testicular atrophy, diabetes)	+	(–)

+: Typically; (+): sometimes; (–): rarely; –: absent.

in a zink finger protein 9 gene on chromosome 3q21 for DM2. Thus, muscle biopsy is not necessary for diagnosis of either DM1 or DM2.

In DM1 there is clear evidence of anticipation. The number of repeat expansions increases from the previous to the next generation. This correlates with the clinical severity and the age of onset of the disease. The mild form becomes manifest in late adulthood with often only cataract and slight muscle weakness. The classical form begins in early adulthood and usually shows all the multisystemic symptoms. The most severe form is the congenital DM1 presenting as floppy infant and severe respiratory insufficiency.

Nuclear envelopathies

There are two clinically very similar muscle dystrophies characterized by early muscle contractures, muscle weakness, and cardiomyopathy. In contrast to other muscle dystrophies with contractures, the contractures in these myopathies usually occur before paresis becomes apparent. Both diseases are due to defects of proteins of the nuclear envelope. The autosomal dominant Hauptmann–Thannhauser muscle dystrophy (HTMD) is associated with more than 30 mutations in the lamin A/C gene (LMNA gene). It is interesting to note that other mutations of the LMNA gene are associated with LGMD type 1B and with isolated dilatative cardiomyopathy. The X-linked Emery–Dreifuss muscle dystrophy (EDMD) is associated with more than 100 mutations of the emerin gene. Clinically, HTMD and EDMD can hardly be distinguished, especially due to the great intra- and interfamiliar variability.

Distal myopathies

This topic is discussed in detail in Chapter 64. Distal myopahies are a clinically and genetically heterogeneous group of disorders. In contrast to the more common proximal myopathies, distal myopathies initially present with weakness in the hands and feet. There are autosomal dominant and recessive forms. The clinically defined forms include the distal myopathies types Welander, Marksbery–Griggs, Nonaka, Miyoshi, Udd, and many others. Age of onset in these various forms ranges from childhood to late adulthood. Serum CK is usually between normal and slightly up (three to ten times elevated), and only in the Miyoshi type up to 100 times elevated. Histopathologically there are often dystrophic changes and some forms (e.g., type Nonaka) show characteristic rimmed vacuoles. Recently, mutations in various genes and gene products have been identified in association with the distal myopathy phenotypes.

These include titin, dysferlin, myotilin, myosin, desmin, crystalline, GNE, and ZASP.

The differential diagnoses of distal myopathies are neurogenic disorders such as Charcot–Marie–Tooth disease, distal spinal muscle atrophy, and hereditary motor neuron diseases. Other myopathies with possible predominant distal involvement are myotonic dystrophy Curschmann–Steinert (DM1), FSHD, inclusion body myopathy, and congenital myopathies with structural abnormalities such as central core disease and nemaline myopathy.

Further reading

Muscle dystrophies
Kanagawa M, Toda T. The genetic and molecular basis of muscular dystrophy: roles of cell-matrix linkage in the pathogenesis. *J Hum Genet* 2006; 51: 915–26.

Dystrophinopathies
Muntoni F, Torelli S, Ferlini A. Dystrophin and mutations: one gene, several proteins, multiple phenotypes. *Lancet Neurol* 2003; 2: 731–40.

LGMD
Bushby K, Norwood F, Straub V. The limb-girdle muscular dystrophies – diagnostic strategies. *Biochim Biophys Acta* 2007; 1772: 238–42.

FSHD
Krasnianski M, Eger K, Neudecker S, Jakubiczka S, Zierz S. Atypical phenotypes in patients with FSHD 4q35 deletion. *Arch Neurol* 2003; 60: 1421–5.

Tawil R, van der Maarel SM. Fascioscapulohumeral muscular dystrophy. *Muscle Nerve* 2006; 34: 1–15.

OPMD
Fan X, Rouleau GA. Progress in understanding the pathogenesis of oculopharyngeal muscular dystrophy. *Can J Neurol Sci* 2003; 30: 8–14.

Müller T, Deschauer M, Kolbe-Fehr F, Zierz S. Genetic heterogeneity in 30 German patients with oculopharyngeal muscular dystrophy. *J Neurol* 2006; 253: 892–5.

Myotonic dystrophies
Machuca-Tzili L, Brook D, Hilton-Jones D. Clinical and molecular aspects of the myotonic dystrophies. *Muscle Nerve* 2005; 32: 1–18.

Nuclear envelopathies
Krasnianski, M, Ehrt U, Neudecker S, Zierz S. Alfred Hauptmann, Siegfried Thannhauser, and an endangered muscular disorder. *Arch Neurol* 2004; 61: 1139–41.

Distal myopathies
Udd B, Griggs R. Distal myopathies. *Curr Opin Neurol* 2001; 14: 561–6.

Chapter 119
Familial periodic paralyses

Chokri Mhiri
Habib Bourguiba University Hospital, Sfax, Tunisia

Introduction

Familial periodic paralyses (FPP) are autosomal dominant disorders due to abnormal sarcolemmal excitability secondary to ion channel dysfunction. They are characterized by attacks of flaccid paralysis. FPP are classically classified as hypokalemic (hypoKPP) or hyperkalemic (hyperKPP) according to serum potassium (K^+) level and the response to K^+ administration. Recent advances in molecular biology permit classification of FPP according to the mutated ion channel. However, genotype–phenotype correlations remain imperfect and in some cases the molecular lesion is still unknown. Cardiac arrhythmia observed in a subset of FPP patients (Andersen's syndrome) may be life-threatening. After several attacks the majority of affected individuals develop persistent weakness.

Clinical features

Hypokalemic periodic paralysis (MIM170400)

Although periodic paralysis was described in 1885 by Westphal, hypokalemia was only demonstrated in 1934. HypoKPP is the most common form of FPP, with a prevalence of 1:100000. Inheritance is autosomal dominant with high penetrance. There is a male predominance due to reduced penetrance in woman and it is more frequent in Asia. HypoKPP may be observed in some cases of thyrotoxicosis (acquired hypoKPP). Usually, disease onset is during the second decade of life and manifests by attacks of flaccid paralysis lasting hours to 1 or 2 days (typically 3–4 hours). Episodes of paralysis occur in the night or on awakening in the early morning. Rarely, premonitory signs, such as asthenia, nausea, limb numbness, thirst, and diaphoresis, precede these episodes. Typically there is no muscle pain, but myalgia may be observed in some cases. During attacks, muscles are hypotonic

and deep tendon reflexes are abolished. Muscle weakness is symmetrical, impeding the ability to walk, and can be severe (tetraplegia). Despite the frequency of sensory symptoms, the sensory examination is normal. Recovery, sometimes preceded by diaphoresis or polyuria, occurs over 3–4 hours and begins in the last affected muscles. Attacks are associated with hypokalemia (often ≤2mmol/l). Attack frequency can vary from daily to a few episodes in a lifetime and it often decreases after age 40. Respiratory, bulbar, and ocular motor muscles and the heart are spared.

Episodes of paralysis occur spontaneously or are triggered by one of several intracellular K^+ transfer enhancing conditions or drugs, for example, a carbohydrate-rich meal, rest after vigorous exercise, alcohol ingestion, emotion, exposure to cold, intercurrent infection, menstruation, pregnancy, and specific medications (e.g., beta agonists, corticosteroids, and insulin). Provocation test by hypokalemia reproduces the attack of paralysis, but the inherent risk is great and this test has been abandoned.

With increased age, attacks become fewer and permanent weakness appears, its degree being independent of the frequency and severity of attacks. There is no myotonia.

Muscle biopsy is unnecessary but, when performed, shows vacuolar myopathy. Vacuoles have been shown to be dilated endoplasmic reticulum.

Hyperkalemic periodic paralysis (MIM170500)

Age of onset is earlier in hyperKPP than in hypoKPP, most commonly the first decade. The chief symptom is the occurrence of paralytic attacks. Triggering factors are rest after intensive physical effort or at the end of the day, exposure to cold, and fasting. Paralytic episodes are announced by paresthesia in the peri-oral area and in limbs extremities, mildew smell, and acid taste. Mild muscular exercise and glucose ingestion may relieve paresthesia and prevent paralysis. If not, a few minutes to half an hour later, muscle weakness appears in the lower limbs and spreads upward to the pelvic girdle, upper limbs, shoulder, and cervico-facial muscles. Facial paralysis,

International Neurology: A Clinical Approach. Edited by Robert P. Lisak, Daniel D. Truong, William M. Carroll, and Roongroj Bhidayasiri. © 2009 Blackwell Publishing, ISBN: 978-1-4051-5738-4.

ophthalmoplegia, and oropharyngeal paralysis are rare. Diaphragmatic involvement is uncommon.

At the height of the attack there is flaccid paralysis and areflexia without sensory abnormalities. Usually the attack is limited to a state of generalized weakness, muscle cramps, spasms, agitation, and irritability lasting 10–60 minutes before progressively improving.

During the attack, kalemia is increased (6–7 mmol/l) secondary to K^+ transfer from the intracellular compartment to plasma, notably in veins draining paretic muscles. Urinary excretion of K^+ is also increased. Electrocardiogram (ECG) shows high and sharp T waves.

Attacks can be induced by K^+ overload and reduced by intravenous Ca^{2+}. Glucose intake, with or without insulin, before K^+ overload ameliorates or prevents the attack.

Between attacks, there is myotonia of the small muscles of the hands, eyelids, tongue, and face in about 20% of cases. Myalgia during attacks may persist for several days. Calf hypertrophy is possible.

Muscle biopsy may show fiber size variation, nuclear centralization, target fibers, subsarcolemmal vacuoles rich in glycogen, or tubular aggregates. Ultrastructural changes include sarcoplasmic endothelium dilatation and I-band glycogen deposits.

In childhood, attacks are shorter, resolving in 10–20 minutes but may recur several times a day. At puberty, attacks may be more severe. Attacks are most symptomatic between 15 and 35 years of age, then decrease. In patients over 40 years, a myopathic syndrome may be observed with muscle weakness and wasting predominant in the pelvic girdle and abdominal muscles.

Normo-kalemic periodic paralysis has been demonstrated to be due to a mutation of the *SCN4* gene and is now grouped with hyperKPP. Paramyotonia congenita (PMC) is an allelic disorder of hyperKPP; affected individuals may have attacks of weakness, but the major clinical symptom is of muscle stiffness, worsening with activity and cold temperature.

Andersen's syndrome (MIM 170390)

Andersen's syndrome, an autosomal dominant disorder, has incomplete penetrance and variable clinical expression. It is related to a mutation of the *KCNJ2* gene encoding the K^+ channel Kir2.1. Described by Andersen in 1971, the syndrome is characterized by the triad of periodic paralysis, ventricular arrhythmia, and dysmorphic features. Genetic studies show that the clinical phenotype can be limited to asymptomatic prolongation of the QT interval of the ECG.

Onset is usually in the first or second decade with episodic weakness occurring spontaneously or triggered by rest following exertion or alcohol ingestion. Attack frequency, duration, and severity are variable between and within affected individuals. K^+ levels may be reduced, normal, or elevated. After several years, permanent proximal weakness often develops. There is no clinical or electrical myotonia.

Dysmorphic features include low-set ears, broad nasal root, ocular hypertelorism, mandibular hypoplasia, prognathism, ogival palate, clinodactyly, syndactyly, and short stature.

ECG reveals various types of ventricular arrhythmia: long QT interval (80% of cases), prominent U waves, premature ventricular contractions, ventricular bigeminy, and polymorphic ventricular tachycardia. Many patients with ventricular ectopy are asymptomatic; others present with palpitations, syncope, or rarely cardiac arrest.

Muscle biopsy shows moderate myopathic features with tubular aggregates.

Diagnosis

Diagnosis of FPP is evoked if there are transient episodes of paralysis and family history of similar cases. During an attack, there is diffuse muscle weakness, hypotonia, and abolished reflexes. Determination of kalemia level, during attacks, is important; it is low in primary hypoKPP, but in hyperKPP it is inconstantly elevated and remains within the normal range in up to 50% of cases.

Electrophysiological testing is helpful for the diagnosis of FPP. During an episode of weakness, the compound motor action potential (CMAP) may be reduced and rarely absent, and at stimulation, muscle is unexcitable. On needle examination, myotonic discharges occur in 75% of individuals with hyperKPP and in all patients with paramyotonia congenita, and do not occur in hypoKPP. Electrodiagnostic studies at room temperature and after cooling the extremity may be more sensitive for hyperKPP and PMC.

Interictal EMG is usually normal. Provoking test is useful. It comprises maximal contraction of a muscle for 5 minutes with repetitive recording of CMAP during effort and 30 minutes after. The test is positive if there is a delayed decrement of more than 40%. This test is highly specific of FPP but has poor sensitivity.

ECG must be performed in all cases of FPP, regardless of the presence or absence of developmental abnormalities or cardiac symptoms.

Thyrotoxic periodic paralysis may mimic hypoKPP, so assessment of thyroid status is required particularly in patients presenting after age 20 or without a family history. Measurement of TSH and free T4 or T3 (fT4, fT3) levels is necessary.

Genetics

HypoKPP may be caused by mutations of two genes, calcium channel gene "*CACNL1A3*" (hypoKPP-type 1) and sodium channel gene "*SCN4A*" (hypoKPP-type 2). The *CACNL1A3* gene, situated on chromosome 1, encodes to a 1S subunit of the skeletal muscle L-type calcium channel (dihydropyridines receptor) and is involved in about 70% of hypoKPP cases. The *SCN4A* gene encodes to alpha subunits of the skeletal muscle sodium channel. Mutation of this gene accounts for about 10% of hypoKPP cases and this mutation is different from that observed in hyperKPP and paramyotonia. Type 2 hypoKPP is characterized by myalgia, and acetazolamid induces worsening, so it is contraindicated. A small number of definitely affected kindreds (20%) do not have a mutation in the calcium or sodium channel genes and are not linked to these loci. Mutation of the K channel KCNE3, suspected by some authors, has not been substantiated.

Regardless of the type of mutation, the close mechanism of hypokalemia remains poorly elucidated. One of the evoked hypotheses is activation of membraneous Na/K pump by insulin, producing K transfer from the extracellular into the intracellular compartment.

Most cases of hyperKPP are caused by mutations in the sodium channel gene "*SCN4A*." This gene is also involved in paramyotonia congenita and K-aggravated myotonia (allelic disorders). The most common are the missense mutations, accounting for 75% of affected individuals; other point mutations account for the remainder.

Andersen's syndrome is related in 70% of cases to mutation of the *KCNJ2* gene encoding to potassium channel Kir2.1. It may be a missense mutation or small deletion. Some kindreds are not linked to the *KCNJ2* gene and the molecular lesion has not been identified in about 30% of cases.

Treatment/management

Correction of hypokalemia or hyperkalemia is in general well tolerated, but it should be avoided because it risks reverse rebound, especially when undertaken late during the attack. Correction of dyskalemia may be needed for cardiac intolerance.

In most cases of hypoKPP, acetazolamide (125–1000 mg/day) reduces attack frequency but may induce worsening in some cases (type 2 hypoKPP). Avoidance of precipitating triggers through lifestyle and dietary care is essential including patient education to consume sodium- and glucose-poor meals and ingest 2–7 g of KCl. Some authors recommend the K^+ sparing diuretics

spironolactone and triamterene. Oral administration of 2–10 g of K^+ at the beginning of an attack may alleviate or shorten the episode. During attacks of hyperKPP, several therapeutic approaches can be implemented including continued mild activity, sweet drinks (avoiding fruit juices rich in K^+), intravenous glucose with insulin, calcium gluconate, adrenaline, tolbutamide, and beta agonist inhalers (1–2 puffs of 0.1 mg salbutamol or albuterol). Preventive treatment of paralytic episodes in hyperKPP is based on diuretics that increase urinary excretion of K^+ such as carbonic anhydrase inhibitors (acetazolamide, chlorothiazide, dichlorphenamide, bendroflumathiazide, etc.). Less then 50% of affected individuals are prescribed prophylactic medication.

In Andersen's syndrome, management must consider the double involvement of skeletal and cardiac muscle because some antiarrhythmic drugs worsen muscle weakness and diuretics (acetazolamide, thiazie) may induce hypokalemia and risk cardiac complications. As in hyperKPP and hypoKPP, some isolated reported cases of Andersen's syndrome suggest that carbonic anhydrase inhibitors may be effective in the prevention of attacks of paralysis. Usually, antiarrhythmic drugs have a very limited effect and are insufficient to control the frequent ventricular ectopy manifested by Andersen's patients. Finally there is no clear evidence that beta-blockers alter the frequency of ventricular tachycardia. Implantation of a cardioverter-defibrillator is a prudent option for patients with tachycardia-induced syncope or aborted sudden cardiac death.

Further reading

Andersen ED, Krasilnikoff PA, Overvad H. Intermittent muscular weakness, extrasystoles, and multiple developmental anomalies. A new syndrome? *Acta Paediatr Scand* 1971; 60: 559–64.

Fontaine B, Vale-Santos J, Jurkat-Rott K, *et al*. Mapping of the hypokalaemic periodic paralysis (HypoPP) locus to chromosome 1q31–32 in three European families. *Nat Genet* 1994; 6: 267–72.

Miller TM, Dias da Silva MR, Miller HA, *et al*. Correlating phenotype and genotype in the periodic paralyses. *Neurology* 2004; 63: 1647–55.

Ptacek L. The familial periodic paralyses and nondystrophic myotonias. *Am J Med* 1998; 104: 58–70.

Venance SL, Cannon SC, Fialho D, *et al*. The primary periodic paralyses: diagnosis, pathogenesis and treatment. *Brain* 2006; 129: 8–17.

Chapter 120
Congenital disorders of the muscle

Young-Chul Choi
Yonsei University College of Medicine, Seoul, Korea

Introduction

Congenital disorders of muscle are a diverse group ranging from congenital deformities of muscle to congenital myopathies (CM). Related conditions of congenital deformities are arthrogryposis and amyoplasia (congenital absence of muscle). CM are a clinically, genetically, and pathologically heterogeneous group of skeletal muscle disorders defined by characteristic structural or histological abnormalities on muscle biopsy. They are genetic in origin, frequently apparent at birth, usually non-progressive or slowly progressive, and have overlapping clinical features. In 1956, CM was first described as "central core disease" by Shy and Magee. Many other forms of CM have been reported. Central core disease, nemaline myopathy, and centronuclear or myotubular myopathy were the major conditions identified in this group of disorders. The classification of CM was based on muscle histology. Due to advances in immunocytochemical and electron microscopic techniques, a large number of CM have been identified. Molecular genetic studies have led to the discovery of new mutations of many genes and the increased knowledge of their genetic basis has provided new insights and redefined the boundaries of CM.

Epidemiology

The exact incidence of CM is unknown. It is thought to be rare. The most common form of CM is nemaline myopathy, which occurs in about 1/50 000 live births. Both sexes are affected equally in most CM with autosomal recessive or dominant inheritance.

Pathophysiology

The etiology and pathogenesis of CM is not fully known. The well-established CM are all genetic in origin.

International Neurology: A Clinical Approach. Edited by Robert P. Lisak, Daniel D. Truong, William M. Carroll, and Roongroj Bhidayasiri. © 2009 Blackwell Publishing, ISBN: 978-1-4051-5738-4.

Recent interest in CM has concentrated on defining and classifying the distinct disease entities and identifying defective genes. In some forms of CM, aggregates of mutant proteins accumulate within affected muscle fibers, but the mechanism of mutant protein formation and aggregation is still unknown. Dysfunction of these proteins presumably leads to the specific morphologic changes.

Clinical features

Patients with CM have generalized weakness, hypotonia, hyporeflexia, poor muscle bulk, and dysmorphic features (i.e., chest deformities or high-arched palate) and usually present at birth or in early infancy with a wide variety of symptoms of clinical severity. Muscle weakness is predominantly proximal. In some patients, weakness may involve the axial muscles and face, or even have a distal predominance. A long "myopathic face" is a common feature, particularly in nemaline myopathy, and extraocular muscle involvement occurs in centronuclear myopathy. The weakness is usually non-progressive or mildly progressive. However, severe progressive weakness with fatal outcomes occurs in some patients, as with X-linked neonatal myotubular myopathy. Lordosis, spinal rigidity, scoliosis, and joint laxity are also frequent. Arthrogryposis may occur in some severe cases of nemaline myopathy and central core disease. Abnormalities of the central and peripheral nervous systems do not usually occur. Intelligence is usually normal.

Investigations

Laboratory studies including serum creatine kinase (CK), electrophysiological studies, imaging, muscle biopsy, and genetic studies are useful for diagnosis. The serum CK test is one of the most useful laboratory studies. However, most CM patients have normal CK levels. Electrophysiological studies including nerve conduction studies and electromyography (EMG) should be part of the routine evaluation of suspected CM. These studies rarely help in making a specific diagnosis, but are useful for differentiating CM from other neuromuscular disorders. Imaging muscle with ultrasound, CT, and MRI can detect particular patterns of selective involvement of muscle, which can help diagnosis and selection of biopsy sites. Muscle biopsy is essential for the diagnosis of CM and Western blot and immunocytochemistry can be helpful for the analysis of certain muscle proteins. Because specific molecular genetic defects are known for a large number of CM, mutation analysis using peripheral blood or muscle tissue DNA also aids the diagnosis of CM.

Central core disease

Central core disease (CCD) is a rare congenital myopathy characterized by the presence of a well-limited round area within muscle fibers, called the "core," where there is sarcomeric disorganization, lack of mitochondria, and lack of oxidative activity. The core usually extends along the entire length of the fiber. The incidence is unknown, but it is thought to be rare. It is autosomal dominantly inherited, but autosomal recessive and sporadic cases have also been reported. The clinical features are variable, ranging from asymptomatic to severely affected. Most patients have a non-progressive or slowly progressive proximal muscle weakness and hypotonia during infancy. Skeletal anomalies such as hip dislocation, kyphoscoliosis, and foot deformity are also common findings. Affected adults with CCD may be nearly asymptomatic or may have muscle cramps and myalgia, with a varying degree of proximal weakness that is typically more pronounced in the legs. Diagnosis of CCD is confirmed by the presence of the core in the muscle biopsy. By electron microscopy, the core is a circumscribed lesion within which the myofibrils may show structured or unstructured cores with excessive Z-band streaming. Serum CK is usually normal or mildly elevated. EMG usually has normal or myopathic findings.

CCD is a genetically heterogeneous disease. The main gene associated with this disorder is the ryanodine receptor (*RYR1*) gene at chromosome 19q13.1, which is also linked to malignant hyperthermia (MH). Both MH and CCD are allelic disorders. The *RYR1* gene is one of the largest genes in humans, spanning over 159 kb and consisting of 106 exons. The mutations of *RYR1* are responsible for 47–67% of patients with CCD and *RYR1* gene mutations were found in 90% of Japanese CCD patients. Although seemingly higher in Japanese, there is no significant difference in hotspots in Asians or Europeans. *RYR1* mutations are found in three relatively restricted regions (*N*-terminal, central and *C*-terminal), with an emphasis on the *C*-terminal region (exon 90–103) in CCD.

Multicore (multi-minicore) disease

Multicore disease (MmD) is a slowly developing congenital myopathy characterized by the presence of multiple short-length core lesions (minicores) in both type 1 and 2 muscle fibers. Minicores consist of localized areas of sarcomere disorganization lacking oxidative activity. EM is essential to confirm the presence of a core, which shows disruption of the sarcomeric network. MmD is often inherited sporadically or as an autosomal recessive. On phenotype, MmD was classified into four clinical types. The classic phenotype is the most common and is characterized by weakness of axial and respiratory muscles with spinal rigidity, severe scoliosis, mild cardiac involvement, and facial dysmorphism. These features are similar to those found in congenital muscular dystrophy with early rigid spine syndrome. Both are caused by recessive mutations in the gene for selenoprotein N1 (*SEPN1*). The second phenotype features generalized muscle weakness with external ophthalmoplegia. An *RYR1* gene mutation has been identified. The third clinical phenotype is characterized by hip-girdle weakness and arthrogryposis, showing a clinical pattern observed in CCD patients with an *RYR1* gene mutation. The fourth phenotype shows marked distal weakness and wasting predominantly affecting the upper limbs.

Nemaline (rod) myopathy

Nemaline myopathy (NM) is a rare, clinically and genetically heterogeneous congenital myopathy characterized by the presence of rod-like structures called nemaline (thread-like) bodies in the muscle fibers (Greek *nema* = thread) and was first described in 1963. To date, six different mutations have been identified including alpha-actin gene (*ACTA1*), nebulin gene (*NEB*), tropomyosin 2 gene (*TPM2*), tropomyosin 3 gene (*TPM3*), troponin T gene (*TNNT1*), and Cofilin-2 gene (*CFL2*) (Table 120.1). NM is the most common form of non-dystrophic congenital myopathy. The clinical spectrum ranges from severe cases with antenatal or neonatal onset and early death to adult-onset cases with slow progression. Muscle weakness mostly affects the neck flexor and proximal limb muscles. Extraocular muscles are usually spared. Diagnostic criteria and a clinical classification, based on data from more than 170 patients from various parts of the world, have been proposed by the European Neuromuscular Center (ENMC) workshop on nemaline myopathy. NM has been divided into the following forms: (1) severe congenital form; (2) intermediate congenital form; (3) typical form; (4) mild, childhood-, or juvenile-onset form; (5) adult-onset form; and (6) other forms. The most common form of NM is characterized by onset in early infancy or childhood with hypotonia, generalized muscle weakness,

Table 120.1 The congenital myopathies with known gene defects.

	Gene	Gene locus	Inheritance	Protein
Central core disease	*RYR1*	19q13.1	AD/AR	Ryanodine receptor
Multi-minicore disease	*SEPN1*	1p36	AR	Selenoprotein N1
	RYR1	19q13.1	AR	Ryanodine receptor
Nemaline myopathy	*ACTA1*	1q42.1	AD/AR	Skeletal α-actin
	NEB	2q22	AR	Nebulin
	TPM3	1q22-q23	AD/AR	α-Tropomyosin
	TPM2	9p13.2-p13.1	AD/AR	β-Tropomyosin
	TNNT1	19q13.4	AR	Slow troponin T
	CFL2	14q12	AD	Cofilin-2
Centronuclear myopathy	*DNM2*	19p13.2	AD	Dynamin 2
Myotubular myopathy	*MTM1*	xq28	XR	Myotubularin
Hyaline body myopathy	*MYH7*	14q12	AD/AR	Slow myosin heavy chain
Sarcotubular myopathy	*TRIM32*	9q31-q34.1	AR	TRIM32
Fiber-type disproportion	*ACTA1*	1q42.1	AD	Skeletal α-actin
Cap disease	*TPM2*	9p13.2-p13.1	AD	β-Tropomyosin

AD: autosomal dominance; AR: autosomal recessive.

facial involvement with elongated and expressionless face, tent-shaped mouth, and high-arched palate. Feeding difficulties, severe respiratory impairment, and skeletal involvement (including scoliosis, spinal rigidity, and joint deformities) are frequently seen. The mode of inheritance can be autosomal dominant or recessive, but many sporadic cases have been reported. Among the five different genes identified, *ACTA1* mutations are responsible for about 20% of NM cases, and were found preferentially in severe cases. Over 60 different missense mutations have been identified in the *ACTA1* gene. Up to 50% of cases with NM are due to *NEB* mutations. Mutations in *TPM2*, *TPM3*, and *TNNT1* are less common, accounting for up to 5–10% of cases. The characteristic pathological feature of NM is a rod-like structure, variable in size, number, and location, seen on light microscopy with Gomori trichrome staining (Plate 120.1). The rods are often clustered at the periphery of fibers and near nuclei, and even in the nuclei. The rods are found predominantly in type 1 fibers. Type 1 fiber atrophy and/or predominance are common. With electron microscopy, rods are visible as the electron-dense structures originating from the Z-discs of sarcomeres.

Centronuclear myopathies

Centronuclear or myotubular myopathy is also a clinically and genetically heterogeneous group of disorders characterized by centrally placed nuclei in the muscle fiber, a type 1 fiber predominance, and type 1 fiber hypotrophy. Originally termed "myotubular myopathy," centronuclear myopathy (CNM) is now recognized as a distinct clinical entity. Based on the clinical features, CNM is classified into three forms: the severe neonatal form, the childhood-onset form, and the adult-onset form. The first clinical phenotype is a severe, clinically uniform,

neonatal form with severe hypotonia, muscular weakness, respiratory failure at birth, and early mortality. The muscle fibers are similar to fetal myotubes. There is also a recessive X-linked myotubular myopathy whose defect was identified at Xq28 and is caused by the mutation of the myotubularin (*MTM1*) gene. The second phenotype, the childhood-onset form, is characterized by a slowly progressive diffuse muscular weakness. Histologically the muscle fibers with central nuclei are different from the embryonic myotubes. The third, adult-onset, form manifests fully in the third decade of life, although the incipient clinical signs and symptoms may occur during the first or second decades. Histologically it is identical to the childhood-onset form. In contrast to the severe neonatal form, the inheritance of the latter two forms is not well defined, with most cases being sporadic. Nevertheless, an autosomal dominant inheritance may occur in the adult-onset form. The childhood- and adult-onset forms are currently referred to as CNM. The pathogenesis of CNM is unclear, but mutations of the dynamin 2 (*DNM2*, 19p13.2) gene were shown to cause autosomal dominant CNM.

Pathologically CNM has an increased number of centrally nucleated muscle fibers, variation in muscle fiber diameter, a type I fiber predominance or atrophy, and a central area of the muscle cell negative for adenosine triphosphatase (Plate 120.1).

Congenital fiber-type disproportion

Congenital myopathy with fiber-type disproportion (CFTD) is a form of CM characterized by a nonprogressive childhood neuromuscular disorder that has a relatively good prognosis and type 1 fiber predominance with smallness of the same type. Clinically, patients show hypotonia and delayed motor milestones, often associated with congenital dislocation of the hip, high arched palate, kyphoscoliosis, and contractures of the elbow and knee, associated with hyperinsulinemia and peripheral insulin resistance. CNS abnormalities have been described in some cases of CFTD. EMG changes have been different in reported cases of CFTD. In some, it has been normal, and in others neurogenic or myopathic, but not conclusively diagnostic. The serum CK level is normal or mildly elevated. Rarely, there is an associated cardiomyopathy. The weak muscles include those of the legs, arms, trunk, neck, or face, but pharyngeal and ocular groups are spared. Despite normal sensation, deep tendon reflexes are usually diminished or absent.

Other uncommon forms of congenital myopathy

Many uncommon forms of CM with specific structural changes have been reported. Morphological abnormalities have given their name to these disorders, such as reducing body myopathy, cylindrical spirals myopathy, fingerprint body myopathy, tubular aggregate myopathy, hyaline body myopathy, zebra body myopathy, sarcotubular myopathy, cap disease, trilaminar myopathy, and lamellar body myopathy. The clinical features of these disorders are variable and they do not have specific clinical characteristics. Some but not all are caused by genetic mutations.

Treatment and management

There is no specific treatment for any of the CM. Therapeutic interventions comprise symptomatic physical therapy, orthopedic treatment of associated skeletal abnormalities, and ventilatory support for those with respiratory muscle weakness. The monitoring of developmental state, progression of deficits, and complications is important for early therapeutic management and improvement of quality of life. Genetic counseling and prenatal diagnosis is paramount.

Further reading

Bitounm M, Maugenre S, Jeannet PY, *et al.* Mutations in dynamin 2 cause dominant centronuclear myopathy. *Nature Genet* 2005; 37: 1207–9.

Bruno C, Minetti C. Congenital myopathies. *Curr Neurol Neurosci Rep* 2004; 4: 68–73.

Ferreiro A, Quijano-Roy S, Pichereau C, *et al.* Mutations of the selenoprotein N gene, which is implicated in rigid spine muscular dystrophy, cause the classical phenotype of multiminicore disease: reassessing the nosology of early-onset myopathies. *Am J Hum Genet* 2002; 71: 739–49.

Goebel HH, Warlo IA. Surplus protein myopathies. *Neuromuscul Disord* 2001; 11: 3–6.

Jeannet PY, Bassez G, Eymard B, *et al.* Clinical and histologic findings in autosomal centronuclear myopathy. *Neurology* 2004; 62: 1484–90.

Na SJ, Kim WK, Kim TS, Kang SW, Lee EY, Choi YC. Comparison of clinical characteristics between congenital fiber type disproportion myopathy and congenital myopathy with type 1 fiber predominance. *Yonsei Med J* 2006; 47: 513–18.

Robinson R, Carpenter D, Show MA, Halsall J, Hopkins P. Mutations in RYR1 in malignant hyperthermia and central core disease. *Hum Mutat* 2006; 27: 977–89.

Wallgren-Pettersson C, Laing NG. 138th ENMC Workshop: Nemaline Myopathy, 20–22 May 2005, Naarden, The Netherlands. *Neuromuscul Disord* 2006; 16: 54–60.

Wallgren-Pettersson C, Pelin K, Nowak KJ, *et al.* Genotype–phenotype correlations in nemaline myopathy caused by mutations in the genes for nebulin and skeletal muscle α-actin. *Neuromuscul Disord* 2004; 14: 461–70.

Wu S, Ibarra MC, Malicdan MC, *et al.* Central core disease is due to RYRI mutations in more than 90% of patients. *Brain* 2006; 129: 1470–80.

Chapter 121
Muscle cramps

Raymond L. Rosales[1,2]
[1]University of Santo Tomas, Manila, Philippines
[2]Saint Luke's Medical Center, Quezon City, Philippines

Phenomenology

Muscle cramps are nearly a universal occurrence, yet are mistaken for a number of phenomena. *Muscle contraction* is a complex process by which an electrical current, carried by the muscle membrane along the T-tubules, evokes Ca^{2+} release and subsequent contractile protein interaction and fiber shortening. *Muscle twitching* takes the form of either fasciculations or myokymia. *Fasciculations* are spontaneous muscle twitches resulting from single motor nerve discharges. *Myokymia* is defined clinically as a continuous rippling or undulating of the muscle surface associated with spontaneous repetitive discharges. Both fasciculations and myokymia persist during sleep.

A generic term, *muscle spasm*, refers to any involuntary abnormal muscle contraction, regardless of whether it is painful or not, that cannot be terminated by voluntary relaxation (e.g., hemifacial spasm). *Muscle stiffness* is an involuntary muscle shortening that usually lasts for seconds to minutes, but may be sustained. Sustained muscle contraction may lead to posturing and even pain as seen in tetany, dystonia, spasticity, and contracture. Whereas *tetany* is brisk, short-lived, and associated with paresthesiae, *dystonia* is a slow, directional, more sustained co-contraction of the agonist and antagonist muscles, that may characteristically be task-specific and abolished by "sensory tricks." *Spasticity* in upper motor neuron syndrome is velocity-dependent sustained muscle contraction, resisting muscle stretch and lengthening. *Muscle contracture* or physiological rigor results from repeated muscle contraction associated with limitation of joint movement.

Myotonia is in fact a delayed muscular relaxation, lasting no longer than minutes, that does not occur spontaneously at rest like muscle cramping, but is provoked by activity, percussion, or electrical or mechanical stimulation of muscle. *Pseudomyotonia* differs clinically from myotonia because delayed muscular relaxation increases instead of decreases with repetitive activity and percussion

myotonia is absent. Pseudomyotonia combined with prolonged muscle spasms, fasciculations, and myokymia is termed *neuromyotonia*.

Myalgia refers to muscle pain that if fairly persistent may be described as a deep aching or a feeling of tenseness, pressure, or soreness and may be associated with *tenderness* on palpation. Myalgia can be secondary to ischemia, inflammation, exogenous toxins, and trauma and must be distinguished from joint pain and bone pain. The perceived change in the quality of myalgia, from "soreness" to "tension" to "cramp," reflecting increasing pain severity, simply relates to the intensity of nociceptive stimulation (i.e., types III and IV sensory afferents from the epimysium, perimysium, endomysium, and aponeuroses). *Ordinary cramp* is the sudden onset of palpable muscle contraction, of gradual resolution, relieved by stretching and having residual soreness. Repetitive motor unit firing at high rates (up to 150 Hz) is found electrophysiologically in cramps; the number of motor units activated and the frequency of their discharges increase gradually with an irregular firing pattern toward the end, known as "cramp discharge" (American Association of Neuromuscular and Electrodiagnostic Medicine glossary of terms). *Pathological cramps* are secondary to disorders of the peripheral nervous system up to the spinal cord and higher centers.

The pathophysiology of muscle cramps remains unresolved. It is theorized that unmyelinated branches of the nerve terminal arborization may be susceptible to the excitatory influences of extracellular ions, muscle metabolites, and neurotransmitters, such as acetylcholine. Evidence for a peripheral mechanism was based on the finding that the main clinical phenomena of muscle cramps can occur without the apparent participation of the motor neuron cell bodies or their synaptic inputs.

Clinical approach to muscle cramps

In the history taking for muscle cramps, familial cases, though rare, should be sought (e.g., familial cramp syndrome and familial dwarfism with muscle cramps). The clinical approach to cramps is largely based on

International Neurology: A Clinical Approach. Edited by Robert P. Lisak, Daniel D. Truong, William M. Carroll, and Roongroj Bhidayasiri. © 2009 Blackwell Publishing, ISBN: 978-1-4051-5738-4.

Table 121.1 Disorders of the muscle.

Muscle cramps	Disorders
(A) With episodic muscle weakness	
• Provoked by glucose load	Hypokalemic periodic paralysis
• Provoked by cold temperature	Hyperkalemic periodic paralysis
• Tremors	Thyrotoxic periodic paralysis
(B) With delayed relaxation and percussion myotonia	
• Muscle atrophy	Myotonic dystrophies
• Muscle hypertrophy	Myotonia congenita
• Provoked by cold temperature	Paramyotonia congenita
(C) With exertional myalgia	
• Myoglobinuria	Lipid storage disease (carnitine palmitoyltransforase II deficiency)
• Myoglobinuria and contractures	Myoadenylate deaminase deficiency, glycogenoses (McArdle's disease, Pompe's disease, Taruis disease, DiMauro's disease), Lambert–Brody syndrome
• Pseudohypertrophy	Dystrophinopathy
• Dysmorphism	Mitochondrial disease
(D) With muscle inflammation	
• Focal	Muscle trauma, muscle infarction, focal myositis, sarcoidosis
• Diffuse	Dermatomyositis, polymyositis, fasciomyositis, eosinophilia-myalgia syndrome, infectious myositis
(E) With drug toxicity	Fibrates, statins, chloroquine, cimetidine, colchicine, penicillamine, beta-agonists, neuroleptics, amiodarone, zidovudine, vitamin E (excess/deficiency), ethanol

Table 121.2 Disorders of the neuromuscular junction.

Muscle cramps	Disorders
With tremors, confusion, and muscarinic effects	Organophosphate and carbamate intoxication
	Toxic envenomation
	Acetylcholinesterase inhibitor overdose

Table 121.3 Disorders of the nerve.

Muscle cramps	Disorders
(A) With radiating pain	
• along a root	Radiculopathies
• along a plexus	Plexopathies
• along a motor nerve	Motor neuropathies
(B) With distal paresthesiae	
• and hyporeflexia	Demyelinating and mixed axonal neuropathies
• and normoreflexia	"Small fiber" neuropathies
(C) With fasciculations or myokymia	
• and delayed muscle relaxation	Neuromyotonia (Isaac's syndrome)
• and normal motor examination	Cramp-fasciculation syndrome

Table 121.4 Disorders at or above the spinal cord.

Muscle cramps	Disorders
(A) With fasciculations and muscle atrophy	Motor neuron diseases, Machado–Joseph disease
(B) With continuous muscle contraction	
• Axial stiffness	Stiff person syndrome
• Tetany	Tetanus, strychnine poisoning
(C) With sudden back pain and paraparesis	Myelopathy (Caisson's disease)
(D) With sustained contraction and posturing	
• Gradual/slow/directional	Dystonia
• "Velocity-dependent"	Spasticity
(E) With rigidity, tremor and bradykinesia	Parkinson's disease with motor fluctuations

the following factors: (1) specific muscle/muscle compartments affected; (2) focal or diffuse muscle weakness; (3) presence of limb posturing; (4) provoking conditions; (5) relationship to movement, stretching, and maneuvers; and (6) presence of spontaneous motor and sensory manifestations. Tables 121.1–5 illustrate an approach to muscle cramps based on generator sites. Tetanus, for instance, may start as localized cramps and paresthesiae at the injury site may generalize and may be provoked by sensory stimuli or maneuvers. Sustained facial grimacing ("risus sardonicus") is a classic presentation (Figure 121.1).

Diagnostic approach to muscle cramps

Not to understate the value of an astute physical and neurological examination, the initial work-up of patients with muscle cramps should include electrolyte and

Table 121.5 Miscellaneous conditions with muscle cramps.

Muscle cramps	Disorders
(A) With pain ameliorated by stretching	"Ordinary Cramps"
(B) With exertion ameliorated by rest	Claudication (vascular insufficiency)
(C) With occurrence at night	Nocturnal leg cramps, restless leg syndrome
(D) With volume and electrolyte disturbances	Heat exposure, pregnancy, uremia/dialysis, cirrhosis, malabsorption, hyponatremia, hypocalcemia, hypomagnesemia
(E) With endocrine disturbances	Cushing's syndrome, adrenal insufficiency, hypothyroidism, hypoparathyroidism
(F) With "rippling muscles"	Rippling muscle disease
(G) With malabsorption, alopecia, and skeletal abnormalities	Satoyoshi's disease
(H) With trigger points and taut bands	Myofascial pain syndrome
(I) With multifocal involvement and provoked by emotional stress	Fibromyalgia

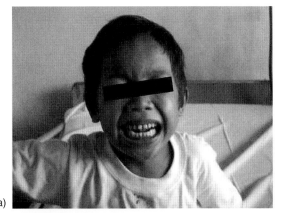

(a)

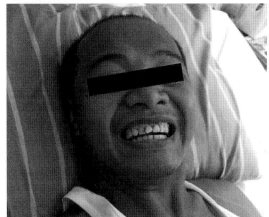

(b)

Figure 121.1 (a) Tetanus in a 5-year-old Filipino boy with "risus sardonicus" due to cramps of the masseter muscles. (b) Tetanus in a 32-year-old Filipino with "risus sardonicus" and cramps of the neck muscles.

metabolic screening and a creatine kinase determination to screen for myopathies. This is followed by electrodiagnosis. Routine nerve conduction velocity studies (NCV) and electromyography (EMG) will sort out the various neuropathies (from root to plexus to peripheral nerve) and motor neuron disease. Aside from being helpful in detecting myopathies, there are certain EMG signatures for myotonia, myokymia, fasciculations, tetanus, and continuous muscle fiber activation. Electrophysiologic cold and prolonged exercise tests are useful in sorting out periodic paralysis, even in the interictal states. The ischemic forearm exercise test is helpful in approaching metabolic myopathies. Muscle biopsy with immunohistochemistry may be the final option for the investigation of various myopathies. Neuroimaging and antibody testing will add credence to the diagnosis.

Therapeutic approach to muscle cramps

Therapeutic approaches are usually geared toward an established diagnosis or origin of the muscle cramp, and toward symptomatology of muscle cramps and spasms. Withdrawal of offending agents, replacement therapy, and immunotherapy are cornerstone treatments. However, symptomatic therapies may be necessary, while the diagnosis is either being sought or not known, and as a complement to therapy based on etiology. Analgesics, muscle relaxants, including benzodiazepines, and physical modalities for symptoms are useful. Quinine sulfate and membrane stabilizers have been beneficial, barring potential adverse events. Botulinum toxin injection and muscle afferent block are therapeutically safe, and effective especially where goals are set prior to treatment.

Acknowledgments

Drs Cabanban and Villarama of the San Lazaro National Infectious and Communicable Disease Hospital in Manila kindly assisted in taking the photos of the tetanus patients, following informed consent. Drs Kimiyoshi Arimura, Arlene Ng, Mildred De Los Santos, and May Christine Malicdan helped in the critical reading of the contents of this chapter.

Further reading

Arimura K, Arimura Y, Ng A, Sakoda S, Higuchi I. Muscle membrane excitability after exercise in thyrotoxic periodic paralysis and thyrotoxicosis without periodic paralysis. *Muscle Nerve* 2007; 36: 784–8.

Arimura Y, Arimura K, Suwazono S, *et al*. Predictive value of the prolonged exercise test in hypokalemic paralytic attack. *Muscle Nerve* 1995; 18: 472–4.

Layzer RB. The origin of muscle fasciculations and cramps. *Muscle Nerve* 1994; 17: 1243–9.

Miller TM, Layzer RB. Muscle cramps. *Muscle Nerve* 2005; 32: 431-42.

Rosales RL, Chua-Yap. Evidence-based systematic review on the efficacy and safety of botulinum toxin therapy in post-stroke spasticity. *Journal of Neural Transmission* 2008; 115: 617-23.

Chapter 122
Dermatomyositis

Marinos C. Dalakas[1,2]
[1]Imperial College, London, UK
[2]Thomas Jefferson University, Philadelphia, USA

Introduction

Dermatomyositis (DM) is one of the three main inflammatory myopathies, the other two being polymyositis (PM) and inclusion-body myositis (IBM). DM is a disease that affects skin and muscle. As a result, it is cared for not only by neurologists but also by rheumatologists and dermatologists. The role of the neurologist is essential to exclude other myopathies and initiate or supervise the immunotherapeutic interventions. The exact incidence of dermatomyositis is unknown. Along with the other two forms of inflammatory myopathy, they occur in approximately 1 in 100 000 adults.

Clinical manifestations

DM occurs in both children and adults. It is a distinct clinical entity because of a characteristic rash that accompanies or, more often, precedes muscle weakness. The skin manifestations include a heliotrope rash (blue–purple discoloration) on the upper eyelids with edema, a flat red rash on the face and upper trunk, and erythema of the knuckles with a raised violaceous scaly eruption (Gottron rash). The erythematous rash can also occur on other body surfaces, including the knees, elbows, malleoli, neck, and anterior chest (often in a V shape), or back and shoulders (shawl shape), and may be exacerbated after sun exposure. The initial erythematous lesions may result in scaling desquamation accompanied by pigmentation and depigmentation, giving at times a shiny appearance. Dilated capillary loops at the base of the fingernails are also characteristic of DM. The cuticles may be irregular, thickened, and distorted, and the lateral and palmar areas of the fingers may become rough and cracked, with irregular, "dirty" horizontal lines, resembling "mechanic's hands." DM in children resembles the adult disease. An early abnormality in children is "misery," defined as an irritable child that feels uncomfortable, has a red flush on the face, is fatigued, does not feel like socializing, and has a varying degree of muscle weakness. A tiptoe gait due to plantar flexion contracture of the ankles is not unusual. In DM the affected muscles are predominantly proximal, but the degree of weakness varies. It can be mild, moderate, or severe, leading to quadriparesis. Patients complain of difficulty getting up from a chair, climbing steps, lifting objects, or combing hair. Fine-motor movements that depend on the strength of distal muscles, such as buttoning a shirt, sewing, knitting, or writing, are affected only late in the disease. In advanced cases, atrophy of the affected muscles takes place. Ocular and facial muscles remain normal even in advanced cases, and if these muscles are affected, the diagnosis of inflammatory myopathy should questioned. The pharyngeal and neck-extensor muscles can be involved, causing dysphagia and difficulty holding the head erect. The tendon reflexes are preserved, but may be absent in severely weakened or atrophied muscles. The respiratory muscles are rarely affected, but respiratory symptoms may not be uncommon due to interstitial lung disease. Myalgia and muscle tenderness may occur early in the disease, especially when DM occurs in the setting of a connective tissue disorder. In patients with DM who have severe muscle pain, involvement of the fascia should be suspected.

Some patients with the classic skin lesions may have clinically normal strength, even up to 3–5 years after onset. This form of DM, referred to as "dermatomyositis sine myositis" or "amyopathic dermatomyositis," has a better overall prognosis. Although in these cases the disease appears limited to the skin, the muscle biopsy shows significant perivascular and perimysial inflammation with immunopathological features identical to those seen in classic DM, suggesting that the "amyopathic" and "myopathic" forms are part of the range of DM affecting skin and muscle to a varying degree.

DM usually occurs alone, but it may overlap with scleroderma and mixed connective tissue disease. Fasciitis and skin changes similar to those found in DM have occurred in patients with the eosinophilia–myalgia syndrome caused by the ingestion of contaminated L-tryptophan, and in patients with eosinophilic fasciitis

International Neurology: A Clinical Approach. Edited by Robert P. Lisak, Daniel D. Truong, William M. Carroll, and Roongroj Bhidayasiri. © 2009 Blackwell Publishing, ISBN: 978-1-4051-5738-4.

or macrophagic myofasciitis. In up to 15% of patients, the DM has a paraneoplastic association. Ovarian cancer is most frequent, followed by intestinal, breast, lung, and liver cancer. In Asian populations, nasopharyngeal cancer is more common. The cancer sites usually correspond to those occurring more frequently at the patient's age. Because tumors are often only discovered at autopsy or on the basis of abnormal findings on medical history and physical examination, blind radiologic searches are rarely fruitful. A complete annual physical examination with breast, pelvic, and rectal examinations (including colonoscopy in high-risk patients), urinalysis, complete blood-cell count, blood chemistry tests, and chest X-ray is usually sufficient and is highly recommended especially during the first 3 years following diagnosis of DM.

In addition to involvement of the muscles and skin, extramuscular manifestations may be prominent in some patients with DM. These include (1) dysphagia, sometimes as prominent as seen in patients with scleroderma; (2) atrioventricular conduction defects, tachyarrhythmia, low ejection fraction, and dilated cardiomyopathy (due to either the disease itself or, more often, hypertension or fluid retention associated with long-term steroid use); (3) pulmonary involvement, resulting from either primary weakness of the thoracic muscles or interstitial lung disease, especially in patients who have anti-Jo-1 antibodies, as discussed later; (4) subcutaneous calcifications, sometimes opening onto the skin and causing ulcerations and infections, especially in children; (5) gastrointestinal ulcerations, due to vasculitis or infections; (6) contractures of the joints, especially in the childhood form; and (7) general systemic disturbances, such as fever, malaise, weight loss, arthralgia, and Raynaud's phenomenon, especially when DM is associated with a connective tissue disorder.

Imunopathogenesis

In DM there is evidence of a humorally mediated process based on immunopathologic studies performed on muscle biopsy. The primary antigenic targets appear to be components of the endothelium of the blood vessels in the endomysium and probably the skin. Alterations in the endothelial cells consisting of pale and swollen cytoplasm with microvacuoles and tubuloreticular aggregates appear early in the disease. The capillaries undergo active focal destruction with undulating tubules in the smooth endoplasmic reticulum of the endothelial cells, leading to vascular necrosis and thrombi. These changes are caused by immune complexes immunolocalized in the endomysial blood vessels along with the C5b-9 membrane attack complex, the lytic component of the complement pathway. The membrane attack complex and the early complement components C3b and C4b are deposited on the capillaries early in the disease and precede the signs of

inflammation or structural changes in the muscle fibers. These complement fragments are also detected in the serum and correlate with disease activity. It is believed that the disease begins when putative antibodies or other factors activate complement C3, C3b, and C4b fragments that lead to formation of the membrane attack complex, which is deposited in the endomysial microvasculature and leads to osmotic lysis of the endothelial cells and capillary necrosis. As a result, there is reduction in the number of capillaries per muscle fiber, impaired perfusion and dilatation of the loop of the remaining capillaries in an effort to compensate for the ischemic process. Larger intramuscular blood vessels are also affected similarly, leading to muscle fiber destruction (often resembling microinfarcts) and inflammation. The perifascicular atrophy often seen in more chronic stages is probably a reflection of the endofascicular hypoperfusion that is prominent distally (Plate 122.1).

The activation of complement induces the release of cytokines and chemokines such as IL-1, IL-6, TNF-α, TNF-β, CXCL4, and CXCL9 which, in turn, upregulate the expression of VCAM-1 and ICAM-1 on the endothelial cells and facilitate the transmigration of activated T cells to the perimysial and endomysial spaces. Immunophenotyping of the lymphocytic infiltrates demonstrates B cells, CD4+ cells, and plasmacytoid dendritic cells in the perimysial and perivascular regions, supporting the view that a humorally mediated mechanism plays the major role in the disease. In the perifascicular regions there is also upregulation of cathepsins and STAT-1, probably triggered by interferon-gamma. Based on gene arrays, a number of adhesion molecules, cytokine, and chemokine genes are upregulated in the muscles of DM patients. Most notable among those genes are the KAL-1 adhesion molecule and genes induced by α/β interferon. The KAL-1 is upregulated by TGF-β and may have a deleterious role in DM by inducing fibrosis. Interestingly, KAL-1 along with TGF-β are downregulated in the muscles of DM patients, who improve after therapy. One of the proteins induced by α/β interferon is the Myxovirus Resistance MxA protein, which is predominantly found in the perifascicular regions. The cellular source of the abundant interferon α/β in DM is probably the large number of plasmacytoid dendritic cells, suggesting that in DM the innate immune response is also involved in a pattern similar to systemic lupus erythematosus. A summary of the immunopathology of DM is shown in Figure 122.1.

The immunopathology of the skin lesions in DM is not fully studied but perivascular infiltrates consisting mainly of CD4+ cells and macrophages along with C5b-9 complement deposits are also noted in the dermis. The basal keratinocytes express CD40 while the neighboring CD4+ T cells express CD40L, suggesting that the CD40–CD40-L system may be involved in the cutaneous manifestations probably via the upregulation of cytokines and

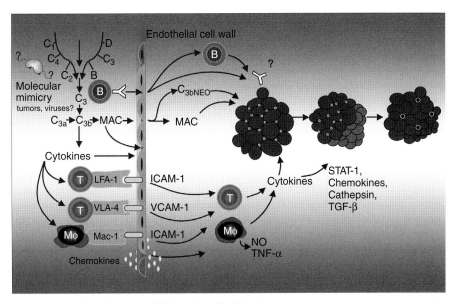

Figure 122.1 The main immunopathologic features of DM, as described in the text.

chemokines, in a pattern similar to the one described for the muscle.

Autoantibodies against nuclear (antinuclear antibodies) and cytoplasmic antigens (ribonucleoproteins involved in translation and protein synthesis) are also found in up to 20% of DM patients. The antibody directed against the histidyl-transfer RNA synthetase, called anti-Jo-1, accounts for 75% of all the antisynthetases and is clinically useful because up to 80% of DM patients with anti-Jo-1 antibodies develop interstitial lung disease. These antibodies are not, however, specific because they also occur in patients with PM and IBM as well as in patients who only have interstitial lung disease without myositis. Patients with the overlap syndrome of DM and systemic sclerosis may have autoantibodies of unclear significance, including the anti-polymyositis/Scl, directed against a nucleolar protein complex, anti-Ku, anti-U2RNP, and others.

Diagnosis

The diagnosis of DM is relatively easy because of the characteristic skin changes that appear unique for DM. The diagnosis is, however, aided by determining the level of serum muscle enzymes and the muscle biopsy.

In the presence of active disease, creatine kinase (CK) can be elevated up to 40 times the normal level. Although CK activity usually parallels disease severity, it can be normal in some patients with untreated disease or when DM is associated with a connective tissue disorder, probably reflecting the predominant involvement of the intramuscular vessels and the perimysium. Along with CK, serum glutamic-oxaloacetic

transaminase, serum glutamic-pyruvic transaminase, lactate dehydrogenase, and aldolase may also be elevated. Needle electromyography (EMG) shows myopathic potentials characterized by short-duration, low-amplitude, polyphasic units on voluntary activation and increased spontaneous activity with fibrillations, complex repetitive discharges, and positive sharp waves. Muscle biopsy is the definitive test to exclude other neuromuscular diseases especially when the skin changes are not clear, and to assess the severity of involvement. The following unique histological features at the light microscopy level are characteristic of DM: (1) endomysial inflammation, predominantly in the perivascular or the interfascicular septa and around rather than within the fascicles; (2) fibrin thrombi (especially in children) and obliteration of capillaries; (3) necrosis, degeneration, and phagocytosis often affecting groups of fibers within a muscle fascicle in a wedgelike shape or at the periphery of the fascicle due to microinfarcts within the muscle; and (4) perifascicular atrophy which is diagnostic of dermatomyositis, even in the absence of inflammation. The skin biopsy also shows the abnormalities mentioned earlier, but routine skin biopsy samples are not helpful.

Although the diagnosis of DM is very rarely in doubt, sometimes muscle strength is normal (dermatomyositis sine myositis), in spite of clear evidence of subclinical muscle involvement in the muscle biopsy. Other times, the rash may be barely detectable (especially in dark-skinned people), and the diagnosis can be made only in retrospect on the basis of subcutaneous calcifications found accidentally or on muscle biopsy when one detects the perifascicular atrophy.

Treatment

The disease is treated with immunosuppressive or immunomodulating agents. Most of the treatment trials have been empirical and non-selective because the specific target antigens are unknown.

The goal of therapy in DM is to improve function in the activities of daily living as the result of improvement in muscle strength, and to improve the skin alterations. Although improvement in strength is usually accompanied by a fall in serum CK, a decrease of serum CK alone without a concomitant improvement in strength has to be interpreted with caution in reference to the efficacy of the given drug. For patients with disease limited to the skin, the use of low-dose steroids or hydroxychloroquine sulfate and avoidance of immunosuppressants until weakness develops is preferred.

Prednisolone is the first-line drug. Because the response to prednisolone, an effective drug for short-term use, determines whether or not stronger immunosuppressive drugs will be needed, an aggressive approach with high-dose prednisolone beginning early in the disease is used by this author, beginning at 80–100 mg/day as a single daily morning dose for 3–4 weeks. Prednisolone is then slowly tapered to an every-other-day dose until the lowest possible dose that controls the disease is reached. Aggressive disease should receive methylprednisolone 1 g intravenously (IV) every day for 3 days first, followed by oral steroid.

Drugs used for "steroid-sparing," when a relapse occurs after attempts to lower the high steroid dosage, include: (1) *azathioprine*, up to 3 mg/kg; (2) *methotrexate*, up to a total of 25 mg weekly; (3) *mycophenolate mofetil*, up to 3000 mg daily; and (4) *cyclophosphamide*, given IV at doses of 0.5–1.0 g/m^2.

If the response to prednisone is limited, *intravenous immunoglobulin (IVIg)* at 2 g/kg has been shown to be effective in DM in a controlled trial. In this double-blind study, IVIg was shown to be effective in patients with refractory DM, not only by improving the strength and the skin rash but also by clearing the underlying immunopathology. The improvement begins after the first infusion and is clearly evident by the second monthly infusion. The benefit, however, is short-lived (not more than 8 weeks), requiring repeated infusions every 6–8 weeks to maintain improvement. In DM, IVIg acts by inhibiting the deposition of activated complement fragments in capillaries and by suppressing cytokines and adhesion molecules at the protein, mRNA, and gene level. If IVIg is not effective, Rituximab, a monoclonal antibody against B cells, appears promising and is being tested in a controlled trial. Plasmapheresis is not effective.

Therefore a recommended approach to the treatment of DM is as follows:

Step 1: High-dose prednisone (oral or intermittent IV in acute cases).

Step 2: Add immunosuppressants, such as azathioprine, methotrexate, or mycophenolate, for steroid sparing effect.

Step 3: If Step 1 fails, try IVIg at 2 g/kg.

Step 4: If the above fail, consider a trial with Rituximab.

Treatment for calcinosis remains difficult; attempts with alendronate, probenecid, or diltiazem are thought to be promising but offer limited benefit.

Prognosis and complications

The natural history of DM is unknown, as most patients nowadays are treated with steroids. The mortality rates reported 20–30 years ago are outdated. Clinical experience indicates that DM responds to therapy more readily than PM. In children, DM may at times be a monophasic disease with infrequent flares once the disease is under control. Patients with interstitial lung disease may have a high mortality rate, requiring aggressive treatment with cyclophosphamide or Tacrolimus. However, there are still a number of patients who do not respond adequately to therapy and remain disabled, especially when subcutaneous calcification has formed because it cannot be dissolved and appears resistant to all treatment. Ulceration, infection, and disfiguring scars result when they protrude through the skin.

Further reading

Dalakas MC. Polymyositis, dermatomyositis, and inclusion-body myositis. *N Engl J Med* 1991; 325: 1487–98.

Dalakas MC. Therapeutic targets in patients with inflammatory myopathies: present approaches and a look to the future. *Neuromuscul Disord* 2006; 16: 223–36.

Dalakas MC, Hohlfeld R. Polymyositis and dermatomyositis. *Lancet* 2003; 362: 1762–3.

Dalakas MC, Illa I, Dambrosia JM, et al. A controlled trial of high-dose intravenous immunoglobulin infusions as treatment for dermatomyositis. *N Engl J Med* 1993; 329: 1993–2000.

Engel AG, Hohlfeld R. The polmyositis and dermatomyositis syndrome. In: Engel AG, Franzini-Armstrong C, editors. *Myology*. New York: McGraw-Hill; 2005, pp. 1335–83.

Greenberg SA. Proposed immunologic models of the inflammatory myopathies and potential therapeutic implications. *Neurology* 2007; 69(21): 2008–19.

Mastaglia FL, Garlepp MJ, Phillips BA, Zilko PJ. Inflammatory myopathies: clinical, diagnostic and therapeutic aspects. *Muscle Nerve* 2003; 27: 407–25.

Chapter 123
Polymyositis

Marinos C. Dalakas[1,2]
[1]Imperial College, London, UK
[2]Thomas Jefferson University, Philadelphia, USA

Introduction

Polymyositis (PM) is one of the three main subsets of inflammatory myopathies, the other ones being dermatomyositis (DM) and inclusion body myositis (IBM). As a stand-alone entity, PM is not a common disease and some even doubt its existence. The exact frequency is unknown, but all three forms occur in approximately 1 in 100 000 adults. PM is the least common of the three. It is often misdiagnosed and requires a careful review of the clinical features, muscle histopathology, and immunopathology to ensure that toxic, metabolic, mitochondrial, or dystrophic muscle diseases are not missed and that a common entity, that of IBM, is not overlooked.

Clinical manifestations

PM has no unique clinical features, and it is a diagnosis of exclusion. It is best defined as an inflammatory myopathy of subacute onset (weeks to months) and steady progression that occurs in adults who do not have the typical DM rash on the face, trunk, or fingers, involvement of eye and facial muscles, family history of a neuromuscular disease, endocrinopathy history of exposure to myotoxic drugs or toxins, or other myopathies such as dystrophy, metabolic myopathy, or IBM. Unlike DM, in which the rash secures early recognition, the actual onset of PM cannot be easily determined, and the disease may exist for months before the patient seeks medical advice.

Patients with PM commonly present with proximal and often symmetric muscle weakness that is rarely acute. An acute onset should raise the suspicion of a necrotizing myopathy. Patients complain of difficulty getting up from a chair, climbing steps, lifting objects, or combing hair. Fine-motor movements that depend on the strength of distal muscles, such as buttoning a shirt, sewing, knitting, or writing, are affected only late in the disease. If these muscles are affected from the outset or early in the course of the disease, IBM should be suspected. In advanced cases, atrophy of the affected muscles takes place. Ocular muscles remain normal even in advanced cases, and if these muscles are affected, the diagnosis of inflammatory myopathy should be doubted. In contrast with IBM, where the facial muscles are affected in the majority of patients, in PM the strength of the facial muscles remains normal except for rare advanced cases. The pharyngeal and neck-extensor muscles can be involved, causing dysphagia and a dropped head state. Tendon reflexes are preserved, but may be absent in severely weakened or atrophied muscles. The respiratory muscles are rarely affected, but respiratory symptoms are common due to interstitial lung disease. Myalgia and muscle tenderness may occur early in the disease, especially when PM occurs in the setting of a connective tissue disorder. In patients with PM who have severe muscle pain, involvement of the fascia should be suspected even without overt signs of skin induration and thickness.

Cardiac abnormalities due to myocarditis related directly to PM are rare. Most often, cardiac abnormalities appear to be secondary to hypertension associated with long-term treatment with steroids or due to pulmonary hypertension related to interstitial lung disease. Interstitial lung disease may occur in up to 10% of patients, half of whom have anti-Jo-1 antibodies or antibodies to various ribonucleoproteins. Associated general systemic disturbances, such as fever, malaise, weight loss, arthralgia, and Raynaud's phenomenon, suggest the presence of a connective tissue disorder.

PM is extremely rare in childhood, and if a diagnosis is made in patients younger than 16 years, a careful review is needed to exclude another disease, especially an inflammatory dystrophy.

Association conditions

PM appears to be a syndrome of diverse causes. As an isolated clinical entity, it is rather uncommon. It is more frequently seen in association with connective tissue disorders, systemic autoimmune diseases, or viral infections,

International Neurology: A Clinical Approach. Edited by Robert P. Lisak, Daniel D. Truong, William M. Carroll, and Roongroj Bhidayasiri. © 2009 Blackwell Publishing, ISBN: 978-1-4051-5738-4.

such as Sjögren's syndrome, rheumatoid arthritis, Crohn's disease, vasculitis, sarcoidosis, primary biliary cirrhosis, adult celiac disease, chronic graft-vs-host disease, discoid lupus, ankylosing spondylitis, Behçet's disease, myasthenia gravis, acne fulminans, dermatitis herpetiformis, psoriasis, Hashimoto's disease, granulomatous diseases, agammaglobulinemia, hypereosinophilic syndrome, Lyme disease, Kawasaki disease, autoimmune thrombocytopenia, hypergammaglobulinemic purpura, hereditary complement deficiency, IgA deficiency, and AIDS. Among viruses, HIV and HTLV-I are the only ones convincingly associated with PM. Claims that other viruses, such as enteroviruses, can be causally connected with PM are unproven. PM is not more frequently associated with cancer compared to other chronic autoimmune disorders treated with immunosuppressants. Cancer is, however, more frequently associated with DM.

Several animal parasites, such as protozoa (*Toxoplasma*, *Trypanosoma*), cestodes (*Cysticerci*), and nematodes (*Trichinae*), may produce a focal or diffuse inflammatory myopathy known as "parasitic polymyositis." In the tropics, a suppurative myositis known as "tropical polymyositis" or "pyomyositis" may be produced by *Staphylococcus aureus*, *Yersinia*, *Streptococcus*, or other anaerobes. Pyomyositis, previously rare in the West, has now be seen in patients with AIDS. Certain bacteria, such as *Borrelia burgdorferi* of Lyme disease and *Legionella pneumophila* of Legionnaires' disease, may infrequently be the cause of PM.

Drugs do not cause PM. The only drug that could trigger PM is *D*-penicillamine. Zidovudine and the cholesterol-lowering drugs can be myotoxic, but they cause a mitochondrial or a necrotizing myopathy that lacks the features of primary endomysial inflammation seen in PM. In these cases, muscle fibers demonstrate prominent mitochondrial or necrotic features.

Immunopathogenesis

PM may be one of the best studied or prototypic T cell-mediated disorders where cytotoxic T cells directed against previously unidentified muscle antigens form an immunological synapse with the MHC-1 class antigen expressed on the surface of muscle fibers.

The cytotoxicity of the autoinvasive T cells has been supported by the presence of perforin granules which are directed towards the surface of the muscle fiber and lead to muscle fiber necrosis upon their release. The specificity of the T cells has been further examined by studying the gene rearrangement of the T cell receptors of the autoinvasive T cells. In patients with PM, as well as IBM, only certain T cells of specific T cell receptor alpha and T cell receptor beta families are recruited to the muscle from the circulation. Cloning and sequencing of the amplified endomysial T cell receptor gene families has demonstrated a restricted use of the *J-beta* gene with conserved amino acid sequence in the CDR3 region, the antigen-binding region of the T cell antigen receptor (TCR), indicating that CD8+ cells are specifically selected and clonally expanded *in situ* by muscle-specific autoantigens. Studies combining laser microdissection, immunocytochemistry, polymerase chain reaction, and sequencing of the most prominent T cell receptor families have shown that only the auto-invasive, not the perivascular, endomysial CD8+ cells are clonally expanded. Comparison of the T cell receptor repertoire between PM and DM with spectra-typing has confirmed that perturbations of the T cell receptor families occur only in PM. Further, among the circulating T cells, clonal expansion occurs only in the cytotoxic CD8+ cells that express genes for perforin and infiltrate the MHC-1-expressing muscle fibers.

The clonally expanded CD8+ T cells form immunological synapses with the muscle fibers they invade, as supported by the co-expression of costimulatory molecules B7-1, B7-2, BB1, CD40, or ICOS-L on the muscle fibers and the respective counter-receptors CD28, CTLA-4, CD40L, or ICOS on autoinvasive T cells. Cytokines, chemokines, and metalloproteinases are all upregulated in the muscle tissue. Some of these cytokines, such as γ-interferon, ILI-1β, and TNF-α, may exert a direct cytotoxic effect on the muscle tissue. Unique to muscle is the observation that the various cytokines and chemokines can also stimulate the muscle fibers to produce endogenously proinflammatory cytokines, such as γ-interferon, which enhances and perpetuates the immune response. Recently, plasma cells and myeloid dendritic cells, which are potent antigen-presenting cells, have been seen among the endomysial infiltrates. Although the myeloid dendritic cells may be candidate cells for antigen presentation to surrounding T cells, their role remains elusive. Based on their immunoglobulin gene isotype, however, the plasma cells appear to mature and expand *in situ*, implying an antigen-driven response (Figure 123.1).

In PM, MHC-1 is expressed in all fibers, even in those not invaded by T cells, often throughout the course of the disease. Such chronic MHC-1 upregulation may be deleterious, exerting a stress effect on the endoplasmic reticulum (ER) of the myofiber, independent of T cell-mediated cytotoxicity. The assembly and folding of MHC-1 occurs in the ER and matures only when it binds to an antigenic peptide synthesized in the cytosol. A system of chaperone proteins, including calnexin, calreticulin, GRP94, GRP78, and ERP72, that form the MHC-loading complex, ensures the proper maturation of MHC for antigen processing. If the "MHC-class-1 loading complex" does not bind to suitable antigens, the heavy chain glycoprotein is misfolded and removed from the ER to the cytosol for degradation. In PM as well as IBM,

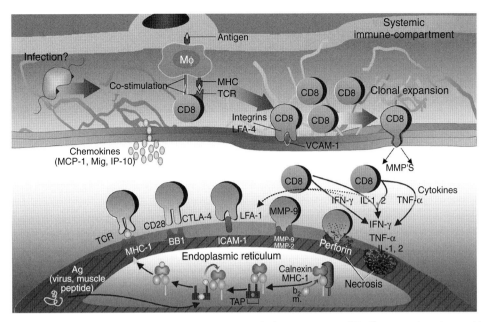

Figure 123.1 The main immunopathological features of polymyositis, including activation of T cells, transmigration, and invasion of MHC-I-expressing muscle fibers.

the muscle fibers are overloaded by MHC molecules and the antigenic peptides cannot undergo proper conformational change to bind to MHC-1 complex, leading to ER stress. This contention is supported by upregulation of the chaperone proteins and the activation of NF-kB, a means by which the cells protect themselves from ER stress. Such stressor effects are also seen in MHC-1 transgenic mice, suggesting that continuous overexpression of MHC-1 alone may be sufficient to induce ER stress and lead to persistence of the chronic inflammatory response.

Factors triggering the T cell-mediated process in PM remain unclear. Viruses may be responsible for breaking tolerance, but only the retroviruses HIV and HTLV-I have been etiologically connected with the disease in infected individuals. These viruses do not, however, directly infect the muscle fibers; instead, they are only present on some of the infiltrating macrophages. Some of the autoinvasive T cells are viral-specific, carrying viral peptides as demonstrated with tetramers, and may play a role in the disease by cross-reacting with antigens expressed on the surface of muscle fibers.

Various serum autoantibodies directed against nuclear or cytoplasmic ribonucleoproteins involved in translation or protein synthesis are detected in as many as 20% of patients with PM. Among them, the antibody directed against the histidyl-transfer RNA synthetase, called anti-Jo-1, accounts for 75% of all the antisynthetases and it is a clinically useful marker because up to 80% of these patients may develop interstitial lung disease. The pathogenic role of Jo-1 antibodies in facilitating or inducing muscle fiber injury remains unknown.

Differential diagnosis

Because PM is a diagnosis of exclusion, all diseases that cause an acquired myopathy should be considered before the diagnosis is established. The following myopathies mimic PM and need to be excluded: (1) hereditary neuromuscular diseases, especially inflammatory muscular dystrophies such as dysferlinopathies, fascioscapulohumeral dystrophy, Becker's muscular dystrophy, and calpainopathies; (2) metabolic myopathies, endocrinopathies, electrolyte disturbances, and mitochondriopathies; (3) any systemic medical illness, including malabsorption syndromes, alcoholism, cancer, vasculitis, systemic infections, sarcoidosis, granulomatous disease, and treatment with various known myotoxic drugs or combinations of unknown but potentially myotoxic drugs or toxins; (4) neurogenic muscular atrophies and neurogenic conditions; (5) biochemical muscle diseases such as McArdle's disease excluded by muscle enzyme histochemistry; (6) IBM; and (7) necrotizing myopathy, which has a rather acute onset and is characterized by infiltration of macrophages, rather than T cell infiltrates, abundant necrotic fibers, and very scattered expression of MHC-1 class antigen.

Diagnosis

In PM the serum muscle enzymes are elevated as much as 30 times higher than normal. Although creatine kinase (CK) usually parallels disease activity, it can be normal in chronic PM and only slightly elevated in PM associated with connective tissue disease, reflecting the preference of the pathologic process for the intramuscular vessels and the perimysium. Along with CK, serum glutamic-oxaloacetic transaminase, serum glutamic-pyruvic transaminase, and lactate dehydrogenase, (but not gamma-GT) may also be elevated. Needle electromyography (EMG) shows active myopathic discharges which have no unique specificity for PM. The definitive diagnosis of PM is established with muscle biopsy.

In PM, the presence of inflammation is the histological hallmark of the disease (Plate 123.1a). The endomysial infiltrates are mostly in foci within the fascicles surrounding healthy muscle fibers, leading eventually to muscle fiber necrosis. Sometimes the inflammatory infiltrates may be so localized and multifocal that they are missed in a small biopsy. Occasionally, inflammation can be better seen in longitudinal sections. As in IBM, the inflammation is primary, a term used to indicate that CD8+ cells invade histologically healthy fibers that express MHC-1 antigen. This lesion is termed the "CD8/MHC-1 complex" and it is considered to be a specific lesion for PM that secures the histological diagnosis (Plate 123.1b). Eosinophils are rare, but, if abundant, the diagnosis of eosinophilic myositis should be considered. When the disease is chronic, the connective tissue is increased. In PM, there should be no vasculitis, or vacuolated fibers with cytoplasmic inclusions, as seen in IBM. A primary intramuscular inflammatory response is an invariable feature of PM and absence of inflammation early in the illness should raise a critical concern about the diagnosis.

The following diagnostic criteria have been proposed. The diagnosis of PM is definite when a patient has: (1) an acquired, subacute myopathy fulfilling the exclusion criteria described earlier and lacking the distribution of weakness typically seen in IBM; (2) elevated CK; and (3) a muscle biopsy with the histologic features of PM, including the MHC-1/CD8 lesion. The diagnosis is probable if the muscle biopsy shows non-specific myopathic features but widespread MHC-1 expression without apparent T cell infiltrates or vacuoles. A repeat muscle biopsy from another site possibly directed by MRI may prove informative in these cases.

Therapy

Treatment remains empirical, and separate, large-scale, prospective, controlled clinical studies have not been performed.

The goal of therapy is to improve functional activities in daily living by improving muscle strength. Although improvement in strength is usually accompanied by a fall in CK, decreases of CK alone need to be interpreted with caution because most immunosuppressive therapies lower serum muscle enzyme levels without necessarily improving muscle strength. Unfortunately, this has been misinterpreted as "chemical improvement" rather than monitoring muscle strength and has led to unnecessary prolongation of immunosuppressive treatment.

Commonly used drugs are:

Steroids and non-steroidal immunosuppressive agents. Because the initial response to prednisolone determines whether or not stronger immunosuppressive drugs will be needed, an aggressive approach with high-dose prednisone early in the disease is preferred, with a single daily morning dose of 80–100 mg for an initial period of 3–4 weeks. Prednisolone is then tapered to an every-other-day program. If after 2–3 months there is no objective increase in muscle strength the patient should be considered unresponsive to prednisolone and the tapering accelerated. In such circumstances, the diagnosis should be reconsidered, because the majority of patients with PM respond to steroids to some degree and for some period of time. For those patients responding to steroids, a "steroid-sparing"-drug is needed to avoid the long-term steroid complications and prevent the relapse that can occur each time the steroid dosage is lowered. The following therapies are used as steroid-sparing agents:
- Azathioprine, up to 3 mg/kg.
- Methotrexate, starting at 7.5 mg weekly for the first 3 weeks and increasing up to a total of 25 mg weekly.
- Mycophenolate mofetil, which has the advantage of working faster than azathioprine; it is well tolerated up to 2500 mg/day.
- Tacrolimus, which has been promising in difficult cases, especially those with interstitial lung disease.

Plasmapheresis, cyclophosphamide and cyclosporine have been disappointing.

Intravenous immunoglobulin (IVIg). IVIg is effective in patients with refractory DM and in the majority of PM patients, although a controlled study in PM has not been performed. Because of its safety and efficacy IVIg is used as second-line therapy after steroid use.

New agents. These are mostly in the form of monoclonal antibodies. These biological drugs appear promising but need control trial evidence. Among them, Rituximab, a B cell-depleting monoclonal antibody, is currently in phase III controlled clinical trial.

When treatment response is suboptimal, the patient should be re-evaluated and the muscle-biopsy specimen re-examined. A second biopsy might be considered to confirm the diagnosis. Disorders commonly misdiagnosed as PM include: IBM; sporadic limb-girdle muscular dystrophy, which is suspected when the disease has a slow onset and progression and the muscle biopsy specimen does not show primary inflammatory features; metabolic myopathy (e.g., myophosphorylase deficiency); endocrinopathy; and neurogenic muscular atrophies.

Prognosis

The natural history of PM is unknown because steroids are almost universally applied early after diagnosis. Occasional cases that present as severe acute myositis, often after viral infection or in association with cancer, are not typical cases of PM; instead, they represent cases of myositis which is resistant to many therapies. In general, older age, interstitial lung disease, and frequent pneumonias due to esophageal dysfunction are factors associated with poor prognosis. There are still patients with PM who do not adequately respond to therapies and remain disabled; in these circumstances it is unclear whether the disease is bona fide PM or another disorder misdiagnosed as PM.

Further reading

Dalakas MC. Polymyositis, dermatomyositis, and inclusion-body myositis. *N Engl J Med* 1991; 325: 1487–98.

Dalakas MC. Signaling pathways and immunobiology of inflammatory myopathies. *Nature Clin Pract Rheumatol* 2006a; 2: 219–27.

Dalakas MC. Therapeutic targets in patients with inflammatory myopathies: present approaches and a look to the future. *Neuromuscul Disord* 2006b; 16: 223–36.

Dalakas MC, Hohlfeld R. Polymyositis and dermatomyositis. *Lancet* 2003; 362: 1762–3.

Engel AG, Hohlfeld R. The polmyositis and dermatomyositis syndrome. In: Engel AG, Franzini-Armostrong C, editors. *Myology*. New York: McGraw-Hill; 2004, pp. 1335–83.

Mastaglia FL, Garlepp MJ, Phillips BA, Zilko PJ. Inflammatory myopathies: clinical, diagnostic and therapeutic aspects. *Muscle Nerve* 2003; 27: 407–25.

Wiendl H, Hohlfeld R, Kieseier BC. Immunobiology of muscle: advances in understanding an immunological microenvironment. *Trends Immunol* 2005; 26: 373–80.

Chapter 124
Inclusion body myositis

Frank L. Mastaglia[1] and Merrilee Needham[2]
[1]University of Western Australia, Perth, Australia
[2]Royal North Shore Hospital, Sydney, Australia

Introduction

Sporadic inclusion body myositis (sIBM) is the most common myopathy in Caucasians over 50 years of age and occasionally also affects younger people. It is traditionally classified as an inflammatory myopathy, but also has myodegenerative features with abnormal protein aggregation and inclusion body formation. The aetiology is unknown, but probably involves a complex interplay between genetic and environmental factors and aging.

Epidemiology and genetic susceptibility

The frequency of sIBM varies in different populations, being low in Korean, Polish, Mesoamerican, African-American, Middle Eastern, and southern Mediterranean populations as compared with northern European, North American Caucasian, and Australian populations in which prevalence figures of $4.9–14.9 \times 10^{-6}$ have been reported. This contrasts with a prevalence of only approximately 1×10^{-6} in Istanbul, Turkey.

Genetic susceptibility was first linked to HLA-DR3 and the 8.1 MHC ancestral haplotype (AH) in a West Australian cohort, and has since been confirmed in the Netherlands, Germany, and North America. Other associations are with HLA-DR52 and B35-DR1, and with the 52.1AH (B*5201 and DRB1*1502) in Japanese. The importance of genetic factors is also emphasized by the rare occurrence of IBM in twins and in families with more than one affected individual. Familial IBM differs from the "hereditary inclusion body myopathies" (hIBM), a heterogeneous group of autosomal dominant or recessive disorders with variable clinical phenotypes and some pathological features resembling sIBM, including rimmed vacuoles and intranuclear and cytoplasmic filamentous inclusions, but lacking inflammatory

changes. The prototypic recessive form first described in Iranian Jews as a "quadriceps-sparing" myopathy is caused by mutations in the UDP-N-acetylglucosamine-2-epimerase/N-acetylmannosamine kinase (*GNE*) gene, and is allelic with the Japanese form of distal myopathy with rimmed vacuoles. However, *GNE* mutations have not been found in sIBM.

Pathology and pathogenesis

Pathologically sIBM is characterized by: (1) a CD8+ T-cell predominant inflammatory infiltrate, with invasion of MHC-1 expressing non-necrotic muscle fibres; (2) rimmed vacuoles, congophilic inclusions, and filamentous protein aggregates; and (3) ragged-red and cytochrome *c* oxidase (COX)-deficient fibers which harbour clonally expanded mtDNA deletions and mutations. In addition to β-amyloid and amyloid precursor protein (APP), a variety of other "Alzheimer's-type" proteins including phosphorylated tau, α-synuclein, prion protein, and apolipoprotein E are present in the inclusions.

There is continued debate as to whether the primary process is inflammatory or myodegenerative. Recent research has highlighted the importance of both processes, but how they interact remains uncertain. Upregulation of the pro-inflammatory cytokines interleukin-1 (IL-1), tumor necrosis factor (TNF-α), and interferon (IFN-γ) could be an early upstream event causing both the inflammatory and degenerative changes. By causing upregulation of MHC-1, pro-inflammatory cytokines could exert a stressor effect on the endoplasmic reticulum (ER), causing NFκB upregulation and further enhancing MHC-1 class assembly activity, and leading to a self-sustaining T-cell response. Pro-inflammatory cytokines (particularly IL-1), as well as NFκB, increase APP transcription and β-amyloid production, and could initiate a cascade of ER stress, proteasomal dysfunction, and protein accumulation. Alternatively, increased APP transcription could be an early upstream event causing ER stress, oxidative stress, and a T-cell response to peptides derived from the accumulating proteins.

International Neurology: A Clinical Approach. Edited by Robert P. Lisak, Daniel D. Truong, William M. Carroll, and Roongroj Bhidayasiri.

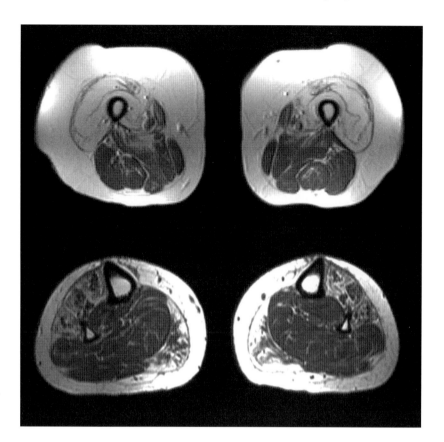

Figure 124.1 MRI scans showing preferential involvement of the quadriceps femoris (upper panel) and medial gastrocnemius and anterior tibial muscle groups (lower panel) in two patients with sIBM.

Clinical features

Sporadic IBM affects males more often than females. This diagnosis is often delayed and the condition may be misdiagnosed as motor neurone disease, polymyositis, or arthritis. The most common presentation is with insidious onset of quadriceps weakness, resulting in difficulty rising from chairs, climbing stairs, and falls, and less commonly with weakness of the fingers, foot-drop, or dysphagia. The weakness is often asymmetric, and more severe on the non-dominant side. Dysphagia occurs in over 50% of cases. Clinical examination typically reveals a selective pattern of weakness and atrophy of the quadriceps femoris and forearm muscles, with the flexor digitorum profundus and flexor pollicis longus being preferentially affected. Other muscle groups are also affected as the condition progresses. Atypical presentations include "dropped head" or camptocormia due to weakness of the neck extensors and paraspinal muscles. It is not known whether the clinical phenotype varies in different ethnic groups.

Investigations and diagnosis

The serum CK level may be normal or mildly elevated (up to 10 times normal). The condition may be associated with a monoclonal gammopathy, with various autoantibodies or another autoimmune or connective tissue disease, or with HIV-1 or HTLV-1 infections, which should be screened for in at-risk populations. Electromyography demonstrates a combination of short- and long-duration motor unit potentials with spontaneous activity which may lead to a mistaken diagnosis of a neurogenic disorder such as motor neurone disease. Some cases also have a subclinical peripheral neuropathy. MRI demonstrates selective involvement of the quadriceps femoris muscles in the thighs (Figure 124.1), medial gastrocnemius in the calves, and flexor muscles in the forearms.

Definitive diagnosis requires a muscle biopsy. The most suitable muscle is the vastus lateralis, or, if too severely atrophied, the deltoid, biceps brachii, or tibialis anterior. In addition to routine stains, stains for β-amyloid (crystal violet or Congo red viewed with Texas red filters) and immunostaining for T-cell subsets and MHC-1 expression should be performed. Electron microscopy is required to demonstrate the characteristic 16–20 nm filamentous cytoplasmic or intranuclear inclusions but is not essential for diagnosis.

Treatment and management

There is currently no therapy that stops progression of the disease (see review by Needham and Mastaglia). The protracted natural history has made the results of drug trials difficult to interpret, as few trials have been of adequate duration or sufficiently powered.

Glucocorticoids and cytotoxic agents

Uncontrolled trials of glucocorticoids reported stabilization or short-term improvement in some cases. However, in a prospective trial of high-dose prednisone, muscle strength continued to deteriorate in spite of a fall in CK level, and repeat biopsies after 6–12 months showed an increased number of fibers with vacuoles and amyloid deposits, despite a reduction in T-cells. Azathioprine, cyclosporine, cyclophosphamide, and methotrexate are usually ineffective. Mycophenolate is beneficial in rare cases.

Immunotherapy

Intravenous immunoglobulin therapy (IVIG) may provide short-term benefit in selected cases. A 3-month double-blind placebo-controlled trial showed mild improvement in lower limb strength and swallowing. In another 3-month double-blind study the addition of prednisone did not enhance the effect of IVIG. A 12-month double-blind trial, although not finding a significant improvement in strength, arrested progression of weakness in 90% of patients. Some patients with severe dysphagia have a good response to IVIG therapy.

A 12-month trial of antithymocyte globulin (ATG) with methotrexate showed a 1.4% increase in muscle strength, compared with 11.1% loss in the control group receiving methotrexate alone. A larger randomized trial of ATG, and of monoclonal antibodies targeting T-cells (e.g., alemtuzumab), may therefore be worthwhile.

Two randomized trials of interferon-β1a did not find any significant improvement. A pilot trial of the TNF-α blocker etanercept showed only a slight improvement in grip strength after 12 months of treatment.

Other therapies

Coenzyme Q_{10}, carnitine, clenbuterol, and oxandrolone may provide symptomatic benefit in some patients. In addition to IVIG, swallowing function can be restored by a bougie dilatation, cricopharyngeal myotomy, or botulinum toxin injection into the upper esophageal sphincter in patients with severe dysphagia. Strength training and aerobic conditioning can improve or stabilize muscle strength and functional performance without increasing CK levels or histological changes. However, exercise programs need to be individualized to avoid muscle overloading. Knee-locking braces may be helpful in preventing falls and ankle-foot orthoses if foot-drop is a problem. In patients with severe finger weakness it may be possible to restore opposition of the thumb and index finger by transferring the tendons of the extensor carpi radialis and brachioradialis muscles to the more severely affected flexor tendons.

Conclusions

Sporadic IBM is the most important myopathy associated with aging. The etiology is poorly understood, but there is strong evidence that genetic susceptibility factors play a role. There are considerable geographic differences in the prevalence of the disease and further surveys in different countries and ethnic groups are required to document these differences more fully and determine whether they are due to genetic or environmental influences. Whether sIBM should continue to be classified as a primary inflammatory myopathy or a myodegenerative disease is still hotly debated. Further clarification of the molecular pathogenesis may lead to the development of more effective therapies targeting the immune response and mechanisms of abnormal protein aggregation.

Further reading

Dalakas MC. Sporadic inclusion body myositis – diagnosis, pathogenesis and therapeutic strategies. *Nature Clin Practice* 2006; 2(8): 437–45.

Needham M, Mastaglia F. Pathogenesis of sporadic inclusion body myositis: trying to put the pieces of the puzzle together. *Neuromuscul Disord* 2008; 18: 6–16.

Needham M, Mastaglia F. Inclusion body myositis: current pathogenetic concepts and diagnostic and therapeutic approaches. *Lancet Neurol* 2007; 6(7): 620–31.

Needham M, Mastaglia FL, Garlepp MJ. Genetics of inclusion-body myositis. *Muscle Nerve* 2007; 35(5): 549–61.

Oldfors A, Lindberg C. Inclusion body myositis. *Curr Opin Neurol* 1999; 12(5): 527–33.

Serdaroglu P, Deymeer F, Parman Y. Prevalence of sporadic inclusion body myositis (s-IBM) in Turkey: a muscle biopsy-based survey. *Neuromuscul Disord* 2007; 17: 849.

Chapter 125
Myoglobinuria

John Vissing
University of Copenhagen, Rigshospitalet, Copenhagen, Denmark

Introduction

The term myoglobinuria is used when there is an increased urinary excretion of myoglobin. Under normal circumstances, myoglobin is excreted in minimal amounts in the urine (less than 5 ng/ml). The excretion becomes visible when it exceeds 100–200 µg/ml, a load that corresponds to the myoglobin present in approximately 50–100 g of muscle. The urine then takes on an appearance of dark tea or Coca Cola. Myoglobin is a small protein (17.8 kDa) that consists of 153 amino acids, and the gene encoding myoglobin consists of just three exons. Because of the small size of the molecule, a rise in plasma myoglobin precedes elevations of the four-times-larger creatine kinase (CK) molecule during muscle injury. Myoglobin is composed of eight helical segments, and with its single heme group has a higher affinity for binding oxygen than hemoglobin. It is well established that myoglobin plays an important role in cellular oxygen supply, but it is not crucial for oxygen metabolism. Thus, adult transgenic mice lacking myoglobin expression have normal life expectancy and can exercise, due to adaptive responses such as increased vascularity and overexpression of hypoxia-inducible transcription factors. Rhabdomyolysis is often used interchangeably with myoglobinuria and describes the dissolution or disruption of striated muscle that leads to loss of muscle proteins, including myoglobin, to the extracellular space.

Irrespective of the mechanism underlying myoglobinuria, it is associated with acute muscle injury, muscle necrosis, swelling of affected muscles, myalgia, and sometimes weakness. Common to all etiologies of myoglobinuria is direct injury to the sarcolemma or failure of energy supply to maintain sarcolemmal transport functions, which inevitably will lead to a rise in intracellular calcium. This will trigger muscle contraction and the need for more energy, while calcium-dependent proteases and phospholipidases will start to break down essential protein structures of the muscle, and lysosomes will digest the protein debris. Thus, disruption of sarcolemmal integrity starts a vicious circle that may end with disintegration of the muscle fiber.

Causes of myoglobinuria

Myoglobinuria has many intrinsic as well as extrinsic causes. They are commonly divided into genetic and acquired causes. Table 125.1 gives an overview of the many etiologies, indicating the main mechanisms responsible and the most common cause(s) for each mechanism. In distinguishing between acquired and hereditary cases, it is helpful to know whether a case of myoglobinuria is recurrent or a first-time incident. Hereditary cases tend to be recurrent, whereas acquired cases usually occur just once, unless they are coupled with episodic triggering mechanisms, such as generalized epileptic seizures or drug/alcohol abuse. In neuromuscular clinics there is a bias towards seeing patients who have recurrent episodes of myoglobinuria due to a genetic disorder, but acquired cases occurring just once probably constitute the bulk of cases with myoglobinuria. Thus, in a study of 77 patients with myoglobinuria seen in a non-specialized clinic, nearly all had acquired causes, alcohol being the most common cause, followed, in order of frequency, by limb immobilization with compression, generalized seizures, direct trauma, and drug abuse.

A number of factors may predispose to myoglobinuria. Low physical fitness decreases the duration and intensity of exercise that can be sustained without muscle injury. Hypokalemia and hypophosphatemia predispose to myoglobinuria, probably by depolarization of the muscle membrane. Hypo- or hyperthermia and infections, which occasionally may produce myoglobinuria alone, also act as potentiating factors.

Hereditary causes
Recurrent myoglobinuria is the hallmark of metabolic myopathies affecting glucose/glycogen metabolism and fatty acid oxidation (FAO). In 77 muscle biopsies from patients with mostly recurrent myoglobinuria, studied in

International Neurology: A Clinical Approach. Edited by Robert P. Lisak, Daniel D. Truong, William M. Carroll, and Roongroj Bhidayasiri. © 2009 Blackwell Publishing, ISBN: 978-1-4051-5738-4.

a neuromuscular clinic, 47% had an identifiable enzyme deficiency compatible with a metabolic myopathy, when obvious extrinsic factors had been ruled out.

Disorders of carbohydrate metabolism

The characteristic symptom preceding myoglobinuria in disorders of muscle carbohydrate metabolism is painful muscle contractures, provoked by sudden vigorous exercise. The most common disorder in this group is myophosphorylase deficiency (McArdle's disease). The enzyme defect in this condition, and in the rarer phosphofructokinase deficiency, is almost always complete, and therefore exercise capacity is severely reduced. The other glycolytic defects are associated with some residual enzyme activity, and consequently the exercise intensity that provokes myoglobinuria is much higher than in McArdle's disease.

Disorders of FAO

These disorders now comprise more than 25 enzyme deficiencies of fat metabolism, but many primarily give rise to hepatic manifestations with hypoglycemia, encephalopathy, and seizures. Less than 10 of the disorders give rise to myopathic symptoms with myoglobinuria. Myoglobinuria evoked by these disorders can be distinguished from McArdle's disease by (1) not having overt contractures, but rather muscle stiffness/tightness and pain, (2) normal plasma CK levels between episodes, (3) close to normal maximal work capacity, and (4) symptoms provoked by exercise of long duration, and worsened or provoked by emotional stress, cold-shivering, fever, and fasting. Like glycolytic defects, muscle integrity may be disturbed by lack of sufficient adenosine triphosphate (ATP) production, but, in addition, accumulated non-metabolized fat intermediates behind the metabolic block may also have a direct toxic effect on the sarcolemma. The most common disorder of FAO with myopathic symptoms is carnitine palmitoyltransferase II deficiency. It is also the most common cause of recurrent myoglobinuria, although very long-chain acyl-CoA dehydrogenase and trifunctional protein deficiencies probably have a higher propensity to cause myoglobinuria.

Mitochondrial disorders

Besides the specific mitochondrial disorders mentioned in Table 125.1, myoglobinuria is very rare in patients with mitochondrial myopathy. The underlying mechanism is probably energy failure, as in other metabolic myopathies, but the low incidence of myoglobinuria in these conditions indicates that other organ dysfunction often prevents patients from muscular overexertion. This is supported by the occurrence of myoglobinuria, preferentially in patients with isolated, primary mitochondrial defects of skeletal muscle.

Table 125.1 Causes of myoglobinuria.

Hereditary

Disorders of muscle carbohydrate metabolism
Myophosphorylase deficiency (McArdle's disease)
Phosphorylase *b* kinase deficiency
Phosphofructokinase deficiency
Phosphoglycerate kinase deficiency
Phosphoglycerate mutase deficiency
Lactate dehydrogenase deficiency

Disorders of fatty acid oxidation
Carnitine palmitoyltransferase II (CPTII) deficiency
Trifunctional protein deficiency
Very long-chain acyl-CoA dehydrogenase (VLCAD) deficiency
Long-chain acyl-CoA dehydrogenase (LCAD) deficiency
Short-chain *L*-3-hydroxyacyl-CoA dehydrogenase (SCHAD) deficiency
Electron transfer flavoprotein (ETF) deficiency

Disorders of mitochondrial respiratory chain function
Cytochrome *c* oxidase deficiency (COX I and III mutations)
Complex III deficiency (cytochrome *b* gene mutations)
Coenzyme Q10 deficiency
A number of mutations in mtDNA tRNA genes
Succinate dehydrogenase deficiency

Malignant hyperthermia susceptibility

Brody's myopathy (sarcoplasmic Ca^{2+}-ATPase deficiency)

Muscular dystrophies
Limb girdle muscular dystrophy type 2I
Sarcoglycanopathies
Dystrophinopathies

Acquired

Toxins (including drugs)
Neuroleptic malignant syndrome
Drugs inducing hypokalemia (thiazides, kaliuretics, laxatives, theophylline, amphotericin)
Cholesterol-lowering drugs (statins, bezafibrate, clofibrate)
Other drugs (antidepressants, anticholinergics, oxprenolol, opiates, amphetamines, pethidine, methylenedioxymethamphetamine (ecstasy), lithium, cocaine, barbiturates, antihistamines, vecuronium, succinylcholine, colchicines, cimetidine, zidovudine)
Alcohol, carbon monoxide, arsenic, ethylene glycol, gasoline, solvents, detergents, herbicides, snake venoms, methanol

Extreme exertion
Epileptic seizures
Electric shock
"March" myoglobinuria
Status asthmaticus
Delirium

Crush/trauma
Prolonged immobility (coma, surgery)
Certain forms of torture
High-impact deceleration/acceleration trauma

Ischemia
Compartment syndrome
Disseminated intravascular coagulation
Arterial occlusion

Extreme temperatures
Fever
Burns
Hypothermia

(Continued)

Table 125.1 Contd.

Metabolic causes
Hypokalemia
Hypothyroidism
Diabetic ketoacidosis or hyperosmolar state
Hyper-/hyponatremia
Hypophosphatemia

Infectious causes
Viral (adeno, coxsackie, influenza, measle, cytomegalo, HIV)
Bacterial (*Campylobacter, Clostridia, E. coli, Listeria, Salmonella, Staphylococcus, Streptococcus*)
Other (*Toxoplasma, Trichinella, Aspergillus*)

Inflammatory muscle disease (rare cause of myoglobinuria)
Poly- and dermatomyositis
Vasculitis

Muscular dystrophies

Recurrent myoglobinuria is being increasingly recognized in a variety of muscular dystrophies, particularly with the advent of better molecular characterization of these muscle diseases. Recurrent myoglobinuria was first recognized in the dystrophinopathies (see also Chapters 58 and 159), and may in Becker's muscular dystrophy be the presenting symptom. However, myoglobinuria may also be the presenting symptom in 20% of patients with limb girdle muscular dystrophy type 2I, and has also been observed in sarcoglycanopathies. In our clinic, recurrent myoglobinuria due to muscular dystrophy is now just as common as that caused by metabolic myopathies.

Acquired causes of myoglobinuria

Drugs and toxins

Drugs and toxins probably account for more than 75% of all cases of myoglobinuria in adults. The most common compounds involved are alcohol, drugs (particularly amphetamines, methylenedioxymethamphetamine (ecstasy), cocaine, opiates), and cholesterol-lowering agents (particularly statins).

Trauma

Myoglobinuria is unfortunately still a major factor in natural and manmade disasters involving compression of musculature. This includes trauma sustained during traffic accidents, falls, war, or other violence. It also includes compression after long immobility, and therefore overlaps with alcohol abuse and compression after

prolonged, severe, generalized seizures, and as a result of compartment syndromes, which may be either traumatic or exercise-induced.

Infections

A number of viral and bacterial agents may cause myoglobinuria (Table 125.1). The most common etiology is influenza virus A and B, streptococci, staphylococci, legionella, and salmonella. The pathogenesis of myoglobinuria is still unclear, but may include direct invasion of myocytes by the infectious agent, toxic effects, hyperthermia, and drug therapy in critically ill patients, particularly those that are being treated with muscle relaxants and steroids.

Treatment and prevention

The mainstay in any case of myoglobinuria is to avoid renal failure. It is therefore important to maintain sufficient blood pressure and avoid hypovolemia. Thus, saline infusion is important to maintain urine output and also as a means to dilute toxic products released from the necrotizing musculature. Myoglobin crystallizes at low pH, and it may therefore be necessary to alkalize the urine. If renal failure occurs, hemodialysis must be commenced. Disturbances of plasma calcium, phosphate, or potassium levels must be corrected, and if a compartment syndrome is present, a fasciotomy may be needed.

After the acute treatment, it is important to identify the correct diagnosis to be able to counsel the patient, and initiate prevention against repetition. Besides being careful about engaging in high-intensity exercise in patients with glycolytic defects or exercise of long duration in those with FAO defects , a diet high in carbohydrate may protect against muscle injury in both groups of disorders. For acquired causes, it is a matter of discontinuing the noxious stimulus, that is, the drug or toxin, if possible.

Further reading

Gabow PA, Kaehny WD, Kelleher SP. The spectrum of rhabdomyolysis. *Medicine* 1982; 61: 141–52.

Sveen ML, Schwartz M, Vissing J. High prevalence and phenotype–genotype correlations of limb girdle muscular dystrophy type 2I in Denmark. *Ann Neurol* 2006; 59: 808–15.

Tonin P, Lewis P, Servidei S, DiMauro S. Metabolic causes of myoglobinuria. *Ann Neurol* 1990; 27: 181–5.

Chapter 126
Genetics in neurology

Karen P. Frei

The Parkinson and Movement Disorder Institute, Fountain Valley, USA

Introduction

Inherited traits have long been of interest. Since the time Gregor Mendel described the heritability of traits in pea plants, we have pursued a modern understanding of our genetic underpinnings. The Human Genome Project, completed in 2003, greatly enhanced this process, providing a comprehensive reference, mapping the whole genome. Many neurological disorders appear to be inherited. Others, such as multiple sclerosis and Parkinson's disease, are thought to be multifactorial in origin with one or more genes involved as part of their etiology. As the subject of genetic disorders in neurology is so vast, this chapter attempts to describe the basics of genetics using selective neurological diseases as an example and the reader is referred to the specific chapters covering these disorders for further discussion of these disease states. The neurocutaneous disorders that are not covered in other chapters are discussed below.

The basics

Deoxyribonucleic acid (DNA) is the chemical that comprises the genetic blueprint. DNA is wound up in chromosomes. There are 43 pairs of chromosomes (22 autosomal and 1 sex) in the human genome. The sex chromosomes are designated X and Y, with females containing two X chromosomes and males one X and one Y chromosome. One set of chromosomes is inherited from each parent. A genome is the entire collection of genes for an organism. Genes are pieces of DNA that code for the controlled production of proteins. Genes are transcribed or copied into RNA and then protein is translated based upon the genetic sequence of RNA. A gene usually contains a promoter region, which allows the transcription of the gene; introns, which are not transcribed; exons, which are the transcribed DNA of the gene; and

International Neurology: A Clinical Approach. Edited by Robert P. Lisak, Daniel D. Truong, William M. Carroll, and Roongroj Bhidayasiri. © 2009 Blackwell Publishing, ISBN: 978-1-4051-5738-4.

a termination codon, which ends the transcription. Mutations are abnormalities seen within the DNA of a gene. There are different types of mutations including substitutions of one base for another, and additions or deletions of DNA. Mutations can produce no change in the protein or they can produce an abnormal or truncated protein. Disease states can be caused by mutations which are then passed on through to the next generation.

Mendelian genetics

Gregor Mendel, known as the father of modern genetics, first described the inheritance of traits in pea plants in 1865. He noted that inheritance of traits follows particular laws. These laws apply to traits such as hair and eye color as well as to disease states resulting from a mutated gene.

Autosomal dominant inheritance
A single mutated gene on one of the non-sex chromosomes that is expressed despite the presence of a normal gene inherited from the other parent is required for an autosomal dominant inheritance disease state to be expressed. This means that the disease is present in one of the parents and in 50% of the children. Examples of autosomal dominant inheritance include neurofibromatosis type 1.

Autosomal recessive inheritance
Two copies of the mutated gene on one of the non-sex chromosomes are required for this disease state to be expressed. Both parents are carriers of the disease and usually are not affected with the disease. Most of the metabolic single enzyme deficiency disease states are inherited through autosomal recessive transmission. An example is Gaucher's disease, which is caused by deficiency of the lysosomal enzyme beta glucocerebrosidase. Gaucher type 3 has neurological features including seizures and myoclonus.

X-linked dominant inheritance
A single mutation occurring on the X chromosome causes this disease state. Females inherit an X chromosome from

each of their parents and males inherit one X chromosome from their mother and one Y chromosome from their father. Because only one chromosome with the mutation is required to develop the disease state, males and females with a mutation are equally likely to have the disease. However, if the father has the mutation, only his daughters will be affected since he passes his unaffected Y chromosome to his sons. Rett's syndrome is an example of the X-linked dominant inheritance pattern. Rett's syndrome consists of autism, developmental delay, severe speech and communication impairment, microcephaly, seizures, and stereotypic non-functional hand movements.

X-linked recessive inheritance

Since males have only one X chromosome, a recessive mutation can result in a disease state. Thus, males are more commonly affected than females. Affected fathers will have heterozygous or carrier daughters and normal sons. Carrier mothers will have carrier or normal daughters and affected sons. Duchenne's muscular dystrophy and the metabolic disorder Fabry's disease are inherited in this manner. Fabry's disease which produces telangiectasias, intestinal disorders, and neuropathy is caused by a mutation in the alpha galactosidase A gene.

Codominant inheritance

Codominant inheritance involves more than one form of a gene (allele). Each allele is expressed and has an influence on the outward expression (phenotype). Blood types are one example of this type of inheritance with A, B, and O alleles.

Many disorders are inherited through a complex interaction between several genes and/or the environment. The genetics of these disorders are more difficult to determine. Alzheimer's dementia, dystonia, and Parkinson's disease are examples of these multifactorial disorders. What follows are some of the genetic interactions and other factors influencing the effects of mutations that have been identified.

Reduced penetrance

Penetrance refers to the proportion of people with a mutation who exhibit signs and symptoms of a genetic disorder. Sometimes some of the people who have inherited the mutation do not develop the disease. In this instance, the genetic pattern is said to have reduced penetrance. Reduced penetrance is seen commonly in autosomal dominantly inherited traits. Examples include dystonia due to the *DYT1* gene and Parkinson's disease due to the *LRRK2* gene. Intuitively, reduced penetrance can create difficulties in determining the genetic pattern of a disease state. It is probably due to several influential factors that are unknown.

Variable expressivity

The range of signs and symptoms occurring in people with the same genetic condition is referred to as variable expressivity. Similar to reduced penetrance, variable expressivity also tends to be seen more often in association with autosomal dominant inheritance pattern; it is likely due to several unknown influential factors and can also interfere with diagnosis of the genetic pattern of the disorder.

An example of reduced penetrance and variable expressivity is the inheritance of dystonia. Oppenheimer's dystonia (DYT1) is inherited in an autosomal dominant pattern with reduced penetrance and variable expressivity. Only approximately 30% of those who inherit this mutation actually show signs of the trait and among family members inheriting the same mutation there is often variability in the types and severity of the dystonia. For example, one family member may have focal dystonia such as writer's cramp and another can have generalized dystonia reflecting the variable expressivity of the trait.

Trinucleotide repeats

A trinucleotide repeat is a series of three nucleotides occurring repetitively in a gene. When at an abnormal number of repeats, the gene is unstable and the number of these repeat sequences can change as the gene is passed from parent to child. When the number of repeats enlarges with each generation it is referred to as trinucleotide repeat expansion. The disease state results when the number of repeats enlarges past a certain number and the gene is no longer functioning normally. With each generation the number of repeats grows, resulting in more severe symptoms and onset of the disease state at an earlier age. This is referred to as *anticipation*. Anticipation is seen in several neurodegenerative diseases including Huntington's disease, Friederich's ataxia, myotonic dystrophy, fragile X syndrome, and spinocerebellar ataxia (SCA). See Table 126.1 for a list of known neurodegenerative diseases with trinucleotide repeats and anticipation.

Genomic imprinting

Each person inherits two copies of their genes, one from their mother and the other from their father. Most of the time, both copies of the gene are functional. Sometimes, however, only one copy is functional and the copy that is functional is dependent on the parent of origin. Some genes are functional only when inherited from the mother and others only when inherited from the father. This phenomenon is referred to as genomic imprinting and is

Table 126.1 Neurological diseases with trinucleotide repeats and anticipation.

Disease name	Mode of inheritance	Trinucleotide repeat	Gene	Protein
Huntington's chorea	Autosomal dominant	CAG	4p16.3 *IT15*	Huntingtin
Dentatorubralpallidoluysian atrophy	Autosomal dominant	CAG	12p13.31 *ATN 1*	Atrophin 1
SCA 1	Autosomal dominant	CAG	6p22.3 *ATXN 1*	Ataxin 1
SCA 2	Autosomal dominant	CAG	12q24.13 *ATXN 2*	Ataxin 2
Machado–Joseph disease SCA 3	Autosomal dominant	CAG	14q32.12 *ATXN 3*	Ataxin 3
SCA 6	Autosomal dominant	CAG	19p13.13 *CACNAIA*	CACNAIA
SCA 7	Autosomal dominant	CAG	3p14.1 *ATXN 7*	Ataxin 7
SCA 17	Autosomal dominant	CAG	6q27 *TBP*	TBP
Kennedy's syndrome	X-linked recessive	CAG	Xq21.3–22	Androgen receptor
Fragile X syndrome	X-linked	CGG	Xq27.3 *FMR1*	FMR1
Friederich's ataxia	Autosomal recessive	GAA	9q13 *FRDA*	Frataxin
Myotonic dystrophy DM1	Autosomal dominant	CTG	19q13.3 *DMPK*	Myotonic dystrophy protein kinase
Myotonic dystrophy DM2	Autosomal dominant	CCTG	3q21 *ZNf9*	Zinc finger protein 9

related to the presence of methyl groups which "mark" the parent of origin. Methylated genes are non-functional and both addition and removal of methyl groups can be used to control the gene activity. Imprinting is seen in a small percentage of human genes and imprinted genes tend to cluster together in the same regions of chromosomes. Two major clusters of imprinted genes have been identified in humans, one on the short (p) arm of *chromosome 11* (at position 11p15) and another on the long (q) arm of *chromosome 15* (in the region 15q11 to 15q13). A classic example of genomic imprinting occurs in the inheritance of Prader–Willi and Angelman's syndrome. Both disorders involve the same imprinted region of chromosome 15q11–13.

Angelman's syndrome consists of developmental delay, ataxia, hypotonia, myoclonic epilepsy, absence of speech, and unusual facies; it is due to loss of the maternal contribution of the imprinted region. Prader–Willi syndrome consists of obesity, hypotonia, mental retardation, short stature, and hypogonadism and is inherited through deletion of the paternal contribution. Imprinting is also seen in the inheritance of myoclonus-dystonia. The epsilon sarcoglycan gene located at 7q21 is maternally imprinted. Mutations in this gene result in a marked difference in penetrance depending on the parental origin of the

gene mutation, with most clinical disease occurring with paternal transmission.

Mitochondrial disorders

The mitochondria contain their own DNA. Each cell contains many mitochondria existing in the cytoplasm. The mitochondria are not inherited according to Mendelian genetic patterns but are inherited solely from the mother, being contained in the oocyte. Inheritance patterns may appear to be familial, may occur in each generation, but are not inherited from the father. Mitochondria are self-replicating. Not only are mitochondria responsible for the production of adenosine triphosphate (ATP), but they are also involved in apoptosis and the production of cholesterol and heme. Mutations occurring in mitochondrial DNA may result in defects of oxidative phosphorylation or production of transfer RNA (tRNA) or ribosomal RNA (rRNA). Disease states resulting from mitochondrial DNA mutations depend upon the number of mitochondria containing the mutation. Well-known neurological mitochondrial disorders include Melas, Merrf, and Leber's optic neuropathy. Table 126.2 lists some of the more well-known mitochondrial disorders.

Table 126.2 Common neurological mitochondrial disorders.

Disease name	Mitochondrial defect	Symptoms
Leigh syndrome	Complex I, II, III, IV, V, pyruvate dehydrogenase complex	Early onset developmental delay, deafness, hypotonia
Kearns–Sayre syndrome	mDNA deletion or tRNA point mutation	Progressive external ophthalmoplegia, cardiomyopathy, and retinitis pigmentosa
Leber's hereditary optic neuropathy	Complex I, III, IV defect in the respiratory chain	Central visual loss leading to central scotoma
Mitochondrial encephalopathy, lactic acidosis and stroke-like episodes (Melas)	Heterogeneous mitochondrial DNA mutations	Myopathy, encephalopathy, lactic acidosis, seizures, hemiparesis, hemianopsia, cortical blindness, and episodic vomiting
Myoclonic epilepsy with ragged red fibers (Merrf)	Heterogeneous mitochondrial DNA mutations	Myoclonic epilepsy

Neurocutaneous disorders

The neurocutaneous disorders, also known as phako-matoses disorders involving the skin and brain. Neuro-fibromatosis, Von Hippel–Lindau disease, tuberous sclerosis, Sturge–Weber syndrome, xeroderma pigmentosum, and incontinentia pigmenti are considered to be neurocutaneous disorders.

Neurofibromatosis

There are two forms of neurofibromatosis: type 1 and type 2. Neurofibromatosis type 1 (NF1), also known as Von Recklinghausen disease, predominantly affects the skin and peripheral nerves. Cutaneous features include café-au-lait spots, freckling, and neurofibromas. Café-au-lait spots are areas of skin discoloration and can be seen anywhere on the body. Six or more café-au-lait spots are supportive of the diagnosis. Skin freckling usually occurs in areas of skin folds or increased friction. Neurofibromas are tumors of the peripheral nerve sheath. Cutaneous and subcutaneous neurofibromas occur mostly in the trunk or upper extremities. Central nervous system (CNS) tumors are usually astrocytomas with a predilection for the optic pathway. Cerebral and spinal cord tumors also occur with a greater frequency in NF1. The gene involved in NF1 is located on chromosome 17q11.2.7 and is thought to be a tumor suppressor gene. The gene product is known as neurofibromin. An individual with NF1 has a copy of the mutation in all cells. A second somatic mutation in the normal is required before the gene becomes non-functional. There is a high spontaneous mutation rate at this site and it has complete penetrance.

Neurofibromatosis type 2 (NF2) consists of mainly CNS tumors. The hallmark of NF2 is bilateral acoustic neuromas: tumors of the Schwann's cells surrounding cranial nerve VIII. Deafness is the main clinical feature of NF2. Skin involvement is variable, with less frequent café–au-lait spots and infrequent neurofibromas. Other CNS tumors are common and include meningiomas, spinal nerve root schwannomas, trigeminal nerve schwannomas, gliomas, and ependymomas. NF 2 is inherited as an autosomal dominant trait and the gene is located on chromosome 22q11.2. The gene product is known as MERLIN, of which dysfunction has been associated with sporadic meningiomas, sporadic schwannomas, and breast and colon cancer. Treatment of neurofibromatosis is palliative and consists of tumor removal.

Von Hippel–Lindau disease

There is an inherited susceptibility to cerebellar and spinal cord hemangioblastomas in Von Hippel–Lindau disease (VHL). Other features include retinal angiomas, bilateral renal cell carcinoma, pheochromocytoma, and multiple cysts mainly located in the kidneys, pancreas, and ovaries. Death usually results from renal cell carcinoma. VHL is inherited in an autosomal dominant manner and the gene is located at the tip of chromosome 3. There are three classifications of VHL: type 1 without pheochromocytoma, type 2a with pheochromocytoma, and type 2b with pheochromocytoma and renal cell carcinoma. Sporadic forms of renal cell carcinoma have been found to have mutations in the VHL gene.

Tuberous sclerosis

Cutaneous symptoms of tuberous sclerosis (TS) include hypomelanotic macules, shagreen patch, ungual fibromas, and facial angiofibromas. Hypomelanotic macules, also known as ash leaf spots, occur in the majority of patients with TS. The shagreen patch is an irregular raised or textured lesion most commonly found on the back or flank. Ungual fibromas are found underneath or adjacent to the nails. Facial angiofibromas are hamartomas of the vascular and connective tissue elements and are found on the face, predominantly around the nose. Facial angiofibromas, also known as adenomatous sebaceum, are considered to be specific for TS; however, only approximately 75% of patients have these lesions, which may become present later in life. Neurological manifestations of TS include developmental delay and seizures. Giant cell astrocytomas may occur and are usually located in the anterior horn of the lateral ventricle. Calcified subependymal nodules are characteristic findings on neuroimaging studies. MRI may reveal cortical and subcortical white matter lesions which correspond to hamartomas, gliotic areas, and neuronal migration defects. Cardiac rhabdomyomata, also considered hamartomas, and renal angiomyolipomas, often a cause of death, may be found in over half of patients with TS. There are two genes associated with TS: *TSC1* found on chromosome 9q34 and *TSC2* found on chromosome 16. These genes are thought to be tumor suppressor genes and a mutation in both genes is required for tumor formation. TS is inherited in an autosomal dominant manner with variable penetrance. Treatment is palliative with seizure control.

Sturge–Weber syndrome

Unilateral facial angioma or port wine stain involving the first branch of the trigeminal nerve is the hallmark of Sturge–Weber syndrome (SW). Seizures and developmental delay are neurological manifestations. Oftentimes developmental delay follows intractable seizures. Leptomeningeal vascular malformations occur and produce characteristic neuroimaging findings. Ocular involvement may occur with vascular malformations occurring in the conjunctiva or choroid and glaucoma in the eye ipsilateral to the port wine stain. SW is a sporadic disorder with unknown cause. Treatment of the port wine stain with the argon laser has been successful and seizure control can help to preserve intellectual function.

Xeroderma pigmentosum

Xeroderma pigmentosum (XP) is a rare recessively inherited disorder involving the ability to repair mutated or damaged DNA. There is a striking photosensitivity, with sun burn occurring first followed by freckling and then telangiectasia and skin atrophy of exposed areas, usually beginning in infancy. Half of affected children have skin cancer by 14 years of age. Corneal scarring, keratitis, and carcinoma can result in vision loss at an early age. Approximately 20% of patients have some form of neurological involvement which can include progressive neurological deterioration, dementia, abnormal ocular motility, choreoathetosis, ataxia, sensorineural deafness, spasticity, and microcephaly. Olivopontocerebellar degeneration may be seen on neuroimaging studies. Treatment is aimed at early diagnosis and protection from UV exposure through clothing, glasses, and sunblock.

Incontinentia pigmenti

Cutaneous features dominate incontinentia pigmenti (IP) and consist of four phases. The first phase occurs within the first month of life and consists of skin lesions occurring in a whorled, linear, or splash like pattern over the trunk, scalp, and proximal and flexor surfaces of the limbs. The rash resolves within a few weeks. The second phase can reoccur during infancy and consists of acanthotic, dyskeratotic lesions in the same distribution as in the first phase. Resolution occurs within a few weeks with some residual atrophic changes. The third phase consists of melanin deposition outside and within melanophores of the upper dermis, result in striking patterns of variable pigmentation in streaks, whorls, and patterns located in the lateral trunk and proximal extremities and oftentimes in areas not previously involved. These characteristic lesions fade in the second and third decade of life. The fourth phase consists of hypopigmented, hairless, atrophic regions. Seizures, spastic paralysis, and developmental delay are neurological manifestations that occur in approximately 33% of patients. Dental anomalies and strabismus may also occur. Inheritance is thought to be X-linked dominant transmission with male hemizygote lethality. Two loci, Xp11.21 and Xq28, are thought to be responsible for IP. Treatment is symptomatic and can include dental repair, photocoagulation, cryotherapy of ocular neovascularization, and seizure control.

Further reading

National Library of Medicine and National Institutes of Health. *Genetics Home Reference*: www.ncbi.nlm.nih.gov/ and *Genes and Disease*, an online book: www.ncbi.nlm.nih.gov/books (accessed April 10, 2008).

Online Mendelian Inheritance in Man, OMIM (TM). McKusick-Nathans Institute of Genetic Medicine, Johns Hopkins University (Baltimore, MD) and National Center for Biotechnology Information, National Library of Medicine (Bethesda, MD): http://www.ncbi.nlm.nih.gov/omim/ (accessed April 10, 2008).

Rosenberg RN, Prusiner SB, Di Mauro S, Barchi RL, editors. *The Molecular and Genetic Basis of Neurological Disease*. Boston: Butterworth-Heineman; 1997.

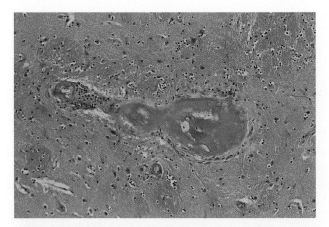

Plate 4.1 Lipohyaline mural change in a caudate nucleus arteriole, with possible microaneurysm formation (haematoxylin and eosin stain × 200).

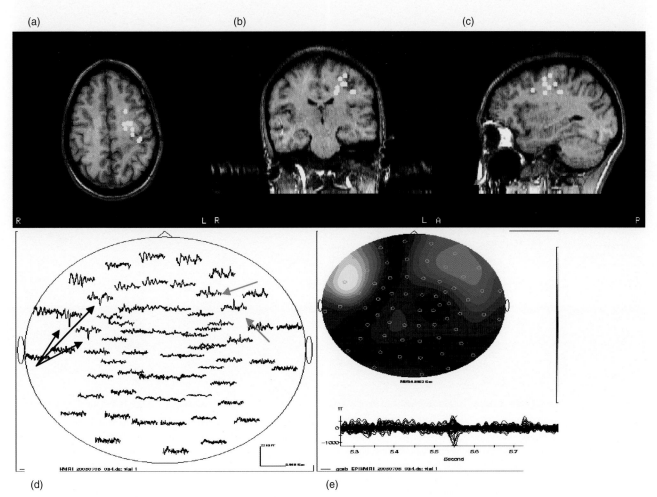

(a)　　　　　　　　　　　　(b)　　　　　　　　　　　　(c)

(d)　　　　　　　　　　　　(e)

Plate 32.1 Magnetoencephalography showing spike waves in axial (a), coronal (b), and sagittal (c) views, superimposed onto MRI. These appeared generalized on electroencephalography (EEG). (d) The spike waveforms on raw magnetoencephalography (MEG) (*black arrows*; *red arrows* show contralateral reflection. (e) Surface current density view of source (*yellow*) and sink (*blue*). (Courtesy of Ernst Rodin and Barbara Swartz.)

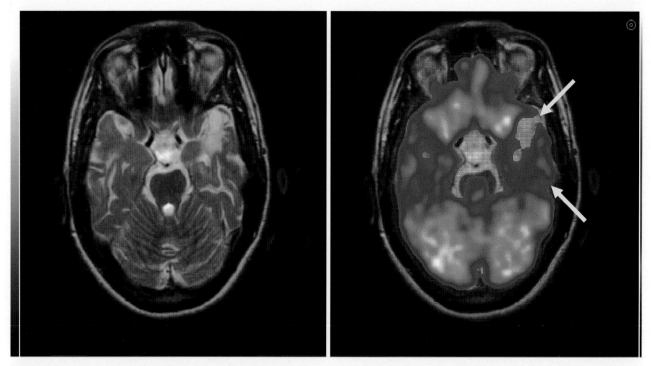

Plate 32.2 Coregistration of an MR image and the corresponding FDG-PET slice show improved anatomical identification of structures on PET. The area of encephalomalicia (*top arrow*) is clear, but, in addition, PEt demonstrates unexpected dysfunction in temporal cortex (*bottom arrow*) as well as the contralateral temporal lobe. (Courtesy of Barbara Swartz.)

(a)

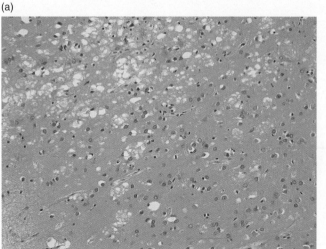

(b)

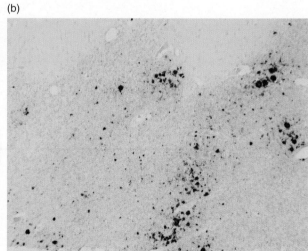

Plate 38.1 Neuropathological picture of CJD. (a) Prominent spongiform changes; neuronal loss and astrocytosis in the frontal cortex in the case of sCJD. Standard hematoxylin and eosin (H&E) staining; original magnification 200×. (b) Diffuse synaptic and focal perivacuolar (patchy) positivity of PrP^{Sc} with some small kuru-like plaques in the cerebellar cortex in the case of fCJD. Immunohistochemical reaction with mouse monoclonal anti-PrP antibody; clone 6H4 (original magnification 200×).

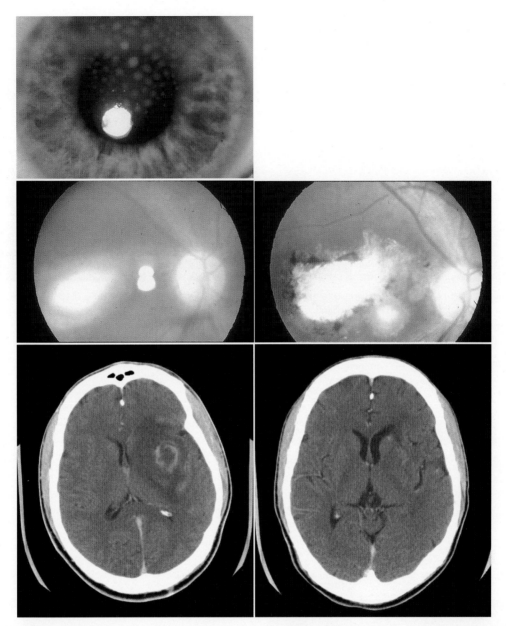

Plate 79.1 Ocular and cerebral toxoplasmosis. Anterior uveitis with mutton-fat keratic precipitates (top). (Courtesy of Caygill Ophthalmic Library, Department of Ophthalmology, University of California, San Francisco.) Toxoplasmosis retinochoroiditis after 6 months (middle left) and after 2 years (middle right). The central exposed white area of each image is the sclera, seen after necrosis of the retina and choroid. Proliferation of the pigmented layer at margins of the lesion is noted with more advanced disease, and the healed lesion is densely pigmented with irregular borders and central atrophy (middle right). (Courtesy of Caygill Ophthalmic Library, Department of Ophthalmology, University of California, San Francisco.) Toxoplasmosis cerebral abscess. CT scans with contrast from an AIDS patient presenting with seizures, aphasia, contrast-enhancing CT lucency, and *Toxoplasma* titers that were positive (lower left). During treatment, 25 days later, there is resolution of the abscess (lower right). (Courtesy C. Jay, Department of Neurology, University of California, San Francisco.)

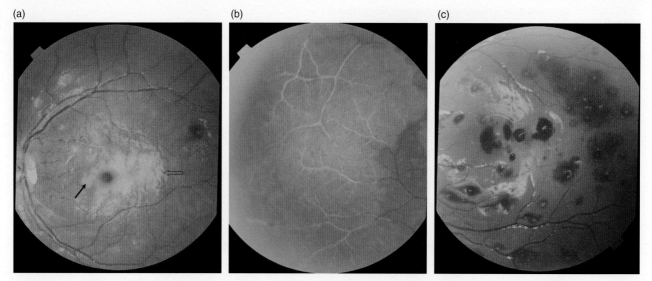

Plate 80.1 (a) Severe macula whitening (*solid arrow*) completely surrounding the foveola of a child with cerebral malaria. Papilledema is present as well as a white-centered hemorrhage temporal to the macula and cottonwool spots above the superior temporal arcade. The *open arrow* indicates glare. (© Beare NAV, *et al. Am J Trop Med Hyg* 2006; 75: 790–7, with permission.)

(b) White retinal vessels in an area of confluent peripheral retinal whitening. (© Beare NAV, *et al. Am J Trop Med Hyg* 2006; 75: 790–7, with permission.) (c) Large number of retinal hemorrhages in a child with cerebral malaria. (© Beare NAV, *et al. Am J Trop Med Hyg* 2006; 75: 790–7, with permission.)

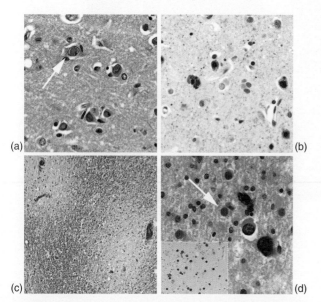

Plate 90.1 Measles inclusion body encephalitis: intranuclear eosinophilic inclusion bodies (a, hematoxylin–eosin, *arrow*) and viral antigen demonstrated by immunohistochemistry (b). PML: focal areas of demyelination (c, luxolfast blue); homogeneous amphophilic nuclear inclusions in oligodendrocytes (*arrow*) and large, bizarre astrocytes (d, haematoxylin–eosin). Detection of JC virus by immunohistochemistry (*inset*).

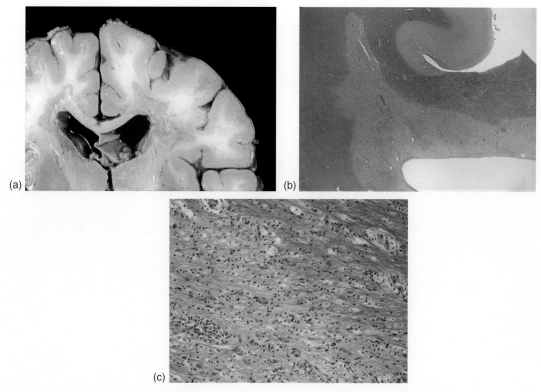

Plate 100.1 (a) Whole brain gross demonstration of several large plaques including those in periventricular regions. (b) Large periventricular plaque (hematoxylin & eosin (H&E) and luxol fast blue (LFB); low power). (c) Perivascular lesions within plaque (high power). (Courtesy of Dr William Kupsky.)

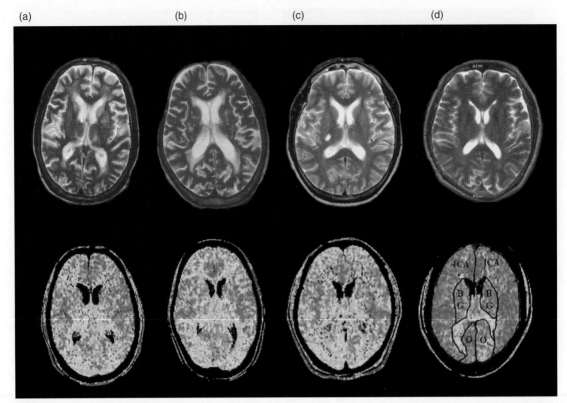

(a) (b) (c) (d)

Right

Plate 106.1 Brain MRI T2-weighted images (*upper row*) of three patients with CS₂ intoxication (a–c) and a normal control (d). The images show multiple high signal intensity lesions in the subcortical white matter and basal ganglia. Brain CT perfusion scan with a regional mean transit time (MTT) map (*lower row*) in three patients with CS₂ intoxication (a–c) and a normal control (d). The images show a statistically significant prolongation of MTT in the brain parenchymal area and basal ganglia (ICA: internal carotid artery; BG: basal ganglia; O: occipital area).

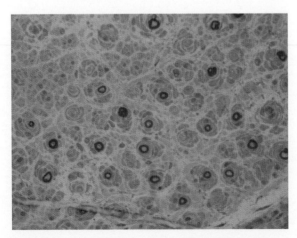

Plate 111.1 Sural nerve biopsy from a patient with CMT1A demonstrates individual nerve fibers surrounded by prominent Schwann's cell proliferation resulting in "onion bulbs".

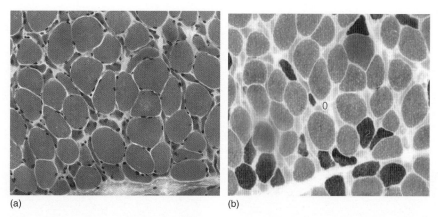

(a)   (b)

Plate 117.1 Critical illness myopathy. Muscle biopsy: H&E stain (a) and myosin ATPase pH 9.4 stain (b). Note the numerous atrophic, angular, and basophilic fibers with large nuclei (a). Atrophic fibers lose their myosin ATPase stain (b – 0) compared to normal stain in type I (b – 1) and type II (b – 2) muscle fibers. This is most apparent at pH 9.4 where the involved muscle fibers stain less intensely than either the type I or type II muscle fibers. Type II muscle fiber atrophy may also occur.

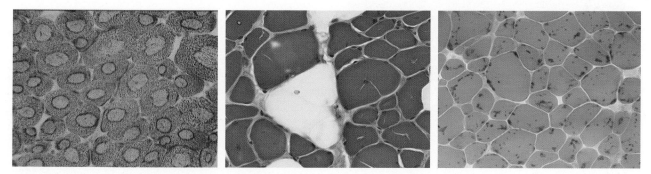

Plate 120.1 The characteristic histological features of congenital myopathies; central core disease (left, NADH-Tr, ×400), centronuclear myopathy (middle, H&E, ×400), and nemaline myopathy (right, Gomori trichrome, ×200).

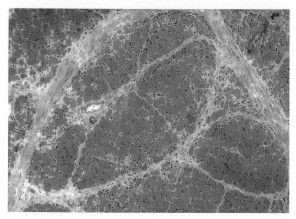

Plate 122.1 Perifasicular atrophy, a classic histopathological feature of DM, as seen in a cross section from a patient's muscle biopsy.

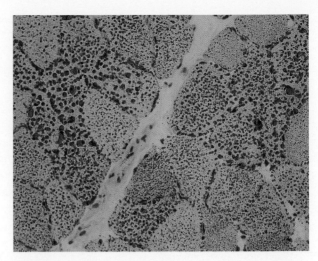

Plate 160.1 Pathologic lipid storage in muscle. Intermyofibrillar accumulation of fatty acids as seen in lipid storage diseases, mitochondrial myopathies, and fatty acid oxidation disorders (Oil red-O staining).

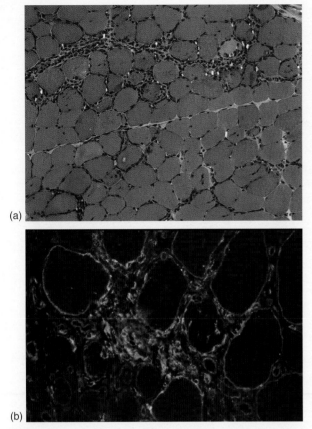

Plate 123.1 (a) Cross section of a muscle biopsy from a patient with PM, demonstrating lymphocytes invading non-necrotic muscle fibers. These cells are CD8+ and surround MHC-I-expressing muscle fibers, as shown in (b).

Chapter 127
Neuro-otology

Kevin A. Kerber
University of Michigan Health System, Ann Arbor, USA

Introduction

Neuro-otology is a multidisciplinary specialty with primary training stemming from either otolaryngology or neurology. The specialty is primarily concerned with evaluating patients who present with dizziness, balance disturbance, or auditory symptoms. While neurologists focus on the clinical evaluation, diagnosis, and non-surgical management of patients with these symptoms, otolaryngologists emphasize surgical approaches to disorders of the ear. The specialty is relatively new, but serves an important purpose because these types of symptoms are extremely common.

Epidemiology

Relatively few epidemiological studies of dizziness have been performed. A recent population-based telephone survey in Germany showed that nearly 30% of the population have experienced moderate to severe dizziness. Although most affected persons reported non-specific forms of dizziness, nearly a quarter had true vertigo. Dizziness is more common among females and older people. Because of this association with age, the presentation of dizziness is only expected to increase with the aging of the population that is taking place in a number of countries. In the United States, the National Centers for Health Statistics has reported that 7.5 million annual ambulatory visits to physicians' offices, hospital outpatient departments, and emergency departments are for vertigo-dizziness, making it one of the most common principal complaints.

More is known about the prevalence of hearing loss worldwide, because it is a leading cause of burden of disease in high-income countries. Hearing loss affects approximately 16% of adults (age >18 years) in the United States. Men are more commonly affected than women, and prevalence increases dramatically with age so that by age 75 nearly 50% of the population reports at least some degree of hearing loss. The most common type of hearing loss is sensorineural, and both idiopathic presbycusis and noise-induced forms are common etiologies. Tinnitus is less frequent in the US population with about 3% reporting it, although this increases to about 9% in subjects older than 65. Among subjects with hearing loss, nearly 75% also experience tinnitus. The most common type of tinnitus is a high-pitched ringing in both ears.

International considerations in patients with neuro-otologic disorders

When considering international factors regarding neuro-otologic symptoms and disorders, one must consider the tremendous variability in how patients of different geographic locations, language backgrounds, and cultures describe their symptoms, particularly the symptom of dizziness. In the United States, the symptom of dizziness is generally felt to infer to either a spinning sensation (vertigo), some other type of "head" sensation (i.e., lightheadedness, wooziness), or imbalance (unsteadiness when walking). However, some patients reporting dizziness will instead describe a visual phenomenon, general ill feeling, anxiety, or another symptom. Other important international factors are genetic disorders and communicable diseases which vary from region to region. As a result, it can be important to identify the patient's geographic and ethnic background.

Clinical approach to patients with dizziness

The most important processes of care when clinically approaching patients with dizziness are obtaining a detailed history and appropriate examination. The information gathered is key for formulating the case, localizing the lesion, generating a differential diagnosis, and planning the management. Numerous studies have shown that tests do not discriminate non-categorized dizziness from normal controls.

International Neurology: A Clinical Approach. Edited by Robert P. Lisak, Daniel D. Truong, William M. Carroll, and Roongroj Bhidayasiri. © 2009 Blackwell Publishing, ISBN: 978-1-4051-5738-4.

Table 127.1 Key components to the examination of the dizzy patient.

Examination component	Description
General medical examination	
Vital signs	Blood pressure, orthostatic blood pressure, pulse rate
Head and neck examination	External ear vesicles, external auditory canal
Cardiac examination	Heart rhythm
General neurological examination	
Mental status testing	Level of alertness, orientation, concentration, memory
Cranial nerves	Cranial nerves 2–12 in details
Motor	Tone, strength
Sensory examination	Distal sensory loss, reflexes
Neuro-otologic examination	
Ocular motor	Spontaneous movements (nystagmus, saccadic intrusions), gaze testing, smooth pursuit, saccades, optokinetic nystagmus, fixation suppression of the vestibular-ocular reflex
Vestibular nerve	Head thrust test, doll's eye test
Positional testing	Head-hanging positions (Dix–Hallpike), supine positional testing
Fistula testing	Pneumatoscopy, Valsalva's maneuver, tragal compression
Gait assessment	Gait initiation, heel strike, stride length, base width, tandem gait, Romberg position
Auditory evaluation	Whisper test, tuning forks, finger rub

History of present illness

The first step is to ask patients to describe the symptoms in their own words. If the patient is unable to adequately describe the symptom, then the patient should be asked to classify the dizziness into one of the following categories: vertigo (spinning of the environment), presyncope (feeling of near faint), lightheadedness or wooziness (abnormal "head" sensation but without presyncope), or imbalance (feeling of unsteadiness when walking without an abnormal "head" sensation). Once the type of dizziness has been determined, the clinician then should obtain information about the characteristics of the dizziness. Patients should be specifically queried about whether the symptom is constant or episodic, whether it came on gradually or suddenly, and about any other accompanying symptoms (particularly auditory symptoms, neurological symptoms, or palpitations). The patient should also be asked about the duration and frequency of the symptom, aggravating or alleviating factors, and identifiable triggers. Obtaining details about the temporal profile is also important. Because many people have difficulty describing or even categorizing the symptom, descriptive characteristics are often the most important information.

A detailed past medical history, list of medications and allergies, social history, and family history should also be obtained. Medication side effects are one of the most common causes of dizziness in general. Many times a specific medicine cannot be identified, but clearly the more medications patients take, the more likely side effects become. A complete family history is now known to be a key part of the dizziness evaluation. Many types of dizziness, including benign recurrent vertigo, chronic forms of dizziness, and ataxia syndromes, are now known

to be genetic disorders or to have important genetic components.

General medical examination

Details of examination components are listed in Table 127.1. A general medical examination is important in the dizzy patient because medical disorders such as metabolic, endocrine, or cardiac disorders are common causes of non-vertiginous types of dizziness. Orthostatic blood pressure measurements can provide important information in patients who report features of presyncope. Measurement of visual acuity may also provide important information because poor vision can contribute to or even cause types of dizziness. Arthritis or joint deformity, chronic lung disease, angina, cardiac failure, or peripheral vascular disease can be important factors in balance disorders.

General neurological examination

A mental status examination helps to exclude cognitive impairment as a feature of the patient's presentation. The cranial nerves should be thoroughly inspected. The examiner should determine whether the patient has full ocular movements. A test of the facial nerve strength and symmetry is important because of the close anatomical relationship between the seventh and eighth cranial nerves. Examining palatal elevation, tongue bulk and protrusion, and the trapezius and sternocleidomastoid muscles helps exclude lower cranial nerve involvement. During the motor examination, the tone should be closely assessed because increased tone or cogwheel rigidity can be the manifestations in patients with early neurodegenerative disorders. The peripheral sensory examination is also important because various forms of peripheral neuropathy can cause non-specific dizziness or imbalance. Reflexes should be tested for their presence and symmetry. However, normal elderly patients often have reduced distal vibratory sensation and absent ankle jerks. Coordination is an important part of the neurological examination in patients with dizziness because disorders characterized by ataxia can present with the principal symptom of dizziness. Ataxia of the limbs, however, may be very subtle or even absent in other ataxic disorders that mainly affect midline cerebellar structures.

The neuro-otological examination
Ocular motor function testing
Assessment of eye movements is a critical part of the evaluation of dizzy patients. Abnormalities found may point to a specific localization and even specific syndromes, whereas normal ocular motor function excludes many neurological disorders. The first step is to search for spontaneous involuntary movements of the eyes, mainly nystagmus or saccadic intrusions. Nystagmus is characterized by a slow and fast phase component that can be classified as spontaneous, gaze evoked, or positional. An important type of nystagmus to recognize is the peripheral vestibular pattern of nystagmus. This pattern is readily apparent in acute disorders as a horizontal greater than torsional, unidirectional nystagmus that can be suppressed with fixation. The nystagmus increases when the patient looks in the direction of the fast phase of nystagmus and decreases or stops when the patient looks toward the opposite side. On the other hand, nystagmus that changes direction on gaze testing (e.g., converts from a left beating nystagmus to a right beating nystagmus) is a central finding. Some patients may be able to suppress the nystagmus when in a well-lit room, but when fixation is removed the spontaneous component becomes apparent. Techniques to block fixation include evaluating the patient in a darkened environment, using Frenzel glasses, blocking the vision of one eye during a fundoscopic examination of the other, or simply placing a blank sheet of paper up to the patient's nose and observing the eyes from the side.

Saccadic intrusions are spontaneous, non-volitional, fast eye movements (i.e., saccades) that do not have the rhythmic fast and slow phases like nystagmus. The most common type of saccadic intrusion is square wave jerks, which are small-amplitude involuntary saccades that take the eyes off target, followed after a characteristic intersaccade delay by a corrective saccade that brings the eyes back on target. Square wave jerks are frequently seen in various neurologic disorders, such as cerebellar ataxia syndromes, Huntington's disease, or progressive supranuclear palsy. Another type of saccadic intrusion is a saccadic oscillation which consists of back-to-back saccadic eye movements without an intersaccadic interval. When a burst of saccades occurs in the horizontal plane,

the term ocular flutter is used. When vertical or torsional components are also present, the term opsoclonus is used. Ocular flutter and opsoclonus are pathological findings typically encountered in several types of central nervous system diseases that involve the brainstem and cerebellar pathways. Paraneoplastic disorders should be considered in patients who present with these saccadic oscillations.

Gaze testing
After searching for spontaneous movements of the eyes, the examiner should search for gaze-evoked nystagmus by instructing the patient to look in each direction. Many normal patients have a few beats of non-sustained nystagmus with gaze greater than 30° off-center, and this is called end-gaze nystagmus. The most common cause of gaze-evoked nystagmus is due to a medication adverse effect, typically an antiepileptic drug. However, brainstem and cerebellar disorders are also common causes of gaze-evoked nystagmus.

Smooth pursuit
When patients track objects that move in their visual field back and forth, the eye movements should be smooth as long as the target is not moving too quickly. This movement of the eyes is called smooth pursuit and it is a central nervous system function. This type of eye movement serves to keep moving objects on the fovea to maximize vision; however, it inevitably breaks down when the target moves at high enough velocity. Patients with impaired smooth pursuit will be observed to have frequent small saccades when trying to keep up with the target. Because of this characteristic, the term saccadic pursuit is used to describe this type of impairment. Abnormalities of smooth pursuit can occur as a result of disorders throughout the central nervous system and also with the use of tranquilizers or alcohol. Patients with early or mild cerebellar degenerative disorders often complain of dizziness (typically imbalance), and usually have impaired smooth pursuit even when truncal and/or limb ataxia is minimally apparent.

Saccades
Saccadic eye movements are fast eye movements that are used to bring the image of an object quickly onto the fovea. These movements are generated by the burst neurons of the pons (horizontal movements) and the midbrain (vertical movements). A lesion or neuronal degeneration of these regions will lead to slow saccades. Slow saccades can occur with lesions of the ocular motor neurons or extraocular muscles. Severe slowing can be readily appreciated at the bedside by instructing the patient to look back and forth from one target to another. When testing saccades, the examiner observes both the velocity of the saccade and the accuracy. Overshooting saccades (hypermetric saccades, missing the target by passing it) typically

indicate a lesion of the cerebellum. Undershooting sacca-des (hypometric saccades) are less specific and to a small degree will occur even in normal persons.

Optokinetic nystagmus and fixation suppression of the vestibular ocular reflex

Optokinetic nystagmus (OKN) and fixation suppression of the vestibular ocular reflex (VOR) can also be informa-tive when examining dizzy patients at the bedside. OKN combines both saccadic and smooth pursuit movements. Though it is best tested using a full field stimulus, mov-ing a striped cloth in front of the patient can approximate OKN at the bedside. Fixation suppression of the vestibulo-ocular reflex (VOR suppression) can be tested at the bedside by having the patient sit in a swivel chair with an arm extended in the "thumbs up" position out in front. The patient is instructed to focus on the thumb and to allow the extended arm to move with the body so that the visual target (i.e., the patient's thumb) remains directly in front of the patient. The chair is then rotated from side to side and the patient's eyes are observed. Normally patients should be able to suppress the nystagmus that is stimulated by the rotation of the chair. If nystagmus is observed during the rotation movements, then there is an impairment of VOR suppression, which is analogous to impairment of smooth pursuit.

Vestibular nerve examination

The head thrust maneuver is a bedside test that directly assesses the VOR. The physiology involved in this test is analogous to that of the test for an afferent pupillary defect. To perform the head thrust maneuver, the physi-cian stands directly in front of the patient seated on the examination table. With the patient's head held in the examiner's hands, the patient is instructed to focus on the examiner's nose. The head is then quickly moved about 5–10° to one side. In patients with an intact VOR, the eyes will move in the direction opposite of the head movement. Therefore the patient's eyes will remain fix-ated on the examiner's nose after the sudden movement. The test is then repeated in the opposite direction. If the examiner observes a corrective saccade required to bring the patient's eyes back to the examiner's nose after the head thrust, impairment of the VOR in the direction of the head movement is identified. Though the doll's eye test can also assess the VOR, this test is not specific to the VOR because fully conscious patients can generate compensa-tory slow movements of the eyes in response to the slow rotation of the head by using the smooth pursuit system. However, the smooth pursuit system does not operate at a high velocity which is why the head thrust test is con-sidered to be a specific test of the VOR. Assessing smooth pursuit, the doll's eye test, the head thrust test, and the VOR suppression test can be helpful in identifying impair-ment of the smooth pursuit system, VOR, or both.

Positional testing

Though typically only thought of in terms of triggering benign paroxysmal positional vertigo (BPPV), positional testing can be extremely helpful in identifying central causes of dizziness. BPPV is caused by free-floating calcium carbonate debris, usually in the posterior semi-circular canal but occasionally in the horizontal canal or rarely the anterior canal. To test for posterior canal BPPV, the patient is taken from the sitting position to the head hanging left or head hanging right position (Dix–Hallpike test) (Figure 127.1). If BPPV is present, a burst of upbeat-torsional nystagmus is triggered on the side that is involved. The nystagmus usually lasts less than 30 sec-onds. If the patient is then brought back up to the sitting position, the debris will move in the opposite direction in the canal so that a burst of downbeat-torsional nystagmus will be seen. Placing these patients through the modified

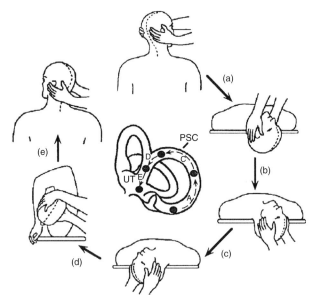

Figure 127.1 Treatment maneuver for benign paroxysmal positional vertigo affecting the right ear. The procedure can be reversed for treating the left ear. The drawing of the labyrinth in the center shows the position of the debris as it moves around the posterior semicircular canal (PSC) and into the utricle (UT). The patient is seated upright, with head facing the examiner, who is standing on the right. (a) The patient is then rapidly moved to head-hanging right position (Dix–Hallpike test). This position is maintained until the nystagmus ceases. (b) The examiner moves to the head of the table, repositioning hands as shown. (c) The head is rotated quickly to the left with right ear upward. This position is maintained for 30 seconds. (d) The patient rolls onto the left side while the examiner rapidly rotates the head leftward until the nose is directed toward the floor. This position is then held for 30 seconds. (e) The patient is rapidly lifted into the sitting position, now facing left. The entire sequence should be repeated until no nystagmus can be elicited. Following the maneuver, the patient is instructed to avoid head hanging positions to prevent the debris from re-entering the posterior canal. (Adapted from Rakel RE, editor. *Conn's Current Therapy*. Philadelphia: WB Saunders; 1995, p. 839 with permission from Elsevier.)

Epley maneuver is a highly effective therapy for patients with posterior canal BPPV, comparing to controls or sham procedures. If the debris is in the horizontal canal, a horizontal nystagmus is triggered by either the head hanging position or turning the patient's head to either side while the patient lies supine. The nystagmus of this variant can be either paroxysmal geotropic (beating toward the ground) or persistent apogeotropic (beating away from the ground). Importantly, a characteristic of the horizontal canal variant is that the nystagmus will change direction after the patient's head is turned to the opposite side. The side with the stronger nystagmus is typically the side with the debris in the horizontal canal. Various techniques have been reported to be effective in removing the debris in the horizontal canal, including rolling the patient toward the normal side and instructing the patient to lie on the normal side for several hours.

Central types of nystagmus can also be triggered by positional testing. Chiari malformations, mass lesions of the posterior fossa, or cerebellar ataxia syndromes are among the most common central nervous system disorders that can present with positional nystagmus. The most common pattern of central positional nystagmus is a persistent downbeat nystagmus which is readily distinguished from BPPV patterns of nystagmus, though the very rare anterior canal variant of BPPV can closely mimic this central pattern of nystagmus. Positional nystagmus may also be observed in patients with migraine-associated dizziness or multiple sclerosis.

Fistula testing
In patients reporting sound- or pressure-induced dizziness, testing for a defect of the bony capsule of the labyrinth can be performed by pressing and releasing the tragus and observing the eyes for brief associated deviations. Pneumatoscopy or Valsalva's maneuver performed against pinched nostrils or closed glottis can also trigger associated eye movements. The direction of the triggered nystagmus helps identify the location of the fistula.

Gait assessment
Since imbalance frequently occurs in patients with complaints of dizziness, a formal gait assessment is a critical part of the evaluation in these patients. The patient's casual gait is closely observed for ability to initiate gait, heel strike, stride length, base width, and general steadiness. The Romberg test and tandem walking are also important tests. A wide-based gait with the inability to tandem walk is considered to be a characteristic feature in patients with truncal ataxia due to midline cerebellar lesions. Patients with acute vestibular loss are unsteady and often veer or fall toward the side of the affected ear for several days after the event. The ability to walk unassisted may be an important discriminator in patients presenting with acute vertigo due to stroke versus vestibular

neuritis. A parkinsonian gait is characterized by small shuffling steps, narrow-based, flexed posture, reduced arm swing, en bloc turns, festination, and postural instability. Patients with peripheral neuropathy or bilateral vestibulopathy may be unable to stand in the Romberg position with eyes closed.

Auditory examination
The external auditory canal and tympanic membrane can be visualized during otoscopy. Since the advent of antimicrobial medications, pathology beginning in the external or middle ear only rarely extends into the inner ear, resulting in dizziness. The Ramsay–Hunt syndrome is a viral disorder caused by the varicella-zoster virus. In addition to vestibular nerve and facial nerve involvement, patients with this disorder usually have vesicles around the outer ear or in the external auditory canal. A fresh vesicle can be unroofed and the base of the vesicle can be swabbed. The cellular material is then rolled onto a sterile glass slide and tested for viral antigens using direct immunofluorescence.

The bedside hearing examination is not very sensitive when used as a screening tool for hearing loss, but it can provide important information. The whisper test has been shown to be the most sensitive test in picking up hearing loss at the bedside. Tuning fork tests, such as the Weber and Rinne tests, are commonly used at the bedside to test for sensorineural or conductive hearing loss. Simply asking patients to judge a difference in hearing quality on one side compared to the other using either finger rub or a tuning fork can also be informative. However, a standard audiogram is much more sensitive in picking up all types of hearing loss due to its ability to assess the wide spectrum of the auditory system.

Common presentations of dizziness

An effective strategy for diagnosing causes of dizziness is to first place patients into specific categories of dizziness based on information obtained from the history and physical examination (Table 127.2). The management of the patient, including testing and treatment, can be directed by the category of dizziness.

Vertigo
Acute severe vertigo
The patient presenting with new onset severe vertigo probably has vestibular neuritis, a presumed viral/post-viral disorder analogous to Bell's palsy, but stroke should also be a concern. An abrupt onset with accompanying focal neurological symptoms or signs suggests an ischemic stroke. Studies now demonstrate how closely a small stroke can mimic vestibular neuritis. Making the proper diagnosis is important because the management is drastically different, and because stroke is a potentially

Table 127.2 Important categories of dizziness and common causes.

Type of dizziness	Characteristics	Common causes
Vertigo	Visualized spinning	
Acute severe		Vestibular neuritis, stroke, Ramsay–Hunt syndrome
Recurrent attacks		Ménière's disease, transient ischemic attacks, migraine, vestibular paroxysmia
Recurrent positional vertigo		Benign paroxysmal positional vertigo, Chiari malformation, posterior fossa tumor, cerebellar degeneration
Presyncope	Near-faint	Orthostatic hypotension, vaso-vagal episodes, cardiac arrhythmia
Non-specific dizziness	Lightheadedness, motion intolerance, floating, internal spinning sensation, other "head" sensation	Medication side effect, cardiac arrhythmia, anxiety, metabolic disturbance, migraine, small vessel ischemic disease
Imbalance	Unsteady when walking without abnormal "head" sensation	Sensory loss syndromes, musculoskeletal causes, cerebellar disorders, parkinsonian syndrome, frontal cortex and subcortical white matter lesions, fear of falling

life-threatening disorder. The patient's age and accompanying risk factors for stroke should be considered. If no abnormalities are noted on the general neurological examination, attention should be directed to the neuro-otological evaluation. The clinician should search for spontaneous nystagmus and if none is observed, a technique to block visual fixation should be applied. The characteristics of the nystagmus should be noted and the effect of gaze on the nystagmus should be assessed. If a peripheral vestibular pattern of nystagmus is identified, a positive result on the head thrust test localizes the lesion to the vestibular nerve. In patients that are not at risk for stroke, the diagnosis can be presumed to be vestibular neuritis. On the other hand, in patients at risk for stroke, acute ischemia of the vestibular nerve, vestibular labyrinth, or even portions of the central vestibular pathway should be considered. When the head thrust test is negative, the possibility of a small brainstem or cerebellar stroke increases significantly. If hearing loss accompanies the episode, labyrinthitis is the most likely diagnosis, but auditory involvement does not exclude a vascular cause, because the anterior inferior cerebellar artery supplies both the inner ear and the brain. When hearing loss and facial weakness accompany acute onset vertigo, the examiner should closely inspect the outer ear for vesicles, caused by varicella-zoster viral infection (Ramsay–Hunt syndrome). An acoustic neuroma is a slow-growing tumor and thus does not typically cause acute onset vertigo. Migraine can mimic vestibular neuritis, although the diagnosis of migraine-associated vertigo hinges on recurrent episodes and lack of progressive auditory symptoms.

Recurrent attacks of vertigo

In patients with recurrent attacks of vertigo, the key diagnostic information lies in the details of the attacks. Ménière's disease is characterized by recurrent attacks of vertigo that generally last hours in duration and are associated with unilateral auditory symptoms. If Ménière-like

attacks manifest in a fulminant fashion, the diagnosis of autoimmune inner ear disease should be considered. Transient ischemic attacks (TIA) should be suspected in patients who report brief episodes (minutes) of vertigo, particularly when the patient is at risk for stroke and when other neurological symptoms, such as dysarthria, are reported. Spontaneous recurrent attacks of vertigo lasting seconds may be caused by scarring, compression, or irritation of the vestibular nerve on one side, a condition referred to as vestibular paroxysmia. Benign recurrent vertigo, characterized by recurrent episodes of vertigo without prominent hearing loss or auditory features, is considered to be a migraine equivalent because patients with this presentation typically have a history of other migraine features, normal findings on examination, a positive family history of migraine headaches, or other features characteristic of migraine.

Recurrent positional vertigo

Positional vertigo syndromes are characterized by the symptoms that are triggered, not simply worsened, by certain position changes. The typical history of a patient with BPPV is recurrent brief (less than 1 minute) episodes of vertigo that are triggered by rolling over in bed to one side, getting in and out of bed, or tilting the head back (top-shelf vertigo). The general medical and neurological examinations are normal in these patients and the neuro-otological examination is normal until positional testing uncovers the positionally triggered nystagmus. The posterior canal is the most commonly involved canal in BPPV and is readily treated by the Epley maneuver. Other potential causes should be considered when the findings are not typical of BPPV or when the patient does not respond to the treatment. However, central causes of positional vertigo generally do not have a burst of nystagmus and the nystagmus is typically down-beating in the head hanging position. If the head hanging tests (Dix–Hallpike testing) are negative, the examiner should search for horizontal canal variant of BPPV. Central positional nystagmus occurs as the result of disorders (e.g., tumors, cerebellar degeneration, Chiari malformation, or multiple sclerosis) that involve posterior fossa structures. The positional nystagmus of these disorders typically is down-beating and persistent, although pure torsional nystagmus may also occur. Finally, migraine can also mimic BPPV. Patients with migraine as the cause typically report a longer duration of symptoms once the positional vertigo is triggered, and the nystagmus may be of a central or peripheral type.

Non-specific dizziness

Non-specific dizziness refers to types of dizziness other than vertigo, imbalance, or presyncope. Because patients may have a difficult time describing their dizziness, characterizing the symptoms and performing a thorough examination are important processes because central vestibular or peripheral vestibular disorders can be identified even when the patient denies true vertigo.

When the symptom is episodic, one should consider a similar differential diagnosis to patients that have recurrent episodes of vertigo. However, anxiety or panic attacks should also be strongly considered. Patients with panic attacks can present with non-specific dizziness accompanied by other symptoms such as a sense of fear or doom, palpitations, sweating, shortness of breath, or paresthesiae. A patient's medication list should be thoroughly reviewed when the complaint is non-specific dizziness because medication side effects can cause episodes of dizziness or constant dizziness. Other medical conditions such as cardiac arrhythmias or metabolic disturbances, such as hypoglycemia, can also cause non-specific episodes of dizziness. Chronic types of dizziness commonly occur in patients who also have migraine headaches or other migraine features. Though the underlying mechanisms leading to migraine-associated dizziness are not yet clear, evidence suggests it can stem from either peripheral or central disturbances. In the elderly, confluent white matter hyperintensities have a strong association with dizziness and balance problems. Presumably the result of small vessel arteriosclerosis, decreased cerebral perfusion has been identified in these patients even when blood pressure taken at the arm is normal. Patients with dizziness associated with white matter hyperintensities typically have impaired balance and they usually feel better sitting or lying down.

Imbalance

Common causes of imbalance include sensory loss syndromes, musculoskeletal causes, cerebellar disorders, parkinsonian syndromes, frontal cortex and subcortical white matter lesions, and fear of falling. Loss of somatosensory, vestibular, and/or visual systems comprise sensory loss syndromes because impairment of any of these afferent systems leads to reduced information about the position of the head and body in space. Because so many genetic causes of hearing loss are now known, bilateral vestibular loss due to genetic causes is probably underrecognized. Musculoskeletal disorders remain a major cause of imbalance simply based upon the prevalence of arthritis and injuries. Abnormalities of the joints can usually be identified and patients typically have an antalgic gait. However, spinal stenosis, caused by degenerative changes in the cervical spine, can lead to cervical spondylotic myelopathy (CSM) in which patients can predominantly present with imbalance. Patients with CSM usually have increased reflexes and may have other signs of spasticity, including increased tone and a spastic gait; however, sensory findings are variable and incontinence is surprisingly rare. Cerebellar causes of imbalance usually have an obvious ataxic gait pattern and associated with ocular motor signs including spontaneous vertical nystagmus, gaze-evoked nystagmus, central positional nystagmus, saccadic dysmetria, and impaired smooth pursuit. When ataxia is acute in onset a stroke of the cerebellum should be considered. When an ataxic presentation is subacute in onset but rapidly progressive, an autoimmune ataxia, postinfectious cerebellitis, paraneoplastic disorder, cerebellar tumor, or even the Brownell–Oppenheimer variant of Creutzfeldt–Jakob disease should be considered. The spectrum of genetic ataxias continues to expand. There are now 30 autosomal dominant spinocerebellar ataxia (SCA) syndromes that have been reported or have a designation reserved. Significant overlapping features among these disorders are common and variability also occurs even in patients with the same mutation. Most of the SCA subtypes have so far been described in single families. SCA1, SCA2, SCA3, SCA6, and SCA7 are the most common autosomal dominant subtypes worldwide, but some SCA types aggregate in certain geographical locations. Other important genetic causes of ataxia include Friedreich's ataxia and the fragile X-associated tremor–ataxia syndrome.

Parkinsonian syndromes which may present with non-specific dizziness or imbalance include Parkinson's disease, progressive supranuclear palsy, and multiple systems atrophy. However, over time other features including a characteristic gait disorder, ocular motor abnormalities, and autonomic failure will develop so that a more specific classification can be made. Frontal gait disorders are similar to parkinsonian disorders, but the gait is characterized by impaired initiation and a magnetic-type gait. In addition, these patients typically do not have rest tremor or cogwheel rigidity. The most common cause of this disorder is probably the multi-infarct syndrome. Patients with this syndrome will have prominent and confluent white matter hyperintensities on brain MRI and presumably these hyperintensities interrupt long loop reflexes that are important for gait and balance. Patients with this syndrome typically have cardiovascular risk factors, but genetic factors likely play a major role in subgroups without prominent cardiovascular risk factors. Patients with normal pressure hydrocephalus (NPH) can also present with a frontal type of gait disturbance. These patients also typically have cognitive impairment and urinary incontinence. A required finding for the diagnosis of NPH is enlargement of the lateral ventricles out of proportion to the degree of generalized atrophy. Finally, fear of falling is common among older people and studies have demonstrated an association between the fear of falling and poor balance performance. Though many of these patients likely have an underlying reason for the fear of falling (e.g., a previous injury from a fall), some individuals who have never fallen and who do not demonstrate impaired balance have high levels of fear of falling.

Management of the patient with dizziness

Symptomatic dizziness can be reduced with the use of medications such as meclizine, benzodiazepines, or antiemetics. These medicines are generally only effective in reducing the symptom and are not preventative.

The management of the patient with dizziness must be driven by the information gathered from the history and physical examination. When a specific disorder is identified treatments should be directed toward that disorder. Patients with vestibular neuritis may benefit from a brief course of corticosteroids. Patients with stroke or TIA should undergo an appropriate assessment to identify the cause and also to prevent a recurrence. Patients with Ménière's disease may improve with a low-salt diet. Though diuretics are usually tried, the benefit of diuretics has yet to be shown in Ménière's disease. Benign recurrent vertigo or chronic dizziness that is presumed to be a migraine phenomenon should first be addressed by instructing the patient in lifestyle modifications such as adequate sleep, stress reduction techniques, regular exercise, and identifying and avoiding any food triggers. If these measures are ineffective, medications for migraine prophylaxis may then be considered, but formal clinical trials of these medicines for treating dizziness are lacking. The repositional maneuvers are highly effective in treating benign paroxysmal positional vertigo.

Patients with non-specific chronic dizziness who are taking several medications should probably undergo trials of reducing the number of medications as an initial step. Anxiety or panic attacks can be treated with general lifestyle measures, combined with serotonin-acting medications. Patients with cardiac arrhythmias causing dizziness should be evaluated by their general internist or a cardiologist. No specific treatment is known to help improve the symptoms of dizziness in patients with severe white matter hyperintensities, but since a flow-related phenomenon could be a factor, patients taking blood pressure lowering medications may note reduced dizziness when those medications are lowered.

Patients with imbalance demonstrated on examination will usually benefit from a formal physical therapy program. Patients with a parkinsonian syndrome may benefit from a trial of levodopa, but this medication has not been shown to improve balance performance and any benefit in patients other than those with Parkinson's disease are generally short-lived. Treating painful joints can help improve the balance of patients who have arthritis as the cause of the gait disorder. Some patients with cervical spondylotic myelopathy will improve or stabilize after surgery to correct it. Patients with a presumed autoimmune ataxia have the potential to benefit from treatments aimed at reducing the immune response, though formal trials are lacking. There is no known treatment for patients who have spinocerebellar ataxia syndromes. These patients should be instructed in fall prevention strategies, encouraged to exercise regularly, and stay as healthy as possible.

Tests

Tests in clinical medicine should be selected based on the patient's clinical presentation and the likelihood of identifying a clinically relevant finding. If neither a positive nor a negative result of a test will change management, the test is probably not warranted. For both new and old tests, properly designed studies are critical for determining the range of normal results, diagnostic accuracy, variability, and the potential role of the testing clinical medicine.

Imaging studies

Imaging studies are the gold standard for identifying and often diagnosing structural lesions of the brain. Though computerized tomography (CT) can rule out a large mass, small lesions and acute ischemia cannot be excluded by CT because of artifacts and poor resolution in the posterior fossa. Because of these limitations, MRI is the imaging modality of choice but is expensive and may not be readily available in many areas. Determining which patients should have an MRI can be difficult. Patients diagnosed with BPPV, vestibular neuritis, or Ménière's disease do not require an imaging study. Patients with normal neurologic and neuro-otologic examinations who report dizziness dating back more than several months are unlikely to have a pertinent abnormality on MRI. In patients experiencing focal neurological symptoms, having unexplained neurological deficits, or an otherwise rapid unexplained progression of symptoms, an MRI may be the critical factor in identifying a tumor or other structural disorder. MRA should be considered in patients who have recurrent attacks of dizziness suspicious for transient ischemic attacks, because a focal narrowing in the posterior circulation may be amendable to endovascular treatments if medical treatment fails. MRI of the cervical spine is the test of choice when cervical spondylosis is suspected, though plain radiographs, CT of the cervical spine, or CT myelogram could also provide the key information.

Vestibular laboratory tests

Vestibular laboratory testing can help to identify and quantify a unilateral or bilateral vestibulopathy and ocular motor abnormalities. Usefulness of the test is highly dependent upon test administration, patient cooperation, and test interpretation. Artifacts are common and there is generally a wide range of normal values. Abnormal findings on these tests must be put in the context of the patient's presentation and clinical findings. Vestibular testing does not add additional information in patients with BPPV, patients diagnosed with vestibular neuritis having a positive head thrust test, or in patients with bedside central nervous system findings, unless quantifying the abnormality is important. The caloric test is the most sensitive and readily available laboratory test for identifying and quantifying a unilateral vestibulopathy. The rotational chair test is the test of choice for identifying and quantifying a bilateral vestibulopathy.

Auditory testing

Because of well-established standards and formal certified training programs, audiograms are a reliable and reproducible test. Audiograms are not subject to as many artifacts and subjective interpretations of vestibular testing. Because the hearing and balance organs are close in proximity, connected as part of the labyrinth, share overlapping vascular supply, and have key nervous system components in close proximity with a common trunk entering the brain stem, a lesion of one system generally affects the other. For patients complaining of vertigo, with or without hearing loss, obtaining an audiogram may be helpful in making a diagnosis or at least in establishing the patient's baseline hearing for later comparison. Although Ménière's disease is characterized by hearing loss in addition to vertigo and tinnitus, the auditory symptoms may not develop in the early stages or patients may not perceive the hearing loss.

Common presentations of hearing loss

Patients with the primary complaint of hearing loss do not generally present to neurologists for an evaluation; however, hearing loss can be an important finding in patients who complain of dizziness or imbalance. Therefore it is important for the neurologist to be familiar with common types of hearing loss.

Asymmetrical sensorineural hearing loss

Evaluation of patients identified as having asymmetrical hearing loss is primarily the search for a tumor in the area of the internal auditory canal or cerebellopontine angle, or more rarely other lesions of the temporal bone or brain. Unfortunately, there is no simple validated rule for deciding when a brain image should be performed in a patient with asymmetrical hearing loss, so clinical judgment is required. A history of gradually progressive unilateral loss and a large difference between the two sides is highly suggestive of a structural lesion. When the hearing loss is in the low frequencies and the patient also has recurrent episodes of vertigo, a diagnosis of Ménière's disease can be made.

Sudden sensorineural hearing loss

The etiology of sudden sensorineural hearing loss is similar to that of both Bell's palsy and vestibular neuritis. A viral cause is presumed in the majority of cases, but proof of a viral pathophysiology in a given case is difficult to obtain. The hearing loss in this situation is generally unilateral and it usually evolves over several hours. Sudden sensorineural hearing loss can result in permanent severe hearing loss, though some patients will regain normal hearing. Focal ischemia affecting the cochlea, cochlear nerve, or the root entry zone can also cause abrupt loss of hearing over several minutes. In a patient at risk for stroke, this should be considered early because it can be the harbinger of basilar artery occlusion.

Hearing loss with age

Presbycusis is the bilateral hearing loss commonly associated with advancing age. It is not a distinct entity but rather represents multiple effects of aging on the auditory system. It may include conductive and central dysfunction, but the most consistent effect of aging is on the sensory cells in the neurons of the cochlea. The typical audiogram appearance in patients with presbycusis is that of symmetrical hearing loss, with the tracing gradually sloping downward with increasing frequency. The most consistent pathological condition associated with presbycusis is a degeneration of sensory cells and nerve fibers at the base of the cochlea.

Genetic hearing loss

Genetic research into hearing loss is probably among the most advanced research in any genetic condition. Likely because of a sensitive marker (i.e., audiogram) and also a phenotype that can be associated with disability, affected families are readily identifiable and phenotypable. Most hereditary hearing loss disorders are autosomal recessive, but autosomal dominant causes are common, and X-linked and mitochondrial forms are also described. Much heterogeneity exists among the many genetic causes and some variability also occurs among patients with the same genetic cause. The non-syndromic hereditary hearing loss disorders typically present with sensorineural hearing loss that can persist in a mild form or progress to profound deafness. Autosomal recessive types typically are severe to profound deafness, prelingual and non-progressive, whereas autosomal dominant types are usually postlingual and progressive from mild to severe.

Common presentations of tinnitus

Tinnitus is a noise in the ear that usually is audible only to the patient, although occasionally the sound can be heard by the examining physician. It is a symptom that can be associated with a variety of disorders affecting the ear or the brain. The most important piece of information is whether the patient localizes it to one or both ears, or whether it is not localizable. Tinnitus that localizes to one ear has a much higher likelihood of having an identifiable cause than tinnitus that localizes to both ears or that is non-localizable. The characteristics of the tinnitus can provide helpful information. For example, the typical tinnitus associated with Ménière's disease is described as a roaring sound, like listening to a seashell. The tinnitus associated with an acoustic neuroma typically is a high-pitched ringing or resembles the sound of steam blowing from a tea kettle. If the tinnitus is rhythmic, the patient should be asked whether it is synchronous with the pulse or with respiration. Recurrent rhythmic or even non-rhythmic clicking sounds in one ear can indicate stapedial myoclonus. The most common form of tinnitus is a bilateral high-pitched sound that is usually worse at night with less background noise to mask it. It may worsen when the patient is under stress, or with the use of caffeine.

Conclusion

Neuro-otologic symptoms are among the most common reasons for a patient to seek medical care and accordingly have been shown to be highly prevalent in population-based studies. A detailed description of the patient's symptoms must be obtained because patients often use the dizziness terms interchangeably and will use "dizziness"' to report any ill feeling. When considering international aspects of dizziness, delineating the terms that are used in various geographical locations and cultures is of paramount importance. Similar terms may radically differ in their connotations from one region to another. The examination is also of critical importance because it localizes the lesion. From this information, the management can be determined.

Further reading

Adams PF, Hendershot GE, Marano MA. Current estimates from the National Health Interview Survey, 1996. *Vital Health Stat* 1999; 10(200): 1–203.

Aw ST, Todd MJ, Aw GE, McGarvie LA, Halmagyi GM. Benign positional nystagmus: a study of its three-dimensional spatio-temporal characteristics. *Neurology* 2005; 64: 1897–905.

Baloh RW, Honrubia V. *Clinical Neurophysiology of the Vestibular System*, 3rd ed. New York: Oxford University Press; 2001.

Colledge N, Lewis S, Mead G, Sellar R, Wardlaw J, Wilson J. Magnetic resonance brain imaging in people with dizziness: a comparison with non-dizzy people. *J Neurol Neurosurg Psychiatry* 2002; 72: 587–9.

Fife TD, Tusa RJ, Furman JM, *et al.* Assessment: vestibular testing techniques in adults and children: report of the Therapeutics and Technology Assessment Subcommittee of the American Academy of Neurology. *Neurology* 2000; 55: 1431–41.

Gouw AA, Van der Flier WM, van Straaten EC, *et al.* Simple versus complex assessment of white matter hyperintensities in relation to physical performance and cognition: the LADIS study. *J Neurol* 2006; 253: 1189–96.

Hajioff D, Barr-Hamilton RM, Colledge NR, Lewis SJ, Wilson JA. Is electronystagmography of diagnostic value in the elderly? *Clin Otolaryngol Allied Sci* 2002; 27: 27–31.

Halmagyi GM, Curthoys IS. A clinical sign of canal paresis. *Arch Neurol* 1988; 45: 737–9.

Lee H, Sohn SI, Cho YW, *et al.* Cerebellar infarction presenting isolated vertigo: frequency and vascular topographical patterns. *Neurology* 2006; 67: 1178–83.

Lethbridge-Cejku M, Rose D, Vickerie J. Summary statistics for US adults: National Health Interview Survey, 2004. National Center for Health Statistics. *Vital Health Stat* 2006; 10(228): 1–154.

Neuhauser HK, von Brevern M, Radtke A, *et al.* Epidemiology of vestibular vertigo: a neurotologic survey of the general population. *Neurology* 2005; 65: 898–904.

von Brevern M, Zeise D, Neuhauser H, Clarke AH, Lempert T. Acute migrainous vertigo: clinical and oculographic findings. *Brain* 2005; 128: 365–74.

Chapter 128
Clinical approaches in neuro-ophthalmology

Anuchit Poonyathalang
Ramathibodi Hospital, Bangkok, Thailand

Introduction

Neuro-ophthalmology, a subspecialty of both ophthalmology and neurology, deals with disorders of the visual, ocular motor, and pupillary systems. The treatment of the purely ophthalmologic disorders should be carried out by ophthalmologists, ophthalmologic specialists, or neuro-ophthalmologists.

Clinical approach to visual loss

Transient visual loss

Patients with transient visual loss should be approached by characterizing the visual loss, including duration and pattern of visual obscuration, the patient's age, and associated symptoms and signs (Table 128.1).

Duration

Binocular visual loss for less than 10 seconds may occur in papilledema with or without postural change. Visual field tests reveal enlarged blind spots with normal visual acuity and normal color vision in the early phase. In the late stage, there is peripheral constriction of the visual field. True edema of the optic nerve head can be confirmed by MRI or ocular ultrasonography. Disc anomalies such as optic disc drusen, high myopia, and coloboma are sometimes confused with edema. In optic disc drusen, discs are scalloped but have a clear edge, are elevated but small in diameter, with whitish-yellow refractile bodies without vascular congestion. Visual field tests often show enlarged blind spot or arcuate scotoma. Ultrasound examination of the optic nerve head and fundus fluorescein angiography (FFA) are usually used to confirm the buried drusen. Optic disc drusen is rare in some countries, such as Thailand. Orbital tumor especially optic nerve sheath meningioma can compress the nerve when the eye moves in a certain direction and cause visual loss with specific directions of gaze. Mild proptosis, subtle relative afferent pupillary defect (RAPD), visual field loss, optociliary shunt vessels, and choroidal fold are common findings. Imaging studies help differentiate the lesion. Young patients with migraine or vasospasm may have visual disturbances lasting seconds to hours. Scintillating scotoma in migraine usually lasts about 15–30 minutes. Headache and nausea are common associated symptoms. Retinal migraine has been reported on rare occasions; transient monocular visual loss with demonstrated visual field defect and correlated retinal artery spasm were temporary findings. Amaurosis fugax, with visual loss lasting for several minutes to half an hour, are caused by retinovascular and cerebrovascular disorders. Platelet or cholesterol emboli can be found in retinal arteries, commonly at bifurcations. Carotid bruit may be audible, but plaque and degree of stenosis should be confirmed by carotid ultrasound and Doppler, Magnetic resonance arteriography (MRA), computerized tomographic arteriography (CTA), or angiography.

Pattern of visual loss

Pattern of visual loss and recovery of vision can be useful in defining the cause of the lesion. An altitudinal pattern with black shade closing down the vision and gradually lifting up while returning vision over several minutes is seen with carotid artery disease (emboli from the proximal carotid artery). Gradual constriction of visual field resembling a camera diaphragm closing in and then opening out from the center during recovery is associated with cardiac arrhythmia or severe stenosis of the great vessels. In patients with vascular risk factors, usually in individuals over 50 years of age, the amaurosis fugax may also precede non-arteritic ischemic optic neuropathy or central retinal artery occlusion. Investigation and preventive treatment should be carried out in those patients. Younger patients may develop brief episodes of binocular visual loss from involvement of the occipital cortex commonly associated with migraine. In patients with migraine, visual loss usually involves a partial field defect during the attack, while in other disorders there is usually loss of the entire visual field. Rarely in patients with frequent recurrent episodes of migraine the visual field defect may become permanent. MRI should be performed

International Neurology: A Clinical Approach. Edited by Robert P. Lisak, Daniel D. Truong, William M. Carroll, and Roongroj Bhidayasiri. © 2009 Blackwell Publishing, ISBN: 978-1-4051-5738-4.

Table 128.1 Clinical aspects of transient visual loss.

	Optic nerve head disorders		Cardiovascular disorders	Migraine	Vasospasm
	Papilledema	Drusen			
Period of visual loss	<10 seconds	10–30 seconds	Few minutes to half an hour	20–30 minutes	Seconds to 1 hour
Laterality	Bilateral	Asymmetrical (bilateral ~80%)	Ocular: unilateral Brain: bilateral	Ocular: unilateral Brain: bilateral	Bilateral
Pattern of visual field loss	Enlarged blind spot	Enlarged blind spot or arcuate scotoma	Shading down and up, iris diaphragm	Scintillating scotoma	Blackout of all fields
Age of patient	Any age	Average 22 years (7–70 years)	>50 years	<50 years	
Fundus findings	Large, blurred, congested disc	Scalloped edge, normal vessels	Emboli, cotton wool spot, hemorrhage	Retinal artery spasm or normal	Normal or cherry-red spot
Laboratory	Ultrasound 30° test	Ultrasound, high spike	FFA delayed filling	—	Nail capillaries
Treatment	Reduce ICP	None	Antiplatelets, carotid surgery	Tryptans for acute attack, etc.	Vasodilator

FFA: fundus fluorescein angiography; ICP: intracranial pressure.

to rule out cerebral arteriovenous (AV) malformations. Vasoconstriction of retinal vessels and transient loss of vascular supply of the optic nerve and visual pathways have been reported. Other systemic vascular related disorders that may decrease blood supply to the eye include systemic lupus erythematosus (SLE), antiphospholipid syndrome, hyperviscosity syndrome, hypercoagulable disorders, and, in patients over 60 years old, extracranial giant cell arteritis. Cortical transient ischemic attacks characterized by symmetrical bilateral fleeting blindness associated with ataxia, vertigo, or double vision occur with vertebrobasilar insufficiency.

Ocular disorders

Ocular disorders causing transient visual loss can be painless or painful. Painful transient visual loss can be found in acute episodes of closed angle, acute uveitis, and glaucomatocyclitic crisis. Visual losses in those patients are described as foggy or blurry; visual deficits are not entirely dark as in vascular obstruction. Non-painful ocular disorders that can cause transient visual loss include vitreous floaters in which the area of decreased visual field moves with the eye movement, corneal punctuate epithelial erosion, or dry spots on the cornea, which improve by blinking or topical tears supplement. Other causes include recurrent hyphema in uveitis–glaucoma–hemorrhage syndrome; here the patient usually describes blurred red vision. In macular-retinal diseases blurring after exposure to bright light is reported. Patients who have central retinal vein occlusion (CRVO), venous stasis retinopathy, or ocular ischemic syndrome can also experience amaurosis fugax. The fundus of patients with CRVO may have an appearance mimicking papilledema.

Venous stasis retinopathy and ocular ischemic syndromes may have fundus resemble diabetic retinopathy. Fundus fluorescein angiogram (FFA) is a helpful diagnostic aid. Investigation to detect any underlying compromise of circulation such as hypertension, dural arteriovenous malformations (DAVM), or carotid artery stenosis, should be performed. Patients with DAVM usually have low flow vascular reversal and a small number of patients may also have venous stasis retinopathy.

Sudden visual loss
Monocular sudden visual loss

Patients with sudden visual loss may experience their symptoms when they awaken or while awake. A common disorder is anterior ischemic optic neuropathy (AION). AION typically presents with profound painless monocular visual loss. In patients over 60 years of age, AION from giant cell arteritis, although less common (5–10% of all AION), must be considered until proven otherwise. This disorder is covered in Chapter 15. Since 20% of patients with AION have no systemic symptoms, investigations should be carried out in every AION patient over 55 years of age. Another form of AION is non-arteritic anterior ischemic optic neuropathy (NAION). NAION is less severe than arteritic AION; the usual patient is younger, 50–60 years of age. Altitudinal blindness on waking up is a common presentation. Associated risk factors are hypertension, diabetes mellitus (DM), dyslipidemia, and smoking. Nocturnal hypotension, sleep apnea syndrome, and treatment with sildenafil or related medications are reportedly associated factors. Altitudinal pale segment with a partly hyperemic swollen disc, cotton wool spot, flame-shaped hemorrhage, and attenuated retinal vessels are typical fundus findings. The fellow eye usually has a disc at risk that is characterized by a small ratio of disc-vein width, diameter less than 1500 μm and no physiologic cup. Visual field tests demonstrate an altitudinal field defect in the affected eye and a small blind spot in the fellow eye. FFA demonstrates delay and slow filling of the optic nerve head without choroidal ischemia. There is no proven effective treatment for the affected eye. A combination of high-dose corticosteroids, aspirin, and pentoxyphylline has been associated with significant improvement of the visual field but not visual acuity. Cause and effect have not been demonstrated. Prevention of an attack in the second eye by aspirin during the subsequent 2 years has been reported. NAION in younger patients (around 40–50 years old) has similar presentation and similar risk factors, but antiphospholipid syndrome has been proposed as an additional risk factor.

Central retinal artery occlusion (CRAO) typically presents as painless monocular blindness. Profound visual loss is common, with visual acuity reduced to hand motion or even no light perception. Markedly impaired pupillay light reaction, RAPD, pale optic disc, pale and edematous retina with foveal sparing (so-called cherry-red spot), and retinal vessel attenuation with possible emboli are typical findings. Associated severe headache and neck pain should raise the possibility of carotid dissection. Common sources of emboli are from the carotid artery and heart. Rare entities such as vasospasm, hypercoagulability, and antiphospholipid syndrome may be the etiology. Emboli are visible in about 10% of cases, compared to 70% in branch retinal artery occlusion (BRAO). Systemic vasculitis and giant cell arteritis should be considered (see Chapter 15). Immediate treatment is required. Anterior chamber paracentesis, ocular massage, sublingual vasodilator, antiglaucoma medications, and anticoagulants are employed, but proof of efficacy is limited. There is no established period to retinal ischemia in humans.

Cortical occipital or subcortical lesions are common causes of sudden binocular loss of vision. Symptoms are homonymous visual field loss, typically congruous homonymous hemianopia; other patterns are tubular visual field, checkerboard, and key-hole appearances. The homonymous hemianopia from the occipital cortical lesion has a sharp vertical midline and a symmetrical pattern rather than asymmetrical tilted hemianopia of the optic tract lesion. Pituitary apoplexy can cause sudden bitemporal hemianopic visual field loss by acute compression of the optic chiasm.

Acute to subacute visual loss

Visual loss, progressing for days or weeks, is acute to subacute. Etiologies are inflammation with or without degeneration, acute compression, and toxins.

Optic neuritis

Optic neuritis is one of the most common causes of acute to subacute visual loss. Visual acuity is variable, from 20/20 to no light perception. In the Optic Neuritis Treatment Trial (ONTT) 77% of patients were female, between the ages of 20 and 50 years, with a mean age of 32 years. A large central scotoma is common and patients may describe preservation of peripheral vision. In the ONTT study the most common reported visual field defect was a diffuse scotoma. Dyschromatopsia is also noted by patients; objects appear as if there is a gray filter in front of the object, or red becomes orange or pink or rarely black or white. Optic neuritis causes demyelination and axonal loss and results in type 2 red–green defect that is more accurately detected by special tests. The degree of poor pupillary reaction to light and dyschromatopsia is often out of proportion to the degree of visual loss. Orbital pain or supraorbital pain particularly with eye movement is characteristic. Prolonged latency time of visual evoked potential (VEP) confirms the decreased ability of nerve conduction by demyelination and can be useful to determine prior optic neuritis (ON) in the uninvolved eye. Based on location, there are two types of ON: anterior or papillitis and retrobulbar. About two-thirds of patients with ON have retrobulbar ON. Since retrobulbar ON is a common presentation of demyelinating diseases, MRI scan of the brain to detect white matter lesions should be performed. The risk of multiple sclerosis (MS) is higher in patients with than without white matter lesions. In some non-Western countries, the risk of MS is still considered low using available criteria. Atypical ON is considered if there is lack of improvement in 3 months or if there is severe pain, ocular inflammatory signs, or disc swelling with exudates. In atypical ON laboratory tests for collagen vascular disease and vasculitis (anti-DNA, antinuclear antibody, erythrocyte sedimentation rate (ESR), Lupus-erythematosus-cell (LE) preparation), syphilis (Venereal Disease Research Laboratory (VDRL) the fluorescent treponemal antibody absorbed (FTAABS) test) and sarcoidosis (chest X-ray or CT scan, gallium scan, serum angiotensin-converting enzyme) should be performed. Other rare causes of optic neuritis are Devic's disease, HIV, cytomegalovirus, herpes virus, *Cryptococcus*, toxoplasmosis, tuberculosis, aspergillosis and Dengue virus. Bilateral ON is common in children; infection and post-viral reaction are more likely etiology than an attack of MS. In children with bilateral or unilateral retrobulbar ON, imaging study of the sphenoid and ethmoid sinuses should be performed. Treatment of idiopathic demyelinating ON is based on visual acuity of the affected and the fellow eye, systemic disorder, and pain. With initial visual acuity better than 20/40 visual outcome is generally excellent, and thus no treatment may be required. When the patient has more severe visual loss, involvement of the only functional eye, or severe discomfort, intravenous methylprednisolone 1 g/day for 3–5 days and possibly oral corticosteroid taper should be strongly considered. Benefits of methylprednisolone treatment are shortening the time of visual recovery and perhaps reduction of clinical definite MS development in the first 2 years. Systemic disorders such as poorly controlled diabetes, systemic infections, active peptic ulcer disease, marked gastresophageal reflux disease (GERD) and early pregnancy may be relative contraindications.

Leber's hereditary optic neuropathy (LHON)

Another cause of acute to subacute central visual field loss is LHON. Males (80–90%) are affected more than females. It occurs mainly in the second or third decade of life. Apart from some reports of associated disorders such as cardiac conduction abnormalities or muscle anomalies, most of the patients are otherwise healthy. This painless visual loss usually reduces vision to 20/200–5/200 with a subtle decrease of pupillary light reaction. The interval between first and second eye involvement is weeks to months. In this period between attacks, RAPD may be present. Deep small central scotoma (about 10–15 degrees) on visual field testing helps to differentiate LHON from malingering with tubular visual field defects. Two-thirds of male patients have typical disc appearance of disc swelling without fluorescein leakage (pseudoedema) on FFA, peripapillary telangiectasia, dilated surface capillaries, tortuosity of medium-sized retinal arterioles, and haziness of nerve fiber layers. Genetic mitochondrial transmission passes from mother to offspring. High percentages of mutated mitochondrial DNA cause overt clinical disease (heteroplasmy). Why males should have more clinical occurrence than females is unknown (see Chapter 159). Patients with mutation at 14 484 are less common than those with mutation at 11 778 but have a better chance of some recovery of vision. Overall, partial visual recovery is about 10–20%. No treatment has been proved effective.

Neuro-retinitis

Neuro-retinitis is inflammation of the disc and the retina with a macular star on examination. Fluid leakage from optic disc capillaries accumulates and forms a white streak radiating sunburst pattern of exudates around the fovea within 1–2 weeks. Visual defects include acuity of 20/40–20/200, decreased color vision, and visual field defect. RAPD and vitreous cells are frequently present. Infections such as syphilis, toxoplasmosis, Lyme disease, and cat scratch disease should be ruled out.

Idiopathic orbital inflammatory syndrome (IOIS)

IOIS or orbital pseudotumor causes visual loss by three mechanisms. First, diffuse inflammation compresses the proximal optic nerve. In this setting, patients may experience combinations of acute pain, vascular

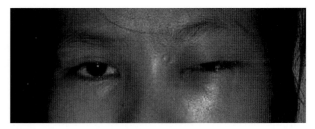

Figure 128.1 External appearance of orbital apex syndrome from gnathostomiasis with optic nerve compression.

congestion, chemosis, lid swelling, ptosis, violaceous injection, limitation of eye movements, proptosis, and optic disc swelling. Second, a posterior scleritis can cause visual loss by associated papillitis, choroiditis, uveitis, or exudative retinal detachment. Inflammation of the optic nerve sheath (perioptic neuritis) is the third mechanism. In this setting, optic nerve sheath inflammation results in disc swelling and retinal vascular congestion. Other disorders that can cause perioptic neuritis are syphilis, *Cryptococcus*, tuberculosis, and carcinomatous meningitis. MRI and ultrasound can be useful for diagnosis. Treatments include high-dose systemic steroids in early phases along with medications for associated infections. Systemic steroid and immunosuppressive agents are used for tapering; long-term low doses are used in recurrent disease. In children, orbital cellulitis is more common than IOIS. Infection usually spreads from adjacent sinuses, and from root canal abscess. Rarely parasitic infection can cause orbital cellulitis with optic neuropathy (Figure 128.1).

Thyroid-associated orbitopathy (TAO)

In the inflammatory form of TAO, acute optic nerve compression can occur and present with the orbital apex syndrome or solely optic nerve dysfunction. Acute central scotoma or diffuse visual field defect along with optic disc edema and RAPD can be observed. Other signs of TAO such as lid retraction, limitation of upward gaze, mild proptosis, lid edema, and conjunctival chemosis help confirm diagnosis. MRI may show the so-called four-leaf-clover-like enlargement of the four rectus muscles, compressing the optic nerve. Intravenous high-dose steroid should be administered on an urgent basis. Orbital radiation or orbital decompression is considered if the steroid treatment is ineffective. After recovery and tapering of steroids, if the optic neuropathy recurs, antithyroglobulin antibody and other thyroid antibodies should be tested to rule out thyroid-associated autoimmune optic neuropathy. Long-term steroid treatment is indicated.

Acute glaucoma

Patients usually present with very painful, acute to subacute as opposed to sudden visual loss. Some complain of severe headache with pain-induced hypertension, and may be mistakenly thought to have headache associated with hypertension or stroke. Foggy vision, corneal haziness, semidilated fixed pupil, ciliary injection, very high ocular pressure, and contralateral shallow anterior chamber are clues to the diagnosis. Urgent treatment by an ophthalmologist is critical.

In a patient with monocular visual loss described as a shade slowly coming down, the pupil should be dilated to search for retinal detachment. Flashing lights and floaters are common preceding symptoms. Presence of loss of visual acuity depends on the area of detachment, with macular involvement causing the greatest deficit. RAPD may not be present if the detached area is small. Examination by direct ophthalmoscope reveals a pale wavy retina, but with shallow detachment the retina may appear normal. With opaque media, ultrasound is always used to detect the obscured retinal detachment.

Radiation optic neuropathy (RON)
RON also presents with subacute severe painless visual loss. Symptoms may develop from 18 months to 10 years, with an average of 1 year, after radiation treatment of sella and parasellar tumors, nasopharyngeal, or intraocular tumors. Anterior RON shows disc edema and radiation retinopathy with cotton wool spots and hemorrhages. Retrobulbar RON is difficult to differentiate from recurrent tumor or empty sella syndrome. Treatment with high-dose systemic steroid is commonly employed, but efficacy is still unproven.

Methanol toxicity
Methanol ingestion can cause profound visual loss even with ingestion of small amounts. Vomiting, abdominal pain, bilateral visual loss, reduced level of consciousness, or coma may develop over 18–48 hours. Patients usually have a history of consuming homemade alcoholic beverages. Since the marked bilateral disc swelling resembles papilledema, increased intracranial pressure should be ruled out. Treatment includes dialysis, bicarbonate for metabolic acidosis, and intravenous ethanol to interfere with methanol metabolism.

Chronic visual loss
Ocular disorders
Cataract
Cataract causes opacity of the lens causing subtle decline of vision over years. The majority of cases can be detected by penlight, except for posterior subcapsular cataract (PSC). PSC has a thin layer of opacity deep in the lens and can be missed even with a slit lamp. Visual acuity of PSC in bright light is far worse than in room light. After pupillary dilation this type of cataract can be detected more easily. Decreased red reflex through the direct ophthalmoscope is an important clue. However, vitreous hemorrhage with dense brown or black cataract (cataract nigra) can also give a very dark red reflex. Ultrasonography is generally

used to differentiate the nature of opacity, whether the opacity is in the anterior or posterior segment.

Glaucoma
Chronic open angle glaucoma is an optic neuropathy caused by slowly increasing intraocular pressure (IOP), ganglion cell death, and nerve fiber layer loss. Enlarged optic disc cup in glaucoma is more likely to be vertical than horizontal. Visual field defects begin with arcuate scotomas; double arcuate scotomas may result in a tubular field of vision in late stages. The optic disc rim is not pale in glaucomatous optic neuropathy. Normal-tension glaucoma occurs in patients who do not have increased intraocular pressure. Several mechanisms are proposed such as chronic ischemia and compression by a dolichoectatic carotid artery.

Toxic and nutritional optic neuropathy
Early symptoms of toxic or nutritional optic neuropathy are very subtle, with blurring or clouding of the fixation point which can be confirmed by Amsler grid. Rapid progressive painless bilateral symmetrical central visual loss and/or dyschromatopsia is a common presentation. Common reported substances that induce toxic optic neuropathy are ethambutol, isoniazid, chloramphenicol, hydroxyquinolones, disulfiram, cisplatine, and vincristine. In ethambutol ON, the earliest symptom is dyschromatopsia, commonly in the blue–yellow axis. Visual acuity is usually around 20/200. Cecocentral and central scotoma are the most common visual field defects; bitemporal field defect is also observed. The disc and retina are usually normal at first, or temporal optic atrophy develops in later stages. Toxicity is dose-related and body-weight-related. Renal function should be monitored, along with the D 15-hue color vision test, AOHRR (American Optical Hardy–Rand–Rittler) color plate, and visual field test. Treatment is immediate cessation; no other treatment has proved effective. Prognosis is unpredictable. In reversible cases, the period of recovery usually starts in 3–8 months, with slow improvement.

Nutritional optic neuropathy
Pernicious anemia, some gastrointestinal disorders, and rarely poor nutrition lead to vitamin B_{12} deficiency. Symptoms and signs are visual acuity loss, central or cecocentral scotoma, and pale discs. Optic neuropathy secondary to thiamine (vitamin B_1) deficiency occurs in patients who are generally malnourished such as alcoholics, and those on starvation diet, dialysis, and chronic parenteral diet without sufficient vitamin supplements and gastric plication. With severe B_1 depletion patients develop Wernicke's syndrome which includes encephalopathy, eye movement disorders, and gait ataxia. Optic nerves usually are normal, but swelling occurs in some cases. With parenteral administration of hydroxycobalamin

(in the case of B$_{12}$ deficiency) and thiamine (in the case of B$_1$ deficiency) early in the course of the disease, vision may return in one to a few days.

Orbital tumor
Orbital tumors slowly compress the optic nerve resulting in disc pallor, usually without disc swelling, retinochoroidal (optociliary) shunt vessels, mild proptosis, and RAPD. Visual field defect can be central, arcuate, or diffuse.

Optic nerve sheath meningioma
Optic nerve sheath meningioma is the second most common primary optic nerve tumor. Women are affected three times more than men, with the most frequent age of onset between 40 and 50 years of age. Because of the very slow growth of the tumor, patients usually notice their visual loss when a large portion of their visual field has already been lost. Because optic nerve sheath meningiomas begin around the optic nerve, the compression leads to a progressively constricted visual field defect. Imaging generally leads to the diagnosis. Bilateral optic nerve sheath meningioma suggests neurofibromatosis. Stereotactic conformal radiation is the treatment of choice when a patient still has vision. Surgical excision is indicated when a patient has no useful vision, with cosmetic concern, and to prevent involvement of the contralateral optic nerve or pressure on the frontal lobes.

Optic nerve gliomas
Optic nerve gliomas are uncommon orbital tumors, but they are the most common primary optic nerve tumor. Most of the cases present in childhood and adolescence. In children with proptosis, leukocoria, monocular nystagmus, and RAPD, optic nerve glioma should be differentiated from retinoblastoma. Because optic gliomas originate from the nerve, visual loss is early and becomes severe by the time proptosis is prominent. Optic nerve gliomas are very slow growing or self-limited. The diagnosis can be made by MRI; typically fusiform enlargement, elongation of optic nerve kinking, smooth sheath margin, and no calcification are typical. Biopsy is not suggested because optic glioma has similar pathology to nerve sheath and biopsy can cause further damage to the nerve. Twenty-five percent of cases occur in patients with neurofibromatosis. Many regimens for chemotherapy have been studied. Chemotherapy helps delay radiation treatment which may affect intellectual, neurological, and endocrine function. Surgical excision is indicated when there is no useful vision, with unpleasant proptosis, or with extension towards the chiasm or brain.

Cavernous hemangiomas
Cavernous hemangiomas are the most common benign orbital tumors in adults. Progressive proptosis, hyperopia, retinochoroidal striae, increased intraocular pressure, strabismus, and optic nerve compression may be present. It is more common in women than men, commonly starting in middle age. Imaging studies such as CT and MRI can help confirm the diagnosis. Unlike capillary hemangioma in children this tumor has limited feeders from the systemic circulation; thus angiogram or venogram is not necessary or helpful. Treatment by surgical excision is indicated when ocular functions are disturbed.

Metastases and tumor invasion
Local invasions from sinuses are not uncommon, with squamous cell carcinoma from maxillary sinuses the most common epithelial tumor invading the orbit. Patients present with proptosis, globe displacement, limitation of eye movement, pain, and compressive optic neuropathy. Differential diagnoses are orbital pseudotumor, orbital apex syndrome, or orbital cellulitis. Imaging studies and tissue biopsy are diagnostic. Treatment includes surgical excision combined with irradiation or chemotherapy in some cases. Mucormycosis presents with violaceous hue of skin and rapid progression of orbital inflammation, more often with pain in diabetics. Tissue biopsy demonstrates fungus invasion of blood vessel walls which confirms the diagnosis. Treatment by wide local excision and amphotericin B is required but with a poor survival rate.

Retinal vascular disorders
Presenting symptoms and signs of CRVO are divided into two types, ischemic and non-ischemic. In the non-ischemic presentation patients may have vague complaint of mild to moderate visual dullness or blurring, with uncertain onset. Examination of the fundus shows venous engorgement and tortuosity and retinal hemorrhage with or without macular edema. In ischemic presentation, visual acuity is more acute, with severe visual loss. Retinal vein engorgements are more severe, there are flame shaped and dot hemorrhages, and cotton wool spots are numerous and obscure most of the macula area. FFA demonstrates areas of retinal capillary non-perfusion causing retinal infarction. Branch retinal vein occlusion usually presents with a strip of black shadow. Visual field tests confirm partial arcuate visual field loss. With macular edema, visual acuity may drop.

Carotid artery and cavernous sinus fistulas (C-C fistulas)
C-C fistulas usually present with corkscrew arterialized conjunctival blood vessels, proptosis, and hearing sounds within the head. Eyelid vessels are engorged; in some cases the pulsating superior orbital vein can be palpated. Bruit is common in high flow type that is usually associated with severe head trauma. Vision can deteriorate due to optic nerve compression, venous stasis retinopathy, choroidal effusions, or glaucoma. DAVM connect the carotid artery

to the cavernous sinuses through small collateral vessels of cavernous sinus wall. Clinical presentations of DAVM are less severe and some may spontaneously close. Treatment for low flow DAVM depends on the severity and findings of angiographs. Self carotid-compression (Higashida technique) is recommended in some cases. Most cases of direct C-C fistula and DAVM can be successfully treated with endovascular embolization.

Central visual field loss from macular disorder
Central serous chorioretinopathy (CSCR)
CSCR is most common in young adults, especially men, and is often associated with stress, lack of sleep, and excessive use of vision. Visual loss is subtle to mild, usually 20/30–20/50, rarely less than 20/70. Examination of the fundus demonstrates a round swelling of retina in the macular area with fluid retention, causing a change of refractive power to mild hyperopia. This macular edema is difficult to detect by monocular viewing ophthalmoscope. The Amsler grid is a very useful test. Color vision is normal. Pupil reaction to light is normal and RAPD is generally absent. Optical coherence tomography (OCT) is a convenient instrument to detect the fluid in different retina layers. In CSCR, fluid is confined in space between the retinal pigment epithelium (RPE) and retina. FFA is also helpful in demonstrating fluid leakage to subretinal space, identifying the point of leakage, which can be treated with laser therapy and may shorten the course of the disorder. CSCR is self limiting in the majority of patients.

Macular edema
Macular edema is a swelling of the central retina caused by accumulation of fluid and blood components leaking from retinal vessels. Diabetic macular edema is one common form of maculopathy, found in the preproliferative stage of diabetic retinopathy. Other disorders that can cause macular edema are uveitis, CRVO, postoperative ocular surgery, neuroretinitis, and optic neuritis. Visual loss is slowly progressive with variable severity. If this edema does not resolve after treating the underlying disease, laser photocoagulation should be performed.

Age-related macular degeneration (AMD)
AMD is a common retinal lesion in older patients. Soft drusen and geographic atrophy of RPE are typical findings in the dry type, and RPE detachment, choroidal neovascularization, and disciform scar indicate the wet type. AMD is now one of the leading causes of blindness in the elderly. Ultraviolet (UV) exposure and smoking are risk factors. Presenting symptoms are blurred vision, metamorphopsia, and central acuity loss. Investigations include FFA, indocyanine green angiography (ICGA), and OCT. The aim of various newer treatments is to inhibit new vascular formation and reduce subretinal neovascular membrane.

Cone and cone-rod dystrophy
Cone dystrophy is a progressive central visual loss with only cone functions affected. Autosomal dominant transmission, autosomal recessive transmission, and sporadic cases have been reported. Mild visual loss with decreased color vision is a common early presentation, with photophobia and day blindness, making it difficult to diagnose. The most common age of presentation is in the first and second decades of life. Visual acuity in the late phase is usually reduced to about 20/400. The macular and disc are normal at first, with late macular depigmentation, areolar atrophy of RPE, and bull's eye appearance. Multifocal ERG is very useful for diagnosis. Differential diagnoses include sick RPE syndrome, central choroid dystrophy, and Stargardt's disease.

Macular hole
Macular hole is a full-thickness round loss of the retina layer in the fovea region. Early thin and elevated retina is difficult to observe at the onset. OCT of the macular can aid in the demonstration of the early phase of a macular hole. After slow thinning of the retina, a full-thickness macular hole develops. The visible underlying choroid is relatively red compared to the yellow-white-colored surrounding retina.

Paraneoplastic syndromes
Cancer-associated retinopathy (CAR) is an autoimmune disorder of the photoreceptors associated with autoantibodies. The antigen identified in most CAR patients is recoverin. Patients usually complain of bilateral dark peripheral vision and difficult night adaptation over weeks to months. Ring scotoma (paracentral scotoma) is confirmed in 120-degree visual field test. Appearance of the fundus appears normal in the early phase, ERG demonstrate markedly decreased amplitudes, while multifocal ERG may give more details. In the late phase, there is a mottling pattern of the retina in the paracentral area developed with attenuated vessels and optic atrophy. CAR precedes identification of the occult cancer. Small cell carcinoma of the lung, and breast, colon, uterine, and cervical cancer have been reported. Treatment includes systemic corticosteroids, intravenous immunoglobulins, and plasmapheresis, with poor prognosis for recovery.

Clinical approach to double vision

There are some steps to help evaluate the patient with double vision (diplopia). First, cover each eye; if diplopia persists the open eye may have one of the following optical problems: corneal disorder, cataract, lens dislocation, large iris hole, or retinal irregularities. Second, ask the patient if the diplopia is vertical or horizontal. With horizontal diplopia, either lateral rectus (CN sixth nerve) or medial rectus function is impaired. If the patient has vertical diplopia, a helpful clue is the presence or absence of ptosis. Without ptosis, the superior oblique may be suspected. Third, if there is variable or intermittent diplopia, myasthenia gravis should be considered.

Horizontal diplopia

Isolated lateral rectus palsy is likely most commonly caused by *ischemia*. Patients who have systemic risks for ischemia such as diabetes, hypertension, hypercholesterolemia, or vasculitis are most at risk. Improvement is generally seen in 6 weeks to 3 months and no further studies are needed, although non-invasive imaging is frequently performed where available. *Increased intracranial pressure* may cause unilateral or bilateral sixth nerve palsies with optic disc edema. Sixth nerve palsy with intermittent diplopia suggests *Duane's retraction syndrome*. Co-contraction of the lateral rectus with adduction causes retraction of the globe and narrowing of the palpebral fissure which resembles ptosis. Isolated medial rectus weakness with ptosis often points to *myasthenia gravis* which can be confirmed by ice pack compression over the ptotic eyelid for 2 minutes (ICE) test (improvement of ptosis or reversal of diplopia). Additional testing is described in Chapter 114. Isolated medial rectus weakness (slow saccades) that improve with convergence with or without abducting nystagmus represents *internuclear ophthalmoplegia (INO)*. MRI scan demonstrated a lesion in the brainstem. MS is a common cause during the second through the fifth decades of life, particularly with bilateral INO.

Horizontal diplopia with other neurological symptoms

Sixth nerve palsy that is associated with facial palsy, facial hypoesthesia, and anterior tongue dysgeusia is caused by intra-axial lesions, so-called Foville syndrome. Millard–Gubler syndrome consists of contralateral hemiplegia, ipsilateral facial palsy and sixth nerve palsy. Sixth nerve palsy with Horner's syndrome suggests a lesion in the cavernous sinus.

Vertical diplopia
Vertical diplopia without ptosis

In *vertical diplopia without ptosis*, if the patient cannot look up, *restrictive myopathy* of the inferior rectus should be confirmed by force duction test. With lid retraction and painless exophthalmos, *thyroid associated orbitopathy (TAO)* should be suspected. With a history of trauma, *fracture orbital floor* or intramuscular hemorrhage are possible diagnoses. A CT scan is recommended to evaluate such patients. Another cause of vertical diplopia without ptosis is *fourth nerve palsy*. Patients usually complain of diplopia when walking down stairs or reading. Superior oblique muscle has rather a small range of contraction; its normal function is best observed when the patient has a complete

third nerve palsy. In fourth nerve palsy, slight asymmetry of eye movement is found when the paretic eye looks down and in. Since the etiologies of isolated fourth nerve palsy are usually benign, some suggest imaging studies should be done when the condition persists longer than 3 months. On rare occasions bilateral fourth nerve palsies can be caused by compression from pineal tumors.

Vertical diplopia with ptosis

Presentation of *vertical diplopia with ptosis* from isolated third nerve is a common syndrome. *Third nerve palsy* can present with complete or incomplete paralysis of the medial, inferior, or superior rectus, levator palpebrae, and inferior oblique muscle. with or without paralysis of the iris sphincter and ciliary muscles. Complete ptosis and large angle exotropia are the typical appearance of a complete palsy. *Third nerve palsy with pupil involvement* is not common. Aneurysms from a posterior communicating artery and internal carotid artery can compress the third nerve either before or after it ruptures. Pupil involvement may develop as much as 7–10 days later. Therefore a third nerve palsy with initial spared pupil must be closely observed and investigated early. Pupil involvement includes dilated fixed pupil, slow reaction to light, or slow consensual light reflex without dilatation. CT angiogram or MR angiogram are effective in detecting small aneurysms ($\geq$2–3 mm). *Third nerve palsy with pupil sparing* is commonly caused by ischemia including that associated with DM. After close observation for 7–10 days (every day for younger patients 20–40 years old without DM or hypertension), if the complete or incomplete third nerve palsy is still pupil-sparing, some feel no imaging is needed. Pain around the eye to the head can happen in both diabetic ophthalmoplegia and aneurysms. If a patient does not improve in 2 months, a compressive lesion should be ruled out by an imaging study. Another indication for imaging is aberrant regeneration; the paretic muscle is reinnervated by the wrong branch. Ischemic third nerve palsy does not cause aberrant degeneration. Other disorders that can lead to vertical diplopia and ptosis are myasthenia gravis, orbital pseudotumor, Tolosa–Hunt syndrome, orbital tumor, infiltrative lesions of cavernous sinuses and the orbital apex, Fisher syndrome, and carotid-cavernous fistula.

Vertical diplopia with bilateral ptosis

On rare occasions, the third nerve nuclei are involved causing bilateral ptosis, bilateral superior rectus paresis, and ipsilateral paresis of the medial and inferior rectus and inferior oblique.

Vertical diplopia with other neurological disorders

Brainstem lesions that involve the third nerve fascicles can cause ipsilateral third nerve palsy with other neurological findings. Associated disorders are contralateral hemiparesis in Weber's syndrome, contralateral hemiparesis with tremor in Benedickt's syndrome, contraleral tremor in Claude's syndrome and skew deviation, and ocular torsion with head tilt in ocular tilt reaction.

Clinical approach to pupillary abnormalities

Examination of the pupil should include size, functions, and shape. The resting size of the pupil becomes smaller with age. Average pupil size is between 4 and 6 mm. Pupils smaller than 4 mm and larger than 6 mm may require attention.

Small pupil

An "occluded" pupil is a condition when synechia from the iris occlude the pupil. The pupil is very small and filled in with synechia that attach from the iris to the lens. Because of severe synechia, pupils do not react to either light or near objects. In early uveitis, a patient may have intense photophobia, ciliary injection, decreased vision, and ocular pain. The small pupil is helpful in distinguishing uveitis from acute glaucoma which has similar symptoms except for the presence of a semi-dilated fixed pupil.

Unilateral small pupil

Visible physiologic anisocoria is common, from 0.4–1 mm. The differences are unchanged in dim light and bright light. In dim light, if the smaller pupil does not dilate or slowly dilates, pathologic anisocoria should be suspected. These pupils can be more easily observed in the dark using a blue or green filter covering a penlight. Horner's syndrome, or oculosympathetic disruption, has more anisocoria in dim light because the fellow normal pupil will fully dilate. Clinical presentations include miosis, ptosis, and an elevated lower lid, and in some cases anhydrosis. Lighter iris color indicates the congenital type, which is usually benign. Cocaine test (topical 10% cocaine eye drops into both eyes) confirms Horner's syndrome when the difference in pupil diameter is 1 mm or more after 60–90 minutes. After 24–48 hours, one can help localize the site of oculosympathetic disruption by 1% hydroxyamphetamine eye drops. If the pupil fails to dilate and anisocoria increases by 1 mm or more, a postganglionic lesion is present. Since false positive and false negative tests of the hydroxyamphetamine test have been reported, other clinical findings should be used to localize the lesion in Horner's syndrome. First-order neuron lesions can be lesions in the brainstem or cervical spinal cord based on other findings. Second-order neuron lesions may be caused by apical lung tumor. Postganglionic (third-order neuron) lesions are often benign, especially the isolated one. Horner's syndrome with involvement of cranial nerves III, IV, and/or VI or second or third divisions of the fifth nerve indicate lesions in the cavernous sinus. MRA, MRI, and CT may be needed to define the nature of the lesion. Acquired childhood Horner's syndrome can be associated with neuroblastoma. In conclusion, patients who have Horner's syndrome accompanied by severe or chronic pain, pulmonary symptoms, cranial nerve abnormalities, or cancer-related symptoms require imaging studies of the suspected locations.

Bilateral small pupils

Bilateral small pupils are commonly found in older individuals, DM, and patients treated with eye drops for glaucoma. Pupils get smaller with age, from 6–7 mm in teenages to 5–6 mm in middle age, and 4–5 mm around age 60. About two-thirds of diabetic patients have smaller pupils than the average for their age; however, a pupil size of 3 mm or less is uncommon. One-third of diabetic patients have sluggish pupils, which is otherwise rare in patients under 40 years old. Pilocarpine or phospholine iodide, now rarely prescribed antiglaucoma drugs, usually cause very small pupils (about 2 mm or less) with very poor light or near reaction. Argyll Robertson's (AR) pupils are very small pupils, often irregular, with light and near dissociation (*loss* of *light* reflex but *normal near* reflex AR pupils are suggestive of tertiary neurosyphilis). Another common bilateral small pupil syndrome, accommodative spasm, is now commonly found in computer vision syndrome (CVS). With prolonged use of a computer, accommodative reflexes are sustained, and patients may have temporary myopia, small pupils, and dull eye pain. Similar to muscle cramp, ciliary muscles and dilator muscles are unable to relax. When patients then change their sight from computer to distance, their vision becomes blurred. This improves with a minus lens. Mydriatic drops at bed time and periodic rest after 45–60 minutes' use of a computer are recommended. Others causes of bilateral small pupils are hypothalamic lesions, pontine lesions, metabolic encephalopathies, and opiate use.

Large pupil
Unilateral large pupil

Differential diagnoses of large pupils with normal or mildly reduced vision include compressive third nerve palsy, internal ophthalmoplegia, Adie's pupil, iris trauma, and instillation of mydriatic eye drops. Patients with large pupil may have visual symptoms such as photophobia and difficulty focusing, especially near focusing. Acute closed angle glaucoma can also cause a large pupil and mid-dilated fixed positions are common. Patients present with marked visual loss, severe eye pain, nausea, and vomiting, and see a halo around light with very high intraocular pressure.

Adie's pupil is a tonic pupillary disorder and occasionally occurs in healthy individuals. Young women are more affected. Patients may complain about a unilateral large pupil in their photographs, photophobia (without pain), or blurred near vision. This large tonic pupil has poor reaction to light, slow redilatation, and light-near dissociation. The lack of constrictions in paralytic segments cause pupils to appear oval or scalloped. Tonic relaxation can also cause difficulty in distance refocusing and far objects become blurred after reading. This tonic pupil is called Adie's syndrome when it is accompanied with absence of deep tendon reflexes. Injuries to parasympathetic ganglions and dorsal root ganglia may be the cause. Topical low concentration (0.1%) pilocarpine is used to confirm diagnosis. Denervation hypersensitivity facilitates pupil constriction with the diluted solution compared to the normal pupil. Treatment of Adie's pupil is with 0.1% pilocarpine to reduce photophobia. In accommodative paresis, plus lenses are needed to aid in near visual tasks specifically in bilateral cases (10% of cases). Laboratory workups are directed to find systemic causes especially in bilateral tonic pupils. Orbital trauma, viral infections, vasculitides, tumor, and orbital surgery are possible etiologies for Adie's pupil. Autonomic dysfunction may occur. The Fisher variant of the Guillian–Barre syndrome, cancer, amyloidosis, and other autoimmune disorders have been reported as rare associated factors.

Trauma-related large pupil

Blunt trauma and ocular surgery can injure the iris sphincter. Pupils are irregularly dilated with poor or no response to miotic drops. Iris pigments can be lost, causing transillumination or iris holes. In certain ocular surgeries such as corneal graft implantation or refractive surgery such as LASIX, patients may experience pupil dilatation with or without accommodative paralysis. Ciliary nerve injuries by laser photocoagulation treatment for diabetic retinopathy, orbital trauma, and strabismus surgery have also been reported to cause dilated pupils. The pupil may be fixed and non-reactive to light or near stimulations.

RAPD are reductions of pupil reaction to light in the affected eye compared to the normal fellow eye. RAPD can be classified into four grades. In a 1+ RAPD the pupil is initially constricted with subsequent dilatation; 2+ means there is no initial constriction followed by subsequent dilatation; 3+ is immediate dilatation; and 4+ means the pupil is totally deafferented and the eye is completely blind. The correct method to test RAPD involves the subject looking in the distance, with dim room illumination, and a oblique light source. Then carry out a swinging flashlight test, allowing 3–5 seconds of light shining on the first side, allowing the pupil to complete its cycle. Repeated tests in one direction, starting from the patient's right eye moving to the left eye, are less confusing. Then reverse the direction of the tests to confirm the site and characteristsics of

the pupillary defect. RAPD may be mildly positive with amblyopia or retina lesions and usually obvious in optic nerve lesions especially in optic neuritis. In monocular cataract patients, RAPD may be found positive in the fellow eye, possibly caused by light diffusion or reduced retinal sensitivity in the cataract eye. In rare occasions, optic tract lesions can cause contralateral RAPD. Homonymous incongruous visual field defects and bow tie disc atrophy are associated findings in such lesions.

In the emergency room, unconscious patients with a unilateral dilated pupil are problematic. With traumatic mydriasis, a small level of hyphema or uveitis may be present. The pupil may have notches and does not respond to miotic drops. Normal contralateral RAPD helps rule out afferent loop trauma. Prominent relative afferent defect (3+ and 4+ RAPD) with a history of trauma around the forehead may suggest traumatic optic neuropathy (TON). If CT scan of the optic canal demonstrates fracture of the adjacent bony structures, optic nerve compression should be performed. Unilateral pupil enlargement and an altered level of consciousness with associated brainstem signs such as negative oculocephalic or progressive third nerve involvement require emergency imaging studies to detect uncal herniation.

Many types of mydriatic eye drops are commonly used in ophthalmologic therapy. Tropicamide is a short-acting (4–5 hours of dilatation) mydriatic agent, which produces mydriasis and accommodative paresis. It is used in outpatient clinics for fundus examinations. Pupil dilatation and paralysis of accommodation are more pronounced and prolonged (7–10 days of dilatation) with atropine, which is often prescribed in uveitis patients to prevent synechia. Cyclopentolate is preferred in childhood refraction because it has more blocking effect on accommodation than dilatation. Phenylephrine and adrenaline have potent effects on ocular sympathetic systems, resulting in large pupils, increased palpebral fissures, and conjunctival vasoconstriction, without affecting accommodation. Phenylephrine and neosynephrine are commonly used for preoperative ocular surgery. Any contamination with these eye drops can cause pharmacologic mydriasis that does not respond to light or near stimulation and is unable to be reversed by miotic eye drops.

Bilateral large pupils

Bilateral large pupils can be caused by bilateral blindness from ocular disorders, anoxic brain injury from midbrain ischemia, generalized tonic–clonic seizures, and other syndromes including the aforementioned Adie's pupil.

Abnormal shape of pupils

Congenital anomalies that cause irregular-shaped pupils are iris coloboma, corectopia, aniridia, anterior chamber cleavage syndrome, ectropion uvea, polycoria, congenital miosis, and persistent pupillary membrane. Acquired disorders resulting in abnormal pupillary shapes include uveitis and iritis, idiopathic or secondary infections or infestations, traumatic iridodialysis, traumatic pupillary tear, surgical iridectomy, tonic pupils, tadpole pupils, iris tumor, laser photocoagulation, laser iridoplasty, and ruptured cornea with anterior synechia.

Further reading

Alvarez E, Wakakura M, Khan Z, Dutton GN. The disc–macula distance to disc diameter ratio: a new test for confirming optic nerve hypoplasia in young children. *J Pediatr Ophthalmol Strabismus* 1998; 25: 151–4.

Chuenkongkaew WL, Lertrit P, Limwongse C, *et al*. An unusual family with Leber's hereditary optic neuropathy and facioscapulohumeral muscular dystrophy. *Eur J Neurol* 2005; 12: 388–91.

Laksanaphuk P, Yarnwit T, Tirakunwichcha S, *et al*. Indications and accuracy of ophthalmic ultrasonography in King Chulalongkorn Memorial Hospital. *Chula Med J* 2005; 49: 459–65.

Poonyathalang A, Boon-gasem B. Treatment of AION by megadose steroid plus ASA and pentoxifylline. *Neuro-ophthalmol Jpn Asian Section* 2002; 19: 369–74.

Poonyathalang A, Preechawat P, Laothammatat J, Charuratana O. Four recti enlargement at orbital apex and thyroid associated optic neuropathy. *J Med Assoc Thai* 2006; 89: 468–72.

Poonyathalang A, Suksuratchai M. Optic neuritis in Ramathibodi Hospital. *Thai J Ophthalmol* 1996; 10: 139–46.

Preechawat P, Poonyathalang A. Bilateral optic neuritis after dengue viral infection. *J Neuroophthalmol* 2005; 25: 51–2.

Preechawat P, Sukawatcharin P, Poonyathalang A, Leksakul A. Aneurysmal third nerve palsy. *J Med Assoc Thai* 2004; 87: 1332–5.

Preechawat P, Wongwatthana P, Poonyathalang A, Chusattayanond A. Orbital apex syndrome from gnathostomiasis. *J Neuroophthalmol* 2006; 26: 184–6.

Sitathanee C, Dhanachai M, Poonyathalang A, Tuntiyatorn L, Theerapancharoen V. Stereotactic radiation therapy for optic nerve sheath meningioma; an experience at Ramathibodi Hospital. *J Med Assoc Thai* 2006; 89: 1665–9.

Toyama S, Wakakura M, Chuenkongkaew WL. Optic neuropathy associated with thyroid-related auto-antibodies. *Neuro-ophthalmol* 2001; 25: 127–-34.

Chapter 129
High grade astrocytomas

Olivier L. Chinot
Université de la Méditerranée, Marseille, France

Introduction

High grade astrocytomas (HGA), which include anaplastic astrocytomas (AA) and glioblastoma multiforme (GBM), are the most frequent and devastating diseases among other brain tumors and cancers. Despite poor prognosis, progress in the care of patients with GBM has been more firmly established than in other gliomas that share a better prognosis and a greater sensitivity to treatment. Although the role of biology, imaging, and oncologic treatment is increasing as in other cancer types, neurological characteristics and the impact on patient status play a central role in the management of patients.

Epidemiology

HGA accounts for 2% of all adult tumors, with an incidence rate of 5/100 000 adults per year. This rate is slightly higher in men (sex ratio male/female of 1.5). While the peak of incidence of GBM is observed around 65–74 years of age, this peak is observed one decade earlier for AA. Increases of brain tumor incidence up to 100% per decade in the last three decades have been described, primarily in the elderly population. Whether this should only be attributed to improvement of diagnostic procedures or is in part related to environmental factors is unknown. Variation of HGA incidence has been observed across countries and ethnicities, but appears to be lower than the variation of many other cancer types. Glioma incidence tends to be higher in countries with more developed medical care and higher rates of glioma have been observed in Caucasians than in Africans, Hispanics, and Chinese in the United States. These variations have been mainly attributed to differences in access to medical care or diagnostic practices. However, considering that in United States, the glioma rate is higher in Caucasians than in African Americans while meningioma rates are similar between these two populations, limits the potential impact of medical care access to explain these differences. Even in Europe, glioma incidence rate may vary from 5 per 100 000 in France and United Kingdom up to 10 per 100 000 in Sweden and Denmark, suggesting that other factors including genetics may influence these differences.

Hereditary genetic syndromes account for less than 5% of glioma and include Li–Fraumeni syndrome (*TP53* gene), Turcot's syndrome (*HMLH1* and *HPSM2* genes), and neurofibromatosis type 1 (*NF1* gene). Other potential risk factors have been examined including exposure to electromagnetic fields, nitrosamines, pesticides, synthetic rubber, and petrochemicals, but no definite conclusion can be made from contradictory results obtained to date.

Clinical features

Symptoms of HGA may include an increase in intracranial pressure (ICP), seizures, and focal deficits related to tumor mass effect or infiltration. Kinetics and the magnitude of clinical symptoms generally reflect tumor aggressiveness. However, tumor location influences not only the type of focal deficit but also the timing of symptoms. For example, intracranial hypertension may be observed rapidly in the evolution of deep tumors that can obstruct cerebrospinal fluid flow or be delayed for tumors located in silent areas.

Headache occurs in approximately 75% of patients with malignant glioma and constitutes the initial symptom in 40% of patients. Headaches are generally more pronounced in the morning, improve or resolve later in the day, and tend to increase with time. Headache can result from an increase of ICP or traction on pain-sensitive structures such as meninges or blood vessels.

Increases in ICP may result from cerebral edema (related to tumor infiltration), vasogenic edema (produced by leakage of the blood–brain barrier), or obstruction of cerebrospinal fluid (CSF) or venous flow. Clinical symptoms of ICP include headache, nausea, vomiting, drowsiness, and visual abnormalities such as

International Neurology: A Clinical Approach. Edited by Robert P. Lisak, Daniel D. Truong, William M. Carroll, and Roongroj Bhidayasiri. © 2009 Blackwell Publishing, ISBN: 978-1-4051-5738-4.

papilledema or diplopia. Intensity of drowsiness and presence of visual symptoms are warning signs of a critical level of ICP that may lead to tentorial, subfalcine, or tonsillar herniation.

Incidence of seizures at presentation is lower in HGA (30%) than in low grade glioma (90%). Both generalized and focal seizures are observed; temporal lesions often result in simple or complex partial seizures.

Focal neurological signs are dependent on tumor location and may include motor or sensory deficits, dysphasia, cognitive deficits, and/or personality change. Typically these deficits increase in intensity and number in relation to increases in tumor volume. Sudden onset of symptoms may suggest a vascular event or seizures.

Investigations

Radiological assessment

Magnetic resonance imaging (MRI) with gadolinium administration is the standard method to determine location, extension, infiltration, edema, and mass effect, and is superior to computed tomography (CT), except when acute hemorrhage is suspected. Typical appearance of GBM is a mixed heterogeneously-enhancing mass associated with extensive vasogenic edema. Infiltration of the corpus callosum is frequently observed, and better identified in T2- or fluid-attenuated inversion recovery (FLAIR) sequences. Hemorrhage is frequently observed (10–20%). While the majority of GBM are solitary lesions, multifocal (multiple connected masses observed on T2 and FLAIR sequences) or multicentric (multiple tumors without any macroscopic or microscopic connection) may account for 5% of GBM. Anaplastic astrocytomas present as infiltrative tumors with indistinct margins with more homogeneous enhancement than GBM. Other imaging techniques such as MRI with perfusion, diffusion, spectroscopy, or positron emission tomography (PET), although not clearly established in the management of brain tumors, may help to differentiate HGA from brain abscess or other non-tumoral process and may also contribute to evaluation of treatment efficacy and potential iatrogenic effects such as radionecrosis.

Pathology and molecular biology

Despite progress in multimodal imaging, histological examination of tumor tissue is required and may correct the suspected diagnosis of glioma to a brain abscess, a solitary metastase, or even a lymphoma. Due to the intrinsic heterogeneity of HGA, appropriate classification and grading are still challenging. HGA includes AA (grade III) and GBM (grade IV). According to revised World Health Organization (WHO) classification (2007), grade III gliomas also include anaplastic oligodendroglioma and mixed anaplastic oligoastrocytoma, while grade IV also includes the newly identified GBM with oligodendroglial component (GBMO). GBM can be observed *de novo* or be secondary to the progression of a lower grade glioma. Despite defined histologic criteria, profound inter- and intra-observer variability in the classification of HGA, particularly in grade III tumors, has been observed. Such difficulties may be solved in part by integrating molecular markers into the classification of gliomas.

Genetic instability is common in HGA and the combination and timing of these events reflect distinct patterns of progression. Alterations of epidermal growth factor receptor (EGFR) that include gene amplification (40%), overexpression (60%), and expression of a truncated constitutionally-activated receptor (EGFRvIII) are observed in *de novo* GBM. These EGFR alterations are mutually exclusive from *TP53* mutations, an early genomic event in glioma progression, observed in 50% of low grade astrocytoma and secondary GBM. Overexpression of platelet-derived growth factor (PDGF) ligands and receptor, amplification of cyclin-dependent kinase 4 (CDK4), and mutations of the retinoblastoma gene are early events in astrocytoma progression and may be observed in secondary GBM. Other frequent alterations common to both patterns of progression include loss of heterozygosity on chromosome 10q (80% of GBM), homozygous deletion of the P16/CDKN2A gene (50%), and mutations of the PTEN/MMAC tumor-suppressor gene (20%). Codeletion of chromosomes 1p and 19q characterizes a significant proportion of oligodendroglial tumors with better prognosis and chemosensitivity and has been described in a limited subset of GBM without an oligodendroglial component, where this codeletion is associated with longer survival. Among all the biological markers described in HGA, MGMT (O6-methylguanine-DNA-methyltransferase) status appears to be the strongest marker related to prognosis and therapeutic impact. MGMT repairs chemotherapy-induced lesions and confers a resistant phenotype to alkylating agents. Epigenetic silencing of MGMT by promoter methylation has been observed in almost half of GBM cases and is associated with loss of MGMT expression; this has been correlated to longer survival irrespective of treatment modalities.

Prognostic factors

Overall, survival of GBM is poor, with a median survival of about 10 months and a 2-year survival rate of 10%. Survival associated with AA is slightly better, with a mean survival that varies by as much as 2–5 years, reflecting variability in the diagnostic criteria of AA. Behind histological grade, age and functional performance status are the strongest prognostic factors in HGA. Age may be considered as a continuous variable, although different limits have been proposed, the first between

45 and 50 years, the second between 65 and 70 years. Performance status is generally evaluated according to the Karnofsky Performance Score (KPS) scale, with distinct risk groups defined by a limit of 70 or 80. Mental status as evaluated by the Mini Mental Status Exam scale (normal versus abnormal) also appears to influence survival. While tumor location does not clearly impact survival, patients with tumors that cross or deviate (more than 0.5 mm) the middle line appear to have a shorter survival. The benefit of extent of resection is not clearly determined and there are no large prospective studies that take into account an objective radiological evaluation of residual disease. However, a consensus exists to consider the benefit of extensive resection as compared to biopsy, while the benefit of partial removal is still under debate. Some of the molecular events described previously appear to significantly impact survival. MGMT status appears to exhibit the strongest and most reproducible impact on survival, independent of therapeutic factors. Moreover, in a retrospective analysis of a subset of patients included in the pivotal European Organization for Research and Treatment of Cancer–National Cancer Institute of Canada (EORTC–NCIC) study that defined chemoradiation with temozolomide as the new standard of care in GBM, methylation of the MGMT promoter gene appeared to predict the benefit of adding chemotherapy to radiotherapy (RT). However, studies are needed to define the best technique for assessing MGMT status and to prospectively validate as a marker. Although the prognostic value of EGFR alterations, including amplification, is under debate, it has been suggested that co-expression of EGFRvIII and PTEN could be associated with response to therapeutic agents that target EGFR, that is, EGFR kinase inhibitors.

In order to define the appropriate prognostic group in glioma, two recursive partitioning analyses (RPA) have been proposed, the most widely used elaborated by the Radiation Therapy Oncology Group (RTOG) for all gliomas, while the other is restricted to GBM. The RTOG approach created a regression tree according to prognostic variables including age, KPS, histology, Mini Mental Status, and extent of surgery, and classified patients into a homogeneous subset by survival. Six classes have been defined associated with median survival time which ranges from 4.6 to 58.6 months. At the time of recurrence, expected median survival of AA and GBM is poor, about 30 weeks. The proportion of patients free of progression at 6 months (APF6) is the consensus target endpoint in clinical trials. Histology (GBM versus AA), age (>40 years versus ≤40 years), KPS, and number of salvage therapies including surgery are identified as the most important prognostic factors. Expected APF6 is about 15% in GBM and 30% in AA. It should be noted that these analyses were performed in populations included in clinical trials, and likely do not reflect survival rates of the general HGA population.

Treatment

The treatment challenge for patients with HGA is to increase survival and maintain or improve functional status without affecting the quality of life of patients.

Symptomatic treatments are important throughout the course of the disease. Steroids that control cerebral vasogenic edema improve clinical symptoms within a few hours or days. Dose should be adapted to the clinical situation and decreased as appropriate to minimize negative side effects. Although clinical status is the most relevant reason for steroid use, mass effect as analyzed on imaging should be taken into account. Finally, it should be considered that contrast enhancement on imaging, and therefore evaluation of tumor response, may be altered by an increase in dosage of steroids within 7–10 days before the imaging. Although widely used, antiepileptics should be restricted to patients with a history of seizure, since to date no studies have proven benefit in patients without prior seizures. When antiepileptics have been administered during the peri-operative period, the drugs should be tapered for patients without history of seizures. When anticonvulsants are required, non-enzyme-inducing drugs are preferred in order to avoid interactions with many chemotherapeutic regimens. Because of a high incidence (20%) of thromboembolic events in patients with HGA, anticoagulants are justified and do not appear to increase the risk of intratumoral hemorrhage. Except for cases of gliomatosis meningitis that often require analgesic treatment, pain is rare in HGA; steroids are generally sufficient in the case of headache related to intracranial hypertension. Rehabilitation must be considered and adapted to physical, cognitive, and speech disorders.

Surgery provides material for diagnosis, tissue for evaluation of molecular markers, and relief of neurological symptoms. Improvements in surgical techniques have led to an increasing role for surgery in the management of glioma even at recurrence. Development of local therapies such as biodegradable polymer or convection-enhanced delivery is increasing the role of neurosurgery in the management of HGA. To date, only carmustine implant has proven some efficacy in the management of HGA as part of first-line therapy, combined with RT, or at recurrence. The benefit of adding this chemotherapeutic agent to the new standard of care in patients with GBM has not been proven.

Radiotherapy has been, until recently, the only treatment that significantly improved survival in patients with HGA. A total dose of 58–60 Gray delivered in 30–35 fractions of 1.8–2.0 Gray on a focal volume adapted to infiltrative and residual tumor evaluated after surgery defined the optimal schedule. Toxicity of RT includes acute (during RT), delayed (2–3 months from the end of RT), and late (over 1 year after RT) reactions. The risk of toxicity, particularly for late reaction, is increased by protracted schedules, large volume, and increased doses, as well as age and vascular risk history of the patient. Increased median survival (from 8.5 months to 12 months) for patients treated with RT as exclusive first-line treatment has been observed in studies performed in the last 30 years, likely reflecting improvements in surgery, RT, treatment at recurrence, as well as general management. Recently, RT as exclusive first-line treatment has been proven to increase survival without affecting functional status or quality of life in elderly patients (over 70 years) with a good performance score (KPS ≥70).

Chemotherapy has recently been firmly established as part of the initial management of patients with GBM. Results from a large controlled study concluded that adding chemotherapy (temozolomide) as concomitant and adjuvant treatment to RT improved median survival from 12 to 14.5 months. This survival advantage, although more pronounced in patients with better prognosis, was also observed in patients with poor prognostic characteristics. Moreover, this benefit was observed with a prolonged follow-up with the percentage of survival at 3 and 4 years up to 16% and 12% respectively. This regimen is under evaluation for AA in which RT may still be considered as the first-line standard of care, despite numerous uncontrolled data that underline the greater chemosensitivity of this tumor type. Tumor evaluation by MRI appears to be more complex with this chemoradiation regimen particularly in the 3 months that follow treatment, since a significant proportion of patients may develop clinical and neuroradiological symptoms of apparent progression (so-called "pseudo-progression") that resolve in the following months without treatment modification. At the time of recurrence, while conventional chemotherapy (i.e., nitrosourea, platinum regimen) has limited efficacy, with response rates of about 5–10%, recent data suggest a role for anti-angiogenic agents that are associated with a high (over 50%) response rate. However, duration of response is variable and patterns of progression appear to be more complex.

Evaluation of response to treatment is becoming challenging in HGA and justifies careful monitoring of clinical status and imaging. Macdonald response criteria are based on neurological status, steroid dosage, and tumor volume restricted to the enhancing component. With the increasing role of new therapeutic modalities, including anti-angiogenic agents and other targeted therapies, these criteria will have to be adapted to take into account the whole tumor volume, including the non-enhancing infiltrative component. The place of metabolic imaging and other potential circulating tumor markers deserves further study.

Conclusion

New techniques in biology and imaging and new treatments including targeted therapies have profoundly modified the care of patients with HGA. The marked increase in interest in these tumors will generate further research and data that must integrate the whole complexity of gliomas in order to have prolonged clinical impact. The increased survival observed in recent years has encouraged the development and evaluation of new therapeutics and combinations, but raises the importance of appropriate evaluation with prolonged follow-up of treatment benefit, including analysis of treatment efficacy, later toxicities, and impact on quality of life.

Further reading

Behin A, Hoang-Xuan K, Carpentier A, Delattre JY. Primary brain tumors in adults. *Lancet* 2003; 361: 323–31.

Curran W, Scott CB, Horton J, *et al*. Recursive partitioning analysis of prognostic factors in three radiation therapy oncology group malignant glioma trials. *J Natl Cancer Inst* 1993; 85: 704–10.

Hegi ME, Diserens AC, Gorlia T, *et al*. MGMT gene silencing and benefit from temozolomide in glioblastoma. *N Engl J Med* 2005; 352(10): 997–1003.

Keime-Guibert F, Chinot O, Taillandier L, *et al*. Association of French-speaking neuro-oncologists. Radiotherapy for glioblastoma in the elderly. *N Engl J Med* 2007; 356(15): 1527–35.

Macdonald DR, Cascino TL, Schold SC, Cairncross JG. Response criteria for phase II studies of supratentorial malignant glioma. *J Clin Oncol* 1990; 8: 1277–80.

Mellinghoff IK, Wang MY, Vivanco I, *et al*. Molecular determinants of the response of glioblastomas to EGRF kinase inhibitors. *N Engl J Med* 2005; 353: 2012–24.

Stupp R, Mason WP, van den Bent MJ, *et al*. Radiotherapy plus concomitant and adjuvant temozolomide for glioblastoma. *N Engl J Med* 2005; 352(10): 987–96.

Chapter 130
Low grade astrocytoma

Martin J. van den Bent
Erasmus University Medical Center, Rotterdam, The Netherlands

Introduction

According to the World Health Organization (WHO) classification, low grade astrocytoma (grade II) is an astrocytic neoplasm, with a high degree of cellular differentiation, slow growth, and diffuse infiltration of neighboring brain. Most textbooks lump grade II astrocytoma with oligoastrocytoma and oligodendroglioma. The rationale is that these tumors pose similar clinical problems and share a better prognosis than their anaplastic counterparts, and, perhaps most importantly, guidelines on the treatment of these tumors are obtained from studies that included all three histologies. Despite their former naming as "benign glioma," low grade astrocytomas are not benign tumors. With 2- and 5-year survival rates of 80–85% and 50–55% in large prospective trials most patients die of recurrent disease, at which time 65% of tumors have transformed into high grade tumors. Little is known about the cause of astrocytomas and most cases are sporadic, although familial predispositions exist.

Epidemiology and clinical features

Astrocytomas constitute about 5–15% of all diffuse glioma and have a peak incidence at the age of 30–40 years. The clinical presentation is dependent on tumor location and growth rate. Many low grade glioma patients present with seizures only. With larger lesions or lesions interfering with cerebrospinal fluid (CSF) flow, signs of raised intracranial pressure or focal deficits may arise.

Pathology and molecular biology

Three histological subtypes of grade II astrocytoma are recognized: fibrillary, gemistocytic, and the rare protoplasmic astrocytoma. This distinction has little clinical relevance, although gemistocytic astrocytoma appears to have a more aggressive course than the more common fibrillary astrocytoma. A caveat in the diagnosis of (all) gliomas is the subjectivity of the criteria for both tumor grading and classification. In patients who are diagnosed after biopsy only, sampling error may easily lead to the erroneous diagnosis of an astrocytoma, while a tumor of oligodendroglial lineage or an anaplastic tumor is actually present. Trisomy or polysomy 7 (or 7q) occurs in 50–65% of grade II astrocytomas and has been correlated with poor survival. About 60% of cases have *TP53* mutations and this figure may be higher in gemistocytic astrocytoma. The simultaneous overexpression of platelet-derived growth factor receptor (PDGFR) and its ligand PDGF is also frequent. Most mixed oligoastrocytomas carry either typical oligodendroglial genetic lesions (1p/19q loss) or *TP53* mutations suggestive of an astrocytic lineage. Thus, there is compelling evidence that mixed oligoastrocytomas are not true mixed tumors but are either of astrocytic or of oligodendroglial lineage.

Investigations

On CT scan, low grade astrocytomas present as low density lesions with or without mass effect and can easily be mistaken for ischemic vascular lesions or white matter disease. Lesions are often hypointense on T1 MRI and hyperintense on T2-weighted images (Figure 130.1). The margins on T2 may be either sharp or somewhat diffuse. Although the area with abnormal signal often appears rather homogeneous, this is not invariable. Most astrocytomas arise supratentorially and do not show enhancement, but exceptions occur. Still, if histological examination of an enhancing tumor suggests a grade II astrocytoma this should be doubted. Many clinicians tend to treat these patients as a high grade tumor, especially if the diagnosis was obtained by biopsy. Radioactively labeled amino acid (methionine, tyrosine) positron emission tomography (PET) imaging may help to guide biopsies, and identify patients with a poor prognosis and rapid dedifferentiation. However, series that investigated PET

International Neurology: A Clinical Approach. Edited by Robert P. Lisak, Daniel D. Truong, William M. Carroll, and Roongroj Bhidayasiri. © 2009 Blackwell Publishing, ISBN: 978-1-4051-5738-4.

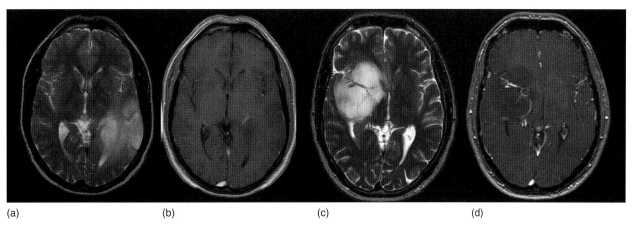

(a) (b) (c) (d)

Figure 130.1 T2 weighted images (a, c) and T1 weighted images after contrast administration (b, d) of patient A (a, b) and patient B (c, d). Both young patients presented with seizures and were followed for years before initiation of treatment, were diagnosed with a grade II astrocytoma at the time of progression, and responded well to radiotherapy. The MR scans are typical for low grade astrocytoma: lesions with limited mass effect, high signal intensity on T2 images either diffuse (a) or more circumscribed (c), and low signal intensity on T1 weighted imaging without enhancement (b, d). T2 weighted images provide superior tumor delineation compared to T1 weighted images.

imaging are rather small, and its clinical relevance needs confirmation. The final diagnosis of a low grade glioma always rests on the histological diagnosis obtained by biopsy or resection.

Prognosis

Large phase III studies on low grade glioma identified astrocytic histology (versus oligodendroglial or mixed), more than 6 cm tumor diameter, midline involvement, presence of neurological deficits, and age above 40 years as poor prognostic factors. In the presence of three or more factors, survival decreased to 3–4 years but was more than 7 years in patients with less than three factors present. These studies included oligodendroglial tumors, and the size and extension of the tumor were assessed with CT. Other studies identified cognitive function, tumor enhancement, and extent of resection as prognostic factors. A more recent prospective study on low grade glioma with an observation-only arm for patients under 40 years of age who had undergone a gross total resection identified both tumor diameter more than 4 cm and astrocytic histology to be poor prognostic factors for progression. After 2 and 5 years of follow-up, only 67% and 34% of patients, respectively, with an astrocytoma more than 4 cm in diameter were still free from progression.

Treatment and management of astrocytoma

The optimal treatment of low grade astrocytoma is controversial, with debate about treatment of good-prognosis patients: young and presenting with seizures only. Because these patients may do well for long periods of time without treatment, many physicians defer diagnostic procedures and treatment, while others advocate early resection with or without adjuvant radiotherapy. Arguments against early treatment including surgery are derived from the observation that many patients remain asymptomatic (apart from the seizures) for prolonged time periods and may deteriorate following treatment. Arguments for early treatment are uncertainty about the diagnosis and potentially better survival after early treatment. Moreover, even so-called stable untreated low grade gliomas show a constant tendency to grow over time (on average 4 mm/year). With respect to clinical decision making two situations must be distinguished: (1) patients presenting with a presumed low grade glioma, and (2) patients with histologically proven astrocytoma. For the management of these patients several issues must be considered, as presented below.

What is the reliability of the neuroradiological diagnosis of "presumable low grade glioma?"

In large series about one-third of patients with unenhancing intra-axial lesions are diagnosed after surgery with a high grade glioma (usually an anaplastic astrocytoma), and patients over 40 years of age may have a greater likelihood of carrying a high grade lesion. Vice versa, 30% of anaplastic astrocytoma and even some glioblastoma were non-enhancing on contrast enhanced CT. This could be an argument for early histological verification, but the assumption that early diagnosis (and treatment) will improve outcome has never been demonstrated in clinical trials. Moreover, regular neuroradiological follow-up will identify those patients with progressive lesions requiring treatment.

What evidence is available to decide at what moment diagnosis should be obtained and treatment initiated?

Small retrospective studies have suggested that early treatment including radiotherapy of young patients with seizures only does not improve outcome and may actually decrease quality of life and cognition. A larger study on cognitive deficits in low grade glioma patients using several non-glioma control groups did not find such an association provided the radiotherapy was given in fractions of 2 Gy or less. Cognitive deficits were found in patients treated with fraction size exceeding 2.0 Gy, and in patients on anti-epileptic drugs. Whether this was due to the seizures or the use of anti-epileptic drugs remains to be established. A randomized trial comparing early radiotherapy versus radiotherapy at the time of progression showed that early radiotherapy improves progression free survival without affecting overall survival. Thus with respect to survival, delaying radiotherapy does not adversely affect outcome.

Which patients should undergo early diagnosis and treatment?

In young patients with an unenhancing intracerebral lesion suspected to be a low grade glioma without mass effect or signs other than well-controlled seizures, a wait-and-see policy can be followed provided the patient is carefully monitored. A first follow-up scan should be obtained within 2–3 months to detect early progression of an unenhancing but high grade tumor. In cases that are being followed, histological confirmation can be postponed until treatment is clinically indicated. Clear radiological progression or new, even if subtle, enhancement provides an indication for treatment, as this may herald focal deficits or a rise in intracranial pressure. Also, tumors that grow relatively rapidly during follow-up are more likely to dedifferentiate early. Intractable seizures may constitute an indication for treatment, as treatment may improve seizure control. In view of the worse prognosis, the higher risk of malignant transformation, and that an unenhancing lesion may be a high grade tumor in elderly patients, most physicians recommend treatment in patients more than 45–50 years of age with presumed or proven low grade glioma. Patients with focal deficits, raised intracranial pressure, or lesions showing mass effect also require treatment without undue delay.

Surgery

In addition to histologic confirmation, surgery in astrocytoma can improve the neurological condition and improve survival by preventing progression and malignant transformation. There are no randomized trials though on the significance of the extent of resection in low grade glioma with regard to survival. Several large retrospective series identified the extent of resection in multivariate analysis as an important prognostic factor, but others were unable to confirm this. Resected low-grade glioma patients with a residual lesion of more than 2 cm had a higher risk of radiological progression than those with a smaller residual lesion, but this did not affect overall survival. However, survival in low grade glioma is better in smaller tumors, not crossing the midline, a subset of patients that is much more likely to undergo extensive surgery. Thus, one might argue that the improved outcome of more extensively operated tumors is due to patient selection. Still, in view of the observed improved outcome in some series it is advisable that once surgery is considered the resection should be as extensive as safely possible.

Radiation therapy

A large randomized trial showed that early radiotherapy increased time to progression from 3.4 years for patients that were observed (and not irradiated until the time of progression) to 5.3 years for patients treated with early radiotherapy. However, early radiotherapy did not improve overall survival, because of the efficacy of salvage radiotherapy in the control arm. The overall picture is that the timing of radiotherapy is less relevant as long as it is given. In addition, at 1 year seizures were better controlled in the radiotherapy arm. Another prospective trial observed a clear radiological response to radiotherapy in almost one-third of low grade glioma patients, and small retrospective surveys have suggested improvement of neurological function or improved seizure control after radiation. Higher dosages of radiotherapy (59–64 Gy) do not lead to a better tumor control and may cause more toxicity. It is generally advised to treat these tumors to a dose of 50–54 Gy in fractions of 1.8 Gy.

Chemotherapy

The results of a randomized study on adjuvant chemotherapy (procarbazine, lomustine, and vincristine) after radiotherapy in low grade glioma suggested an increase in progression free survival without improving overall survival. The subset analysis on astrocytoma is pending. In small phase II trials favorable response rates to temozolomide were also obtained in astrocytic tumors, either at first diagnosis or at recurrence. The role of temozolomide chemotherapy in newly diagnosed low grade astrocytoma is being evaluated in phase III studies; until results are available this treatment must be considered experimental for newly diagnosed astrocytoma. For progressive astrocytoma after radiotherapy, chemotherapy is often the only remaining treatment option and trials have shown a 30–60% response rate to temozolomide. This compound is obviously the drug of choice; other drugs either have not been systematically evaluated or have been proven to be inactive.

Further reading

Klein M, Heimans JJ, Aaronson NK, *et al*. Effect of radiotherapy and other treatment-related factors on mid-term to long-term cognitive sequelae in low grade gliomas: a comparative study. *Lancet* 2002; 360: 1361–8.

Pignatti F, van den Bent MJ, Curran D, *et al*. Prognostic factors for survival in adult patients with cerebral low-grade glioma. *J Clin Oncol* 2002; 20: 2076–84.

Shaw E, Arusell RM, Scheithauer B, *et al*. A prospective randomized trial of low versus high dose radiation in adults with a supratentorial low grade glioma: initial report of a NCCTG–RTOG–ECOG study. *J Clin Oncol* 2002; 20: 2267–76.

van den Bent MJ, Afra D, De Witte O, *et al*. Long term results of EORTC study 22845: a randomized trial on the efficacy of early versus delayed radiation therapy of low-grade astrocytoma and oligodendroglioma in the adult. *Lancet* 2005; 366: 985–90.

Chapter 131
Low grade and anaplastic oligodendroglioma

Ayman I. Omar[1,2] *and Warren P. Mason*[1,2]
[1]Princess Margaret Hospital, Toronto, Canada
[2]University of Toronto, Toronto, Canada

Introduction

Oligodendroglial tumors are a subset of gliomas that typically arise within the supratentorial and much less frequently the infratentorial compartment including the brainstem and spinal cord. According to the World Health Organization (WHO) grading system, these tumors are classified into low grade oligodendrogliomas (OD; WHO grade II) and anaplastic oligodendrogliomas (AOD; WHO grade III). Occasionally, low grade and anaplastic oligodendroglial tumors have histologic features of both oligodendrogliomas and astrocytomas and these tumors are known as low grade oligoastrocytomas (OA) and anaplastic oligoastrocytomas (AOA), respectively.

Oligodendroglial tumors consist of uniform cells with rounded nuclei and are classified as malignant if cytoplasmic and nuclear pleomorphism and frequent mitoses are noted. In addition, oligodendroglial tumors frequently harbor a distinct genetic fingerprint, namely loss of heterozygosity (LOH) on the short arm of chromosome 1 (1p) and the long arm of chromosome 19 (19q). This genetic alteration is found in 60–80% of OD and AOD, and less frequently in OA and AOA. Tumors with combined 1p and 19q LOH are especially sensitive to chemotherapeutic agents and carry a far better prognosis compared to tumors with intact 1p and 19q.

The optimal initial management of OD and AOD is one of the most controversial areas in neuro-oncology. Based on current data, OD is best managed by maximal feasible resection and either immediate postoperative radiotherapy (RT) or deferred RT given at the time of progression. Because of the potential neurocognitive decline that may follow the use of RT, many neuro-oncologists are increasingly deferring RT initially and prescribing chemotherapy as primary therapy after surgery or at the time of progression; this is particularly the case for tumors with 1p and 19q LOH.

AOD is similarly managed by maximal feasible surgical resection, but the use of immediate postoperative RT is advocated. The role of adjuvant (after RT) or neoadjuvant (before or concurrent with RT) chemotherapy in this setting remains the subject of debate. Two prospective randomized trials have demonstrated that while chemotherapy prolonged time to tumor progression, it did not confer an overall survival advantage over delayed chemotherapy for management of progression following radiotherapy failure.

Epidemiology and prognosis

Incidence

The incidence of oligodendrogliomas is between 4% and 25% of all intracranial gliomas depending on the series examined. This wide variation may be due in part to interobserver variability among neuropathologists. The incidence of OD peaks between the second and fourth decade of life and is slightly more common in males. AOD represents approximately 3.5% of anaplastic gliomas and approximately 15% of all oligodendroglial tumors. They also have a slight male predominance but typically peak in older populations between the fifth and sixth decades of life.

Prognostic factors

The single most important predictor of outcome for patients with oligodendroglial tumors is the histological grade. AOD have a worse prognosis and shorter median overall survival compared to the lower grade OD tumors. The median overall survival for AOD is approximately 4–5 years compared to 10–15 years for low grade OD. Furthermore, the presence of an astrocytic component is associated with a worse prognosis when compared with that of pure oligodendrogliomas. Tumors with one or both deletions on chromosomes 1p and 19q carry a more favorable outcome compared with tumors lacking this deletion. It appears that tumors with 1p and 19q LOH have low levels of the DNA repair enzyme methylguanine-DNA-methyltransferase (MGMT), an association that

International Neurology: A Clinical Approach. Edited by Robert P. Lisak, Daniel D. Truong, William M. Carroll, and Roongroj Bhidayasiri. © 2009 Blackwell Publishing, ISBN: 978-1-4051-5738-4.

might in part explain the more chemosensitive nature of these tumors to DNA alkylating agents and consequently a more favorable overall prognosis.

Other factors contributing to prognosis include age at diagnosis, with younger patients generally living longer than older patients, and the presence of neurologic deficits at the time of diagnosis which is associated with worse outcome. Interestingly, long-standing seizures are a favorable prognostic indicator especially when they are the only manifestation of disease. The extent of surgical resection has also been shown to be associated with better outcome.

Pathology and molecular biology

Microscopic appearance

Microscopically, low grade ODs contain sheets of rounded cells with a perinuclear halo (an artifact of fixation) that gives the tumor a classic "fried-egg appearance." Tumor cells are occasionally clustered around blood vessels and neurons, a phenomenon described as perivascular and perineuronal satellitosis, respectively. Frequently, areas of microcalcifications are encountered and a dense meshwork of capillaries can be seen, a feature described as "chicken-wiring." AOD are composed of a more dense and hypercellular tumor mass with a high mitotic index, nuclear pleomorphism, endothelial proliferation, and focal tumor necrosis.

Molecular biology

More than 60% of oligodendroglial tumors have loss of heterozygosity of 1p and/or 19q and this alteration was shown to be associated with a high response rate to a combinational chemotherapy regimen (procarbazine, lomustine vincristine (PCV)). These discoveries initiated a shift in the pathological classification of oligodendroglial tumors from that based on histological features to one based on genetic markers. For example, AOD with intact 1p and 19q are increasingly being segregated with anaplastic astrocytomas, despite the differences in histology, since both tumors have a similar biological behavior as well as prognosis. Other alterations seen in oligodendroglial tumors include LOH of chromosomes 4, 9p, and 10, but these molecular genetic abnormalities occur with much less frequency than 1p and 19q LOH.

Clinical picture

The presentation of a patient with an oligodendroglial tumor depends on tumor location within the central nervous system. Since low grade OD are slow growing tumors, they may remain asymptomatic for years. Occasionally, patients treated for long-standing

"idiopathic" seizures are diagnosed with low grade OD when appropriate imaging is performed. Tumors arising from eloquent brain regions are commonly diagnosed early because neurological deficits develop rapidly. Those deficits may range from language dysfunction to motor weakness or sensory changes, depending on the region involved. Anaplastic tumors because of their relatively faster rate of growth frequently present with signs of increased intracranial pressure such as headaches, nausea, vomiting, and blurring of vision.

Imaging

Oligodendroglial tumors are most often located in the supratentorial compartment where the frontal lobe is the most frequent region to harbor such a tumor. On computed tomography (CT), low grade OD appears as a hypodense mass that is typically non-enhancing, although areas of minimal enhancement may be present. In addition, CT may reveal areas of calcification within low grade OD. AOD similarly appears as a hypodense mass on CT but with a higher degree of contrast enhancement, mass effect, and peritumoral vasogenic edema. AOD can also be associated with focal areas of necrosis as well as hemorrhage within the tumor mass.

On magnetic resonance imaging (MR scans), OD appears as a hypointense mass on T1-weighted imaging and lacks contrast enhancement following gadolinium-DTPA administration. On T2-weighted imaging, both OD and AOD appear as hyperintense masses. Arguably, the fluid-attenuation inversion recovery (FLAIR) sequence provides the best resolution for the detection of low grade tumors. Both OD and AOD may appear as hyperintense masses that are easily distinguished from the less intense cerebrospinal fluid (CSF) and surrounding brain parenchyma.

Treatment

Oligodendroglial tumors are perhaps the most responsive of gliomas to both RT and chemotherapy. Despite this sensitivity the best management approach, its timing, and sequencing remains the subject of intense debate.

Management of OD
Surgery
When surgery is indicated, maximal feasible resection is always the goal for low grade OD. Surgical cure cannot usually be achieved because of microscopic infiltration of tumor cells within the normal brain parenchyma. Surgery, however, may alleviate neurological deficits and improve overall quality of life (QOL). Because of the lack of prospective, randomized trials comparing the efficacy of

resection versus best medical management, it is difficult to ascertain whether surgery positively impacts overall survival among OD patients. Several retrospective analyses have concluded that the extent of surgical resection correlates with improved outcomes in this patient population. The role of surgical resection in patients presenting with a large OD with mass effect, signs of increased intracranial pressure, and neurological deficits is more clearcut than for those with indolent and asymptomatic masses. Surgery may be deferred for those patients presenting with small tumors and no neurological deficits until the time of tumor progression. Open resection is superior to stereotactic biopsy as it provides adequate tissue sampling in order to make an accurate pathological diagnosis and assessment of tumor grade. The use of stereotactic biopsy may be the only option in some instances, as in the case of deep-seated tumors or those involving eloquent brain regions.

Radiation therapy

Although RT is an effective treatment modality for controlling gliomas, the timing as well as optimum dosing is still the subject of debate. The European Organization for the Research and Treatment of Cancer (EORTC) conducted several prospective randomized trials to address these two important questions. One EORTC trial concluded that there was no difference between low dose (45 Gy) and high dose (59.4 Gy) RT, both in terms of progression free survival (PFS) and overall survival (OS). A subsequent trial to address the question of the optimal timing of RT concluded that early postoperative RT resulted in a longer median PFS as opposed to deferred RT given at the time of tumor progression, but overall survival was similar in both early and deferred RT groups. It is not known, however, whether this increase in median PFS as a result of early RT translates into better QOL, as this was not addressed. Many neuro-oncologists prefer to defer RT until the time of tumor progression especially given the potential long-term consequences associated with RT. The best timing for RT (early versus delayed) should be decided on a case-by-case basis. For example, there appear to be some prognostic variables that if present carry an unfavorable prognosis and shorter overall survival. These include (1) patients over 40 years of age, (2) tumor size greater than 6 cm, (3) a tumor crossing the midline, (4) astrocytic morphology, and (5) the presence of neurological deficits. Patients with two or more of these variables are considered high-risk for tumor progression while those with less than two variables are low-risk patients. Consequently, early RT may be considered a reasonable option for such high-risk patients.

Chemotherapy

There have been several recent trials examining the role of postoperative chemotherapy either before or after RT

for the treatment of low grade OD. Several early reports describe favorable responses for OD and AOD patients treated with PCV, although cumulative toxicities such as myelosuppression, hapatotoxicity, seizures, and encephalopathy limit its use. The newer alkylating agent temozolomide has a more favorable toxicity profile and is being increasingly utilized for the first-line treatment of OD and AOD (Figure 131.1). Recent data indicate that upfront temozolomide is effective for the treatment of low grade gliomas, especially those whose tumors harbor 1p and 19q LOH.

Temozolomide was also evaluated for the treatment of low grade OD and OA after PCV failure and was shown to be active in this population. Tumors with 1p and 19q LOH have hypermethylated (silenced) MGMT promoters and low MGMT expression levels. Since MGMT is a DNA repair enzyme that essentially reverses temozolomide DNA alkylating action, low levels of MGMT are associated with a higher degree of chemosensitivity to temozolomide. Theoretically therefore, tumors with 1p and 19q LOH are expected to respond favorably to temozolomide. This makes the use of upfront temozolomide an attractive alternative to RT for the treatment of OD, especially the subset of tumors with 1p and 19q LOH. To investigate the validity of this approach, the EORTC is conducting a phase III trial where patients with low grade OD will be randomized to receive either RT or temozolomide at the time of tumor progression. Patients will be stratified based on their 1p and 19q LOH status in order to dissect differential response to treatment among those tumor subsets.

Management of AOD
Surgery and radiation therapy

The initial management of AOD patients includes maximal safe resection. The use of immediate postoperative RT is advocated because these tumors are aggressive and grow rapidly without further therapy following resection.

Chemotherapy

Historically, surgery and RT were the only treatment modalities available for the treatment of AOD. In 1988, Cairncross and McDonald provided the first evidence that AOD was responsive to PCV. They subsequently tested an intensified PCV regimen (PCV-I) for the treatment of AOD at the time of recurrence and showed a response rate of approximately 75% with a median response duration of 14 months. Subsequently these investigators demonstrated that tumors with 1p and 19q LOH were associated with higher chemosensitivity and better overall prognosis. These early studies demonstrating chemosensitivity of AOD stimulated further trials attempting to define the best timing and chemotherapeutic agent for the treatment of AOD.

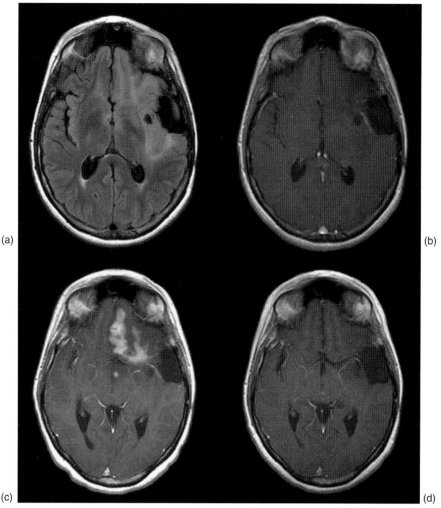

Figure 131.1 Response to temozolomide in recurrent oligodendroglioma. This patient was diagnosed with a left frontotemporal low grade OD. After a partial tumor resection and postoperative RT, an MR scan revealed evidence of residual disease, as can be noted by hyperintense FLAIR signal abnormality adjacent to the resection bed (a). Note that the T1-weighted MR scan shows no contrast enhancement of the tumor following gadolinium-DTPA administration (b). A follow-up T1-weighted MR scan performed approximately 4 years after diagnosis showed marked contrast enhancement following gadolinium-DTPA administration, indicating tumor progression and likely anaplastic transformation (c). Following three cycles of temozolomide, a complete radiographic response was achieved (d).

The role of chemotherapy in the adjuvant and neoadjuvant setting has been recently evaluated in two large phase III randomized controlled trials. A North American trial concluded that the addition of (neo)adjuvant chemotherapy to standard RT resulted in an increased time to tumor progression but overall survival was unaffected even among tumors with 1p and 19q LOH. An EORTC study comparing RT alone versus RT followed by adjuvant PCV (up to six cycles) in AOD reached similar conclusions. These two trials provide valuable information but fell short of defining a new standard of care that included early chemotherapy for AOD for several reasons. First, it is unclear whether prolonging the time to tumor progression among AOD patients translated into a better QOL since this outcome was not examined. Second, most patients who progressed in the RT arm subsequently received chemotherapy and thus the early advantage in PFS achieved by the group randomized to chemotherapy and RT was diminished by the subsequent administration of chemotherapy at the time of progression for patients randomized to RT alone.

The role of chemotherapy in the management of AOD at the time of recurrence has been demonstrated clearly in several studies. The use of PCV or PCV-I for the treatment of recurrent AOD is associated with a response rate of approximately 80% and a median response duration of 1.0–1.5 years. However, given the toxicity associated with PCV, temozolomide is currently being evaluated as a first-line chemotherapeutic agent for AOD with some early encouraging results especially among tumors with 1p LOH.

Conclusions

Despite the chemo- and radiosensitivity of oligodendroglial tumors, their optimal management remains highly controversial. Several recent trials have provided answers to some important long-standing questions such as the use of early versus late RT for the treatment of low grade OD, and the value of PCV chemotherapy when used in the neoadjuvant and adjuvant setting for AOA.

The development of temozolomide as a chemotherapy for gliomas and the use of this agent concurrently with RT and adjuvantly thereafter have been demonstrated to provide survival advantage for patients with newly diagnosed glioblastoma. Using temozolomide in this way for patients with newly diagnosed AOD, while an intuitively appealing option, needs to be established by carefully conducted clinical trials, which are in development. These trials will likely replace histologic diagnosis by molecular criteria, with 1p and 19q LOH as a necessary criterion for enrollment.

Oligodendroglial tumors remain incurable and it is unlikely that further refinement of RT and chemotherapy will cure these neoplasms or render them chronic diseases. While better initial and salvage chemotherapy regimens are needed for the treatment of recurrent tumors, a deeper understanding of the molecular pathogenesis of these tumors may eventually result in the development of targeted therapies that alone or combined with chemotherapy will confer a meaningful survival advantage for patients.

Further reading

Cairncross JG, Macdonald DR. Successful chemotherapy for recurrent malignant oligodendroglioma. *Ann Neurol* 1988; 23(4): 360–4.

Karim ABMF, Maat B, Hatlevoll R, *et al*. A randomized trial on dose-response in radiation therapy of low grade cerebral glioma: European Organization for Research and Treatment of Cancer (EORTC) study 22844. *Int J Radiat Oncol Biol Phys* 1996; 36: 549–56.

van den Bent MJ, Afra D, de Witte O, *et al*. Long-term efficacy of early versus delayed radiotherapy for low-grade astrocytoma and oligodendroglioma in adults: the EORTC 22845 randomised trial. *Lancet* 2005; 366(9490): 985–90.

Chapter 132
Brain stem glioma

Ira J. Dunkel[1] and Mark M. Souweidane[1,2]
[1]Memorial Sloan-Kettering Cancer Center, New York, USA
[2]New York Presbyterian Hospital, Weill-Cornell Medical College, New York, USA

Introduction

Brain stem tumors are heterogeneous. They range from the diffuse pontine tumors which are almost invariably fatal despite all known therapies, to lower grade focal or exophytic tumors that often have a very good prognosis with surgery or observation only.

Diffuse pontine tumors, while rare, are a significant contributor to mortality among pediatric oncology patients. Diagnosis in typical cases is made via MRI scan, without biopsy. No highly effective standard treatment exists and so inclusion of eligible patients in well-designed clinical research studies is extremely important. If an appropriate trial is not available, conventionally fractionated external beam radiation therapy can provide good short-term palliation to a significant proportion of patients. Finally, autopsy should be considered for patients who die of diffuse pontine tumors with the goal of obtaining tumor tissue for biological studies that may in the future lead to novel therapies.

Epidemiology

About 30 000–40 000 children worldwide develop brain tumors each year. Data from the population-based German Childhood Cancer Registry reveal that 1 in 2500 children will be diagnosed with a central nervous system tumor within the first 15 years of life, and from their data we can estimate that about 1 in 23 000 children will develop a diffuse pontine tumor by 15 years of age.

While rare, diffuse pontine tumors represent a significant portion of the deaths due to childhood cancer. The German Registry included 16 826 pediatric oncology patients enrolled over a 10-year period. If we assume that 75% of the children were cured, then about 4200 children died of all forms of cancer. There were 351 patients with tumors of the brain stem (not otherwise specified) and

pons, and if we assume that 90% of those died, then they represent about 8% of the total deaths due to childhood cancer.

Clinical features

Patients with diffuse pontine tumors usually present with a short history (weeks) of signs or symptoms. The most common symptoms include double vision and gait instability. Physical examination typically reveals long tract signs, ataxia, and cranial neuropathies, particularly afflicting the sixth cranial nerve.

While this chapter focuses on diffuse pontine tumors, it is important to realize that there are other types of brain stem tumors that should not be categorized with the highly lethal diffuse pontine tumors. Cervicomedullary, dorsally exophytic, and focal brain stem tumors are usually low grade and associated with a better prognosis. Similarly, tumors in patients with a longer antecedent history of signs or symptoms and brain stem lesions in patients with neurofibromatosis type 1 often behave less aggressively.

Investigations

Brain MRI scan with and without gadolinium typically reveals infiltrative expansion of the pons, with high signal on T2- and fluid-attenuated inversion recovery (FLAIR) weighted images, little or no enhancement, and no significant exophytic component. Cystic changes are infrequently seen, while envelopment of the basilar artery is commonly present.

Treatment/management

While treatment aims, of course, to provide a cure, the reality to date has been that therapy for diffuse pontine tumors has almost always been palliative only. The current extremely poor prognosis of patients with diffuse pontine tumors suggests that autopsies should be

International Neurology: A Clinical Approach. Edited by Robert P. Lisak, Daniel D. Truong, William M. Carroll, and Roongroj Bhidayasiri.

strongly considered to obtain tumor tissue that may allow us to improve our understanding of biological features of the tumor that may translate into new biologically based therapies.

Surgery

Diffuse pontine tumors are not surgically resectable and even diagnostic biopsy is not indicated for patients presenting with typical signs and symptoms and unequivocal MRI evidence of such a tumor. Prior to the advent of MRI, biopsy was performed, with the majority of tumors being World Health Organization (WHO) grade III or IV fibrillary astrocytomas. Autopsy series have demonstrated that at the time of death diffuse pontine tumors are usually high grade astrocytomas.

In contrast, biopsy should be considered if there is any suspicion that the lesion has atypical characteristics for a diffuse pontine tumor. Exophytic primary neuroectodermal tumors of the brain stem and focal low grade brain stem tumors are two examples that would demand a different therapeutic approach.

Radiation therapy

External beam radiation therapy is the standard therapy for diffuse pontine tumors, but several cooperative group trials published in the early 1990s indicated that only approximately 10% of patients achieve 3-year survival despite dose escalation as high as 7800 cGy via hyperfractionation.

Pediatric Oncology Group (POG) 9239 was a phase III trial of conventional radiation therapy versus hyperfractionated radiation therapy in children with newly diagnosed diffuse intrinsic brain stem tumors. Conventionally-treated patients received 5400 cGy in 180 cGy daily fractions, while patients on the experimental arm received 7020 cGy in 117 cGy fractions administered twice daily. Two-year survival rates were 7.1% and 6.7%, respectively.

Accelerated fractionation (conventional fraction doses administered twice daily, resulting in shorter total treatment duration) was studied in the United Kingdom. While the treatment was tolerable, it was also associated with very poor survival.

Multiple agents have been used in conjunction with radiation therapy, often as putative radiation sensitizers. Recent examples include high-dose tamoxifen, topotecan, and etandizole. None has yet been demonstrated to be superior to radiation therapy alone, but clinical research in this area continues. There is some evidence that the combined use of external beam radiation therapy and radiosensitizers may actually be worse than radiation therapy alone. POG investigators non-randomly compared patients with diffuse pontine tumors treated with hyperfractionated radiation therapy alone (7020 cGy) on POG 8495 with those treated with the same radiation therapy plus concurrent cisplatin on POG 9239. A strong trend towards inferior 1-year survival amongst patients treated with combined therapy was noted.

We strongly support the participation of all children with diffuse pontine tumors in well-designed clinical research trials that may allow progress to be made to improve the very inadequate therapies currently available. Outside of a clinical research protocol, standard radiation therapy should be considered as single daily fractionated treatment (about 180 cGy/day) to a dose of approximately 5400–5940 cGy.

Chemotherapy

Conventional-dose chemotherapy (usually administered in conjunction with external beam radiation therapy) has not been effective for diffuse pontine tumors. Children's Cancer Group (CCG) 9941 was a randomized phase II trial of two intensive pre-radiation chemotherapy regimens for children with newly diagnosed diffuse pontine tumors. Thirty-two patients received regimen A: vincristine (1.5 mg/m^2/day), carboplatin (600 mg/m^2/day × 2), and etoposide (167 mg/m^2/day × 3). Thirty one received regimen B: vincristine (1.5 mg/m^2/day), cisplatin (100 mg/m^2), cyclophosphamide (1500 mg/m^2/day × 2), and etoposide (167 mg/m^2/day × 3). Regimen A resulted in a 10% (±5%) objective response rate (≥25% decrease in two-dimensional tumor size) while regimen B resulted in a 19% (±8%) objective response rate. All patients then received hyperfractionated radiation therapy (7200 cGy) and 2-year event-free survival for the entire group was only 6%.

High-dose thiotepa-based chemotherapy with stem cell rescue has been investigated and has not proven to be effective for diffuse pontine tumors.

Emerging therapies

The blood–brain barrier presents a significant obstacle to achieving high tissue concentrations of therapeutic agents delivered systemically. Interstitial infusion, also referred to as convection-enhanced delivery (CED), is a method of local delivery that bypasses the blood–brain barrier. CED is typically accomplished by inserting a small-bore cannula directly into a tumor, followed by infusion through the cannula. Experimental studies have revealed that local drug concentration exceeds that achieved with systemic administration by several thousand-fold, while systemic exposure by way of efflux into the vasculature is negligible. CED can also be used for the delivery of large macromolecules such as monoclonal antibodies or targeted toxins, a feat not possible by systemic administration.

A number of laboratories have investigated using CED in the brain stem. Given the highly unique nature of the brain stem and the potential mechanical considerations, CED has first been tested in naïve rats and primates as well as in brain stem xenographic tumor models in the rat. These preclinical investigations have revealed that

CED appears to be safe, but clearly a rigorous preclinical evaluation of any candidate agent must be performed prior to implementing a human clinical trial. The authors have assessed conventional chemotherapeutic agents such as carmustine and carboplatin, a targeted toxin (IL13PEQQR), and a monoclonal antibody (8H9) in rats, and are designing phase I clinical studies that will assess the surgical technique, parameters of infusion, the timing of treatment, and the method of assessing distribution.

Further reading

Albright AL, Packer RJ, Zimmerman R, Rorke LB, Boyett J, Hammond GD. Magnetic resonance scans should replace biopsies for the diagnosis of diffuse brain stem gliomas: a report from the Children's Cancer Group. *Neurosurgery* 1993; 33: 1026–30.

Fisher PG, Breiter SN, Carson BS, *et al*. A clinicopathologic reappraisal of brain stem tumor classification. Identification of pilocystic astrocytoma and fibrillary astrocytoma as distinct entities. *Cancer* 2000; 89: 1569–76.

Mandell LR, Kadota R, Freeman C, *et al*. There is no role for hyperfractionated radiotherapy in the management of children with newly diagnosed diffuse intrinsic brainstem tumors: results of a Pediatric Oncology Group phase III trial comparing conventional vs. hyperfractionated radiotherapy. *Int J Radiat Oncol Biol Phys* 1999; 43: 959–64.

Chapter 133
Intracranial ependymoma

Sajeel Chowdhary[1] and Marc Chamberlain[2]
[1]University of South Florida, Tampa, USA
[2]University of Washington, Seattle, USA

Introduction

Ependymomas arise from the ependymal cells of the cerebral ventricles, the central canal of the spinal cord, and cortical rests. Ependymomas constitute 8–10% of brain tumors in children and 1–3% of brain tumors in adults. Sixty percent of ependymomas occur in children under 16 years of age and 25% occur in children less than 4 years of age. Tumors arising in the supratentorial compartment (50–60% of adult ependymomas; 30% of pediatric ependymomas) most often are hemispheric or occur in relation to the third ventricle. Posterior fossa tumors either are seen in a midline fourth ventricular location (40–50%) or are located in the cerebellopontine angle (50–60%). The World Health Organization (WHO) classification of tumors separates ependymomas into subependymomas (grade 1), myxopapillary ependymomas (grade 1), ependymomas (grade 2), and anaplastic ependymomas (grade 3). Ependymoblastomas are considered a different type of tumor, classified under embryonal primitive neuroectodermal tumors (PNET).

Approximately 30% of all intracranial ependymomas are anaplastic, though the prognostic significance of anaplasia is controversial. Part of this uncertainty relates to the lack of uniform histological criteria for diagnosing anaplastic ependymomas. Defining tumors as anaplastic based on proliferation indices such as Ki67 staining more than 1% may permit stratification of patients at high risk for recurrence and decreased survival.

Cerebrospinal fluid (CSF) dissemination occurs in 3–12% of all intracranial ependymomas and is most frequent with infratentorial anaplastic ependymomas. Because a small but measurable risk for CSF dissemination exists for all patients with newly diagnosed ependymoma, an extent of disease evaluation including CSF cytology and craniospinal MRI is mandated following surgery. Staging permits stratification of patients into those with (M+) or without (M_0) metastasis and with or without residual disease following surgery, the two most important clinical parameters affecting outcome.

Little is known about the genetic alterations of ependymomas. Tumors in adults frequently have loss of chromosome 22q (not involving the NF2 gene) whereas in children, chromosomal loss is more commonly seen on chromosomes 1, 17p, and 6q. Loss of p14^{arf} has been correlated with increasing anaplasia.

Treatment

Surgery

Intracranial ependymomas often present with signs and symptoms of raised intracranial pressure (headache, alteration in level of consciousness, nausea/vomiting, diplopia, gait instability, papilledema, menigismus) due to either tumor mass or obstructive hydrocephalus. Treatment is primarily surgical, as essentially all analyses have determined that completeness of surgical resection is the most important covariant affecting progression free and overall survival. As a consequence, if initial surgery is found to be incomplete or at time of tumor recurrence, reoperation is advocated assuming complete resection is achievable.

Postoperative complications are not uncommon and should be anticipated. It has been estimated that about 33% of adult patients develop new cranial nerve abnormalities after resection of infratentorial ependymomas, often with dysphagia requiring gastrostomy tube placement. Most deficits resolve with time and support. The posterior fossa syndrome (cerebellar mutism) following an infratentorial craniotomy in children is a well-defined yet infrequent complication.

Following surgery, the issue of how often to image patients is unclear. It is generally accepted that surveillance neuroimaging can reveal asymptomatic recurrences and its use favorably impacts survival and subsequent treatment, in particular, the ability to perform a reoperation with complete resection.

Radiotherapy

After resection, radiotherapy represents the most frequently utilized adjuvant treatment for ependymomas

International Neurology: A Clinical Approach. Edited by Robert P. Lisak, Daniel D. Truong, William M. Carroll, and Roongroj Bhidayasiri. © 2009 Blackwell Publishing, ISBN: 978-1-4051-5738-4.

Table 133.1 Chemotherapy trials in newly diagnosed and recurrent ependymoma. (Adapted from Chowdhary, *et al. Curr Treat Options Neurol* 2006; 8: 309–18.)

No. of patients	Chemo regimen	PFS	OS
66	CYC+VCR/CDDP+VP16	41% at 1year	NR
19	CBDCA+VCR/IFOS+VP16	74% at 5 years	NR
32	Randomized to CCNU+VCR+PRED or "8 in 1" regimen	50% at 5 years	64% at 5 years
73	PCZ+CBDCA/VP16+CDDP/VCR+CYC	22% at 4 years	59% at 4 years
83	PCZ+CBDCA/VP16+CDDP/VCR+CYC	48% at 5 years, 46% at 10 years	68% at 5 years, 47% at 10 years
8	CYC+VCR+VP16	13% at 3 years	32% at 3 years

No. of patients	Chemo regimen	RR	SD
12	PCV	15%	NR
16	HDC+ABMT	0%	63%
5	Etoposide	40%	NR
15	HDC+ABMT	0%	0%
16	Platinum or nitrosurea	67% and 25%	30% and 50%
12	Etoposide	17%	30%
13	Paclitaxel	6%	37%
10 (SCE)	Etoposide	20%	50%
13	Cisplatin	30%	46%

PFS: progression free survival; OS: overall survival; NR: not reported; CYC: cyclophosphamide; VCR: vincristine; CDDP: cisplatin; VP16: etoposide; CBDCA: carboplatin; IFOS: ifosfamide; CCNU: lomustine; PRED: prednisone; 8 in 1 regimen: VP16+CBDCA+PCV+MOPP (mechlorethamine+vincristine+prednisone+procarbazine) alternating with CYC+VCR+CDDP+VP16+ABMT (autologous bone marrow transplantation); PCZ: procarbazine; RR: response rate; SD: stable disease; PCV: procarbazine, CCNU, and vincristine; NR: not reported; HDC: high-dose chemotherapy; ABMT: autologous bone marrow transplantation; SCE: spinal cord ependymoma.

despite the lack of a randomized clinical trial showing benefit and the belief that ependymomas are radioresistant. Furthermore, there are no data regarding a dose–response relationship in ependymomas and, as such, total tumor dose has varied. By consensus, many radiation oncologists believe a tumor dose exceeding 45 Gray (Gy) is necessary and most advocate a dose of 54–55 Gy for ependymomas and 60 Gy for anaplastic ependymomas. Because of the possibility of CSF spread, one controversy regarding the radiotherapeutic management of ependymomas is the volume of brain that needs to be treated. Notwithstanding early enthusiasm for craniospinal irradiation (CSI), several recent studies support limited-field radiotherapy for M_0 tumors and reserve CSI for M+ tumors. There are advocates for observation only following complete resection for supratentorial ependymomas (withholding radiotherapy); however, this is based on case series and has not been rigorously evaluated. Conformal radiotherapy including stereotactic radiotherapy is increasingly utilized despite few studies showing survival or quality of life benefits. A radiotherapy boost following conventional radiotherapy (most often administered by linear accelerator (LINAC) radiosurgery, gamma knife, or cyberknife) is increasingly utilized outside of clinical trials. This is based on the assumption that the radio-resistance of ependymomas is

relative and that by increasing dose to the tumor, radioresistance may be overcome. Also, in that the majority of ependymoma treatment failures are local, augmenting tumor radiotherapy dose may improve long-term control. Despite an appealing construct, the lack of an established dose response relationship for ependymomas following radiotherapy and the empiric observation that measurable neuroradiographic responses are rare suggest more is not necessarily better.

Chemotherapy

The role of chemotherapy in the management of ependymomas is controversial (Table 133.1). In newly diagnosed adults or children, most studies suggest either no additional benefit after surgery and CSI or only modest efficacy. Patients who received postsurgical chemotherapy in lieu of radiation have poorer survival than those who received adjuvant radiation, also supporting the absence of a primary role for chemotherapy in this disease.

Recurrent ependymoma

The management of recurrent ependymoma has not received much attention despite the fact that nearly

50% of patients will recur. In general, median time to recurrence is about 3 years and in the majority of cases the relapse is local, with a small percentage having local recurrence with concomitant distant metastasis. Reoperation should be considered followed by radiation, if possible. Most patients will also receive chemotherapy at relapse. Numerous regimens have been explored, with cisplatin often felt to be the most active agent amongst the four commonly used chemotherapeutics (cisplatin, procarbazine, 1-(2-chloroethyl)-3-cyclohexyl-1-nitrosourea (CCNU), and vincristine).

Summary

Optimal management of ependymomas includes surgical resection and evaluation of the extent of central nervous system (CNS) involvement using both cerebrospinal fluid (CSF) cytology and craniospinal contrast-enhanced magnetic resonance imaging (MRI). In patients not considered for further surgery and with residual disease, limited-field radiotherapy is usually administered. The role of craniospinal irradiation in patients with local disease and no evidence of metastasis is controversial because the majority of tumor recurrences are local and at the site of the primary tumor. No clear role for adjuvant chemotherapy has been demonstrated. Recurrent ependymomas are managed by reoperation of tumors that are surgically accessible, by radiotherapy if not previously administered, and by salvage chemotherapy.

Further reading

Chowdhary S, Green MR, Chamberlain M. Ependymomas. *Curr Treat Options Neurol* 2006; 8: 309–18.

Merchant TE, Fouladi M. Ependymoma: new therapeutic approaches including radiation and chemotherapy. *J Neurooncol* 2005; 75: 287–99.

Paulino AC, Wen BC, Buatti JM, *et al.* Intracranial ependymomas: an analysis of prognostic factors and patterns of failure. *Am J Clin Oncol* 2002; 25: 117–22.

Chapter 134
Nerve sheath tumors

Nathan J. Ranalli and Eric L. Zager
Hospital of the University of Pennsylvania, Philadelphia, USA

Introduction

Nerve sheath tumors may affect any peripheral, cranial, or autonomic nerve and can be separated into two broad categories: (1) benign nerve sheath tumors, which include schwannomas and neurofibromas, and (2) malignant peripheral nerve sheath tumors (MPNSTs). Although most nerve sheath tumors are solitary lesions arising from single nerves, they may be associated with genetic disorders, such as neurofibromatosis type 1 (NF-1) or type 2 (NF-2), in which case there may be multiple tumors involving different nerves. The introduction of the operative microscope and intraoperative neurophysiologic monitoring has contributed significantly to improved surgical outcomes.

Epidemiology and pathophysiology

Benign nerve sheath tumors
Schwannomas
Schwannomas are one of the two most common histological types of benign nerve sheath tumors. These lesions occur at any age but are most common in the third to sixth decades. They represent 5% of all benign soft-tissue neoplasms. Over 50% of schwannomas are located in the head and neck and they may originate from any of the cranial, peripheral, or autonomic nerves. Most schwannomas are indolent and generally painless, though patients may present with a radiculopathy or paresthesias secondary to compression of an adjacent nerve. Schwannomas arise from Schwann cells, occurring within the endoneurium, and are surrounded by a capsule of perineurium and fibrous epineurium; they do not contain axons. Most schwannomas are solitary, though multiple or plexiform schwannomas may be found in association with neurofibromatosis and schwannomatosis. Microscopically, these tumors are composed of Schwann cells arranged

into Antoni A (sheets and palisades of spindle-shaped cells within pathognomonic Verocay bodies) and Antoni B (loose myxoid matrix with collagen fibrils, rare spindle cells, and lymphocytes) areas.

Neurofibromas
The neurofibroma is the other common nerve sheath tumor, having a peak incidence in the third to fifth decades. These lesions arise from the perineurial cells of the nerve sheath and are not encapsulated. They may occur in isolation but are frequently multiple, especially in cases associated with NF-1. Solitary neurofibromas can occur on peripheral nerves throughout the body and are often visible as small subcutaneous nodules. Generally, neurofibromas can be divided into three subtypes: localized, diffuse, and plexiform. The first of these represents nearly 90% of all neurofibromas in patients without NF-1. Diffuse neurofibromas are rare and occur almost exclusively in children and young adults. Plexiform neurofibromas, which have the appearance of a thick, convoluted, bulbous mass, are pathognomonic for NF-1. Histologically, neurofibromas are composed of intercalated bundles of fusiform, elongated cells with darkly staining nuclei surrounded by a matrix containing collagen fibrils, mucoid deposits, lymphocytes, and xanthoma cells.

Malignant peripheral nerve sheath tumors (MPNSTs)
MPNSTs are highly malignant, rare tumors and more than 50% of patients with MPNSTs have NF-1. MPNSTs are a form of soft tissue sarcoma and account for 5–10% of these tumors. The World Health Organization (WHO) defines MPNSTs as any malignant tumor arising from a peripheral nerve or exhibiting nerve sheath differentiation, excluding those originating from the epineurium or peripheral nerve vasculature. Older terms for MPNSTs include neurofibrosarcoma, malignant neurilemmoma, malignant schwannoma, and neurogenic sarcoma. These neoplasms usually present as a painful, enlarging mass, typically located deep in the trunk, extremities, or head and neck region. Risk factors for developing MPNSTs include NF-1 and a history of radiation. Patients with NF-1 typically develop tumors in the third and fourth decades, while

International Neurology: A Clinical Approach. Edited by Robert P. Lisak, Daniel D. Truong, William M. Carroll, and Roongroj Bhidayasiri.
© 2009 Blackwell Publishing, ISBN: 978-1-4051-5738-4.

those with sporadic MPNSTs are frequently affected in the fifth and sixth decades. The average latency period for development of a radiation-induced MPNST is 15 years. Microscopically, most MPNSTs are comprised of spindle cells with markedly increased cellularity, nuclear pleomorphism, mitotic figures, hemorrhage, and necrosis.

Neurofibromatosis

Neurofibromatosis is one of the most common genetic disorders. The disease can be classified based on gene locus and associated characteristics into two major subtypes: NF-1 (Von Recklinghausen's disease) and NF-2.

1 NF-1 has an incidence of 1 in 2500 at birth regardless of gender and accounts for 90% of all neurofibromatosis patients. The syndrome can be caused by an inherited or new gene mutation of the *NF-1* gene. NF-1 is characterized by neurocutaneous findings (café-au-lait spots, axillary freckling), superficial neurofibromas, and iris hamartomas (Lisch nodules). This disease also has a variety of effects on the ocular, musculoskeletal, endocrine, and vascular systems. Nearly all individuals with NF-1 will develop peripheral neurofibromas (any of the three subtypes) and are at increased risk for MPNSTs, optic gliomas, and childhood leukemia.

2 NF-2 is much less common than NF-1, occurring in 1 in 33 000 live births. The NF-2 tumor suppressor gene resides on chromosome 22 and its inactivation leads to the generation of multiple neural tumors. The diagnostic hallmark of NF-2 is the presence of bilateral eighth cranial nerve schwannomas, which occur in over 95% of NF-2 cases. These patients often have multiple cranial and spinal schwannomas as well as meningiomas; spontaneous malignant transformation of a schwannoma to an MPNST rarely occurs.

Diagnosis of nerve sheath tumors

The signs and symptoms of a nerve sheath tumor depend on the location of the tumor and extent of nerve compression. Presenting complaints include local or radiating discomfort, paresthesias, weakness, autonomic dysfunction, and cosmetic deformity. Key features of the history include the rate of growth, presence of neurologic complaints or severe pain, a personal or family history of neurofibromatosis or any of its stigmata, and the presence of other masses or systemic diseases. Physical examination should focus on the size and location of the tumor, the extent of tenderness and ease of mobility, Tinel's sign (which can be present in both benign and malignant processes), and neurological deficit. Pigmentary abnormalities such as café-au-lait spots and skinfold freckling are the most obvious clinical features of NF-1. A rapidly enlarging, deep, or very painful lesion is suggestive of a malignant tumor, particularly in the presence of significant neurological deficits.

MRI is currently the most useful imaging modality and is particularly helpful in delineating the relationships among the lesion, the nerve of origin, and the surrounding vessels, bone, and soft tissues. Neurofibromas frequently show inhomogeneous enhancement with gadolinium while small schwannomas tend to enhance uniformly. Degenerative cyst formation may be seen in schwannomas; this finding does not necessarily indicate malignancy. In some cases the ragged, invasive margin of an MPNST can be demonstrated on MRI, but this finding is not reliably present. A recent modification of MRI, known as MR neurography, can be useful in discriminating between intraneural and perineural masses. Preoperative electromyography (EMG) may provide evidence of nerve involvement. Ultrasonography (US) can reveal a nerve sheath tumor as a hypoechoic lesion with well-defined contours, but it is usually not as helpful as MRI in providing anatomic detail. For deep nerve sheath tumors, intraoperative ultrasound can localize the lesion for incision placement.

Treatment of nerve sheath tumors

Options for the treatment of nerve sheath tumors include conservative management, surgical resection, radiation, and chemotherapy. Small, non-painful, indolent tumors that cause neither neurologic dysfunction nor cosmetic concern can be observed. For patients with neurofibromatosis or schwannomatosis, asymptomatic tumors should be monitored with serial MRI studies, typically on an annual basis. Surgery is indicated for lesions that cause deficits or pain, or for any rapidly growing tumors that raise a suspicion of malignancy. Surgical resection is the treatment of choice for most benign nerve sheath tumors and complete resection usually results in a cure. Surgical goals include the resolution of pain, preservation of neurological function, correction of a cosmetic deformity and attainment of a diagnosis. Maximal efforts are made to preserve the nerve of origin and to avoid additional nerve injury. If a functional nerve fascicle has to be sacrificed during tumor removal, grafting should be considered to achieve good functional recovery (or, alternatively, a small portion of tumor should be left in place and followed in order to preserve nerve function). Sacrifice of an entire nerve segment should virtually never occur in the setting of a benign tumor. Benign solitary symptomatic neurofibromas and schwannomas can usually be completely resected and result in a cure, especially with the refinement of microsurgical techniques. MPNSTs carry a high risk of local invasion, recurrence, and metastasis to lung, liver, bone, and soft tissue. Therefore, if a lesion is suspicious for malignancy, the recommended procedure is an open biopsy to obtain a tissue diagnosis and to guide further therapy. Percutaneous needle biopsy is also a viable option, but has problems with sampling error, obtaining non-diagnostic tissue, nerve injury, and exquisite pain during and/or after the procedure. If the diagnosis of MPNST is confirmed, treatment involves wide resection (occasionally including appendicular amputation) followed or preceded by adjuvant chemotherapy and radiation to help provide local control and delay the onset of recurrence. In the future, biological therapies directed at relevant genetic alterations and new pharmaceutical agents will ultimately lead to novel therapeutic strategies to treat these difficult tumors.

Further reading

Artico M, Cervoni L, Wierzbicki V, D'Andrea V, Nucci F. Benign neural sheath tumours of major nerves: characteristics in 119 surgical cases. *Acta Neurochir* 1997; 139: 1108–16.

Perrin RG, Guha A. Malignant peripheral nerve sheath tumors. *Neurosurg Clin N Am* 2004; 15: 203–16.

Pilavaki M, Chourmouzi D, Kiziridou A, Skordalaki A, Zarampoukas T, Drevelengas A. Imaging of peripheral nerve sheath tumors with pathologic correlation: pictorial review. *Eur J Radiol* 2004; 5: 229–39.

Tiel R, Kline D. Peripheral nerve tumors: surgical principles, approaches and techniques. *Neurosurg Clin N Am* 2004; 15(vi): 167–75.

Chapter 135
Meningiomas

Laurie Rice and Jeffrey Raizer
Northwestern University, Chicago, USA

Introduction

Meningiomas are typically slow-growing dural-based tumors arising from arachnoid cells. They are frequently an incidental finding when an MRI or CT scan of the brain has been ordered for other neurologic evaluations or are found on autopsy. Meningiomas are the most common type of all primary intracranial tumors. Although the vast majority of these tumors are benign, they can recur and can cause significant morbidity depending on location. Rates of recurrence increase with increasing grade. Survival decreases with increased grade; grade I meningiomas are cured in most cases, while patients with grade III meningiomas survive less than 2 years after diagnosis. In a large series of patients the 5-year survival rate for patients with all grades of meningioma was 69%. The recurrence rate for benign (grade I) meningiomas is 7–20%, 29–40% for atypical (grade II) meningiomas, and 50–78% for anaplastic (grade III) meningiomas.

Epidemiology

The overall incidence of intracranial meningiomas is 2–6/100 000 with this representing 13–26% of all primary intracranial tumors in adults. Spinal meningiomas make up about 10% of all meningiomas and 70–80% are seen in women. Meningiomas occur predominately in patients in their fifth to eighth decade of life and are twice as common in women than men. Multiple meningiomas are seen in approximately 8% of patients. The etiology of meningiomas is not clearly understood, but patients who have had prior cranial radiation seem to be at risk; usually they present after a pronged latency with multiple meningiomas and are of increased grade. Patients with some familial and genetic disorders, in particular neurofibromatosis (NF) type 2 (NF2), are also at risk.

International Neurology: A Clinical Approach. Edited by Robert P. Lisak, Daniel D. Truong, William M. Carroll, and Roongroj Bhidayasiri. © 2009 Blackwell Publishing, ISBN: 978-1-4051-5738-4.

Pathophysiology

Genetics

The most frequent genetic abnormality in meningiomas is loss of the chromosomal region (22q,12.2) of the NF2 gene seen in patients with NF but also those with sporadic meningiomas. This gene codes for a protein called Merlin or Schwannomin, a member of the protein 4.1 family, which regulates cell growth and motility. Other genetic aberrations and alterations in the signaling pathways are well described and are more prevalent with higher grade meningiomas; importantly these genetic changes are part of the transformation that occurs from a grade I to a grade III meningioma.

Gonadal hormones

The control of cell growth and multiplication is controlled by growth factors, hormones, and their receptors. The role of gonadal steroid hormones in meningioma development and growth is implied by the higher incidence in females. Meningiomas frequently increase in size during pregnancy and increased incidence has been seen in women who use hormone replacement therapy. Low concentrations of estrogen receptors are seen in approximately 30% of meningiomas and 70% have progesterone receptors. Progesterone receptors tend to decrease in meningiomas that undergo malignant transformation. Somatostatin receptors are also found in 70–100% of meningiomas; their role is unknown.

Histology

The World Health Organization (WHO) has distinguished 15 histologic variants of meningiomas based on architectural patterns, which often dictate tumor grade more than histologic changes. WHO grade I (benign meningiomas) account for approximately 90% of cases; they have occasional mitotic figures and pleomorphic nuclei. WHO grade II (atypical meningiomas) make up 5–7% of meningiomas and this grade is based on architectural pattern or greater than four mitoses per high-powered field (HPF). If the mitotic rate is not elevated, then at least three of the following other characteristics are required for a grade II diagnosis: increased cellularity, high nuclear to cytoplasmic ratio, prominent nuclei, sheet-like growth pattern, or geographic necrosis. WHO grade III (anaplastic meningiomas) account for 1–3% of these tumors. Again, certain architectural patterns are considered anaplastic and these tumors often have more than 20 mitoses per HPF. The recent WHO classification does not have brain invasion as a criterion of malignancy despite this often being present in higher grade meningiomas.

Clinical presentation

The most common presenting symptom is seizures in 30–70% of patients. The location of the meningiomas determines the neurological symptoms. Tumors compressing the cerebrum can cause focal symptoms such as weakness or a visual field defect and those compressing the cerebellum may cause ataxia or symptoms of raised intracranial pressure. Meningiomas of the skull base can cause cranial neuropathies or visual loss.

Investigations

The histologic diagnosis is based on biopsy or resection of the lesion. The typical meningioma on CT is a well-defined extra-axial mass that displaces normal brain tissue. The lesions may have calcification, a smooth contour, and show uniform bright enhancement with contrast. The presence of indistinct margins, marked edema, or deep parenchymal infiltration suggests aggressive behavior or higher grade. Invasion of underlying bone is uncommon. MRI is the preferred method of imaging because it may illustrate the dural origin of the tumor (Figure 135.1). Meningiomas are usually iso-intense to gray matter in T1 MRI images and hyperintense in T2-weighted images. There is homogeneous enhancement when gadolinium is used. Characteristic signs of most meningiomas are marginal thickening that tapers to form a dural "tail." MR venogram may show occlusion when a meningioma abuts a dural sinus. Catheter-based angiography may show a tumor blush.

Treatment

Surgery
For tumors that are deemed non-resectable, biopsy may be done for histologic confirmation. Surgical resection, partial or complete, is preferred for large benign meningiomas with mass effect and those causing progressive neurologic symptoms. For large vascular meningiomas, an angiogram with embolization of the tumor is often done to minimize bleeding. The complete removal of the tumor cures most patients with benign meningiomas. Patients with a grade III meningioma should have as much tumor removed as is feasible, given the very high rate of recurrence.

Radiation therapy
Radiation therapy (RT) should be used after surgery to treat all grade III meningiomas. For grade II meningiomas, postoperative RT is used for incompletely resected tumors, but for patients with complete resection observation can be used. Grade I meningiomas are usually not treated with RT unless they progress after initial resection. Radiation can either be external beam RT or radiosurgery. Radiosurgery allows higher doses to be used, providing better control rates, but it is limited by lesion size.

Chemotherapy
To date there is no widely used effective chemotherapy for meningiomas. As there are hormonal receptors

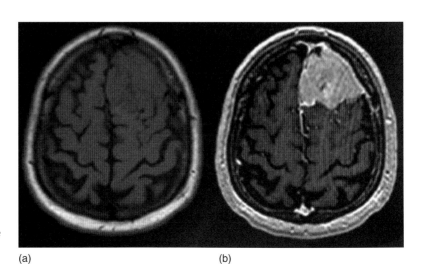

Figure 135.1 (a) Axial T1 precontrast MR image showing a left frontal meningioma that is iso-intense to brain. (b) Axial T1 postcontrast MR image showing a homogeneously enhancing meningioma with dural thickening.

(a)   (b)

in meningiomas, antihormonal agents have been evaluated without large success (i.e., tamoxifen and RU486). Chemotherapies have also been used without marked activity. The most widely used agent is hydroxyurea; other agents such as a combination of cyclophosphamide, adriamycin, and vincristine (CAV), or interferon also have had limited success. Newer agents such as temozolomide and irinotecan (CPT-11) have had no appreciable activity.

With the increased understanding of meningiomagenesis, a move toward biologic agents has started. Several of these agents have been evaluated in clinical trials, with others under investigation. Platelet-derived growth factor receptors (PDGFR) and epidermal growth factor receptors (EGFR) are both tyrosine kinase receptors expressed in meningiomas. Agents such as imatinib (targets PDGFR) and erlotinib (targets EGFR) have been evaluated in clinical trials, but when used as single agents neither has impacted outcome or had major evidence of activity. Since meningiomas are vascular tumors, agents that inhibit vascular endothelial growth factor (VEGF) may be a rational approach and trials of these agents are in process. As more cellular and intracellular targets in meningiomas are identified, targeted agents can be developed and tested. Some of these agents may prove to be effective alone, in combination, or combined with chemotherapy.

Further reading

Simon M, Bostrom JP, Hartmann C. Molecular genetics of meningiomas: from basic research to potential clinical applications. *Neurosurgery* 2007; 60: 787–98.

Wen PY, Drappatz J. Novel therapies for meningiomas. *Expert Rev Neurother* 2006; 6: 1447–64.

Whittle IR, Smith C, Navoo P, Collie D. Meningiomas. *Lancet* 2004; 363: 1535–43.

Chapter 136
Medulloblastoma

Regina I. Jakacki
Children's Hospital of Pittsburgh, Pittsburgh, USA

Overview

Medulloblastomas (MB) or primitive neuroectodermal tumors (PNET) of the cerebellum comprise 20% of all pediatric brain tumors. In contrast, they account for only 1–2% of primary brain tumors in adults, and rarely occur after the fifth decade of life. They have a bimodal distribution in children, peaking at 3–4 years of age and then again at 8–9 years. They are densely cellular, highly malignant, small, round, blue, cell tumors named after the elusive and now known to be non-existent "medulloblast," thought to be a precursor cell for both glia and neurons. It is now believed that they develop from progenitor cells within the external granular layer of the cerebellum. Although MB are chemosensitive and radiosensitive tumors, they are difficult to treat for several reasons. First, they have a propensity to disseminate throughout the craniospinal axis, necessitating the administration of craniospinal irradiation (CSI) to optimize the likelihood of cure. Second, CSI results in irreversible dose-related deleterious effects on neurocognitive processing, endocrine function, and bone and soft tissue growth, especially in younger children. Third, these tumors are biologically diverse, and some will behave aggressively despite favorable clinical features. While tremendous strides have been made in the overall treatment and prognosis of children with MB, the optimal chemotherapeutic and radiotherapeutic regimens that will maximize the likelihood of cure and minimize the late effects of treatment have yet to be determined for individual subgroups.

Presentation

Patients typically present with signs and symptoms of obstructive hydrocephalus and/or cerebellar dysfunction. Papilledema and morning headache, often associated with vomiting, are present in the majority of patients at the time of diagnosis. Symptoms are not usually present for more than 3 months and can be intermittent early in the course. As the tumor increases in size, progressive truncal ataxia usually develops. Sixth nerve palsies are common, and are usually the result of increased intracranial pressure. Infants with an open fontanelle often develop massive hydrocephalus prior to diagnosis, manifesting as increasing head circumference, with more non-specific symptoms such as irritability and intermittent vomiting.

Diagnosis and surgery

Most children are diagnosed when either a computed tomography (CT) scan or magnetic resonance imaging (MRI) of the brain is obtained. Medulloblastomas are typically hyperdense on CT, making it fairly easy to identify tumor even without intravenous (IV) contrast (Figure 136.1). The sensitivity of MRI is far superior to that of CT, particularly for detecting subarachnoid spread, and can assist the neurosurgeon by providing information about the tumor's invasion of and proximity to adjacent structures. Surgery should be undertaken with the goal of removing as much of the primary tumor as possible, guided by the anatomy of the tumor involvement. Approximately 30% of patients will have persistently elevated intracranial pressure after surgery, requiring placement of a ventriculoperitoneal shunt.

Staging evaluation

Approximately 25–35% of patients will have identifiable metastatic disease at the time of diagnosis, although they are not typically symptomatic. An MRI of the spine with intravenous gadolinium contrast, preferably with images obtained in both the axial and sagittal planes, is essential to adequately evaluate for spinal metastases. Obtaining the spinal MRI *prior* to surgical resection is optimal, as it is not uncommon to see postoperative blood and/or other changes within the spine, limiting the ability to detect leptomeningeal "sugar coating." The amount

International Neurology: A Clinical Approach. Edited by Robert P. Lisak, Daniel D. Truong, William M. Carroll, and Roongroj Bhidayasiri. © 2009 Blackwell Publishing, ISBN: 978-1-4051-5738-4.

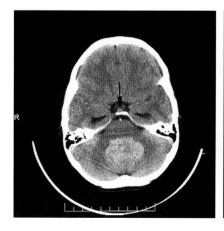
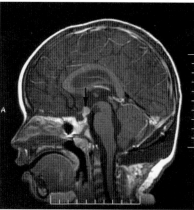

Figure 136.1 Non-contrast CT scan of a 3-year-old girl presenting with a several week history of morning headache and vomiting, along with worsening ataxia. She was brought to the emergency room after becoming obtunded during an airline flight. The CT scan done prior to being taken emergently to the operating room shows the hyperdense midline posterior fossa mass causing obstructive hydrocephalus, as well as a suprasellar metastasis that was later verified on postoperative MRI scan.

Table 136.1 Risk stratification for children older than 3 years of age.

Factors	Average risk	High risk
Extent of disease	Posterior fossa only	Dissemination within the central nervous system or extraneural disease
Extent of resection	Total or near-total resection	Biopsy only; minimal resection; >1.5 cm² residual
Histologic	Classic/non-anaplastic Desmoplastic	Anaplastic/large cell variant
Biologic	High expression Trk-C/neurotrophin 3; immunoreactivity for beta-catenin	MYC-C amplification; high expression ErbB2; isolated 17p loss

Trk-C is the oncogene that encodes the neurotrophin-3 receptor; ErbB2 is a class I receptor tyrosine kinase that is part of an important signal transduction pathway that regulates the growth of cells; MYC-C is an oncogene that acts to increase cell proliferation.

of residual disease in the brain should be assessed on a postoperative MRI scan performed within 24–48 hours of surgery to minimize postoperative artifact. Cerebrospinal fluid (CSF) to evaluate for microscopic tumor should be obtained from a lumbar puncture performed either at the conclusion of the surgical resection or no sooner than 2 weeks after surgery. Bone marrow examinations and bone scans are no longer considered part of routine screening, as the incidence of extraneural dissemination at the time of diagnosis is very low.

Prognostic factors (Table 136.1)

Clinical risk factors
The results of previous cooperative group trials have defined clinical prognostic factors used to stratify patients more than 3 years of age into two risk groups, with higher doses of radiation given to those considered high risk. The presence of metastatic (M+) disease (Table 136.2) is clearly the most powerful predictor of outcome, making a complete staging evaluation crucial

Table 136.2 M (metastatic) stage.

M-0	No evidence of metastases
M-1	Microscopic tumor cells found in cerebrospinal fluid
M-2	Gross nodular seeding in the intracranial subarachnoid space or in the third or lateral ventricles
M-3	Gross nodular seeding in the spinal subarachnoid space
M-4	Extraneural metastases

for accurate determination of risk status. The prognostic importance of other risk factors defined in the pre-MRI era have either been invalidated or diminished by the results of more recent studies. Brainstem involvement is no longer considered a negative prognostic factor. Whether the amount of postoperative residual tumor is a significant risk factor particularly in children who receive radiation therapy, is controversial. Although a Children's Cancer Group (CCG) study found that the presence of residual tumor on postoperative CT scans (arbitrarily defined as larger than 1.5 cm²) was an important prognostic factor in patients with localized disease, this has not been validated in studies done in the MRI era. Regardless, the current risk stratification in the Children's Oncology Group (COG) for children more than 3 years of age defines "low risk" (also known as "average risk") patients as those with less than $1.5\,cm^2$ residual tumor and no evidence of tumor dissemination (M0). High risk patients are those with more than $1.5\,cm^2$ residual tumor or tumor dissemination (M+).

Children less than 3 years of age (infants) are considered "high-risk" by virtue of their age. Their generally poor outcome is felt to be related more to the reluctance to use radiation therapy in this patient population, given the prohibitive side effects of CSI at a very young age. There are subgroups of patients, however, whose prognosis may be reasonably good even without radiation therapy. Cooperative group infant studies have found desmoplastic histology to be a strong positive predictor of outcome. The German Oncology group found that patients with desmoplastic MB enjoyed an 85 + 8% 4-year progression free survival versus 34 + 10% for those with classic MB.

Histologic features

Histologic differentiation along glial, neuronal, and/or ependymal lines has not consistently shown prognostic significance. The degree of anaplasia, however, has been associated with more aggressive behavior, particularly the large cell variant. Anaplastic medulloblastomas contain cells with large nuclei, which are markedly atypical with coarse chromatin and irregular shapes. Large cell medulloblastomas contain large, round neoplastic cells with prominent nucleoli intermixed with the more common small cells. COG studies in both low-risk M0 patients and high-risk patients with metastatic disease found severe anaplasia to be an independent negative predictor of outcome. Based on these findings, all patients with anaplastic tumors should be considered high risk, regardless of clinical stage.

Biology

Molecular studies have revealed that histologically similar tumors are comprised of distinct subgroups with vastly different prognoses. Although clearly important, the ability to predict outcome using the current clinically defined prognostic factors to determine "risk" is suboptimal. Many molecular markers have been evaluated and growth factors that are both powerful negative and positive predictors of outcome have been identified. Increased expression of the receptor tyrosine kinase ERBB2 and the presence of isochromosome 17q within the tumor have been shown to be powerful negative predictors of outcome. Conversely, high levels of the neurotrophin-3 receptor (TrkC), which are present on mature cerebellar granular cells, are associated with a favorable outcome.

The COG is prospectively analyzing these markers in the current standard-risk medulloblastoma study.

Treatment

Medulloblastomas are not curable with surgery alone, but are fortunately quite responsive to both radiation and chemotherapy. Radiation therapy remains the single most effective treatment for medulloblastoma. It has to be assumed that even M0 patients have micrometastases, since the omission of CSI results in a dramatic increase in the frequency of disseminated relapses. Therefore, standard treatment for children older than 3 years of age includes CSI with a boost to the primary tumor site. For many years a craniospinal dose of 36 Gy delivered in 1.8 Gy fractions was administered to all MB patients. However, as the number of survivors increased, so did the awareness of the severity of the late effects. Once it became clear that medulloblastomas were chemosensitive tumors and a randomized study showed that the addition of chemotherapy to radiotherapy improved the outcome in high-risk patients, clinical trials were undertaken to determine whether the addition of chemotherapy could allow reductions in the CSI dose, hopefully decreasing the late cognitive sequelae. Indeed, the CCG-9961 study showed that 23.4 Gy CSI along with adjuvant chemotherapy resulted in a 5-year overall survival of 86 ± 9% in low-risk patients. Prospective studies are underway to determine whether the craniospinal dose can be reduced further. Whether this approach can decrease late effects without compromising survival remains to be seen, for although the whole brain dose of RT is usually considered the major culprit in terms of neurocognitive sequelae, the role that the tumor, surgery, and the radiotherapy boost play in the final neurocognitive outcome should not be underestimated. There is increasing evidence that the cerebellum plays a significant role in cognitive functioning, particularly in the areas of attention, visual-spatial domains, and executive functioning.

Historically, patients with high-risk disease have had 5-year survival rates of less than 50% following treatment with CSI and adjuvant chemotherapy. More recent studies utilizing new chemotherapy strategies as well as radiotherapy boosts to the areas of metastatic disease have resulted in a significantly improved prognosis, particularly for patients without anaplasia. Standard dose chemotherapy is not sufficient to allow a reduction in the craniospinal dose for patients with disseminated disease, with survival rates of 20–40% when this has been attempted.

A variety of different chemotherapeutic agents have shown activity as single agents against MB, including cisplatin, cytoxan, oral VP-16, and carboplatin.

Frequently used multi-agent regimens include cisplatin, 1-(2-chloroethyl)-3-cyclohexyl-1-nitrosourea (CCNU), cytoxan, and vincristine. Pre-irradiation chemotherapy has not been shown to be of benefit and may result in inferior outcomes. The optimal regimen and duration of treatment has yet to be determined.

Further reading

Packer RJ, Gajjar A, Vezina G, *et al.* A phase III study of craniospinal radiation therapy followed by adjuvant chemotherapy for newly diagnosed average risk medulloblastoma. *J Clin Oncol* 2006; 24: 4202–8.

Chapter 137
Primary central nervous system lymphoma (CNSL)

Deborah T. Blumenthal[1,2]
[1]Tel-Aviv University, Tel-Aviv, Israel
[2]University of Utah, Salt Lake City, USA

Introduction

Primary central nervous system lymphoma (CNSL) is a relatively rare brain neoplasm that is of growing importance due to its increased incidence and favorable response to conventional treatments. Although CNSL is similar histologically to systemic large B-cell lymphomas, it has a different biology and natural history, and its location in the central nervous system dictates a different approach in both diagnostic work-up and therapy.

Epidemiology

The incidence of CNSL has increased from rates of 1% before the 1980s to 3–8% in the 1990s and 2000s. Part of the increased incidence is related to the AIDS epidemic, but there is also a less understood increase seen in the "immune-competent" population. There are several hypotheses to explain this increase in incidence, including observation bias, population shift towards the elderly, and increased use of immunosuppressive regimens. Unlike the varied histologic classification in systemic lymphoma, the classification of CNSL is typically that of diffuse large B-cell origin, with a much smaller percentage (2% to as high as 8% reported in Japan) being T-cell. Histologic examination usually reveals a vasocentric neoplasm with invasion of the perivascular spaces.

As the apparent biology of the CNSL differs from most systemic lymphomas, so does its appearance and its treatment. Mass lesions involving the deep parenchyma of the brain are more likely to be primary versus systemic lymphoma. While primary CNSL can also involve the cerebrospinal fluid (CSF), nervous system metastasis of systemic lymphoma typically follows a subdural-meningeal pattern and/or dissemination via the leptomeninges.

International Neurology: A Clinical Approach. Edited by Robert P. Lisak, Daniel D. Truong, William M. Carroll, and Roongroj Bhidayasiri.
© 2009 Blackwell Publishing, ISBN: 978-1-4051-5738-4.

Investigations

Since CNSL is a treatment-sensitive tumor, surgical intervention, with its inherent risks, should be restricted to biopsy for the purpose of definite diagnosis. Outcomes are also not improved by an aggressive resection. Additionally, as CNSL typically responds to treatment, but also grows quickly, it is imperative to begin therapy as soon as the diagnosis is definite. The longer the neurologic symptoms worsen, the more the patient is at risk for suffering irreversible neurologic deficits. Post-treatment imaging may show excellent response to therapy, but the patient may remain disabled by neurologic damage if therapy is delayed.

A caveat in securing the definite diagnosis is performing the biopsy without exposure to steroids. Steroids are tumor cell-lytic in the case of lymphoma, and steroid-exposure can cause the enhancing mass to disappear completely, rendering a biopsy non-diagnostic.

The work-up of CNSL also includes consideration of the systemic immune status of the patient. A thorough history should be taken for any auto-immune disorder or exposure to immune-suppressive treatment or environmental agents. It is recommended to stop the immune-suppressive agent in question, which may assist in managing the CNSL. It is standard practice to check for HIV status even if the patient is without obvious risk factors.

MRI, the imaging study of choice, assists greatly in making the diagnosis of CNSL. Lymphoma typically appears densely contrast enhancing (on CT or MRI). The exception is central, "ring-enhancing" necrosis, which can be seen in HIV-associated CNSL. As the tumor is densely cellular, T2 MR images are typically hypointense in the area of the lesion while diffusion-weighted sequences show hyperintense signal. More than 30% of CNSL lesions are multicentric, often appearing in a periventricular pattern, involving the deep white matter parenchyma. The more commonly involved brain regions are frontal, temporal, deep nuclei, occipital, and cerebellar. Slightly more than 50% of cases are solitary enhancing lesions with either measurable borders (Figure 137.1) or more diffuse in nature. Only 10% of patients present with seizures, as most

535

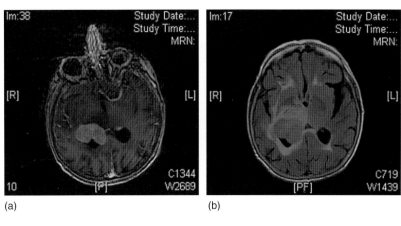

Figure 137.1 Primary CNSL. (a) Axial T1 gadolinium-enhanced MRI shows a densely enhancing solitary mass in the area of the right temporal trigone. (b) Axial fluid-attenuated inversion recovery (FLAIR) MRI shows a hypointense mass (due to increased cellular density), with some surrounding (hyperintense) edema.

lesions involve the deeper white matter. Microscopically, although a lesion may appear well-defined on imaging, lymphoma cells are known to infiltrate widely throughout apparently radiographically uninvolved brain areas. More extensive disease than would be suspected by MRI has been confirmed histologically and correlated with autopsy. Hence, CNSL should be treated as a diffuse, not focal, disease. MRI of the spine is indicated in patients who have spinal or radicular symptoms. Primary spinal lymphoma has been reported but is an exceedingly rare entity. Unless there is a pressure-related threat of tonsillar or uncal herniation, a spinal tap should be performed for examination of the CSF and for cytology and flow cytometry. The finding of monoclonal lymphocytes in the CSF is diagnostic for CNSL. Tests for protein, cell count and differential, and glucose can be supportive but not specific for CSF involvement. Lowered glucose, increased protein, and pleocytosis are usually seen if the CSF is involved. Elevated lactic dehydrogenase (LDH) isoenzymes and β-2 microglobulin are suggestive of CNSL involvement of the CSF but can also be seen in infections and other illnesses. Slit lamp examination by an ophthalmologist should be performed in the initial evaluation as intraocular involvement of CNSL occurs in 10–25% of patients at presentation. There is debate regarding the need for body computed tomography (CT) scanning as primary CNSL is not expected to metastasize outside of the CNS. Bone marrow analysis is unlikely to be revealing in the work-up of primary CNSL. A complete systemic evaluation is recommended if histology of the nervous system lesion is other than large B-cell.

Prognosis and treatment

The prognosis of CNSL without treatment is dismal, with survival less than 4 months, although some individual patients can respond for extended periods with steroid treatments alone. Increased age (above 60), decreased Karnofsky performance status (KPS, less than 70), and spread of disease outside of the hemispheres (CSF, orbits)

impact negatively on prognosis. Unlike gliomas, the initial KPS at diagnosis should not dictate the decision to treat, as if started in a timely fashion, CNSL therapy may lead to a rapid clinical recovery.

Until the 1980s, whole brain radiation treatment (WBRT) was the accepted standard therapy for CNSL. Tumors responded quickly in almost all cases but invariably recurred in a resistant fashion within 12 months. Furthermore, most patients whose tumors were controlled often suffered from disabling neurotoxicity, in some cases beginning less than a year after their treatment.

The standard chemotherapy regimens used for high-grade systemic lymphoma are not efficacious in CNSL, likely due to the poor CNS penetration of the active agents in contrast to methotrexate (MTX)-based regimens due to its high rate of CNS penetration. Therefore most accepted chemotherapy regimens for CNSL today include methotrexate often combined with alkylators, antimetabolite agents, monoclonal antibodies (e.g., rituximab, a monoclonal anti-B-cell antibody), and at times radiation. The leading data support this multimodality approach with median overall survival of over 3 years. Careful selection of patients and adherence to a rigorous hydration and alkalinization regimen prevents most methotrexate associated toxicity. Intrathecal chemotherapy for patients with newly diagnosed disease is less frequently recommended, especially if the CSF is initially negative, as similar outcomes with decreased toxicity may be obtained with high doses (up to $8\,g/m^2$) of systemic methotrexate. For patients who cannot tolerate methotrexate, other chemotherapy regimens can be considered. Recent small series have showed responses to lower doses of methotrexate ($3\,g/m^2$) in combination with oral temozolomide.

Anecdotal responses have been seen by the author in elderly, frail candidates with reduced dose WBRT (24 Gy) combined with low dose ($50\,mg/m^2$) of temozolomide. The regimen of temozolomide and rituximab also seems to have activity for CNSL. In cases of leptomeningeal involvement intrathecal chemotherapy is recommended. Intrathecal rituximab may be useful in this setting and is currently under study in several trials.

There is some controversy regarding the optimal treatment of ocular disease in CNSL; if detected after initial chemotherapy, direct treatment of the eye (ocular radiation or intraocular chemotherapy) should be considered. Even with initial response to systemic chemotherapy, relapse in an initially involved eye is high. High-dose systemic methotrexate can bring responses in intraocular disease, but with relapse seen in half the cases. Most centers rely on direct radiation to the orbits to treat retinal-choroidal disease that does not respond to initial systemic intravenous therapy. Radiation therapy is used routinely to address intraocular disease, but not without serious treatment-related side effects; complications of radiotherapy can include cataracts, dry eyes, punctate keratopathy, radiation retinopathy, and optic atrophy. Intravitreal injection of methotrexate may also be an important treatment option for intraocular disease. Initial studies show possibly improved responses with less morbidity than seen with radiation to the orbit. Intraocular methotrexate injections may result in better long-term ocular outcome and freedom from local disease. Such treatment should be performed at a center with an experienced ophthalmologist, to minimize side effects. Lastly, systemic chemotherapy with ifosfamide and trofosfamide has shown promising results for ocular CNSL.

Salvage therapy

Salvage regimens for recurrent CNSL disease may include repeated treatment with high-dose methotrexate if sufficient time has elapsed (early recurrence suggests methotrexate resistance). The use of temozolomide and rituximab for salvage appears to have a role and patients can respond to further therapy after recurrence. WBRT alone is an option or at a reduced dose with temozolomide, although data are only anecdotal. Topotecan has been studied as a salvage agent, but can cause significant myelosuppression. High-dose chemotherapy with hematopoietic cell transplantation has been studied, but its use has not been supported by results of initial trials, arguably due to inferior induction agents.

Treatment-related toxicity

It was recognized in the late 1980s/1990s that a significant proportion of CNSL patients who survived 6 months or longer developed a neurologic degenerative syndrome characterized by progressive dementia, gait apraxia, and incontinence. Imaging shows atrophy and white matter changes. Although it is felt that all patients suffer some degree of radiation-induced neurotoxicity, increased patient age is associated with a more significant risk. Also, concurrent treatment with methotrexate or treatment shortly following WBRT increases the syndrome's severity. Intrathecal chemotherapy can also cause leukotoxicity independently, and increases the neurologic damage from radiation. Some patients with this syndrome have responded at least temporarily to ventriculo-peritoneal shunt placement.

HIV/AIDS-related CNSL

CNSL is recognized as one of the AIDS-defining illnesses in an HIV-positive patient. CNSL affects advanced HIV patients whose CD4 count is $50\,mm^3$ or less.

There have been anecdotal reports of regression of CNSL after combination highly active antiretroviral therapy (HAART) is initiated and the lymphocytic immune status restored. The AIDS patient is usually more susceptible to the toxic effects of chemotherapy, and although the tumor may respond radiographically, the patient may succumb to a myriad of infectious complications from overly aggressive chemotherapy. Hence, the approach to CNSL in this setting is often palliative and median survival for AIDS-CNSL is 4 months. Standard treatment involves WBRT. There are small series that support the use of chemotherapy (although not the standard high-dose intravenous regimens used for immunocompetent patients).

AIDS-related CNSL is an example of a true "oncovirus," in that Epstein–Barr virus (EBV) incorporates itself cellularly and triggers a clonal expansion of the neoplasm. The definitive diagnosis of CNSL in the case of a suspicious mass in an HIV-postive patient can be made by CSF DNA analysis. The sensitivity and specificity of EBV polymerase chain reaction (PCR) in such a patient is 80% and 100% respectively.

Treatment guidelines, clinical trials, and future direction

CNSL is sensitive to chemotherapy and radiation. It should be approached with a multimodality, preferably methotrexate-based chemotherapy regimen, with radiation used judiciously on a case-by case basis (e.g., initial consolidation versus salvage, reduced dose radiation). Initial data using reduced dose WBRT with immunochemotherapy appear promising, showing improved survival responses and decreased neurotoxicity. A small series of patients treated with immunochemotherapy (rituximab, carboplatin, and methotrexate) and blood–brain barrier disruption shows promising early results.

Current phase II clinical trials are evaluating several key controversial issues including the benefit of adding rituximab, the efficacy of temozolomide, and reduced dose radiation (36 Gy given in hyperfractionated twice-daily doses).

Further reading

Doolittle ND, Jahnke K, Belanger R, *et al*. Potential of chemo-immunotherapy in relapsed primary central nervous system (CNS) lymphoma. *Leuk Lymphoma* 2007; 48: 1712–20.

Gerstner E, Batchelor T. Primary CNS lymphoma. *Expert Rev Anticancer Ther* 2007; 7: 689–700.

Hoffmann C, Tabrizian S, Wolf E, *et al*. Survival of AIDS patients with primary central nervous system lymphoma is dramatically improved by HAART-induced immune recovery. *AIDS* 2001; 15: 2119–27.

Wong ET. Salvage therapy for primary CNS lymphoma with a combination of rituximab and temozolomide. *Neurology* 2004; 63: 901–3.

Chapter 138
Brain metastases

Silvia Hofer[1,2] and Michael Brada[1]
[1]The Institute of Cancer Research and The Royal Marsden NHS Foundation Trust, London and Sutton, UK
[2]University Hospital Zürich, Zürich, Switzerland

Introduction

Brain metastases are a common manifestation of malignancy, affecting 10–20% of patients with solid tumors. The majority develop in the context of known primary or metastatic disease and a small proportion of patients present with intracranial lesions as the first feature of malignancy. The approach to management has consisted of corticosteroids, brain irradiation, and surgery for solitary lesions. With developments in radiotherapy and systemic treatment the range of treatment options has increased even though the evidence base for management alternatives is limited.

Incidence

The frequency of brain metastases reflects the incidence of primary malignancy as well as the propensity for central nervous system (CNS) dissemination. The overall risk of developing brain metastases in patients with solid tumors is about 10%. The reported incidence for patients with lung cancer is 20%, melanoma 7%, renal carcinoma 7%, breast cancer 5%, and colorectal cancer 2%. Patients with breast cancer aged 20–39 years have the highest proportional risk of brain metastases.

Presentation and diagnosis

Patients may present with any sign or symptom associated with a brain tumor and therefore any patient with known malignant disease presenting with features indicating an intracranial problem requires CT or MRI with and without contrast.

Brain metastases are typically iso- or hyperdense on CT and iso- or hyperintense on MRI, usually with surrounding low density assumed to represent edema and usually

enhance with intravenous contrast. The difficulty in differential diagnosis arises in the presence of hemorrhage into the lesion, which does not allow for visualization of the underlying tumor. While the majority of brain metastases lie within the brain parenchyma, they may occasionally mimic tumors such as meningioma or acoustic neuroma.

In the presence of known systemic malignancy and metastatic disease, there is no indication for biopsy of intracranial lesions unless there is a high index of suspicion for an alternative diagnosis such as an atypical infection. In patients presenting with lesions in the brain, without previous history of primary malignancy, histological confirmation is generally required preferably from an extracranial site.

Prognosis

Median survival in patients with multiple brain metastases is 3–4 months, with 10–15% 1-year survival. Prognostic factors for survival are Karnofsky performance status (KPS), age, and the presence and activity of systemic disease. Patients with all three favorable factors (KPS > 70, age < 65, and absence of extracranial metastases with controlled primary tumor) have a median survival in the region of 7 months. In the presence of one adverse factor, the median survival is 4 months, and if KPS score is below 70 the median survival is just over 2 months.

The prognostic factors for survival in patients with solitary brain metastases are the same as in patients with multiple brain metastases. The dominant adverse prognostic factor for survival is performance status; patients with poor performance status and marked disability have survival similar to patients with multiple brain metastases.

Medical management

The aim of treatment is to improve neurological deficit and quality of life (QoL) and to prolong survival. Mass effect and deficits assumed to be due to surrounding edema

International Neurology: A Clinical Approach. Edited by Robert P. Lisak, Daniel D. Truong, William M. Carroll, and Roongroj Bhidayasiri. © 2009 Blackwell Publishing, ISBN: 978-1-4051-5738-4.

are treated with corticosteroids. Oral dexamethasone is generally the drug of choice and can be administered in a single daily dose. One randomized trial compared daily dexamethasone doses of 4–12 mg. Improvement in function at 1 week was the same regardless of dose, with patients receiving higher doses experiencing more severe side effects. In patients with features of increased intracranial pressure, higher loading doses are recommended. After clinical benefit has been achieved, the dose should be gradually titrated to the lowest necessary to maintain improvement. Corticosteroids should be reduced and discontinued after definitive treatment to avoid Cushingoid side effects. In patients with no or minimal symptoms, corticosteroids should not be automatically administered. Corticosteroids are not recommended as a prophylactic treatment prior to cranial irradiation or chemotherapy.

The management of seizures in patients with brain metastases is the same as that of patients with any brain tumor. There is no evidence for benefit of prophylactic anticonvulsants. If chemotherapy is part of the management it is preferable to avoid enzyme-inducing anticonvulsants which increase the metabolism of many oncologic agents, leading to lower effective doses.

Specific treatment modalities

Surgery

Surgery is the appropriate treatment for accessible solitary brain metastases in non-eloquent areas. In patients with multiple brain metastases, surgical excision is generally not indicated, unless one easily accessible lesion is responsible for the majority of symptoms. Although resection of multiple brain metastases has been recommended by some, the apparent favorable survival seen was most likely due to patient selection rather than the efficacy of surgery.

The survival benefit of surgical resection of solitary brain metastasis has been tested in three small randomized trials comparing surgery and whole brain radiotherapy (WBRT) with WBRT alone. Two studies showed prolongation in survival that was not confirmed in the third study. The consensus opinion is that surgery is appropriate for patients with a solitary brain metastasis. Radical excision should be reserved for patients with favorable prognostic factors, particularly without progressive systemic disease.

Radiotherapy

Whole brain irradiation has been the mainstay of treatment of patients with brain metastases. Only one randomized trial compared supportive care (corticosteroids alone) with WBRT and showed a small improvement in median survival in patients receiving WBRT. No randomized studies have shown benefit for more intensive radiation dosing. The preferred WBRT for patients with multiple brain metastases is 20 Gy in five fractions or 30 Gy in 10 fractions.

It is generally accepted that patients with good performance status and reasonable prognosis may benefit from WBRT both in terms of survival and neurological function/QoL. The value of radiotherapy in patients with marked disability and poor performance status is unclear.

Patients with brain metastases from chemosensitive tumors are appropriately treated with chemotherapy. Because of presumed residual microscopic disease following completion of chemotherapy, patients are usually offered consolidation WBRT, although randomized studies assessing the additional value of irradiation are not available.

In diseases with high incidence of intracranial dissemination, brain irradiation is used as prophylaxis. Prophylactic cranial irradiation (PCI) improves intracranial tumor control and survival in patients with limited and advanced stage small-cell lung cancer (SCLC) who achieve complete or good partial remission, although the magnitude of gain in life expectancy is not large. There is no proven benefit of PCI in patients with other solid tumors.

Radiation therapy and radiosensitizers

A number of radiation sensitizers have been tested in addition to radiotherapy, but none to date has demonstrated benefit in randomized studies.

Radiosurgery

Stereotactic radiotherapy delivers localized radiation for lesions less than 4 cm in diameter. Following single fraction radiosurgery to a dose of 15–25 Gy, the probability of reduction in the size of a solitary metastasis is 80–90%; complete disappearance is uncommon. In patients with MRI proven solitary brain metastasis, the addition of radiosurgery to WBRT improves survival and tumor control. Radiosurgery does not prolong survival in patients with two or more brain metastases. The present recommendation is to offer radiosurgery to patients with a solitary brain metastasis and good performance status.

The role of WBRT following surgery or radiosurgery is currently debated. One small randomized study has shown that the addition of WBRT prolonged intracranial disease control but did not offer a survival benefit. Our policy is not to offer WBRT following successful local treatment and continue close monitoring, although routine addition of WBRT is a reasonable alternative approach. Patients considered for radiosurgery as primary treatment often have initial WBRT as a rapid initial therapy, allowing time for more technologically intensive radiosurgery.

Systemic treatment

The blood–brain barrier (BBB) has been considered a bar to the delivery of systemic agents which are not lipid soluble. Nevertheless, the administration of water-soluble drugs, which cannot cross an intact BBB, results in regression of brain metastases. Therefore the BBB should not be considered the reason for withholding potentially effective chemotherapy, particularly as enhancing brain metastases are likely to have impaired BBB.

Response rate of brain metastases to chemotherapy tends to reflect the chemoresponsiveness of the malignancy. In patients with brain metastases from untreated chemosensitive tumors such as non-Hodgkin's lymphoma, SCLC, and germ-cell tumors the appropriate first-line treatment is chemotherapy.

Chemotherapy has been considered as an additional treatment to WBRT, although several randomized phase II studies showed no additional survival benefit and at best a small difference in response rate and progression free survival.

Management in common solid tumors

Non-small-cell lung cancer (NSCLC)

The actuarial 2-year cumulative risk of developing brain metastases in patients with locally advanced stage III adenocarcinoma and squamous cell carcinoma following combined modality treatment is 22% and 10% respectively and nearly half present within 4 months of completion of treatment. Chemotherapy reduces the risk of extracranial failure but has no effect on the incidence of CNS relapse. In patients with locally advanced NSCLC, PCI may reduce the risk of developing disease in the brain, but the overall benefit is not clear.

Patients with brain metastases from NSCLC tend to be heavily pretreated and therefore have less chance of responding to second- or third-line agents and should receive short palliative WBRT as the treatment of choice. The response rate of brain metastases to platinum-based chemotherapy is as would be expected in systemic NSCLC. In asymptomatic chemo-naïve patients not in need of immediate radiotherapy, chemotherapy can be considered as an alternative, particularly in the presence of disseminated or locally advanced and progressive disease, with radiotherapy reserved for progressive intracranial disease.

Small-cell lung cancer (SCLC)

The incidence of brain metastases is particularly high in SCLC. In patients with limited disease who achieve complete/good remission, PCI has become part of the initial treatment. PCI decreases the incidence of brain metastases and has a modest survival benefit. Even in responding patients with extensive disease, PCI reduces the incidence

of brain metastases and improves survival, albeit at a cost of some acute toxicity. Although there is concern regarding the impact of PCI on QoL and cognitive function, there is no consistent difference between patients with or without PCI.

Intracranial metastases from SCLC respond to chemotherapy as disease at other sites. In newly diagnosed chemo-naïve patients the response of brain metastases to chemotherapy (without irradiation) is 70–80%, while at relapse it is 40–50%. The use of additional WBRT does not translate into improved survival, suggesting that extracranial disease is the major determinant of outcome in these patients.

Breast cancer

Because of the high incidence of the disease, nearly a quarter of patients presenting with brain metastases have underlying breast cancer. The risk of developing brain metastases is higher in younger patients with negative estrogen receptor status, grade 3 disease, and large tumors, and is also more common in the presence of visceral metastases, especially lung. Patients with human epidermal growth factor receptor 2 (HER-2) overexpressing tumors are more prone to developing brain metastases and the incidence is not reduced by the HER-2 monoclonal antibody trastuzumab. The dual epidermal growth factor receptor (EGFR) and HER-2 tyrosine kinase inhibitor lapatinib which penetrates the BBB may be effective in these patients.

Breast cancer is both chemo- and radio-responsive. WBRT remains the standard of care in the majority of symptomatic patients. Patients who have chemosensitive tumors particularly with metastatic disease at other sites can be considered for systemic chemotherapy and if they have hormone-responsive disease for hormone therapy. Capecitabine has shown activity in the brain while temozolomide has minimal activity.

Malignant melanoma

Although radiotherapy is perceived to be poorly effective, patients with melanoma brain metastases have not been identified as having significantly worse survival and WBRT remains the treatment of choice. Chemotherapy with dacarbazine (DTIC), temozolomide, or fotemustine results in brain response rates of 7%. Although a more aggressive approach with platinum and DTIC combined with IL-2 and interferon may result in marginally better response rates and occasional complete responses it does not prevent the development of brain metastases. Replacing DTIC with temozolomide in immunochemotherapy has been claimed to reduce the incidence of CNS progression, but did not result in improved survival.

Germ-cell tumors

Approximately 10% of all patients with advanced gonadal germ-cell tumors present with brain metastases.

CNS disease may also appear as part of systemic relapse. The primary treatment in patients with brain metastases is chemotherapy as in advanced nonseminoma. Despite high response rate, WBRT is recommended as adjuvant treatment.

Conclusion

Nearly a quarter of patients with malignant disease develop brain metastases and this is generally a hallmark of incurable disseminated disease. In this context the primary aim of management is palliative and this can be achieved with symptomatic management and a range of oncological treatments, of which WBRT remains the most effective. More aggressive treatment with surgery, radiosurgery, and combined therapies is best reserved for patients with solitary brain metastases with minimal neurological deficit and absent or static systemic disease. Intensive local treatments are inappropriate for patients with multiple brain metastases particularly in the context of other metastatic disease. The development of targeted systemic therapies has so far had minimal impact on the natural history and treatment options in the majority of patients with brain metastases.

Palliative care services play an important and often primary role in the care of patients affected by brain metastases and their families. The aim in all patients with brain metastases should be to allow symptom-free independent life at home or in a palliative care setting and this must focus on support and not oncological treatment alone.

Further reading

Andrews DW, Scott CB, Sperduto PW, *et al*. Whole brain radiation therapy with or without stereotactic radiosurgery boost for patients with one to three brain metastases: phase III results of the RTOG 9508 randomised trial. *Lancet* 2004; 363(9422): 1665–72.

Barnholtz-Sloan JS, Sloan AE, Davis FG, *et al*. Incidence proportions of brain metastases in patients diagnosed (1973 to 2001) in the Metropolitan Detroit Cancer Surveillance System. *J Clin Oncol* 2004; 22: 2865–72.

Lagerwaard FJ, Levendag PC, Nowak PJ, *et al*. Identification of prognostic factors in patients with brain metastases: a review of 1292 patients. *Int J Radiat Oncol Biol Phys* 1999; 43: 795–803.

Sperduto PW, Berkey B, Gaspar LE, Mehta M, Curran W. A new prognostic index and comparison to three other indices for patients with brain metastases: an analysis of 1960 patients in the RTOG database. *Int J Radiat Oncol Biol Phys* 2008; 70(2): 510–4.

Vecht CJ, Wagner GL, Wilms EB. Interactions between antiepileptic and chemotherapeutic drugs. *Lancet Neurol* 2003; 2: 404–9.

Chapter 139
Leptomeningeal metastases

Elizabeth R. Gerstner[1] and Tracy T. Batchelor[1,2]

[1]Massachusetts General Hospital, Boston, USA
[2]Harvard Medical School, Boston, USA

Introduction and epidemiology

Leptomeningeal metastasis (LM), the spread of cancer to the leptomeninges, is being diagnosed more frequently as patients live longer with systemic cancer. Approximately 4–15% of patients with cancer will develop symptomatic LM. The most common tumors associated with LM spread are breast cancer, lung cancer, and melanoma. Less frequently gastrointestinal tumors or adenocarcinoma of unknown primary cause can metastasize to the leptomeninges. The incidence of LM in patients with breast cancer may be increasing as these patients now have prolonged survival and the central nervous system (CNS) may serve as a sanctuary site for tumor cells. Drugs such as trastuzumab do not readily cross the blood–brain barrier so tumor cells may survive within the CNS.

Pathogenesis

Systemic cancer typically reaches the leptomeninges and cerebrospinal fluid (CSF) by hematogenous spread, direct extension from intraparanchymal tumors, perineural spread via peripheral/cranial nerves, or iatrogenic spread during neurosurgical procedures. Once cancer cells gain access to the CSF, they can disseminate throughout the neuraxis by bulk flow. Tumor cells typically settle in the basal cisterns, posterior fossa, and cauda equina because of slow flow in these areas. These deposits then become sources for continuous shedding of malignant cells into the CSF.

Diagnosis

LM usually present when the systemic cancer is widely disseminated but can also appear when the cancer is under good control or even in remission. For this reason,

a high index of suspicion must be maintained whenever evaluating a cancer patient with neurological complaints. Patients with LM can present with signs of obstructed CSF flow, multifocal neurological signs, or altered mental status. CSF obstruction occurs when tumor cells block flow or reabsorption of CSF, leading to signs and symptoms of increased intracranial pressure. The hallmark of LM, though, is multiple focal neurological complaints. Any new occurrence of focal numbness/weakness, headache, back/radicular pain, or incontinence should prompt consideration of LM. The oculomotor nerve, followed by the facial, optic, and auditory nerves are the most commonly involved cranial nerves. Loss of one or more deep tendon reflexes is seen in up to 70% of patients so a careful neurological examination is warranted. Rarely, LM can present as a diffuse encephalopathy possibly from alteration of underlying brain metabolism or competition between tumor cells and normal brain for necessary metabolites.

MRI

Following a history and physical examination searching for the symptoms and signs mentioned above, magnetic resonance imaging (MRI) with and without gadolinium is the next diagnostic step. Computed tomography (CT) scan with contrast can be performed as well but is not as useful as MRI in detecting tumor deposits. Imaging should focus on the origin of the symptoms, but scanning the brain and entire spine often identifies asymptomatic lesions, and brain imaging is usually recommended prior to diagnostic lumbar puncture. Neuroimaging is abnormal in approximately 50% of patients. Suggestive findings include enhancement of the leptomeninges or communicating hydrocephalus. However, it is important to keep in mind that leptomeningeal enhancement can also be seen in patients with infection, inflammation, or trauma, or following lumbar puncture – one reason why neuroimaging is important prior to performing a lumbar puncture in this setting.

Lumbar puncture (LP)

CSF examination is the most informative investigation to confirm LM. Opening pressure, cell count, protein,

International Neurology: A Clinical Approach. Edited by Robert P. Lisak, Daniel D. Truong, William M. Carroll, and Roongroj Bhidayasiri. © 2009 Blackwell Publishing, ISBN: 978-1-4051-5738-4.

glucose, and cytology should be tested. Flow cytometry is useful if hematological malignancy is suspected. CSF pressure and protein are elevated in at least 50% and 80%, respectively, of patients. Glucose less than 40 mg/dl is found in 24–40% of patients and is highly suggestive of LM. The LP may have to be repeated since the yield of cytology increases from 50% to 85% by the third LP. CSF biomarkers such as carcinoembryonic antigen (CEA) or lactate dehydrogenase have limited utility because of a lack of specificity and sensitivity. Vascular endothelial growth factor and tPA have had early promising results, but more studies are needed to confirm their value.

Treatment

Unfortunately, LM carries a poor prognosis with a median survival of only 4–6 weeks without treatment. Some indolent tumors such as breast cancer or lymphoma can have longer survival. The main goal of treatment is palliation and prevention of new neurological deficits, as fixed deficits usually do not improve. Patients who are most likely to benefit from aggressive treatment are those who have slow-growing tumors, good functional status, encephalopathy, minimal/absent systemic disease, and no CSF flow abnormalities. Treatment for LM involves radiation with or without chemotherapy. Surgery plays little role in the management of LM other than ventriculoperitoneal shunting for hydrocephalus or placement of an Ommaya reservoir for intrathecal chemotherapy.

Radiation therapy (RT)

RT is typically given focally to symptomatic areas or sites of bulky disease that chemotherapy is unable to penetrate well. Craniospinal irradiation is usually too toxic to the typical LM patient who has often received multiple prior chemotherapy agents and is at high risk for bone marrow suppression. RT may help to relieve obstructed CSF flow, allowing for improved distribution of chemotherapy. Whole brain irradiation at a dose of 30 Gy is customarily delivered in 10 fractions over 2 weeks. This leads to pain relief and stabilization of neurological deficits but uncommonly results in clinical improvement.

Chemotherapy

Intrathecal (i.t.) chemotherapy is administered to eradicate microscopic disease and cancer cells circulating in the CSF that could form new leptomeningeal deposits. The blood–brain barrier (BBB) and blood–CSF barrier prevent most systemic chemotherapeutics from entering the CNS, so direct delivery into the CSF is advisable. Intrathecal chemotherapy is most effectively delivered through a ventricular catheter such as an Ommaya reservoir rather than through repeated LP procedures. During an LP as much as 10–15% of the drug does not reach the subarachnoid space and the procedure can be uncomfortable for patients.

Problems of distribution arise with intraventricular chemotherapy as well, however, because of abnormal CSF flow that is observed in up to 70% of LM patients. Flow can be obstructed at the ventricular outlet and impaired along the spinal cord or over the convexities of the hemispheres, leading to uneven distribution of chemotherapeutics and increasing the risk of neurotoxicity. It is also important to recognize that there may be discordant cytology results between CSF samples obtained from the ventricle versus the lumbar cistern. Consequently, an LP may still be needed to confirm clearance of CSF during treatment.

Currently, there are three standard chemotherapeutics that are given via the i.t. route. Methotrexate, a folate antagonist, is given twice weekly with oral folic acid supplementation such as leucovorin. Leucovorin does not cross the BBB so it does not interfere with methotrexate-induced cytotoxicity in the CNS but can mitigate extraneural side effects such as myelosuppression. The main side effects from i.t. methotrexate are arachnoiditis, altered mental status, nausea, vomiting, and rarely seizures. Success with methotrexate is limited, with only approximately half of patients treated having stabilization of their disease for longer than 1 month.

Cytarabine is an antimetabolite given twice weekly, while a newer, liposomal formulation of cytarabine can be given every 2 weeks. Liposomal cytarabine has a half-life of 141 hours vs. 3.4 hours for cytarabine. Arachnoiditis is a common side effect from liposomal cytarabine and dexamethasone is give prophylactically the day of and for 4 days following instillation of the drug. Headache is also commonly seen with liposomal cytarabine. In one small study, liposomal cytarabine had an improved response rate when compared with standard cytarabine.

The alkylating agent thiotepa is also available for i.t. administration. However, the half-life of the drug in CSF is very short, questioning the viability of this agent when administered only twice a week. The most concerning side effect with thiotepa is leukoencephalopathy, which can vary from asymptomatic white matter changes to progressive dementia that appears approximately 6 months after treatment.

More recent studies have begun to explore alternative treatment options. Use of systemic chemotherapy to treat LM is limited to agents that penetrate the BBB. High-dose intravenous methotrexate has been used with promising results, but many solid tumors are not sensitive to methotrexate alone. A phase I trial of i.t. rituximab in patients with lymphomatous meningitis identified the maximum tolerated dose (25 mg twice per week) and produced responses in 6 out of the 10 patients treated. Trastuzumab, a humanized antibody to human epidermal growth factor receptor 2 (HER2) which does not cross the BBB when given systemically, the subject of a case report in which a patient with LM from a HER2 over-expressing breast cancer survived for 11 months during i.t. therapy with trastuzamab. Future studies are likely to focus on the identification of new and existing drugs that can be administered via the i.t. route. For example, microcrystallized temozolomide is now being studied as an i.t. injection in animal models. Safe, more effective i.t. therapeutics are desperately needed for this patient population.

Conclusion

Leptomeningeal metastases will become an increasingly important challenge in cancer treatment as systemic therapies improve survival. The protected environment of the CNS shields malignant cells from many systemically administered agents, allowing the tumor to grow without interference. New and multifocal neurological symptoms in a cancer patient should prompt an evaluation for LM that should include contrast-enhanced cranial MRI followed by lumbar puncture if the latter can be performed

safely. Treatment involves whole brain irradiation or focal irradiation to symptomatic areas or sites of bulky disease. Intrathecal chemotherapy through an Ommaya reservoir remains a standard part of the therapeutic approach to this patient population, although new drugs are desperately needed.

Further reading

Glantz MJ, Cole BF, Recht L, *et al.*High-dose intravenous methotrexate for patients with nonleukemic leptomeningeal cancer: is intrathecal chemotherapy necessary? *J Clin Oncol* 1998; 16(4): 1561–7.

Rubenstein JL, Fridlyand J, Abrey L, *et al.* Phase I study of intraventricular administration of rituximab in patients with recurrent CNS and intraocular lymphoma. *J Clin Oncol* 2007; 25(11): 1350–6.

Sampson JH, Archer GE, Villavicencio AT, *et al.* Treatment of neoplastic meningitis with intrathecal temozolomide. *Clin Cancer Res* 1999; 5(5): 1183–8.

Stemmler HJ, Schmitt M, Harbeck N, *et al.* Application of intrathecal trastuzumab (Herceptintrade mark) for treatment of meningeal carcinomatosis in HER2-overexpressing metastatic breast cancer. *Oncol Rep* 2006; 15(5): 1373–7.

Chapter 140
Spinal epidural metastases

Lee I. Kubersky and David Schiff
University of Virginia Health System, Charlottesville, USA

Introduction

This chapter outlines the epidemiology, pathophysiology, presentation, diagnostic workup, treatment, and prognosis of epidural metastases (metastatic epidural spinal cord compression, MESCC) and discusses the broad differential diagnosis from an international perspective.

Epidemiology

The incidence of MESCC is approximately 5% of patients with cancer. While metastatic tumor from any primary site can produce ESCC, cancers of the lung, breast, and prostate are the most common culprits. Although epidural disease arises most often in patients known to have systemic cancer, ESCC is the initial manifestation of malignancy in up to 30% of patients. This is most often seen in cancers of unknown primary origin, myeloma, lung cancer, and non-Hodgkin's lymphoma.

Cancers of the prostate, breast, lung, and colon dominate in much of North America, Europe, and Australia. Stomach and cervical cancer predominate in Central and South America, whereas cancer of the liver, bladder, and Kaposi's sarcoma are commonly found in Africa. Countries of southern and southeastern Asia have significantly higher incidences of esophageal, stomach, and liver carcinoma. Nasopharyngeal cancer, common in southwest Asia and the Mediterranean basin, commonly metastasizes to the bony skeleton.

Pathophysiology

Since the 1940s, cancer cells have been thought to enter the vertebral column through Batson's vertebral venous plexus. However, recent studies suggest that arterial seeding of the vertebrae may be a more common mechanism. This occurs largely in the hematopoietic bone marrow, and thus the posterior vertebral body is invaded first, followed by the pedicle and laminae. Less commonly,

tumors such as lymphomas spread from the paraspinal region through the intervertebral neural foramen.

Clinical presentation

Approximately 70% of spinal epidural metastases occur in the thoracic vertebrae, 20% in the lumbosacral spine, and 10% in the cervical spine. Multiple metastatic lesions are reported in about one-third of patients.

Early recognition of ESCC is crucial, as treatment success is directly related to the severity of neurologic deficits at presentation. Studies have shown that overall survival is directly related to ambulatory status at diagnosis, but unfortunately about two-thirds of patients are not ambulatory at diagnosis of ESCC.

In over 90% of patients, pain is the initial symptom. Back pain from epidural metastases is often aggravated with recumbency, Valsalva maneuver, or spinal percussion. Radicular pain is less common than local pain; however, thoracic epidural lesions can produce a band-like sensation around the anterior trunk.

ESCC produces upper motor neuron weakness if localized at or above the conus medullaris, manifested by hyperreflexia, hypertonicity, extensor plantar responses, and symmetric weakness of the lower extremities. Proximal leg weakness is most severe with thoracic ESCC.

Sensory symptoms are almost as common as motor findings at diagnosis. Early symptoms include ascending numbness and paresthesias. If a spinal sensory level is found, it is usually one to five levels below the site of cord compression. Cauda equina lesions may produce saddle anesthesia. Autonomic dysfunction is a late finding and most often manifests as painless urinary retention.

Diagnosis

In addition to the clinical diagnosis, radiologic confirmation is necessary for treatment planning, while contrast-enhanced magnetic resonance imaging (MRI) is generally accepted as the most sensitive and specific diagnostic tool for MESCC. Plain radiographs are easily available and can

International Neurology: A Clinical Approach. Edited by Robert P. Lisak, Daniel D. Truong, William M. Carroll, and Roongroj Bhidayasiri.
© 2009 Blackwell Publishing, ISBN: 978-1-4051-5738-4.

demonstrate classic signs of ESCC such as vertebral body collapse or pedicle erosion. However, they have an unacceptably high false negative rate (up to 17%) because 50% of cortical bone must be destroyed before the radiograph becomes abnormal. Similarly, radiation ports planned on the basis of radiographs alone are commonly insufficient.

Radionuclide bone scanning is more sensitive than plain radiographs but less specific in detecting bone metastasis correctly and predicting the presence and location of epidural spinal lesions in about two-thirds of patients. However, there is evidence that patients with cancer who present with back pain but who have negative bone scans and spinal radiographs have a very low incidence of ESCC.

Myelography, often combined with postmyelogram CT, can define the level and extent of epidural compression. Early studies comparing myelography to MRI showed roughly equal sensitivities and specificities for ESCC. However, myelography is invasive, may not visualize paravertebral soft tissue involvement, and can rarely precipitate neurologic deterioration in patients with complete spinal subarachnoid block above the level of lumbar puncture ("spinal coning"). For these reasons, MRI has replaced myelography as the gold standard. MRI can also detect intramedullary metastases and multiple epidural lesions, which if present may alter the treatment plan. Therefore, most experts agree that patients with suspected MESCC should undergo MRI of the entire spine, or at least the thoracic and lumbosacral spine, as asymptomatic epidural deposits are rarely found in the cervical spine.

Differential diagnosis

The differential diagnosis of back pain with or without neurologic dysfunction in patients with cancer includes malignant and non-malignant etiologies. In patients with systemic cancer, vertebral metastases with or without epidural extension can be differentiated from intramedullary spinal cord metastases (ISCM) via neuroimaging. Other complications to consider include leptomeningeal metastases and neoplastic plexopathy. Radiation myelopathy usually follows treatment by approximately 1 year and presents with ascending sensory deficits, weakness, and hemicord symptoms. This can be distinguished from ESCC by MRI.

A detailed discussion of specific infections is beyond the scope of this section; however, a few key regional infections are important to consider in the differential diagnosis of ESCC. Risk factors for spinal epidural abscesses (SEA) include intravenous drug use, diabetes, and spinal trauma, while fever, back pain, spinal tenderness, and peripheral leukocytosis should raise clinical suspicion. Localization is most often thoracic, followed by cervical.

The diagnostic method of choice is contrast-enhanced MRI, while cultures often yield a microbiologic diagnosis. *Staphylococcus aureus* is the most common bacterial infection causing ESCC worldwide.

Spinal involvement with *Mycobacterium tuberculosis* (Pott's disease) can include discitis, epidural abscess, or osteomyelitis. An estimated 8 million people worldwide develop tuberculosis each year; however, less than 1% will have spinal disease. Nonetheless, tuberculosis (TB) spondylitis is the most common cause of non-traumatic paraplegia in developing countries. TB myelopathy is characterized by its predominantly thoracic location, painless leg weakness, and frequent co-occurrence with human immunodeficiency virus (HIV). Plain radiographs are often but not always abnormal.

With 40 million people worldwide infected with HIV and the largest number of affected people in sub-Saharan Africa, HIV-associated myelopathy (HAM) is an important entity to consider. Patients present with slowly progressive painless spastic paraparesis, urinary incontinence, and gait ataxia. MRI is typically normal, and HAM is a diagnosis of exclusion. HIV infection predisposes to bacterial SEA, bone metastases from Kaposi's sarcoma, intramedullary lymphoma and radiculomyelitis from cytomegalovirus (CMV), herpes simplex virus (HSV), varicella zoster virus (VZV), and human T-cell lymphotropic virus (HTLV), among others.

Acute viral myelitis presents with motor weakness, sensory loss, and autonomic dysfunction evolving over days, but rarely involves pain. Etiologies include HSV-1 and 2, VZV, CMV, Epstein–Barr virus (EBV), enteroviruses, West Nile Virus, and Japanese B encephalitis. Poliovirus presents with proximal greater than distal flaccid areflexic paralysis. Despite nearly worldwide eradication, close to 1500 cases were reported in India in 2002.

HTLV-associated myelopathy/tropical spastic paraparesis (HAM/TSP) develops in less than 5% of the estimated 20 million people worldwide infected with the retrovirus. HAM/TSP presents similarly as HIV-associated myelopathy. Contrasted MRI may or may not show abnormal enhancement and spinal cord edema at affected sites.

Schistosomiasis is endemic to Africa, the Middle East, and southeast Asia. In sub-Saharan Africa, neuroschistosomiasis causes 1–5% of non-traumatic spinal cord lesions. Schistosomal myelopathy most commonly involves *Schistosoma mansoni* localized to the conus medullaris and presents with flaccid paraplegia, lumbar radiculopathy, and autonomic dysfunction weeks to months after initial infection. Eosinophilia and the schistosomal ova in biopsy specimens lead to the diagnosis.

Brucella species cause 2–5% of all spondylodiscitis in Mediterranean countries, most often localized to the lumbar region. Complaints of systemic brucellosis dominate early and include fever, malaise, and polymyalgia. Unlike spinal tuberculosis, brucella infection preserves the vertebral architecture despite diffuse spondylodiscitis.

Lyme neuroborreliosis causing acute painful radiculoneuritis is more common in Europe than in North America. The tapeworm *Echinococcus granulosus*, endemic to the Mediterranean basin, Middle East, central Asia, and eastern Africa, spares the intervertebral discs and usually remains confined to one vertebral body. *Coccidioides immitis* preferentially affects the thoracic spines of Filipinos, African-Americans, and the elderly of the southwest United States, Central America, and parts of South America, while *Blastomyces dermatitidis* is found in the Mississippi and Ohio River basins of the United States. Neurocysticercosis very rarely involves the spine by causing inflammation in the subarachnoid space leading to cerebrospinal fluid (CSF) obstruction. Neurosyphilis can cause either thrombosis of spinal vessels, resulting in a syndrome similar to transverse myelitis, or tabes dorsalis, which manifests years to decades after initial infection. Rarely, osteomyelitis has been attributed to *Aspergillus* species, *Salmonella typhi*, and *Bartonella henselae*.

Treatment

The treatment of MESCC focuses on pain control, minimizing complications, and stabilizing or improving neurologic function. Pain control often requires opiate analgesics. Anticoagulation should be considered in non-ambulatory patients to prevent venous thromboembolism. Corticosteroids reduce vasogenic edema and improve pain scores and clinical outcome. Dosages of between 16 and 96 mg of dexamethasone as an initial bolus are acceptable, usually followed by 16 mg daily in divided doses, tapered over days to weeks.

Definitive therapy includes radiation therapy (RT) with or without surgery. External beam RT in divided fractions is preferred for most patients with a radiation port extending two levels above and below the symptomatic lesion. While pretreatment neurologic function is the strongest predictor of outcome, tumor histology is an important prognostic factor. Radiosensitive tumors such as breast, prostate, small cell lung cancer, lymphoma, and myeloma (as opposed to the more radio-resistant melanoma and renal cell carcinoma) portend a better prognosis. Median survival in patients undergoing RT for ESCC is approximately 3–6 months, with non-ambulatory patients faring significantly worse. Recurrence rates after RT range from 7.5% to 20%, and almost half of recurrences will be at a site distant from the initial lesion.

Surgery is currently reserved for when the diagnosis is in doubt, for spinal instability, when vertebral body collapse has caused bony impingement on the cord or nerve roots, for local recurrence after spinal radiotherapy, or for particularly radio-resistant tumors. Historically, posterior approaches including decompressive laminectomy were utilized; however, this method often further destabilizes the spinal column. Given that the anterior vertebral elements are most often involved in MESCC, vertebral corpectomy with instrumentation via an anterior approach is becoming more commonplace. In a recent prospective study of RT versus RT plus surgery, significantly more patients undergoing combined therapy regained or maintained ambulatory status and required lower doses of corticosteroids and opiates.

Systemic chemotherapy has been shown to be effective for ESCC caused by chemosensitive tumors such as Hodgkin's and non-Hodgkin's lymphoma, germ cell tumors, neuroblastoma and breast cancer. Hormonal therapy has been employed successfully in ESCC secondary to prostate and breast cancer. Other avenues that have been explored recently include embolization, stereotactic radiosurgery, and brachytherapy.

Prognosis

The overall median survival following diagnosis of ESCC is between 3 and 6 months. However, survival is closer to 4 weeks in those patients who remain non-ambulatory after treatment. Prognosis appears to be best in breast and prostate cancer, and significantly worse in lung cancer or in cases of multiple epidural spinal cord metastases. If radiotherapy is initiated while patients are still ambulatory, the majority of these patients will maintain the ability to walk. However, fewer than 1 in 10 paraplegics will regain ambulation despite adequate treatment. Therefore, prompt diagnosis and initiation of treatment before permanent neurologic sequelae develops from MESCC is key.

Pediatric epidural metastases

The most common pediatric tumors associated with MESCC include sarcoma (especially Ewing's sarcoma), neuroblastoma, germ-cell neoplasms, and Hodgkin's disease. Neurologic complications of neuroblastoma and non-Hodgkin's lymphoma are not uncommonly the initial manifestation of systemic malignancy. Plain radiographs of pediatric epidural metastases are often normal because the mechanism is usually invasion of the epidural space through vertebral foramina, forming paravertebral masses without producing bony lesions. Overall, prognosis is thought to be better than in adults due to the radio- and chemosensitivity of neuroblastoma, germ cell tumors, and Hodgkin's lymphoma.

Further reading

Loblaw DA, Perry J, Chambers A, Laperriere NJ. Systematic review of the diagnosis and management of malignant extradural spinal cord compression: the Cancer Care Ontario Practice Guidelines Initiative's Neuro-Oncology Disease Site. *J Clin Oncol* 2005; 23(9): 2028–37.

Posner JB. *Neurologic Complications of Cancer*. Philadelphia: FA Davis; 1995.
Scheld WM, Marra CM, Whitley RJ, editors. *Infections of the Central Nervous System*. Philadelphia: Lippincott Williams & Wilkins; 2004.

Chapter 141
General approach to the diagnosis and treatment of paraneoplastic neurologic disorders

Myrna R. Rosenfeld and Josep O. Dalmau
University of Pennsylvania, Philadelphia, USA

Introduction

Paraneoplastic neurologic disorders (PND) are immune-mediated disorders that may affect any part of the nervous system. The concept is that the expression of neuronal proteins by a tumor provokes an immune response against both the tumor and the nervous system. This hypothesis is supported by the frequent detection in the serum and cerebrospinal fluid (CSF) of antibodies reacting with antigens expressed by the tumor and nervous system. Some antibodies appear to have a direct pathogenic role in causing the neurologic dysfunction, while other antibodies occur in association with cytotoxic T-cell responses that are the main effectors of the neuronal degeneration.

Diagnosis

The diagnosis of PND is based on recognizing the neurologic syndrome, demonstrating the presence of an associated cancer, and detecting serum and CSF paraneoplastic antibodies (Table 141.1). Recognizing the syndrome can be difficult since PND precede the cancer diagnosis in about 60% of patients and similar syndromes may occur in the absence of cancer. Some syndromes (e.g., acute or subacute cerebellar dysfunction in an adult or opsoclonus-myoclonus in a child) are highly characteristic and so often associate with cancer that their presence should immediately lead to the suspicion of a paraneoplastic etiology. Other syndromes (e.g., brainstem dysfunction, myelopathy), may result from paraneoplastic mechanisms but occur more frequently in the absence of cancer and therefore require a more extensive differential diagnosis. An initial clue is the mode of onset, as most PND present in an acute or subacute manner compared with

International Neurology: A Clinical Approach. Edited by Robert P. Lisak, Daniel D. Truong, William M. Carroll, and Roongroj Bhidayasiri.
© 2009 Blackwell Publishing, ISBN: 978-1-4051-5738-4.

Table 141.1 Paraneoplastic syndromes and antibody associations.

Syndromes of the central nervous system (possible antibody associations)
- Paraneoplastic cerebellar degeneration (anti-Hu, anti-CV2/CRMP5, anti-Yo, anti-Ri, anti-Tr, anti-Zic4, anti-VGCC in association with LEMS)
- Paraneoplastic encephalomyelitis (anti-Hu, anti-CV2/CRMP5)
- Limbic encephalitis (anti-Hu when associated with encephalomyelitis, anti-NMDAR; anti-Ma proteins; anti-VGKC)
- Paraneoplastic opsoclonus-myoclonus (anti-Ri)
- Stiff-man syndrome (anti-amphyphysin)

Syndromes of the peripheral nervous system
- Paraneoplastic sensory neuronopathy
- Vasculitis of the nerve and muscle
- Subacute and chronic sensorimotor neuropathies
- Sensorimotor neuropathy associated with plasma cell dyscrasias and B-cell lymphoma
- Peripheral nerve hyperexcitability (anti-VGKC)
- Autonomic neuropathy (anti-nAChR)
- Brachial neuritis
- Acute polyradiculoneuropathy (Guillain–Barré syndrome)

Syndromes of the neuromuscular junction and muscle
Lambert–Eaton myasthenic syndrome (anti-VGCC)
Myasthenia gravis (anti-AChR)
Dermatomyositis
Acute necrotizing myopathy

Paraneoplastic visual syndromes
- Retinopathy (antirecoverin; antibipolar cell)
- Optic neuritis
- Uveitis (usually in association with encephalomyelitis) (anti-CV2/CRMP5)

the chronic progression of non-inflammatory neurodegenerative disorders.

PND usually develop at early stages of cancer and therefore the tumor (or its recurrence) may be difficult to demonstrate. In most instances, the tumor is revealed by CT of the chest, abdomen, and pelvis. Combined CT and 18-fluorodeoxyglucose positron emission tomography (FDG-PET) are useful in demonstrating occult neoplasms; cancer serum markers are also helpful. Patients with a neuropathy of unclear etiology should be examined for a monoclonal gammopathy in the serum and urine, and if positive should undergo a skeletal survey and bone marrow biopsy.

The specificity of paraneoplastic antibodies for certain PND or some types of cancer makes them useful diagnostic tools. In the appropriate clinical context the detection of a paraneoplastic antibody helps diagnose the PND and focus the search for the neoplasm. For antibody positive patients, if a cancer is not discovered, the presence of an occult neoplasm is assumed. Although almost any cancer can associate with PND, the tumors most commonly involved are small cell lung cancer (SCLC), cancers of the breast, ovary, thymoma, and neuroblastoma, and plasma cell tumors.

The diagnosis of PND is more difficult in patients who develop less characteristic symptoms (e.g., brainstem dysfunction, myelopathy), especially if no antibodies are found. In a patient known to have cancer, metastases and non-metastatic neurological complications of cancer should be considered and can often be ruled out with neuroimaging. The CSF of patients with PND of the central nervous system (CNS) often suggests an inflammatory process: pleocytosis, increased protein concentration, intrathecal synthesis of immunoglobulin G, and oligoclonal bands. Biopsy of an abnormal brain region identified by MRI or FDG-PET may be considered if a neoplastic process is suspected or if the clinical, CSF, and MRI findings are unusual. Abnormalities supporting, but not specific to PND, include infiltrates of mononuclear cells, neuronophagic nodules, neuronal degeneration, microglial proliferation, and gliosis.

For patients in whom no cancer is found but the suspicion of a PND remains high, periodic cancer screening for at least 5 years is recommended, keeping in mind that in 90% of patients the underlying tumor will be uncovered within the first year of PND symptom onset. Patients whose cancer is in remission and who develop PND should be examined for tumor recurrence.

Treatment

The first approach for treating any PND is to promptly identify and treat the tumor. Based on the syndrome and associated immune responses, for treatment purposes PND can be divided into those in which the paraneoplastic antibodies are pathogenic and those in which cytotoxic T-cells are the likely mediators of the neurologic dysfunction. In the former category are disorders such as Lambert–Eaton myasthenic syndrome associated with antivoltage-gated calcium channel (VGCC) antibodies, myasthenia gravis with anti-acetylcholine receptor (AChR) antibodies, neuromyotonia associated with antivoltage-gated potassium channel (VGKC) antibodies, and a subset of autonomic neuropathies with antibodies

to the ganglionic AChR. Since the antibodies are pathogenic their removal with plasma exchange or modulation of the immune response with intravenous IgG (IVIg) often results in neurologic improvement.

For those PND that are likely T-cell mediated, immunosuppression or immunomodulation is recommended. For patients who may simultaneously be receiving chemotherapy, corticosteroids, IVIg, or plasma exchange may be considered. Patients with progressive symptoms who are not receiving chemotherapy should be considered for more aggressive immunosuppression that may include cyclophosphamide, tacrolimus, cyclosporine, or rituximab.

The remainder of this chapter briefly describes four syndromes that are highly characteristic and so frequently associate with cancer that their identification should lead to an immediate suspicion of a paraneoplastic etiology.

Specific syndromes

Paraneoplastic cerebellar degeneration (PCD)

PCD usually presents with dizziness, gait unsteadiness, and oscillopsia, and evolves in a few days or weeks to severe cerebellar dysfunction. Most patients become wheelchair bound, with dysarthria, dysphagia, blurry vision, or diplopia, and absent or very mild impairment of sensation and reflexes. Cognitive functions are usually preserved, but about 25% of patients show mild impairment. Almost all well-characterized paraneoplastic antibodies have been reported in association with PCD. Serological markers that associate with "pure" PCD include Yo, Tr, VGCC, and infrequently Zic4 and Ma2 antibodies. Between 30% and 40% of patients with PCD do not have detectable paraneoplastic antibodies; in these patients the diagnosis relies on the exclusion of other etiologies and demonstration of the cancer. PCD rarely responds to treatment. An exception is the group of patients with anti-Tr antibodies and Hodgkin's lymphoma; approximately 20% show improvement after tumor treatment and corticosteroids, IVIg, or plasma exchange.

Paraneoplastic encephalomyelitis (PEM)

Patients with PEM may develop dysfunction of any part of the CNS, dorsal root ganglia (causing paraneoplastic sensory neuronopathy), and autonomic nerves. Symptoms develop rapidly and progress over weeks or months until stabilization or death. The CSF usually shows a mild to moderate lymphocytic pleocytosis, increased protein and normal glucose concentrations, and oligoclonal bands or increased IgG index. Brain MRI often shows fluid-attenuated inversion recovery (FLAIR) or T2 sequence hyperintensities in involved and at times clinically silent regions. Patients with PEM and SCLC often have anti-Hu, and less frequently anti-CV2/CRMP5 antibodies, or both.

The management of PEM is based on prompt treatment of the tumor along with immunosuppression. Although the standard of care remains to be established, the use of corticosteroids and IVIg combined with chemotherapy may help to stabilize or improve the neurologic symptoms during the period of time that the tumor is treated. Afterwards, if the neurologic symptoms have stabilized or improved, patients should be considered for prolonged treatment with immunosuppressants that target not only the antibodies but also the T-cell immunity (e.g., cyclophosphamide combined with corticosteroids, among other strategies).

Limbic encephalitis (LE)

Patients with paraneoplastic LE present with anxiety, depression, confusion, delirium, hallucinations, seizures, or short-term memory loss. In approximately 80% of patients the MRI T2 and FLAIR sequences show hyperintense abnormalities in one or both medial temporal lobes. Almost all patients have an abnormal electroenchephalogram (EEG) that includes uni- or bilateral temporal lobe epileptic discharges, or slow background activity. Two main phenotypes of LE have been described based on the associated immune responses. These are LE associated with antibodies to intracellular antigens and LE associated with antibodies to cell surface membrane bound proteins, receptors, or ion channels. LE associated with antibodies to intracellular antigens (e.g., Hu, Ma2, CV2/CRMP5) is likely mediated by cytotoxic T-cell responses and in general these disorders are poorly responsive to treatment. An exception is patients with Ma2 antibodies, in which 30% respond to treatment of the tumor and immunotherapy (corticosteroids and IVIg).

LE associated with antibodies to cell surface proteins, receptors, or ion channels (e.g., VGKC) represent a varied group of disorders. The location of the target antibodies, response to IgG depleting strategies, and limited numbers of cytotoxic T-cell inflammatory infiltrates in pathologic specimens from some of these patients support a direct pathogenic role of the antibodies in mediating the neurologic dysfunction. Patients with LE associated with antibodies to the *N*-methyl-*D*-aspartate receptor (NMDAR) are mostly young women between 15 and 45 years of age. The syndrome is highly characteristic with prominent subacute psychiatric manifestations at presentation. Patients become confused, restless, or agitated, with frequent paranoid or delusional thoughts. While often admitted to psychiatric centers most will develop seizures, decreased level of consciousness, autonomic instability, severe dyskinesias, and central hypoventilation prompting medical intervention and often a need for prolonged mechanical ventilation. Evaluation of the CSF usually reveals pleocytosis or increased protein concentration supporting an inflammatory or immune-mediated neurological process. The majority of patients will harbor an ovarian teratoma that may appear as a benign ovarian cyst and be considered unrelated to the disorder. Rarely, an extra-ovarian teratoma has been found and recent studies show that it can occur in men or patients without teratoma. While this disorder can be fatal, prompt identification and removal of the tumor in association with immunotherapy abrogates progression to severe complications and shortens symptom duration.

Patients who develop LE and anti-VGKC antibodies may present with the typical features of LE, but when compared with other immunotypes are more likely to develop hyponatremia and less likely to have CSF abnormalities. Only 20% of patients with VGKC antibodies have an underlying tumor (usually SCLC or thymoma). Approximately 80% of patients with LE and VGKC antibodies respond to treatment, including corticosteroids, plasma exchange, or IVIg. Some patients have spontaneous improvement of symptoms. Other than LE, patients with VGKC develop peripheral nerve hyperexcitability, autonomic dysfunction, hyperhydrosis, rapid eye movement sleep behavior abnormalities, and seizures.

There are a group of patients who develop classic signs and symptoms of LE and who have antibodies to unknown extracellular antigens that are highly expressed in the hippocampus and cerebellum. Whether there are a limited or large number of antigenic targets is unclear at this time. The detection of these neuronal cell surface-reacting antibodies supports the use of immunotherapy, and carries a better prognosis for neurological improvement than when antibodies to intracellular antigens are detected. A cancer association has been found in just over half of the patients with these antibodies, including thymic carcinoma, lung cancer (SCLC and adenocarcinoma), thymoma, ovarian fibrothecoma, melanoma, and Hodgkin's lymphoma.

Paraneoplastic sensory neuronopathy (PSN)

PSN results from an immune attack against the neurons of the dorsal root ganglia. Patients develop pain, numbness, and sensory deficits that can affect the limbs, trunk, and cranial nerves. The presentation is frequently asymmetric, associated with decreased or abolished reflexes, and relative preservation of strength. All types of sensation can be affected, but loss of proprioception is often predominant, resulting in sensory ataxia and pseudoathetoid movements of the extremities (predominantly the hands). PSN may occur in isolation, but often precedes or coincides with the development of PEM. Prompt treatment of patients with corticosteroids and IVIg along with treatment of the tumor may result in stabilization or mild improvement of the dorsal root ganglia dysfunction.

Further reading

Graus F, Delattre JY, Antoine JC, *et al.* Recommended diagnostic criteria for paraneoplastic neurological syndromes. *J Neurol Neurosurg Psychiatry* 2004; 75: 1135–40.

Rosenfeld MR, Dalmau J. Current therapies for paraneoplastic neurologic syndromes. *Curr Treat Options Neurol* 2003; 5: 69–77.

Tuzun E, Dalmau J. Limbic encephalitis and variants: classification, diagnosis and treatment. *Neurologist* 2007; 13: 261–71.

Chapter 142
Insomnia

Colin A. Espie[1] and Delwyn J. Bartlett[2,3]

[1]University of Glasgow Sleep Centre, Scotland, UK
[2]Woolcock Institute of Medical Research, University of Sydney, Sydney, Australia
[3]Royal Prince Alfred Hospital, Sydney, Australia

Introduction

Insomnia is frequently observed in a number of medical, neurological, and psychiatric disorders, representing a considerable public health concern. Insomnia is the repeated difficulty in initiating sleep (greater than 30 minutes), maintaining sleep (greater than 30 minutes), or waking early, which is chronically non-restorative despite adequate sleep opportunity. Within the neurological field, insomnia may present as a hypersomnia such as narcolepsy and/or as a sleep-related movement disorder including restless legs syndrome (RLS) and period limb movement (PLM) (Table 142.1).

Epidemiology

Insomnia affects one-third of adults occasionally, and 9–12% on a chronic basis. It is more commonly reported in women, shift workers, and patients with medical and psychiatric disorders. Among older adults, prevalence has been estimated at 25%, although co-morbid conditions and hypnotic drugs are factors in this increased prevalence.

Pathophysiology

Sleep disruption is often unreported until insomnia is well established. It is unclear whether the physiological changes associated with insomnia precede onset or are a consequence. High-frequency electroencephalogram (EEG) activity is exaggerated in individuals with insomnia. These findings suggest a central nervous system arousal, supporting previous research that found increased cortisol and adrenocorticotrophic hormones. This could also reflect an adaptation to poor quality sleep, as objective performance is not necessarily impaired.

Clinical features

Subjectively, sleep is non-restorative and daytime functioning is impaired. Individuals are overwhelmingly concerned about sleep onset, returning to sleep, and the unpredictability of sleep. Severity is judged by frequency (three or more times per week), with a minimum duration of 1 month. The clinical presentation is commonly one of a frustrated patient trapped in a vicious circle of anxiety and poor sleep, reporting having "tried everything," and generally unable to "down-regulate" arousal levels at bedtime.

Insomnia also causes daytime impairments, including fatigue, inattention, and mood changes, with anxiety and irritability. Less frequently, cognitive and performance abilities may be affected. The presence of excessive daytime sleepiness (EDS) is unusual in insomnia. When EDS is a prominent complaint, investigations for other sleep disorders should be considered, including obstructive sleep apnea syndrome (OSA), narcolepsy, periodic limb movement disorder (PLM), and restless legs syndrome (RLS). Additionally, head injury or depression may be causes of EDS.

Insomnias due to a drug or substance can include hypnotic-dependent sleep disorder – commonly associated with benzodiazepine (BZ) drugs, where withdrawal exacerbates the primary problem, reinforcing hypnotic dependency. Psychiatric conditions, particularly affective disorders, have associated sleep symptomatology. When the diagnostic criteria for DSM-IV Axis I or Axis II disorders are fulfilled, a primary diagnosis of psychophysiological insomnia cannot be made. Sleep disturbances often precede depression, being an independent risk factor for a first episode or recurrence of depression. Insomnia due to medical conditions arises from an identified medical cause (orthopedic, neurologic, pulmonary, cardiac, etc.) and may vary with the condition. The natural history of insomnia is not clear. It is known that sleep quality is reduced with increasing age. Circadian rhythm

International Neurology: A Clinical Approach. Edited by Robert P. Lisak, Daniel D. Truong, William M. Carroll, and Roongroj Bhidayasiri.
© 2009 Blackwell Publishing, ISBN: 978-1-4051-5738-4.

Table 142.1 Diagnosis and differentiation of the insomnias – International Classification of Sleep Disorders (ICSD-2).

Classification	Sleep disorder	Essential features Complaint of insomnia plus …
Insomnias	Psychophysiological insomnia	Learned sleep-preventing associations, conditioned arousal, "racing mind" phenomenon
	Paradoxical insomnia	Complaint of poor sleep disproportionate to sleep pattern and sleep duration
	Idiopathic insomnia	Insomnia typically begins in childhood or from birth
	Insomnia due to a mental disorder	Course of sleep disturbance concurrent with mental disorder
	Inadequate sleep hygiene	Daily living activities inconsistent with maintaining good-quality sleep
	Insomnia due to a medical disorder	Course of sleep disturbance concurrent with mental disorder
	Insomnia due to drug or substance	Sleep disruption caused by prescription medication, recreational drug, caffeine, alcohol or foodstuff
	Adjustment insomnia	Presence of identifiable stressor; insomnia resolves or is expected to resolve when stressor is removed

disorders, shift work, parasomnias, and inadequate sleep hygiene can all be triggers for insomnia.

Investigations

A thorough history incorporating questions regarding mood, lifestyle, restlessness, limb movements, and breathing is important. Sleep diary monitoring is a useful form of assessment in addition to questionnaires on beliefs and moods. Wrist actigraphy estimates sleep-wakefulness based upon body movement for up to 10 consecutive 24-hour periods and can identify paradoxical insomnia, along with circadian anomalies. Polysomnography (PSG) is undertaken only when another sleep disorder is suspected.

Treatment and management

Drug therapy
BZ compounds superseded barbiturates and, although effective short term, were found to cause potential problems with tolerance and withdrawal. Contemporary hypnotic therapy includes BzRAs ("z" drugs) and, more recently, melatonin receptor agonists (MeRAs), which have yet to become established. BzRAs offer fewer adverse effects; however, long-term effectiveness is less clear. Increasingly (off-label) sedative antidepressants are being used.

Melatonin, the pineal hormone, triggers sleep onset by lowering core body temperature and is a useful chronobiotic for reducing sleep latency in delayed sleep phase syndrome (DSPS).

Psychological and behavioral therapy
Psychological treatment with cognitive behavioral therapy (CBT) has demonstrated large-effect size changes in primary outcomes and is maintained at long-term follow-up. CBT is also effective in general practice and can be adapted for other settings.

Management strategies

Educating the patient about sleep is an important aspect of treating insomnia. Understanding what sleep is, how sleep changes with age, good sleep hygiene practices (reducing caffeine and alcohol, etc.), and some facts about sleep loss are starting points for self-management.

Bright light is a potent marker for human circadian rhythm, resetting sleep-times in advanced sleep phase syndrome (ASPS) and DSPS. Sleep initiation insomnia is improved with morning light and avoidance of evening light.

Exercise can positively influence sleep quality, particularly in the late afternoon or early evening. Morning exercise with light exposure suppresses melatonin, enhancing circadian rhythm and setting a constant waking time. Sleeping in a safe environment includes minimizing disruption from external factors (heating, noise, violence, others) and internal factors relating to previous experiences.

Stimulus control

Stimulus control is a reconditioning treatment forcing discrimination between daytime and sleeping environments. For the poor sleeper, the bedroom triggers associations with being awake and aroused. Treatment involves removing all stimuli that are potentially sleep-incompatible (reading and watching television) and excluding sleep from living areas. The individual is instructed to get up if not asleep within 15–20 minutes or when wakeful during the night.

Sleep restriction therapy

Sleep restriction relates to the ratio of time asleep with time in bed, and involves recording average nightly sleep duration. The aim is to slowly reduce time in bed to match recorded sleep duration, increasing sleep efficiency and confidence.

Cognitive control

Intrusive thoughts need to be addressed before bedtime. Setting aside 15–20 minutes before bedtime to rehearse the day and to plan for tomorrow allows the day to be put to rest. Thought-stopping attempts to interrupt the flow of thoughts via "blocking" techniques, such as repeating the word "the" every 3 seconds, occupying the short-term memory store (used in processing information), potentially allowing sleep to happen. Cognitive restructuring challenges faulty beliefs that help maintain both wakefulness and helplessness.

Relaxation methods include progressive relaxation, imagery training, biofeedback, meditation, hypnosis, and autogenic training, with little evidence to indicate superiority of any one approach. At the cognitive level, these techniques may act by distraction.

Paradoxical intention

Attempting to remain wakeful rather than "trying" to fall asleep (decatastrophizing technique) strengthens the sleep drive and reduces performance effort.

Treatment of insomnia should include assessment for known extrinsic causes of certain sleep disorders including alcohol, stimulants, and proprietary drugs, which interfere with sleep. Individuals need to be encouraged to seek advice early rather to than self-administer treatment. Avoiding the use of hypnotic agents would substantially reduce the number of iatrogenic cases of chronic insomnia.

Further reading

ICSD. *The International Classification of Sleep Disorders Revised: Diagnostic and Coding Manual.* American Sleep Disorders Association; 2005.

Morin C, Espie C. *Insomnia: A Clinical Guide to Assessment and Treatment.* New York: Kluwer Academic/Plenum; 2003.

NIH. State-of-the-Science Conference Statement on Manifestations and Management of Chronic Insomnia in Adults. State-of-the-Science Conference; 2005.

Perlis M, Lichstein K. *Treating Sleep Disorders: Principles and Practice of Behavioral Sleep Medicine.* Chichester: Wiley; 2003.

Smith M, Perlis M, Park A, *et al.* Comparative meta-analysis of pharmacotherapy and behavior therapy for persistent insomnia. *Am J Psychiatr* 2002; 159: 5–11.

Chapter 143
Narcolepsy

Marcel Hungs[1] and Emmanuel Mignot[2]
[1]University of California, Irvine, USA
[2]Stanford University Center for Narcolepsy, Palo Alto, USA

Introduction

Narcolepsy is a common sleep disorder characterized by excessive daytime sleepiness, cataplexy (episodes of muscle weakness triggered by emotions), hypnagogic hallucination, sleep paralysis, fragmented night sleep, and automatic behaviors. It is generally separated into two pathophysiological subtypes: narcolepsy with or without cataplexy (defined as sleepiness with rapid sleep onset into rapid eye movement (REM) sleep). Narcolepsy was first reported by Westphal in 1877 and was coined "narcolepsy" by Gélineau in 1880. Narcolepsy, along with obstructive sleep apnea (OSA) and idiopathic hypersomnia, is one of the leading causes of excessive daytime sleepiness (EDS). The discovery in 1999 that narcolepsy with cataplexy was caused by a hypocretin/orexin deficiency in the hypothalamus led to a major advancement not only in the insights related to this condition, but also in the general understanding of the sleep–wake system. In contrast, much less is known regarding narcolepsy without cataplexy.

Epidemiology

The prevalence of narcolepsy with cataplexy in North America and Europe averages 0.02–0.05%. Similar prevalence estimates have been reported in Hong Kong. Prevalence data from other countries suggest a higher prevalence in Japan (0.16%) and a lower prevalence in Israel (0.002%), although these figures may be confounded by differences in epidemiological methods and other factors such as reduced access to healthcare and limited awareness of healthcare providers regarding sleep disorders. Incidence data are limited; one US study reports an incidence rate of 0.74 per 100 000 person-years for narcolepsy with cataplexy.

Few studies have reported the prevalence of narcolepsy without cataplexy due to the requirement of a sleep study for diagnosis. In one study, the prevalence of diagnosed cases was observed to be 0.02% with an incidence of 1.37 per 100 000 person-years. However, many cases meeting the diagnostic criteria may go undiagnosed. In two studies, where sleep studies were performed in a population-based sample, approximately 2–4% of the population met international criteria for narcolepsy without cataplexy.

Pathophysiology

When cataplexy is present, narcolepsy in humans is almost always caused by a deficiency of hypocretin (also called orexin), a neurotransmitter produced by 50 000–100 000 neurons located in the posterior hypothalamus. Hypocretin receptors are located in various areas of the brain, including the cerebral cortex, hypothalamus, brainstem, and spinal cord. Input from the limbic system and interaction with metabolic signals such as leptin and glucose allow hypocretin neurons to play a role in emotion, energy homeostasis, reward, addiction, and arousal. The hypocretin system has effects on midbrain dopaminergic systems other than the nigral–striatal pathway. Interestingly, patients with hypocretin deficiency are less susceptible to stimulant abuse, suggesting a role for hypocretin in the regulation of drug addiction. Hypocretin neurons interact with the cholinergic and monoaminergic systems, which modulate the sleep–wake cycle. In narcolepsy, it is suggested that the loss of excitatory hypocretin input to monoaminergic cell groups mediates sleepiness and short REM sleep latency. This parallels the observation that indirectly stimulating monoaminergic transmission, using amphetamine-like compounds and antidepressants, improves narcolepsy symptoms.

The occurrence of narcolepsy involves genetic predisposition and environmental triggers. Multiplex families are rare, but a 10- to 40-fold increase in relative risk is reported in first-degree relatives. The strong association of narcolepsy with the human leukocyte antigen (HLA)

International Neurology: A Clinical Approach. Edited by Robert P. Lisak, Daniel D. Truong, William M. Carroll, and Roongroj Bhidayasiri.
© 2009 Blackwell Publishing, ISBN: 978-1-4051-5738-4.

system suggests an autoimmune mechanism responsible for hypocretin cell loss. Most patients with typical cataplexy carry HLA-DQB1*0602, an HLA subtype found in 12% of Japanese, 25% of Caucasians, and 38% of African-Americans. The HLA association and associated hypocretin deficiency is robust (>90%) in patients with definite cataplexy. In patients without cataplexy, a weaker HLA association is observed, with approximately 40% of patients positive for DQB1*0602.

Clinical features

Narcolepsy can be best described as a disorder of wakefulness, sleep consolidation, and abnormal REM sleep. Narcolepsy typically begins in adolescence and early adulthood, although late adult onset or onset in prepubertal children is described in approximately 10% of cases. The following symptoms are the primary clinical features of narcolepsy.

Excessive daytime sleepiness
Excessive daytime sleepiness is often the first symptom of narcolepsy and is frequently the presenting complaint requiring medical attention. Sleepiness in narcolepsy is often severe. It frequently culminates with sudden sleep attacks (an overwhelming urge to sleep within minutes). The resulting sleep episode is usually brief, often associated with dreaming, and, in contrast to naps in other sleep disorders, frequently refreshing. When severe, sleep attacks may be associated with automatic behaviors in which there is a semiautomatic continuation of activities, with multiple mistakes and no memory of the event. Sleepiness in narcolepsy is not always distinguishable from sleepiness due to other sleep disorders in that it typically occurs after lunch or in the absence of external stimulation.

Cataplexy
When cataplexy is present in combination with sleepiness, the diagnosis of narcolepsy is almost certain, and confirmatory tests are optional, although still advisable. Cataplexy is characterized by sudden and transient episodes of bilateral loss of muscle tone, without loss of consciousness, often triggered by an emotional stimulus such as laughter, surprise, anger, fear, or humorous situations. Early in the course of narcolepsy, cataplexy may only affect facial muscles or cause knee buckling. Severe cataplectic attacks can lead to falls and temporary loss of striated muscle tone in the extremities. The events can last from seconds to minutes. Other clinical events that can cause falls (such as syncope, sleep attacks, or generalized seizures) can be differentiated from cataplexy as they are associated with a loss of consciousness. In true cataplexy, the episodes of muscle weakness are reasonably frequent

(more than once a month), and are often triggered by strong emotions such as laughter or joking.

Sleep paralysis
Patients with narcolepsy often experience sleep paralysis and an inability to move for seconds (or even longer) at the onset of sleep or upon waking. Sleep paralysis is considered normal REM sleep atonia that occurs without other features of REM sleep. Sleep paralysis can occur in normal individuals when sleep deprived or upon waking from a dream. It can also be associated with depression in patients without narcolepsy.

Half-asleep hallucinations
Hypnagogic (while falling asleep) or hypnopompic (upon awakening) hallucinations occur in narcolepsy. They are usually visual, sometimes tactile or auditory, and reflect an immediate transition from wake to dreaming, without loss of consciousness. In severe cases, hallucinations can occur while drowsy, and can be difficult to distinguish from reality. Hypnagogic hallucinations can also occur in individuals without narcolepsy. In these cases, however, they are often less vivid in nature.

Sleep fragmentation
Individuals with narcolepsy usually lack the difficulty of falling asleep at bedtime but experience frequent nocturnal awakenings. Spontaneous micro-arousals lead to sleep fragmentation and reduced deeper sleep stages. Sleep fragmentation contributes to non-restorative overnight sleep, the severity of cataplexy, and EDS. Periodic leg movements (PLM), REM behavior disorder, and nightmares are also frequent in narcoleptic patients.

Diagnosis

Narcolepsy with cataplexy can often be diagnosed based on a detailed history and physical examination of the patient. The interview must focus on the detection and confirmation of typical cataplexy, if present. Narcolepsy without cataplexy requires a sleep study (International Classification of Sleep Disorders (ICSD-2) diagnostic criteria for narcolepsy were recently published (Table 143.1)). In some cases, a biochemical determination of low cerebrospinal fluid (CSF) hypocretin-1 can also provide a definitive diagnosis.

The most common differential diagnoses are sleep apnea, insufficient sleep, psychiatric hypersomnia, and circadian rhythm sleep disorders. Further, a combination of these diagnoses is not infrequent, further confusing the picture. Assessments for these diagnoses are included in Chapters 144–147. Anemia, hypothyroidism, infection, or various cardiovascular problems should be ruled out. A careful interview of the patient may reveal history of a brain trauma, central nervous system (CNS) infection, medication effects from drugs such as sedatives, anxiolyics, and antihistamines (such as those used in decongestants), and encephalopathy due to various causes including renal or liver dysfunction.

Once clinical suspicion of narcolepsy is raised, confirmatory testing including overnight polysomnogram (PSG) and a Multiple Sleep Latency Test (MSLT) should be completed to identify comorbid sleep disorders causing fragmented sleep. The MSLT, used to objectively quantify daytime sleepiness, consists of five 20-minute daytime naps at 2-hour intervals. Sleep latency along with the occurrence of REM sleep should be recorded.

Table 143.1 International Classification of Sleep Disorders (ICSD-2) diagnostic criteria for narcolepsy.

Narcolepsy with cataplexy

1. Excessive daytime sleepiness occurring almost daily for at least 3 months
2. Definite history of cataplexy
3. Confirmed by nocturnal PSG followed by an MSLT:
   (a) mean sleep latency on MSLT ≤8 minutes
   (b) ≥2 or more sleep onset REM periods (SOREMPs)
   (c) sufficient nocturnal sleep (6 hours) the night before the test
4. Alternatively, hypocretin-1 levels in the CSF ≤110 pg/ml

Narcolepsy without cataplexy

1. Excessive daytime sleepiness occurring almost daily for at least 3 months
2. No definite history of cataplexy
3. Confirmed by nocturnal PSG followed by an MSLT:
   (a) mean sleep latency on MSLT ≤8 minutes
   (b) ≥2 or more SOREMPs
   (c) sufficient nocturnal sleep (6 hours) the night before the test
4. The hypersomnia is not better explained by another sleep disorder, medical or neurological disorder, psychiatric disorder, medication use, or substance use disorder

A mean sleep latency (MSL) of less than 8 minutes and two or more sleep onset REM periods (SOREMPs) is diagnostic for narcolepsy. If there is no cataplexy, an MSLT (preceded by PSG) is indispensable. Special considerations in arranging the MSLT are as follows:

• The MSLT should be preceded by a PSG to rule out other causes of short MSL or SOREMPs such as sleep apnea, insufficient sleep, or delayed sleep phase syndrome.

• Psychotropic medications that affect REM sleep, especially antidepressants, should be avoided for 2 weeks prior to the study.

• In the 15% of patients with cataplexy in whom the MSLT is not diagnostic, measurement of CSF hypocretin-1 levels may assist in diagnosing narcolepsy. Low CSF hypocretin-1 levels (less than or equal to 110 pg/ml or one-third of mean normal values) are found in over 90% of patients with narcolepsy with cataplexy and almost never in controls or in patients with other pathologies.

• A urine toxicology screen may be used to screen for sedatives, stimulants, and antidepressants that may influence PSG and MSLT.

Treatment/management

The management and treatment of narcolepsy includes life-modifying interventions and medications targeting the most disabling symptoms, typically EDS and cataplexy (see Table 143.2). Life-modifying interventions include scheduled napping for 20 minutes, once at noon and once in the later afternoon to decrease EDS, minimizing the use of stimulants, and reducing the frequency and severity of cataplexy.

Pharmacological treatment choices for EDS include stimulants and other wake-promoting agents. Commonly

Table 143.2 Pharmacological management of narcolepsy.

Compounds	Daily dosage	Notes
Stimulants		
Armodafinil	150–250 mg	Well tolerated, longer half life than modafinil
Modafinil	100–400 mg	Few sympathomimetic effects and side effects, well tolerated
Methylphenidate	10–60 mg	Short duration of action
Dextroamphetamine	5–60 mg	Variable duration of action
Methamphetamine	5–60 mg	More potent and effective
Anticataplectic compounds		
Venlafaxine	75–225 mg	Slow release formulation, acting on both the serotoninergic and adrenergic systems
Atomoxetine	10–80 mg	Norepinephrine reuptake inhibitor
Protriptyline	5–60 mg	Anticholinergic effects, mild stimulant
Imipramine	10–100 mg	Anticholinergic effects
Desipramine	25–100 mg	Same as imipramine but more adrenergic effects
Clomipramine	10–150 mg	Very effective
Fluoxetine	20–60 mg	Well tolerated, less weight gain
Hypnotic compounds		
Sodium oxybate	4.5–9 g	Short duration of action, resulting anticataplectic effects during daytime, also alleviates daytime sleepiness

prescribed stimulant agents include modafinil, armodafinil, amphetamine, methylphenidate, and pemoline. Side effects include insomnia, hypertension, palpitations, and worsening of psychiatric conditions (such as mania), and very rarely with amphetamines, psychosis. Modafinil is the drug of choice because it is safer than other traditional stimulants and has less potential for abuse.

Hypnagogic hallucinations, sleep paralysis, and cataplexy respond to tricyclic antidepressants and monoamine reuptake inhibitors. A drug of choice is venlafaxine, a dual noradrenergic/serotoninergic uptake inhibitor. These drugs are rapidly effective for cataplexy. It is important to emphasize to patients the need for compliance, as sudden cessation of these drugs leads to a rebound of cataplexy. Atomoxetine, an adrenergic reuptake inhibitor used for attention deficit hyperactivity disorder (ADHD), can be helpful to treat cataplexy and mild daytime sleepiness.

Sodium oxybate, an hypnotic used twice during the night, is now increasingly used to consolidate sleep and reduce sleep fragmentation. It is a drug of choice in narcolepsy/cataplexy, as it can reduce the symptoms of narcolepsy. It is suggested that the increased amount of deep sleep induced by sodium oxybate leads to decreased EDS, reduced frequency and severity of cataplexy, and a reduced need for stimulants. In many cases, sodium oxybate alone or in combination with a small dose of velafaxine and/or modafinil confer adequate coverage for patients with narcolepsy/cataplexy. In patients without cataplexy, typical treatments may involve modafinil or atomoxetine, with careful use of amphetamine-like stimulants, unless hypocretin deficiency is documented.

Further reading

Bassetti C, Billiard M, Mignot E, editors. *Narcolepsy and Hypersomnia.* New York: Informa Health Care; 2007, 697 pp.

Dauvilliers Y, Arnulf I, Mignot E. Narcolepsy with cataplexy. *Lancet* 2007; 369(9560): 499–511.

Hungs M, Mignot E. Hypocretin/orexin, sleep and narcolepsy. *Bioessays* 2001; 23: 397–408.

Lin L, Hungs M, Mignot E. Narcolepsy and the HLA region. *J Neuroimmunol* 2001; 117: 9–20.

Mignot E, Lin L, Finn L, Lopes C, Pluff K, Sundstrom ML, Young T. Correlates of sleep-onset REM periods during the Multiple Sleep Latency Test in community adults. *Brain* 2006; 129(Pt 6): 1609–23.

Morgenthaler TI, Kapur VK, Brown T, *et al.* Standards of Practice Committee of the AASM. Practice parameters for the treatment of narcolepsy and other hypersomnias of central origin. *Sleep* 2007; 30(12): 1705–11.

Chapter 144
Idiopathic hypersomnia

Marcel Hungs[1] and Jed Black[2]
[1]University of California, Irvine, USA
[2]Stanford University, Stanford, USA

Introduction

Idiopathic hypersomnia (IH), along with obstructive sleep apnea (OSA) and narcolepsy, is a frequent neurological condition presenting with excessive daytime sleepiness (EDS). Patients experience difficulty waking in the morning and sleep drunkenness (a difficulty with waking), daytime sleepiness, a frequent urge to nap, and occasionally autonomic dysfunction. The total sleep time at night may be normal or longer than 10 hours. Despite significant impairment in quality of life due to daytime sleepiness, little is known about the epidemiological and pathophysiological background or ethnic and regional variations of IH. Treatment includes education and the use of wake-promoting agents.

Epidemiology

The evolving clinical concept of IH, with the search for a proper clinical and pathophysiological definition, lacks widespread epidemiological data. International studies are lacking, but some researchers suggest that narcolepsy is three times more common than IH.

Pathophysiology

In contrast to narcolepsy, there are no animal models available for IH, and basic science data are limited. Destruction of noradrenergic neurons in cats leads to a hypersomnia resembling IH. There is no HLA-DQB1*0602 association, as seen in narcolepsy, but the possibility of an *HLA-Cw2* and *DR11* association is reported without other evidence of an autoimmune-mediated mechanism. Interleukin-6 and tumor necrosis factor-α are elevated in IH, but are also elevated in other disorders with excessive daytime sleepiness, such as sleep apnea and narcolepsy.

International Neurology: A Clinical Approach. Edited by Robert P. Lisak, Daniel D. Truong, William M. Carroll, and Roongroj Bhidayasiri.
© 2009 Blackwell Publishing, ISBN: 978-1-4051-5738-4.

Cerebrospinal fluid (CSF) studies reveal decreased monoaminergic metabolites and histamine levels, as well as normal hypocretin-1 levels. Brain imaging studies are normal. Although a few studies suggest a genetic relationship in IH, a definitive determination of a mode of inheritance is not substantiated.

Clinical assessment

The symptoms of IH are characterized by excessive daytime sleepiness, with non-refreshing prolonged naps and sleep drunkenness. Historically, IH lacked objective diagnostic approaches (such as an overnight sleep study or Multiple Sleep Latency Test) and absent pathophysiological concepts. IH is often misdiagnosed as narcolepsy, sleep apnea, depression, or circadian rhythm disorder (Table 144.1). Our understanding of IH has primarily emerged in the last decade and is characterized by the following features.

Excessive daytime sleepiness
The hallmark of IH presenting to healthcare providers is excessive daytime sleepiness with prolonged unrefreshing daytime naps. Individuals with IH experience, despite sufficient and sometimes prolonged night sleep, reduced daytime alertness and, upon awakening, feelings of sleep

Table 144.1 Differential diagnoses for idiopathic hypersomnia.

- Narcolepsy (without or with cataplexy)
- Obstructive sleep apnea
- Delayed sleep phase syndrome
- Depression
- Periodic limb movement disorder
- Behaviorally-induced insufficient sleep syndrome
- Hypersomnia due to medical condition, drug, or substance
- Hypothyroidism
- Brain trauma
- Central nervous system infections
- Encephalopathy
- Periodic hypersomnia, e.g., Kleine–Levine syndrome
- Sleeping sickness
- Hypersomnia not due to substance or known physiologic condition

drunkenness (difficulty to completely awake accompanied by confusion, disorientation, poor motor coordination, and slowness). Overnight sleep is rarely refreshing, and individuals with IH tend to doze off in monotonous situations such as dark rooms, offices, or even at traffic lights. Daytime naps are common but non-refreshing and do not increase alertness (in contrast to the refreshing effect of napping in narcolepsy). The detailed history of an individual with IH will reveal that he/she does not experience cataplexy, an element frequently seen in narcolepsy. However, it is difficult to distinguish IH from narcolepsy on the basis of daytime sleepiness patterns alone.

A monosymptomatic form of IH is characterized by isolated sleepiness, while the polysymptomatic (also called classical) form includes other symptoms, such as autonomic dysfunction. The polysymptomatic form of the disorder is rare and is classified as "IH with long sleep time." Nocturnal sleep may or may not be of long duration (10 or more hours). An important feature is that of normal overnight sleep without sleep fragmentation, as seen in sleep apnea or periodic limb movement (PLM).

Autonomic dysfunction
Some patients experience autonomic dysfunction with fainting episodes, orthostatic hypotension, and peripheral vascular complaints of the Raynaud-type. Migraine or tension-type headaches are also observed.

Other features
IH is a life-long disorder without remission or significant fluctuations in the clinical presentation. The onset of EDS is less apparent than in narcolepsy and usually presents in adolescence and before age 30. Sleep paralysis and hypnagogic hallucinations are described in up to 40% of individuals with IH; dreams are less bizarre than in narcolepsy. The socio-economic impact of the disease can be significant, affecting social, academic, and personal achievement.

Differential diagnosis
IH is characterized by EDS, unexplained by other conditions, and is essentially a diagnosis of exclusion (Table 144.1). A main consideration is narcolepsy, a condition with EDS, sleep paralysis, hypnagogic hallucinations, and cataplexy (loss of muscle tone while awake triggered by emotional stimulus). Patients with narcolepsy have a normal overnight sleep test with short sleep latency, two or more rapid eye movement (REM) episodes, and a mean sleep latency ≤8 minutes on the Multiple Sleep Latency Test (MSLT). Insufficient sleep, as seen in chronic sleep deprivation, can be excluded using sleep logs. PLM during sleep, conditions with significant sleep fragmentation, or sleep-disordered breathing (such as obstructive sleep apnea (OSA) or upper airway resistance syndrome) can be identified in an overnight sleep study. EDS associated with conditions such as depression, Parkinson's disease, or post-traumatic stress should be considered.

Diagnostic assessment

While narcolepsy and sleep apnea are marked by well-defined clinical, polysomnographic, or immunogenetic features, IH is not well defined and is mainly diagnosed by exclusion (Table 144.1). The diagnosis of IH with or without long sleep time is suspected clinically after careful review of the patient's history, comorbidities, and physical examination. Normal or prolonged overnight sleep with short sleep latency is an important feature of IH. In an overnight polysomnogram (PSG), normal sleep stage distribution and lack of clear sleep fragmentation are observed. In contrast to narcolepsy, with IH, a mean sleep latency of ≤8 minutes is seen on the MSLT *without* occurrence of two or more REM sleep episodes.

A recent revision of the classification of sleep disorders by the American Academy of Sleep Medicine differentiates between IH with and without long sleep time:
• *IH with prolonged sleep time* is characterized by excessive sleepiness, prolonged non-refreshing naps up to 3 or 4 hours, major sleep episodes of at least 10–14 hours, difficulty waking, and sleep drunkenness.
• *IH without long sleep time* reflects excessive sleepiness and unintended non-refreshing naps, with the major sleep episode less than 10 hours, difficulty waking, and sleep drunkenness.

Treatment/management

In contrast to narcolepsy, naps may not be refreshing for patients with IH; therefore, patients avoid napping. Treatment parallels that of EDS in narcolepsy patients, but the response to medication is variable. The drug of choice is modafinil (100–200 mg in the morning and in the early afternoon) or its successor armodafinil (150–250 mg in the morning). Stimulant drugs, such as dextroamphetamine (5–60 mg), methylphenidate (10–60 mg), and pemoline (20–115 mg), are used, but are often less effective in IH than in narcolepsy.

Further reading

Black JE, Brooks SN, Nishino S. Narcolepsy and syndromes of primary excessive daytime somnolence. *Semin Neurol* 2004; 24(3): 271–82.

Dauvilliers Y. Differential diagnosis in hypersomnia. *Curr Neurol Neurosci Rep* 2006; 6(2): 156–62.

Morgenthaler TI, Kapur VK, Brown T, *et al.* Standards of Practice Committee of the AASM. Practice parameters for the treatment of narcolepsy and other hypersomnias of central origin. *Sleep* 2007; 30(12): 1705–11.

Young TJ, Silber MH. Hypersomnias of central origin. *Chest* 2006; 130(3): 913–20.

Chapter 145
Obstructive sleep apnea

Christine Won[1], Jee Hyun Kim[2], and Christian Guilleminault[2]
[1]University of California, San Francisco, USA
[2]Stanford University, Stanford, USA

Introduction

Obstructive sleep apnea (OSA) is a condition characterized by repeated episodes of upper airway collapse and obstruction during sleep. It is associated with a constellation of symptoms and objective findings.

Epidemiology

Recent population-based studies report a wide range of prevalence estimates for OSA in the adult Western population, from 2% to 28%. Mild OSA likely affects 1 in 5 adults, while 1 in 15 adults has at least moderate OSA. In the adult population, the most significant risk factors are obesity and male gender. Other risk factors for OSA include age between 40 and 65 years, cigarette smoking, use of alcohol, and poor physical fitness.

The prevalence of OSA peaks between the fifth and seventh decades and plateaus thereafter. In the Cleveland Family Study, the prevalence of moderate OSA (apnea-hypopnea index (AHI) ≥15 events per hour) for subjects more than age 60 years was 32% in women and 42% in men. The prevalence in adults less than 60 years of age is 4% for women and 22% for men.

Both epidemiological and sleep clinic-based studies indicate that OSA is generally more common in men. In clinic-based studies, the proportion of men to women with OSA is approximately 8 to 1, while in population-based studies the ratio is closer to 2 to 1. The Wisconsin Sleep Cohort Study evaluated the association between OSA and premenopause, perimenopause, and postmenopause states, and found that the odds ratios for having OSA in perimenopausal women compared to premenopausal women was 1.2 and 2.6 for postmenopausal women, after adjusting for age, body habits, smoking, and other potentially confounding factors. In fact, menopausal women have similar prevalence and incidence of OSA as men.

Reported prevalence rates in different ethnic groups vary. OSA was found to be more prevalent in Black Americans than in the White population after controlling for body mass index (BMI), alchohol use, and tobacco exposure. In the Sleep Heart Health Study, however, the prevalence of OSA was not higher in African-Americans compared to Caucasians, after adjusting for age, sex, and BMI. Unfortunately, there are no data on OSA prevalence in the black population of African countries.

Pacific Islanders and Mexican-Americans have been reported by some to have a higher incidence of OSA than Caucasians. However, a study in New Zealand comparing sleep apnea severity among Maori, Pacific Islanders, and Europeans reported that race was not an important predictor of OSA severity when adjusted for factors such as neck size, BMI, and age.

In a study of middle-aged men in Hong Kong, the estimated prevalence of OSA was approximately 5%, and the prevalence of OSA syndrome (AHI >5 with excessive daytime sleepiness) was estimated to be approximately 4%. Chinese women in Hong Kong have a reported prevalence of 2% for OSA syndrome. In the Singaporian population, sleep apnea affects about 15% of adults. The prevalence of OSA in an Indian population in New Delhi is reportedly 14%. The relatively higher prevalence of OSA in the Asian population, despite their lower prevalence of obesity, suggests the presence of other predisposing factors such as craniofacial anatomy.

Pathophysiology

Sleep-disordered breathing is caused by increased upper airway resistance secondary to narrowing at one or more sites of the upper airway. Locations of narrowing include the nose, retropalatal region, retroglossal region, or, less commonly, the hypoglossal region.

With sleep onset, there is an increase in resistance due to a natural decrease in upper airway muscle tone. In those with narrow airways, the upper airway dilators are unable to oppose the negative pharyngeal intraluminal pressure to maintain minute ventilation and normal gas exchange. In these cases, inspiratory effort is increased. With this

International Neurology: A Clinical Approach. Edited by Robert P. Lisak, Daniel D. Truong, William M. Carroll, and Roongroj Bhidayasiri.
© 2009 Blackwell Publishing, ISBN: 978-1-4051-5738-4.

increase, there is a further decrease in the diameter of the upper airway as upper airway dilators are unable to overcome the inspiratory negative pressure. At some point, an abnormally negative intrathoracic pressure is reached, tidal volume is reduced for one to three breaths, and an arousal response is triggered.

Clinical features

Snoring, witnessed apneas, snorting, and gasping during sleep, recurrent awakenings from sleep, and unrefreshing sleep are the most common nocturnal symptoms of OSA. Loud guttural snoring, at its worst in the supine position, punctuated by choking sounds and followed by cessation of breathing, is virtually pathognomonic. Nocturnal diaphoresis may be seen in association with the increased effort required to inspire against resistance during the night.

Dry mouth or drooling during the night is a sign of mouth-breathing, and is commonly associated with OSA. Many sleep apneics have sleep bruxism, which is often eliminated by continuous positive airway pressure use. Increased intra-abdominal pressure from exaggerated inspiratory attempts against a closed upper airway is thought to contribute to enuresis and nocturnal esophageal acid reflux. Non-rapid eye movement (NREM) parasomnias – such as sleep walking, sleep eating, and nocturnal confusional spells – can be the presenting symptoms in adults as well as in children with OSA.

The cardinal daytime symptom of OSA is excessive daytime sleepiness (EDS), which manifests as a tendency to inadvertently fall asleep during quiet or passive activities, to take intentional naps, or to experience short but repetitive attention lapses while doing monotonous tasks. Such sleepiness is the consequence of sleep fragmentation.

Cognitive complaints from nocturnal hypoxemia and sleep fragmentation are common, and may be the only clue to OSA in those who misperceive their sleepiness. Studies have shown that OSA patients have abnormal neuropsychologic test results in attention, executive function, visuospatial learning, motor performance, and constructional ability.

Investigations

A full-night polysomnography (PSG) study in the sleep laboratory is the main method of evaluation. An entire night of study is generally recommended, as opposed to a partial night, because substantial changes in respiratory disturbances typically occur from one sleep cycle to another across the night. Because rapid eye movement (REM) sleep predominates toward the end of the night,

REM sleep-related respiratory disturbances might easily be missed without a full night of study.

Although a portable study is a convenient, cost effective, and accessible alternative to standard PSG, there are important limitations. The absence of trained personnel to intervene in the event of technical difficulty or medical emergency is one of the primary shortcomings. Concern has also been raised about the precision and accuracy of some portable units for the evaluation of more subtle cases of sleep-disordered breathing, such as those with a predominance of hypopneas or upper airway resistance syndrome. The most recent practice parameters regarding portable PSG studies, published in 2003 by the American Academy of Sleep Medicine, the American Thoracic Society, and the American College of Chest Physicians, conclude that there is insuffienct evidence to recommend the use of portable PSG.

Treatment

Positive airway pressure
Continuous positive airway pressure (CPAP) eliminates upper airway obstruction during sleep and is considered the treatment of choice for OSA. It abolishes obstructive events by increasing the pressure in the pharyngeal airway, thereby eliminating the negative intraluminal pressures that makes airway collapse possible.

A subgroup of sleep apnea patients, even when obstructive respiratory events are eliminated by CPAP, will continue to have increased AHI (mainly because of central apneas or hypopneas) and will also continue to experience significant oxygen desaturation (mainly due to hypoventilation). These patients are considered to have a reduced ventilatory drive, often with daytime hypercapnia, and may benefit from bilevel positive airway pressure ventilation instead of CPAP. Bilevel positive airway pressure is also used to help with patient compliance. Effective bilevel positive airway pressure titration depends on not only appropriate inspiratory pressure (IPAP), but also expiratory pressure (EPAP). Studies show that upper airway resistance increases during end-expiration, particularly during the three to four breaths preceding an apneic or hypopneic event. This narrowing of the airway may be an active, rather than passive, effect of the expiratory pharyngeal constrictor and dilator muscles. Thus, even though IPAP may be equivalent to therapeutic CPAP, inadequate EPAP may result in residual apneas and hypopneas.

Automatic positive airway pressure (AutoPAP) units measure upper airway obstruction by detecting a reduction or flattening of flow, or an increase in airway impedance. Median AutoPAP levels are lower than fixed CPAP levels, while being equally effective at ameliorating sleep apnea and preserving sleep architecture. AutoPAP has been shown to decrease common side effects associated with pressure intolerance and to increase compliance, particularly in patients requiring CPAP greater than 10 cm of water.

Surgery

In general, surgical success for OSA is unpredictable and not as effective as CPAP. Procedures addressing nasal obstruction include septoplasty, turbinectomy, and radiofrequency ablation of the turbinates. These procedures, while providing better nasal breathing, often do not suffice for treating OSA, and are often used in adjunct to CPAP.

Surgical procedures to reduce soft palate redundancy include uvulopalatopharyngoplasty, laser-assisted uvulopalatoplasty, lateral pharyngoplasty, and radiofrequency soft palate ablation. Surgery directly on the pharyngeal tissues is associated with severe pain, hemorrhage, and airway edema in the postoperative period. Such surgeries may also result in permanent velopharyngeal insufficiency, nasopharyngeal stenosis, voice change, and dysphagia.

Surgical options for retrolingual obstruction in patients with OSA include tongue suspension, genioglossal advancement with hyoid suspension, genioglossal advancement with mandibular osteotomy, hyoepiglottoplasty, and radiofrequency tongue ablation. Tongue suspension and genioglossal advancement stabilize the tongue without modifying tongue position or volume, and produce appreciable results when performed on non-overweight patients suffering from severe OSA.

Maxillomandibular advancement, which "pulls forward" the anterior pharyngeal tissues attached to the maxilla, mandible, and hyoid to enlarge the entire velo-orohypopharynx, is the most effective surgical treatment for OSA (excluding tracheostomy, which completely bypasses any upper airway obstructions), with reported success rates in selected patients of over 90%. This procedure requires a multidisciplinary approach with surgeons, sleep specialists, and dentists who need to determine the appropriate degree of advancement while making sure teeth alignment and bite, and aesthetics remain in tact.

Tissue reduction using radiofrequency energy has been the most valuable development in the field of surgery. This procedure has been shown to be effective and minimally invasive. In the last 5 years, other new surgical techniques have not been attempted. Instead, development in this area appears to concentrate on combining previously known methods (so-called multilevel surgery) and optimizing methods of patient selection. Combined surgical procedures can achieve success rates of about 70–95%.

Oral appliances

Oral appliances are a relatively recent development and act by positioning the mandible in a protruded position during sleep. This creates a structural change in the upper pharyngeal anatomy, and enhances the caliber of the airway by triggering stretch receptors which activate the airway support muscles. Up to one-quarter of patients are unable to tolerate this particular device due to temporamandibular joint pain, teeth pain, excessive salivation, dry mouth, gum irritation, and/or next morning occlusion changes. Although this device has been recommended for use in patients with mild to moderate OSA or in those who have failed a trial of CPAP, there is a paucity of data about its effectiveness, utility, and long-term outcome.

Further reading

Young T, Finn L, Austin D, Peterson A. Menopausal status and sleep-disordered breathing in the Wisconsin Sleep Cohort Study. *Am J Respir Crit Care Med* 2003; 167(9): 1181–5.

Young T, Palta M, Dempsey J, Skatrud J, Weber S, Badr S. The occurrence of sleep-disordered breathing among middle-aged adults. *N Engl J Med* 1993; 328(17): 1230–5.

Young T, Peppard PE, Gottlieb DJ. Epidemiology of obstructive sleep apnea: a population health perspective. *Am J Respir Crit Care Med* 2002; 165(9): 1217–39.

Young T, Rabago D, Zgierska A, Austin D, Laurel F. Objective and subjective sleep quality in premenopausal, perimenopausal, and postmenopausal women in the Wisconsin Sleep Cohort Study. *Sleep* 2003; 26(6): 667–72.

Young T, Shahar E, Nieto FJ, *et al.* Predictors of sleep-disordered breathing in community-dwelling adults: the Sleep Heart Health Study. *Arch Intern Med* 2002; 162(8): 893–900.

Chapter 146
Restless legs syndrome

Birgit Högl[1], Birgit Frauscher[1], and Claudio Sergio Podestá[2]
[1]Innsbruck Medical University, Innsbruck, Austria
[2]Neurology Department, Fleni, Buenos-Aires, Argentina

Introduction

Restless legs syndrome (RLS) is a frequent neurological disorder that is often underdiagnosed and undertreated by many neurologists. Approximately one out of eight RLS sufferers who seeks consultation for RLS symptoms is correctly diagnosed. During epidemiological studies, it was found that not one RLS patient was on a first-line RLS treatment and that approximately two out of three were initially misdiagnosed with a vascular disorder.

Epidemiology

RLS occurs one-and-a-half to two times more commonly in women than in men. The prevalence of idiopathic RLS is estimated to be approximately 10% in Europe and North America. Studies in other countries have shown varying prevalence rates, from 0–1% in India, Singapore, and Japan, up to 4% in Korea, and 5% in Japan. Similarly, in South America prevalence estimates range between 2% in native South Americans in Ecuador to 13% in Chile – a population of predominantly European origin. In African-Americans, a prevalence of about 5% has been found. Differences in prevalence may be due to the genetic variability in different ethnic groups or to a lack of consistent diagnostic criteria across studies.

Idiopathic RLS has two phenotypes based on age of onset. In comparison to late-onset RLS, early-onset RLS has a younger age of onset, a slower progression, and frequently a family history of RLS. Secondary RLS is associated with an underlying disorder or condition such as iron deficiency, end-stage renal disease, polyneuropathy, pregnancy, multiple blood donations, spinocerebellar ataxia type 2, and Parkinson's disease – whether these secondary associations are causally related or coincident remains controversial. There are also medications reported to induce or aggravate RLS, including caffeine, dopamine receptor antagonists, estrogens, H2 antagonists, interferon-α, lithium, L-thyroxin, mirtazapine, neuroleptics, tricyclic antidepressants, and selective serotonin reuptake inhibitors. The selective serotonin reuptake inhibitors and venlafaxine have been reported to induce periodic leg movements (PLM).

Pathophysiology

Dopaminergic mechanisms are hypothesized to play a key role in the pathophysiology of RLS. Although dopaminergic drugs are very effective in RLS, a structural dopaminergic deficit has not been found and thus RLS is hypothesized to result from a functional impairment of the dopaminergic system.

Impaired brain iron metabolism is another principal factor in the pathogenesis of idiopathic RLS. MRI and brainstem sonography report correlates of reduced iron in the substantia nigra. In the cerebrospinal fluid (CSF), reduced ferritin levels and increased transferrin levels have been found. In postmortem studies of the substantia nigra in RLS patients, multiple signs of iron deficiency have been reported. Paradoxically, transferrin receptors are decreased instead of being upregulated. This suggests impaired cellular regulation of iron in RLS. Because iron deficiency can affect dopaminergic neurotransmission, it may be that the dopaminergic hypoactivity in RLS is downstream from iron deficiency.

Spinal structures are the final pathway for PLM and the primary input stage for sensory symptoms. RLS and PLM have been reported in patients suffering from spinal cord lesions and spinal cord ischemia, as well as transiently after undergoing spinal anesthesia. Moreover, investigation of the flexor reflex, resembling PLM, suggests increased spinal cord excitability in the pathogenesis of RLS.

In RLS, several studies have reported significant linkage on different chromosomes. Recently, variants in four genomic regions (*MEIS1*, *BTBD9*, *MAP2K5/LBXCOR1*, and *PTPRD*) have been identified, but their actual role in RLS generation remains unknown.

International Neurology: A Clinical Approach. Edited by Robert P. Lisak, Daniel D. Truong, William M. Carroll, and Roongroj Bhidayasiri.
© 2009 Blackwell Publishing, ISBN: 978-1-4051-5738-4.

Clinical features

RLS is diagnosed by history. The neurological examination is normal. The diagnostic criteria of the International Restless Legs Syndrome Study Group (IRLSSG) are given in Table 146.1; all four essential criteria must be fulfilled to diagnose RLS. Supportive clinical features include a positive family history of RLS, response to dopaminergic treatment, and PLM during wakefulness (PLMW) or sleep (PLMS). The natural history of RLS varies. There is usually a very slow progression in early-onset RLS and a faster progression in late-onset RLS. Remissions can occur. Sleep onset or sleep maintenance disturbances are often associated.

The diagnosis of RLS in children or the cognitively impaired elderly can be problematic; often, a typical RLS history is difficult to obtain. In children, a family history of RLS in a first-degree relative, the presence of a sleep disturbance, and a PLM index >5/hour during polysomnography (PSG) can support the diagnosis, although a definite diagnosis requires the child to describe RLS symptoms in her/his own words. In the cognitively impaired elderly, a diagnosis of probable RLS demands the presence of visible or behavioral signs of leg discomfort and excessive motor activity in the lower extremities during periods of inactivity or in the evening.

Periodic leg movements (PLM) and periodic limb movement disorder (PLMD)

PLM are defined as stereotyped limb movements lasting between 0.5 and 10 seconds, an inter-movement interval between 5 and 90 seconds, and at least four movements in a row. Figure 146.1 shows a typical PLM sequence. Although PLM is frequently associated with RLS, it is not specific and is frequently found in normal elderly persons. PLMD can only be diagnosed when PLM is present alongside an additional sleep disturbance or a complaint of daytime fatigue not explained by any other sleep disorder. PLMD can only be diagnosed in the absence of RLS.

Investigations

As mentioned previously, diagnosis of RLS is based on history. Patients with idiopathic RLS do not have neurological findings, such as peripheral neuropathy, but may have comorbid disorders. To exclude secondary causes of RLS, laboratory testing to assess iron status (iron, ferritin, transferrin, and transferrin saturation) is necessary. Additional testing should be done as indicated. PSG is only indicated if there is uncertainty in the diagnosis or a sleep disturbance is suspected.

Table 146.1 Diagnostic criteria of restless legs syndrome.

- An urge to move the legs, usually accompanied with or caused by uncomfortable and unpleasant sensations in the legs (sometimes the arms or other body parts are involved in addition to the legs)
- The urge to move or unpleasant sensations begin or worsen during periods of rest or inactivity such as lying or sitting
- The urge to move or unpleasant sensations are partially or totally relieved by movement, such as walking or stretching, at least as long as the activity continues
- The urge to move or unpleasant sensations are worse in the evening or night than during the day or only occur in the evening or night (when symptoms are very severe, the worsening at night may not be noticeable but must have been previously present)

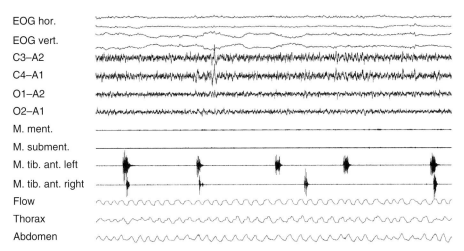

Figure 146.1 A 2-minute PSG example of stage 2 sleep in a patient with symptomatic RLS due to spinocerebellar ataxia type 2. In the tibialis anterior muscles, bilateral periodic leg movements during sleep (PLMS) occur with different periodicity.

Pharmacological treatment/management

Not all patients with RLS need or seek pharmacological treatment. If RLS is associated with a reduced serum ferritin <50 µg/l, iron replacement should be carried out and the possible causes of iron deficiency evaluated. Oral iron replacement is difficult. Ferrous sulfate given with vitamin C one to two times daily between meals for three consecutive months is recommended. In severe iron deficiency, intravenous iron substitution is recommended. Iron studies should be done regularly to avoid iron overload.

If RLS symptoms are frequent and bothersome, treatment is indicated. Dopaminergic agents are considered as first-line therapy in RLS. Large, double-blind, placebo-controlled clinical trials have demonstrated the efficacy of levodopa and dopamine agonists. The ergot dopamine agonists (pergolide and cabergoline) require echocardiographic monitoring due to their association with cardiac valvulopathy. Dopaminergic agents are usually given once per day, in the evening. Dopamine receptor agonists are preferred to levodopa for chronic treatment due to the increased frequency of augmentation with levodopa. For each dopamine agonist, the initial dose should begin low and slowly titrate upward until benefits are reached. Opioids (low dose oxycodone or methadone) and anticonvulsant drugs (gabapentin) are usually considered as second-line therapy.

Augmentation

Augmentation is the major long-term complication of dopaminergic therapy in RLS. Basically, one should always think of augmentation when RLS worsens, despite increasing treatment (paradoxical response). A typical sign of augmentation is the occurrence of RLS symptoms over 4 hours prior to the onset of treatment (in the afternoon versus the evening); or an increase or the spreading of symptoms to previously unaffected body parts, shorter latency to symptoms at rest, etc. Augmentation has been reported frequently with levodopa, as well as with dopamine agonists. To prevent augmentation, the dopamine agonist dosages should be kept low and ferritin levels should be checked regularly. Treatment of augmentation implicates a need to switch to another substance, often a longer acting dopaminergic drug or an opioid. The recently revised criteria for augmentation are given in the Further reading section below.

Further reading

Allen RP, Picchietti D, Hening WA, *et al*. Restless legs syndrome: diagnostic criteria, special considerations, and epidemiology. A report from the restless legs syndrome diagnosis and epidemiology workshop at the National Institutes of Health. *Sleep Med* 2003; 4: 101–19.

Garcia-Borreguero D, Allen RP, Kohnen R, *et al*. Diagnostic standards for dopaminergic augmentation of restless legs syndrome: report from a World Association of Sleep Medicine – International Restless Legs Syndrome Study Group consensus conference at the Max Planck Institute. *Sleep Med* 2007; 8: 520–30.

Hening W, Walters AS, Allen RP, Montplaisir J, Myers A, Ferini-Strambi L. Impact, diagnosis and treatment of restless legs syndrome (RLS) in a primary care population: the REST (RLS epidemiology, symptoms, and treatment) primary care study. *Sleep Med* 2004; 5: 237–46.

Chapter 147
Circadian sleep disorders

Sergio Tufik, Monica L. Andersen, Lia R.A. Bittencourt, and T. De Mello
Universidade Federal de São Paulo (UNIFESP-EPM), São Paulo, Brazil

Introduction

Regularity in sleep timing and duration is a rhythmic behavior regulated by complex physiological and psychological factors. Times selected to go to bed and awaken are clearly influenced by subjective needs, but the tendency to sleep at night and to be active during the day is under physiological control and highly specific to the human species. The pattern of sleeping at night and being awake during the day is referred to as a diurnal pattern.

Because the secretion of melatonin at night occurs at the same time humans need to sleep, the pineal has long been suspected of being involved with sleep. Although melatonin secretion is influenced by the light–dark cycle, the diurnal rhythm of the pineal is directly controlled by an endogenous clock, probably the suprachiasmatic nucleus (SCN) of the anterior hypothalamus. The SCN is the central biological clock of the brain, which synchronizes the overt biochemical, physiological, and behavioral rhythms. Determination of melatonin rhythm may therefore reflect the internal perception of external conditions and provide a means of assessing the temporal organization of the organism.

While circadian rhythms are part of normal physiology, some individuals have an irregular sleep–wake pattern or are fully arrhythmic to it. The arrhythmicity is very disruptive to familial and social life, and to successful employment. Circadian rhythm sleep disorders (CRSD) are characterized by a desynchronization between the timing of the intrinsic circadian clock and the extrinsic light–dark and social/activity cycles, resulting in symptoms of excessive sleepiness and insomnia.

Pathophysiology

According to the International Classification of Sleep Disorders (2005), CRSD is one of eight categories of sleep

International Neurology: A Clinical Approach. Edited by Robert P. Lisak, Daniel D. Truong, William M. Carroll, and Roongroj Bhidayasiri.
© 2009 Blackwell Publishing, ISBN: 978-1-4051-5738-4.

disorders. The main characteristic of this category is that, for optimal sleep, the desired sleep time should match the timing of the circadian rhythm of sleep and wake propensity. Therefore, a recurrent or chronic pattern of sleep disturbance may result from alterations of the circadian timing system, or a misalignment between the timing of the individual's circadian rhythm of sleep propensity and the 24-hour social and physical environments. These disorders may arise when the physical environment is altered relative to internal circadian timing or the circadian timing system is altered relative to the external environment. In addition to physiological and environmental factors, maladaptive behaviors influence the presentation and severity of CRSD.

a *Delayed sleep phase type (DSP)* is characterized by habitual sleep–wake times that are delayed relative to conventional or socially acceptable times. There are some controversies, but prevalence of DSP in the general population is 7–16%.

b *Advanced sleep phase type (ASP)* is a stable advance of the major sleep period, characterized by habitual sleep onset and wake-up times that are several hours earlier, relative to conventional/desired times. The prevalence of ASP in the general population is unknown. Genetic factors may also influence the development of the condition.

c *Irregular sleep–wake type* is characterized by a temporally disorganized sleep–wake pattern so that sleep and wake periods are variable throughout a 24-hour period.

d *Free-running type* is characterized by sleep symptoms that occur because the intrinsic circadian pacemaker is not entrained to a 24-hour period, or is free running with a non-24-hour period. Most individuals presenting non-entrained circadian rhythms are totally blind, and the failure to entrain circadian rhythms is related to the lack of photic input to the circadian pacemaker.

e *Jet lag type* is characterized by a temporary mismatch between the timing of the sleep–wake cycle generated by the endogenous circadian clock and that of the sleep and wake pattern required by a change in time zone.

f *Shift work type* is characterized by complaints of insomnia or excessive sleepiness occurring in relation to work hours that are scheduled during the usual sleep period. In addition to an impairment of performance at work, reduced alertness may be associated with consequences for safety.

g *Due to medical condition:* Etiology of CRSD is an underlying primary medical or neurological condition. Depending on the underlying neurological or medical disorder, patients may present with a variety of symptoms, including insomnia and excessive sleepiness.

h *Other circadian rhythm disorders:* Disorders that (1) satisfy the criteria of a circadian rhythm sleep disorder, (2) are not due to drug or substance, and (3) do not meet the criteria for other CRSD are classified by ICSD-2.

Treatment

Treatment should be tailored to the severity of symptoms, comorbid psychopathology, school schedules, work obligations, social pressures, and the ability and willingness of the patient/family to comply with treatment. Current treatment options for CRSD include sleep hygiene education, timed exposure to bright light and avoidance of bright light (at the wrong time of the day), and pharmacologic approaches, such as melatonin (which is not currently Food and Drug Administration (FDA)-approved for treatment of CRSD).

Conclusions

The detrimental effects caused by the impossibility of reconciling sleep needs with social demands have far-reaching consequences. As a result, scientific productivity in the field has been intense, as sleep loss will most likely continue to be a major affliction. The treatment of CRSD remains a challenge, in part because large multicenter, placebo-controlled clinical studies using phototherapy or pharmacologic agents are scarce.

Further reading

American Academy of Sleep Medicine. *International Classification of Sleep Disorders (ICSD-2): Diagnostic and Coding Manual*, 2nd ed. Westchester, IL: AASM; 2005.

Barion A, Zee PC. A clinical approach to circadian rhythm sleep disorders. *Sleep Med* 2007; 8(6): 566–77.

Dunlap JC, Loros JJ, DeCoursey PJ. The relevance of circadian rhythms for human welfare. In: Dunlap JC, Loros JJ, DeCoursey PJ, editors. *Chronobiology: Biological Timekeeping*. Sunderland, MA: Sinauer; 2004, pp. 325–58.

Pandi-Perumal SR, Smits M, Spence W, *et al*. Dim light melatonin onset (DLMO): a tool for the analysis of circadian phase in human sleep and chronobiological disorders. *Prog Neuropsychopharmacol Biol Psychiatry* 2007; 31: 1–11.

Reid KJ, Zee P. Circadian disorders of the sleep–wake cycle. In: Kryger MH, Roth T, Dement WC, editors. *Principles and Practice of Sleep Medicine*, 4th ed. Philadelphia: WB Saunders; 2005, pp. 691–701.

Chapter 148
Disorders of arousal

Li Ling Lim
Gleneagles Medical Centre, Singapore

Introduction

Disorders of arousal (arousal disorder, AD) belong within the spectrum of parasomnias which refer to undesirable sleep-related movements, behaviors, or experiences which cause sleep disruption and other adverse health effects. Common ADs include confusional arousals, sleepwalking, and sleep terrors. These usually occur in non-rapid eye movement (NREM) slow-wave sleep, but can also occur in stage 2 NREM sleep.

Epidemiology and risk factors

ADs are more common in children than in adults. Childhood prevalence estimates are: confusional arousals 17.3%; sleepwalking 17%; and sleep terrors 1–6.5%. Adult prevalence estimates are: confusional arousals 2.9–4.2%; sleepwalking 2–4%; and sleep terrors 2.2%. In adults, sleepwalking associated with violence is more commonly reported in men. Sleepwalking peaks by age 8–12 years. Sleep terrors peak at about 5–7 years and usually resolve by adolescence.

ADs can be triggered by sleep deprivation, forced awakenings, physical or emotional stress, anxiety, fever, psychotropic drugs, antihistamines, alcohol, environmental stimuli, and primary sleep disorders such as obstructive sleep apnea (OSA). In adults, associated psychiatric problems (depression, anxiety, or bipolar disorder) have been reported, although significant psychopathology is usually not present.

Pathophysiology

AD tends to run in families and is believed to be a result of faulty transitions between slow-wave and lighter stages of sleep, with a sleep–wake state dissociation. This faculty

transition is reflected by episodes of EEG activity comprising of an admixture of slower sleep and faster wake-like frequencies. Other factors contributing to the complex behaviors include dissociation of locomotor centers (from the state of NREM sleep) and inherent instability of slow-wave sleep. Structural lesions in the brain's normal wake centers (posterior hypothalamus and reticular activating system) have been reported to cause AD; however, most cases present with normal brains.

A positive family history in a first-degree relative is found in 60% of children. One study reported the prevalence of sleepwalking and sleep terrors being 10 times higher in first-degree relatives of sleep terror patients than in the general population. The rate of sleepwalking in children with a family history increases to 45% with one parent and 60% with both parents affected.

Clinical features and differential diagnoses

AD patients act out complex behaviors while in deep sleep, typically remaining amnestic of their actions. Episodes tend to occur in the first third of the night when slow-wave sleep predominates. Forced arousals from sleep can also induce episodes.

Confusional arousals occur most frequently in infants and toddlers, but are also seen in young adults (age 15–24 years), decreasing with age. Episodes are characterized by disorientation, slowed mentation, agitation, crying, thrashing, and combative behavior, lasting 5–15 minutes or as long as 30–40 minutes.

Sleepwalking consists of walking around in a state of altered consciousness, either calmly or agitated, after partial arousal from slow-wave sleep. It can vary in duration and complexity. Safety is a main concern, as falls, environmental exposure, and injury may occur.

In contrast to sleepwalking, in which the child usually remains calm, sleep terrors usually begin with a piercing cry or scream, associated autonomic arousal (tachypnea, mydriasis, tachycardia, and diaphoresis), behavioral manifestations of intense fear, and prominent motor activity (running or hitting). The child is typically

International Neurology: A Clinical Approach. Edited by Robert P. Lisak, Daniel D. Truong, William M. Carroll, and Roongroj Bhidayasiri.

inconsolable and difficult to arouse, and may later recall feeling threatened or scared.

Sleep disorders that cause recurrent arousals – such as OSA and periodic limb movement disorder (PLMD) – can trigger AD. Physical examination is usually normal, but should include a comprehensive evaluation of clinical features of associated conditions.

The diagnosis of childhood arousal parasomnias can usually be made by the witnessed description of events (given by a parent). Movements and behaviors, when they occur shortly after sleep onset, can be recorded in sleep diaries and on home videos. Conditions that mimic AD include nocturnal seizures (frontal lobe epilepsy and complex partial seizures), sleep-related movement disorders, panic attacks, and nightmares.

Investigations

Polysomnography (PSG) is not routinely required for AD, but is useful in providing corroborative documentation as well as excluding associated primary sleep disorders. If epilepsy is suspected, an expanded EEG montage is required (ideally with time-synchronized video-EEG recording). Multiple arousals from slow-wave sleep are classic PSG findings in AD. EEG may show a mixture of alpha, theta, and delta waves, reflecting the sleep–wake state dissociation characteristic of AD.

Management

Parents should be reassured that ADs are common and generally benign. Often, therapy is not required; however, sensible safety precautions should be discussed, such as padding the bedroom environment, securing doors and windows, and installing alarm/monitoring systems. Using good sleep hygiene, avoiding sleep deprivation, and discontinuing stimulants (caffeine and triggering medications) should also be recommended. Parents should be advised not to wake the child during an episode, or to discuss the events of the night with the child. If episodes become predictably recurrent, scheduled awakenings just before the typical time of a sleepwalking episode have been reported to successfully eliminate sleepwalking. Relaxation therapy may also be useful.

Parasomnias that pose a risk of injury to the patient (or bed partner) and those that are triggered by treatable conditions (OSA and PLMD) require specific therapy. For frequent or potentially injurious arousal parasomnias, benzodiazepines and tricyclic antidepressants are helpful. Clonazepam has been used successfully, starting at low doses (0.25 mg at bedtime) and titrating according to effect and tolerability.

Clinical course

Pediatric parasomnias are generally benign and self-limited, and usually do not persist into late adolescence or adulthood. Confusional arousals decrease after the age of 5 years, but may progress to sleep walking in adolescence. The adult variant may persist and is associated with sleep-related injury and impaired performance.

Summary

Classic arousal parasomnias form a spectrum of common features, including abnormal transition from slow-wave sleep, complex automatic behaviors, and amnesia following episodes. Management should focus on accurate diagnosis, exclusion of treatable associated conditions, and simple behavioral interventions to reduce the risk of physical injury and psychosocial problems.

Further reading

Frank NC, Spirito A, Stark L, Owens-Stively J. The use of scheduled awakenings to eliminate childhood sleepwalking. *J Pediatr Psychol* 1997; 22(3): 345–53.

Kales A, Soldatos CR, Bixler EO, *et al.* Hereditary factors in sleepwalking and night terrors. *Br J Psychiatry* 1980; 137: 111–18.

Mahowald M, Schenck C, Basetti C, *et al.* Parasomnias. In: Sateia M, editor. *The International Classification of Sleep Disorders.* 2nd ed. Westchester, IL: American Academy of Sleep Medicine; 2005, pp. 137–47.

Ohayon MM, Guilleminault C, Priest RG. Night terrors, sleepwalking, and confusional arousals in the general population: their frequency and relationship to other sleep and mental disorders. *J Clin Psychiatry* 1999; 60(4): 268–76.

Chapter 149
REM behavior disorder (RBD)

Li Ling Lim
Gleneagles Medical Centre, Singapore

Introduction

Rapid eye movement (REM) sleep behavior disorder (RBD) is the most common REM sleep parasomnia. RBD is characterized by the absence of muscle atonia, which permits acting out of dreams, often resulting in physical injury. RBD was first described as a distinct clinical entity in a series of adults manifesting violent behaviors while acting out dreams during sleep and injuring themselves or their spouses in the process. RBD is characterized by a loss of normal REM atonia, loss of chin muscle atonia, and excessive muscle twitching on polysomnography (PSG). RBD is often associated with neurodegenerative disease and is responsive to clonazepam.

Epidemiology and risk factors

The estimated overall prevalence of RBD is about 0.5%, with a reported range from 0.38% to as high as 0.8%. The majority (approximately 90%) of RBD patients are older men, although any age group or gender can be affected.

RBD has been associated with a range of neurologic conditions, most notably parkinsonism and degenerative dementia, often reflecting an underlying synucleinopathy. RBD may precede the onset of parkinsonism or dementia in patients with Parkinson's disease (PD), multiple system atrophy (MSA), or dementia with Lewy bodies (DLB) by years or decades. Thus "idiopathic" RBD may represent the initial manifestation of an evolving neurodegenerative disorder. A higher incidence of RBD is also seen in narcolepsy. This probably reflects the REM sleep-related dyscontrol common to both conditions in which the elements normally regulating REM sleep are not present.

Many commonly used drugs (e.g., selective serotonin reuptake inhibitors (SSRIs), monoamine oxidase inhibitors, and tricyclic antidepressants) can induce or aggravate RBD symptoms in patients at risk.

International Neurology: A Clinical Approach. Edited by Robert P. Lisak, Daniel D. Truong, William M. Carroll, and Roongroj Bhidayasiri. © 2009 Blackwell Publishing, ISBN: 978-1-4051-5738-4.

Pathophysiology

The pathophysiology of RBD is believed to be analogous to that described in animal models in which damage to pontine tegmental pathways mediating REM-atonia (and those structures that normally suppress the phasic locomotor drive in REM sleep) result in complex behaviors as seen in RBD. Positron emission tomography (PET) and single photon emission computed tomography (SPECT) studies have shown dysfunction in the nigrostriatal dopaminergic pathways in patients with idiopathic RBD. In humans, RBD may precede the onset of the motor symptoms of parkinsonism. This suggests that the first clinical symptoms to appear may correspond to the brainstem regions first affected by neuronal degeneration (RBD when beginning in the mesopontine junction or parkinsonism when beginning in the midbrain).

Clinical features and differential diagnoses

RBD typically manifests as complex dream-enacting behaviors that are often vivid, unpleasant, or violent, such as being attacked or chased. Typically, the abnormal movements include vocalizations, flailing, punching, kicking, swearing, gesturing, leaping, and running. These movements lead to sleep disruption and sometimes injuries. The episodes typically occur approximately 90 minutes after sleep onset, coinciding with the timing of the first REM cycle, and may recur with subsequent REM sleep cycles.

RBD is usually a chronic and progressive disorder that is either idiopathic or associated with a range of neurological disorders – including the synucleinopathies such as PD, MSA, and DLB. RBD can also occur with cerebrovascular disease, neoplasm (such as brainstem and cerebellopontine angle tumors), and inflammatory conditions (such as Guillain–Barré syndrome and multiple sclerosis). RBD has been noted in patients with narcolepsy, mitochondrial disorders, Tourette syndrome, autism, normal pressure hydrocephalus, and spinocerebellar ataxia. An acute form of RBD can occur during REM sleep rebound states, such as withdrawal from alcohol or sedative–hypnotic agents, and may be triggered by medications, including serotonergic antidepressants.

The diagnosis of RBD is based on a clinical history of injurious or potentially injurious dream-enacting behavior that disrupts REM sleep. PSG shows REM sleep without atonia, excessive tonic and phasic electromyogram (EMG) activity recorded from the chin, excessive phasic EMG activity in the limbs, and abnormal REM sleep behaviors. This occurs in the absence of EEG epileptiform activity during REM sleep.

Differential diagnoses encompass other causes of abnormal behavior in sleep, such as NREM parasomnias (sleepwalking, sleep terrors), nocturnal epilepsy, and OSA, which may mimic RBD.

Investigations

PSG with time-synchronized video-EEG recording is needed to document the typical PSG features of RBD and to exclude disorders that may mimic RBD. Periodic limb movements of sleep (PLMS) can be seen in about 75% of RBD patients during NREM sleep.

Management

Clonazepam (beginning dose of 0.5 mg at night, increasing to 1 or 2 mg) is very effective in treating RBD and is considered first-line treatment. It is generally well tolerated and produces rapid (within the first week) and sustained (up to several years) improvement in the majority of patients, with little evidence of tolerance or abuse. Beneficial effects may be related to suppression of motor manifestations and partly to clonazepam's serotonergic properties.

Alternatively, melatonin (dosing between 3 and 12 mg at night) works as monotherapy for patients who may not tolerate long-acting benzodiazepines, or who have OSA. The mechanism of melatonin is not well understood, but has been reported to be effective for RBD, especially in patients with low melatonin levels. Studies have reported that melatonin reduces motor activity during sleep and partially restores REM sleep muscle atonia. Postulated mechanisms of melatonin include restoration of RBD-related desynchronization of the circadian rhythm and mechanisms producing REM sleep muscle atonia.

The effectiveness of other drugs including dopaminergic agents (pramipexole or levodopa), acetylcholinesterase inhibitors (donepezil or rivastigmine), and antiepileptic agents (carbamazepine or gabapentin) remains unclear.

Improving sleeping environment safety, removing potentially dangerous objects, and allotting separate sleeping arrangements for bed partners are also useful measures.

Clinical course

RBD is slowly progressive and is rarely associated with spontaneous remissions, though symptoms may subside in the advanced stages of an underlying neurodegenerative condition. Drug-induced RBD should improve upon withdrawal of the offending medication.

Summary

RBD, the most common REM parasomnia, is a striking clinical entity associated with neurodegeneration, affecting primarily older men. Evaluation should include a comprehensive clinical history detailing sleep behaviors and medication use, neurologic examination, and PSG. Prompt recognition is important to reduce potential complications including physical injury and marital discord arising from trauma and sleep disruption. Treatment with clonazepam is safe and effective in the majority of cases.

Further reading

Boeve BF, Silber MH, Ferman TJ. Melatonin for treatment of REM sleep behavior disorder in neurologic disorders: results in 14 patients. *Sleep Med* 2003; 4(4): 281–4.

Boeve BF, Silber MH, Parisi JE, *et al*. Synucleinopathy pathology and REM sleep behavior disorder plus dementia or parkinsonism. *Neurology* 2003; 61(1): 40–5.

Gagnon JF, Postuma RB, Montplaisir J. Update on the pharmacology of REM sleep behavior disorder. *Neurology* 2006; 67(5): 742–7.

Schenck CH, Bundlie SR, Ettinger MG, Mahowald MW. Chronic behavioral disorders of human REM sleep: a new category of parasomnia. *Sleep* 1986; 9(2): 293–308.

Schenck CH, Mahowald MW. Polysomnographic, neurologic, psychiatric, and clinical outcome report on 70 consecutive cases with REM sleep behavior disorder (RBD): sustained clonazepam efficacy in 89.5% of 57 treated patients. *Cleve Clin J Med* 1990; 57(Suppl): S9–23.

Chapter 150
Paroxysmal nocturnal dystonia

Cynthia L. Comella
Rush University Medical Center, Chicago, USA

Introduction

Paroxysmal nocturnal dystonia (PND) is one of a group of clinically heterogeneous disorders included under the category of nocturnal frontal lobe epilepsy (NFLE). The clinical presentation of NFLE includes paroxysmal arousals, partial arousals with sleep walking, sleep terrors or confusional arousals, repetitive stereotypic behaviors, and paroxysmal nocturnal dystonia or dyskinesias. PND was initially described in the early 1980s in five patients. The episodes in these patients were brief (<2 minutes) and stereotypic, occurring nearly every night during non-rapid eye movement (NREM) sleep. Although scalp electroencephalography failed to show epileptiform discharges, all responded to carbamazepine. Whether these episodes were a manifestation of a paroxysmal movement disorder or seizure activity was clarified when sphenoidal and zygomatic electrodes showed epileptic discharges in mesiotemporal and orbital or mesial frontal regions.

Clinical features

NFLE has diverse presentations that have been categorized into four general types. Paroxysmal arousal is a very brief, abrupt, recurrent arousal from NREM sleep. Patients may look around, appear frightened, and have vocalizations. NPD presents as a sudden arousal, with movements that may be dystonic (e.g., twisting of the head, neck, torso, and limbs) or ballistic and last up to 100 seconds. NPD may be preceded by a paroxysmal arousal. Asymmetric bilateral tonic seizures can also occur. Episodic nocturnal wanderings often appear as more violent motor behaviors, such as getting out of bed, screaming, and showing fear. These episodes may last up to 3 minutes. The episodes appear similar in the same patient, but may vary from patient to patient.

International Neurology: A Clinical Approach. Edited by Robert P. Lisak, Daniel D. Truong, William M. Carroll, and Roongroj Bhidayasiri. © 2009 Blackwell Publishing, ISBN: 978-1-4051-5738-4.

Episodes of NFLE are frequent, may occur several times a week, and recur several times a night. During an episode, there is autonomic activation. The age of onset is usually in childhood or adolescence, although onset as late as 64 years of age has been reported. Up to 35% of NFLE patients have occasional seizures during daytime wakefulness. Family history is positive for a parasomnia or daytime epilepsy in 25–40% of patients. Neurological examination and brain imaging are usually normal.

Genetics

Most NFLE is primary, without an underlying cause. In some families, NFLE is autosomal dominant, but with considerable genetic heterogeneity. Mutations include two genes (*DHRNA4* and *CHRNA2*) coding for the α4 and β2 subunits of the neuronal nicotinic acetylcholine receptor, and a locus on chromosome 15q24. However, in many families, these genes have been excluded, indicating the heterogeneity of the disorder despite a similar phenotype.

Differential diagnosis

The differential diagnosis of NFLE includes a variety of parasomnias that occur in NREM and REM sleep. These include confusional arousals, sleep terrors, and sleep walking. REM parasomnias include REM sleep behavior disorder and nightmares. Other disorders that can cause episodic movements during the night include bruxism, sleep starts, and propriospinal myoclonus at sleep onset.

Evaluation

Evaluation of patients with sleep-associated movement disorders includes a careful history from the patients and bed partners. Additional clinical assessments include home video footage showing several occurrences of the nocturnal movements. Video polysomnography (PSG) is the most important diagnostic test. Electroencephalography

(EEG) with scalp electrodes often does not show abnormal activity, even during the ictal period. Deep electrodes (sphenoidal or zygomatic) are more sensitive, but may not always be revealing.

Treatment

NFLE is a chronic disorder with few spontaneous remissions. Treatment of NFLE with carbamazepine may significantly reduce the number and severity of episodes, although 30–50% of patients do not benefit. Topiramate may be more effective in up to 90% of patients. The efficacy of many anticonvulsants has not been assessed.

Further reading

AASM. *Sleep Related Epilepsy. International Classification of Sleep Disorders: Diagnostic and Coding Manual*, 2nd ed. Westchester, IL: American Academy of Sleep Medicine; 2005, pp. 232–5.

De Marco EV, Gambardella A, Annesi F, *et al*. Further evidence of genetic heterogeneity in families with autosomal dominant nocturnal frontal lobe epilepsy. *Epilepsy Res* 2007; 74: 70–3.

Lugaresi E, Cirignotta F. Hypnogenic paroxysmal dystonia: epileptic seizure or a new syndrome? *Sleep* 1981; 4: 129–38.

Oldani A, Manconi M, Zucconi M, *et al*. Topiramate treatment for nocturnal frontal lobe epilepsy. *Seizure* 2006; 15: 649–52.

Provini F, Plazzi G, Montagna P, Lugaresi E. The wide clinical spectrum of nocturnal frontal lobe epilepsy. *Sleep Med Rev* 2000; 4: 375–86.

Provini F, Plazzi G, Tinuper P, *et al*. Nocturnal frontal lobe epilepsy. A clinical and polygraphic overview of 100 consecutive cases. *Brain* 1999; 122(Pt 6): 1017–31.

Tinuper P, Provini F, Bisulli F, *et al*. Movement disorders in sleep: guidelines for differentiating epileptic from non-epileptic motor phenomena arising from sleep. *Sleep Med Rev* 2007; 11(4): 255–67.

Chapter 151
Sleep abnormalities in neurological disorders

Margaret Park and Cynthia L. Comella
Rush University Medical Center, Chicago, USA

Sleep-disordered breathing (SDB)

SDB includes obstructive sleep apnea–hypopnea syndrome (OSA) and central sleep apnea (CSA). Obstructions are absence of airflow despite respiratory effort, hypopneas are reduced airflow despite respiratory effort, and central events represent a complete airflow absence. Polysomnography (PSG) evaluates respiratory events per hour, called the apnea–hypopnea index (AHI); AHI >5 is considered diagnostic for SDB. Continuous positive airway pressure (CPAP) is considered the primary treatment of choice for OSA; oxygen and other ventilation may be useful for CSA. SDB is frequently comorbid to neurological conditions, including the following.

Stroke
SDB is prevalent in stroke, with shared risk factors including hypertension. SDB is both a risk factor and consequence of stroke, but an unclear cause-and-effect relationship exists. SDB in stroke is associated with worsening functional impairment, increased hospital stay, and increased future stroke risk. Studies are needed to determine whether treating SDB reduces stroke risk and improves outcome.

Neuromuscular disease (NMD)
NMD compromises diaphragmatic function, whether due to motor neuron disease (poliomyelitis or amyotrophic lateral sclerosis), phrenic nerve involvement (Guillain–Barré), or neuromuscular junction alterations (myasthenia gravis). NMD generally interferes with rapid eye movement (REM) sleep, as REM sleep is heavily dependent on the diaphragm. However, central respiratory involvement, pharyngobulbar weakness, craniofacial dysmorphisms, and musculoskeletal deformities also compromise ventilation, causing SDB-related nocturnal hypoxemia. Treating SDB improves quality of life in NMD and may prolong the need for intubation or tracheostomy.

This, in addition to the high prevalence of SDB in NMD, warrants a low threshold in obtaining evaluation.

Headache (HA) syndromes
HA syndromes are common in OSA, with an uncertain pathophysiological link. Possible mechanisms include intermittent hypoxia and/or hypercarbia, causing fluctuations in cerebral blood flow and intracranial pressure. In addition to morning HAs, OSA also triggers migraines and cluster headaches, usually during or around REM as opposed to non-REM (NREM) sleep, and particularly after oxyhemoglobin desaturation. HA improvement can occur when OSA is successfully treated.

Restless legs syndrome (RLS) and periodic limb movement disorder (PLMD)

Clinical criteria for RLS include non-specific sensory disturbances, association with an urge to move, relief with movement, and a nocturnal component. PLMD is diagnosed by evaluating periodic limb movements during sleep (PLMS) on PSG. PLMS are repetitive, stereotypical limb movements during sleep and are scored per hour of sleep, called the PLMS index (PLM-I). PLM-I >5 is considered diagnostic for PLMD.

RLS and PLMD are often grouped together because 80–90% of RLS patients also have PLMD. Pathophysiologically, they share presumed dopaminergic dysfunction, with contribution from low ferritin levels. Treatment is primarily with dopaminergic medications, although sedative-hypnotics are often used. In addition to idiopathic/primary forms, RLS/PLMD occurs in neurological disorders, including the following.

Neuropathy
RLS/PLMD is frequently found in neuropathy, possibly due to shared sensorimotor disturbances. Theoretically, abnormal sensory stimuli from small- or large-fiber neuropathy, axonal neuropathy, or radiculopathy inappropriately activate movement generators in the medulla or spinal motor dopaminergic cells. This may explain

International Neurology: A Clinical Approach. Edited by Robert P. Lisak, Daniel D. Truong, William M. Carroll, and Roongroj Bhidayasiri. © 2009 Blackwell Publishing, ISBN: 978-1-4051-5738-4.

why medications that address neuropathic pain can successfully treat RLS/PLMD, although secondary forms of RLS/PLMD may differ in pathophysiology from primary forms.

Parkinson's disease (PD)

RLS/PLMD is frequently found in PD and has assumed a pathophysiologic relationship due to a shared responsiveness to dopamine. Brainstem, rather than spinal cells, may be responsible for PLMS, possibly indicating that PLMS is an early sign of PD brainstem involvement. However, the increased prevalence of RLS in PD may be due to lower ferritin levels in these patients rather than a true pathophysiologic link. Overall, studies are too few to conclude whether physiological differences exist between idiopathic versus PD-related RLS/PLMD, but an inherent relationship is likely.

Parasomnias

Parasomnias are undesirable behavioral phenomena during sleep, classified as NREM or REM, although overlap syndromes frequently occur.

NREM parasomnias (confusional arousals, sleep terrors, or sleep walking) are "arousal disorders" due to their tendency to occur after an arousal from slow-wave sleep. Although generally found in childhood, persistence into adulthood is common. Medication may not be necessary and is left to clinical discretion; however, if episodes are frequent, potentially injurious, cause social dysfunction, or cause excessive daytime sleepiness (EDS), benzodiazepines are generally prescribed. Other sleep disorders, including OSA, PLMD, and nocturnal seizures, are potential causes of arousals and should be treated accordingly. Avoidance of alcohol and sleep deprivation should accompany recommendations.

The most common REM parasomnia is REM-behavior disorder (RBD), characterized by loss of physiological muscle atonia during REM, allowing patients to "act out" dreams, often with injurious results. PSG is diagnostically helpful, even in the absence of laboratory events, as loss of muscle atonia is evident during REM. RBD typically occurs in older adults and is associated with other disorders, including OSA, narcolepsy, and neurodegenerative disorders, particularly synucleinopathies (PD, Lewy body dementia, or multiple systems atrophy). Idiopathic RBD may precede neurodegenerative disorders; thus, frequent follow-up is advised. Clonazepam is considered the treatment of choice; pramipexole and melatonin may be partially beneficial. Avoidance of alcohol and sleep deprivation are recommended, in addition to general safety precautions.

Pathological hypersomnias: narcolepsy and idiopathic hypersomnolence (IH)

Narcolepsy is the instability of sleep–wake states, likely due to mutations in the hypothalamic hypocretin/orexin system. Complaints include EDS, fragmented nocturnal sleep, and REM intrusion into wakefulness (cataplexy, sleep paralysis, or hypnogogic/hypnopompic hallucinations). Diagnostically, PSG and Multiple Sleep Latency Tests (MSLT) show shortened sleep latencies and 2+ sleep-onset REM periods. EDS is typically treated with stimulants and/or frequent napping schedules. REM intrusion can be treated with antidepressants or sodium oxybate. Comorbid sleep disorders often accompany narcolepsy, including OSA, PLMD, and RBD.

IH is characterized by EDS, with non-refreshing sleep despite prolonged sleep episodes. PSG/MSLT shows high sleep efficiency and shortened sleep latencies. Despite attempts to further characterize IH, pathophysiology remains unclear. IH thus remains a diagnosis of exclusion. Treatment with stimulants has variable response and prolonged sleep schedules are generally not beneficial.

Further reading

Avidan A, editor. *Sleep in Neurological Practice.* New York: Thieme; 2005.

Diagnostic Classification Steering Committee of the American Sleep Disorders Association. Thorpy MJ, Chairperson. *The International Classification of Sleep Disorders: Diagnostic and Coding Manual.* Rochester, MN: American Sleep Disorders Association; 1997.

Meir H, Kryger T, Dement W, editors. *Principles and Practice of Sleep Medicine.* Philadelphia: Elsevier; 2006.

Chapter 152
Disc disease

David B. Vodušek[1,2] and Simon Podnar[2]
[1]University of Ljubljana, Ljubljana, Slovenia
[2]University Medical Centre, Ljubljana, Slovenia

Introduction

"Spinal pain" is estimated to be one of the most prevalent morbid conditions, also leading to absenteeism from work and early retirement. Lifetime prevalence of spinal pain both in the neck and lower back has been reported as up to 80%.

The two adjacent spinal vertebrae are joined by paired facet joints and the intervertebral disc, and form the "motion segment." The disc is formed by the collagenous outer annulus fibrosus and the gel-like nucleus pulposus. Only the outer layer of the annulus has nerve and blood supply and the other parts are dependent on diffusion exchange of nutrients. By middle age, the annulus develops fissures, and through these, disc protrusion, prolapse, or even sequestration may occur, with the possibility of mechanical compression of nerve roots, spinal cord, or blood vessels within the spinal canal and the nerve root exit foramina (Figure 152.1). From the second decade onwards, the degeneration process becomes more and more frequent; degeneration of the superior and inferior margins of the vertebral bodies accompanied by the formation of osteophytes, osteoarthritic changes of the facet joints (i.e., spondylosis), and hypertrophy of the longitudinal ligament invariably leads to the extremely prevalent changes seen on plain X-ray, CT, and MRI, which in the majority of patients is asymptomatic. The changes may cause pain without actually involving and injuring nervous system structures. In a minority of patients structural changes damage nerve roots or the spinal cord, through either compression of the nervous tissue or its vascular supply; inflammatory mechanisms possibly contribute.

In adults, the spinal cord occupies the spinal canal to the level of the L1/L2 interface (with some individual variability). The anterior and posterior roots are attached to the spinal cord, the spinal ganglion on the posterior root being situated just before the two roots unite into the spinal nerve. The anterior root and the posterior root with

International Neurology: A Clinical Approach. Edited by Robert P. Lisak, Daniel D. Truong, William M. Carroll, and Roongroj Bhidayasiri. © 2009 Blackwell Publishing, ISBN: 978-1-4051-5738-4.

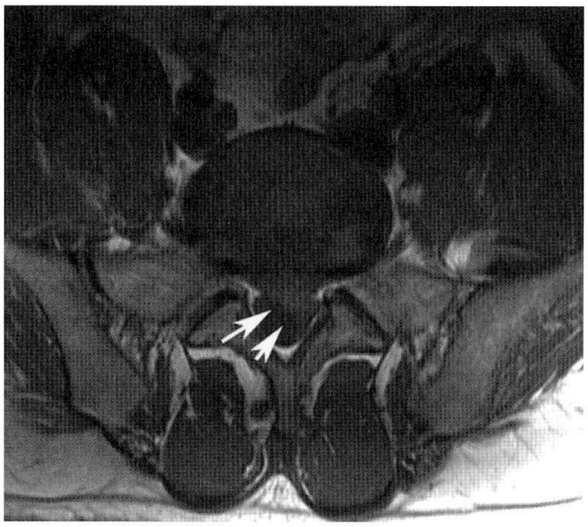

Figure 152.1 Magnetic resonance imaging, axial view, T1 weighted slice at the level of the L5–S1 intervertebral space, demonstrating a partially sequestered herniated disc on the left (*white arrows*) compressing the dural sac and the left S1 root in a 47-year-old man. He presented with acute onset of pain radiating from his back to his left heel, and tingling on the lateral aspect of the left foot. Weakness of left plantar flexion and left ankle areflexia were found. (Courtesy Prim. Miha Škrbec, MD, Radiology Department, University Medical Centre, Ljubljana, Slovenia.)

the ganglion are intradural, exiting individually and uniting into the spinal nerve extradurally. The anterior and posterior roots join before leaving the spinal canal through the intervertebral foramen. Nerve roots are accompanied by arteries and veins. In the neck, the spinal ganglion lies within the intervertebral foramen. From L2, it moves more medially. The L5 spinal ganglion lies at the inner aperture of the foramen, and the spinal ganglia below that level move into the spinal canal. The cervical roots exit from foramina lying above the respective vertebrae (the C8 root thus being situated above T1). From root C4 downwards the roots have a more and more steep downwards course. They also increase in length, with the lowermost roots reaching a length of 25 cm. The bundle of lumbar and sacral roots below the conus medullaris is called the cauda equina. The steep downwards course of lumbar and sacral roots means that a disc prolapse typically compresses the root of the segment below (the L5–S1 disc prolapse compresses the S1 root; see Figure 152.1);

but also two adjacent roots may be compressed. The cervical (and rarely the thoracic) disc prolapse may injure only the respective root if the direction of prolapse is lateral (mostly postero-lateral) but compresses the spinal cord if it is medial-posterior. In the most commonly affected segments in the back (L4–L5, L5–S1, and L3–L4) postero-lateral protrusion will affect only one or two roots while posteromedial protrusion will compress the cauda equina.

Root compression by disc or spondylosis causes demyelination of the nerve fibers within the root, or axonal injury; in the latter case, axonal degeneration takes place. In the case of the motor axons this will lead to denervation of the respective motor units (a motor unit comprises all muscle cells innervated by a single lower motor neuron). Dorsal root compression may cause preganglionic axonal injury of the primary sensory neuron; this leads to degeneration of the proximal but not the distal neurite.

Pathologic processes affecting the "mobile spinal segment" (even though not compromising the roots) cause pain, and the pain may radiate in the affected segment (known as referred pain). Referred pain does not as a rule irradiate to the most distal segments of the upper or lower limb, and is – of course – not accompanied by segmental neurologic deficit. The distribution of "neurogenic" pain (a typical consequence of root compression) is related to the segmental innervation of skin, muscles, and bones (dermatome, myotome, and the sclerotome).

Cervical disc disease

The most commonly affected segment in the neck is the C5–C6 level (a lateral disc herniation will affect the C6 root). The next most common cervical radiculopathy is C7 (herniation at level C6–C7), and then C5 (herniation at C4–C5). Patients usually complains of neck pain radiating to the shoulder and upper arm (C5) and in many cases into the lower arm and hand into the thumb (C6), or the second, third, and fourth fingers (C7). Root involvement is accompanied by paraesthesiae and dysaesthesiae affecting the dermatome (in the distal part). Motor symptoms are usually not prominent, although needle electromyography (EMG) of the muscles belonging to the particular myotome may show abnormalities (see below). Notably the deltoid will be paretic in the C5 syndrome, the biceps and brachioradialis in the C6 syndrome, the pectoralis major and the triceps muscle in the C7 syndrome. C5 radiculopathy weakens the biceps reflex, which may be absent in C6 radiculopathy. The triceps brachii reflex is affected particularly in the C7 syndrome. Cervical radiculopathy is not accompanied by vegetative symptoms, as autonomic fibers do not leave the spinal cord via cervical roots.

An acute postero-medial disc herniation in the cervical region may lead to spinal cord compression, causing myelopathy. This is clinically manifested by more or less pronounced long-tract signs with paraesthesiae in lower limbs accompanied by a spastic tetra- or paraparesis (according to the level of the lesion) with lower urinary tract, anorectal, and sexual dysfunction. Cervical myelopathy due to cervical spondylosis occurs as a slowly progressive disorder, unless it is precipitated by (minor) neck injury.

Lumbar disc disease

Most commonly affected individuals are middle-aged men, but a functionally significant episode of low back pain may be encountered by up to 80% of the adult population over a lifetime. The typical presentation is with low back pain. This may be accompanied by referred pain. In a minority of patients, there is radicular pain with neurological deficit. The term "sciatica" is used for pain referred to the lower limb, but it is indicative of root involvement only in the case of distal radiation of pain ("proof" of root involvement is paraesthesiae and/or neurological deficit in the appropriate segmental distribution). In the case of radiculopathy, pain may begin in the back and "move" downwards. It may also be restricted to the lower limb. Onset may be spontaneous or associated with mechanical stress to the spine. The pain may be excruciating and make the patient more or less immobile. Radicular neurological deficit may be discrete or prominent, and may occur (or be revealed) after the acute pain episode. Local tenderness to palpation or percussion over the spinous processes may be present, and the patient often adopts a fixed posture, somewhat tilted away from the affected side. Passive hip flexion with the lower limb extended at the knee exacerbates the pain in L5 and S1 root involvement (Lasègue sign), particularly if the foot is passively dorsiflexed when the extended leg is raised. Pain is exacerbated by increases in intra-abdominal pressure (coughing, sneezing, defecating, etc.).

Most commonly the L4–L5 and L5–S1 interspaces are affected, with the L5 or S1 and uncommonly L4 roots being compressed. Other interspaces and other roots are rarely affected. A postero-medial protrusion may affect several roots and lead to a cauda equina syndrome.

L4 radiculopathy leads to pain radiating down the distal lateral thigh and the antero-medial leg. (The pain in L4 root compression is exacerbated by the patient lying on his or her stomach with the knee flexed, and the hip extended.) L5 radiculopathy leads to pain radiating to the antero-lateral leg and the dorsum of the foot and hallux. Pain in the S1 syndrome radiates down the posterior leg to the heel, and the lateral aspect of the foot to the third to fifth toes.

The L4 syndrome may partially weaken the quadriceps, and usually somewhat more the tibialis anterior muscle with hyporeflexia of the knee jerk and sensory loss along the antero-medial leg.

The L5 syndrome leads to weakness of the ankle and big toe dorsiflexion. The ankle jerk may be slightly reduced but may not be particularly affected; the tibialis posterior reflex absence is helpful only in individuals with brisk jerks which will allow the unequivocal demonstration of the contralateral reflex. The L5 dermatome is typically affected only in its distal part – the dorsal foot and the antero-lateral leg.

In S1 radiculopathy walking "on toes" may be affected (due to paretic plantar flexors) and the ankle jerk a- or hyporeflexic. The sensory loss involves the lateral and plantar surface of the foot and the fifth toe.

A cauda equina lesion is recognized by bilateral symptoms (which, however, are as a rule asymmetrical). Pain radiates from the lower back to both legs and paraesthesiae may be bilateral and typically involve the perineal region. Distal lower limb paresis may or may not be present, but ankle jerks are asymmetrically weak or absent. Urinary retention usually precedes urinary incontinence, which is of the overflow type. Urinary symptoms are the leading autonomic dysfunction in the acute stage with anorectal and sexual dysfunction revealed in due course. The sensory deficit involves the affected segments and typically the lower sacral segments. The upper posterior parts of the thighs and buttocks (S2), the perineal and perianal regions, as well as the region overlying the coccygeal bone (S3–S5) are affected. The anal reflex is absent unilaterally or bilaterally. (In most healthy subjects, pricking the perianal skin with a pin causes visible anal sphincter contraction.)

In a patient presenting with bilateral neurological symptoms and signs attributable to sacral segments, the question of a cauda equina versus conus medullaris lesion arises. Conus medullaris presents the lowest part of the spinal cord (sacral segments S3–S5), which is usually positioned behind the L1 vertebral body. Below the conus medullaris the assembly of L2–S4 spinal roots, known as cauda equina, pass to their respective foraminae and contain peripheral nerve fibers passing between the respective spinal cord segments and the target segments. In theory, conus medullaris lesions should demonstrate a combination of upper and lower motor neuron signs, but usually the signs of a lower motor neuron lesion predominate. Cauda equina lesions tend to be more asymmetrical, with radicular pain and more pronounced lower limb deficits. Dissociated sensation, when found, distinctly diagnoses a conus medullaris lesion. Sacral function (bladder, bowel, and sexual) deficits, and saddle sensory loss, are usually found in both. In case of more subtle lesions, difficult or incomplete emptying of the bladder may be the first symptom.

Cauda equina lesions are more common than those of the conus medullaris with estimated annual incidence rates of 3.4 and 1.5 per million, and prevalence rates of 8.9 and 4.5 per 100 000 population, respectively. The most common etiologies are lumbar intervertebral disc herniations for cauda equina lesions, and T11–L1 spinal fractures for conus medullaris lesions.

Natural course of disc herniation

Prognosis of acute disc disease is good and it has been demonstrated by MRI that disc protrusion and prolapse tend to recede with time. The prognosis of root demyelination is excellent. Root lesions of the axonal type probably get little true regeneration of the destroyed axons, but collateral reinnervation of the partially denervated muscle from remaining axons can result in good functional recovery.

Diagnosis

The clinical picture of acute neck pain radiating to one upper limb with neurological deficit should be readily recognizable. The clinical examination defines the neurological deficit and thus the particular root syndrome. Plain radiography only helps to exclude serious disease (malignant, infectious), the readily and expectedly demonstrable degenerative changes being of no diagnostic relevance. Thus MRI is the diagnostic procedure of choice, but is relevant only if surgery is contemplated (Figure 152.1). In the acute stage electrodiagnostic testing is not indicated – the diagnostically relevant abnormal spontaneous ("denervation") activity detected by needle EMG takes 3 weeks to develop. After the period of acute denervation, reinnervation processes manifest themselves by "remodeling" of motor units. This process is mirrored in the change of motor unit potentials (which become large, polyphasic, and of prolonged duration), as detected by needle EMG. The residual abnormality in radiculopathy is recognized by a myotomal distribution of abnormal EMG findings. In practice, electrodiagnostics is particularly useful to exclude involvement of plexus and limb nerves, often a relevant differential diagnostic consideration, particularly since therapy for a median neuropathy at the wrist (carpal tunnel syndrome), for instance, if promptly instituted will abolish the symptoms.

Treatment

The generally good prognosis of disc disease dictates conservative treatment as the primary approach. Emergency surgery is indicated in acute spinal cord compression and the cauda equina syndrome. Similarly, early surgery may be contemplated in acute radiculopathy with a severe and functionally relevant motor deficit.

Treatment approaches to radiculopathy vary considerably in different centers and countries, and there are no generally agreed guidelines. In many hospitals (delayed) surgery is commonly performed and for a variety of indications. A common indication is the situation when the symptoms (with significant pain) do not recede in weeks or months. However, there are no large-scale controlled clinical trials demonstrating surgery to be superior to other treatments in the long term .

Conservative treatment comprises an explanation of the usual benign and self-limiting course of the disease, and appropriate analgesia (primarily with non-steroid anti-inflammatory drugs), which may be combined with (temporary) striated muscle relaxants. Relative immobilization in the acute stage may be necessary, but the patient should remain mobile as much as possible. Physical therapy to abate pain and physiotherapy to improve mobility may be helpful. Appropriate positioning in bed (at night-time) is important. Nightly soft neck immobilization is often appropriate and necessary in the acute stage. Ventral or ventrolateral positioning in bed (with appropriate positioning of cushions) is often helpful in the patient with severe lumbar radicular pain. Local infiltration with analgesics and steroids has limited and short-term symptomatic benefit. Manual manipulation in the presence of neural system involvement should not be attempted.

Chronic radicular symptoms may occasionally gain a neuropathic pain quality and should be treated as such.

Chronic spinal pain (as a rule without neurological symptoms) is the more common and much more therapy-resistant problem, which may require a multidisciplinary approach with behavioral treatment, and is often only complicated by surgery.

Cervical spondylosis

Symptoms due to cervical spondylosis develop mostly after middle age and more commonly in men. Although the overall clinical picture may be similar to that of disc disease, both the onset and intensity of the symptomatology are less dramatic and sensory-motor deficits are usually less marked. Pain is increased on head movement. Although the morphologic changes are not expected to recede, symptomatology often fluctuates. Repeated exacerbations of symptoms occur, but with a decreased range of spine movement due to progressive spondylotic changes, pain episodes may decrease.

Spondylotic changes may deform the spinal canal and the intervertebral foramina leading to root irritation and radiculopathy. The sixth and seventh cervical roots are most commonly affected; C8 is only occasionally involved.

Spondylotic changes may encroach on the spinal canal. Protrusion of discs, hypertrophy of facet joints, and thickening of the ligamentum flavum leads to both stenotic changes of the intervertebral foramina as well as the spinal canal itself. Below a canal width of 12 mm myelopathy may develop with slowly progressive long tract signs (spastic paraparesis with sensory ataxia), leading to a broad-based uncertain gait. Urinary symptoms may appear. The segmental involvement of cervical spinal cord and concomitant radiculopathy can cause a segmental cervical sensory-motor deficit with muscle atrophy.

MRI is the diagnostic procedure of choice as it demonstrates not only the osseous and non-osseous components of the spinal stenosis but also intramedullary signal intensity changes in the spinal cord (myelopathic change). The progression of the disease is unpredictable and may comprise prolonged static intervals punctuated by episodic deterioration. An expectant conservative approach is appropriate in mild and non-progressive cases, while progressive neurological deficits should be treated early rather than late, because, once developed, functional impairment tends not to recede after surgery.

Lumbar spinal stenosis

Spondylotic changes of the lumbar spine along with other degenerative changes lead – particularly in the presence of a congenitally narrow spinal canal – to encroachment on lumbosacral roots causing radiculopathy or at worst a specific clinical picture – neurogenic claudication (of the cauda equina). It comprises lumbo-sacral discomfort and pain radiating downwards, usually bilaterally, and exacerbated by walking. Pain slowly increases on walking and becomes too uncomfortable to bear after a certain distance. Other sensory symptoms in the lumbar and sacral segments may appear (numbness, paraesthesia). Motor weakness and occasionally autonomic symptoms (urinary incontinence, but also urgency of micturition and persistent penile erection (priapism), due probably to lower sacral root irritation, occasionally occur. If the patients are followed up, the distance they can walk without symptoms gets shorter. Typically walking downhill is more difficult for the patient than uphill, because it is the extension of the lumbar lordosis that causes buckling of the ligamentum flavum and leads to an up to 20% additional narrowing of the spinal canal. Typically these patients may cycle for long distances even though being unable to walk even short distances without becoming symptomatic. Symptoms can also appear during prolonged standing in the upright position (such as during funerals, etc.), and particular in a "back leaning" position of the body (such as reaching to shelves above the head).

Typically in most patients the neurological examination during rest will not reveal significant abnormalities, and EMG may be non-informative.

In mild cases, conservative/expectative treatment (ensuring that the patient understands the nature of the problem) is appropriate. Patients may remain reasonably mobile with a rational alteration of their lifestyle. With progressive problems and if the limitation of their mobility is unacceptable, surgery will relieve the symptoms, particularly if there is discrete and focal narrowing of the spinal canal.

Paget's disease

In Paget's disease there is excessive bone resorption coupled with abnormal new bone formation resulting in altered bone structure, increased vascularity, and mechanical weakness. The disease has a predilection for the axial skeleton. Back pain has been described in up to 43% of patients with spinal Paget's disease. The involved vertebrae are increased in width and reduced in height. Particularly (mid) lumbar (58%), low thoracic (42%), and cervical (14%) segments are involved. The disease manifests itself in the elderly, affecting up to 3% of the population above 55 years of age in Europe and North America. In up to 14% of patients there is a family history, but the etiology is poorly understood. Although changes may be prominent, most patients are asymptomatic. Most commonly local pain occurs though the overlying skin, which may be warmer due to increased bone vascularization. The pain is typically worse at rest. Fractures may occur. Creeping neurological symptoms may develop due to encroachment of the changed bone on the spinal canal, compressing either single roots, spinal cord, or cauda equina. Acute neurological syndromes may occur with pathological fractures. Neural compromise may occur also through vascular causes; epidural hematoma causing acute compressive myelopathy has been described.

Spinal stenosis occurs in 10–20% of patients with Paget's disease. Extradural ossification of the ligamentum flavum and epidural fat may result in spinal cord or root compression, but myelopathy and the cauda equina syndrome may occur without evidence of direct compression on neuroimaging. Because neurological symptoms respond to medical treatment with calcitonin (which reduces the abnormal skeletal blood flow to normal), an arterial "steal phenomenon" has been suggested as a cause in such instances.

The diagnosis is usually made by imaging, finding of increased serum alkaline phosphatase, and increased urinary hydroxyproline. However, alkaline phosphatase levels have been described as normal in almost one-third of patients with Paget's disease and spinal stenosis. Radionuclide scans localize disease activity.

The treatment of choice for symptomatic spinal stenosis is medical (calcitonin or a biphosphonate) and results in improvement of myelopathy or cauda equina syndrome. Unfortunately, relapses occur, but may be treated by repeating the therapy. Oral biphosphonates are recommended for patients with slowly progressive symptoms and intravenous biphosphonates are indicated in rapidly progressive neurological deterioration before surgery to minimize bone hemorrhage. Surgical treatment of spinal disease is difficult also because involvement is often at multiple levels. Clinical monitoring of neurological function with repeated imaging, serum alkaline phosphatase, and urinary hydroxyproline determinations every 6–12 months have been recommended if surgery can be delayed.

Fibrous dysplasia

Fibrous dysplasia of bone is a mesenchymal disease affecting single or multiple bones, in most cases already diagnosed in childhood. It is caused by activating missense mutations of the *GNAS1* gene, encoding the α subunit of the stimulatory G-protein, $G_s\alpha$. These mutations are postzygotic, are not inherited, and result in a mosaic state. Diagnosis is established based on clinical, radiographic, and histopathological features. Markers of bone turnover are usually elevated. Total body bone scintigraphy determines the extent of bone involvement.

In the polyostotic form, fibrous dysplasia may be accompanied by pigmented skin areas (patches) and endocrinological abnormalities (much more frequently in girls).

The disease may appear and progress in adults and uncommonly affects the lumbar and thoracic vertebrae. Scoliosis occurs in approximately 50% of patients with the polyostotic form of the disease. In addition to deformity, pain may be prominent and pathological fractures occur, as do neurological complications, often due to compression. Expansion of either the vertebral body, the arches, or the articular processes has been described, with the potential to involve nerve roots and spinal cord.

Therapy is surgical if warranted by symptoms. Treatment with biphosphonates has been advocated, but there have been no controlled studies.

Other compressive disorders and their investigation

In the spinal canal there is little free space outside the cord and the nerve roots. Neural compression most often arises anteriorly, particularly from the intervertebral joint and disc which, through mechanical stress of the mobile segments of the lower cervical spine and the weight-bearing lumbar spine, develop degenerative changes. The clinical picture of spinal pain with root or spinal cord symptoms may of course occur with any type of compressive, traumatic, or inflammatory lesion. Trauma usually has a clearcut history, and will not be further discussed, but minor injuries can lead to a severe neurological deficit in patients with cervical stenosis, and from pathological vertebral fractures of any cause including osteoporosis (osteoporotic fractures are by no means always "benign").

Infection will usually but not always give additional symptoms and cause "atypical" local pain. Root compression with pain may be caused by an extradural tumor, such as secondary carcinoma, reticulosis, and neurofibroma. Posteriorly located tumors may at first cause only a sensory deficit. Intradural extramedullary tumors (meningioma, neurolemmona) commonly arise within the vicinity of dorsal roots and cause radicular pain. They progress and compress both roots and spinal cord. In other locations tumor(s) will cause a different sequence of neurological deficit. Intradural intramedullary tumors (glioma, ependymoma) rarely cause radicular pain but may cause a neuropathic burning or dull more diffuse pain in the segments below the lesion. Tumors, especially typically neurolemmona may grow in the intervertebral foramen, achieving an "hourglass" shape and compressing first the root and then the spinal cord. Rarely an extradural hematoma (particularly in patients with defects in coagulation) gives rise to a local pain syndrome with neurological deficit.

In addition to these diverse compressive pathologies which may cause both a pain syndrome (local and irradiating referred pain) and radiculopathy (without or with myelopathy), the most common differential diagnostic considerations to discopathic or spondylotic radiculopathy are pain syndromes originating in one of the structures of the mobile spinal segment itself. These are (if not malignant or inflammatory) rather trivial as far as the medical issues involved, but may cause prolonged and recidivant symptoms.

A final important diagnostic consideration is that of painful clinical conditions accompanied by localized neurologic symptoms, arising from involvement of structures peripheral to the root.The diagnostic possibilities range from plexus involvement – of different aetiologies – to distal neuropathy, which is most commonly caused by entrapment.

In considering the differential diagnosis of discopathic and spondylotic radiculopathy, two basic clinical syndromes can be conceptualized: on the one hand, there is the "typically" localized pain syndrome without (clinically obvious) neurological involvement and, on the other hand, there is a "localized" neurological syndrome accompanied (or not) by pain. In the first, it is necessary to rule out malignant and infectious spinal disease (pyogenic epidural abscess, tuberculous abscess, acute discitis), and

readily curable disease such as carpal tunnel syndrome (which may not be accompanied by any neurological deficit even in patients with bothersome symptoms). The other group comprises patients with clinically relevant (and particularly progressive) neurological symptomatology with (or without) pain. These patients usually need more diagnostic attention to clarify the problem. (A typical situation would be a patient with irradiating pain from the shoulder to the fifth finger and paraesthesia, in whom in due course a Pancoast tumor compressing the lower brachial plexus is demonstrated.)

Generally speaking the investigations recommended for suspected spinal compressive disorders are blood tests (full blood count, sedimentation rate, C-reactive protein, fasting glucose, serum proteins, calcium phosphatase) and a spinal tap for cerebrospinal fluid testing (for infection/inflammation). MRI is excellent for cord and root lesions, combined with gadolinium enhancement for neoplastic and inflammatory processes. CT is very good for osseous lesions, and if MRI is not possible or available. Isotope scans are helpful for bone metastases and infective lesions.

Electrodiagnostic testing is helpful to extend and refine the clinical examination and to follow up peripheral nervous system involvement. EMG helps to diagnose recent denervation and reinnervation in muscles. It helps to distinguish between the radicular, plexus, and nerve syndromes, and generalized disease, particularly if appropriately combined with testing parameters of conduction in both proximal and distal parts of the motor nerve fibers, and recording sensory neurograms. Nerve conduction studies help to diagnose compression neuropathy and other neuropathies. Evoked potential studies have limited value in the diagnosis of compressive and inflammatory lesions, because the nervous system involvement is mostly characterized by axon loss, and is thus less easy to demonstrate with conduction studies.

Ischemic and congestive myelopathies

Acute ischemic myelopathy
Ischemic cord infarction is a rare and devastating condition when compared to all acute myelopathies (5–8%), as well as all vascular neurological pathologies (1–2%). Therefore pathogenesis and natural history of this disorder have been little studied. Basic knowledge of the spinal cord vascular supply is essential for understanding spinal vascular disorders. The spinal cord is supplied by a single anterior and a pair of posterior spinal arteries, whose rostral origin is from the vertebral arteries and which anastomose caudally at the level of the conus medullaris. The spinal arteries anastomose with the pial plexus, and the posterior spinal arteries may be linked together. At each level the anterior spinal artery provides

central arteries entering the spinal cord and supplying the anterior horn and the anterior part of the lateral columns. The spinal arteries also receive supply from the radicular arteries, thus forming several functional regions of the spinal cord: C1–T3 (vertebral artery branch at C3 level, and a branch from ascending cervical arteries at C6–C7 level), T3–T7 (sometimes a branch from the intercostal artery), and T8-conus medullaris (a branch from the intercostals artery at T9–T12 level – artery of Adamkiewicz, and sometimes a conus feeding artery originating from the internal iliac artery most often at L5 level – artery of Desproges-Gotteron).

In patients with acute ischemic myelopathy, symptoms usually develop in less than 2 minutes but can in some extend to several hours. Clinical symptoms and findings include motor, spinothalamic, and lemniscal sensory deficits depending on the spinal level and the pattern of ischemic myelopathy. In general, in clinically and radiologically proven anterior spinal artery (uni- or bilateral) and posterior spinal artery (uni- or bilateral) occlusions, central and transverse patterns are observed. Unilateral patterns are explained by the duplication of the anterior system and by the incomplete linking of the posterior systems.

Typical is the neurological deficit arising with the anterior spinal artery syndrome, which as a rule involves the anterior parts of the cord bilaterally and exhibits the following: segmental lower motor neuron lesion with flaccid paresis in involved myotomes, pyramidal tract signs below the segmental lesion with spastic paraparesis (and also bladder and bowel dysfunction), and damage to decussating anterior spinothalamic tracts with analgesia and thermanalgesia in the involved dermatomes (the so-called dissociated sensory loss, as commonly there is no loss of fine touch and other dorsal column sensibility). Anterior spinothalamic tract lesions in the affected segments cause dissociated sensory loss in body parts below the lesion. Unilateral anterior spinal artery territory infarcts occur, and also spare lemniscal sensory fibers within the dorsal columns of the spinal cord.

Due to separate perfusion by anterior and posterior spinal arteries, vascular cord lesions generally do not result in a hemicord or Brown–Sequard syndrome (which includes ipsilateral segmental lower motor neuron signs, ipsilateral pyramidal involvement, and ipsilateral lemniscal sensory deficits below the level of the lesion, combined with a contralateral spinothalamic sensory deficit). This syndrome is most often due to trauma, but may be also caused by demyelination plaque, tumor, disc herniation, and so on.

Only a minority of patients, such as those with ischemia of the cervical cord, report identical previous transitory symptoms – transient ischemic attacks (TIAs). At the onset of symptoms patients often report back or neck pain localized to the level of the spinal cord lesion (59% in one study), with a radicular component in the majority of these patients (81%). Paraesthesiae are rare and, as with pain, usually resolve spontaneously within a few days.

Laboratory studies are usually normal, with the exception of increased cerebrospinal fluid protein concentration in a proportion of patients (up to 44%). MRI often shows a well-demarcated area of increased signal on T2 weighted images, corresponding to the involved arterial territory, and may be mirrored by restriction on diffusion-weighted imaging.

The aetiology of the spinal cord ischemia is unclear in most patients, as only a small proportion usually have vascular risk factors (e.g., diabetes, hypertension). Profound and prolonged arterial hypotension usually results in central and transverse spinal cord lesions, caused by global hypoperfusion of the spinal cord. Due to high motor neuron density and the high prevalence of atherosclerosis in the aorta and iliac arteries, the thoracolumbar region is particularly at risk. The other commonly observed factor found in these patients is mechanical stress. The spinal arteries run along a mobile spinal column, which makes them prone to mechanical damage. Patients have a variety of spinal conditions, and ischemic symptoms often occur immediately after some movement. Intervertebral disc herniation at the appropriate levels is also sometimes observed. Central herniations may compress the anterior spinal artery, and lateral herniations may occlude radicular arteries. A special case of the latter is occlusion of the cone (Desproges–Gotteron) artery by intervertebral disc at L4–L5 or L5–S1 level. The condition may result in a conus medullaris syndrome, which may be reversible.

In spite of the general belief in the ominous prognosis of spinal cord ischemia, the outcomes are not always unfavourable. Complete or incomplete recovery occurs in a high proportion of patients (70% in one study), with about half of patients having significant gait impairment on leaving the hospital. Motor deficits show better recovery than sensory and sacral deficits. Thus, long-term prognosis depends largely on the degree of conus medullaris involvement. Neuropathic pain may appear following hypesthesia after several months.

To improve the patients' outcome a variety of medications (antiplatelet agents, anticoagulants, corticosteroids) and interventions (hyperbaric therapy) have been tried. However, none of these or a variety of experimental drugs so far has had any proven clinical effect. No prospective therapy trials have so far been published.

Congestive myelopathy

The condition was described by Foix and Alajouanine in 1926; it is rare (annual incidence rate, 5–10/million). It has been shown to be due to venous hypertension resulting from a dural arteriovenous fistula – a tiny connection between a radicular artery and vein which impedes venous drainage of the spinal cord. Congestive edema develops, followed by necrosis, predominantly of the spinal cord gray matter. Damage most often starts at the conus medullaris, and spreads slowly up the spinal cord to the level of the fistula. The resulting clinical picture is a chronic progressive myelopathy. The mechanism by which the arteriovenous fistula itself forms remains unclear, but it is assumed to be an acquired condition. Most often arteriovenous fistulas are intradural, occurring in the intervertebral foramen on the dorsal surface of the dural root sleeve, where the radicular vein and dural branch(es) of the radicular artery pierce the dura. Most fistulas are located in the thoracolumbar region, but they can occur at any cranio-spinal level, including intracranially.

This type of myelopathy occurs more commonly in men than women (ratio 5:1), with a peak age of 55–60, and very rarely before 30 years of age. It usually presents with gait difficulties (50–81%), paraesthesiae in one or both feet, diffuse or patchy sensory loss (sensory disturbances, 17–72%), radicular pain (13–64%), and micturition (4–75%) and defecation (0–38%) problems. The condition progresses slowly, often has a "claudicatory" component, and it usually takes 1–3 years before it is diagnosed. On examination, both central or anterior sensory and upper motor neuron signs are found in the lower limbs. The condition is probably underdiagnosed as it is rare and presents with non-specific symptoms.

Apart from history and clinical neurological examination, MRI and catheter angiography are most useful in making the diagnosis. Homogenous changes in the signal intensity (hypo on T1 and hyper on T2 weighted images) extending over an average of five to seven vertebrae, often occurring in the spinal cord center with peripheral sparing, which may extend to involve the conus medullaris, are most characteristic. Lesions may show some enhancement, most often 45 minutes after gadolinium injection. "Flow void phenomena" over the surface of the spinal cord are also characteristic, which MR angiography typically shows to be serpentine perimedullary dilated venous structures in up to 100% of patients, which may also give an indication about the level of fistula. This is important for planning catheter angiography, which remains the "gold standard" for the diagnosis. It must, furthermore, determine whether the arterial feeder is only a dural branch or also a tributary to the anterior spinal artery. The latter situation prohibits endovascular therapy, which is otherwise becoming increasingly popular. Although endovascular embolization using liquid polymers is less invasive than surgical ligation, the outcome of surgery still seems to be better. The outcome of both methods depends on the success of occlusion of the vein draining the fistula. The main determinant of the patient's outcome is pretreatment disability, but neurological deficit

may improve after early successful treatment. Gait difficulties and muscle strength respond better than micturition, pain, and muscle spasms. Gait improved in 64% and muscle strength in 56% of patients in one recent study.

Most neurologists will see only a few patients with congestive myelopathy during their career, but the condition should be recognized and duly incorporated into differential diagnosis of progressive myelopathy, particularly in older men.

Further reading

Disc disease

Armon C, Argoff CE, Samuels J, Backonja M-M. Assessment: use of epidural steroid injections to treat radicular lumbosacral pain. Report of the Therapeutics and Technology Assessment Subcommittee of the American Academy of Neurology. *Neurology* 2007; 68: 723–9.

Healy JF, Healy BB, Wong WH, Olson EM. Cervical and lumbar MRI in asymptomatic older male lifelong athletes: frequency of degenerative findings. *J Comput Assist Tomogr* 1996; 20: 107–12.

Mulleman D, Mammou S, Griffoul I, Watier H, Goupille P. Pathophysiology of disk-related sciatica. I. Evidence supporting a chemical component. *Joint Bone Spine* 2006; 73: 151–8.

Podnar S. Epidemiology of cauda equina and conus medullaris lesions. *Muscle Nerve* 2007; 35: 529–31.

Paget's disease

Ooi CG, Fraser WD. Paget's disease of bone. *Postgrad Med* 1997; 73: 69–74.

Siris ES, Lyles KW, Singer FR, Meunier PJ. Medical treatment of Paget's disease of bone: indications for treatment and review of current therapies. *J Bone Miner Res* 2006; 21: P94–8 (doi: 10.1359/JBMR.06S218).

Fibrous dysplasia

Collins MT, Bianco P. Fibrous dysplasia. In: Favus M, editor. *Primer on Metabolic Bone Diseases*. Philadelphia/Washington: Lippincott Williams & Wilkins/American Society for Bone and Mineral Research; 2003, pp. 466–70.

Leet AI, Magur E, Lee JS, Wientroub S, Robey PG, Collins MT. Fibrous dysplasia in the spine: prevalence of lesions and association with scoliosis. *J Bone Joint Surg* 2004; 86: 531–7.

Ischemic and congestive myelopathy

Aminoff MJ, Barnard RO, Logue V. The pathophysiology of spinal vascular malformations. *J Neurol Sci* 1974; 23: 255–63.

Jellema K, Tijssen CC, van Gijn J. Spinal dural arteriovenous fistulas: a congestive myelopathy that initially mimics a peripheral nerve disorder. *Brain* 2006; 129: 3150–64.

Nedeltchev K, Loher TJ, Stepper F, et al. Long-term outcome of acute spinal cord ischemia syndrome. *Stroke* 2004; 35: 560–5.

Novy J, Carruzzo A, Maeder P, Bogousslavsky J. Spinal cord ischemia: clinical and imaging patterns, pathogenesis, and outcomes in 27 patients. *Arch Neurol* 2006; 63: 1113–20.

Chapter 153
Syringomyelia

Alla Guekht
Russian State Medical University, Moscow, Russia

Introduction

The term syringomyelia was suggested in 1827 by the French physician Ollivier d'Angers after the Greek *syrinx* (a cavity of tubular shape) and *myelos* (marrow). Later, the term *hydromyelia* was used to indicate a dilatation of the central canal, and syringomyelia referred to cystic cavities separate from the central spinal canal. Syringomyelia today is recognized as a chronic disorder characterized pathologically by the presence of long cavities, surrounded by gliosis, situated in the central part of the spinal cord and sometimes extending up into the medulla (syringobulbia). These cavities are filled with the fluid that is identical or similar to cerebrospinal (CSF) and extracellular fluid (ECF).

Epidemiology

Syringomyelia occurs in approximately 8 of every 100000 individuals. The pathological condition is probably more common, since the widespread availability of MRI identified that some individuals can have small asymptomatic syrinxes. The onset is most commonly observed between ages 25 and 40 years, but symptoms can appear at any age between 10 and 60 years. Males are affected more often than females. The condition has been described in more than one member of a family and other congenital malformations, including spina bifida, have been found in families containing affected members.

No geographic difference in the prevalence of syringomyelia is known, and the occurrence of syringomyelia in different races is also unknown.

Pathophysiology

The typical pathological changes are most frequently found in the lower cervical and upper thoracic regions of the cord. Extension to the medulla is common and, rarely, the process may reach the pons. The affected region of the cord may be enlarged, mainly in the transverse plane. Transverse section of the cord reveals a cavity surrounded by a zone of translucent gelatinous material which, microscopically, contains glial cells and fibers. The expanding cavity and surrounding gliosis affect the less-resistant gray matter more severely than the dense white matter and invade the anterior horns of the gray matter, thus causing injury and loss of anterior horn cells and degeneration of their axons in the ventral roots and peripheral nerves.

Four main types of syringomyelia are described in descending order of frequency: (1) associated with Chiari I malformations, (2) associated with vertebral trauma, (3) associated with basilar invagination, and (4) associated with hydrocephalus.

The pathophysiology of syringomyelia is not fully understood.

Syringomyelia is regarded as a state, where ECF is trapped in the spinal cord due to CSF flow obstruction, spinal cord tethering, or an intramedullary tumor. Extracellular space and subarachnoid space are two parts of a single fluid compartment, and the only anatomical barriers between the two are the pia mater on the surface of the central nervous system and the ependymal cells of the ventricles or central canal. Depending on local flow resistances, ECF may accumulate predominantly in the central canal or in the extracellular space spinal cord itself.

Clinical features

Segmental amyotrophy, suspended (segmental) dissociated sensory disturbances, paresis and spasticity, bladder dysfunction, scoliosis, and pain have been reported in patients with syringomyelia. The onset is usually insidious. Occasionally, the first symptoms may follow an episode of coughing, sneezing, or straining. Wasting and weakness of the small muscles of the hands are common early symptoms, but, alternatively, the patient may notice loss of temperature appreciation in the hands or the resulting

International Neurology: A Clinical Approach. Edited by Robert P. Lisak, Daniel D. Truong, William M. Carroll, and Roongroj Bhidayasiri. © 2009 Blackwell Publishing, ISBN: 978-1-4051-5738-4.

injuries. Less often, pain or trophic lesions first appear. Attention may be drawn to the disorder by the appearance of scoliosis in childhood (a 50% incidence of scoliosis in patients with syringomyelia is reported).

Sensory disturbances are usually the most prominent and can be explained as the consequence of the progressive lesion in the central region of the spinal cord. At the earliest stage there is a predominantly unilateral syrinx in the central gray matter, extending longitudinally through several segments, usually in the lower cervical and upper thoracic cord. It interrupts decussating sensory fibers derived from several consecutive dorsal roots. As these fibers conduct pain, heat, and cold sensitivity, these forms are impaired while others are preserved (dissociated sensory loss). At some point a "half-cape" distribution of sensory loss commonly develops. When the lesion is situated centrally, or has extended from one side of the cord to the other, the area of dissociated sensory loss is bilateral. When the syrinx reaches the upper cervical segments, it may involve the spinal tract and nucleus of the trigeminal nerve, with the formation of an area of dissociated sensory loss extending in a concentric manner from the periphery to the center of the face.

The progressive extension of the spinal lesion later causes compression of the lateral spinothalamic tracts on one or both sides, leading to loss of appreciation of pain, heat, and cold over the lower parts of the body. Thermoanesthesia and analgesia exposes the patient to injuries, especially burns to the fingers, which, being painless, go unnoticed at the time.

Pain is a prominent feature in 50–90% of adult patients with syringomyelia. Patients often present with complaints of radicular pain (often in a capelike distribution), headache, neck, or interscapular pain. In addition to the more common clinical pain syndromes, approximately 40% of patients with syringomyelia experience significant dysesthetic pain, which is variously described as a burning sensation, pins and needles, or stretching of the skin. Other common characteristics include dermatomal patterns of hypersensitivity, as well as trophic changes such as hyperhydrosis, glossy skin, coldness, and pallor.

The earliest *motor manifestations* are usually muscular weakness and wasting of the intrinsic hand muscles due to compression or destruction of the anterior horn cells. As the lesion extends, the wasting spreads to involve the forearms and later the arms, shoulder girdles, and upper intercostals. In contrast to motor neuron disease, fasciculation and severe wasting are uncommon. Contractures may develop, especially in hand and forearm muscles. Extension of the lesion to the posterolateral medulla often involves the nucleus ambiguus, causing paresis of the soft palate, pharynx, and vocal cord, occasionally giving laryngeal stridor. Compression of the corticospinal tracts in the spinal cord causes weakness, with slight spasticity and extensor plantar responses in most cases in the later stages. The tendon reflexes are exaggerated in the lower limbs, but are diminished and lost early in the upper limbs, particularly on the side of the dissociated anesthesia. In some patients the combination of mixed upper and lower motor neurone signs may be present.

Lower cranial nerve involvement becomes apparent with development of syringobulbia.

Impairment of *autonomic pathways* can cause Horner's syndrome, trophic changes of skin, and neurogenic bladder. Cutaneous trophic changes include cyanosis and hyperkeratosis. Loss of sweating or excessive sweating may occur, usually over the face and upper limbs.

Twenty percent of patients exhibit neuropathic osteoarthropathy (Charcot joints) commonly at the shoulders and elbows. Ulceration, whitlows, and necrosis of bone are not uncommon. The scars of former injuries are usually evident upon the palmar surface of the fingers.

Investigations

MRI is the leading investigative tool used in the diagnosis of syringomyelia. T1-weighted sagittal and axial spin-echo images reveal the low-signal central cavity in the spinal cord. When the syrinx is associated with a Chiari malformation, the latter is also readily demonstrated on sagittal T1-weighted images at the level of the foramen magnum. Where the differential diagnosis includes intrinsic spinal cord tumor, gadolinium may identify enhancing tumor tissue (enhancement is not seen in syrinxes). Myelography, followed by immediate and delayed CT, is used now only if MRI is contraindicated or unavailable.

The CSF usually shows no abnormality unless the cavity is large enough to cause a block, when the protein content of the fluid is raised.

Involvement of anterior horn cells in the cervical segments can be demonstrated by needle electromyography (EMG).

Treatment/managment

Symptomatic treatment for pain and spasticity may be required. Protection of analgesic areas and early treatment of cutaneous lesions in order to promote healing are essential. Physical therapy may be needed to maximize muscular function.

Surgical treatment remains problematic and is aimed at stopping the progression of spinal cord injury by an enlarging syrinx. Duraplasty and syringoperitoneal shunts may be considered in such cases. Surgery is more likely to be performed if there is an identifiable mass compressing the spinal cord. In cases associated with a Chiari malformation, surgery has been undertaken to provide more space for the descending cerebellar tonsils and cerebellum at the base of the skull and upper cervical spine.

Successful surgery should ideally stabilize the condition and perhaps gain a modest improvement in symptoms. Surgical intervention may also be indicated to correct spinal deformities and relieve various appendicular deficits and complications.

Further reading

Greitz D. Unraveling the riddle of syringomyelia. *Neurosurg Rev* 2006; 29(4): 251–63.

Klekamp J. The pathophysiology of syringomyelia – historical overview and current concept. *Acta Neurochir (Wien)* 2002; 144(7): 649–64.

Klekamp J, Samii M. *Syringomyelia: Diagnosis and Treatment.* New York: Springer Verlag; 2001.

Miller D. Spinal cord disorders. In: Donaghy M, editor. *Brain's Diseases of the Nervous System*, 11th ed. New York: Oxford University Press; 2001, pp. 601–30.

Ravaglia S, Bogdanov EI, Pichiecchio A, Bergamaschi R, Moglia A, Mikhaylov IM. Pathogenetic role of myelitis for syringomyelia. *Clin Neurol Neurosurg* 2007; 109(6): 541–6.

Chapter 154
Pediatric neurotransmitter diseases

Stephen Deputy
Louisiana State University School of Medicine, New Orleans, USA

Introduction

The pediatric neurotransmitter disorders represent a challenging group of rare neurometabolic disorders classified on the basis of alterations in neurotransmitter metabolic pathways. The disorders are currently classified into disturbances of monoamines (dopamine, serotonin, and norepinephrine) and gamma-aminobutyric acid (GABA) metabolism. One of the challenging aspects of these disorders is their varied clinical presentations ranging from mental retardation to epilepsy to movement disorders. Another challenging aspect is their diagnosis which often relies on measuring neurotransmitter metabolites in the cerebrospinal fluid (CSF), as analysis of amino acids in the plasma and organic acids in the urine is uninformative. Disorders that fall under the spectrum of GABA metabolism include succinic semialdehyde dehydrogenase deficiency, pyridoxine-dependent epilepsy, and GABA-transaminase deficiency. Disorders of monoamine metabolism include guanosine triphosphate (GTP)-cyclohydrolase deficiency, tyrosine hydroxylase deficiency, aromatic *L*-amino acid decarboxylase deficiency, and sepiapterin reductase deficiency.

Pathophysiology

Figure 154.1 shows the normal synthesis and metabolism of the monoamine neurotransmitters serotonin, dopamine, and norepinephrine and their analyzable metabolites. Figure 154.2 shows the synthesis and metabolic pathways of GABA.

International Neurology: A Clinical Approach. Edited by Robert P. Lisak, Daniel D. Truong, William M. Carroll, and Roongroj Bhidayasiri.
© 2009 Blackwell Publishing, ISBN: 978-1-4051-5738-4.

Monoamine neurotransmitter disorders

GTP cyclohydrolase I deficiency (GCH-I deficiency, Segawa disease)

This autosomal dominant inherited form of dystonia was first described by Masaya Segawa in 1971 as a hereditary progressive basal ganglia disease with marked diurnal fluctuation. It is caused by heterozygous mutations of the guanosine triphosphate cyclohydrolase I gene located on 14q22–q22.2. There is a female:male ratio of 3:1.

Clinical symptoms usually begin with monomelic postural dystonia (often pes equinovarus) beginning in early school age, which then expands to all limbs over the next 10–15 years. There is a marked diurnal fluctuation of the dystonia severity at the onset of the disease which diminishes over time. A superimposed postural tremor often begins around 10 years of age. On physical examination, deep tendon reflexes are exaggerated with flexor plantar responses. Linear growth is often impaired whereas cognitive function is usually spared. There is also a marked, sustained improvement of all neurological deficits to low doses of orally administered *L*-dopa. Prolonged use of *L*-dopa does not tend to produce dyskinesias as it often does with Parkinson's disease. Neuroimaging studies are normal.

The pathophysiology of GCH-I deficiency is caused by reduced levels of dopamine within the striatum without destruction of the dopamine nerve terminals. Tyrosine hydroxylase activity is markedly reduced within the striatum. Reduced activity of GTP cyclohydrolase results in reduced formation of neopterin and biopterin which are essential cofactors for tyrosine, tryptophan, and phenylalanine hydroxylases.

The diagnosis of GCH-I deficiency is strongly suggested by reduced levels of tetrahydrobiopterin, neopterin, homovanillic acid, and 5-hydroxyindolacetic acid in the CSF. The disease can also be confirmed in 60% of patients by finding heterozygous mutations in the *GCH-I* gene. A significant reduction in the degree of dystonia following low-dose *L*-dopa is also highly suggestive of the disease.

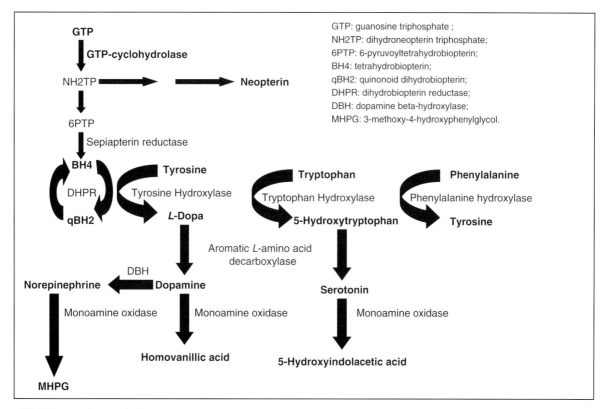

Figure 154.1 Monoamine metabolism.

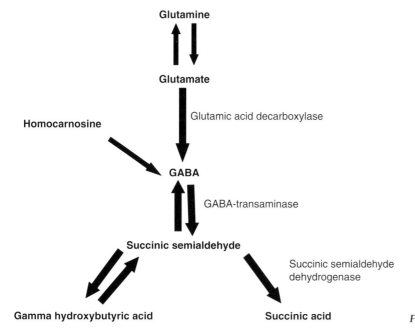

Figure 154.2 GABA metabolism.

Tyrosine hydroxylase (TH) deficiency

TH catalyzes the hydroxylation of tyrosine to *L*-dopa (see Figure 154.1). It is the rate-limiting step in the biosynthesis of the catecholamines dopamine, norepinephrine, and epinephrine. The *TH* gene has been mapped to chromosome 11p15.5.

Children with autosomal recessive TH deficiency often present in the first year of life with an infantile encephalopathy consisting of progressive psychomotor retardation along with pyramidal and extrapyramidal signs. Early in the course of the disease, many infants are found to be quite hypotonic, though brisk deep tendon reflexes and extensor plantar responses point to a central cause. Oculogyric crises are common but may go unrecognized. Life-threatening paroxysmal periods of lethargy, sweating, and drooling are common. Between 2 and 5 years of age, muscle tone increases and contractures may develop. Unlike Segawa's syndrome, treatment with *L*-dopa may affect modest improvement of the dystonia and usually takes months before the full benefit is achieved. *L*-Dopa treatment, however, does not improve other aspects of the encephalopathy.

Diagnosis of TH deficiency may be suggested by elevated serum prolactin levels (due to reduced dopaminergic inhibition of prolactin secretion). Diagnosis is confirmed by the findings of low or undetectable levels of homovanillic acid and 3-methoxy-4-hydroxyphenylglycol (MHPG) with normal 5-hydroxyindolacetic acid in the CSF reflecting the selectively reduced tyrosine hydroxylase enzymatic activity.

Aromatic *L*-amino acid decarboxylase (AADC) deficiency

AADC, which requires pyridoxine (vitamin B$_6$) as a cofactor, is responsible for decarboxylating *L*-dopa and 5-hydroxytryptophan into dopamine and serotonin, respectively (see Figure 154.1). AADC deficiency results in a combined catecholamine and serotonin deficiency. The disorder is transmitted in an autosomal recessive pattern with the *AADC* gene mapped to chromosome 7p11.

Children with AADC deficiency share a characteristic movement disorder that is present by 6 months of age and consists of intermittent oculogyric crises with limb dystonia and athetosis. Ocular convergence spasm, myoclonic jerks, orofacial dystonia, limb tremor, blepharospasm, and breath-holding spells have been frequently reported. Autonomic dysfunction, including paroxysmal sweating, impaired gastric motility with reflux, hypothermia, sudden cardiorespiratory arrest, and abnormal sympathetic modulation of heart rate and systolic blood pressure have been reported. All children reported have variable degrees of mental retardation and several have epilepsy. Treatment with dopamine receptor agonists and monoamine inhibitors has been reported to reduce the frequency of paroxysmal spells and to improve voluntary movements, though many patients suffer from dyskinesias. All patients are treated with supplemental pyridoxine, though no obvious direct benefit has been reported.

Diagnosis is based on the findings of low levels of homovanillic acid and 5-hydroxyindolacetic acid, elevated levels of *L*-dopa, 5-hydroxytryptophan, and 3-*O*-methyldopa levels, and normal pterin levels in the CSF. Many patients have also been noted to have markedly increased urinary secretion of *L*-dopa, 5-hydroxtryptophan, and 3-methoxytyrosine.

Sepiapterin reductase (SR) deficiency

Only 12 known cases of SR deficiency have been reported in the literature. All have shown dystonia with spasticity and psychomotor retardation. SR is responsible for the conversion of 6-pyruvoyltetrahydrobiopterin to tetrahydrobiopterin which is an essential cofactor for tyrosine, tryptophan, and phenylalanine hydroxylase enzymes. Hence, diagnosis of SR deficiency rests on the presence of elevated biopterin and dihydrobiopterin in the presence of reduced levels of 5-hydroxyindolacetic acid and homovanillic acid in the CSF. The disorder is felt to be transmitted in an autosomal recessive pattern and the SR gene has been mapped to chromosome 2p14–p12. Treatment has been attempted with *L*-dopa and 5-hydroxytryptophan with variable success.

GABA neurotransmitter disorders

Succinic semialdehyde dehydrogenase (SSADH, 4-hydroxybutyric aciduria) deficiency

SSADH is necessary for the degradation of GABA (see Figure 154.2). In SSADH deficiency, GABA is preferentially metabolized to gamma-hydroxybutyric acid (GHB) which accumulates and becomes the primary neurotoxic metabolite in this disorder. This disorder is transmitted in an autosomal recessive manner and the gene for SSADH has been mapped to chromosome 6p22.

Presenting clinical features may vary, though the most consistent clinical findings are those of developmental delay and hypotonia. Ataxia is frequent and generally improves slightly over time. Absence and convulsive seizures have been reported in about half of patients, despite elevated GABA levels. MRI has revealed in some patients an increased T2 signal within the globus pallidus and subcortical white matter bilaterally and MR spectroscopy has shown elevated peaks of GABA and GABA metabolites when they have been looked for.

Diagnosis is based on the presence of elevated levels of GHB on urinary organic acid analysis. Other GABA metabolites, such as 3,4-dihydroxybutyric acid, 3-oxo-4-hydroxybutyric acid, and glycolic acid may also be identified. Unlike other disorders of organic acid and fatty acid metabolism, metabolic acidosis and hypoglycemia are not features of SSADH deficiency. CSF analysis has shown significant elevations of GHB and free GABA.

Treatment has been attempted with vigabatrin, an irreversible inhibitor of GABA transaminase, which should theoretically inhibit the formation of succinic semialdehyde and therefore GHB. The treatment response has been limited at best, however. Symptomatic treatment of epilepsy and behavior with a wide variety of medications has been attempted. There is a theoretical contraindication to valproate use as it may inhibit residual SSADH activity.

Pyridoxine-dependent epilepsy (PDE)

Most children with PDE present in the neonatal period with frequent seizures that are unresponsive to traditional anticonvulsant medications. The diagnosis of definitive PDE has been suggested by the complete cessation of seizures within 7 days of pyridoxine administration, the recurrence of seizures following withdrawal of pyridoxine, and the subsequent remission of seizures when pyridoxine is re-administered. While most children present in the newborn period, convincing cases with epilepsy onset as late as 7 years of age have been reported. While the full spectrum of clinical symptomatology has not been fully elucidated, some children with PDE appear to be cognitively normal whereas others have been reported to have autism or mental retardation.

Diagnosis of PDE is suggested by normalization of the interictal electroencephalogram (EEG) and cessation of seizures following 50–100 mg injection of intravenous pyridoxine. Pyridoxine is an essential cofactor for glutamic acid decarboxylase and is necessary for the conversion of glutamic acid into GABA (see Figure 154.2). Patients with PDE who are treated with intravenous pyridoxine may become hypotonic and apneic due to the sudden increase in CSF GABA concentrations, and artificial respiration may be required. There are, however, cases of PDE who do not immediately respond to intravenous pyridoxine but who do gradually but completely respond to ongoing oral pyridoxine administration.

More recently, several patients with PDE have been found to have point mutations in the *antiquitin* gene on chromosome 5q31. This gene encodes the enzyme alpha-aminoadipic semialdehyde dehydrogenase which is part of the cerebral lysine degradation pathway. Dysfunction of this enzyme leads to accumulations of alpha-aminoadipic semialdehyde (AAAS) as well as delta-1-piperidine-6-carboxylate (P6C) and L-pipecolic acid. P6C inactivates pyridoxalphosphate which is the active form of pyridoxine. Several children with PDE have been found to have significant elevations of pipecolic acid in the serum prior to administration of pyridoxine treatment and milder elevations that persisted once treatment was begun. Likewise, significant elevations of serum and urine AAAS have been reported in PDE even after treatment.

Once a diagnosis of PDE is confirmed (either through pyridoxine treatment criteria or by documenting elevated levels of serum pipecolic acid or AAAS), ongoing maintenance therapy with oral pyridoxine at dosages ranging from 10 to 200 mg/day or more should be instituted. The dosage should be titrated upwards until all seizures stop. Titrating the dosage until there is normalization of CSF glutamate levels has also been suggested.

GABA transaminase (GT) deficiency

GT deficiency is a very rare disorder of GABA catabolism that has been reported in only two families. The affected children had early-onset generalized convulsions that were unresponsive to treatment, along with lethargy, feeding problems, central hypotonia, and hyperreflexia. The EEGs showed a burst supression pattern. CSF analysis revealed elevated levels of GABA and homocarnosine (see Figure 154.2). The disease was fatal by 2 years of age in all three patients.

Further reading

De Vivo D, Johnston MJ, editors. Pediatric neurotransmitter diseases. *Ann Neurol* 2003; 54(6): S1–109.

Plecko B, Paul K, Paschke E, *et al.* Biochemical and molecular characterization of 18 patients with pyridoxine-dependent epilepsy and mutations of the antiquitin (ALDH7A1) gene. *Hum Mutat* 2007; 28(1): 19–26.

Chapter 155
Neonatal neurology

Mary Payne[1] and Ann Tilton[2]
[1]Marshall University, Huntington, USA
[2]Louisiana State University Health Sciences Center, New Orleans, USA

Introduction

Modern improvements in neonatal intensive care worldwide have improved the survival rate of premature infants and ill term infants. Thus many children who have suffered intracranial hemorrhage, asphyxia, infection, and seizures survive to be cared for by the neurologist.

Hypoxic ischemic encephalopathy

Perinatal asphyxia occurs in premature and term newborns. Diagnosing asphyxia is based on cord blood acidosis, low Apgar scores, or other metabolic abnormalities that may suggest damage to other organs besides the brain (heart, liver, kidneys). Asphyxia exposes the brain to low oxygen, decreased blood flow, and hypercarbia. In a state of prolonged hypoxic-ischemic injury, cardiac output fails, systemic hypotension occurs, and cerebral blood flow decreases. Healthy brain vasculature is able to compensate by autoregulation to maintain adequate blood flow to the brain. However, premature brains and infants with cardio-respiratory illness have poor autoregulation. The cerebral circulation is pressure-passive, meaning that a fluctuating arterial blood pressure causes an associated fluctuating pattern of cerebral blood flow velocity due to the poor ability of the cerebral vessels to compensate for these alterations. As a result, levels of many neurotransmitters are unbalanced, including glutamate, excitatory amino acids, and aspartate, and there may be an influx of sodium, calcium, and chloride in cells. Cell death then occurs.

Sequelae of hypoxic-ischemic injury are determined by the extent and area of ischemia. A global hypoxic-ischemic injury produces infarction in the watershed areas of the brain, whereas a more focal injury from localized vascular compromise leads to focal infarction. Affected white matter causes spasticity in corresponding limbs. Often, the basal ganglia, a region in which active metabolism increases susceptibility to periods of relative ischemia, is injured and may produce a concomitant movement disorder such as dystonia or athetosis with spasticity. Gray matter damage causes seizures and cognitive dysfunction.

Intraventricular hemorrhage

Periventricular and intraventricular hemorrhage (IVH) are most likely to occur in the infant born before 32 weeks gestational age. The incidence has been reported to be as high as 50% in the United States for births less than 35 weeks gestational age. Internationally, the incidence of hemorrhage is directly related to the incidence of prematurity. The germinal matrix is very cellular and highly vascularized and supports the differentiation of glial cells until about 32 weeks gestation. The capillary bed in the subependymal germinal matrix is composed of thin endothelial-lined vessels lacking a developed adventitia. The combination of poor autoregulation and fragile vessels predisposes premature infants to intraventricular and periventricular hemorrhage in this area. Bleeds range in severity as listed in the table below.

Grade I	Blood in subependymal region
Grade II	Blood extends into lateral ventricles
Grade III	Blood extends into lateral ventricles with ventricular dilatation
Grade IV	Intraparenchymal hemorrhage

IVH is frequently accompanied by global hypoxic-ischemic injury and periventricular leukomalacia, as these diseases also occur in the setting of variable pressure changes (most notably low pressure states leading to ischemia) and occur more frequently in infants with cardiorespiratory illness. The periventricular white matter adjacent to the germinal matrix becomes ischemic from hypoperfusion and hemorrhagic from ventricular blood impairing venous drainage.

IVH causes hydrocephalus from decreased absorption of cerebral spinal fluid due to blockage of blood and debris in the arachnoid villi. Chronic obstruction from arachnoiditis impairs outflow of the fourth ventricle, causing hydrocephalus.

International Neurology: A Clinical Approach. Edited by Robert P. Lisak, Daniel D. Truong, William M. Carroll, and Roongroj Bhidayasiri.
© 2009 Blackwell Publishing, ISBN: 978-1-4051-5738-4.

Infection

Infection may occur in the prenatal, perinatal, or postnatal period. Prenatal infections acquired by the mother and transmitted to the fetus that cause brain damage include cytomegalovirus, toxoplasmosis, rubella, HIV, varicella zoster virus, parvovirus B19, and syphilis. Brain calcifications are commonly seen in cytomegalovirus and toxoplasmosis. Microcephaly, seizures, and thrombocytopenia are common in all of these infections. Mental retardation is a common outcome, as well as sensorineural hearing loss (most common in congenital rubella).

Herpes, *Listeria*, *Escherichia coli*, group B streptococcus (GBS), and other Gram-negative or Gram-positive organisms present in the birth canal may be transmitted to the newborn during birth. Infection with these organisms may lead to meningoencephalitis with seizures, coma, cerebral edema, ventriculitis, and infarction. Chronic changes resulting from these insults include encephalomalacia, hydrocephalus, and gray and white matter atrophy.

Inborn errors of metabolism

Inborn errors of metabolism include disorders of amino acids, organic acids, and carbohydrates, and present in the neonatal period with seizures, encephalopathy, and poor feeding. Metabolic acidosis, hyperammonemia, and hypoglycemia are indicators of a deficient metabolic enzyme.

Hyperbilirubinemia occurs in hemolytic disease and from inherited defects of conjugation. It is more common in infants of Asian or Hispanic descent. Neurons are particularly sensitive to high levels of bilirubin. Extracellular bilirubin is unconjugated and binds to phospholipids on the plasma membrane of cells, forming a complex with the cell membrane. Bilirubin then enters the cell and binds to mitochondria and the nucleus. Ligandin is an intracellular substance that binds to the bilirubin complex and removes its toxicity; neurons do not contain ligandin. Thus, neuronal cell death occurs. Therefore, acute bilirubin encephalopathy is associated pathologically with bilirubin staining of neurons, or "kernicterus." A later finding is neuronal necrosis. Premature infants are more susceptible to kernicterus at a lower level of total bilirubin compared to term infants.

Infants that survive kernicterus have severe neurologic sequelae including movement disorders such as chorea, ballismus, dystonia, and tremor. Also seen are gaze abnormalities, hearing loss, and cognitive deficits.

Seizures

Seizures occurring within 48 hours after birth are most likely from hypoxic-ischemic encephalopathy, intracranial hemorrhage, or hypoglycemia. Seizures occurring later are usually symptomatic seizures in the setting of infection, metabolic disturbance, pyridoxine deficiency, or inborn error of metabolism. Several types of seizures occur in the neonate and include tonic, clonic, myoclonic, and fragmentary. Fragmentary (or subtle) seizures may be challenging to manage since they are frequently associated with electro-clinical dissociation. Neonates may have focal or generalized seizures; however, because the neonatal brain is not yet myelinated, generalized seizures consist of spread of focal activity, not the type of generalized convulsion that is seen in older age groups.

Other etiologies to consider include fifth-day fits, in which the seizures begin on the fifth day of life, are multi-focal clonic activity, and disappear by 20 days of life. Familial neonatal seizures are recognized by the autosomal dominant family history of neonatal seizures.

Treatment of neonatal seizures consists of lorazepam in the acute setting and phenobarbital and/or fosphenytoin load for status epilepticus and for daily maintenance therapy.

Further reading

Al Otaibi SF, Blaser S, MacGregor DL. Neurological complications of kernicterus. *Can J Neurol Sci* 2005; 32(3): 311–15.

Bada HS, Korones SB, Perry EH, *et al*. Mean arterial blood pressure changes in premature infants and those at risk for intraventricular hemorrhage. *J Pediatr* 1990; 117(4): 607–14.

Ellenberg JH, Nelson KB. Cluster of perinatal events identifying infants at high risk for death or disability. *J Pediatr* 1988; 113(3): 546–52.

Klein J, Remington J. Current concepts in infections of the fetus and newborn. In: Remington J, Klein J, editors. *Infectious Diseases of the Fetus and Newborn Infant*. Philadelphia: Saunders; 2001, pp. 1–24.

Sheth RD, Hobbs GR, Mullett M. Neonatal seizures: incidence, onset, and etiology by gestational age. *J Perinatol* 1999; 19(1): 40–3.

Chapter 156
Floppy infant syndrome

Jong-Hee Chae
Seoul National University Children's Hospital, Seoul, Korea

Introduction

Floppy infant syndrome is a disease in which infants present with generalized hypotonia at birth or early infancy. There are many possible etiologies, which make a specific diagnosis difficult. The expanding knowledge of genetic disorders has made non-invasive genetic testing available for specific diagnoses. Therefore, it is very important for clinicians to use a systematic approach for the investigation of such children. This chapter reviews the many possible etiologies of the floppy infant syndrome, and proposes a systematic approach for the evaluation of this disorder.

Clinical evaluation

Floppy infants usually demonstrate a characteristic "frog-leg posture," excessive joint mobility, and profound weakness. These babies may also have limp and drooping limbs when they are held by the trunk, and a prominent head lag when traction is delivered. Muscle stretch reflexes are diminished or absent in floppy infants with neuromuscular disorders, whereas in those with central causes, these reflexes are usually present or even exaggerated. Floppiness can have a variety of causes, which can affect the brain and any part of the motor units. It can be clinically useful to classify the syndrome into central and peripheral disorders (Table 156.1). For appropriate and cost-effective investigations, it is essential to document the prenatal and perinatal history of infants in detail as well as carry out careful physical and neurological examinations. Any history of gestational drug or teratogen exposure, breech presentation, reduced fetal movements, presence of polyhydramnios, or maternal diseases (e.g., diabetes, myotonic dystrophies, myasthenia gravis, or epilepsies) should be assessed. In addition, any family history of neuromuscular diseases and details of perinatal birth event such as birth trauma, birth asphyxia, or low APGAR scores should be included. The presence of associated malformation of other organs and facial dysmorphic features can provide important clues to make a diagnosis: for example, Down syndrome or Prader–Willi syndrome. More than two-thirds of floppy infants have primary causes of central nervous system (CNS) disorders. If floppy babies have seizures, impairment of consciousness level, apnea, or delayed intellectual and language milestones, these suggest CNS disorders. Among those with central hypotonia, axial weakness is characteristic and prominent in early life, and this changes to hyperreflexia over time. Usually, these findings can allow clinicians to make a diagnosis readily without unnecessary electrophysiological studies or the need for muscle biopsies.

The presence of profound weakness with diminished or absent deep tendon reflexes suggests peripheral causes of this syndrome. Such children also show low-pitched weak crying, poor sucking power, and decreased spontaneous movements. A high arched palate and typical myopathic face are often noted in infants with neuromuscular diseases. In addition, they are usually alert with bright eyes, compared to infants with central disorders. However, sometimes it is difficult to make a clear distinction, because infants with lower motor neuron disorders may have suffered perinatal asphyxia caused by abnormal uterine presentation or severe respiratory muscle weakness immediately after birth. Moreover, some disorders such as metachromatic leukodystrophy and Pelizaeus–Merzbacher disease have pathologies that affect both the central and peripheral nervous systems.

Laboratory investigations

The next step in the differential diagnosis is a cost-effective use of laboratory investigations. For infants with causes suggestive of central disorders, cytogenetic study and a neuroimaging study (brain computer tomography or magnetic resonance imaging) are

International Neurology: A Clinical Approach. Edited by Robert P. Lisak, Daniel D. Truong, William M. Carroll, and Roongroj Bhidayasiri. © 2009 Blackwell Publishing, ISBN: 978-1-4051-5738-4.

Table 156.1 Possible causes of floppy infant syndrome.

Central disorders	Chromosomal abnormalities	Down syndrome Turner syndrome Prader–Willi syndrome (PWS)
	Inborn error of metabolism	Aminoacidopathy Hyperammonemia Lipid storage diseases Hypoglycemia Neurodegenerative diseases
	Hypoxic ischemic encephalopathy	Birth asphyxia Perinatal trauma Cerebral palsy
	Congenital malformation of brain development	Lissencephaly
	Spinal cord disorders	Syringomyelia Spinal hypoxia
Peripheral disorders	Motor neuron	Spinal muscular atrophy (SMA)
	Nerve	Peripheral neuropathy (e.g., Dejerine–Sottas, CMT 1A, CMT 4E)
	Neuromuscular junction	Congenital myasthenic syndrome Infantile botulism
	Muscle	Congenital myopathies (e.g., myotubular myopathy or nemaline myopathy) Congenital muscular dystrophies Metabolic myopathies (e.g., Pompe's disease) Congenital myotonic dystrophies

CMT: Charcot–Marie–Tooth disease.

recommended. Screening for inborn errors of metabolism should also be included for infants with multisystem involvements in addition to hypotonia. Classical laboratory tests including the evaluation of muscle enzymes, electromyography (EMG), nerve conduction studies (NCS), and muscle biopsies with enzyme histochemistry, immunohistochemistry, and electron microscopy are usually helpful for the diagnosis of peripheral neuromuscular disorders. In general, EMG is useful to differentiate between denervation and myopathy. However, in early infancy within a few weeks or in infants with mild weakness, EMG and muscle pathology is sometimes not concordant. So, even if the electrophysiological studies and muscle enzymes prove normal, muscle biopsies should be considered, especially in the diagnosis of suspected congenital myopathies and congenital muscular dystrophies.

The congenital myopathies are classified into classic myopathies, such as nemaline myopathy, central core disease, centronuclear or myotubular myopathy, and other myopathies such as congenital fiber type disproportion, multicore disease, and cytoplasmic body myopathy. Although recent advances make it possible to clarify genetic etiologies and pathogenetic mechanisms, morphologic diagnosis by muscle pathology still plays a crucial role in the diagnosis of congenital myopathies and most genetic tests are only performed

for research purposes. Congenital muscular dystrophies (CMD) are genetically heterogeneous disorders, which usually present severe weakness at birth and early joint contractures with mildly increased creatinine kinase (CK) level and dystrophic features in muscle pathology. They are typically classified into two categories: classic CMD (CMD without mental retardation or nonsyndromic CMD) and CMD with mental retardation (syndromic CMD). In classic CMDs, they are divided into two groups depending on the presence of merosin (laminin α2): merosin-deficient form and merosin-positive form. The merosin-deficient form CMD is prominent in Western countries but rare in the Asian population. The most striking feature of merosin-deficient CMD is leukodystrophy with normal cognition. Merosin-positive groups tend to have a wide spectrum of severity, progression, and associated features of rigid spine or severe distal joint laxity in Ullrich disease. The other form, syndromic CMD, including Fukuyama type, Walker–Warburg syndrome, and muscle-eye brain diseases, have variable involvements of eye abnormalities and brain structural anomalies with mental retardation. In CMDs, brain MRI is quite useful for classification and further genetic research.

In several neuromuscular disorders such as spinal muscular atrophy and congenital myotonic dystrophy, rapid genetic tests are available (*SMN* and *DM1*,

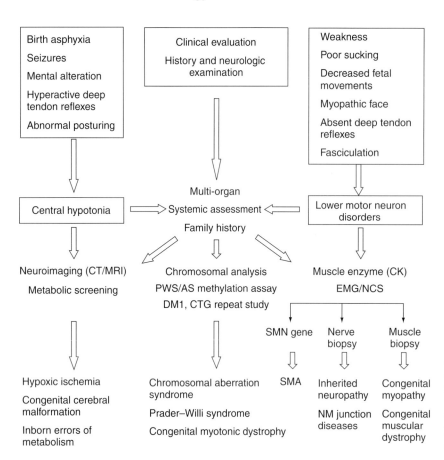

Figure 156.1 Proposed algorithm for the diagnosis of floppy infant syndrome. PWS: Prader–Willi syndrome; AS: Angelman syndrome; DM1: Myotonic dystrophy type 1; CK: creatine kinase; EMG: electromyography; NCS: nerve conduction study; SMA: spinal muscular atrophy.

respectively). Spinal muscular atrophy (SMA) is an autosomal recessive disorder involving the anterior horn cells, almost 95% of all of the spinal muscular atrophy patients is responsible for the SMN1 gene, located on chromosome 5q13. The presence of tongue fasciculation with striking proximal weakness suggests spinal muscular atrophy. If the child shows tented lips with facial weakness, severe respiratory muscle weakness with diaphragmatic eventuration, and foot deformities such as talipes, these features are strongly suggestive of congenital myotonic dystrophy. Therefore, an examination of the mother's face, particularly evidence of eyelid closure weakness and grip myotonia, are needed. These clinical situations will often confirm the clinical suspicion of a genetic disorder, and confirmation using DNA analysis and genotyping can then proceed without invasive diagnostic investigations.

Although neuromuscular junction disorder is not a common cause of floppy infant syndrome, it must be differentiated in the clinical setting. In mothers with myasthenia gravis, acetylcholine (Ach) receptor antibodies cross the placenta to the baby, resulting in blocked neuromuscular transmission (transient myasthenic syndrome)

and floppiness of the baby, which is usually reversible in about 6 weeks. Congential myasthenic syndromes are genetic defects of neuromuscular transmission, such as ion channels, acetylcholine receptor, or the recyling mechanism for Ach itself, which often present with easy fatigability of ocular, bulbar, and limb muscles, with family history in later infancy.

Diagnostic approach

As mentioned above, the diagnostic approach to the investigation of the floppy infant syndrome has significantly changed, thanks to the advances of DNA-based diagnostic tests. The internet link http://geneclinics.org gives updated information of available genetic tests in various inherited neuromuscular disorders. These allow clinicians to make rapid and sensitive diagnoses and decrease the need for unnecessary electrophysiological studies or invasive muscle biopsies. Therefore, an algorithm for the systemic evaluation of infants with hypotonia is available for pediatric neurologists and neonatologists (Figure 156.1).

Conclusion

Floppy infant syndrome has highly variable etiologies, including central and peripheral nervous system disorders. Thorough history taking and careful clinical evaluation is important for the proper diagnosis and management of patients.

Further reading

Swaiman KF, Ashwal S, Ferriero DM. *Pediatric Neurology, Principles and Practice*, 4th ed. Philadelphia: Mosby; 2006.

Volpe JJ. *Neurology of the Newborn*, 4th ed. Philadelphia: WB Saunders; 2001.

Chapter 157
Storage disorders

Jeffrey Ekstrand[1] and Raman Sankar[2]
[1]University of Utah School of Medicine, Salt Lake City, USA
[2]David Geffen School of Medicine at UCLA, Los Angeles, USA

Introduction

Storage disorders consist of a clinically diverse group of individually relatively rare disorders that collectively constitute a significant medical burden to society. In most cases they result from a genetic mutation which causes an enzymatic defect in the catabolic process of large macromolecules. Historically, each subclassification of the various storage disorders was named based on the type of macromolecule being degraded. For example, the glycogenoses are a group of storage disorders that have a defect in the catabolic pathway of glycogen. However, there are also examples (e.g., the leukodystrophies) where the disease classification name is based on criteria previously established before a complete understanding of the disorders' biochemistry was achieved. Most of the storage disorders can be characterized as lysosomal diseases because many of the macromolecules are catabolized in this structure. The molecular defect is not always a primary degradative enzyme. Instead, a wide variety of protein functions including but not limited to trafficking of macromolecules to specific organelles, transmembrane protein receptor targets, and chaperone molecules can impact the catabolic process.

The geographical regional differences observed for some of these disorders almost certainly result from the different distribution of ethnic populations with particular genetic endowments. This chapter is limited to describing such differences when relevant, along with descriptions of the clinical characteristics, current diagnostic tools, and treatments if available of the more commonly observed conditions. It is not meant to be exhaustive, nor is it intended to describe the often very complicated biochemical molecular genetics. For these features, the reader is referred to the Further reading section and the OMIM website (www.ncbi.nlm.nih.gov/omim/).

Lipidoses

The lipidoses are storage diseases that are characterized by a defect in the metabolism of lipids, including lipoproteins or glycolipids. This results in the accumulation in cells of incompletely metabolized lipid intermediate products in a variety of tissues including the brain, peripheral nervous system, liver, and bone marrow. There are a number of subcategories of lipid storage disorders that are named based on the starting complex macromolecule being metabolized, although each has a lipid component. These are neuronal ceroid lipofuscinosis, gangliosidosis, sphingomyelinosis, cerebrosidosis, and mucolipidosis. Other lipidoses that are not classified under this nomenclature include Fabry's disease, abetalipoproteinemia, and Tangier disease. Finally, although Krabbe's disease and metachromatic leukodystrophy are lipid storage diseases, they are discussed separately with the other leukodystrophies.

Neuronal ceroid lipofuscinosis (NCL)

The NCLs are a group of neurodegenerative disorders that are characterized by the accumulation of autoflourescent lipopigment material within neuronal lysosomes. This results in a heterogenous clinical picture, although motor and mental deterioration with visual dysfunction is commonly seen. Historically, the NCLs were separated into four subclassifications based on age of presentation and electron microscopic appearance of the inclusions. More recently at least eight genetically distinct forms have been described. The childhood NCLs are inherited in an autosomal recessive fashion, while the adult disorder can be either recessive or dominant.

The infantile form (Santavouri–Haltia disease or CLN1) usually presents between age 6 and 24 months with rapid mental deterioration, microcephaly, failure to thrive, and myoclonus. Visual impairment occurs with a brownish pigmentation of the macula, hypopigmentation of the fundi, and optic atrophy. Ultrastructural examination of neuronal and other tissue demonstrates granular osmiophilic deposits. The gene defect is a lysosomal enzyme, palmitoyl-protein thioesterase 1 (PPT1) mapped to chromosome 1p32. This defect has also been occasionally seen

International Neurology: A Clinical Approach. Edited by Robert P. Lisak, Daniel D. Truong, William M. Carroll, and Roongroj Bhidayasiri. © 2009 Blackwell Publishing, ISBN: 978-1-4051-5738-4.

in later-onset disease. Although observed worldwide, this disorder is particularly prevalent in Finland, with an incidence of 1 in 13 000 and an estimated carrier rate of 1 in 70. This disease progresses rapidly with death usually occurring in early childhood.

The primary late infantile form (also called Jansky–Bielschowsky disease or CLN2) usually presents between age 2 and 4 years with cognitive decline, ataxia, and either myoclonic or generalized seizures. Progressive visual decline usually follows. Typically development is normal for the first 2 years of life, although in retrospect some mild clumsiness can be recalled after the diagnosis becomes apparent. The gene defect is a lysosomal enzyme, tripeptidyl-peptidase 1 mapped to chromosome 11p15.5. Ultrastructure examination shows a characteristic pattern of curved stacks of lamellae called curvilinear bodies. The disease has been observed worldwide with an incidence of 0.46 per 100 000 live births. There is also a variant of this more common late infantile form (Finnish-Variant Late Infantile NCL or CLN5) which is prevalent in Finland with an incidence of 1 in 21 000. The gene defect encodes a transmembrane protein of unknown function which maps to chromosome 13q21.1–q32. Other variants of this form have been even less well characterized and include CLN8 in Finland and CLN7 in Turkey as well as CLN6 in multiple geographic areas (Costa Rica, South America, Portugal, and the United Kingdom). Death usually occurs by the end of the first decade.

The juvenile form (Batten disease, Spielmeyer–Vogt disease, CLN3) usually presents between age 5 and 8 years with progressive visual loss, seizures, and ataxia. Although it has been described worldwide, the incidence is enriched in Finland with an incidence of 1 in 21 000. The gene defect is a transmembrane lysosomal protein of unknown function that maps to chromosome 16p12.1. Ultrastructure examination shows a "fingerprint" lamellae pattern distinct from the curvilinear bodies seen in CLN2. Death occurs in the late teens or early twenties.

The adult form (also called Kufs' disease or CLN4) usually presents before age 30 and is characterized by a more slowly progressive course. Visual dysfunction is not a frequent feature. The gene defect has not yet been characterized.

When the clinical suspicion for an NCL is present, the definitive diagnosis can be achieved by an enzymatic assay or morphological electron microscopy examination of sweat gland tissue showing the distinctive ultrastructure characteristics. Treatment is symptomatic and prognosis is poor.

Gangliosidoses

The gangliosidoses are a group of disorders characterized by the impaired breakdown of specific plasma membrane lipid marcromolecules primarily found in the gray matter of neuronal tissue ganglion cells. These macromolecules

are composed of sphingosine, fatty acids, hexose, hexosamine, and neuraminic acid. The three most important gangliosidoses are Tay–Sachs disease, Sandhoff disease (both part of the GM2 gangliosidoses), and generalized GM1 gangliosidosis. All three are autosomal recessive with no sex predilection.

Tay–Sachs disease is the most common of the gangliosidoses and results from an enzyme defect in the alpha subunit of beta-hexosaminidase A. This defect is 100 times more common in Ashkenazi Jewish populations than in non-Jewish groups. The incidence is approximately 1 per 360 000 newborns in the general population, as opposed to 1 per 2500–3600 in Ashkenazi Jewish populations. There also appears to be an increased frequency of this disease (comparable to that in the Ashkenazi Jewish population) in the Cordoba region of Argentina, French Canadians of the eastern St Lawrence river valley, and isolated population groups of Cajuns in Louisiana. Although less than what is observed in Ashkenazi Jewish populations, there is an increased frequency in non-Ashkenazi Jewish groups in both Morocco and Iraq. Initially, children with this disease develop normally for the first few months of life. Clinical symptoms usually begin between ages 3 and 10 months with developmental arrest or regression, hyperacusis (resulting in an exaggerated startle reflex), and generalized hypotonia. Examination of the fundus will invariably reveal the presence of the cherry red spot which is due to the sparing of the red choroid of the fovea surrounded by white, lipid-laden ganglion cells. The disease progresses with hearing loss, blindness, severe spasticity, seizures, and macrocephaly. Diagnosis is made initially on clinical grounds and confirmed with an assay for hexosaminidase from serum. This assay is also used as a carrier screening tool in very high risk ethnic groups. There is no effective treatment for this disorder. Anti-epileptic and antispasticity medications are used for symptomatic treatment. Death usually occurs by the age of 4 years.

Sandhoff disease results from an enzyme defect in the beta subunit of both beta-hexosaminidase A and beta-hexosaminidase B. The incidence is approximately 1 per 310 000 newborns worldwide, and there is no increased frequency of this disease among Ashkenazi Jewish populations. An increased incidence of this disease has been observed in Creoles of northern Argentina, Metis Indians of northern Saskatchewan, and individuals of Lebanese heritage, and there is a very high carrier rate in a small Maronite community in Cyprus. It shares the same clinical symptoms and progression as Tay–Sachs disease. Additional symptoms include organomegaly, skeletal abnormalities, doll-like facies, and cardiac murmur. As with Tay–Sachs disease, there is no effective treatment for this disorder. Death usually occurs by age 4.

The generalized GM1 gangliosidoses result from an enzyme defect in beta-galactosidase. It is a rare disorder occurring worldwide, with an unusually high incidence (1 in 3700 births) in the population of Malta. There are three forms based on the age of presentation. The early infantile GM1 presents before 1 year, often at birth. Symptoms include hypotonia, neurologic degeneration, seizures, hepatosplenomegaly, coarsening of facial features, dermal melanocytosis, skeletal abnormalities, and abnormal startle reflex. In approximately half the cases a cherry red spot is seen on fundal examination. The disease is rapidly progressive and death usually occurs by age 3. Late infantile GM1 presents between ages 1 and 3 years. Symptoms include ataxia, pronounced hyperacusis, seizures, slowly deteriorating mental function, and difficulties with speech. Adult GM1 occurs between ages 3 and 30. Symptoms include progressive intellectual deterioration, ataxia, spasticity, and progressive athetosis or dystonia. Bony abnormalities, organomegaly, and the presence of cherry red spots are not usually present in these two late occurring forms. Diagnosis is usually made by showing the absence of beta-galactosidase activity from conjunctival biopsy. Treatment is symptomatic.

Sphingomyelinoses
The sphingomyelinoses are disorders associated with the accumulation of sphingomyelin, a macromolecule composed of sphingosine, fatty acid, phosphoric acid, and choline, which is found abundantly in the spleen and is a major constituent of myelin. In this section the various types of Niemann–Pick diseases will be discussed. At least six types of Niemann–Pick disease have been described (types A–F), although the four most important types (types A–D) can be grouped into two broad biochemical pathological processes, described further below. Types E and F are not well characterized adult forms, have minimal to no neurological symptoms, and will not be discussed further. All are autosomal recessive with no clear sex predilection.

Niemann–Pick types A and B result from a defect in the lysosomal enzyme sphingomyelinase which is responsible for the initial cleaving of sphingomyelin into phosphatidylcholine and ceramide. Type A is found in all ethnic groups with an estimated incidence of 1 in 264 000 live births. The rate is higher (1 in 40 000) in Ashkenazi Jewish populations. Type B is also pan-ethnic with the highest incidence occurring in individuals of Turkish, Arabic, and North African descent, but does not show a higher incidence among Ashkenazi Jewish populations. Niemann–Pick type A disease begins during infancy and presents with hepatosplenomegaly, growth retardation, hypotonia, and progressive neurodegeneration. The disease rapidly progresses with loss of motor development, increasing spasticity, and sometimes seizures. Death usually occurs by age 3. Niemann–Pick type B disease presents with hepatosplenomegaly, growth retardation, and problems with increased lung infections. There are little

to no neurologic problems and individuals usually survive into adulthood. The different clinical course between these two diseases is believed to be due to the relative residual activity of sphingomyelinase present with each enzymatic defect.

Niemann–Pick diseases types C and D result from a disruption of cholesterol transport from endosomes to the plasma membrane. Both diseases show accumulations of intracellular cholesterol and sphingomyelin. Type C is further subdivided into C1 and C2 categories based on genotype. C1 represents 95% of the cases of Niemann–Pick type C disease. Type D has now been shown to be an allelic variant of type C1 that was initially described in patients of Nova Scotia Acadian ancestry. The incidence of this disorder (combined C1, C2, and D) is estimated to be 1 in 150 000 births. The disease occurs with a much higher frequency in people of French-Acadian descent in Nova Scotia and Cajuns in Louisiana, with an estimate of 1% of the population (heterogenetic carrier frequency between 10% and 26%). The clinical features can be quite heterogenous, with the initial presentation ranging from infancy to adulthood; however, the more common course is relatively normal development in the first 2 years of life, followed by mild organomegaly, progressive neurologic decline, ataxia, weakness, and vertical gaze palsy. Death often occurs by age 20.

Niemann–Pick types A and B can be diagnosed by demonstrating deficient sphingomyelinase activity in leukocytes and skin fibroblasts. Types C and D are diagnosed by showing increased amounts of unesterified cholesterol in fibroblasts. Another method is to show sea-blue histiocytes in the bone marrow. There is no established treatment other than symptomatic treatment for this disorder.

Cerebrosidoses
The cerebrosidoses are disorders of degradation of cerebrosides, which are glycosphingolipids that consist of a ceramide with a single sugar residue at the 1-hydroxyl moiety. The sugar residue can be either glucose (glucocerebrosides) or galactose (galactocerebrosides). The primary cerebrosidosis that will be discussed in this section is Gaucher's disease which results from an enzyme defect in the breakdown of glucocerebrosides. The disorder resulting from the defect for galactocerebrosides (Krabbe's disease) will be discussed with the other leukodystrophies.

Gaucher's disease is the most prevalent lipid storage disorder. The primary defect results from a deficiency in the lysosomal enzyme glucocerebrosidase. There are three specific clinical subtypes based on the presence of neuronal symptoms and rate of progression. All are autosomal recessive with no sex predilection. Type 1, the non-neuronopathic form, is the most common with an estimated incidence of 1 in 40 000. It is even more common in Ashkenazi Jewish populations with a disease frequency of 1 per 855. It often presents in childhood with progressive hepatosplenomegaly, pancytopenia, and skeletal problems. There are no neurological manifestations. Type II Gaucher's disease is an acute neuronopathic form with initial presentation in infancy. It has an estimated incidence of 1 in 100 000 births. Patients are usually normal at birth but develop hepatosplenomegaly, developmental regression, eye movement disorders, spasticity, and seizures. Death occurs by age 2. Type III Gaucher's disease is the subacute neuronopathic form. It has a general estimated incidence of 1 in 100 000 births; however, it is observed with greater frequency in Swedish patients from the Norrbotten region with an incidence of 1 in 50 000 births. It is characterized by more slowly progressive and milder symptoms compared to the type II form. Symptoms can begin in early childhood or adulthood and include hepatosplenomegaly, intellectual deterioration, ataxia, spasticity, skeletal abnormalities, horizontal supranuclear gaze palsy, anemia, and respiratory problems. Death often occurs by age 30.

Presumptive diagnosis can be made by detection of Gaucher's cells in bone marrow aspirates in the correct clinical context. Definitive diagnosis can be made with an assay of glucocerebrosidase in leukocytes and fibroblast cultures. There has been promising success with treatment for this condition using enzyme replacement therapy and substrate reduction therapy to treat the systemic effects of this disease. However, because these methods lack an effective mechanism to transport through the blood–brain barrier, their effect on neurologic symptoms is more marginal.

Mucolipidoses

The mucolipidoses are composed of four distinct clinical conditions (designated type I–IV) that result from the accumulation of lipid and carbohydrate molecules due to specific lysosomal enzyme defects. All are autosomal recessive with no sex predilection. Mucolipidosis type I, also referred to as sialidosis, results from an enzymatic defect in sialidase which is involved in the initial cleavage of the sialic acid residue in glycoproteins. The incidence has been estimated at 1 in 2 175 000 individuals, and there has not been any documentation of regional or ethnic predilections. Symptoms present within the first year of life and include progressive mental retardation, myoclonus, ataxia, seizures, hypotonia, coarse facial features, corneal opacifications, macroglossia, hepatosplenomegaly, and skeletal malformations. Diagnosis is made by demonstrating deficient alpha-N-acetyl neuraminidase activity measured in leukocytes and fibroblasts. Treatment is symptomatic, and most infants die before the age of 1 year. Mucolipidosis type II is also referred to as inclusion cell (I-cell)

disease. The defect is in UDP-N-acetylglucosamine:N-acetylglucosaminyl-1-phosphotransferase, an enzyme that contributes to the marking of enzymes so they are correctly targeted to lysosomes. In the absence of this step, lysosomal enzymes are incorrectly routed into the extracellular space. This disorder is rare, with an estimated incidence of 1 in 640 000 births, although it may be higher in Saguenay-Lac-St Jean, a French Canadian isolate. Symptoms present at birth and include hypotonia, coarse facial features, gingival hyperplasia, and skeletal abnormalities, and progressive mental deterioration and microcephaly occur over time. This condition is diagnosed by the presence of inclusion bodies in bone marrow cells and cultured fibroblasts. Death occurs in childhood. Treatments are limited for this disorder, although bone marrow transplantation has shown some promise. Mucolipidosis type III, also called pseudo-Hurler polydystrophy, is a milder form of type II likely due to partially retained enzymatic activity with the defect. Symptoms do not occur until after age 2. Patients are generally of normal intelligence or have mild mental retardation. Other symptoms include short stature, coarse facial features, skeletal abnormalities, and corneal clouding. Prolonged survival into late adulthood is possible. Mucolipidosis type IV is due to a defect in mucolipin 1, a transmembrane protein that is involved in endosomal transport within the cell. Its relative incidence worldwide is unknown, although Ashkenazi Jewish populations are believed to have a higher frequency with a carrier rate of 1 in 100 individuals. Symptoms include developmental delay, corneal clouding, hypotonia, achlorhydria with abnormal stomach pH, and hypoplastic corpus callosum.

Fabry's disease

Fabry's disease results from an enzyme defect in alpha-galactosidase A which is necessary for the degradation of glycosphingolipids. As a result, globotriaosylceramide accumulates in blood vessels and other organ tissues. It has an X-linked recessive inheritance pattern, although heterozygous female carriers can sometimes also be affected likely because of X-inactivation patterns during development. It is more common than many of the other lipid storage disorders, with an incidence of 1 in 40 000. Symptoms present in early childhood or adolescence with anhidrosis, angiokeratomas, and burning pain of the extremities especially with warm weather, fever, or exercise. Ocular corneal whirling and vortex keratopathy may also occur. Renal and cardiac complications are other systemic manifestations. The diagnosis in males is confirmed by observing a deficiency of alpha-galactosidase A in plasma or serum leukocytes or cultured skin fibroblasts. Female patients must be diagnosed by mutation testing. Treatment has been relatively successful with enzyme replacement therapy.

Mucopolysaccharidosis

This group of lysosomal disorders results from a defect in the catabolism of mucopolysaccharides. There are now six major classifications (types I–IV and VI–VII), some with subtypes based on genetic enzyme defect. Mucopolysaccharides, also now more commonly referred to as glycosaminoglycans, are large polymers composed of a core protein with carbohydrate branches. Different polymers are important constituents found in bone, cartilage, connective tissue, skin, and cornea. Not surprisingly, in many cases these organ structures are affected to various degrees in each of the subtypes of the disorders.

Mucopolysaccharidosis type I (Hurler's syndrome – type IH, Scheie's syndrome – type IS, and Hurler–Scheie syndrome – type IH/S)

Mucopolysaccharidosis type I results from an enzymatic defect in alpha-*L*-iduronidase which is essential for the metabolism of two glycosaminoglycans, heparan sulfate and dermatan sulfate. It is divided into three subtypes based on severity of clinical symptoms. All are autosomal recessive with no ethnic, regional, or sex predilection.

The most severe form is Hurler's syndrome (mucopolysaccharidosis type IH). It has an estimated incidence of 1 in 144 000 births. Affected children initially appear normal, although they may have frequent ear infections and an increased incidence of inguinal or abdominal hernia. Clinical symptoms usually present by 1 year with developmental delay, dystosis multiplex, hepatosplenomegaly, cardiomegaly, corneal opacifications, and retinal degeneration. The typical child is small with a large head and coarse facial features. The bony deformities result in short stature (usually less than 4 ft in height), a wide barrel chest, kyphosis, and short fingers prone to contractures. The face is dysmorphic with wide eyes, a depressed nasal bridge, large lips, and frontal bossing. Diagnosis can often be suspected based on these clinical characteristics, but can be confirmed either by demonstrating increased mucopolysaccharides output in urine or by assaying for alpha-*L*-iduronidase in lymphocytes or cultured fibroblasts. Untreated, the disease progresses, and death often occurs by age 10 from respiratory complications or congestive heart failure. Current treatment options have been improved by the use of bone marrow transplantation in children less than 2 years of age if the mental regression has not become severe. Enzymatic replacement therapy has also been used.

Scheie's syndrome (mucopolysaccharidosis type IS) represents the least severe clinical manifestation in the continuum of alpha-*L*-iduronidase deficiency. It has an estimated incidence of 1 in 500 000 births. Symptoms commonly occur after age 5 and are often so mild that the diagnosis is not considered until adulthood. Affected individuals have stiff joints, clouding of the cornea, and a predisposition for aortic regurgitation and carpal tunnel syndrome. Intellectual deterioration and bony abnormalities are not present and individuals live to late adulthood.

Some individuals have a clinical course and symptoms intermediate between the severity of Hurler's and Scheie's syndromes. These cases are referred to as mucopolysaccharidosis type IH/S and it has an estimated incidence of 1 in 115 000 births. Symptoms present between age 3 and 8 years with short stature, corneal clouding, joint stiffness, bony abnormalities, and hepatosplenomegaly. Although these features are shared with Hurler's syndrome, symptoms tend to be milder and progress more slowly. There is also little to no intellectual deterioration, and survival into adulthood is typical.

Mucopolysaccharidosis type II (Hunter's syndrome)

Mucopolysaccharidosis type II, also referred to as Hunter's syndrome, results from an enzyme defect in iduronate sulfatase. Like alpha-*L*-iduronidase in mucopolysaccharidosis type I, this enzyme is important in the metabolism of dermatan sulfate and heparan sulfate. Mucopolysaccharidosis type II is the only X-linked mucopolysaccharidosis. It has an estimated incidence of 1 in 110 000–165 000 male births; however, there may be a slightly higher incidence in Jewish populations in Israel. Because of its X-linked recessive inheritance, it is almost exclusively found in males, but females may present with the disease due to inactivation of the paternal allele. The disorder is divided into two subgroups (types IIA and IIB) based on the severity of the disease and the presence of mental retardation. The most severe form, type IIA, usually presents between age 2 and 4 years with mental deterioration, coarse facial features, skeletal deformities, short stature, joint stiffness, hepatosplenomegaly, seizures, hearing loss, and respiratory complications. Although retinal degeneration is present, corneal clouding (as seen in mucopolysaccharidosis type I) is usually not observed. Death from respiratory complications or cardiovascular failure usually occurs by age 15. The more mild form, type IIB, presents with more mild facial features in early childhood. Short stature, skeletal abnormalities, hepatosplenomegaly, hearing loss, retinal degeneration, cardiomegaly, and respiratory complications are usually seen but are less severe and more slowly progressive than type IIA. Intellectual deterioration is not observed, and although premature death can occur due to respiratory and cardiac dysfunction, many individuals live into the fifth decade. Diagnosis is made by demonstrating deficient enzyme activity in serum, lymphocytes, or fibroblasts. Unlike mucopolysaccharidosis type I, bone marrow transplantation does not prevent mental retardation.

Mucopolysaccharidosis type III (Sanfilippo's syndrome)

Mucopolysaccharidosis type III, also referred to as Sanfilippo's syndrome, results from a dysfunction in the catabolism of heparan sulfate. The disorder is divided into four subtypes (IIIA–D) based on distinct enzymatic gene defects. However, they are virtually indistinguishable clinically, except for possibly a slightly more severe course for type IIIA. Type IIIA results from a defect in heparan-*N*-sulfatase. Type IIIB results from a defect in *N*-acetyl-alpha-*D*-glucosaminidase. Type IIIC results from a defect in acetyl CoA alpha-glucosaminide acetyltransferase. Type IIID results from a defect in *N*-acetylglucosaminide 6-sulfate sulfatase. All are autosomal recessive with no ethnic, regional, or sex predilection. All combined subtypes have an estimated incidence of 1 in 58 000 births, making them the most common mucopolysaccharidoses. Symptoms usually present between age 2 and 5 years with developmental delay and/or regression, coarse facial features, and mild hepatosplenomegaly. Growth retardation and corneal clouding are not typically observed. As the mental deterioration progresses, aggressive behavior and sleep disturbances become a prominent feature in many cases. Diagnosis can be made in suspected clinical cases by demonstrating urinary excretion of heparan sulfate, although definitive confirmation by enzymatic assay from serum, skin fibroblasts, or lymphocytes is often needed. Death usually occurs before the age of 20 years, and bone marrow transplantation does not appear to offer any benefit.

Mucopolysaccharidosis type IV (Morquio's syndrome)

Mucopolysaccharidosis type IV, or Morquio's syndrome, results from a defect in the metabolism of keratin sulfate and chondroitin-6-sulfate. There are two subtypes that are distinguished based on the specific enzymatic defect. Type IVA results from a defect in *N*-acetylgalactosamine-6-sulfate sulfatase. Type IVB results from a deficiency of beta-galactosidase and, despite a very different clinical presentation, is an allelic variant with GM1 gangliosidosis (see below). Type IVA was previously believed to represent a more severe form, but with genetic analysis there now appears to be more overlap between the two subtypes. Both forms are autosomal recessive with an estimated incidence of 1 in 200 000, although the incidence may be higher in Northern Ireland. Symptoms usually present between age 1 and 3 years with corneal clouding, skeletal dysplasia, short stature, joint stiffness, and predisposition for spinal odontoid hypoplasia. Neurologic complications do not occur except secondarily to spinal compression from the skeletal abnormalities. Intelligence is not affected. The diagnosis is made by the presence of keratin sulfate in

urine or enzymatic assay from leukocytes or fibroblasts. In the most severe cases, individuals generally do not live past the third or fourth decade.

Mucopolysaccharidosis type VI (Maroteaux–Lamy syndrome)

This disorder results from an enzymatic deficit in arylsulfatase B. This enzyme is important for the catabolism of dermatan sulfate and chondroitin-4-sulfate. It is an autosomal recessive disorder with no ethnic, regional, or sex predilection. Its estimated incidence is 1 in 320 000 births. Clinical presentation varies widely, but the most severe form is similar to Hurler's syndrome except that intellectual function is preserved. It is diagnosed by demonstrating dermatan sulfate without heparan sulfate in the urine or by enzymatic assay. Treatment includes enzymatic replacement therapy.

Mucopolysaccharidosis type VII (Sly syndrome)

Mucopolysaccharidosis type VII, also known as Sly syndrome, results from an enzymatic defect in beta-glucuronidase which is involved in the metabolism of heparan sulfate and dermatan sulfate. It is an autosomal recessive disorder with an estimated incidence of 1 in 250 000 births. Clinical presentation varies widely, with the most severe form causing *hydrops fetalis* at birth. Others are less affected, with mild to no mental retardation, hepatosplenomegaly, and skeletal and facial abnormalities. Most children with mucopolysaccharidosis type VII live into the teenage or young adult years. Diagnosis is made with enzymatic assay from serum, leukocytes, or fibroblasts.

Glycogenoses

The glycogenoses refer to a group of disorders that result from a defect in the metabolism of glycogen. At least nine diseases have been enzymatically characterized. The three most prominent (types I, II, and V) are discussed below. All show an autosomal recessive inheritance pattern.

Glycogen storage disease type I (von Gierke's disease)

This disorder is also referred to as von Gierke's disease and it results from an enzymatic deficiency in glucose-6-phosphatase. The incidence of this disorder has been estimated at 1 in 100 000–200 000 births, without regional or ethnic predilections. Clinical symptoms usually present by the age of 2 years and include hypoglycemia, lactic acidosis, hepatomegaly, hyperlipidemia, growth failure, and joint problems. Neurologic complications include seizures and chronic brain damage usually provoked by episodes of hypoglycemia. Definitive diagnosis is made with liver biopsy. Treatment involves preventing hypoglycemia by providing a frequent source of carbohydrate.

Glycogen storage disease type II (Pompe's disease)

Pompe's disease results from a defect in acid alpha-glucosidase. It is the only glycogen storage disease that is a true lysosomal disease. It has an estimated incidence of 1 in 40 000 births; however, the highest frequency occurs in the African American population (1 per 14 000 for infantile category). Other regional areas with less well characterized common mutations have been documented in Taiwan, southern China, and the Netherlands. The pathological process is due to progressive accumulation of glycogen in skeletal muscle, heart, liver, and central nervous system (CNS). Three subgroups have been described based on age of presentation. The infantile form presents in the first months of life with feeding problems, poor weight gain, muscle weakness, and hypotonia. Development is initially normal for the first few months but slowly declines as the disease progresses. The heart is grossly enlarged due to the excess accumulation of glycogen (restrictive cardiomyopathy) and most infants die from cardiac or respiratory problems by 2 years of age. Glycogen accumulation results in progressive macroglossia which can interfere with swallowing. In the juvenile form, symptoms appear in early to late childhood. Both this form and the adult form are characterized by progressive weakness of respiratory and other skeletal muscles. While the heart may be affected, it is generally not enlarged. Intelligence is also not affected. Diagnosis is made by muscle biopsy. The current treatment is with enzyme replacement therapy. In 2006, the drug alglucosidase alfa (Myozyme) received approval from the Food and Drug Administration (FDA) for the treatment of Pompe's disease.

Glycogen storage disease type V (McArdle's disease)

This disorder, also termed McArdle's disease, is due to a deficiency in myophosphorylase. It has an estimated incidence of 1 in 100 000 births. Although it is an autosomal recessive disorder, more males have been documented. No studies have shown any regional or ethnic preference for the disorder. The disease primarily presents in the second or third decade of life, although an infantile form has been described. Symptoms include intermittent muscle pain, cramping, myogloniuria, and weakness, often relieved by rest. Differential diagnoses include Tarui disease (phosphofructokinase deficiency, glycogen storage disease type VII) and the myopathic form of carnitine palmitoyltransferase II deficiency. Muscle biopsy shows increased glycogen and deficiency in muscle phosphorylase activity. The diagnosis can also be made by nuclear MR spectroscopy.

Leukodystrophies

The leukodystrophies are a group of inheritable disorders that primarily affect the white matter of the CNS. Defects causing delayed myelination, dysmyelination, or demyelination have all been observed.

Pelizaeus–Merzbacher disease

Pelizaeus–Merzbacher disease is an X-linked recessive disorder of dysmyelination. The defect is in proteolipid protein (PLP1), which results in myelin not forming properly. The incidence has not been well described, but has been estimated at 1 in 500 000 births. It is found worldwide without any regional or ethnic predisposition. Symptoms present in infancy, usually before age 3 months, with a distinctive rotatory nystagmus. Hypotonia, poor head control, and delayed motor and cognitive development are also seen. Eventually, spasticity, optic atrophy, and mental retardation occur. Diagnosis is made based on X-linked inheritance in the right clinical setting with abnormalities of white matter on MRI. The diagnosis can be confirmed with fluorescent *in situ* hybridization using a planar langmuir probe (PLP). There is no effective treatment for this condition.

Cockayne's syndrome

Cockayne's syndrome is an autosomal recessive demyelinating leukodystrophy that results from a defect involved in transcription regulated DNA repair. There are at least two variants (types I and II) based on genotype. It is rare, with an estimated incidence of less than 1 in 250 000 births, with no specific regional or ethnic predilection. It is a progressive disorder characterized by abnormal facial features of large ears and sunken eyes, premature aging, failure of growth starting by age 2, progressive intellectual deterioration, pigmentary retinal degeneration, and hypersensitivity of skin to sunlight. There is no effective treatment other than symptomatic care. Death usually occurs in adolescence, although survival into adulthood is possible.

Alexander's disease

Alexander's disease results from a defect in glial fibrillary acidic protein (GFAP). The infantile form accounts for 80% of cases, although juvenile and adult forms can be present. It is very rare, with less than 300 cases reported, and no studies have suggested a regional or ethnic predilection. Most cases are sporadic, although an autosomal dominant inheritance pattern can also be seen, especially in the adult form. In the infantile form, symptoms usually present by 6 months with macrocephaly (see Canavan's disease, below), seizures, spasticity, and psychomotor and cognitive decline. MRI imaging shows extensive cerebral white matter signal changes with a frontal predominance. Histopathologic examination shows a distinctive pattern of Rosenthal fibers. Diagnosis is made by a combination of neuroimaging and gene analysis in the correct clinical context. There is no effective treatment for this disorder and death usually occurs by the first decade.

Canavan's disease

Canavan's disease is an autosomal recessive leukodystrophy that results from a defect in the enzyme aspartoacylase which hydrolyzes *N*-acetylaspartic acid to *L*-aspartic acid. The disorder is present worldwide, but is more common in Ashkenazi Jewish populations where carrier rates as high as 1 in 40 have been observed. There may also be a higher incidence in families from Saudi Arabia, although this is less well documented. Symptoms present usually by 3–6 months with macrocephaly (see Alexander's disease, above), hypotonia, optic atrophy, and psychomotor and mental retardation. Over time, seizures and progressive spasticity occur. Diagnosis is confirmed by demonstrating increased *N*-acetylaspartic acid in plasma, urine, or brain (by MR spectroscopy). There is no effective treatment. Death usually occurs by the age of 4 years, although some children survive into the second and third decade.

Krabbe's disease (globoid cell leukodystrophy)

This is an autosomal recessive leukodystrophy resulting from a defect in degrading galactocerebrosides. It also can be categorized as a cerebrosidosis, but is included here because of its specific pattern of white matter pathology. The specific enzymatic defect is galactosylceramidase (galactocerebroside-beta-galactosidase). It has an estimated worldwide incidence of 1 in 100 000 births, although in an isolated Druze community in Israel a much higher incidence of 6 in 1000 births has been reported. The incidence may also be slightly higher in Sweden, with a reported incidence of 1.8 in 100 000 births. The most common presentation occurs in infancy, although juvenile and adult forms also occur. The infantile form is characterized by onset before 6 months, with irritability, decreased psychomotor and cognitive development, seizures, muscle weakness, spasticity, deafness, and optic atrophy. Diagnosis is made by typical white matter changes on neuroimaging (deep white matter signal abnormalities in cerebrum and cerebellum: increase in T2, decrease in T1) and showing near absence of beta-galactosidase activity in leukocyte or skin fibroblasts. Peripheral nerve involvement in the infantile form seems to be very early and is demonstrable by electrodiagnostics. Histopathological analysis also shows distinctive globoid cells near blood vessels of altered white matter. Untreated, the prognosis for the infantile form is poor with death usually occurring before age 2. The prognosis has improved somewhat with early bone marrow transplantation and umbilical cord transplantation although the best outcomes have occurred in the more mild juvenile and adult forms.

Metachromic leukodystrophy

Metachromic leukodystrophy results from a defect in the enzyme arylsulfatase A which is required to hydrolyze sulfatides to cerebrosides. The disorder has an estimated worldwide incidence of 1 in 40 000 births, making it one of the more common leukodystrophies. Higher incidences have been reported in the western region of the Navajo nation, with an incidence of 1 in 2520 births, and also less well described isolated Arab groups in Israel. The most common form occurs in infancy, although juvenile and adult forms also have been characterized. In the infantile form symptoms present with psychomotor retardation, developmental delay, muscle wasting, progressive loss of vision, and seizures. Death usually occurs by age 5. Diagnosis is confirmed by demonstrating reduced arylsulfatase-A activity in leukocytes. Peripheral nerve involvement is common, and the nomenclature for this disease reflects the early observation of metachromasia (failure to stain "true" with a given stain, brown coloration with cresyl violet in this case) in peripheral nerve biopsy specimens. There have been some promising results of delaying the progression of this disorder with bone marrow transplantation.

Adrenal leukodystrophy

Adrenal leukodystrophy is an X-linked peroxisomal disorder resulting in a defect in catabolism of very long chain fatty acids (VLCFA). The gene responsible is that for the D1 subtype of the ATP-binding cassette (ABCD1) which encodes a protein, ALDP, which is a member of the ATP-binding cassette transport system family. This protein is involved in the transport of fatty acids into peroxisomes. Because of the defect, fatty acid chains with 24–30 carbon atoms cannot undergo beta-oxidation and accumulate in a variety of tissues. This disease is the most common sudanophilic leukodystrophy, with an incidence of 1 in 20 000 individuals. There is no regional or ethnic predilection. Three forms have been described based on age and severity of neurologic symptoms. The most common form occurs between the ages of 5 and 10 years and presents with behavioral changes (either withdrawal or increased aggression), developmental regression, ataxia, seizures, adrenal insufficiency, and degeneration of visual and auditory systems. It is rapidly progressive and if untreated usually results in death or vegetative state by an early age. The second form, termed adrenomyeloneuropathy (AMN), has its onset in the third or fourth decade and is characterized by slowly progressive paraparesis. The third form is Addison's disease and usually presents in adulthood as isolated adrenal insufficiency without neurologic symptoms. Diagnosis is made by measuring high levels of VLCFA in serum and cultured fibroblasts. In classic X-liked ALD, MRI shows pathognomonic increased T2 signal bilaterally in the occipital white matter. The disease is treated with either bone marrow transplantation or dietary modification with Lorenzo's Oil. The discovery of this dietary supplement was described in the popular film of the same name.

Refsum's disease

Refsum's disease (hereditary motor sensory neuropathy IV) results from a defect in phytanoly-coenzyme A hydroxylase which is involved in degrading phytanic acid. It is a rare disorder, with only 60 published cases worldwide, and no specific regional or ethnic predilections have been reported. It typically presents in children aged 2–7 years with peripheral neuropathy, increased night blindness due to retinal degeneration, anosmia, cerebellar degeneration, itchthyosis, skeletal abnormalities, and cardiac arrythmias. Diagnosis is made by demonstrating a high level of phytanic acid in serum. Treatment involves diet restriction of all foods with high levels of phytanic acid including beef, lamb, and fatty fish.

Other lipidoses

There are two specific lipidoses that are often considered separately from the lysosomal lipid storage diseases. Rather than resulting from an enzymatic defect in a specific lysosomal degradative enzyme, these disorders result from a more fundamental error in lipid metabolic processing.

Abetalipoproteinemia

Abetalipoproteinemia, also termed Bassen–Kornzweig syndrome, is a rare autosomal recessive disorder that results in the complete lack of serum beta-lipoproteins. This is due to a decreased function in a microsomal triglyceride transfer protein that mediates the transfer of lipid molecules in the endoplasmic reticulum to nascent lipoprotein particles, including chylomicrons, very low density lipoproteins, and low density lipoproteins. As a consequence, absorption of fat and fat-soluble vitamins is deficient. The incidence of this condition has not been well established, although the carrier rate in one Ashkenazi Jewish population is 1 in 131 individuals. Symptoms present in the first year of life with failure to thrive, abdominal distention, diarrhea, and steatorrhea. Peripheral blood smears will show acanthocytosis. Neurologic symptoms usually present between the age of 2 and 17 years. Initially patients present with ataxia, proprioceptive loss, muscle weakness, and retinal degeneration resulting in night blindness. Imaging shows progressive combined posterior column degeneration. Approximately one-third of patients will develop mental retardation. The neurologic symptoms are primarily due to the resultant vitamin E deficiency. Treatment involves supplementing vitamin E (100 mg/kg/day orally) to prevent the development or progression of neurologic or retinal deficits.

Tangier disease

Tangier disease is a rare autosomal recessive disorder characterized by a deficiency in high-density lipoprotein. Only 50 cases have been identified worldwide. The name is derived from the island off the coast of Virginia where the first two patients were discovered; however, the disorder has now been observed in other countries as well. The defect responsible for this disease is the ATP-binding cassette transporter 1 (ABCA1) transporter which is responsible for transporting cholesterol and phospholipids from inside the cell into the bloodstream. The most distinct symptom is the enlargement of the tonsils which appear orange or yellow. Other symptoms include hepatosplenomegaly, early atherosclerosis, corneal clouding, retinitis pigmentosa, and peripheral neuropathy.

Further reading

Kolter T, Sandhoff K. Sphingolipid metabolism diseases. *Biochim Biophys Acta* 2006; 1758(12): 2057–79.

Lyon G, Fattal-Valevski A, Kolodny EH. Leukodystrophies: clinical and genetic aspects. *Top Magn Reson Imaging* 2006; 17(4): 219–42.

Meikle PJ, Hopwood JJ, Clague AE, Carey WF. Prevalence of lysosomal storage disorders. *JAMA* 1999; 281(3): 249–54.

Menkes JH, Sarnat HB, Maria BL, editors. *Child Neurology*, 7th ed. Baltimore: Lippincott Williams and Wilkins; 2006.

Mole SE, Williams RE, Goebel HH. Correlations between genotype, ultrastructural morphology and clinical phenotype in the neuronal ceroid lipofuscinoses. *Neurogenetics* 2005; 6(3): 107–26.

Muenzer J. The mucopolysaccharidoses: a heterogeneous group of disorders with variable pediatric presentations. *J Pediatr* 2004; 144(5 Suppl): S27–34.

Poorthuis BJ, Wevers RA, Kleijer WJ, *et al.* The frequency of lysosomal storage diseases in the Netherlands. *Hum Genet* 1999; 105(1–2): 151–6.

Chapter 158
Disorders of amino acid, organic acid, and ammonia metabolism

Stephen Cederbaum
University of California, Los Angeles, USA

Introduction and general principles

Inborn errors of amino acids and organic acids are a subgroup of genetic disorders that involve the transformation of metabolites in the body. Amino acid and organic acid pathways involve small molecules that generally are ingested in the diet or are the result of tissue breakdown during the catabolism that accompanies a variety of acute intercurrent illnesses. These disorders are generally inherited in an autosomal recessive manner, although some are sex-linked. Like all genetic diseases, their severity is dependent on the degree of enzyme deficiency caused by the specific mutation, and the input of other genetic and environmental influences that are difficult to identify and quantify.

Neonatal disorders

Maple syrup urine disease
Introduction

Maple syrup urine disease, sometimes referred to as maple syrup disease, is caused by a genetic deficiency in branched-chain keto acid decarboxylase, an enzyme complex that is responsible for the decarboxylation of the keto acids of the three branched-chain amino acids, leucine, isoleucine, and valine. Its name derives from the odor given off by a byproduct of isoleucine accumulation that has the sweet smell which to North Americans resembles the smell of maple syrup. The odor may be particularly apparent on the skin and in the earwax. The three branched-chain amino acids accumulate in the body with leucine predominating, and the symptoms appear to correlate most closely with the level of leucine, although the precise pathogenic mechanism is not known.

Epidemiology

The disorder is infrequent (1 per 180 000 newborns) in a randomly mating population, but has a higher prevalence

International Neurology: A Clinical Approach. Edited by Robert P. Lisak, Daniel D. Truong, William M. Carroll, and Roongroj Bhidayasiri. © 2009 Blackwell Publishing, ISBN: 978-1-4051-5738-4.

in some inbred groups such as the Old Order Amish and their Mennonite brethren who migrated from Switzerland and Germany in the eighteenth century.

Clinical presentation

In the most severe form, onset occurs in the neonatal period and symptoms progress rapidly, due to complete or nearly complete enzymatic deficiency. The infants appear normal at birth but then begin to deteriorate neurologically and become flaccid, alternating with hypertonicity and eventually with opisthotonic posturing. The cry becomes high pitched and the patients become unresponsive and are dependent completely on intravenous or enteral tube feeding. Seizures and lethargy can be accompanied by severly abnormal electroencephalogram (EEG). Spikes, polyspikes, triphasic waves, severe slowing, and even bouts of a burst–suppression pattern may be seen. It is in these more severely affected patients where the odor of maple syrup is most likely to occur.

With greater residual enzyme activity onset may be delayed for weeks or months and the severity of the neurological illness may be diminished. The most mildly affected patients may go undiagnosed and be asymptomatic for years or suffer from such mild episodes of intoxication that they are likely to be ascribed to some non-genetic cause. Despite this, severe catabolism can cause a sufficient accumulation of leucine so that the brain edema that results can be fatal. It is noteworthy that specialists in inborn errors are not infrequently confronted with healthy infants who have an odor resembling maple syrup. Their plasma amino acid levels are normal and the condition appears to be due to something in their environment, as least one of which is the herb fenugreek.

Diagnosis

If not picked up in the new, expanded newborn screening by tandem mass spectrometry (MS/MS), the diagnosis is relatively easy to make. Plasma amino acid determination reveals high levels of leucine, isoleucine, and valine, the former sometimes rising as high as 3000–4000 μM (normal value below 300 in all laboratories). An isomer of isoleucine, alloisoleucine, is present in virtually all patients and is pathognomonic for the disorder. Organic

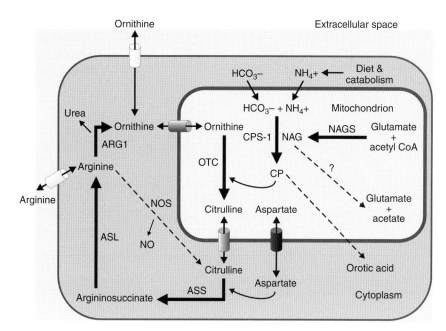

Figure 158.1 The urea cycle. Depicted are the six enzymes of the urea cycle in bold arrows. The first three enzymes, NAGS (*N*-acetylglutamate synthase), CPS-1 (carbamylphosphate synthase-1) and OTC (ornithine transcarbamylase) all function in the mitochondrion, whereas the next three, ASS (argininosuccinate synthase), ASL (argininosuccinate lyase) and ARG1 (arginase 1) function in the cytosol. Two distinct transporters are known, those for ornithine and aspartate, each of which are depicted and deficiency of which causes symptomatic disease. The mode of citrulline egress from the mitochondrion is uncertain, but may utilize the ornithine transporter. There is no known disorder of citrulline egress from the mitochondrion. Other compounds moving in or out of the cell and the mitochondrion are depicted as well.

acid analysis of urine reveals the keto acids of these three amino acids as the proximate product behind the site of the block. Ketones are detected in the urine during routine urinalysis.

Treatment

Acute episodes occurring in the immediate postnatal period or periodically thereafter are medical emergencies. It is essential that plasma levels of leucine be reduced rapidly and effectively. This is accomplished in two ways used separately or together. The first and usually quite reliable method is to feed an amino acid mixture lacking the branch-chain amino acid precursors of the deficient enzyme step. This should be undertaken with the help of a metabolic disease specialist to prevent catabolic consequences.

The second approach to lowering the amino acid levels is hemodialysis, dialysis that effectively removes the excess branch-chain amino acids (as well as the others present in normal amounts) from the body fluid space. The most effective method of dialysis is hemodialysis. This must be used in conjunction with proper nutritional support or else body protein catabolism will occur and the salutary effect will be lost.

Treatment of intercurrent catabolic episodes or of those patients presenting later in life is simpler. These events can often be managed with fluid and electrolyte support and administration of non-branch-chain amino acids. As with the treatment of all inborn errors, attention to adequate caloric intake, the prevention of constipation, and special intervention during intercurrent illness are required.

Urea cycle disorders
Introduction

The urea cycle (Figure 158.1) is an eight-step cycle consisting of six enzymes operating sequentially and two transporters, all of which are essential for the conversion of ammonia, generated from either endogenous or exogenous amino acids, to urea.

The six enzymes are *N*-acetylglutamate synthase, carbamylphosphate synthase I, ornithine transcarbamylase (OTC), argininosuccinate synthase, argininosuccinate lyase, and arginase. The two transporters are both in the mitochondrial membrane, one transporting ornithine and the other transporting aspartate into the mitochondrion. Complete absence of any of the first five enzymes in the cycle results in severe neonatal hyperammonemia, rapid neurological deterioration, coma, and then death. Like other inborn errors of metabolism, it cannot be distinguished from a variety of other acute conditions of the neonatal period such as sepsis or perinatal hypoxia. A plasma ammonia determination which if elevated, accompanied by relatively normal electrolyte balance, is highly suggestive of such a disorder.

Epidemiology

Seven of the eight disorders of the urea cycle are inherited in an autosomal recessive manner, whereas ornithine transcarbamylase deficiency is inherited in a sex-linked codominant manner. A moderately large minority of female carriers of OTCD have protein intolerance or worse and some may die or suffer permanent brain damage from hyperammonemia, particularly during parturition. With

Table 158.1 Neurological manifestations of urea cycle disorders. (Adapted from Gropman AL, Summar M, Leonard JV. Neurological implications of urea cycle disorders. *J Inher Metab Dis* 2007; 30: 865–9.)

Classic proximal urea cycle defects	Partial enzyme deficiencies
Anorexia	Protein aversion
Vomiting	Hyperactive behavior
Cognitive and motor deficits	Self-injurious behavior
Lethargy	Stroke-like episodes
Ataxia	Psychiatric symptoms
Asterixis	
Brain edema	
Cytotoxic and vasogenic edema	
Hypothermia	
Seizures	
Coma	

the possible exception of deficiency of the aspartate transporter (citrin deficiency) which may be more prominent in people of Japanese ethnicity, none of the disorders has any particular ethnic or geographic predilection.

Clinical presentation
Patients may present with ataxia, tremors, asterixis, slurred speech, or seizures and may progress to lethargy and obtundation. Those with partial deficiencies may exhibit learning disabilities, hyperactivity, and psychiatric disorders. Sometimes a history of protein aversion may be elicited (see Table 158.1).

Pathophysiology and treatment
Severe neonatal hyperammonemia constitutes a medical emergency and must be addressed immediately. The ammonia and glutamine levels (which are in approximate equilibrium) must be reduced as rapidly as possible and prior to any determination of the precise site of the block. The most effective means of carrying this out is by hemodialysis, which is more effective than peritoneal dialysis and certainly more effective than exchange transfusion which has little utility or efficacy. In some larger centers, intravenous sodium benzoate combined with sodium phenylacetate is available and may be used to divert the ammonia from the urea cycle and to be excreted as benzoylglycine and/or phenylacetylglutamine. The resynthesis of glycine and glutamine in the body will then utilize one or two molecules of ammonia destined for the urea cycle in this synthetic reaction. Nutritional support with guidance by a metabolic specialist can prevent the development of a catabolic state during treatment.

Hyperammonemia is the cause of the brain damage, possibly acting through glutamine with which it is in equilibrium. The most obvious and visible effect of ammonia intoxication is cerebral edema, although a number of

other pathological mechanisms may be operating simultaneously. The degree of neurologic damage correlates best with the length of time the patient spends in coma and to a much lesser degree with the level of ammonia. Few patients escape severe neonatal hyperammonemia without permanent neurologic injury.

Chronic treatment consists of adequate calories and fluids, and a diet low in natural protein and supplemented by essential amino acid formula and sodium phenylbutyrate. Phenylbutyrate is metabolized quite rapidly to phenylacetate which is then conjugated to glutamine as described above. In developing countries phenylbutyrate may prove to be too expensive or otherwise unavailable, but sodium benzoate, readily available and inexpensive, may be a suitable, albeit less effective, substitute.

Propionic and methylmalonic *acidemia*

Introduction
These two disorders involve sequential steps in the disposition of the carbon skeletons of four amino acids, threonine, methionine, isoleucine, and valine. Defects in either propionyl CoA-carboxylase or methylmalonyl CoA mutase cause the propionic acid or methylmalonic acid to accumulate behind the site of the block. Because propionic acid is a precursor of methylmalonic acid it accumulates as well in methylmalonic acidemia. These metabolites are toxic to the brain, heart, and bone marrow and can cause severe illness and death in their most severe form. Methylmalonyl CoA mutase requires an activated form of vitamin B_{12} as a cofactor. This B_{12} gets to the site of action only after having undergone a series of metabolic steps. Inherited defects in any of these steps may also cause methylmalonic acidemia. The most common of these defects is referred to as cobalamin C deficiency and is characterized by elevated body fluid levels of both methylmalonic acid and homocysteine. Remethylation of homocysteine to methionine also requires an activated form of vitamin B_{12} and shares many metabolic steps with that which serves as a cofactor for the mutase reaction.

Epidemiology
Like any autosomal recessive disorder, forms of propionic and methylmalonic acidemia may be found in increased frequency in population isolates and/or in populations that practice cousin marriage as a social custom. No large ethnic predilection has been described for either condition.

Pathophysiology and clinical features
The largest number of patients with both disorders have severe enzyme deficiencies and present in the newborn period. Initial symptoms include decreased suck, poor feeding, irritability, hypotonia, seizures, and lethargy

which progresses to stupor and coma. In the past when these conditions were poorly recognized, death ensued in most instances. Other manifestations include bone marrow depression, acidosis, hyperammonemia, hypotonia, and cardiac failure. The signs and symptoms may mimic neonatal sepsis and the neonatologist should be alert to the possibility of conditions like this, particularly in suspected cases of sepsis that are atypical in one or another of their manifestations.

In those countries and jurisdictions in which newborn screening using tandem mass spectrometry (MS/MS) is usual, the majority of patients with these disorders will be ascertained by an elevation in C3 carnitine esters on the dried blood spot. In these jurisdictions, the level of suspicion in patients who have had a successful newborn screen will be altered and the position of these disorders on the list of diagnostic possibilities will be lowered.

Laboratory abnormalities found in these disorders include metabolic acidosis with an increased anion gap, elevated blood lactate, ketonuria, hyperammonemia, and bone marrow depression. Ketonuria in a newborn is exceedingly rare and is a telltale sign of a disorder of organic acid metabolism.

The pathophysiology of these conditions is not known with certainty. The resemblance between propionyl CoA and acetyl CoA is great and propionyl CoA is thought to compete with acetyl CoA for the active site of enzymes using the latter substrate, particularly the biosynthesis of acetylglutamate and activation of the urea cycle.

Treatment and management

In the initial phases of diagnosis, the two disorders may be indistinguishable until the results of newborn screening or diagnostic urinary organic acid analysis becomes available. The treatment will, therefore, be generic, seeking to reduce the level of accumulated toxic metabolite and simultaneously diminishing the production of the offending compound. The most effective way of lowering the levels of either of these readily excreted organic acids, which could accumulate rapidly in the period of catabolism following birth, is by dialysis. The most effective form of dialysis is hemodialysis, but when this is not available peritoneal dialysis is an acceptable alternative. Exchange transfusion is largely ineffective. Treatment should include vitamin B_{12} 1000 mg intramuscularly daily until it is demonstrated that the patient does not have a vitamin B_{12}-responsive form of methylmalonic acidemia. Intravenous carnitine 300 mg/kg is a frequently recommended adjunct to therapy. The usual supportive measures of maintenance of electrolyte balance and hydration are important in these patients and in general follow nursery routine.

Infants rescued from the most acute manifestations of these disorders will often have suffered irreversible neurologic damage and may over a period of years show mental retardation, growth delay, and a variety of neurologic handicaps. Remarkably, some patients who have suffered grievously in the newborn period do remarkably well developmentally and may go on to live normal or near-normal lives. Most patients will, after rescue, continue to make developmental progress and may achieve varying degrees of independence in aspects of daily life. These patients are prone, particularly in infancy and early childhood, to episodes of metabolic deterioration usually caused by intercurrent infection. The cause of these less frequent episodes in later life may not be apparent. Both propionic and methylmalonic acids are "anorectogenic" probably due to chemically-induced pyloric stenosis. As a consequence most patients require some or virtually all of their enteral feeding through a gastrostomy tube, at least in infancy and for the first decade of life.

Adequate calories, a diet limited in the precursors of these organic acids, prevention of constipation, carnitine supplementation, and metronidazole (to decrease the load of gut bacteria which generate propionic acid) are mainstays of long-term therapy.

In all disorders of metabolism, partial enzyme defects due to less severe mutations in the gene may result in attenuated disease. This more mild disease may manifest as chronic low-level intoxication resulting in little to moderate brain damage, may cause later onset severe metabolic deterioration in response to catabolic stress, or may not manifest until later in life in response to such events as pregnancy and parturition. The physician should always be alert to the possibility that a metabolic disorder lies behind undiagnosed cases of developmental delay or recurring episodes of acute encephalopathy.

Progressive diseases of infancy and childhood

In contrast to the disorders described above, a number of metabolic disorders are characterized by the absence of acute manifestations in the newborn period, but rather by progressive or more insidious developmental delay or neurological handicap. This section describes these disorders.

Phenylketonuria (deficiency of phenylalanine hydroxylase)
Introduction
The most common of these metabolic disorders in Western European countries, the United States, Canada, and China, among countries in which accurate statistics are available, is phenylketonuria (PKU), a disorder caused by deficiency of the enzyme phenylalanine hydroxylase. When deficiency of this enzyme is complete or nearly so, plasma phenylalanine rises to levels of 1200 μM or more when the patient is ingesting breast milk or an otherwise

normal diet. This causes no obvious immediate symptoms but the intoxicating effect is insidious. Depending on the individual patient and the astuteness of the parent and/or the physician, manifestations become apparent between 6 months and 1 year of age, by which time some degree of irreversible neurologic damage has occurred.

Lesser degrees of enzyme deficiency lead to lower levels of plasma phenylalanine accumulation and correspondingly lower levels of jeopardy for short- or longer-term neurologic damage. Although normally newborn phenylalanine levels in blood fall rapidly to the adult ones of 100 μM or less, individual patients may tolerate levels up to 600 μM or slightly more without apparent neurologic damage, although there is some suspicion that these individuals may be prone to higher incidence of learning disability or attention deficit disorder.

PKU was the flagship disorder for which newborn screening was developed by Robert Guthrie. When properly carried out, nearly all individuals with PKU can be detected by an elevation in blood phenylalanine and/or by an elevated phenylalanine/tyrosine ratio after 24 hours of age, and pre-emptive therapy can be instituted. Evidence suggests that virtually all of these individuals will be protected from overt neurologic damage and mental retardation and may be allowed to achieve success in professions requiring higher cognitive function such as academics, medicine, law, and others. Evidence also suggests that the brain is continuously vulnerable to high phenylalanine levels and that the therapy (described below) will have to be life-long.

The advent of newborn screening and effective therapy for PKU is one of the great success stories in the field of metabolic disorders. It has taken a disorder in which the incidence of mental retardation was virtually 100% and has reduced it to the background level found in the population. It has raised, however, the specter of maternal PKU. In this disorder, normal women with PKU and high phenylalanine levels are at risk of having children who become intoxicated *in utero* and who suffer a variety of adverse effects including microcephaly, mental retardation (virtually universally), and, in 15% of instances, congenital heart defects. The imperative for female patients to stay on the diet is therefore increased.

Epidemiology
The incidence of PKU varies greatly between countries and ethnic groups. Aside from genetic isolates such as a group of gypsies (travelers) in Great Britain, the frequency varies between about 1 in 4000 births in Ireland, to 1 in 100 000 in Japan, to virtually undetectable levels in Finland and amongst Ashkenazi Jews.

Clinical features
Untreated PKU has become a virtual historical oddity in those places where newborn screening is routine.

A report from Asia described West's syndrome in 10.9% of those who did not receive dietary therapy in the first 3 months, and 15.9% in those whose dietary management was delayed till 12 months of age. MRIs showed delayed myelination and increased T2 signal in the periventricular regions. Even many metabolic specialists are unfamiliar with the clinical features of mental retardation, a withdrawn autistic-like demeanor, spasticity, a "mousey" odor, and pigment dilution in hair and skin. With treatment the average IQ is near normal, but some patients, even when well treated, have an increased incidence of attention deficit disorder and academic difficulties.

Treatment
The diet is simple, effective, and onerous. The maintenance of the diet requires continuous discipline on the part of the family and, as the patient grows older and assumes greater responsibility for his or her own care, on the part of that individual as well. This therapy currently consists almost exclusively of diet. All high-protein foods must be eliminated since the average individual, particularly in countries that ingest a relatively higher protein diet, may consume about three times as much phenylalanine as is required by the body for growth and maintenance. The natural food component of the diet, therefore, consists of fruits and vegetables with low protein content and now special foods such as breads, pastas, and rice from which protein has been removed as well. This diet, if ingested without supplementation of the other amino acids handled normally, would cause malnutrition. The missing nutrients are made up of special amino acid formulas from which phenylalanine has either been removed or to which it has not been added.

More recently, it has been discovered that a fraction of patients with phenylalanine hydroxylase deficiency may respond with increased enzyme activity to the addition of tetrahydrobiopterin (BH$_4$), the natural cofactor in the phenylalanine hydroxylase reaction (see below). This increases phenylalanine hydroxylase activity and increases the degree of tolerance to phenylalanine in these patients. About 10% of patients with severe phenylalanine hydroxylase deficiency may be responsive in whole or in part to this treatment; approximately half with more moderate phenylalanine elevations on a natural diet may be responsive, and the majority of those with phenylalanine levels under 600 μM on a normal diet will respond. This expensive product has been available in Europe and Japan for a number of years and was approved by the Food and Drug Administration in the United States in 2007. All patients detected with elevated phenylalanine in the newborn period will undergo a trial of BH$_4$ prior to the institution of diet and those who are responsive will, in those venues that can afford it, be maintained on this therapy while receiving no special diet or one that is far less stringent.

Homocystinuria (homocystinemia)
Introduction
Classical homocystinuria was first described in 1968, simultaneously in retarded infants and in adults seen in an ophthalmology clinic. The latter are individuals who, for reasons unknown, escaped the retardation that often occurs in homocystinuria due to cystathionine β-synthase deficiency and who only later manifested a characteristic feature of the disorder, lens dislocation. Subsequently, those affected in an intermediate manner manifesting retardation at variable ages were found as well. The cardinal biochemical features are greatly elevated methionine in the blood and greatly elevated homocysteine in the blood and the urine.

Methionine is a critical amino acid in the body, playing a role not only in protein synthesis but also as a major methyl group donor in methylation reactions including the synthesis of neurotransmitters. The product of these methylation reactions is homocysteine which may have two fates in the body. During periods of low or no methionine intake, a fraction of homocysteine that may be high as 50% is remethylated to methionine to allow physiologic methylation reactions to continue. The other variable fraction is metabolized by cystathionine β-synthase, ultimately ending up as cysteine, another important but non-essential amino acid, and the excess as part of the carbon pool and as sulfate. Thus, lower levels of cysteine are a characteristic feature of homocystinuria.

Disorders of remethylation of homocysteine to methionine have been mentioned previously in the discussion of the methylmalonic acidemia. While many, if not most, members of this family of disorders are ascertained by the elevated levels of plasma and urine levels of methylmalonic acid, the others that involve homocysteine accumulation alone must be found through increased levels of this metabolite or sometimes by low methionine levels.

Epidemiology
Cystathionine β-synthase deficiency is far less frequent than PKU and less is known about its population frequency in various countries. Therefore no general ethnic predilection is known.

Clinical manifestations
The symptoms of cystathionine β-synthase deficiency alone will be discussed as they are more distinctive than those of the remethylation defects which share with it only the homocysteine-related predilection for precocious arterial and venous thrombosis. The cardinal clinical manifestations of "classical" homocystinuria are a thin and marfanoid-like habitus, mental retardation in a significant fraction of affected patients, a predisposition to arterial and venous thromboses (elevated risk of stroke), osteopenia, and dislocation of the ocular lenses. It is easily ascertained by the hypermethioninemia, although accurate levels of homocysteine require an independent study in which the sulfhydryl bonds between homocysteine and the plasma proteins are broken. It cannot be reliably diagnosed by MS/MS-based newborn screening.

Treatment
Treatment when ascertained in infancy is a rigid low-methionine diet with supplementation by a dietary product from which this amino acid is excluded. This diet is more rigorous and onerous than those for many other metabolic disorders and long-term compliance is difficult. However, outcome in early treated patients may be quite good. Instituting this rigorous diet in adulthood is extremely problematic and compliance is rarely very good. Because of the tendency toward precocious thrombosis, the use of aspirin and other antiplatelet aggregation medications is indicated. Prophylaxis for venous thrombosis is rarely specifically undertaken. In addition, betaine is useful in providing an alternative pathway from homocysteine back to methionine and may work in an adjunctive fashion to lower the toxic levels of homocysteine. High levels of methionine are far less likely to be intoxicating or cause symptoms. The remethylation defects too respond to treatment with betaine, vitamin B_{12}, and antiplatelet adhesion therapy. Folate supplementation is used in all of the hyperhomocysteinemias.

Disorders of lysine and tryptophan metabolism: glutaric acidemia, type I
Introduction
Although a number of disorders in the breakdown of lysine are known, glutaric acidemia alone appears to have severe clinical consequences. This disorder, due to a deficiency of glutaryl CoA dehydrogenase, may present in the newborn period, but more commonly presents with acute and devastating symptoms at a later stage in infancy and in association with intercurrent infection or less frequently another type of catabolic event. This should be distinguished from glutaric acidemia, type II, which is a disorder resulting from multiple acyl-coenzyme A dehydrogenase deficiency. Biochemically, type I glutaric acidemia is characterized by the accumulation of glutarate, 3-hydroxyglutarate and glutarylcarnitine in blood and glutarate and 3-hydroxyglutarate in the urine. Unfortunately, some patients may have very low plasma and urine levels of these metabolites outside of the times when they are in metabolic crisis. Most but not all affected infants are picked up on newborn screening by MS/MS technology, and pre-emptive therapy is an important factor in eliminating or reducing the pathological

consequences of this disorder. Newborn screening by MS/MS has, however, led to the diagnosis of a number of patients who never experience a metabolic crisis and no apparent intellectual or neurological deficit.

Epidemiology

Like maple syrup disease this disorder appears in high frequency in the Old Order Amish community. It is also more frequent in the Ojibway tribe of Canadian Indians. No other ethnic or national predilection is known.

Pathophysiology and clinical features

Much effort has been invested in understanding the pathophysiology of this condition, but despite the availability of a reasonably faithful knockout mouse model, it remains to be elucidated. Genotype–phenotype correlation is poor and the plasma and urine levels of glutarate do not seem to be an accurate gauge of the severity of clinical symptoms.

The majority of symptomatic patients present with macrocephaly, hypotonia, and a basal ganglia-type injury resulting in dystonia and athetosis. In some, spasticity eventually develops. The patients may be more devastated neurologically than they are cognitively, although many affected individuals are mentally retarded as well. Seizures may occur, although they are not a defining part of the phenotype. In contrast to many other inborn errors of metabolism, there may be a characteristic MRI picture suggesting corticovenous lakes as a prominent feature and perhaps as a contributor to the macrocephaly that occurs. Macrocephaly may occur in asymptomatic patients.

Treatment

Therapy consists of a semisynthetic low-lysine diet and great care in the prevention of acute episodes of deterioration. Families are urged to come to the emergency room very quickly upon the onset of infection and evidence that fluid and food intake are diminishing or that the level of alertness is decreased. Supportive intravenous therapy with 10% glucose and insulin may prevent the development of acute neurologic deterioration. A distinctive feature of this disorder in contrast to many others is the relative immunity to further neurologic damage after emergence from infancy and almost invariably after the age of 5 or 6. Carnitine and riboflavin supplementation is frequently used but has never been subjected to rigorous study.

Biotinidase deficiency
Introduction

Biotin is an essential vitamin whose requirement is mitigated by its reuse in the body. In normal metabolism, biotin is bound covalently to lysine groups on a number of enzymes which carboxylate carbon skeletons; these include propionyl CoA carboxylase, methylcrotonyl CoA carboxylase, pyruvate carboxylase, and acetyl CoA carboxylase. When these enzymes are degraded, the biotinilated lysine or biocytin releases free biotin to be reutilized in a reaction catalyzed by biotinidase. In the absence of biotinidase, the biocytin is lost in the urine and the body becomes biotin deficient.

Pathophysiology

Patients with biotinidase deficiency excrete variable amounts of the precursors of each of the impaired enzymatic reactions and these were thought to be toxic. More recently a far broader role for biotin in the regulation of gene expression has been found, so that the breadth of metabolic derangements that might be involved in the disease pathogenesis has grown.

Clinical features

Biotinidase deficiency rarely presents with symptoms in the neonatal period. The symptoms usually begin in the first few months of life and consist of skin rashes, alopecia, visual difficulties, hearing difficulties leading to deafness, and ultimately a neurologic syndrome, developmental delay, and retardation. In one series, 55% of the symptomatic children had seizures. In 38% of the enzyme-deficient patients, seizures were the presenting symptom. Patients may lose the ability to walk and become mute.

Biotinidase is easy to measure and is now a part of many newborn screening programs. Generally, in individuals with biotinidase activity 10% or more of normal are usually free of symptoms; lesser levels of activity occurring in about 1 in 100 000 in many Western populations are generally required for the development of overt symptoms. In addition to the deficiency of biotinidase in plasma, the enzymatic defects that occur in consequence of deficiency of the normal cofactor for the above-mentioned enzymatic reactions lead to an abnormal acylcarnitine profile in plasma and urinary organic acid abnormalities in which metabolites of propionyl CoA carboxylase, of methylcrotonyl CoA carboxylase and pyruvate carboxylase accumulate. Unfortunately, the accumulation of these metabolites is variable and occurs after infancy and is not a reliable means of ascertaining this disorder by MS/MS technology.

Treatment

Biotinidase deficiency is readily treated by administering 10–20 mg biotin/day, resulting in complete protection from neurologic damage. The adequacy of therapy may be monitored by urinary organic acid analysis and more recently acylcarnitine analysis. Biotin therapy results in the rapid control of medically-refractory seizures in these patients, accompanied by improvement in the EEG.

Further reading

Blau N, *et al.*, editors. *Physicians Guide to the Treatment and Followup of Metabolic Diseases*. New York: Springer-Verlag; 2006.

Fernandes J, editor. *Inborn Metabolic Diseases: Diagnosis and Treatment*, 4th ed. New York: Springer-Verlag; 2006.

McKusick VA. *Mendelian Inheritance in Man*. URL: http://www3.ncbi.nlm.nih.gov/Omim.

Scriver CR, Beaudet AL, Sly WS, *et al.*, editors. *The Metabolic and Molecular Basis of Inherited Disease*, 8th ed. New York: McGraw-Hill; 2001 (available online at www.genetics.accessmed.com).

Chapter 159
Mitochondrial encephalomyopathies

Stacey K.H. Tay[1] and Salvatore DiMauro[2]
[1]National University of Singapore, Singapore
[2]College of Physicians and Surgeons, New York, USA

Introduction

Mitochondrial diseases are a heterogeneous group of disorders characterized by impaired mitochondrial function. Because of the ubiquitous distribution of mitochondria in tissues, clinical phenotypes involve multiple organ systems and often encompass a bewildering variety of symptoms. Mitochondrial function is especially important in tissues with high energy requirements such as brain and skeletal muscle, so it is not unusual for symptoms to primarily affect brain and muscle. Given the functional complexity of the nervous system, the neurological manifestations of mitochondrial diseases are diverse and include seizures, cognitive regression or dementia, ataxia, myoclonus, strokes, migraine, myopathy, and peripheral neuropathy. However, some patients may have isolated organ involvement, most frequently isolated myopathy, whereas others have multisystemic disorders that may progressively involve more organ systems with age. Because many respiratory chain disorders involve both the brain and skeletal muscle, they are also known as "mitochondrial encephalomyopathies," and they are the scope of this chapter.

Given the complexity of phenotypes, it is not surprising that mitochondrial diseases are often considered in the differential diagnosis of "difficult patients." Nonetheless, there are important clinical clues that can orient clinicians towards the correct diagnosis. This chapter aims to give an overview of current knowledge and recent advances in the genetics of mitochondrial diseases affecting both central and peripheral nervous systems.

Mitochondrial genetics

Genomic organization

Mitochondria are relics of bacterial intruders that developed a symbiotic relationship with proto-eukaryotic cells over a billion years ago. A positive consequence of this "invasion" is that mitochondria have conferred on these cells the ability to meet cellular energy requirements by using oxygen as a substrate. This unusual relationship also resulted in mitochondria retaining their original circular DNA (mtDNA), which now encodes only 13 of the approximately 90 proteins of the respiratory chain (Figure 159.1). Thus, the mitochondria are "slaves" of the nuclear genome because most proteins of the respiratory chain and all other proteins needed for mtDNA maintenance and replication are encoded by nuclear DNA (nDNA). Together, the 13 mtDNA-encoded and the 75-plus nDNA-encoded proteins of the respiratory chain are assembled into five enzyme complexes embedded in the inner mitochondrial membrane (IMM), where electron transfer and proton translocation generate adenosine triphosphate (ATP) through the action of a magnificent "turbine," complex V (ATP synthase).

The human mitochondrial genome is a double stranded circle of 16 569 base pairs and contains only 37 genes, of which 13 encode essential polypeptides and the rest form the ribosomal machinery necessary for protein translation: 2 ribosomal RNAs (12S and 16S rRNA) and 22 transfer RNAs (tRNAs). As mentioned above, the 13 polypeptides are subunits of the respiratory chain: seven subunits of complex 1 (NADH dehydrogenase (ND) 1, 2, 3, 4, 4L, 5, and 6), one subunit of complex III (cytochrome *b*), three subunits of complex IV or cytochrome *c* oxidase (*COXI*, *COXII*, and *COXIII*), and two subunits of ATP synthase (ATPase 6 and ATPase 8). To date, about 200 pathogenic point mutations of mtDNA have been described, and the number of nuclear gene mutations is expected to be much greater and is rapidly escalating.

MtDNA replication, transcription, and translation

Not too surprisingly, some features of mtDNA replication are reminiscent of bacterial DNA replication. Replication of mtDNA is controlled by a combination of RNA and DNA polymerases that synthesize the daughter strands simultaneously in a bidirectional fashion. The mitochondrial replisome is thought to consist of several proteins: polymerase γ (POLG), Twinkle (with 5' to 3' helicase

International Neurology: A Clinical Approach. Edited by Robert P. Lisak, Daniel D. Truong, William M. Carroll, and Roongroj Bhidayasiri.

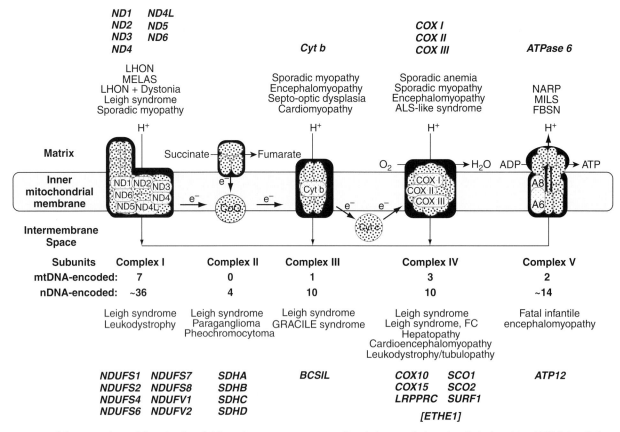

Figure 159.1 Schematic view of the mitochondrial respiratory chain, showing subunits encoded by nuclear DNA (nDNA) in ⋮⋮⋮ and subunits encoded by mitochondrial DNA (mtDNA) in ⬭. As electrons (e⁻) flow down the electron-transport chain, protons (H⁺) are pumped from the matrix to the intermembrane space through complexes I, III, and IV, then back into the matrix through complex V (ATP synthetase). Coenzyme Q (CoQ) and cytochrome c (Cyt c) are electron carriers. The genes responsible for mitochondrial disorders are listed above or below the clinical entities. FBSN: familial bilateral striatal necrosis; LHON: Leber's hereditary optic neuropathy; MELAS: mitochondrial encephalomyopathy, lactic acidosis, and stroke-like episodes; MILS: maternally inherited Leigh syndrome; NARP: neuropathy, ataxia, retinitis pigmentosa; GRACILE: growth retardation, aminoaciduria, iron overload, lactic acidosis, early death; ALS: amyotrophic lateral sclerosis; Leigh syndrome, FC: Leigh syndrome, French-Canadian type.

activity), and a mitochondrial single-stranded binding protein. Replication ends with the formation of a pair of circles, each containing a double helix of one "parent" strand and one "daughter" strand. This pair of catenated circles is then separated by topoisomerase II.

MtDNA transcription is also reminiscent of the bacterial system, because the mtDNA genes are transcribed in two giant 16-kb polycistronic precursor transcripts, cleaved precisely from precursor RNAs, and processed to produce individual tRNA and mRNA molecules.

Translation of the mitochondrial mRNAs takes place on mitochondrial ribosomes and involves the mtDNA-encoded 12S and 16S rRNAs as well as imported ribosomal proteins. The mtDNA genetic code differs from the "universal code" of nDNA at four of the 64 triplet positions: adenine–uracil–adenine (AUA) specifies methionine instead of isoleucine; uracil–guanine–adenine (UGA) specifies tryptophan instead of stop

codon; adenine–guanine–adenine (AGA) and adenine–guanine–guanine (AGG) encode stop codons instead of arginine.

Mitochondrial DNA inheritance and transmission

Human mtDNA is maternally inherited. A woman transmits her mtDNA to all her children regardless of gender, but only her daughters will pass their mitochondria on to their children. Paternal mitochondria are known to enter the ovum at fertilization, but are destroyed selectively through an unknown mechanism. It was recently reported that a patient with mitochondrial myopathy and a 2-bp pathogenic deletion in the *ND1* gene, had inherited most of his muscle mtDNA (but not the mutation) from his father. However, this appears to be a rare exception and maternal inheritance of mtDNA is still the rule and current genetic counseling still considers that fathers with mtDNA mutations do not risk transmitting the defect to their children.

A mutation in mtDNA can affect all genomes (a situation known as homoplasmy) or only some genomes, resulting in the coexistence of two mtDNA populations (this situation is called heteroplasmy). Neutral mutations (polymorphisms) are usually homoplasmic whereas most – but not all – pathogenic mutations are heteroplasmic. Both homoplasmic and heteroplasmic mtDNA mutations are transmitted to all maternal offspring. Genetic counseling, however, becomes complicated for disorders due to homoplasmic mtDNA mutations because nuclear genetic factors are important in regulating the expression of the disease. In Leber's hereditary optic neuropathy (LHON), for example, only 50% of males and 10% of females develop impaired vision, implying an X-linked genetic modifier. Environmental factors are also important in the expression of diseases associated with homoplasmic mtDNA mutations. For example, the 12S rRNA A1555G mutation causes sensorineural hearing loss only following exposure to aminoglycoside antibiotics.

Heteroplasmy and the threshold effect

Each mitochondrion contains two to ten copies of mtDNA, and each cell contains hundreds of mitochondria, depending on oxidative demands. In conditions of heteroplasmy, mutant mtDNAs coexist with wild-type genomes, and the clinical features of the corresponding mitochondrial disease depend on several factors. First, the proportion of pathogenic mtDNA mutation: if and when this exceeds the tissue "threshold," it will result in clinically evident mitochondrial dysfunction. The threshold for disease is lower in tissues that are highly dependent on oxidative metabolism, such as the brain, heart, skeletal muscle, retina, renal tubules, and endocrine glands, explaining why patients with the same heteroplasmic mutation may have variable tissue involvement and variable overall clinical severity. The T8993G mutation illustrates this concept nicely. Patients with a mutation load of about 70–90% present with neuropathy, ataxia, and retinitis pigmentosa (NARP) syndrome, while those with a mutation load of more than 90% present with maternally inherited Leigh syndrome (MILS), a more severe form of infantile encephalomyopathy.

Second, the distribution of the mutation may vary in different tissues, thus affecting the clinical expression. In patients with large-scale single mitochondrial deletions, infants may present with Pearson syndrome, a severe sideroblastic anemia, when most deleted mtDNA is in bone marrow stem cells. If these children survive the original hematological dysfunction, they usually develop a multisystem mitochondrial disorder, Kearns–Sayre syndrome (KSS), in which deleted mtDNA is present in multiple tissues, including skeletal, cardiac muscle, and the central nervous system, thus explaining the typical KSS phenotype: external ophthalmoplegia, ptosis, cardiac conduction block, and pigmentary retinopathy.

Segregation

The random redistribution of organelles at cell division can change the proportion of mutant mtDNAs received by daughter cells; if and when the pathogenic threshold in a previously unaffected tissue is surpassed, the phenotype can also change. This explains the age-related, and even tissue-related, variability of clinical features frequently observed in mtDNA-related disorders.

The number of organelles and their mtDNA content may also vary among cells and tissues, as well as during development and aging. Certain conditions that increase the oxidative demands of a tissue may also increase its mitochondrial content, including acclimatization to high altitude or endurance training. Conversely, aging may result in progressive accumulation of mitochondrial mutations, leading to a progressive decline in mitochondrial function.

Genetic and functional classification

Disorders of mtDNA

Disorders of mtDNA can be classified according to the type of genetic defect: large-scale rearrangements, such as mitochondrial deletions or duplications, or point mutations (Table 159.1). A functional classification divides mutations that affect mitochondrial protein synthesis *in toto*, for example, large-scale rearrangements characteristic of KSS, or tRNA mutations typically seen in MELAS, and mutations that affect protein-coding genes, for example, those causing Leber's hereditary optic neuropathy (LHON). Below, we describe eight of the most common mtDNA syndromes.

Kearns–Sayre syndrome (KSS)

KSS is a multisystemic disorder characterized by an obligate triad of progressive external ophthalmoplegia, pigmentary retinopathy, and onset before 20 years of age, as well as at least one of the following features: conductive cardiac block, cerebrospinal fluid (CSF) protein above 100 mg/dl, and cerebellar ataxia. Other supportive findings include short stature, hearing loss, dementia, limb weakness, dysphagia, and various endocrinopathies. Large-scale deletions of mitochondrial DNA have been found in over 90% of KSS patients, and large-scale duplications in some. Although KSS is multisystemic, a muscle biopsy is ideal to confirm the presence of mtDNA deletions, which are often undetectable in blood. Deletions vary in size and location within the mitochondrial genome, but there is a deletion hotspot between nucleotides 8469 and 13 147. This 4.9-kb "common deletion" accounts for one-third of cases of KSS.

Table 159.1 Classification of mtDNA disorders according to the underlying genetic defect.

Functional defect	Genetic defect	Disorder	Inheritance
Mutations in protein synthesis genes	Large-scale rearrangements MtDNA deletions	Kearns–Sayre syndrome (KSS) Progressive external ophthalmoplegia (PEO) Pearson syndrome (congenital pancytopenia with sideroblastic anemia, and intestinal malabsorption)	Usually sporadic
	Point mutations (tRNA genes)	Mitochondrial encephalomyopathy, lactic acidosis, and stroke-like episodes (MELAS) Myoclonic epilepsy with ragged-red fibers (MERRF)	Usually maternally inherited
Mutations in protein coding genes	Point mutations (protein coding genes)	Leber's hereditary optic neuropathy (LHON) Neuropathy, ataxia, retinitis pigmentosa (NARP) syndrome Maternally inherited Leigh syndrome (MILS)	

Blood creatine kinase (CK) may be modestly elevated, but lactate and pyruvate levels are more substantially increased. As already mentioned, CSF protein is greatly elevated, usually above 100 mg/dl. MRI of the brain often shows cerebral and cerebellar atrophy, and, more commonly, abnormal T2-weighted signal in the subcortical white matter. Electrocardiogram (ECG) characteristically shows cardiac conduction defects and should be performed at regular intervals because timely placement of a pacemaker is often life-saving.

Ophthalmological evaluation shows pigmentary retinopathy and electroretinography (ERG) may show retinal degeneration. Sensorineural hearing loss should be assessed with brainstem auditory evoked responses. Muscle biopsy usually demonstrates "ragged-red fibers" (RRF, due to subsarcolemmal aggregates of abnormal mitochondria) on the modified Gomori trichrome stain. Using COX (cytochrome *c* oxidase) histochemistry, most RRF (and many non-RRF) are COX-deficient.

This condition is progressive, but several measures can improve quality of life. First, patients with cardiac conduction block should have a pacemaker inserted to prevent complete heart block. Second, management of ptosis (eyelid "crutches," blepharoplasty, or frontalis muscle-eyelid sling placement) improves vision and cosmetics. Third, aerobic exercise may improve strength and avoid deconditioning, despite the concern that oxidative stress may increase the percentage of deleted mtDNA in exercising muscle. Dysphagia may be treated with cricopharyngeal myotomy or gastrostomy feeding.

Progressive external ophthalmoplegia (PEO)
PEO is one of the most common clinical manifestations of mitochondrial myopathy. It may appear in isolation or in association with other features suggestive of a specific mitochondrial syndrome such as KSS or MNGIE (see below). PEO may be sporadic, maternally inherited (mtDNA disorder), or subject to Mendelian in inheritance

(nDNA disorder). Sporadic PEO is most frequently due to a single large-scale mtDNA rearrangement, as in KSS, of which, in fact, this is the muscular variant, characterized by progressive bilateral ptosis, ophthalmoplegia, exercise intolerance, and muscle weakness.

Diagnosis has to be made by muscle biopsy because the mtDNA deletions are not found in blood. Electroretinography and visual-evoked potential testing are usually normal.

Pearson syndrome (PS)
PS is the most severe of the conditions associated with large-scale mtDNA rearrangements. This infantile disorder includes sideroblastic anemia, exocrine pancreatic dysfunction with malabsorption, chronic diarrhea, failure to thrive, lactic acidemia, and various endocrine abnormalities. PS is almost universally fatal, and the few patients who survive the initial severe sideroblastic anemia tragically develop the multisystemic symptoms of KSS later on in life.

Mitochondrial encephalopathy, lactic acidosis, and stroke-like episodes (MELAS)
MELAS is a relatively common multisystemic mitochondrial disorder characterized by the following:
1 stroke-like episodes before 40 years of age,
2 encephalopathy, with seizures and/or psychomotor retardation/regression,
3 myopathy with ragged-red fibers,
4 lactic acidosis.

The stroke-like episodes are often occipital in location (resulting in cortical blindness), do not correspond to vascular territories, and involve predominantly the cortex and adjacent white matter, sparing the deeper white matter. These stroke-like episodes may not be due to acute ischemia, but rather to a combination of metabolic dysfunction with decreased oxidative phosphorylation and altered cerebrovascular autoregulation. Other neurological features of MELAS include ataxia, myoclonus, episodic encephalopathy, optic nerve atrophy, sensorineural hearing loss, retinopathy, ophthalmoplegia, and migraine-like headaches. Psychiatric disturbance such as depression or schizophrenia may also be present. Non-neurological features include cardiac dysfunction with cardiomyopathy (sometimes the presenting and predominant manifestation), arrhythmias or conductive heart block, endocrine dysfunction with diabetes mellitus, short stature, gastrointestinal dysfunction with dysmotility, and renal dysfunction with nephropathy.

The age at onset varies and the disease sometimes starts in infancy or early childhood with developmental delay, seizures, learning disability, failure to thrive, and exercise intolerance. However, in many patients a stroke-like episode is the first presentation, which may occur in childhood, adolescence, or, less frequently, later in life.

Point mutations in mtDNA are almost always underlying MELAS. This syndrome illustrates one of the key concepts of mitochondrial genetics, namely, genotypic diversity. The most common mutation is A3243G in the $tRNA^{Leu(UUR)}$ gene, which is seen in about 80% of patients, but many mutations have been described in other tRNA genes, including $tRNA^{Leu}$, $tRNA^{Val}$, $tRNA^{Phe}$, and $tRNA^{Glu}$, as well as mutations in protein-coding genes, such as complex I (*ND1*, *ND4*, *ND5*, *ND6*) and complex IV (*COXIII*) genes. Interestingly, mutations in *ND1* (G3376A) and *ND5* (G13513A, A13045C, and A13084T) often cause overlap phenotypes of MELAS, LHON, and Leigh syndrome.

Lactic acidosis is a hallmark of the syndrome and increased lactic acid levels in the CSF and in the brain parenchyma can be appreciated by magnetic resonance spectroscopy (MRS). Abnormal neuroimaging findings include the following: (1) stroke-like lesions with increased signal in T2-weighted or fluid attenuation inversion recovery (FLAIR) images; (2) increased signal on diffusion-weighted images (DWI), with normal or increased apparent diffusion coefficient (ADC) values suggestive of vasogenic edema; (3) relatively normal angiograms; (4) basal ganglia calcifications; (5) variable cerebral atrophy; and (6) as already mentioned, increased lactate in the ventricular CSF and in the brain parenchyma on MRS. Positron emission tomography (PET) may reveal reduced cerebral metabolic rate for oxygen. Single photon emission computed tomography (SPECT) often shows decreased tracer accumulation in acute and subacute lesions, possibly due to focal loss of metabolically active cells.

Blood screening for the common mtDNA mutations is usually diagnostic. However, in oligosymptomatic or asymptomatic relatives of MELAS patients, the mutation is often undetectable in blood while it is readily detectable in another easily accessible tissue, urinary sediment. Muscle biopsy shows scattered ragged-red fibers (which are positive for COX activity) and blood vessels with increased succinate dehydrogenase (SDH) and COX stainings. Biochemical analysis of the respiratory chain enzymes suggests partial defects in the activities of complexes containing mtDNA-encoded subunits (I, III, and IV), contrasting with normal activities of the nDNA-encoded complex II (succinate dehydrogenase) and citrate synthase.

Treatment of MELAS includes "cocktails" of vitamins and dietary supplements, symptomatic management of seizures and other medical complications (e.g., diabetes mellitus), and avoidance of metabolic stressors. Patients with severe neurosensory hearing loss may need cochlear implants. *L*-arginine, a nitric oxide precursor that may favor vascular dilatation, has been shown to improve outcome in stroke-like episodes when used acutely within the first 3 hours after onset of the event, as well as to decrease the frequency and severity of stroke-like episodes when administered in between episodes.

Myoclonus epilepsy and ragged-red fibers (MERRF)

MERRF is a multisystemic mitochondrial disorder dominated by myoclonus, which is often the first symptom, followed by generalized epilepsy, ataxia, weakness, and dementia. Onset is usually in childhood, although adult onset has been described. Other common findings include sensorineural hearing loss, short stature, optic atrophy, and cardiomyopathy with Wolff–Parkinson–White (WPW) syndrome. Occasionally, pigmentary retinopathy and multiple lipomatosis may be observed. The presence of multiple lipomas in the context of a mitochondrial disorder is virtually pathognomonic of MERRF.

Neuropathological studies have demonstrated degeneration of the cerebellum, brainstem, and spinal cord, which may explain the prominent ataxia in some patients. In addition, there is significant cortical hyperexcitability resulting in cortical reflex myoclonus.

The mitochondrial $tRNA^{Lys}$ gene is a hotspot for mutations causing MERFF (A8344G, T8356C, G8361A, G8363A) although MERRF-like syndromes have also been associated with point mutations in $tRNA^{Phe}$, $tRNA^{Ser(UCN)}$, $tRNA^{His}$, and $tRNA^{Leu\,(UUR)}$. The most common mutation (seen in 80% of cases) is the A8344G point mutation in $tRNA^{Lys}$, which may easily be screened in blood of suspected MERFF patients. In the absence of the common mutations, however, muscle biopsy is useful because the presence of COX-negative RRF confirms the suspicion of a mitochondrial disorder. It should also be noted that several $tRNA^{Lys}$ mutations (A8344G, T8356C, G8363A) cause symptoms overlapping with MELAS and Leigh syndrome.

Treatment is supportive, and there are no comparative studies of relative efficacy of different anticonvulsants. Myoclonus was reported to improve in several patients with the use of levetiracetam.

Leber's hereditary optic neuropathy (LHON)

LHON is an mtDNA disorder causing subacute visual loss predominantly in young men. There is a rapid and painless loss of central vision, which affects both eyes simultaneously in 50% of cases, and within the space of 6 months in the rest. During the acute phase, there is loss of central vision as well as fading of colors. Fundoscopy reveals peripapillary telangiectasia, microangiopathy, and disc pseudoedema (from swelling of the nerve fiber layer around the disc). This is followed by the atrophic phase, when there is progressive optic atrophy and decline in visual acuity.

In 95% of cases, LHON is caused by homoplasmic mutations in one of three ND genes, G11778A (*ND4*), G3460A (*ND1*), and T14484C (*ND6*). However, only 50% of men and 10% of women harboring LHON mutations actually develop the symptoms of LHON, stressing the role of mitochondrial or nuclear modifier genes. Several patients with mutations in *ND5* have shown overlap with MELAS symptoms, while patients with mutations in *ND4* or *ND6* may show, in addition to LHON, basal ganglia degeneration and symptoms of dystonia and spasticity. The clinical course may also vary depending on the mutation: more patients with the T14484C mutation show recovery compared with those with the G11778A mutation (71% vs. 4%).

Neuropathy, ataxia, retinitis pigmentosa (NARP)

NARP is a maternally inherited mitochondrial disorder of young adulthood, defined by the presence of sensory neuropathy, ataxia, and retinitis pigmentosa. This is caused by either a T8993G or a T8993C mutation in the mitochondrial ATP synthase subunit 6 gene (ATPase6). The diagnosis of NARP is suggested by peripheral neuropathy, which may be sensory or sensorimotor axonal, ataxia with cerebellar atrophy, and retinitis pigmentosa, plus seizures and dementia. The retinopathy usually has a "salt and pepper" appearance, although a more severe appearance with classical bone spiculae may also be seen. Optic atrophy may appear later in the course of the disease. It should be noted that muscle biopsy does not show RRF.

Patients with NARP typically have mutation loads ranging between 70% and 90%, but this appears to be part of a continuum because patients with higher mutation loads (above 90%) are affected by MILS (see below).

Maternally-inherited Leigh syndrome (MILS)

MILS is characterized by progressive psychomotor degeneration, signs and symptoms of brainstem and/or basal ganglia abnormalities, and raised lactate in both blood and CSF. Both neuroimaging and pathology show the hallmarks of LS, that is, symmetrical necrosis of the basal ganglia, thalamus, and brainstem. About 40% of patients with MILS also have retinitis pigmentosa, tipping off

the clinician to the underlying molecular defect, because retinitis pigmentosa is rarely, if ever, seen in other forms of LS. Adult-onset MILS has been described in association with tRNA^{Val} mutations, and MILS with spinocerebellar ataxia with tRNA^{Lys} mutations.

Disorders of nDNA

The nuclear genome encodes hundreds of mitochondrial proteins that are essential for various mitochondrial functions besides maintenance and replication of mtDNA (intergenomic signaling). Mitochondrial diseases may result therefore from a plethora of abnormalities, affecting mitochondrial motility, fission, or fusion, protein importation, and membrane composition, with or without direct involvement of the respiratory chain (Table 159.2).

Clinical syndromes due to nDNA mutations tend to be more stereotyped than those due to mtDNA mutations, as they are not subject to variable mutation load and differential tissue distribution of mutant mtDNA. Several common syndromes are discussed below.

Leigh syndrome (LS)

LS is a condition of subacute necrotizing encephalomyelopathy with typical pathological findings of symmetrical foci of spongiform degeneration in the basal ganglia, thalami, brainstem, dentate nuclei, and optic nerves. Most patients with LS present in infancy with psychomotor regression, although onset in childhood or even adolescence has also been reported. Other features include hypotonia, progressive visual impairment, progressive external ophthalmoplegia, hearing impairment, nystagmus, ataxia, and seizures. Respiratory insufficiency is fairly common and is an important cause of mortality. Clinical criteria were proposed by Rahman *et al.* in 1996:

- Progressive neurological disease with motor and intellectual developmental delay.
- Signs and symptoms of brainstem and/or basal ganglia disease.
- Raised lactate concentration in blood and/or CSF.
- One or more of the following:
  ○ Characteristic features of LS on neuroimaging: symmetrically increased signal in the basal ganglia and brainstem on T2-weighted or FLAIR images.
  ○ Typical neuropathologic changes: multiple symmetric foci of degeneration and necrosis with capillary proliferation, demyelination, and gliosis in the basal ganglia, brainstem, thalamus, cerebellum, and spinal cord.
  ○ Typical neuropathology or neuroimaging findings in a similarly affected sibling.

LS is genetically heterogeneous because it may be caused by mtDNA mutations (see MILS) or nDNA mutations and therefore be maternally inherited, autosomal recessive, or X-linked. LS is caused by nDNA mutations in genes encoding for subunits of the pyruvate dehydrogenase complex (PDHC), genes encoding respiratory chain

Table 159.2 Classification of nDNA disorders according to the underlying biochemical and genetic defects.

Functional defect	Biochemical/genetic defect	Defective gene	Disorder	Inheritance
Mutations in structural components of the respiratory chain	Complex I	*NDUFS2, NDUFS4, NDUFS8, NDUFV1, NDUFS1, NDUFS7*	Leigh syndrome	AR
		NDUFS2, NDUFV2	Cardioencephalomyopathy	AR
	Complex II	Flavoprotein subunit of *SDH*	Leigh syndrome	AR
		SDHB, SDHC, SDHD	Hereditary paraganglioma or phaeochromocytoma	AD
	Complex II	*UQCRB*	Hypoglycemia, lactic acidosis	AR
Mutations in ancillary proteins of respiratory chain	Complex	*B17.2L*	Early onset progressive encephalopathy	AR
	Complex II	*BCS1L*	Encephalopathy, tubulopathy, hepatopathy	AR
	Complex IV	*SURF1*	Leigh syndrome	AR
		SCO2, COX15	Infantile cardioencephalomyopathy	AR
		SCO1	Infantile hepatoencephalomyopathy	AR
		COX10	Infantile nephroencephalomyopathy	AR
		LRPPRC	French-Canadian Leigh syndrome	AR
	Complex V deficiency	*ATPAF2*	Early onset encephalopathy, lactic acidosis	AR
Defects of intergenomic communication	Multiple mtDNA deletions	Thymidine phosphorylase (*ECGF1*)	MNGIE	AR
		POLG	AD-PEO, AR-PEO, Alpers' syndrome, SANDO syndrome	AR/AD
		ANT1, Twinkle helicase (*C10ORF2*)	AD-PEO	AD
	MtDNA depletion	*TK2*	Infantile myopathy	AR
		dGK	Infantile hepatopathy and encephalopathy	AR
Defects of mitochondrial membrane function	Cardiolipin defect	Tafazzin (*G4.5*)	Barth syndrome	XLR
	CoQ10 deficiency	*COQ2, PDSS2*	Infantile encephalomyopathy with nephropathy	AR
Defects of mitochondrial protein synthesis	Translation defect	*EFG1*	Severe hepatoencephalopathy and lactic acidosis	AR
		EFTu	Severe infantile leukodystrophy and polymicrogyria	AR
Defects of mitochondrial import		*Tim 8/9 (DDP)*	Deafness-dystonia (Mohr–Tranebjaerg syndrome)	XLR
Defects of mitochondrial motility, fission and fusion	Impaired motility	*OPA1*	AD-optic atrophy	AD
		KIF5A	Hereditary spastic paraplegia	AD
	Mitochondrial fusion	Mitofusin (*MFN2*)	Charcot–Marie–Tooth disease (CMT2A)	AD
Defects of iron homeostasis	Iron storage	Frataxin (*FRDA*)	Friedreich's ataxia	AR
	Iron transport	*ABC7*	X-linked sideroblastic anemia with ataxia	XL
Defects of mitochondrial metabolism	Pyruvate dehydrogenase E1α subunit	*PDHA1*	X-linked Leigh syndrome	XL
	Ethylmalonic acid metabolism	*ETHE1*	Encephalopathy, ethylmalonic aciduria	AR
Others	Chaperone function	*SPG7*	Spastic paraplegia	AR

AR: autosomal recessive; AD: autosomal dominant; XLR: X-linked recessive; XL: X-linked.

components of complex I (*NDUFS2, NDUFS4, NDUFS8, NDUFV1, NDUFS1, NDUFS7*) or complex II (*SDHA*), or genes encoding proteins needed for the assembly or maintenance of respiratory chain function (*SURF1, COX10, COX15, SCO1, SCO2, LRPPRC*). Underlying all these diverse genetic defects, however, is the unifying problem of impaired adenosine triphosphate (ATP) synthesis.

Autosomal dominant or recessive progressive external ophthalmoplegia (PEO)

PEO is a mitochondrial myopathy with droopy eyelids, paralysis of the extraocular muscles, and variably severe proximal limb weakness. It may be isolated or associated with other clinical features of mitochondrial syndromes. Autosomal dominant (adPEO) and autosomal recessive (arPEO) PEO are associated with multiple mtDNA deletions, have onset in adolescence or in early adulthood, and are usually slowly progressive. The genes responsible for adPEO include *POLG* (encoding polymerase gamma, the only mtDNA polymerase), *ANT1* (encoding the muscle-specific isoform of mitochondrial adenine nucleotide translocator), and *PEO1* (encoding Twinkle, a helicase involved in mtDNA replication). *POLG* mutations have also been described in arPEO. However, clearly other genes remain to be identified because several adPEO and arPEO families do not have mutations in the above genes. *POLG* mutations appear to have more severe symptoms and often complex clinical manifestations, including sensory ataxia, dysphagia, dysphonia, and – less frequently – parkinsonism, cerebellar ataxia, chorea, gastrointestinal dysmotility, and psychiatric disturbances. In contrast to adPEO conditions, arPEO tends to begin in childhood or adolescence, and may be part of multisystemic disorders like MNGIE or autosomal recessive cardiomyopathy and ophthalmoplegia (ARCO).

Mitochondrial neurogastrointestinal encephalomyopathy (MNGIE)

MNGIE is an autosomal recessive disorder associated with mtDNA depletion, multiple deletions, and site-specific point mutations, and is caused by mutations in the thymidine phosphorylase (*TP*) gene that regulates the mitochondrial nucleotide pools (although the TP protein is predominantly cytosolic). This condition is characterized by PEO, severe gastrointestinal dysmotility and cachexia, peripheral neuropathy, and leukoencephalopathy. The peripheral neuropathy is demyelinating in half of the patients and axonal in the other half. The leukoencephalopathy shown by MRI is usually asymptomatic. Relative sparing of the corpus callosum has been reported in some individuals.

Allogeneic stem cell transplantation has been performed as a therapeutic approach and has normalized the biochemical features in one patient, who is alive and subjectively improved 18 months after the transplant. However, overall clinical efficacy remains to be assessed.

Alpers' syndrome

Alpers' syndrome is an autosomal recessive disorder of infancy or early childhood characterized by encephalopathy, intractable seizures, and liver failure. Neuronal loss, spongiform degeneration of the cerebral cortex and basal ganglia, and astrocytosis of the visual cortex are typical neuropathological findings. Hepatic microvesicular steatosis, proliferation of the bile ducts, and cirrhosis are typically seen on liver biopsy. Abnormal mitochondria were previously demonstrated in the cerebral neurons, suggesting a mitochondrial pathology. Indeed, it was recently confirmed that depletion of mtDNA in most patients is associated with pathogenic mutations in the *POLG* (polymerase gamma) gene.

Coenzyme Q10 (CoQ10) deficiency

CoQ10 is an important quinone that transfers electrons from complex I and II to complex III of the respiratory chain. Deficiency of CoQ10 has been associated with myopathy, ataxia, or infantile encephalomyopathy and nephropathy. Defects in CoQ10 biosynthesis have recently been identified in patients with infantile CoQ10 deficiency with encephalopathy and nephropathy, and mutations in three biosynthetic genes have been reported (*COQ2*, PDSS2, and *PDSS2*).

Secondary forms of CoQ10 have been associated with mutations in the aprataxin gene (*APTX*) in patients with ataxia and oculomotor apraxia (AOA1) syndrome, although the relationship between aprataxin and CoQ10 deficiency is not clear. The pathogenic relationship between CoQ10 deficiency and genetic defect is less obscure in patients with lipid storage myopathy and mutations in the gene encoding the enzyme electron transport flavoprotein dehydrogenase (ETFDH) because ETFDH normally discharges electrons from the beta-oxidation pathway to CoQ10 in the respiratory chain. From the practical point of view, it is important to keep in mind that for all of these conditions, oral supplementation with CoQ10 is beneficial, highlighting the importance of early diagnosis.

Neurodegenerative disorders

There is little question that mitochondrial dysfunction (oxidative stress) plays a role in apoptosis and in the pathogenesis of neurodegeneration. Late-onset neurodegenerative disorders, including Parkinson's disease (PD), Huntington's disease (HD), Alzheimer's disease (AD), and amyotrophic lateral sclerosis (ALS), have been associated with oxidative stress as an important pathogenetic step. Nonetheless, the relative contributions of nDNA, mtDNA, and various environmental factors on the aging process remain to be clearly defined.

Epidemiology

Epidemiological evidence suggests that mutations in mtDNA are not uncommon. Collective numbers have been hard to collate previously as most patients with mitochondrial disorders are seen by a variety of specialists. Nonetheless, a series of population studies have yielded some useful epidemiological information. For example, the common MELAS A3243G mutation is estimated at 16.3 in 100 000 persons in north Finland where a total of 245 201 adults were studied. LHON is the most common mtDNA disorder, with a minimum prevalence of 11.82 in 100 000 mtDNA LHON mutations in the population of northeastern England. In northeastern England, the cumulative frequency of mtDNA mutations in adult and child populations was estimated to be 12.48 in 100 000. Overall, the minimum prevalence of mtDNA mutations is at least 1 in 5000, underlining the fact that mitochondrial disorders as a group are not rare.

Neurological manifestations

The range of neurological manifestations of mitochondrial disorders is vast. In the central nervous system (CNS), they include fluctuating encephalopathy, cognitive decline, loss of motor skills, psychiatric disturbance, migraine-like headaches, stroke-like episodes, seizures, movement disorders (dystonia, myoclonus), spasticity, ataxia, dysarthria, dysphagia, hypotonia, and visual problems. In the peripheral nervous system, symptoms include myopathy or neuropathy (demyelinating or axonal neuropathy).

Some patients may have a constellation of symptoms or signs typical enough to allow recognition of specific mtDNA syndromes (Table 159.3). Certain disorders affect a single organ, such as aminoglycoside-induced deafness or pure myopathies, while others involve multiple organ systems but often with predominant neurological or neuromuscular features.

Abnormalities of the CNS may also be secondary to mitochondrial dysfunction in other organs: thus, endocrine dysfunctions may cause Hashimoto's or diabetic encephalopathy, and liver/kidney failure may cause hepatic or uremic encephalopathy. It should also be remembered that specific drugs may worsen or unmask symptoms of mitochondrial disorders. For example, valproic acid may cause hepatic failure in patients with Alpers' syndrome, and statin drugs may cause rhabdomyolysis in patients with MELAS.

Diagnosis

Because of the bewildering heterogeneity of clinical phenotypes, the diagnosis of mitochondrial diseases is fraught with difficulty even for the most experienced neurologist. In general, mitochondrial disorders should be suspected in the differential diagnosis of any multisystemic disorder. The diagnosis is more challenging when a single organ is involved. Specific "red-flags" should be looked for in the history and on clinical examination, and a judicious range of investigations chosen to document mitochondrial dysfunction.

History

A careful and detailed history of the patient's symptoms is essential to obtain an accurate diagnosis. "Red-flags" in the history include exercise intolerance, migraine headaches, diabetes mellitus, short stature, hearing loss, neuropathy, hypertrophic cardiomyopathy, and, in children, unexplained developmental delay or failure to thrive. Family history is also important in distinguishing maternal from Mendelian forms of inheritance. Maternal family members in a pedigree with mtDNA mutations may have mild symptoms of headaches or early onset diabetes mellitus, and careful screening of "red-flags" in the extended pedigree is necessary. Consanguinity is, of course, suggestive of an autosomal recessive nDNA disorder.

A history of mid-trimester or late pregnancy loss and infant deaths (often with a dubious label of "sepsis") should also be sought. While mitochondrial disorders may manifest at any age, it is useful to remember that, in general, nuclear DNA abnormalities tend to appear in infancy and childhood, while mtDNA abnormalities often present in late childhood or adult life. Exposure to drugs such as aminoglycosides, valproic acid, and other drugs known to compromise mitochondrial function should also be carefully recorded.

Physical examination

A careful physical examination may yield clues to the diagnosis. Failure to thrive in a child or short stature in a young person or adult may be significant. Ptosis and external ophthalmoplegia are telltale signs of mitochondrial dysfunction after myasthenia gravis has been excluded in a young patient and autosomal dominant oculopharyngeal muscular dystrophy (OPMD) has been excluded in an old individual. Multiple lipomatosis is a typical feature of MERFF. Fundoscopy may show a pigmentary retinopathy (often with "salt and pepper" appearance) in KSS, NARP, MILS, and, less commonly, MELAS and MERFF. Peripheral neuropathy is typical of NARP, but may also be present in MELAS and MERFF, and – among the Mendelian conditions – it is very common in AD or AR PEO with *POLG* mutations and in patients with MNGIE.

Investigations

An extensive evaluation is necessary in patients with a complex neurological picture or with a single neurological symptom but other organ involvement. The strategy for

Table 159.3 Clinical features of mitochondrial diseases associated with mtDNA mutations.

Tissue	Symptom/sign	Δ-mtDNA		tRNA		ATPase	
		KSS	Pearson	MERRF	MELAS	NARP	MILS
CNS	Seizures	–	–	+	+	–	+
	Ataxia	+	–	+	+	+	±
	Myoclonus	–	–	+	±	–	–
	Psychomotor retardation	–	–	–	–	–	+
	Psychomotor regression	+	–	±	+	–	–
	Hemiparesis/hemianopia	–	–	–	+	–	–
	Cortical blindness	–	–	–	+	–	–
	Migraine-like headaches	–	–	–	+	–	–
	Dystonia	–	–	–	+	–	+
PNS	Peripheral neuropathy	±	–	±	±	+	–
Muscle	Weakness	+	–	+	+	+	+
	Ophthalmoplegia	+	±	–	–	–	–
	Ptosis	+	–	–	–	–	–
Eye	Pigmentary retinopathy	+	–	–	–	+	±
	Optic atrophy	–	–	–	–	±	±
	Cataracts	–	–	–	–	–	–
Blood	Sideroblastic anemia	±	+	–	–	–	–
Endocrine	Diabetes mellitus	±	–	–	±	–	–
	Short stature	+	–	+	+	–	–
	Hypoparathyroidism	±	–	–	–	–	–
Heart	Conduction block	+	–	–	±	–	–
	Cardiomyopathy	±	–	–	±	–	±
GI	Exocrine pancreatic dysfunction	±	+	–	–	–	–
	Intestinal pseudo-obstruction	–	–	–	–	–	–
ENT	Sensorineural hearing loss	–	–	+	+	±	–
Kidney	Fanconi's syndrome	±	±	–	±	–	–
Laboratory	Lactic acidosis	+	+	+	+	–	±
	Muscle biopsy: RRF	+	±	+	+	–	–
Inheritance	Maternal	–	–	+	+	+	+
	Sporadic	+	+	–	–	–	–

Boxes denote the most common symptoms or signs characteristic of the particular mitochondrial disorder. AID: aminoglycoside-induced deafness; Δ-mtDNA: mitochondrial DNA large scale deletion; tRNA: transfer ribonucleic acid; ATPase: adenosine triphosphate synthase 6; KSS: Kearns–Sayre syndrome; MERRF: myoclonic epilepsy with ragged-red fibers; MELAS: mitochondrial encephalomyopathy, lactic acidosis, stroke-like episodes; NARP: neuropathy, ataxia, retinitis pigmentosa; MILS: maternally inherited Leigh syndrome; CNS: central nervous system; ENT: ear, nose and throat system; GI: gastrointestinal system; PNS: peripheral nervous system.

evaluation is greatly simplified when the clinical picture is typical of a specific mitochondrial syndrome (such as KSS, MELAS, or MERRF) because studies of blood mtDNA can be targeted to the appropriate mutations, starting with the most common. Should the clinical picture be non-specific, but still suggestive of a mitochondrial condition, simpler laboratory tests should be performed first.

Basic laboratory tests
Laboratory evaluation should include routine blood tests, including full blood count, renal and liver function tests, lactate, and pyruvate. Lactate and pyruvate are often elevated at rest in mitochondrial diseases and may increase further with exercise. In general, the lactate/pyruvate ratio of mitochondrial patients should be greater than 30:1. However, lactate may not be raised in conditions like NARP, and often repeated lactate levels are necessary to confirm the lactic acidosis. Creatine kinase (CK) is usually mildly elevated in mitochondrial disorders, but may be markedly raised in the myopathic form of mtDNA depletion. Should there be a suggestive history, other investigations may be considered, such as fasting blood glucose for diabetes mellitus or hormonal tests for thyroid, parathyroid, and pituitary function.

CSF studies are not always performed, but may be useful to demonstrate cerebral lactic acidosis. CSF protein may be raised in MELAS and KSS (especially KSS, where protein is often more than 100 mg/dl), and oligoclonal bands may also be present in a number of patients. Lactate may be raised during or following stroke-like events or generalized seizures.

Electrocardiogram (ECG) may reveal conductive heart block in KSS or MELAS, and pre-excitation in MELAS and MERFF. 2D-echocardiography may confirm hypertrophic cardiomyopathy in some patients.

Neuroimaging

Computed tomography (CT) scans of the brain in patients with mitochondrial disorders may show non-specific findings, such as white matter and basal ganglia hypodensity, calcification of the cortex and basal ganglia, atrophy of the pons and cerebellum, or hypotrophy of the corpus callosum. Magnetic resonance imaging (MRI) of the brain is extremely useful to demonstrate certain characteristic patterns in specific syndromes. For example, the diagnosis of LS is dependent on bilateral symmetrical signal hyperintensity of the basal ganglia and brainstem. Acute stroke-like events in MELAS are demonstrated on MRI as lesions with increased signal on T2-weighted and FLAIR images, with no conformation to large vessel territories, and affecting the cortex and adjacent white matter. These lesions also show increased diffusion weighted signal with normal or increased ADC values, typical of vasogenic edema rather than cytotoxic edema. Other common findings on MRI include diffuse signal abnormalities of the central white matter (KSS, MERRF, MNGIE, PEO), basal ganglia calcifications (KSS, MELAS), supratentorial cortical atrophy (PEO, MNGIE), and cerebellar atrophy (KSS).

Proton MRS is useful to reveal lactate accumulation in ventricular CSF and in various areas of the brain. In fact, MRS reveals abnormal lactate peaks in oligosymptomatic carriers of the A3243G mutation. Lactate peaks may even precede stroke-like lesions in MELAS patients.

Neurophysiological studies

Electroencephalography (EEG) may show focal or diffuse slowing and various focal and generalized epileptiform discharges. Visual evoked potentials (VEP) may show prolonged P100 latencies, especially in patients with LHON and retinopathy, but sometimes also in the absence of clear morphological changes. Brainstem auditory evoked responses (BAER) are used to demonstrate sensorineural hearing loss, which may be present even in asymptomatic individuals.

Exercise physiology

Formal exercise testing with near-infrared spectroscopy and measurement of oxygen consumption is available in specialized centers. These tests assess the respiratory chain function non-invasively, and are abnormal in patients with mitochondrial disorders. While useful, these tests may not be applicable to young infants and children because of the need for the patient's active cooperation.

Muscle biopsy

Muscle biopsy is performed with two main objectives: histochemistry (comprising modified Gomori trichrome, SDH, and COX staining) and enzyme biochemical assays to assess the various complexes of the respiratory chain (Table 159.4). Histological and ultrastructural studies may show mitochondrial proliferation, enlarged mitochondria with disorganized cristae, or abnormal mitochondrial inclusions. The RRF seen with the modified Gomori trichrome staining have abnormal subsarcolemmal (and, less prominently, intermyofibrillar) collections of mitochondria. SDH, NADH-TR (nicotinamide dehydrogenase-tetrazolium reductase), and COX stains can also demonstrate excessive mitochondrial proliferation (fibers hyperintense with the SDH stain have been dubbed "ragged-blue"), and may also identify isolated enzyme defects. Disorders of protein synthesis usually have COX-negative RRF, with the exception of MELAS, where there may be relative preservation of COX staining. Certain conditions such as LHON and NARP usually do not cause abnormal histology and do not show any respiratory chain enzyme defects.

Biochemical assays of respiratory chain function may be performed either in isolated mitochondrial fractions or in whole tissue homogenates. The following assays are usually performed: NADH-cytochrome *c* reductase (complexes I + III); NADH-CoQ reductase (complex I); NADH dehydrogenase (complex I); succinate-cytochrome *c* reductase (complexes II + III); reduced CoQ-cytochrome *c* reductase (complex III); cytochrome *c* oxidase (complex IV); succinate dehydrogenase (complex II); and citrate synthase, a matrix enzyme of the Krebs cycle. Citrate synthase, which is encoded by nDNA, is a good marker of mitochondrial abundance, and we refer the activities of respiratory chain enzymes to those of citrate synthase to correct for increased (more rarely decreased) numbers of mitochondria. Conditions with multiple deletions or depletion of mtDNA usually have multiple partial defects of the respiratory chain enzymes, although in some cases these defects may not be apparent. Isolated defects of complex I, II, or IV activity suggest mutations in mtDNA genes encoding subunits of that complex, or in nDNA genes encoding subunits or assembly proteins of the same complex. Enzyme assays should always be interpreted in the light of the clinical presentation and caution should be used in assessing data in very young and very old patients.

Table 159.4 Summary of clinical syndromes, genetic and pathological classification, and associated lactic acidosis (LA), type of ragged-red fibers (RRF) (with cytochrome *c* oxidase (COX) staining), and patterns of respiratory chain complex deficiencies in the muscle.

Genetic defect	Functional defect	Clinical features	LA	RRF	Muscle biochemistry
mtDNA mutations	Defects of protein synthesis	KSS; PS; CPEO; MELAS; MERRF	+	COX–	I + III + IV
	Protein coding genes mutations	LHON; NARP/MILS	–	–	I; V
		MELAS overlaps	±	–	
		Myopathy	+	COX+	I; III; IV
Intergenomic signaling defects (nDNA)	Multiple mtDNA deletions	AD-PEO; AR-PEO; ARCO; MNGIE; SANDO	+	COX–	I + III + IV
	mtDNA depletion	Hepatocerebral; myopathic; Alpers' syndrome	+	COX–	I + III + IV
	Defects of mtDNA translation	Hepatocerebral; generalized; MLASA	+	COX–	I + III + IV
Other nDNA mutations	RC subunits	LS	+	–	I; II
	Assembly proteins	LS; LSFC; EE; GRACILE	+	–	I; III; IV; V
	Fusion/fission/motility	AD-optic atrophy; CMT2A; HSP	±	–	?
	Lipid milieu	Barth syndrome	–	+	IV

Question mark denotes variable muscle biochemistry defects. KSS: Kearns–Sayre syndrome; PS: Pearson syndrome; CPEO: chronic progressive external ophthalmoplegia; MELAS: mitochondrial encephalomyopathy, lactic acidosis, stroke-like episodes; MERRF: myoclonic epilepsy with ragged-red fibers; LHON: Leber hereditary optic neuropathy; NARP: neuropathy, ataxia, retinitis pigmentosa; MILS: maternally inherited Leigh syndrome; AD-PEO: autosomal dominant-progressive external ophthalmoplegia; AR-PEO: autosomal recessive–progressive external ophthalmoplegia; ARCO: autosomal recessive cardiopathy and ophthalmoplegia; MNGIE: mitochondrial neurogastrointestinal encephalomyopathy; SANDO: sensory ataxic neuropathy dysarthria and ophthalmoplegia; MLASA: mitochondrial myopathy and sideroblastic anemia; LS: Leigh syndrome; LSFC: Leigh syndrome, French-Canadian type; EE: ethylmalonic encephalopathy; GRACILE: growth retardation, aminoaciduria, iron overload, lactic acidosis, early death; AD-optic atrophy: autosomal dominant-optic atrophy; CMT2A: Charcot–Marie–Tooth disease 2A; HSP: hereditary spastic paraplegia.

Molecular genetic testing

The choice of the appropriate DNA test is a complex decision that requires review of the clinical features, histology, and biochemical results. If a mitochondrial syndrome such as MELAS, MERRF, NARP, MILS, or NARP is evident, the appropriate mutations can be screened in blood, starting from the most common. Other easily accessible tissues may also be used, such as urinary sediment, buccal mucosa, hair follicles, or cultured skin fibroblasts. If there is a history suggestive of PEO or KSS, Southern blot to detect single or multiple mtDNA deletions should be performed. In pure sporadic myopathy, muscle is the tissue of choice as the mutant mtDNA is not found in other tissues. Patients with the MNGIE phenotype should be screened for thymidine phosphorylase activity in leukocytes and the diagnosis genetically confirmed by screening the *TP* gene.

Leigh syndrome is a particularly difficult condition to define because of its striking biochemical and genetic heterogeneity. Certain clinical features may be useful, for example, retinitis pigmentosa is almost pathognomonic for MILS due to the T8993G mutation in the ATPase6 gene. X-linked transmission suggests mutations in the PDHC E1 subunit. In the presence of a history suggestive of autosomal recessive inheritance, biochemical analysis of muscles may reveal a specific complex deficiency for which the specific genes can then be screened (Table 159.2).

Therapy

Therapy for mitochondrial diseases is woefully inadequate. To date, treatments have been palliative or have involved the use of vitamins, cofactors, and antioxidants, with the aim of mitigating, postponing, or circumventing the potential damage to the respiratory chain. Because of the clinical diversity of mitochondrial disorders and their unpredictable clinical course, rigorous, controlled therapeutic trials have not been performed very often, and therefore most interventions are not evidence-based. Commonly used laboratory measures such as lactic acid, neurophysiological responses, MR spectroscopy, or muscle strength testing may not adequately reflect the efficacy of treatment. Class 1 evidence is therefore unlikely to be obtained in evaluating treatments of mitochondrial disorders.

Symptomatic therapy

Treatment of specific symptoms is important in patients with mitochondrial encephalomyopathies. Seizures usually respond to anticonvulsants, although valproic acid should be used with caution because it inhibits carnitine uptake (which could worsen myopathy) or trigger fulminant hepatic failure in patients with Alpers' syndrome. PEO can be treated with surgery for ptosis and sensorineural hearing loss with cochlear implants. Episodes of recurrent myoglobinuria should be treated aggressively with fluid hydration and urine alkalinization.

Exercise training may benefit patients not only by improving their oxidative capacity, but also potentially by inducing regeneration of muscle fibers that have lower amounts of mutant mtDNA than mature muscle fibers.

In general, most anesthetic and surgical procedures are well tolerated by patients with mitochondrial disorders. Problems with anesthesia are usually related to pre-existing clinical conditions, for example, seizures, respiratory compromise, and cardiac arrhythmias. Careful pre-operative assessment is necessary and patients with myopathy should avoid the use of inhalational agents and depolarizing muscle relaxants that may trigger malignant hyperthermia.

Dietary measures such as the ketogenic diet may be useful in selected conditions, such as PDHC deficiency, and potentially even in KSS, where ketogenic treatment has been shown to decrease deleted mtDNA in cell cultures, although this has not yet been explored in clinical trials.

Pharmacological therapy
Removal of noxious metabolites
Dichloroacetic acid (DCA) is a pyruvate dehydrogenase kinase inhibitor, which keeps PDH in the active form and favors lactic acid oxidation, thereby decreasing lactic acidosis. While it is useful for treatment of acute lactic acidosis, the side effects of chronic therapy, specifically peripheral neuropathy, suggest that DCA should not be used over extended periods of time.

Administration of electron acceptors
Primary CoQ10 deficiency can be treated with CoQ10 supplementation. High-dose oral CoQ10 supplementation (300–1500 mg/day) was shown to be beneficial in the severe infantile encephalopathic as well as the myopathic forms of primary CoQ10 deficiency. Patients with the ataxic form tended to respond less well, probably due to irreversible cerebellar damage.

Administration of vitamins and cofactors
Various cocktails of vitamins (riboflavin, thiamine, folic acid) and cofactors (CoQ10, L-carnitine, creatine, and lipoic acid) have been used based on anecdotal reports. Some of these compounds may be decreased in patients (e.g., carnitine deficiency secondary to partial impairment of -oxidation), warranting supplementation, while others are considered to be neuroprotective because they supposedly favor ATP production and counteract free radical generation and apoptosis. Anecdotal evidence

also supports the use of folinic acid in patients with KSS because of abnormal CSF:serum folate ratio.

Alteration of nitric oxide (NO) homeostasis is thought to underlie the endothelial dysfunction in MELAS patients, resulting in stroke-like episodes. Intravenous administration of L-arginine (0.5 g/kg) during the acute phase and interictal oral administration (0.15–0.3 g/kg/day) diminished the frequency and severity of stroke-like episodes in open-label trials.

Administration of oxygen radical scavengers
In order to decrease free radical damage in energy-challenged cells, several oxygen radical scavengers have been used, such as vitamin E, CoQ10, idebenone, glutathione, and dihydrolipoate. Idebenone, which is an analogue of CoQ10, was shown to improve cardiac function in patients with Friedreich's ataxia.

Gene therapy
Gene therapy for mtDNA disorders is not available, mainly because no investigator has been able to transfect DNA into mitochondria in a heritable fashion. Currently, one of the most promising strategies is to force a shift in heteroplasmy, reducing the ratio of mutant to wild-type genomes. This can be achieved by inhibiting replication of mutant genomes with peptide nucleic acids, importing RNAs into the mitochondria, importing polypeptides into mitochondria, selecting for respiratory function, inducing muscle regeneration, and inducing mitochondrial fusion. Most of these approaches have shown promising results *in vitro*, but none is readily applicable to patients.

Gene therapy for nDNA disorders is similar to that for other Mendelian disorders. Proof of principle studies have been performed by inserting transgene ANT1 protein into the mitochondrial inner membrane of transgenic *Ant1* mutant mice, ameliorating their muscle pathology.

Conclusions

The nervous system is one of the most frequently affected organs in mitochondrial diseases and therefore should be extensively investigated if mitochondrial disease is suspected. While therapy for mitochondrial disorders is woefully inadequate at present, rapidly increasing knowledge of different molecular defects and their pathogenic mechanisms may allow individualized treatments in the near future.

Further reading

Barragan-Campos HM, Vallee JN, Lo D, *et al.* Brain magnetic resonance imaging findings in patients with mitochondrial cytopathies. *Arch Neurol* 2005; 62(5): 737–42.

Carelli V, Barboni P, Sadun AA. Mitochondrial ophthalmology. In: DiMauro SH, Hirano M, Schon EA, editors. *Mitochondrial Medicine*. Oxford: Informa Healthcare; 2006, pp. 105–42.

DiMauro S, Hirano M, Schon EA. Approaches to the treatment of mitochondrial diseases. *Muscle Nerve* 2006; 34(3): 265–83.

DiMauro S, Quinzii CM, Hirano M. Mutations in coenzyme Q10 biosynthetic genes. *J Clin Invest* 2007; 117(3): 587–9.

Gempel K, Topaloglu H, Talim B, *et al.* The myopathic form of coenzyme Q10 deficiency is caused by mutations in the electron-transferring-flavoprotein dehydrogenase (ETFDH) gene. *Brain*, published online April 5, 2007.

Kaufmann P, Shungu DC, Sano MC, *et al.* Cerebral lactic acidosis correlates with neurological impairment in MELAS. *Neurology* 2004; 62(8): 1297–302.

Koga Y, Akita Y, Junko N, *et al.* Endothelial dysfunction in MELAS improved by l-arginine supplementation. *Neurology* 2006; 66(11): 1766–9.

Majamaa K, Moilanen JS, Uimonen S, *et al.* Epidemiology of A3243G, the mutation for mitochondrial encephalomyopathy, lactic acidosis, and stroke like episodes: prevalence of the mutation in an adult population. *Am J Hum Genet* 1998; 63(2): 447–54.

Rahman S, Blok RB, Dahl HH, *et al.* Leigh syndrome: clinical features and biochemical and DNA abnormalities. *Ann Neurol* 1996; 39(3): 343–51.

Schaefer AM, Taylor RW, Turnbull DM, Chinnery PF. The epidemiology of mitochondrial disorders – past, present and future. *Biochim Biophys Acta* 2004; 1659(2–3): 115–20.

Shanske S, Pancrudo J, Kaufmann P, *et al.* Varying loads of the mitochondrial DNA A3243G mutation in different tissues: implications for diagnosis. *Am J Med Genet A* 2004; 130(2): 134–7.

Taivassalo T, Gardner JL, Taylor RW, *et al.* Endurance training and detraining in mitochondrial myopathies due to single large-scale mtDNA deletions. *Brain* 2006; 129(Pt 12): 3391–401.

Chapter 160
Fatty acid oxidation disorders

Thomas Wieser[1] and Thomas Deufel[2]

[1]Krankenhaus Göttlicher Heiland, Vienna, Austria
[2]University Hospital Jena, Jena, Germany

Introduction

Carbohydrates and fatty acids comprise the major energy supply in the mammalian organism. Glucose, the main carbohydrate fuel, is stored as glycogen in liver and muscle; fatty acids are stored as triglycerides and as other lipids. In general, there is a hierarchy of usage for these substrates, with glucose as the primary fuel for short-term demands, its constant level maintained by glycogenolysis. Depletion of liver glycogen stores, for example, during prolonged fasting, triggers a systemic switch to lipolysis and, consequently, oxidation of fatty acids which predominantly occurs as β-oxidation in mitochondria.

This hierarchy of energy substrate use constitutes the connection between any disturbances of carbohydrate and fatty acid metabolism: if the use of carbohydrates is restricted by a disorder of glucose metabolism, the inability to maintain glucose supply from glycogen breakdown or a failure to create glycogen stores, the dependence on fatty acid oxidation is increased. Conversely, disturbances in the oxidation or restrictions in the availability of fatty acids, for example, in decreased lipolysis or disturbances in their transport into cells and across the mitochondrial membrane to the site of β-oxidation, will immediately increase the dependence on carbohydrate supply which is both short term and quickly exhausted, for example, during fasting.

Striated muscle and brain both have specific features of energy substrate usage that make them specifically, yet in different ways, vulnerable to any disturbance of energy metabolism. In muscle it is the essential use of fatty acids in long-term exercise; for the brain it is the unique dependence on glucose and ketone bodies, the latter formed as an end product of β-oxidation, which can neither be stored nor produced in the brain itself.

The brain requires a stable blood level of both low molecular substrates. This can be maintained only when liver metabolism is intact. If a shortage of these substrates occurs *secondary* to a disturbance in hepatic fatty acid oxidation, the central nervous system (CNS) is readily affected and so-called "hepatocerebral crises" will occur. The clinical symptomatology is characterized by severe metabolic derangement with hypoketotic hypoglycemia, hyperammonemia, lethargy or reduced consciousness, seizures, and, potentially, cerebral edema.

A completely different situation is found in skeletal muscle and heart. Muscle cells possess the complete enzymatic apparatus required to form and break down both glycogen and triglycerides and, therefore, can utilize the entire range of fuels. While glycolysis and glycogenolysis are able to stave off acute peaks of energy demand, the main energy supply is through oxidation of fatty acids, especially during long-term exercise and fasting. With this unique feature of energy production, muscle and heart are *primarily* and predominantly affected whenever fatty acid oxidation is disturbed. Clinically, chronic muscle weakness, myopathy, hypotonia, cardiomyopathy, arrhythmia, and heart block can result from chronic disruption of muscular function.

Muscle symptoms can be permanent as well as progressive, as exemplified in primary carnitine deficiency where there is a defect of delivery of fatty acids at the site of β-oxidation and, consequently, triglyceride accumulation in the cytosol. On the other hand, patients with carnitine palmitoyl transferase II (CPT II) deficiency are, in general, without symptoms and have normal muscle strength but are prone to painful episodes of rhabdomyolysis and weakness provoked by prolonged exercise or fasting.

Epidemiology and genetics

Fatty acid oxidation disorders rarely occur, with only a few cases reported for each enzyme defect. An exception is medium chain acyl-CoA dehydrogenase (MCAD) deficiency, for which the incidence in Europe is reported to be 1 in 10 000–16 000. Disease-causing mutations in the MCAD gene on chromosome 1p31 are known; notably, there is a common mutation 985A>G (*K304E*), which can be found on 54–90% of mutant alleles.

International Neurology: A Clinical Approach. Edited by Robert P. Lisak, Daniel D. Truong, William M. Carroll, and Roongroj Bhidayasiri. © 2009 Blackwell Publishing, ISBN: 978-1-4051-5738-4.

Screening for primary carnitine deficiency (PCD) revealed a prevalence of 1 in 40 000 births in the Akita prefecture in Japan and 1 in 37 000–100 000 in Australia. Epidemiological data for other areas are not available. PCD is caused by mutations in the *SLC22A5* gene on chromosome 5q31.1 encoding the sodium-dependent carnitine transporter OCTN2.

Carnitine palmitoyltransferase II (CPT II) deficiency, which, like all other disorders of fatty acid oxidation, is inherited in an autosomal recessive mode, has been described in about 300 patients to date. Mutations are found in the CPT II gene on chromosome 1p32, with a "common" mutation (*S113L*) found in approximately 60% of mutant alleles. There is consistent genotype–phenotype correlation where missense mutations are associated with the muscle form (including the common S113L mutation) and therefore these are called "mild" mutations, truncating mutations are frequently associated with the lethal neonatal forms and therefore are considered "severe" mutations.

Clinical features and pathophysiology

Acyl-CoA dehydrogenase deficiencies

The first step in mitochondrial β-oxidation is the dehydrogenation of acyl-CoA to enoyl-CoA; this is catalyzed by different acyl-CoA dehydrogenases with distinct but somewhat overlapping substrate specificity (short chain, medium chain, and very long chain, as well as branched chain fatty acids); the long chain activity is not mitochondrial and does not seem to play a role as a genetic defect.

Defects of this first step frequently result in abnormal lipid accumulation in muscle and carnitine deficiency, because intramitochondrial-accumulated acyl-CoA ester are buffered as carnitine-ester which can permeate the mitochondrial membrane and are then excreted by the kidneys. Lipid accumulation in muscle, as seen, for example, in MCAD deficiency, is shown in Plate 160.1. Typically, when medium or very long chain activities are affected, there is also an increased bypass to ω-oxidation; the resulting dicarboxylic acids are diagnostic when detected in urine analysis or as carnitine esters in blood.

The clinical symptomatology varies depending on the age of onset. Manifestation in childhood usually presents with multi-organ involvement, including the liver, heart, and kidneys. CNS and muscular symptoms are not prominent. Manifestations in adolescence or early adulthood produce almost exclusively muscular symptoms. Important to bear in mind is the significant, often even intrafamilial, clinical heterogeneity seen in these disorders. A sufficient explanation for this variability is still lacking.

The most common of these defects is MCAD deficiency (see section on Epidemiology). Children with this defect seem normal at birth and manifestation is between 3 and 24 months, but occasionally manifestation may occur in adulthood. A previously healthy child develops hypoketotic hypoglycemia, vomiting, and lethargy triggered by a common illness or fasting. More than 18% of affected children die during their first metabolic crisis. However, once the defect is known, prognosis is usually good, and the crisis is reversed by intravenous glucose. Liquid chromatography-tandem mass spectrometry (LC-tandem MS) newborn screening now facilitates early detection of the disease.

Carnitine deficiency

Long-chain fatty acids are transported across the inner mitochondrial membrane with the help of the carnitine shuttle. Carnitine, which is actively transported into the muscle cells using the sodium-dependent carnitine transporter (OCTN2), is esterified with long-chain acyl residues transferred from acyl-coenzyme A esters by CPT 1, translocated as acylcarnitines across the inner mitochondrial membrane by carnitine-acylcarnitine translocase (CAT) and then transferred back to coenzyme A by CPT II to enter the β-oxidation cycle. The functioning of this shuttle is dependent on sufficient free carnitine in the cells which is derived from both the diet (especially meat and dairy products) and biosynthesis in the liver, with 90% of body carnitine found in muscle.

Mutations in the OCTN2 carnitine transporter gene cause primary carnitine deficiency. In most patients hepatocerebral crises occur characterized by Rye-like symptoms with reduced consciousness, tonic–clonic seizures, hepatomegaly, hypoglycemia, acidosis, liver failure, and skeletal and cardiac myopathy. Age of onset varies between 8 months and early adulthood. Early recognition and treatment with high doses of oral carnitine can be life saving.

Carnitine palmitoyltransferase deficiency

The CPT system mediates the transport of long-chain fatty acids into the mitochondrial matrix. This system includes two different enzymes: CPT I, located in the outer leaf of the inner mitochondrial membrane, and CPT II, located in the inner aspect of the inner membrane, which catalyzes the exchange of acyl groups between acyl-coenzyme A (CoA) and acylcarnitine. Only a few cases are described, with CPT I deficiency presenting with severe episodes of hypoketotic hypoglycemia usually occurring after fasting or illness, with onset in infancy or early childhood. CPT II deficiency, on the other hand, is probably the most common defect in muscle fatty acid metabolism. Consistent epidemiological data are not available, yet more than 300 cases have been described to date. Three distinct clinical presentations occur. The first is the "lethal neonatal" form manifesting within days after birth as liver failure with hypoketotic hypoglycemia, cardiomyopathy, cardiac arrhythmias, and seizures; it is often accompanied by malformations (facial and neuronal migration defects, among others). Onset during the first year of life is characteristic of the "severe hepato-cardiomuscular" form; liver failure, cardiomyopathy, seizures, hypoketotic hypoglycemia, abdominal pain, and peripheral myopathy are the main clinical features. Probably the most common presentation is the "adult onset muscular" form, with age of onset between the first and sixth decade of life. It is characterized by recurrent attacks of myalgia accompanied by myoglobinuria precipitated by prolonged exercise, especially after fasting; it may also be triggered by cold exposure or stress. Muscle weakness during attacks is possible. Characteristically there are no signs of myopathy (weakness, myalgia, elevation of serum creatine kinase concentration) between attacks and patients are healthy and completely normal in neurological examination between attacks.

The infantile as well as the adult cases have been shown to be associated with a decreased amount of steady-state CPT II protein. The lethal neonatal as well as the severe infantile forms are characterized by reduced CPT II enzyme activity in multiple organs, reduced serum concentrations of total and free carnitine, and increased serum concentrations of long-chain acylcarnitines and lipids. For adult onset type, reduced enzyme activity can also be measured. However, using the "isotope forward assay" normal enzyme activity is found; patients can be distinguished from controls because inhibition of enzyme activity by malonyl-CoA, a natural regulator of this pathway, is significantly greater. This has led to the hypothesis that in adult onset muscular type CPT II deficiency, not the catalytic activity but the regulation to this system is impaired.

Investigations

While obtaining a patient's history, one should focus on episodes of rhabdomyolysis, myoglobinuria, hypoglycemia, and encephalopathy, and Rye-like symptoms. Family history regarding myopathy, encephalopathy, and sudden infant death is also of eminent importance.

Routine management should include echocardiography, sonography, and neurophysiology. Laboratory tests should include blood sugar, pH, liver enzymes, urea, aldolase, lactate dehydrogenase, and creatine kinase, as well as plasma acylcarnitines, plasma fatty acid (free or total) profile, urine organic acids, and urine acylglycines.

For the diagnosis of fatty acid oxidation disorders tandem mass spectrometry is the method of choice. Findings suggestive of a defect in mitochondrial β-oxidation can be obtained not only in plasma or serum but also in dried blood spots. Ultimately, measurement of the respective enzyme activities reveals the enzymatic defect. Mutation analysis in index patients may be performed to facilitate early or prenatal diagnosis, but often is mainly of research interest.

Management

In contrast to other metabolic diseases such as glycogenoses or defects of the respiratory chain, effective treatment is possible for fatty acid oxidation disorders. Therapeutic strategies include dietary recommendations as well as medications. Published recommendations are based on limited experience and thus have to be treated with caution; close clinical monitoring and the implementation of individual regimens are warranted.

"Low fat, high carbohydrate" diets are recommended (70% carbohydrate, less than 20% fat), preferably with multiple small meals and the avoidance of fasting. Catabolic states that may easily precipitate severe crisis should be avoided at any rate; timely application of intravenous glucose is important in any situation where supply of carbohydrate fuels might be impaired, such as during infections, diarrhea, or fasting. A high rate of glucose intake not only normalizes the plasma glucose level but also efficiently suppresses lipolysis, diminishing the production of toxic long-chain acylcarnitines in the case of long-chain fatty acid oxidation defects and probably the production of other toxic metabolites such as octanoate in the case of medium-chain or short-chain defects. Long-term exercise should be avoided.

Carnitine supplementation has produced mixed results. In primary carnitine deficiency, administration of carnitine (100 mg/kg/day) is necessary and successful. Interestingly, despite clinical improvement in some cases, carnitine levels have stayed low.

Prenatal diagnosis

Prenatal diagnosis of fatty acid disorders can be offered to all parents with an increased familial risk. All enzymes of mitochondrial fatty acid oxidation are expressed in chorionic villi biopsies as well as cultured chorionic villous fibroblasts and amniocytes. When the molecular defect of the index patient is known, direct analysis of the genetic mutation can be performed.

Further reading

Deschauer M, Wieser T, Zierz S. Muscle carnitine palmitoyltransferase II deficiency. *Arch Neurol* 2005; 62: 37–41.

Matter D, Rinaldo D. Medium chain acyl coenzyme A dehydrogenase deficiency. In: *GeneReviews at GeneTests: Medical Genetics Information Resource 2000* (updated 2005); Copyright University of Washington, Seattle 1997–2006, available at http://www.genetests.org.

Wanders RJA, Vreken P, Den Boer MEJ, Wijburg FA, Van Gennip AH, Ijlst L. Disorders of mitochondrial fatty acyl-CoA β-oxidation. *J Inherit Metab Dis* 1999; 22: 442–87.

Chapter 161
Disorders resulting from transporters

David Gloss
Tulane University School of Medicine, New Orleans, USA

Introduction

Transporter defects comprise a set of diseases, mostly rare, that span many areas of neurology. This chapter describes some of the best understood and most well-known transporter defects (Menkes' disease, Wilson's disease, and carnitine O-palmitoyltransferase 2 deficiency), as well as two very rare disorders (GLUT-1 deficiency and hereditary folate malabsorption), to give readers an idea of the range of deficits involved in transporter defects.

Menkes' disease

Menkes' disease was first described by Menkes in 1962. It is an X-linked recessive disorder with onset at 1–2 months after birth, with a relentless course ending in death by age 1–2. The disorder is characterized by scant, white, silver, or gray, stubby, kinky hair (the disease is also known as kinky hair disease); skin pallor; growth retardation; hypothermia with acute illness; long bone metaphyseal demineralization; tortuosity of cerebral vessels; and diffuse cerebral atrophy with subdural fluid collections. Seizures often complicate the picture.

There seem to be several different variants of the disease, but the paucity of cases makes it hard to know if these are truly related or not. There are some Japanese cases which do not show the hair distortions. There is an occipital horn syndrome with occipital exostoses that do not develop until age 3 or 4 with skin laxity, dysarthria, and chronic diarrhea. Late-onset and asymptomatic cases have also been described.

The disease is due to a defect of the *ATP7A* gene on chromosome Xq13.3. This gene codes for an ATPase that is integral to transmembrane copper transport. It is present in the brain, intestines, kidneys, and other organs, but not present in the liver. Variation among the types of mutations on the *ATP7A* gene may produce some of the variety of clinical manifestations. A large deletion or a frame-shift mutation is thought to cause infantile-onset Menkes' disease, while mutations causing either reduced levels *ATP7A* or reduced function of *ATP7A* cause the occipital horn syndrome. The ATP7A protein transports copper and is located on the trans-Golgi network. When intracellular copper levels become too high, the protein translocates to the cell membrane to excrete the copper. This explains, in part, why there is deficient transport of dietary copper in the intestine but accumulates in the duodenum, kidney, pancreas, placenta, and skeletal muscle.

The symptoms of Menkes' disease can be explained by the effect of the gene mutation on the essential enzymes that need copper to function. The loss of hair and skin pigment may be explained by tyrosinase dysfunction. Arterial defects are due to defects in collagen cross-linking from lysyl oxidase dysfunction. Kinky hair comes from monoamine oxidase dysfunction. Hypothermia may be explained by cytochrome c oxidase dysfunction. The long bone demineralization may come from ascorbate oxidase.

Diagnosis is generally clinical, with confirmation by low serum copper and ceruloplasmin levels (if after 6 weeks of age), high placental copper levels, or abnormal catecholamines. The latter two can be tested at birth.

The treatment for Menkes' disease is subcutaneous administration of copper chloride and L-histidine, in an attempt to restore normal copper levels to the body. Within 6 weeks, responders will have normal blood and cerebrospinal levels of copper, with a regression of symptoms, except for the connective tissue problems. Neurologic symptoms may or may not respond. Some children do not respond. It is thought that copper administration may work only for those children with some functioning *ATP7A*.

Wilson's disease

Dr Wilson first described this disease in 1912 in England. Wilson's disease is relatively common, with a carrier frequency of 1 in 100. It is the most common cause of childhood liver disease. It is an autosomal recessive disorder that has a broad range of ages of presentation, with typical cases presenting at ages 6–20. The main features of

International Neurology: A Clinical Approach. Edited by Robert P. Lisak, Daniel D. Truong, William M. Carroll, and Roongroj Bhidayasiri. © 2009 Blackwell Publishing, ISBN: 978-1-4051-5738-4.

the disease are cirrhosis and neuropsychiatric phenomena. Typically, if the presentation is before age 10, it occurs with fulminant hepatic failure without symptoms of neurologic impairment. If the presentation is after age 10, the opposite is often true.

The initial symptoms often include abnormal gait, speech, and behavioral disturbances. These initial symptoms will worsen without treatment, and with development of bulbar dystonia including dysarthria and risus sardonicus, parkinsonism, dysdiadochokinesia, or other dystonias. Nearly all patients with neurologic impairment will have a brownish-yellow discoloration of the limbus, called a Keyser–Fleischer ring. Copper deposition in Wilson's disease can also cause renal damage, greenish-gray pigmented cataracts, and cardiomyopathy. There are some cases of hidranitis supporativa, rhabdomyolysis, and hypoparathyroidism associated with the disease.

The disease arises from a defect in the *ATP7B* gene on chromosome 13q14.3–q21.1. Like *ATP7A*, *ATP7B* is a transmembrane ATPase that mediates copper excretion and transport, allowing copper to be excreted in the bile. With *ATP7B* dysfunction, copper buildup leads to liver damage, and copper eventually spills into the bloodstream. This excess copper binds to neuromelanin, causing copper deposits in the putamen and globus pallidus. The excess copper is also thought to be the cause of the damage to eyes, kidneys, and heart.

Diagnosis is typically screening with a low serum copper and serum ceruloplasmin concentration. This is usually followed up by a 24-hour urinary copper determination and a slit lamp examination for Keyser–Fleischer rings.

Treatment is with life-long copper chelation. Typically chelation is accomplished with penicillamine. Trientene has not been studied as well, but, based on preliminary data, it appears to work just as well with fewer side effects. Some patients may have initial worsening of symptoms, as copper is released into the urine, but this should not be a reason to discontinue treatment, and patients should be warned that this may happen. Pyridoxine should be administered to prevent deficiency. Chelation is often verified with a second 24-hour urinary copper excretion measurement. After chelation, zinc is often used to interfere with intestinal absorption of copper. Some use vitamin E as adjunctive therapy, as there are reports of symptomatic improvement in some patients. Low serum levels of vitamin E have been shown in both serum and liver in Wilson's disease.

Carnitine *O*-palmitoyltransferase 2 deficiency

Carnitine *O*-palmitoyltransferase 2 deficiency is the most common metabolic disorder of skeletal muscle. It has an autosomal recessive pattern of inheritance. There are three different manifestations of this disorder. The neonatal form is universally fatal with non-ketotic hypoglycemic encephalopathy, respiratory failure, seizures, and an irregular heart beat leading to cardiac arrest. These neonates often display dysmorphic features. The second form typically presents between 6 months and 2 years of age with significant problems during infections or fasting. During times of stress, the infant will lose consciousness and may have seizures due to hypoglycemia. For unknown reasons, this form is sometimes accompanied by hepatomegaly. The best known form typically presents in the teen to young adult years, with muscle pain and swelling after either fasting or sustained exercise. There is increased risk of malignant hyperthermia in patients with this deficiency. There are significant differences in penetrance in the disease even among members of the same family. There is some evidence that peripheral neuropathy and migraines may develop.

The gene locus for the disease is 1p32. Carnitine *O*-palmitoyltransferase 2 is present on the inner membrane of mitochondria. While not a transporter per se, it is a necessary part of a three enzyme group: itself, acetyl-CoA synthase, and carnitine/acylcarnitine translocase, which allow fatty acids to be transferred into mitochondria to undergo oxidation.

Diagnosis is accomplished by measuring creatine phosphokinase (CPK) and urinary myoglobin after exercise. Muscle histology is typically normal during attacks. Muscle biopsy with carnitine *O*-palmitoyltransferase 2 level measurement confirms the diagnosis.

Treatment is supportive. A diet with carbohydrate loading during meals can be protective. Prolonged exercise is avoided. A small amount of data suggest that prolonged exercise may be safe with intravenous glucose during exercise, but this seems hardly practical. Carnitine supplementation may help if migraines develop.

GLUT-1 deficiency

GLUT-1 (facilitated glucose transporter-1) deficiency was first described by De Vivo in 1991, and is sometimes called De Vivo's disease. It is thought to be transmitted by autosomal dominant inheritance, although most cases seem sporadic. The typical manifestations of the disease include infantile seizures, acquired microcephaly, spasticity, and encephalopathy, with a wide variety of additional manifestations. There are two other less common presentations. One includes hypotonia, choreoathetosis, dysarthria, dystonia, and developmental delay. The other includes ataxia, dysarthria, dystonia, and developmental delay.

The gene locus is 1p31–p35. GLUT-1 is present in all tissues at low levels. It has its highest concentration in the erythrocytes and in cerebral capillary endothelial cells, such as those that represent an aspect of the blood–brain barrier. This causes normal serum glucose, low or normal cerebrospinal fluid lactate, and otherwise unexplained hypoglycorrhacia, with typical values being approximately one-third of the serum values. This lack of metabolic energy substrate affects brain development.

Diagnosis has not been standardized. It can be accomplished through appropriate cerebral spinal fluid studies, performed after a 4-hour fast. Most reported cases do not have brain magnetic resonance abnormalities, but there is one reported case of delayed myelination.

Treatment is through a ketogenic diet. Acetoacetate and β-hyroxybutyrate are products of fatty acid metabolism that can be transported across the blood–brain barrier. The brain is well adapted to utilize ketone bodies as fuel. The ketogenic diet has been shown to treat the seizures associated with this condition. Antiseizure medications have been ineffective. Some, including diazepam and phenobarbital, may actually exacerbate the condition. Others, such as phenytoin and carbamazepine, do not seem to worsen the condition. If seizures cannot be controlled with a ketogenic diet, judicious use of selected anticonvulsants may be effective. The diet may also improve associated motor symptoms, and, to some extent, the developmental delay. In the one reported case of delayed myelination, 6 months of the ketogenic diet improved the myelination, which may explain why the developmental delay is ameliorated.

Hereditary folate malabsorption

Hereditary folate malabsorption was first described in 1965. Neither the gene nor the transporter has been identified. Patients have developmental delay, megaloblastic anemia, and seizures. Some have ataxia; others have athetosis. In some patients, there are basal ganglia calcifications and/or diarrhea. Most of the reported cases have parental consanguinity. Many children with this disorder may die in the first few months of life without the disorder being recognized.

Diagnosis is made by the clinical constellation of megaloblastic anemia with seizures. Confirmation of folate deficiency in each of the serum, red blood cells, and cerebrospinal fluid demonstrates the disorder.

Folate treatment will cure the anemia and diarrhea if it is present. Seizures seem to variably respond to folate supplementation. Seizures may be controlled with a combination of folate, cyanocobalamin, and methionine. Intermittent folic acid supplementation seems to have ameliorated the symptoms of one child.

Further reading

Jebnoun S, Kacem S, Mokrani C, Chabchoub A, Khrouf N, Zittoun J. A family study of congenital malabsorption of folate. *J Inherit Metab Dis* 2001; 24: 749–50.

Klepper J, Voit T. Facilitated glucose transporter protein type 1 (GLUT1) deficiency syndrome: impaired glucose transport into the brain – a review. *Eur J Pediatr* 2002; 161: 295–304.

Menkes JH. Kinky hair disease: twenty five years later. *Brain Dev* 1988; 10: 77–9.

Scheinberg IH, Jaffe ME, Sternlieb I. The use of trientine in preventing the effects of interrupting penicillamine therapy in Wilson's disease. *N Engl J Med* 1987; 317: 209–13.

Vladutiu GD, Bennett MJ, Fisher NM, *et al.* Phenotypic variability among first-degree relatives with carnitine palmitoyltransferase II deficiency. *Muscle Nerve* 2002; 26: 492–8.

Chapter 162
Lesch–Nyhan disease

Allison Conravey and Ann Tilton
Louisiana State University Health Sciences Center, New Orleans, USA

Introduction

Lesch–Nyhan disease (LND) was first described in 1964 in a 4-year-old boy with neurological abnormalities and hematuria. It presents as hyperuricemia with a distinct neurobehavioral phenotype that includes mental retardation, motor disabilities such as spasticity and choreoathetosis, and self-injurious behavior.

Epidemiology

LND has been described in all parts of the world. The incidence of LND is thought to be 1 in 10 000 males. Because it is X-linked, LND is almost exclusively expressed in boys. However, there have been six females described with the disease.

Pathophysiology

LND is a recessive disorder caused by an inborn error of purine metabolism. The gene (HPRT1) is mapped to Xq26–q27.2. It codes for the purine salvage enzyme hypoxanthine guanine phosphoribosyltransferase (HGPRT). More than 200 mutations have been reported. Patients whose enzyme activity is less than 1.5% of normal demonstrate classic LND. A number of patients with 2–10% residual enzyme activity display partial features of the syndrome.

HGPRT normally catalyzes the conversion of hypoxanthine and guanine to their respective nucleotides. HGPRT deficiency causes hypoxanthine to be converted instead to xanthine and uric acid. Serum, cerebrospinal fluid (CSF) and urine uric acid levels are greatly elevated. The excretion of other purines is also increased.

It is unclear how this disordered purine metabolism causes the neurological abnormalities associated with LND. A principal hypothesis concerns abnormalities in neurotransmitters. An abnormality of dopaminergic function in the basal ganglia has been well documented. This is thought to be caused by a loss of dopaminergic fibers projecting to the basal ganglia. Loss of striatal dopamine in adults usually results in parkinsonism; however, in children it most often causes dystonia. The self-injurious behavior, which is the hallmark of LND, is thought to be due to developmental loss of dopaminergic fibers and exacerbated to exposure to dopamine agonists. There is also good evidence for problems with norepinephrine turnover and a diminution of striatal cholinergic neurons. Increased activity of the serotonergic system has also been demonstrated, which may explain some of the behavioral abnormalities seen in LND.

Clinical features

Patients with HGPRT deficiency fall into three groups. The first is classic LND. These are the most severely affected individuals. A second group has neurological manifestations and hyperuricemia. The final group has isolated hyperuricemia and renal symptoms but lacks neurological deficits.

Affected children appear normal at birth, and usually develop normally for the first few months of life. Most infants present at 3–9 months of age with neurological symptoms, typically hypotonia and the inability to sit. However, hypertonia has also been reported. Most patients eventually develop spasticity. Deep tendon reflexes are frequently increased and toes are sometimes up-going on the Babinski test. Choreoathetosis is a major motor feature. Dystonia is also almost universal, starting between 6 and 24 months of age. Abnormal movements are relatively minor at rest, becoming worse with voluntary movement and stress.

Symptoms progress until the age of 5 or 6, and then stabilize. Patients cannot walk or sit unsupported. Speech is delayed in all patients, and some never gain the ability to speak at all. When speech does occur, it is almost always

International Neurology: A Clinical Approach. Edited by Robert P. Lisak, Daniel D. Truong, William M. Carroll, and Roongroj Bhidayasiri.

dysarthric. Patients with LND also have problems with chewing and swallowing, sometimes requiring a gastrostomy tube.

Most patients with LND have severe cognitive impairment with IQs of approximately 60. However, patients with normal cognition have been reported.

Self-injurious behaviors, believed to be a form of compulsion, begin to emerge by age 3. There is a wide variation in severity, with most patients having a waxing and waning course. The classic manifestation of this behavior is self biting. Patients bite their lips, fingers, arms, shoulders, and sometimes even their toes. Head banging and eye poking are often seen. Patients are only limited in self injury by their disability, and most have to be restrained. Teeth removal is often necessary. Some patients may also try to injure others. Remarkably, sensation in LND is normal and pain is felt. Patients are relieved and happy when self-mutilation is prevented. Perhaps not surprisingly, LND patients have a large amount of anxiety. These behaviors seem to worsen with stress.

Other neurological disorders are often seen with LND. Seizures occur in 50% of cases. Electroencephalographies (EEGs) are usually normal. Tics are also common. Nystagmus, strabismus, optic atrophy, and recurrent coma have been reported.

Hyperuricemia is another regular feature of LND. Orange sand in the diaper may be the first clinical sign of the disease. This hyperuricemia results in gouty arthritis, renal calculi, hematuria, urate tophi, and urate nephropathy. Uricemia can be prevented with treatment. Untreated patients will die of renal failure.

Investigations

Diagnosis can be made solely on clinical presentation. Serum uric acid is usually from 6 to 10 mg/dl. A better test is the urinary uric acid to creatinine ratio. A ratio of greater than 3:1 is diagnostic. There is an assay for HGPRT which can be done on erythrocytes, cultured skin fibroblasts, or other tissue. The test can be run on amniotic fluid cells and chorionic villus samples for prenatal diagnosis.

Imaging abnormalities are seen, but are not diagnostic for LND. Atrophy is the most common abnormality seen on brain CT scan or MRI. Volume loss is most notable in the basal ganglia, especially the caudate.

Treatment/management

The mainstay of treatment is allopurinol. Allopurinol is a xanthine oxidase inhibitor that blocks the last steps of uric acid synthesis. It treats the renal and arthritic manifestations of the disease but has no effect on the neurologic ones. The usual dose is 20 mg/kg/day. The goal is to keep the serum uric acid levels at less than 3 mg/dl.

Dopaminergic drugs have been tried to treat both the dystonia and the self-mutilating behaviors with disappointing results. Spasticity has been treated with benzodiazepines, baclofen, and botulinum toxin. Botulinum toxin is also helpful for localized areas of painful dystonia. Neurosurgical procedures such as thalamotomy and deep brain stimulation have been tried with mixed results. Bone marrow transplantation is not effective. Orthopedic treatments are also ineffective.

Many drugs have been proposed for treatment of the self-mutilating behaviors. These include serotonin agonists, dopaminergic agonists, dopaminergic antagonists, risperidone, benzodiazepines, carbamazepine, and naltexone. These medicines have been effective in a few cases, have not helped in some, and have made symptoms worse in others. Larger trials are necessary. The only effective treatments at this time are physical restraints and removal of teeth.

Further reading

Christie R, Bay C, Kaufman IA, Bakay B, Borden M, Nyhan WL. Lesch–Nyhan disease: clinical experience with nineteen patients. *Dev Med Child Neurol* 1982; 24: 293–306.

Jinnah HA, Visser JE, Harris JC, *et al*. Delineation of the motor disorder of Lesch–Nyhan disease. *Brain* 2006; 129: 1201–17.

Menkes J, Wilkox WR. Inherited metabolic diseases of the nervous system. In: Menkes JH, Sarnat HB, Maria BL, editors. *Child Neurology*, 7th ed. Philadelphia: Lippincott Williams and Wilkins; 2006, pp. 118–19.

Nyhan WL. The recognition of Lesch–Nyhan syndrome as an inborn error of purine metabolism. *J Inherit Metab Dis* 1997; 20: 171–81.

Nyhan WL. Inborn errors of metabolism II: disorders of purine and amino acid metabolism. In: David RB, editor. *Child and Adolescent Neurology*, 2nd ed. Richmond: Blackwell; 2005, pp. 371–3.

Schretlen DJ, Ward J, Meyer SM, *et al*. Behavioral aspects of Lesch–Nyhan disease and its variants. *Dev Med Child Neurol* 2005; 47: 673–7.

Visser JE, Bar PR, Jinnah HA. Lesch–Nyhan disease and the basal ganglia. *Brain Res Rev* 2000; 32: 449–75.

Yoshiaki S, Sacio T. Neurotransmitter changes in the pathophysiology of Lesch–Nyhan syndrome. *Brain Dev* 2000; 22: S122–31.

Chapter 163
The porphyrias

Frank J.E. Vajda[1,2] and Carlo Solinas[1,3]
[1]Monash University and Medical Centre, Clayton, Australia
[2]University of Melbourne, Melbourne, Australia
[3]University of Siena, Siena, Italy

Introduction and overview

Porphyria comprises of a group of largely inherited disorders which are inborn errors of metabolism due to deficiency of enzymes involved in the production of heme molecules along a complex pathway. These enzyme deficiencies form the preferred basis of classification. Porphyrias are overproduction syndromes, with potentially toxic metabolites causing clinical disease.

Porphyrias have been classified as either hepatic or erythropoietic, based on the site of the metabolic defect, but may be classified into acute types of porphyric attacks contrasting clinically with the production of chronic skin disorders.

There are seven types of porphyria, of which three, acute intermittent porphyria (AIP), variegate porphyria (PV), and hereditary coproporphyria (HCP), commonly give rise clinically to neuropsychiatric syndromes. AIP does not give rise to skin manifestations, but HCP and PV can do so. Two erythropoietic porphyrias manifest as skin disorders, as does porphyria cutanea tarda (PCT). The condition of amino-levolinic dehydratase (ADL) deficiency or plumboporphyria is excessively rare.

The prevalence of hepatic porphyrias varies between 1/20500 and 1/12500 of the population. Porphyria tends to be underdiagnosed. It may be potentially serious, even life threatening. The diagnosis is corroborated by knowledge of relatives being affected. In the presence of otherwise unexplained neurological symptoms, biochemical and genetic testing must be performed rapidly on the relatives, to identify asymptomatic carriers.

Treatment depends on the specific disorder, but it is also individually variable, depending on differences in precipitating factors, which must be avoided. Ascertainment of porphyria is often incidental. Neurological complications may precede the definitive biochemical diagnosis. The clinical picture is often complex and heterogeneous. Neurological complications are common, but the clinical picture may be transient, often initially disregarded. A family history and recurrence of otherwise unexplained neurological symptoms should alert the clinician to a possible diagnosis of porphyria.

Biochemical aspects The biochemical steps of heme synthesis are shown in Figure 163.1.

Classification

Classification is based on the clinical syndromes indicating the enzyme deficiency and the chromosomal location of the genetic defect. The inheritance for most of the syndromes is autosomal dominant, except for congenital erythropoietic porphyria (CEP) and ALA dehydratase deficiency porphyria (see Table 163.1).

Geographic and epidemiological considerations

The overall prevalence and incidence of porphyrias is geographically variable. The hepatic form appears far more frequently than the erythropoietic.

The acute syndromes have a higher prevalence in Scandinavia and the United Kingdom. AIP has been estimated to have a prevalence of 1/10000 in Sweden.

PCT has a prevalence of 1/25000 in the British population. In contrast, a prevalence of 1/125000 has been reported in Argentina, whereas in the same country PV had a prevalence of 1/600000. An update on the molecular diagnosis of porphyrias was produced in Italy, together with a flow chart to facilitate the identification of mutations in heme biosynthetic genes. The molecular analysis permitted identification of the molecular defect underlying the disease in 66 probands with different porphyrias (AIP, PV, PCT, and erythropoietic protoporphyria (EPP)). No Italian patients with defects in the coproporphyrinogen oxidase gene, responsible for HCP, have been detected.

The rarity of AIP in Africans has been emphasized by various authors. An increasing number of cases have recently been reported from Nigeria. Most of them have

International Neurology: A Clinical Approach. Edited by Robert P. Lisak, Daniel D. Truong, William M. Carroll, and Roongroj Bhidayasiri. © 2009 Blackwell Publishing, ISBN: 978-1-4051-5738-4.

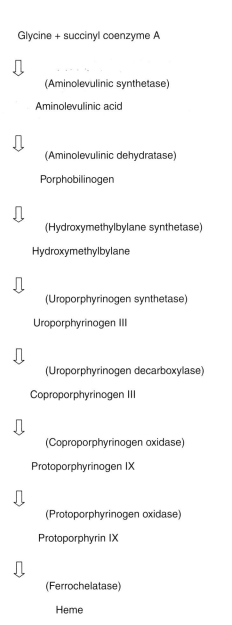

Glycine + succinyl coenzyme A

⇩   . . . . .

(Aminolevulinic synthetase)

Aminolevulinic acid

⇩

(Aminolevulinic dehydratase)

Porphobilinogen

⇩

(Hydroxymethylbylane synthetase)

Hydroxymethylbylane

⇩

(Uroporphyrinogen synthetase)

Uroporphyrinogen III

⇩

(Uroporphyrinogen decarboxylase)

Coproporphyrinogen III

⇩

(Coproporphyrinogen oxidase)

Protoporphyrinogen IX

⇩

(Protoporphyrinogen oxidase)

Protoporphyrin IX

⇩

(Ferrochelatase)

Heme

Figure 163.1 Biochemical steps of heme synthesis. The synthesis of heme, a complex molecule, proceeds from the amino acid glycine through a series of eight steps (indicated by arrows), denoting the enzyme responsible for the next intermediate product.

initially been misdiagnosed and later found to be cases of AIP. Doctors working among African populations should be alerted about this disease. A simple Watson–Schwartz test for porphobilinogens will save many patients from the unnecessary hazards of treatment.

Genetic heterogeneity is also a prominent feature of some porphyrias. The mutation R116W, which has a high prevalence in Dutch and Swedish population, was found on three different haplotypes in three Norwegian families and five Swedish families.

Congenital porphyrias are exceedingly rare. Only 15% of the carriers of mutations develop clinical syndromes and more than 30% of patients have no family history. However, in China, of a total of 145 cases, 75.2% were EPP (109 cases), but only 19.3% (28 cases) were PCT.

This prevalence differs from that in other parts of the world. Early diagnosis of EPP using the fluorescence microscopic test for determination of red blood cell (RBC) protoporphyrin is important. The complication of hepatobiliary aspects in PCT and EPP was noted. Liver disease seems to be an important precipitating factor in China.

The clinical picture

Erythropoietic porphyrias (EP), including X-linked sideroblastic anemia, congenital erythropoietic porphyria (CEP), and EPP, are rare. CEP has been documented in just 150 cases in the literature. The clinical picture is characterized by hemolytic anemia, severe photosensitivity, and epidermal bullae. The latter is caused by accumulation of porphyrins in the skin derived from bone marrow erythrocytes, with consequent phosphosensitization. Chronic liver failure is occasionally observed, due to the protoporphyrin accumulation.

Hepatic porphyrias are characterized by a systemic involvement, comprising gastrointestinal symptoms and, rarely, chronic liver failure, cardiovascular involvement, a diffuse erythematous reaction, and subsequent vesicles. Sideroblastic anemia is the most common hematological complication. Several commonly used medications may

Table 163.1 Classification of porphyric syndromes, inheritance, and enzyme defects.

Clinical condition	Enzyme deficiency	Chromosome location	Inheritance
Congenital erythropoietic porphyria (CEP)	Uroporphyirinogen III synthetase	10q25.2–q26.3	Autosomal recessive
Erythropoietic protoporphyria	Ferrochelatase	18q21.3	Autosomal dominant
ALA dehydratase deficiency porphyria	ALA dehydratase	9q34	Autosomal recessive
Acute intermittent porphyria (AIP)	Hydroxymethylbylane synthetase	11q23.3	Autosomal dominant
Hereditary coproporphyria	Coproporphyrinogen oxidase	3q12	Autosomal dominant
Variegate porphyria	Protoporphyrinogen oxidase	1q23	Autosomal dominant
Porphyria cutanea tarda (PCT)	Uroporphyrinogen decarboxylase	1p34	Variable
Hepatoerythropoietic porphyria	Uroporphyrinogen decarboxylase	1p34	Autosomal recessive

ALA: δ-aminolevulinic acid.

induce or aggravate porphyric attacks. Infections, pregnancy, and menstrual irregularities are also considered potential triggering factors.

Neurological manifestations can affect both central and peripheral nervous systems. Peripheral neuropathy is the most common, affecting predominantly motor nerves, with a rapid onset of symmetrical weakness affecting all limbs, and with cranial nerve involvement, sensory disturbances, consistent pain, and an asymmetrical pattern of weakness, spreading to the trunk and legs, rarely progressing to paresis. Tachycardia and hypotension may be present in the acute phase.

Epilepsy is not infrequent in porphyric patients. The etiology of seizures is multifactorial, attributable to hyponatremia, consequent on vomiting or diarrhea, brain structural pathology, or supposed neurotoxic and epileptogenic effects of some porphyrins. Psychiatric and cognitive disturbances have also been documented. Crimlisk, in an extensive review, described mood disturbances, anxiety, depression, psychosis, restlessness, insomnia, schizophrenic symptoms, impulsive behavior, persecutory delusions, and catatonia. Both transient and permanent brain structural damage has been reported. Cortical or subcortical brain structural damage, radiologically or pathologically defined, may occur. Brain ischemic damage was also reported in a patient showing transient cortical blindness. Bi-occipital MRI lesions were noted in two patients with AIP. Hemiparesis and abnormal brain MRI study were noted in a patient with hepatoerythropoietic porphyria. Transient T2 hyperintensity MRI lesions have also been reported, as well as multiple, reversible cortical lesions, mainly affecting the posterior cortical region.

Seizures are not uncommon during exacerbations of porphyric attacks, showing a prevalence of 2.2% in patients with known AIP and 5.1% among those with manifest AIP. About 30% of teenagers and 10–20% of adults with acute porphyria also suffer from seizures. Seizures may precede the presentation of porphyria by many years. Complex partial seizures are most common; absences, myoclonic and tonic–clonic seizures, and electroencephalogram (EEG) abnormalities have also been recorded.

Precipitating factors comprise a variety of almost 200 drugs, including antiepileptic drugs, sulphonamides, methyldopa, tetracycline, antihistamines, amphetamines, and cocaine, or an excessive quantity of alcohol. Infections may be associated.

In women, pregnancy and premenstrual seizures are considered potential triggering factors for a relapse. Treatment with sex hormones may also precipitate an acute attack of porphyria.

The differential diagnoses to be considered are polyneuropathy, especially acute polyneuritis, Guillain–Barré syndrome, epilepsy, various psychiatric illnesses including cognitive–affective disorders, and neurological syndromes due to vasculits, lupus erythematosus, and polyarteritis.

Extra-neurological manifestations are characterized by acute attacks of abdominal pain, nausea, constipation, vomiting, and gastrointestinal upset. Tachycardia and postural hypotension may occur due to autonomic disturbances.

Cutaneous manifestations associated with PCT (but also present in PV and HCP) are attributed to accumulation of porphyrins in the skin, a burning sensation after exposure to sunlight, followed by diffuse erythema and tense fluid-filled vesicles, fragile skin, pigmentation, and hypertrichosis, which may also present differential diagnostic problems.

Pathogenesis of neurological dysfunction

Neurological dysfunction may underlie not only nervous system-related symptoms but also non-neurological manifestations. Histopathology reveals edema, irregularity of myelin sheaths, axonal vacuolization, and degeneration of autonomic nerves. Evidence from electrophysiological studies discloses muscle denervation and slow nerve conduction.

A possible protective effect was claimed for melatonin, whose urinary excretion was shown to be reduced in AIP non-epileptic patients compared to matched controls.

A possible direct epileptogenic effect of α-aminolevulinic acid (ALA) has been postulated after ALA was shown to interfere with γ-aminobutyric acid (GABA) and, possibly, glutamate activity. ALA neurotoxicity has been demonstrated in chick embryo neuronal and glial cells. Some cases of acute toxic neuropathy, such as lead poisoning, are associated with increased ALA urinary excretion, but a clear causative effect has not been established. Another observation is the potential auto-oxidation of ALA in the presence of iron or other heavy metals, potentially inducing the formation of free radicals, causing oxidative stress on mitochondria and increased Ca^{2+} uptake in cortical neurons. Eight patients affected by end-stage protoporphyric liver disease had neurological manifestations similar to those observed in acute attacks.

Porphyric attacks caused by antiepileptic medications

Many antiepileptic drugs (AEDs) can induce the isoenzyme of cytochrome P_{450} and may worsen or precipitate attacks, of AIP and PCT. Induction of cytochrome P_{450} accelerates catabolism by uroporphyrinogen decarboxylase, hydroxymethylbilane synthetase, and alteration of the feedback mechanism on heme biosynthesis.

A worsening of acute porphyric attacks was seen in patients treated with phenytoin, carbamazepine, phenobarbital, sodium valproate, and lamotrigine. Topiramate and tiagabine can increase liver porphobilinogen content, and the latter has been demonstrated to be potentially porphyrogenic in chicken embryos. Seizures have been successfully treated with gabapentin and oxcarbazepine in patients with acute porphyria, not associated with exacerbation of acute attacks. However, oxcarbazepine can induce hyponatremia, which may induce or complicate porphyric attacks. Levetiracetam was reported to be safe in AIP, HCP, and PCT.

Differential diagnosis

Porphyria has been named as "the little imitator". The differential diagnoses involve various aspects of neurological manifestations ranging from polyneuropathy, autonomic disturbances, seizures, and a wide range of psychiatric disorders as mentioned above. The cutaneous manifestations form a differential diagnosis for photosensitization, bullae, dermatitis, vesicles, and pigmentation. Abdominal crisis and unexplained systemic manifestations complete the spectrum.

Concluding comments

Prompt diagnosis and treatment of porphyria have to date been suboptimal because of underestimation of the clinical picture and lack of recognition of family history, poor availability of biochemical tests, and false negative test results during aymptomatic periods. The clinical picture is often transient and the differential diagnosis is often difficult if porphyria is not considered at the time of the acute symptoms. From the neurologist's viewpoint, there is a difficulty in trying to identify and characterize the psychiatric abnormalities. Better epidemiological data and understanding of the comorbidity of porphyrias are needed.

Identification of metabolic imbalances that can induce seizures during porphyric attacks has been recognized. It is important to perform serum and urinary porphyrin measurements during the attack as their specificities are very high in hepatic porphyrias. Sensitivity of the analysis does not allow a reliable exclusion in asymptomatic AIP patients. The possible neurotoxicity of ALA seems to be contradicted by some *in vivo* experiments. An alternative toxic role of protoporphyrin and porphobilinogen (or other porphyrins) or a neural metabolic failure due to heme deficiency have not been confirmed. Animal models do not explain completely the clinical effects observed.

Some patients appear reluctant to accept the diagnosis of porphyria because of psychiatric implications. A register for porphyric patients, focusing on family history and the results of genetic testing, is gaining acceptance.

Addendum

Lists of over 200 drugs that have been reported to be unsafe in patients with porphyria are available on the internet at www.uq.edu.au/porphyria. Key references are also provided by Prof. Michael Moore of the University of Queensland and at www.drugs-porphyria.org.

Acknowledgments

We thank the Porphyria Association of Australia and our colleagues at St Vincent's Hospital and Monash University.

Further reading

Albers JW, Fink JK. Porphyric neuropathy. *Muscle Nerve* 2004; 30(4): 410–22.

Crimlisk HL. The little imitator – porphyria: a neuropsychiatric disorder. *J Neurol Neurosurg Psychiatry* 1997; 62: 319–28.

Desnick RJ. The porphyrias. In: Braunwald E, Fauci AS, Kasper DL, Hauser SL, Longo DL, Jameson JL, editors. *Harrison's Principles of Internal Medicine*. New York: McGraw-Hill; 2001.

Kauppinen R. Porphyrias. *Lancet* 2005; 365(9455): 241–52.

Solinas C, Vajda F. Epilepsy and porphyria: new perspectives. *J Clin Neurosci* 2004; 11: 356–61.

Chapter 164
Wilson's disease

Peter A. LeWitt[1,2] and Anna Członkowska[3,4]
[1]Henry Ford Hospital, Detroit, USA
[2]Wayne State University School of Medicine, Detroit, USA
[3]Institute of Psychiatry and Neurology, Warsaw, Poland
[4]Medical University, Warsaw, Poland

Introduction

This rare systemic disorder of copper metabolism was described by S.A.K. Wilson in 1912 as *hepatolenticular degeneration*, now known as Wilson's disease (WD). Clinicians need to recognize WD early before it progresses to disability and fatal outcome. Because the brain is diffusely affected in WD, there can be several patterns of neurological impairment simultaneously. Clumsiness and slowness in tasks may be early complaints. Gait disturbance, impaired handwriting, trunk titubation, and muscle cramping are among the non-specific problems that may puzzle a clinician. WD can affect all ages but especially those of pediatric and young adult years. Because of its recessive inheritance, it can appear both in familial and seemingly sporadic forms.

The pathophysiology of WD involves defective packaging and excreting of cellular copper. Dietary copper taken up from the gut needs continuous biliary removal to avoid overload and systemic toxicity. The massive copper deposition in the brain has a propensity for the lenticular nuclei, which can be obliterated by cystic or cavitary degeneration. Extensive degenerative changes are often found also in the thalami, midbrain, pons, and cerebellum, and can appear in white matter or different cortical regions. Characteristic pathological changes involve glia, which proliferate (especially Alzheimer's type II and Opalski cells).

Neurological presentations can be extremely subtle, intermittent, and hard to categorize. Most typically, these involve action tremor or dystonia (especially affecting cranial musculature). Sometimes, typical parkinsonian features are initial presentations. Cerebellar outflow tremor, ataxic speech, and other signs characteristic of white matter disease can also develop. The tremor in WD can be symmetrical or unilateral, and sometimes is paroxysmal. A characteristic form is a coarse, irregular proximal tremulousness with a "wing beating" appearance. Tremor in WD is unresponsive to ethanol or medications used for treating the tremor in Parkinson's disease or essential tremor. It can coexist with generalized ataxia.

Commonly, motor impairment in WD also involves the cranial region. Clinical manifestations include problems such as dysarthria, drooling, and cranial and oropharyngeal dystonia. Wilson described a characteristic facial grimacing with jaw opening and lip retraction. Blepharospasm, tongue dyskinesia, progressive speech disturbance, and drooling frequently occur as WD progresses.

WD can also present with a wide spectrum of behavioral or psychiatric disorders. Sometimes these are the earliest features, preceding motor impairments. The psychiatric features can involve relatively common problems in the general population such as depression, other mood alterations, and anxiety. In childhood WD, the psychiatric manifestations may include declining school performance, personality changes, impulsiveness, and behavioral regression. Memory impairment and other aspects of cognitive decline can also develop. Patients have been described with initial presentations of psychotic features resembling paranoia and schizophrenia. Less common psychiatric presentations have included aggressiveness, suicidal ideation, self-injury, and hypersexuality. In rare instances, WD can manifest as either focal or generalized seizures.

Characteristic ophthalmic involvement in WD produces Kayser–Fleischer (KF) rings, composed of copper – containing granules within Descemet's membrane of the cornea (Figure 164.1). KF rings are usually bilateral and arise around the corneal periphery, especially at its upper pole. Virtually all WD with neurological involvement shows KF rings. Generally identified without magnification, KF rings require a careful slit lamp examination for definitive diagnosis (and many ophthalmologists are unfamiliar with this finding). Also typical of copper deposition is a "sunflower" cataract. WD can show disturbances of smooth pursuit, convergence, and fixation as well as eyelid-opening apraxia.

International Neurology: A Clinical Approach. Edited by Robert P. Lisak, Daniel D. Truong, William M. Carroll, and Roongroj Bhidayasiri.
© 2009 Blackwell Publishing, ISBN: 978-1-4051-5738-4.

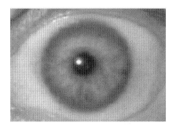

Figure 164.1 A complete Kayser–Fleischer ring in Wilson's disease, with characteristic enhanced pigmentation due to copper accumulation seen in upper and lower peripheral regions of the cornea.

Genetics

WD is an autosomal recessive disorder, localized on chromosome 13q14.3. The gene, *ATP7B*, encodes a copper-transporting P-type ATP-ase. Mutation within the *ATP7B* gene in WD leads to ineffective packaging of copper and ineffective biliary excretion. Thus, the net result is progressive copper accumulation in the hepatocytes and, eventually, extrahepatic tissues. Over 300 *ATP7B* mutations have been identified. Only homozygotes who inherit disease-specific mutations of both alleles of the *ATP7B* gene develop WD. Heterozygote carriers of the mutations are spared any clinical features, although they may manifest a reduced serum ceruloplasmin. Age of onset, site of organ involvement, and other disease characteristics could conceivably have their origins in different *ATP7B* mutations. In general, there is no definite association between *ATP7B* genotype and WD presentation or its subsequent clinical course.

Diagnostics

Neurological WD should be suspected with unexplained extrapyramidal or cerebellar impairments, or psychiatric, cognitive, and behavioral disorders. Asymptomatic siblings need to be tested. Although the first clinical signs and symptoms generally develop in the second to third decades of life, earlier and later WD manifestations have also been reported. Familial WD helps guide diagnostics with known affected siblings. Clinicians should be aware that initial disease manifestations (hepatic or neuropsychiatric) often vary greatly in families.

Beyond screening for KF rings, the clinical diversity in WD always requires diagnostic confirmation by testing for abnormal copper metabolism or gene mutation. Serum ceruloplasmin concentration characteristically is less than 50%, although it can be normal in WD (especially with WD hepatitis). Total serum copper concentration in WD is low, although free copper is elevated. Twenty-four hour urinary copper excretion is more than 100 μg (normal value is less than 50 μg).

With equivocal laboratory findings, and especially in the context of hepatic involvement, liver biopsy is needed for histological study and for measurements of tissue copper content. In WD, hepatic copper is more than 250 μg/g dry tissue. Borderline changes in serum ceruloplasmin and copper concentrations in serum, liver, and urine may be observed in other liver disorders, and *ATP7B* mutation heterozygotes can also demonstrate mild abnormalities. Further investigation can utilize the uptake and distribution of radiolabeled copper. The lack of a "second peak" (indicating labeled copper incorporation into ceruloplasmin) implicates WD.

DNA analysis for *ATP7B* mutation often confirms a diagnosis of WD. However, screening tests targeted at the most frequent mutations in a particular regional population are often inconclusive. In these circumstances, sequencing the entire gene can provide diagnostic confirmation. DNA analysis is especially valuable for diagnosis of presymptomatic relatives of previously diagnosed WD patients. For a definite diagnosis, mutations on both alleles of the WD gene must be found.

Other testing can enhance suspicion of WD. In some instances, neuroimaging can point to WD even with inconclusive copper metabolism and DNA studies. In mild WD, CT brain scans can be normal, though more severe cases have bilateral hypodensities in basal ganglia and other deep structures. Unlike CT, almost all cases of neurological WD have abnormalities on brain MRI (especially high signal intensities on T2-weighted and fluid-attenuated inversion recovery (FLAIR) images, typically in the putamen, globus pallidus, caudate, thalamus, midbrain, pons, and cerebellum) (Figure 164.2a,b). In these structures, T1-weighted images may show hypointensities (Figure 164.2c).

Treatment

Early treatment is necessary for survival of a WD patient and to lessen the impact of copper deposition in brain, liver, and other organ systems. The constant removal of copper, massively increased in even the presymptomatic patient and inevitably present in the diet, is the goal. Although dietary control is inadequate, foods high in copper content should be avoided, along with copper-containing water. Medications achieving a negative copper balance involve different strategies for initial versus maintenance therapy. Pregnant and pediatric patients require different treatment options.

D-penicillamine continues to be most widely used for copper chelation in WD. Though highly effective, *D*-penicillamine is problematic because of many possible adverse effects. It is dosed with meals at up to 1.5 g/day, starting with 125 mg and building up over several weeks by 125 mg increments in order to avoid neurological

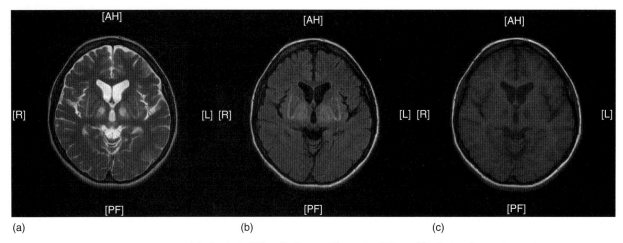

Figure 164.2 Magnetic resonance images of the brain in Wilson's disease, illustrating bilateral high signal intensity in the putamen, pallidum, and thalamus in T2-weighted (a) and FLAIR (b) images, and low intensity in thalamus in a T1-weighted image (c).

deterioration. Urinary copper output guides the choice of dose. Months can elapse before observing clinical improvement. *D*-penicillamine also increases systemic copper mobilization which can worsen neurological function due to entrance of copper into the brain. Worsening of tremor, dystonia, and parkinsonism, and "status dystonicus" can occur.

Adverse effects of chronic *D*-penicillamine therapy include the occurrence of skin disorders (including urticaria, rash, epidermolysis bullosa, subcutaneous bleeding, impaired wound healing, and damage to the skin's elastic properties).

Immunological problems associated with prolonged use may include systemic lupus erythematosus, myasthenia gravis, Goodpasture's syndrome, immunoglobulin deficiency, nephritic syndrome, and immune complex nephritis.

D-penicillamine-treated patients can develop lymphadenopathy, unexplained fever, thrombocytopenia, leucopenia, polyarthritis, and dysgeusia. Pyridoxine supplementation does not avert adverse effects. Though the safety of *D*-penicillamine has not been established for pregnancy, copper chelation therapy must be continued with either this drug or other options.

Another copper-binding drug is trientine (trien). Trien lacks most of the toxicity known to occur with *D*-penicillamine, but can result in lupus nephritis, colitis, duodenitis, proteinuria, iron deficiency, and sideroblastic anemia. Trien is an alternative to *D*-penicillamine and is less likely to produce rapid systemic copper mobilization. Trien is dosed between 0.75 and 2 g/day apart from meal times.

Regular administration of zinc offers another mechanism to achieve a negative copper balance through a mechanism different from chelation. Although slow at

removing copper, zinc is a well-tolerated alternative (but cannot be administered to a patient simultaneously receiving a copper chelator). Although zinc is the treatment of choice for children and during pregnancy, progression of WD can nonetheless occur. Zinc can be administered as either an acetate or a sulfate salt, with a typical dosage of 50 mg of elemental zinc three times a day after meals.

All of the abovementioned pharmacologic options are highly effective for the majority of hepatic and neurological WD patients, leading to a marked clinical improvement. Given to presymptomatic cases (obligatory diagnosis of all siblings), such treatment can prevent development of clinical symptomatology. Of greatest importance is maintaining lifelong treatment. Unfortunately, many patients stop therapy after achieving initial improvement despite the inevitable risk of future deterioration. Recurrence of hepatic or neurological symptoms can be rapid, leading to severe disability or death.

The most effective treatment for WD, though seldom utilized, is liver transplantation. In cases with acute liver failure or progression of liver failure despite pharmacotherapy, liver transplantation is recommended. The potential for improvement of neurological symptoms after transplantation has not been well studied. However, this treatment is associated with a relatively high morbidity and mortality, posed by the procedure itself and long-term immunosuppression.

Further reading

Brewer GJ. Neurologically presenting Wilson's disease: epidemiology, pathophysiology and treatment. *CNS Drugs* 2005; 19: 185–92.

Członkowska A, Gajda J, Rodo M. Effect of long-term treatment in Wilson's disease with D-penicillamine and zinc sulphate. *J Neurol* 1996; 243: 269–73.

Das SK, Ray K. Wilson's disease: an update. *Nat Clin Pract Neurol* 2006; 2: 482–93.

Ferenci P. Pathophysiology and clinical features of Wilson disease. *Metab Brain Dis* 2004; 19: 229–39.

Ferenci P, Caca K, Loudianos G, *et al.* Diagnosis and phenotypic classification of Wilson disease. *Liver Int* 2003; 23: 139–42.

LeWitt P, Pfeiffer R. Neurologic aspects of Wilson's disease: clinical manifestations and treatment. In: Jankovic J, Tolosa E, editors. *Parkinson's Disease and Movement Disorders*, 5th ed. Philadelphia: Lippincott Williams & Wilkins; 2006, Chapter 21, pp. 254–70.

Chapter 165
Traumatic brain injury

Christopher C. Giza
David Geffen School of Medicine at UCLA, Los Angeles, USA

Introduction

Traumatic brain injury (TBI) refers to any biomechanically-induced acquired brain injury. It is the most common cause of death and disability in young persons in many countries, often resulting in chronic neurological, cognitive, and behavioral impairments. TBI occurs in a spectrum from mild to severe, typically classified based on clinical signs as determined by the Glasgow Coma Scale (GCS, Table 165.1). TBI encompasses a range of pathophysiological injuries – from simple concussions to intracranial hematomas to profound cerebral edema with ischemic secondary damage.

Epidemiology

TBI occurs in a trimodal age distribution, with peaks in infancy, adolescence/young adulthood, and senescence. There is a male:female predominance of 2–3:1. Specific mechanisms of injury are quite variable in terms of the biomechanical forces imparted to the brain and the severity of the injury.

The mildest injuries (concussions) typically involve lower forces and may be associated with only transient neurological signs and symptoms. These represent the majority (70–80%) of all TBI. Recurrent mild concussions are most commonly seen in sports-related settings, although the specific sport may differ based on geographic location. Football is by far the biggest contributor to mild TBI in the United States, while in many other countries soccer, rugby, and, to some extent, boxing would be more important causes. In Asia, the various forms of contact martial arts constitute other contributors to mild TBI.

Mechanisms underlying moderate and severe TBI vary by age and geography. Agewise, infants and toddlers are more commonly injured by inflicted TBI (child abuse) and falls. Teenagers and young adults are more often affected

Table 165.1 The Glasgow Coma Scale.

Eye opening (E)	
• Spontaneous	4
• To speech (to shout)	3
• To pain	2
• None	1
Motor response (M)	
• Obeys commands	6
• Localizes pain	5
• Withdraws	4
• Abnormal flexion	3
• Extensor response	2
• None	1
Verbal response (V)	
• Oriented	5
• Confused conversation	4
• Inappropriate words	3
• Incomprehensible sounds	2
• None	1
Verbal response, modified for infants	
• Babbles, coos appropriately	5
• Cries, but consolable	4
• Cries inconsolably	3
• Grunts or moans to pain	2
• None	1

by road traffic accidents (RTAs). Worldwide, in 2002, RTAs resulted in 1.2 million deaths and between 20 and 50 million people becoming disabled. The specific etiologies of RTAs vary considerably by geographic location. In developed countries, the most common types of RTA causing TBI involve automobile-to-automobile crashes. The incidence of these injuries has decreased slightly in recent years due to improved protective measures, such as seatbelts and airbags. In developing countries, RTAs involving pedestrians or motorized scooters are more common and have generally been on the rise. In Thailand, nearly 80% of RTA deaths involve motorized cycles. Malaysia has similarly high rates of cycle-related RTA deaths. In India, Indonesia, and Sri Lanka, motorized cycles are involved in 40% of cases, pedestrians in another 40%. In more developed countries such as the United States and Australia, motorized four-wheeled vehicles

International Neurology: A Clinical Approach. Edited by Robert P. Lisak, Daniel D. Truong, William M. Carroll, and Roongroj Bhidayasiri.
© 2009 Blackwell Publishing, ISBN: 978-1-4051-5738-4.

constitute 80% of RTA-related deaths. These numbers certainly suggest different types of TBI etiology and pathology, and may result in marked differences in the approach to treatment and prevention.

Pathophysiology

The underlying pathophysiology of TBI depends, to a large degree, upon the injury severity; however, some basic neurobiological processes appear to be constant. Acutely, the biomechanical strain on neuronal membranes results in indiscriminate ionic flux and glutamate release in both animal models and human patients. Acute energy demands compromise neuronal function, and, if severe, result in cell death. Subsequently, cerebral glucose metabolism is reduced for 7–10 days in experimental animals and days to months in humans. The duration of metabolic depression appears to be related to injury severity.

Other cellular processes involved in the response to TBI include inflammatory processes, neurotransmitter dysfunction, delayed cell death, gliosis/scarring, and axonal injury. Impairment of neurotransmission may be especially relevant during the recovery period, particularly in children and young people whose brains are still undergoing development. Axonal injury is also an important mechanism that may have unique consequences in terms of neural connectivity during the state of coma and in recovery.

Based upon the understanding of pathophysiology, the most clinically relevant intervention is the detection, avoidance, and treatment of secondary insults. This refers to deleterious physiological events that are distinct from the primary injury itself, such as hypotension/ischemia, hypoxia, seizure, and hyperthermia. The presence of a secondary insult is the single most important treatable factor in improving TBI outcome. The ability to address these remediable conditions varies greatly depending upon geographic location and medical resources. Both pre-hospital care and adequate hospital intensive care are crucial to monitor and treat these important problems. In developed nations, reductions in mortality following severe TBI (as seen in the 1970s and 1980s) can be directly traced to the development of pre-hospital emergency medical services (EMS) systems and to improved monitoring and treatment of complications in the hospital in specialized intensive care units (now, neuro-intensive care units). The establishment and optimal operation of these systems is still a major obstacle in many developing nations and regions undergoing armed conflict.

Clinical features

The hallmarks of TBI are neurological dysfunction and impairment of mental status, but the range of clinical features varies greatly depending upon injury severity. Here it is best to discuss mild TBI/concussion separately from moderate–severe TBI.

Mild TBI/concussion

Concussion has been defined as any transient disturbance of neurological function imparted by injury due to biomechanical forces. This type of injury can occur with any TBI mechanism, but is generally associated with short falls and sports-related head injuries. The most common clinical hallmarks of concussion include: memory impairment, headaches, confusion, nausea, dizziness, and visual disturbances. Loss of consciousness may occur, but is not necessary for a diagnosis of concussion. Most commonly, these disturbances recover relatively rapidly over the course of days up to a few weeks. Mild TBI includes concussions, but is generally defined as TBI with a GCS of 13–15 without evidence of intracranial pathology. The hallmark of mild TBI/concussion is the presence of neurological symptoms in the absence of demonstrable structural brain injury.

Moderate–severe TBI

More severe TBI incorporates a broad range of distinct injury processes and pathology. Moderate TBI is defined by an initial GCS of 9–12, while severe is defined by a GCS of 3–8. The underlying mechanisms here are assault (including inflicted TBI or child abuse), high falls, gunshot wounds, and RTAs. These head injuries are divided into closed head injuries and penetrating injuries. Penetrating injuries will be associated with skull fracture and the primary destruction of brain parenchyma, as well as intracranial hemorrhage and often foreign bodies. Gunshot wounds tend to be more common in urban areas, but, worldwide, can also be attributed to warfare and terrorism. In undeveloped areas, significant penetrating injuries are likely to result in death, as operative interventions and methods to prevent subsequent infection may not be readily available. Closed head injuries are by far more common, and may include non-displaced skull fractures, intracranial hemorrhage (epidural, subarachnoid, and subdural), and parenchymal brain damage such as contusions and diffuse axonal injury.

Blast injuries may represent a unique type of TBI due to proximity to an explosive device as might occur during terrorism or warfare. These injuries may run the range from concussion to severe penetrating injury from shrapnel or bomb fragments. In addition, rapid elevations of intrathoracic pressure are hypothesized to contribute to a diffuse cerebral injury in some patients.

The clinical signs of moderate–severe TBI include altered mental status/coma, amnesia, focal neurological deficits, and seizures. Physical examination may reveal scalp hematomas or lacerations, palpable skull stepoffs (indicating fractures), hemotypanum or otorrhea (associated

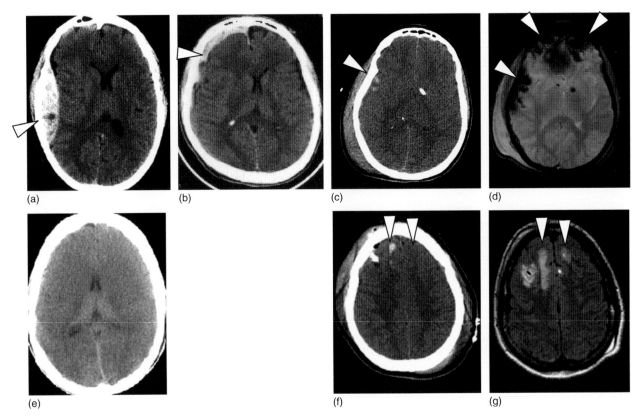

Figure 165.1 Radiographic appearances of acute TBI. Arrows indicate the highlighted pathology. (a) Epidural hematoma; (b) subdural hematoma; (c) cerebral contusion on CT; (d) multiple cerebral contusions evident on MRI done the same day as the CT scan in (c); (e) diffuse cerebral edema; (f) diffuse axonal injury on CT; (g) more extensive diffuse axonal injury evident on MRI done the same day as the CT scan in (f).

with basilar skull fractures), and raccoon eyes or rhinor-rhea (associated with orbitofrontal skull fractures).

Investigations

Most mild TBI/concussion will not require additional diagnostic testing. The routine use of skull X-rays to evaluate mild TBI has not been supported in the literature; however, if there is clinical suspicion of a skull fracture at a facility where head CT is not available, skull X-ray has some clinical utility. In these circumstances, presence of a skull fracture on X-ray strongly suggests the need for transport to a facility with head CT capability, as the risk of intracranial pathology is increased 21- to 80-fold.

Diagnostic evaluation of moderate–severe TBI is best accomplished by a non-contrast head CT. This method can quickly and definitively diagnose conditions requiring neurosurgical intervention, such as space-occupying lesions (epidural and subdural hematomas, and contusions) (Figure 165.1a, b, and c, respectively), and delayed complications of TBI (hydrocephalus and cerebral infarction). MRI is not indicated acutely, but may be valuable subacutely for patients with persistent coma by

identifying the extent of lesions not optimally seen on CT (Figure 165.1c vs d – contusions, Figure 165.1f vs g – diffuse axonal injury).

Treatment/management

Mild TBI/concussion
The foundation of mild TBI management is careful clinical assessment and observation. Determination of risk factors (high force impact, very young or old age, prolonged or continuing alteration in mental status, loss of consciousness, seizure, repeated vomiting, focal neurological signs, or intoxication of patient) is important to properly triage these patients. In the vast majority of cases, a normal or improving neurological examination, in the absence of clinical risk factors, will permit management solely with observation, foregoing the need for neuroimaging. As indicated above, however, there are circumstances where skull X-ray or non-contrast head CT would be prudent.

Moderate–severe TBI
More severe injuries warrant more aggressive intervention – beginning outside of the hospital. Evidence-based

guidelines for the management of severe TBI have been published and recently revised. Pre-hospital management of TBI varies worldwide based on the availability of EMS, but basic care can still significantly impact the outcome by interventions to reduce secondary injuries. This includes immediate assessment of airway, breathing, and circulation (ABC) as well as instituting proper resuscitative efforts. Maintenance of an adequate airway may be achieved using oral or nasopharyngeal airways and proper head position. Careful assessment and immobilization for concomitant cervical spine injury should be undertaken. Supplemental oxygen can be administered as soon as it is available, and intravenous (IV) access should be established for fluid resuscitation to address hypotension and shock, as well as to provide a means of rapid drug delivery.

The mainstay of management for moderate–severe TBI centers on identification and treatment of elevated intracranial pressure (ICP) and maintenance of adequate cerebral perfusion pressure (CPP = mean arterial pressure – ICP). In the initial assessment, elevated ICP and/or impending cerebral herniation may be detected based on clinical signs (declining mental status, unilateral dilated pupil, hemimotor signs, or posturing) or neuroimaging. Increased ICP can occur due to a space-occupying lesion (such as a hematoma; Figure 165.1a,b) or cerebral edema (as occurs adjacent to a contusion or diffusely; Figure 165.1c,e). Surgical intervention is warranted in cases of a significant mass lesion. For severe TBI, ICP monitoring in an intensive care unit should be the standard of care in locations where such resources are available. ICP may be measured via a surface transducer or by a ventriculostomy. The latter is preferred because it allows both measurement of ICP and therapeutic drainage of cerebrospinal fluid (CSF). Medical interventions are important in the management of elevated ICP. It is recommended that these interventions occur in a stepwise fashion, from less aggressive to an increasing intensity of therapy.

The first steps include slight elevation of the head of the bed (15–30°) and maintenance of the head in a neutral position to facilitate jugular venous drainage. Next is sedation and analgesia, followed by neuromuscular blockade. The resulting reduction of intrathoracic pressures can help in lowering ICP, particularly in intubated patients who may struggle against positive pressure breathing. Hyperosmolar agents may be administered intravenously – mannitol (0.25–1 g/kg IV every 3–6 hours) is the agent of choice. Hypertonic saline (3%) may also be used. Finally, controlled ventilation or mild hyperventilation (pCO_2 = 30–35) can be used, but care should be taken not to over-ventilate, which may result in vasoconstriction of cerebral vasculature and secondary ischemic injury. In a setting of clinical herniation, airway control

and hyperventilation are usually the most rapid means of reducing ICP in the absence of a ventriculostomy. IV hyperosmolar agents should follow closely. This process takes slightly longer; however, this results in more sustained ICP reductions and is less likely to result in ischemia.

Second-tier therapies are reserved for refractory elevations of ICP in the absence of a surgical lesion and include: metabolic suppressive therapy, severe hyperventilation, lumbar drain, and decompressive craniectomy. Pharmacological suppression of cerebral activity is typically accomplished with barbiturate coma and continuous electroencephalogram (EEG) monitoring. More aggressive hyperventilation (pCO_2 <30) can be safely implemented if monitoring for cerebral ischemia is available via jugular venous O_2 saturation or newer tissue oxygenation monitors. Systemic hypothermia has not proven effective for TBI, but may be promising in younger patients.

The third set of therapies is considered supportive and include avoidance of hyperthermia, prophylaxis against early post-traumatic seizures, deep venous thrombosis (DVT) prophylaxis, and caloric supplementation. The use of corticosteroids is *not* recommended.

Chronic management of sequelae
TBI results in many persistent neurological sequelae that may fall to neurologists for ongoing management. These include prolonged post-concussive syndrome, persistent headaches, and dizziness in mildly injured individuals. Sequelae of severe TBI include post-traumatic epilepsy, spasticity, and occasionally hydrocephalus. All types of TBI can result in varying degrees of behavioral or cognitive deficits, particularly personality change, impulsivity, poor attention, and memory deficits.

Further reading

Edwards P, Arango M, Balica L, *et al*. Final results of MRC CRASH, a randomised placebo-controlled trial of intravenous corticosteroid in adults with head injury – outcomes at 6 months. *Lancet* 2005; 365(9475): 1957–9.

Guidelines for the Acute Medical Management of Severe Traumatic Brain Injury in Infants, Children and Adolescents, *Pediatr Crit Care Med* 2004; 4(Suppl): s3, available at http://www.braintrauma.org/site/pageserver?pagename=guidelines.

Guidelines for the Management of Severe Traumatic Brain Injury. *J Neurotrauma* 2007; 24(Suppl 1): s1–2, available at http://www.braintrauma.org/site/pageserver?pagename=guidelines.

Madikians A, Giza CC. A clinician's guide to the pathophysiology of traumatic brain injury. *Indian J Neurotrauma* 2006; 3(1): 9–17.

World Health Organization. World Report on Road Traffic Injury Prevention; 2004, available at http://www.who.int/world-health-day/2004/infomaterials/world_report/en/.

Chapter 166
Spinal injury

Enver I. Bogdanov
Kazan State Medical University, Kazan, Russia

Epidemiology

Annual incidence rates of spinal cord injury (SCI) vary considerably from country to country (2.5–57.8 per million population). SCI is most frequent in young adults and often associated with vertebral fracture. The main causes of injuries in the economically developed countries are road traffic and sporting accidents, whereas falling from a height is the most common cause in less developed regions. Injuries due to intentional violence are a relatively common cause of cord injury in particular areas (e.g., parts of South Africa). In Bangladesh, SCI after falling while carrying a heavy load on the head is frequent. Universally, there is a large predominance in males (3–4:1).

Pathophysiology and clinical features

The mechanisms of SCI can be broadly subclassified into five types: dislocation, lateral bending, axial loading, rotation, and hyperflexion/hyperextension, although severe injuries often result from a combination of more than one of these subtypes. Intra- and extramedullary circulatory impairment occurs not only at the initial impact level, but also in the adjacent levels. The presence of constitutional or spondylotic narrowing of the canal seems to predispose to lesions of the cord. In 50% of cases, the cervical spine is affected, followed by the thoracic and lumbosacral spine, respectively.

Spinal shock is characterized by a state of areflexia below the level of the SCI. It is manifested by flaccidity in the legs, which gradually disappears and is replaced by increasing muscle tone. The duration of spinal shock varies from days to a few weeks. Sparing of sensation in lower sacral segments may be the only sign present that indicates some recovery may occur. The onset of some voluntary movement within 72 hours of SCI is a good prognostic sign. Flaccidity remains in lower motor neuron lesions associated with permanent cauda equina damage. Autonomic disturbances are less common and can include bowel and bladder dysfunction. In the setting of acute trauma, hypotension without tachycardia should raise concern for severe SCI. By 6–7 weeks, injury cord-damaged patients present an average of seven contractures.

Approximately 30% of blunt contusive human SCI results in a complete loss of continuity of central nervous system (CNS) tissue that is clinically indistinguishable from spinal cord transection. The neurological completeness/incompleteness of an injury at any stage can be graded according to the American Spinal Injury Association from A to E, as follows: A – complete: no sensory or motor function preserved in S4–5; B – incomplete: sensory but no motor function preserved below the neurological level and extending through S4–5; C – incomplete: motor function preserved below the neurological level, majority of key muscles present a grade <3; D – incomplete: motor function preserved below the neurological level, majority of key muscles presents a grade ≥3; E – normal motor and sensory function.

Incomplete injuries may be classified into four types: anterior spinal syndrome, central cord syndrome (CCS), Brown–Séquard syndrome, and mixed types. The anterior cord syndrome typically results in some degree of paralysis, with a loss of pain and temperature sensation below the level of the lesion and relative sparing of touch, vibration, and proprioception. CCS typically occurs following trauma to the cervical spinal cord and an elderly patient with pre-existing cervical spondylosis is a classic presentation. An associated fracture of a cervical vertebra is uncommon. CCS is characterized by symmetrically incomplete quadriplegia, affecting the upper more than the lower limbs; sensory impairment is variable and urinary retention common. The "burning hands syndrome" is a variant of CCS characterized by burning dysesthesia of the hands and associated weakness in the hands and arms. Most symptoms quickly resolve. Brown–Séquard syndrome consists of ipsilateral weakness and loss of proprioceptive sensation due to disruption of the corticospinal tracts and

International Neurology: A Clinical Approach. Edited by Robert P. Lisak, Daniel D. Truong, William M. Carroll, and Roongroj Bhidayasiri. © 2009 Blackwell Publishing, ISBN: 978-1-4051-5738-4.

dorsal columns. Pain and temperature sensations are lost on the contralateral side due to the affected spinothalamic tract. Traumatic "cauda equina" syndrome consists of sensory disturbance, characteristically in the perineal region, as well as difficulty in walking due to weakness of the legs.

Patients may develop new symptoms several weeks or even years later. Progressive post-traumatic myelomalacic myelopathy (PPMM) and syringomyelia are the well-known "late" post-traumatic complications of SCI. PPMM has been reported in 0.3–3.2% of patients with chronic spinal cord injury and can occur as soon as 2 months and up to 30 years following injury. PPMM is a possible precursor of syringomyelia. Clinically, PPMM and post-traumatic syringomyelia are neurologically indistinguishable; however, MRI can be used to differentiate the two entities. Syringomyelia occurs in 3–4% of cases as early as 8 weeks after injury, or may be delayed in onset for several years. It is caused by cystic degeneration of the injured spinal cord at or near the site of the trauma. The clinical presentation in post-traumatic syringomyelia is non-specific. Most patients present with ascending sensory signs and motor deficit. The treatment consists of shunting, with improvement of the symptoms in the majority of patients. Spinal cord atrophy is a third type of lesion found in the chronic stage of spinal cord injury. It is usually observed many years after the traumatic event and occurs in approximately 15–20% of patients. Occasionally, it is difficult to differentiate atrophy from a subarachnoid cyst with cord compression and from "post-syrinx" syndrome. Pain is a common problem and has a major impact on patients with chronic SCI. It commonly begins in the first 6–9 months post injury, but can start several years after. Several types of pain may occur, which can be divided into musculoskeletal pain, visceral pain, and above-level, at-level, and below-level neuropathic pains indicated by descriptions such as burning, shooting, electric shock-like, and hypersensitivity.

Investigations

The trauma patient who is alert, oriented, and neither sedated nor distracted may or may not have neck pain or tenderness upon clinical examination. The probability of structural injury in such patients is close to zero; it is increasingly recognized that imaging such patients is unnecessary.

A plain, three-view radiograph is usually performed for patients with neurological signs, although multislice CT is usually recommended for initial evaluation of spinal trauma patients, and clarification as to whether a fracture is present. MRI typically serves as a problem-solving technique when CT is unable to adequately assess the cause of neurological deficits, determine acuity of a fracture, or assess the presence of ligamentous injury. MRI can show transection, hemorrhage, contusion, or edema of the spinal cord. It can also demonstrate ligamentous injuries, muscular lesions, facet joint dislocations, and bone marrow edema. The presence of abnormalities on MRI in a patient with a complete cord syndrome is generally a bad prognostic sign. Absence of spinal cord edema is a strong predictor of full recovery in patients with acute central cervical cord injury involving only the upper extremities. Spinal cord injury without radiographic abnormality (SCIWORA) is well known in the pediatric population. SCIWORA can manifest with symptoms that range from transient paresthesiae to complete motor paralysis and sensory loss.

Clinical examination and imaging can be complemented by electrophysiological recordings to deduce the degree of involvement of different spinal pathways. Corticospinal, spinothalamic, dorsal column, and sympathetic pathway functions may be quantifiably measured by motor evoked potentials, laser evoked potentials, somatosensory evoked potentials, and sympathetic skin response techniques, respectively.

Treatment

Trauma patients with SCI should be managed by immobilization to attain anatomical alignment. In the acute setting, initiation of intravenous methylprednisolone treatment as a 30 mg/kg bolus within 8 hours of the injury, followed by 5.4 mg/kg/hour for the ensuing 23 hours is recommended. Subsequent treatments must be individualized and depend on the degree of neurological deficit, spinal level, and severity of deformity. Occasionally, spinal surgery is required (e.g., when there are bony fragments compressing the cord). For a compression fracture of the upper lumbar spine (typically occurring in older osteoporotic patients), the decision between bracing and surgery is based on the degree of initial deformity. Secondary medical complications for acute SCI such as respiratory failure, deep venous thrombosis, and urological complications should be appropriately corrected. Spasticity, pain, autonomic dysreflexia, and contractures are common complications associated with chronic SCI, requiring pharmacological measures and physical therapy.

Further reading

Bogdanov EI, Heiss JD, Mendelevich EG. The post-syrinx syndrome: stable central myelopathy and collapsed or absent syrinx. *J Neurol* 2006; 253: 707–13.

Burt AA. The epidemiology, natural history and prognosis of spinal cord injury. *Curr Orthop* 2004; 18: 26–32.

Hoffman JR, Mower WR, Wolfson AB, *et al.* Validity of a set of clinical criteria to rule out injury to the cervical spine in patients with blunt trauma. *N Engl J Med* 2000; 343: 94–9.

Kramer KM, Levine AM. Posttraumatic syringomyelia: a review of 21 cases. *Clin Orthop Relat Res* 1997; 334: 190–9.

Lee TT, Arias JM, Andrus HL, *et al.* Progressive posttraumatic myelomalacic myelopathy: treatment with untethering and expansive duraplasty. *J Neurosurg* 1997; 86: 624–8.

Chapter 167
Whiplash injury

Anthony Ciabarra
Neurology Center of North Orange County, La Habra, USA

Introduction

Whiplash associated disorders (WAD) are a frequent cause of disability. Acceleration–deceleration forces applied to the neck, particularly with flexion–extension movements, commonly result in whiplash injury. The term "whiplash" should be used to describe an injury mechanism. Whiplash injury results in a mechanical sprain or strain, often with tissue edema or contusion. The posture of the neck and direction of forces dictate the injury sustained. Acceleration strain of the spine may occur in the sagittal plane resulting in extension, flexion, or translational injury; in the frontal plane resulting in lateral inclination or translational injury; or in the axial plane resulting in rotational injury. Neck rotation at the time of impact may correlate with more severe musculo-ligamental strain. More serious injuries may result from whiplash mechanisms, including anterior subluxation, spinous process fractures, facet dislocation, and vertebral compression fractures.

Epidemiology

Considerable variability exists in the frequency and prognosis of whiplash injuries sustained in different geographic regions. This may be partially attributable to societal differences, including such factors as traffic volume, expectations with regards to outcome, as well as the legal and financial ramifications associated with the injury. Reported rates of WAD range from 0.1 to more than 10 per 1000. Women show a greater susceptibility to whiplash injury than men, with a 2:1 ratio. A longer duration of symptoms has been correlated with older age, a past history of neck pain, degenerative changes on radiographs, number of dependents, and a front seat position. The speed limit necessary to produce a whiplash injury is generally considered to be above 6–8 km/hour. Injury

rates with rear-end collisions are approximately twice that of front-end collisions. The utility of head restraints in preventing whiplash injury is controversial; improper adjustment is a factor in determining their effectiveness. The use of seat belts has not been definitively shown to affect the incidence of whiplash injury.

Clinical features

Comparison of findings in clinical studies on WAD has been hampered by non-uniform definitions of whiplash injury. The Quebec Task Force guidelines established grades of WAD in 1995. WAD grade 0 indicates no complaints or physical signs; grade 1 indicates neck pain or stiffness in the absence of physical signs; grade 2 indicates neck complaints and musculoskeletal signs such as decreased range of motion; grade 3 indicates neck complaints and neurological signs including decreased or absent reflexes, sensory loss, or weakness; grade 4 indicates fracture/dislocation. The term whiplash is generally used to refer to grades 1–2.

Whiplash injury can be associated with a variety of physical and psychosocial symptoms. The diagnosis of cervical sprain and strain resulting from a whiplash injury is a clinical one. Pain and stiffness in the neck and shoulders, with limitation in movement, are felt within 24 hours of the injury. Headache, particularly at the occiput, is frequently reported. The injury sustained has not been found to accelerate the development of degenerative changes. The pathophysiology of WAD is controversial. Zygoapophyseal joints are considered to be a significant source of neck pain after WAD, particularly in those who are chronically affected.

Chronic whiplash syndrome (CWS) is defined by the presence of symptoms beyond 6 months. This is controversial and is often accompanied by a combination of symptoms including persistent headache, neck pain and stiffness, paresthesiae and often memory disturbance, fatigue, and anxiety. Some have proposed that CWS is a stress-related disorder caused by the injury or due to psychosocial mechanisms. It is difficult to distinguish whether factors involving financial gain play a significant

International Neurology: A Clinical Approach. Edited by Robert P. Lisak, Daniel D. Truong, William M. Carroll, and Roongroj Bhidayasiri. © 2009 Blackwell Publishing, ISBN: 978-1-4051-5738-4.

role in reported symptoms in individual cases. It is clear that the reported incidence of CWS varies significantly over different geographical regions. Whiplash injury is easy to simulate and difficult to disprove. Observed behavior and the presence of non-physiological sensory loss must be carefully assessed. Settlement of litigation does not always lead to clinical improvement in patients with CWS and lawsuit initiation within the first month of injury has not been found to influence recovery. Nonetheless, preconceived notions regarding whiplash injury may influence outcomes. In Lithuania, for example, where automobile insurance is uncommon, preconceived notions that a whiplash injury will have long-term consequences do not exist, and chronic symptoms from whiplash are infrequent.

Considerable variability has been noted between trials with regard to prognosis, which may be attributable to patient selection methods, definition of whiplash, and societal expectations regarding whiplash injury. After 1 month, most patients improve and 75% perform their regular duties. More than 90% of patients will return to normal daily activities within 1 year. Those suffering from continued pain and inability to work after 1 year are likely to have persistent symptoms. The cervical range of motion test has been found to have a high sensitivity in predicting handicap after whiplash injury.

Management

There is evidence from randomized controlled trials to support mobilization as an effective early intervention for WAD. The efficacy of exercise therapy in CWS is uncertain. Soft collars and rest do not reduce the duration of neck pain. Missed work time is reduced by high-dose methylprednisolone administered within 8 hours of injury. Multimodal programs including exercise, cognitive, and behavioral therapies may be useful, but randomized trials are lacking. Evidence of the benefits of intra-articular steroid injections is conflicting. Botulism neurotoxin A (BoNTA) and traction have not been found to be useful. For those with pain after 6 months, percutaneous frequency neurotomy may be beneficial if a response to local anesthetic injections of facet joints is helpful.

Further reading

Pearce JMS. Polemics of chronic whiplash injury. *Neurology* 1994; 44: 1993–7.

Pettersson K, Toolanen G. High-dose methylprednisolone prevents extensive sick leave after whiplash injury. A prospective, randomized, double-blind study. *Spine* 1998; 23(9): 984–9.

Rodriquez AA, Barr KP, Burns SP. Whiplash: pathophysiology, diagnosis, treatment, and prognosis. *Muscle Nerve* 2004; 29(6): 768–81.

Spitzer WO, Skovron ML, Salmi LR, *et al.* Scientific monograph of the Quebec Task Force on Whiplash-Associated Disorders: redefining "whiplash" and its management. *Spine* 1995; 20(8 Suppl): 1S–73S.

Chapter 168
Decompression sickness

Leon D. Prockop
University of South Florida, Tampa, USA

Introduction

In scuba diving, caisson work, flying, and simulated altitude ascents, rapid reduction in ambient pressure may allow the formation of bubbles from inert gases, especially nitrogen, normally dissolved in body tissues. The relationship between pressure and volume is governed by Boyle's Law, which states that the volume of a fixed mass of gas is inversely proportional to the absolute pressure. The major medical issues are barotrauma, arterial gas embolism (AGE), and decompression sickness (DCS). Barotrauma encompasses disorders related to the overexpansion of gas-filled cavities, such as the lung and inner ear. In the former, lung rupture can occur. In the latter, pain and hearing dysfunction can occur. AGE describes the penetration of gas bubbles into the systemic circulation as a result of pulmonary barotrauma, transpulmonary passage after massive bubble formation (such as chokes), and cardiac shunting. DCS is caused by the growth of gas nuclei in predominantly fatty tissues. The resulting lesions involve the limbs, cardiopulmonary system, and central nervous system (CNS). In divers, DCS primarily affects the spinal cord. Aviators may develop typical musculoskeletal or neurological DCS symptoms while at altitude, with resolution of symptoms frequently occurring on return to sea level. AGE is frequently related to a rapid ascent, and is far more common in diving than in altitude exposure. Other medical problems that may occur during diving and/or flying include nitrogen narcosis, hypoxia, CNS and pulmonary oxygen toxicity, hypercapnia, and hypocapnia.

Epidemiology

The incidence of DCS in divers is between 1% and 30%. Although the spinal cord is the most common site of neurological lesions, encephalopathy is also often described.

Electrophysiological studies, experimental models, and isolated postmortem examinations of patients have shown predominant involvement of the posterolateral and posterior columns in the watershed areas of the thoracic, upper lumbar, and lower cervical cord. Ischemic perivascular lesions are usually confined to the white matter, but subsequent petechial hemorrhage may occur and extend into the gray matter. Lesions result from bubbles occluding vessels or directly disrupting tissue. Coincident intra-arterial embolism may cause cerebral damage.

DCS manifestations include limb pain; itching and skin markings; non-specific constitutional symptoms such as headache, fatigue, malaise, nausea, vomiting, and anorexia; enlarged and tender lymph nodes; vertigo and deafness; and cardiovascular or pulmonary compromise. Neurological signs range from subtle and subjective to unconsciousness or tetraplegia. With cord damage, radicular symptoms are followed by leg paresthesia, paresis, and bladder and bowel dysfunction. When the brain is affected, neurologic signs and symptoms include visual impairment, vertigo, hemiparesis, loss of consciousness, and seizures. Unless recompression is achieved promptly, the signs, including paralysis, may become permanent. Preventive medical clearance and proper scuba diving techniques are essential. Absolute neurological contraindications to scuba diving include a history of any of the following: a seizure occurring other than in childhood, febrile, transient ischemic attack or stroke, and prior DCS with residual deficit. Other neurological conditions of serious concern in preventive evaluation include complicated migraine, head injury, herniated nucleus pulposis, multiple sclerosis (MS), trigeminal neuralgia, and a history of cerebral gas embolism. There are also relative and absolute contraindications for diving in those presenting other body system diseases (such as intracardiac right to left shunt).

Manifestations of DCS, including any neurologic symptoms and signs, are a medical emergency. Current therapy consists of recompression in a hyperbaric chamber and the concurrent administration of 100% oxygen. Results of treatment vary, but the sooner recompression is begun, the better the outcome. Although the use of drugs to improve outcomes is being investigated, no particular

International Neurology: A Clinical Approach. Edited by Robert P. Lisak, Daniel D. Truong, William M. Carroll, and Roongroj Bhidayasiri. © 2009 Blackwell Publishing, ISBN: 978-1-4051-5738-4.

adjunctive pharmacotherapy has been proven effective. Some advise the use of steroids or lidocaine. Intravenous fluids are important. MRI can document the extent of brain and spinal cord damage. For chamber locations and emergency information, US physicians should contact the Divers Alert Network (tel. 919-681-4326, a 24-hour hotline). The following website is for the Diving Division Research Center in Derriford, UK: http://www.ddrc.org. For locations of hyperbaric chambers worldwide, contact http://scuba-doc.com/listchmbr.htm.

Further reading

Cianci P, Slade JB Jr. Delayed treatment of decompression sickness with short, no-air-break tables: review of 140 cases *Aviat Space Environ Med* 2006; 77(10): 1003–8.

Dutka AJ. Long term effects on the central nervous system. In: Brubakk AO, Neuman TS, editors. *Bennett and Elliott's Physiology and Medicine of Diving*, 6th ed. New York: WB Saunders; 2003, pp. 680–99.

Gronning M, Risberg J, Skeidsvoll H, *et al*. Electroencephalography and magnetic resonance imaging in neurological decompression sickness. *Undersea Hyperb Med* 2005; 32 (6): 397–402.

MacDonald RD, O'Donnell C, Allan GM, *et al*. Interfacility transport of patients with decompression illness: literature review and consensus statement. *Prehosp Emerg Care* 2006; 10(4): 482–7.

US Navy Diving Manual. Washington, DC: Naval Sea Systems Command, Edition: Revision 4. http://purl.access.gpo.gov/gpo/lp539797.

Vorosmarti J. Investigation of diving accidents. In: Brubakk AO, Neuman TS, editors. *Bennett and Elliott's Physiology and Medicine of Diving*, 6th ed. New York: WB Saunders; 2003, 718–24.

Chapter 169
Post-traumatic movement disorders

Louis C.S. Tan[1] and Daniel D. Truong[2]
[1]National Neuroscience Institute, Singapore
[2]The Parkinson and Movement Disorder Institute, Fountain Valley, USA

Introduction

Trauma to the central nervous system as a cause of movement disorders has been widely accepted and described in many publications and medical textbooks. However, the occurrence of movement disorders after peripheral injury remains a matter of controversy. The most common post-traumatic movement disorders (PMDs) are tremor, dystonia, and parkinsonism.

Epidemiology

The most common cause of PMDs is head injuries. Studies of individuals presenting with severe head injuries revealed that 13–66% of patients developed movement disorders. Among 221 survivors of severe head injury with a Glasglow Coma Scale (GCS) of 8 or less, PMDs were found in 23%. Among those patients who developed movement disorders, 46% were transient, while the disorder persisted in the remaining patients after a mean follow-up of 4 years. The most common PMD is tremor, followed by dystonia, parkinsonism, and other movement disorders. Among another cohort of 158 patients with mild to moderate head injury (GCS 9–15), 10% were found to have a PMD. These were transient in 75% of the patients and comprised mainly postural/intention tremor.

Pathophysiology

The pathophysiology of movement disorders secondary to trauma of the central nervous system could be attributed to primary damage by direct insult to the basal ganglia and their pathways, as well as secondary mechanisms such as hypoxia, hypotension, and increased cranial pressure. Other factors that could play a role include release of neurotoxins, cytokines, oxidative stress, genetic predisposition, and the restorative process itself which may result in aberrant sprouting, ephaptic transmission, and alterations of neurotransmitter sensitivity.

The role of peripheral trauma in causing movement disorders is controversial, although there are a number of clinical studies supported by animal models that suggest such a notion. It has been postulated that peripheral trauma alters sensory input and induces central cortical and subcortical reorganization, resulting in a movement disorder. Clinical studies investigating such an association are limited by problems with diagnostic criteria, patient selection, and recall bias.

Clinical features, investigations, treatment, and management

Post-traumatic tremor

Tremor is the most common PMD associated with serious head injury and may occur weeks or even months after the injury. It is typically a high-amplitude postural and kinetic tremor that may interfere with motor function. These rhythmic oscillatory movements may be interrupted by irregular jerking movements, leading to a myoclonic appearance, and may even resemble hemiballistic movements. Such tremors are commonly associated with limb and truncal ataxia, cognitive impairments, dysarthria, oculomotor deficits, and residual hemiparesis or tetraparesis. Tremor related to peripheral trauma has been reported following local limb injuries or whiplash-type neck injuries. At times, these may spread to other parts of the body and may be associated with dystonia or reflex sympathetic dystrophy.

Post-traumatic tremors may lessen or resolve spontaneously within 1 year after onset; however, the majority persist. This type of tremor usually does not respond well to medical therapy. Drugs that have been reported to improve post-traumatic tremor include gluthethimide, isoniazid, *L*-tryptophan, propranolol, primidone, benzodiazepines, carbamazepine, levodopa, anticholinergics, and botulinum neurotoxin injections. In patients with disabling tremors, thalamotomy or deep brain stimulation of the thalamus may be performed. The latter is preferred

International Neurology: A Clinical Approach. Edited by Robert P. Lisak, Daniel D. Truong, William M. Carroll, and Roongroj Bhidayasiri. © 2009 Blackwell Publishing, ISBN: 978-1-4051-5738-4.

as it is associated with fewer side effects and allows for adjustment of stimulation parameters, to optimize the results of surgery.

Post-traumatic dystonia

Post-traumatic dystonia has been reported after head injury or peripheral trauma. Hemidystonia is a typical presentation of post-traumatic dystonia secondary to head injury. It often occurs after a short interval of recovery. Dystonia may be accompanied by tremor or myoclonic movements. It may occur at rest, but is usually an action dystonia that is exacerbated by voluntary activity. Rarely, cervical dystonia and segmental axial dystonia may occur after head injury.

Post-traumatic peripherally-induced dystonias are characterized by a fixed posture present at rest, often with underlying contracture, limitation of passive range of movement, absence of sensory tricks, and presence of complex regional pain syndrome. These occur often within a short time after injury. In some patients, direct nerve injury or surgery and electrical injury have been related to the onset of dystonia, which usually develops within the same region of injury. The neck and limbs are most frequently involved; however, blepharospasm and oromandibular dystonias have been reported.

Investigations for post-traumatic dystonia are necessary to detect the site and nature of injury and to exclude structural causes of abnormal posturing, such as atlantoaxial subluxation. Structural causes and entrapment neuropathies should be appropriately treated. The long-term prognosis of post-traumatic dystonia has not been well studied, but seems to be characterized by a slow progression of the movement disorder until stabilized. Fixed contractures often develop when physical therapy and muscle relaxation therapies are delayed. Anticholinergics and botulinum neurotoxin injections are of limited benefit. There is limited experience with surgical interventions.

Post-traumatic parkinsonism

Post-traumatic parkinsonism may occur in the context of a single, significant head injury or as a result of repeated head trauma. Parkinsonism after a single head injury is typically a bradykinetic-rigid syndrome, often unilateral with varying tremor, slowly becoming generalized. Postural instability, gait disorders, headache, psychiatric and cognitive dysfunction, and pyramidal signs are often present. Imaging studies may show structural damage in the basal ganglia or midbrain after the injury. Parkinsonism may also develop from chronic subdural hematomas. "Pugilistic" parkinsonism, which occurs after repeated head injury, is a chronic encephalopathy that results from cumulative effects of subclinical concussions, secondary to rotational acceleration traumas by direct blows to the head. This condition usually develops several years after the end of an active boxing career. The clinical features include ataxia, dysarthria, personality changes, psychosis, rest tremor, and cognitive decline. Imaging studies show generalized brain atrophy often with cavum septum pellucidum. Neuropathological studies have revealed depigmentation of the substantia nigra, but an absence of Lewy bodies. Levodopa may be of benefit and should be tried in all patients with post-traumatic parkinsonism.

Other post-traumatic movement disorders

In addition to tremor, dystonia, and parkinsonism, a variety of other movement disorders have been reported to occur after trauma. Chorea, ballism, paroxysmal dyskinesia, and tics have been reported after head injury. Less commonly described are myoclonus, opsoclonus, palatal myoclonus, stereotypy, and akathisia following head injury. Movement disorders that have been reported after peripheral injury include adult-onset tics, painful legs and moving toes, segmental myoclonus, and hemifacial spasm.

Further reading

Jankovic J. Can peripheral trauma induce dystonia and other movement disorders? Yes! *Mov Disord* 2001; 16: 7–12.

Krauss JK, Jankovic J. Head injury and posttraumatic movement disorders. *Neurosurgery* 2002; 50: 927–40.

Truong DD, Dubinski R, Hermanowicz N, Olson W, Silverman B, Koller W. Posttraumatic torticollis. *Arch Neurol* 1991; 48: 221–3.

Weiner WJ. Can peripheral trauma induce dystonia and other movement disorders? No! *Mov Disord* 2001; 16: 13–22.

Chapter 170
Pain

Guillermo García-Ramos, Bernardo Cacho Díaz, and Bruno Estañol Vidal
National Institute of Medical Sciences and Nutrition, Mexico City, Mexico

Introduction

Pain is defined by the International Association for the Study of Pain (IASP) as "an unpleasant sensory and emotional experience associated with actual or potential tissue damage, or described in terms of such damage." Although its exact etiology is not always found, pain is always pathologic.

Classification of pain disorders

Many classifications of pain have been proposed, including one postulated by Sir Henry Head, who divided pain inputs to the central nervous system (CNS) as either epicritic or protopathic. Epicritic sensation discriminated touch, temperature, and pain, and the protopathic sensation was a poorly localized, long-lasting, unpleasant feeling. This theory was later rejected by Trotter and Davies. Currently, we divide pain into nociceptive, visceral, and neuropathic sensations. Nociceptive pain results from physiologic activity of the normal pain receptors, with no primary dysfunction of the nervous system. Neuropathic pain results from dysfunction of the central or peripheral nervous system and involves two different kinds of pain reflecting several different pathophysiologic mechanisms. Visceral pain will be treated separately.

Mechanisms of pain transmission and modulation

Pain is the consequence of stimulation of pain-sensitive structures (nociceptors) and is often, but not always, a sign of tissue damage. In order to detect a noxious signal as painful, several steps have been identified.

International Neurology: A Clinical Approach. Edited by Robert P. Lisak, Daniel D. Truong, William M. Carroll, and Roongroj Bhidayasiri.
© 2009 Blackwell Publishing, ISBN: 978-1-4051-5738-4.

Transduction

Transduction is recognized as the process by which noxious stimuli are converted to electrical signals by "pain" receptors (nociceptors) that do not have a specialized structure, such as pacinian corpuscles or Merkel disks, and are free nerve endings. Nociceptors do not respond to non-noxious stimuli and do not adapt. Nociceptive afferent fibers come from pseudounipolar neurons, whose bodies reside at the dorsal root ganglia. The neurotransmitters produced by these cells are released at both endings; therefore it has an afferent and efferent neurotransmitter release. The afferent release of neurotransmitters produces the "axon reflex" which leads to peripheral changes that are clinically recognized as indicators of pain (e.g., redness, swelling, and tenderness). The painful stimulus may result in two, not exclusive, reactions: activation and sensitization.

Pain and temperature are sensations mediated at a primary afferent level by fibers of a smaller diameter than those that mediate touch, vibration, and position sense. Cold sensation is transmitted by small, poorly myelinated A-delta fibers; warm sensation is transmitted by unmyelinated warm-specific C-fibers; and pain is mediated by small, myelinated A-delta nociceptors and unmyelinated C nociceptors. The skin, subcutaneous tissues, muscles, and joints are sensitive to a variety of potentially harmful mechanical, thermal, and chemical stimuli. Although the ultrastructural characteristics of pain receptors are not well known, classically two types have been characterized, depending on the fiber characteristics they associate with: unmyelinated C and those associated with A-delta fibers. The third type of cutaneous nociceptor has been described. These nociceptors are activated only during inflammation and modulate information through unmyelinated C fibers. In the absence of inflammation, these receptors usually do not respond even to a high noxious stimulation. These receptors have also been named mechano-insensitive and heat-insensitive (MiHi), and probably mediate hyperalgesia and itch in different populations.

Glabrous and hairy skin is richly innervated by nociceptors with unmyelinated C fibers. These are known as C-polymodal nociceptors (CPNs) because they respond to a variety of noxious stimuli (mechanical, thermal, and chemical). A single CPN innervates an area of skin approximately 1 cm^2. CPNs respond to capsaicin and to temperatures below 15°C.

A-delta nociceptors seem to be stimulated mainly through mechanical provocation and display a smaller, usually punctiform, receptive field and have higher mechanical and heat thresholds than CPNs. Excitation of cutaneous CPNs evokes a pure burning sensation. A-delta nociceptors evoke sharp pain that is projected to a punctiform area. CPNs are also involved in inflammation; its excitation determines the release of algogenic substances from nociceptive terminals in the skin, causing vasodilation and thus local redness of the skin; this reaction spreads some centimeters around the site of stimulation through an axonal reflex that depends on a network of fine dermal afferent fibers, described as a nocifensor system.

Hyperalgesia occurring at the site of injury is defined as primary hyperalgesia and is a characteristic response to heat and mechanical stimuli. Secondary hyperalgesia is hyperalgesia that occurs at a wider area of undamaged surrounding skin. The first type of hyperalgesia is the consequence of sensitization of CPNs at the site of injury, whereas the latter is due to plastic changes in the CNS and probably in the peripheral nervous system. MiHi receptors develop heat and mechanical sensitivity in areas of secondary hyperalgesia.

Transmission

Transmission is the second stage of processing noxious signals. Information from the periphery is relayed to the spinal cord, then to the thalamus, and finally to the cortex. Noxious information is relayed mainly via two types of primary afferent nociceptors. C-fibers are non-myelinated fibers that conduct impulses in the range of 0.5–2 m/s. Nociceptive C-fibers transmit noxious information from a variety of modalities, including mechanical, thermal, and chemical, and thus have been termed C-polymodal nociceptors. As described earlier, they transmit their information through the release of substance P and glutamate. A-delta fibers are thinly myelinated fibers that conduct impulses in the range of 2–20 m/s. All fibers respond to high-intensity mechanical stimulation and are therefore termed high-threshold mechanoreceptors. Some, but not all, receptors respond to thermal stimulus; thus they are named mechano-thermal receptors.

These fibers then synapse on a second-order neuron in the superficial layer of the spinal cord, whose axons are sent across the midline and form the ascending spinothalamic tract, where it reaches a third-order neuron in the thalamus and then projects to the sensory cortex.

The second-order neurons also have the capacity to change their response patterns when a sustained discharge of afferent fibers occurs, e.g., injury. These neurons

then respond to lower thresholds and form inputs over a broader area in the periphery, having expanded receptive fields. This is termed central sensitization and also contributes to the phenomena of hyperalgesia and allodynia.

Once the nociceptive afferents have terminated in the dorsal horn of the spinal cord, they transmit the signal from the periphery by releasing specific neurotransmitters. One of the most important pain neurotransmitters, and the primary afferent, is glutamate, which can interact with both NMDA-type and non-NMDA receptors. Another very important neurotransmitter is substance P, which interacts with the tackynin receptor family (G-protein coupled receptor).

Nociceptive-specific neurons, located mainly in lamina I of Rexed, receive inputs mainly from primary nociceptive afferents. These neurons project to the contralateral spinothalamic tract and their activity is modulated by local interneurons. Wide dynamic range neurons respond more vigorously to inputs from nociceptive afferents, but also discharge in response to non-noxious stimuli; they are predominantly located in lamina V but can be found in laminae I and II. They are thought to project to the contralateral spinothalamic tract. In humans, anterolateral chordotomies abolish pain sensitivity and electrical stimulation of the spinothalamic tract elicits pain. Second-order neurons (nociceptive neurons) also project to higher regions through the spinoreticular, spinomesencephalic, and spinocervical tracts, and some project into the posterior columns. The spinomesencephalic and spinocervical tracts project to the reticular formation, the thalamus, and the periaqueductal gray nuclei.

Third-order neurons are mainly localized in the ventral posterior lateral nucleus. This nucleus receives input from neurons in laminae I and V and projects to the primary somatosensory cortex. The ventral posterior medial nucleus receives input from the second-order nociceptive neurons of the trigeminal nuclei. The intralaminar nuclei receive input from the deep dorsal horn laminae and the reticular formation of the brainstem; this thalamic region is probably concerned with arousal rather than with pain sensation itself. The facial sensations of pain and temperature are carried by cranial nerve V and ascend separately to the thalamus.

In the primary somatosensory cortex, two main types of neurons have been described. One group, which receives inputs from the ventral posterior lateral thalamus, displays a small, contralateral receptive field. The other group comprises neurons that have wide receptive fields, usually bilateral, and probably receive inputs from the medial thalamic nuclei. The thalamocortical projections and the primary sensory cortex in the parietal lobe have a homuncular sensory pattern, in which projections for the face are closest to the sylvian fissure, those for the hand and arm are above, and those for the leg lie near the central sulcus.

Modulation

This third process involves changes in the nervous system's response to noxious stimuli and allows noxious signals received at the dorsal horn of the spinal cord to be selectively inhibited so that the signal transmission to higher centers is modified. An endogenous pain modulation system which inhibits transmission of the pain signal consists of intermediate neurons (superficial layers of the spinal cord) and descending neural tracts. Opiates can act on the presynaptic terminal of the primary afferent nociceptors via *Mu* opioid receptor by indirectly blocking voltage gated calcium channels as well as opening potassium channels, resulting in hyperpolarization and thus in the inhibition of pain neurotransmitter release from these fibers, and hence analgesia. Opioids have the second site of action at the spinal cord, on the postsynaptic neuron; when activated by an opioid, indirectly potassium channels are opened resulting in hyperpolarization of these neurons.

Activation of the cortical descending neural system is thought to involve the supraspinal release of beta-endorphins and enkephalins. These peptides represent two families of endogenous peptides that are associated with pain relief, especially under stress.

Descending modulatory systems

Activation of these systems by endorphins occurs through specific receptors called opioid receptors. These systems are activated in and around the periaqueductal gray mesencephalic (midbrain) region. The neurons project to sites in the medullary reticular formation and the locus ceruleus (the main sources where serotonin and norepinephrine are produced, respectively). The descending fibers then project to the dorsal horn of the spinal cord along a tract called the dorsolateral funiculus, to synapse with the incoming primary afferent neuron, second-order neuron, or interneurons. The descending pain modulatory neurons either (1) release neurotransmitters in the spinal cord, especially serotonin (5HT) and norepinephrine (NE), both of which directly inhibit release of pain transmitters from the incoming nociceptive afferent signal or inhibit the second-order pain transmission cell, or (2) activate small, opioid-containing interneurons in the spinal dorsal horn to release opioid peptides.

Perception of pain is frequently triggered by a noxious stimulus, but it can be elicited by lesions in the peripheral or CNS, for example, diabetic neuropathy or stroke. It is important to realize that pain can occur without nociception. Pain due to nerve injury does not respond to analgesics such as morphine as efficiently as pain caused by tissue damage, indicating the complex relationship that exists between injury and pain. Another relevant issue is that the intensity of chronic pain frequently bears little or no relation to the extent of tissue injury or other quantifiable pathology.

Visceral pain

There are two common principles that apply to all visceral pain. The first is that the neurologic mechanisms of visceral pain differ from those involved in somatic pain, and therefore findings in somatic pain research cannot necessarily be extrapolated to visceral pain. The second principle is that the psychophysics (perception and psychological processing) of visceral pain also differ from that of somatic pain.

Visceral pain has five important characteristics:
1 It is not evoked from all visceral organs. The liver, kidney, most solid viscera, and lung parenchyma are not sensitive to pain.
2 It is not always linked to visceral injury. For example, cutting the intestine causes no pain, whereas stretching the bladder is painful despite no injury.
3 It is diffuse and poorly localized.
4 It is referred to other locations.
5 It is accompanied by motor and autonomic reflexes, such as the nausea, vomiting, and lower back muscle tension present in renal colic.

These features are due to functional properties of the peripheral receptors of the nerves that innervate certain visceral organs and to the fact that many viscera are innervated by receptors that do not evoke conscious perception and, thus, are not sensory receptors in the strict sense. Visceral pain tends to be diffuse because of the organization of visceral nociceptive pathways in the CNS, particularly the absence of a separate visceral sensory pathway and the low proportion of visceral afferent nerve fibers compared with those of somatic origin.

Two distinct classes of nociceptive sensory receptors innervate internal organs. The first class of receptors have a high threshold to natural stimuli (mostly mechanical); high-threshold receptors have been identified in the heart, veins, lung parenchyma and airways, esophagus, biliary system, small intestine, colon, ureters, urinary bladder, and uterus. The second class of receptors are intensity-encoding receptors that have a low threshold to natural stimuli (mostly mechanical) and an encoding function that spans the range of stimulation intensity from innocuous to noxious. These receptors are intensity encoding because they encode the stimulus intensity in the magnitude of their discharges; they have been described in the heart, esophagus, colon, urinary bladder, and testes.

A third nociceptive receptor family – silent receptors – has been increasingly recognized. These receptors are normally unresponsive to stimuli and become activated only in the presence of inflammation. This new class of sensory receptors contributes to the signaling of chronic visceral pain, to long-term alterations of spinal reflexes, and to abnormal autonomic regulation of internal organs. They comprise no more than 40–45% of total afferent visceral innervation of the colon and bladder.

High-threshold receptors and intensity-coding receptors contribute to the peripheral encoding of noxious events in the viscera. Brief, acute visceral pain could be triggered initially by activation of high-threshold afferents. More extended forms of visceral stimulation result in sensitization of high-threshold receptors and bring into play previously unresponsive silent nociceptors. Once sensitized, these nociceptors begin to respond to the innocuous stimuli that normally occur in internal organs. As a consequence, the CNS receives an increased afferent barrage from peripheral nociceptors that is initially due to the acute injury, but that is also influenced by the physiologic activity of the internal organ and persists until the process of peripheral sensitization subsides completely. In this way, the pain is intensified and its duration extended by a central mechanism brought into action by the peripheral barrage.

Damage and inflammation of the viscus also affects its normal pattern of motility and secretion, which produces dramatic changes in the environment that surrounds the nociceptor endings. The altered activity of the viscus further increases the excitation of sensitized nociceptors and may even be sufficient to excite more distant nociceptors that were not affected by the initial insult. Therefore, afferent discharges due to viscus activity after an injury or inflammation may be greater in magnitude and duration than the discharges produced by acute injury, and visceral pain may persist even after the initial injury is on its way to resolution.

Fine caliber unmyelinated primary afferents that innervate somatic and visceral tissues have two distinct biochemical classes: the first class contains neurons that express peptide neurotransmitters, such as substance P and calcitonin-gene-related peptide; the other class does not express these substances. These two classes can be distinguished by various enzymes, such as fluoride-resistant acid phosphatase (non-peptide group), and receptors, such as the nerve-growth-factor receptor, tyrosine kinase A. They also differ with regard to trophic requirements.

The peptide-containing afferents of the somatic system terminate in the outermost layers of the posterior horn, lamina I, outer lamina II, and lamina V, whereas the non-peptide groups terminate in the inner lamina II. In contrast to the somatic fine afferent fibers, most visceral afferent fibers seem to belong to the peptide class that expresses peptide neurotransmitters and does not express carbohydrate group characteristics of the non-peptide class. As with somatic peptide-containing afferents, visceral

afferents also terminate on spinal cord laminae I and V. Peptides seem to have more importance in the transmission of information from the viscera; substance P may have a specific role in visceral hyperalgesia.

Several pathways have been found to be responsible for transmission of visceral pain: traditional crossed anterolateral pathways, mainly the spinothalamic and spinoreticular tracts which were believed to be the only pathways, but the dorsal column pathway, the spino(trigeminal)-parabrachio-amygdaloid pathway, and the spino-hypothalamic pathway have also been demonstrated to transmit pain.

Current information tells us how very complex the visceral pain integration in the brain is. For example: (1) there are descriptions of responses to visceral sensory signals in neurons of the visual cortex that emphasize the convergent nature of most sensory messages but do not deny the primary role of the visual cortex in visual perception; (2) microstimulation of the thalamus can evoke visceral pain experiences, such as angina or labor pain. This observation highlights the integrative role of the thalamus in processing memories of pain and the existence of long-lived neural mechanisms capable of storing painful experience; and (3) enteric representation in healthy volunteers who received acute noxious stimulation of the rectum evoked brain activity in the anterior cingulated cortex, a region associated with the perception of the affective emotional qualities of the pain experience; the precise components of the cingulate cortex activated by visceral stimulus differ from those normally activated by somatic stimulation.

The so-called functional abdominal pain syndromes, which include irritable bowel syndrome, functional dyspepsia, and other conditions, may be the result of sensitization of the peripheral nociceptors or of alterations of central processing that lead to increased activation of visceral nociceptive pathways.

Neuralgias and neuropathic syndromes

Peripheral nerve injury usually results in numbness and a sensory deficit in the territory of the involved nerve; occasionally tingling or pins-and-needles sensation (paresthesias) are reported. Pain as a manifestation of nerve injury is difficult to predict – for instance, up to 50% of diabetics develop neuropathy during the course of their disease, but only 10% of those patients complain of pain.

Three cardinal features of neuropathic pain are usually present in varying degrees. These are as follows:
1 Continuous pain, commonly described as burning, an icy feeling, or intense tightness.
2 Paroxysmal pain, described as lancinations, jabbing, or shooting.

3 Allodynia, defined as an aberrant sensation of pain response to what is normally an innocuous stimulus, for example, light touch.

Physical signs of neuropathic pain include *hyperalgesia*, characterized by an intensely painful response to modest irritation, such as pinprick. *Hyperpathy* is an abnormally prolonged sensation of a stimulus, usually painful, after the stimulus has stopped. *Dysesthesia* is the term for the disagreeably abnormal sensations evoked when an area of abnormal sensation is touched. Abnormal territory sensory disturbances.

After the initial nerve injury, accumulation of sodium channels at the site of neuroma formation, at the axon and at the dorsal root ganglia immediately begins. All these sites are foci of ectopic impulses; in addition to firing spontaneously, these sites may produce prolonged discharges and nearby fibers and inactive fibers respond excessively, generating a broader than normal location of pain distribution.

Classification of painful neuropathies depends on the localization or distribution of affected nerves. Painful neuropathies can be divided into the following:
1 *Symmetrical polyneuropathies*: usually distal areas are affected. Hyporeflexia and trophic changes are seen. These neuropathies result from conditions that have a diffuse effect on the peripheral nervous system. Examples include diabetes mellitus, ethanol abuse, renal failure, toxic, paraneoplastic syndromes, and CIDP.
2 *Focal neuropathies*: affected areas follow a specific nerve territory. Examples include entrapment neuropathies (e.g., carpal tunnel syndrome), tumor infiltration, trigeminal neuralgia, postherpetic neuralgia, and post-traumatic neuralgia.
3 *Multifocal mononeuropathies*: areas affected present as patchy, due to simultaneous or sequential damage to non-contiguous nerves. Some examples include diabetes mellitus, vasculitis, and brachial or lumbar plexitis.
4 *Small fiber neuropathy*: one of the most painful neuropathies. Allodynia and changes in proprioception or vibration along with regional autonomic dysfunction are seen (e.g., abnormal sweating, temperature changes, erythematic). Examples include amyloid neuropathy, diabetes mellitus, idiopathic disorders, Fabry's disease, Tangier disease.

Motor deficits tend to dominate the clinical picture in acute and chronic inflammatory demyelinating neuropathies, multifocal motor neuropathy with conduction block, hereditary neuropathies, neuropathies associated with myeloma, porphyria, lead or organophosphate intoxications, and hypoglycemia. Predominant sensory involvement may be a feature of neuropathies associated with diabetes mellitus, carcinoma, Sjögren's syndrome, dysproteinemia, HIV, vitamin B_{12} deficiency, and cisplatinum or pyridoxine use, among others.

Entrapment neuropathies

Entrapment neuropathies are defined as a group of focal neuropathies caused by mechanical compression or distortion of a nerve in an anatomical tunnel or fibrous canal or, less frequently, by nearby structures such as bone, ligament, or connective tissue.

Compression, constriction, angulation, and stretching are the physical mechanisms that harm the nerve at certain vulnerable areas. The mechanism of harm is induced by morphologic changes that lead the nerve into demyelination, remyelination, or axonal, or, in severe cases, wallerian degeneration. In addition, endoneural inflammation, collagen proliferation, and thickening of perineural structures may be present. All of these changes induce a self-perpetuating cycle of compression–ischemia–edema. The characteristic feature of entrapment neuropathy is either conduction delay or conduction block across the site of entrapment.

Complex regional pain syndromes

Causalgia means burning pain. It is defined by the IASP as "burning pain, allodynia, and hyperpathia, usually in the hand or foot after partial injury of a nerve or one of its major branches." At present, post-injury pain syndromes have been divided into the following: complex regional pain syndrome type I (CRS type 1, reflex sympathetic dystrophy, RSD), and complex regional pain syndrome type II (CRS type 2, causalgia). RSD develops without evidence of nerve injury, whereas causalgia is the result of a traumatic nerve lesion. The sympathetic nervous system has been implicated in the pathogenesis of both; however, this is in question and these broadly used terms are applied to different, unrelated, painful neuropathic disorders. RSD is defined by the IASP as a "continuous pain in a portion of an extremity after trauma, which may include fracture, but does not involve a major nerve, associated with sympathetic hyperactivity. RSD usually involves the distal extremity adjacent to a traumatized area and the main feature is pain described as burning, continuous, exacerbated by movement, cutaneous stimulation, or stress, with onset usually weeks after injury. Therapeutic modalities include sympathetic block and physical therapy with sympathectomy if long-term results are not achieved with repeated blocks."

Central pain

In lesions of the CNS, deafferentation of secondary neurons in the posterior horns or of sensory ganglion cells that terminate on them may cause the deafferented cells to become continuously active and, if stimulated, reproduce pain. The patient with spinal cord transection may have intolerable pain below the level of the lesion that can project to areas disconnected from suprasegmental structures and be exacerbated or provoked by movement, fatigue, or emotion. Loss of descending inhibitory systems seems a likely explanation in lesions of the pons and medulla. This may also explain the pain of the Déjerine–Roussy thalamic syndrome (painful anesthesia).

Pain due to systemic disorders

Pain is a component of many different diseases. It is usually poorly defined and difficult to explore. Examples of diseases accompanied by pain include multiple sclerosis, diabetes, and fibromyalgia.

Pain can be due to an undiagnosed medical disease. The source of this pain is usually peripheral and caused by a lesion that irritates and destroys nerve endings. Carcinomatosis is a good example. Osseous metastases, peritoneal implants, invasion of retroperitoneal tissues or the hilum of the lung, and implication of the nerves of the brachial or lumbosacral plexuses can be extremely painful. It is sometimes necessary to repeat all diagnostic procedures months after a negative investigation in order to reach a diagnosis. Treatment is directed to pain relief and, if possible, stopping progression of the primary disease.

Psychiatric patients often have pain as the predominant symptom. Examples of psychiatric diseases associated with pain are depression, malingering, and hysteria. A psychiatric evaluation is very helpful in diagnosing and treating patients who complain of chronic pain. All other diagnoses should be excluded, however, before deciding that a psychiatric condition is responsible for pain.

Approach to the patient with pain

Many factors cause a stimulus to become painful. Characteristics of the host (e.g., genetics, gender, endogenous pain control, anxiety, depression, coping behavior, cognitive factors, disease history, socialization, lifestyle, traumas, expectations, and roles) play an important part in this transition. In other words, pain is a result of not only physical disorders, but also combinations of physiologic, pathologic, emotional, psychological, cognitive, environmental, and social factors.

Although not always associated with tissue damage, a complete history should be obtained and physical examination must be done before labeling pain as idiopathic. It is important to identify factors that initiate and maintain pain. Because pain is usually accompanied by psychological issues regardless of its etiology, we recommend not using the term psychological pain or conversive pain.

Suffering is a state of severe distress associated with events that threaten the intactness of the person and occurs when the physical or psychological integrity of the person is vulnerable. It is a negative response induced by pain, and also by fear, anxiety, stress, loss of loved objects, and other psychological states. Not all pain causes suffering, and not all suffering expressed as pain, or coexisting with pain, stems from pain. Patients are dynamic psychological and social entities. Thus, suffering is the consequence of perceived impending destruction of the person or of some essential part of the person, and entails a disparity between what one expects of oneself and what one does or is. Vulnerability to suffering depends partially on who one is and what one does in society.

Pain is essentially subjective and the measurement of quality is based on verbal concepts. Several subjective measures of pain based on word descriptions have been developed, including the following:

1 Unidimensional scales:
  a Verbal rating scales use words ranked in order of severity (e.g., none, mild, moderate, severe).
  b Visual analog scales may be continuous or intermittent: colored analog scale, facial anchors, 10 cm unmarked line.
2 Multidimensional scales:
  a The McGill Pain Questionnaire consists of 20 descriptor scales (each containing a variable number of words as a list ranked in intensity), divided into four main dimensions. The patient is asked to choose one word from any relevant list.
  b The short form McGill Pain Questionnaire consists of 11 sensory and four affective descriptor scales scored as none, mild, moderate, or severe.

Therapy

The goal of therapy is to control pain and to rehabilitate the patient so that he or she can function as well as possible.

Treating patients who are in pain should be a multidisciplinary task, in which each member has his or her own role. Physicians, psychologists, nurses, physical and occupational therapists, vocational counselors, and pharmacists should work together with the most important member of the therapeutic team: the patient.

An injury usually unleashes the production of cytokines and chemokines (tumor necrosis factor alpha, growth factors, interleukin-1 beta, interleukin-8), surface antigens, adenosine triphosphate, cannabinoids, and neuropeptides that, in turn, produce the release of excitatory chemicals, including glutamate, bradykinin, cyclo-oxygenase 2, and nitric oxide, producing CNS sensitization as a final pathway.

Table 170.1 Mechanisms, diagnostic features, molecular targets, and drugs proposed for treatment of patients with pain.

Mechanism	Diagnostic features	Molecular target	Drugs proposed
General sodium channels: redistribution or altered expression	Spontaneous pain, paresthesia	Sodium channels sensitive to tetrodotoxin	Local anesthetics, antiepileptics, antiarrhythmics, tricyclic antidepressants
Specific sodium channels	Spontaneous pain	Sodium channels resistant to tetrodotoxin	Selective blockers
Central sensitization	Hyperalgesia (in response to touch, cold, pin prick)	NMDA receptor (glutamate, glycine), neurokinin 1 receptor (bradykynin), neuronal nitric oxide synthase, protein kinase	NMDA antagonist (ketamine, dextromethorphan, memantine), glycine site antagonists, neurokinin 1 receptor antagonists, neuronal nitric oxide synthase inhibitors, protein kinase inhibitors
Peripheral sensitization	Hyperalgesia in response to pressure	Vanilloid receptor	Capsaicin, cannabinoids
	Hyperalgesia in response to thermal stimuli	Neurokinin 1 receptor	Neurokinin 1 receptor antagonist
	Neurogenic inflammation	Nerve growth factor	Nerve growth factor antagonist
Sympathetic activity	Spontaneous pain	Adrenergic receptors (alpha adrenergic), nerve growth factor or trKA	Phentolamine, guanethidine, clonidine, nerve growth factor antagonists
Reduced inhibition	Hyperalgesia	Opioid receptors, GABA transaminase, neurokinin 1, adenosine, purine, kainite, cholecystokinin, acetylcholine (nicotinic)	Morphine, gabapentin

Along with pharmacologic treatment of chronic pain, the physician should:
• Obtain a complete medical history and perform a thorough physical examination.
• Prepare a written treatment plan that states the objectives, such as pain relief and improved physical and psychosocial function, that will be used to assess treatment success.
• Discuss the risks and benefits of each medication with the patient.
• Review the course of treatment. Continuation or modification of therapy should depend on the physician's evaluation of progress toward the stated treatment objectives. The physician should monitor the patient's compliance with the treatment plan.
• Be willing to refer the patient for additional evaluation and treatment to achieve treatment objectives.

When treating patients with acute pain – defined as the normal, predicted physiologic response to an adverse chemical, thermal, or mechanical stimulus associated with surgery, trauma, or acute illness – the physician should: (1) discuss the options for pain control with the patient and provide instruction for simple, cognitive–behavioral techniques; (2) assess pain routinely, just as monitoring vital signs; (3) treat pain as early as possible; (4) use non-drug and drug interventions together; (5) select treatment according to the clinical setting and promptly modify it according to the patient's response; and (6) provide continuity of pain control after discharge. One should identify and treat any causative lesion as soon as possible, remembering that multiple neural and biochemical mechanisms may be operative and multiple modalities and treatments may be required. Multidisciplinary treatment is the better approach.

Depending on their mechanism and diagnostic tests, we can divide pharmacologic treatments as shown in Table 170.1. When patients are suffering from neuropathic pain, it is important to classify peripheral neuropathic pain into stimulus-evoked pain or stimulus-independent (spontaneous) pain.

Opioids

Respiratory depression is kept to a minimum when appropiate, regular doses of opioid are given to patients with chronic pain. Appropriate titration keeps serious adverse effects to a minimum. The medical use of opioids does not create drug addicts, and restricting opioids because this fear may hurt patients.

Common opioids include morphine, diamorphine, meperidine, methadone, hydromorphone, oxycodone, fentanyl, and buprenorphine. All types of pain probably respond equally well to all opioids.

Fast onset of effect is not a critical factor if the patient is receiving continual analgesics for chronic pain, but it may be relevant for patients who are taking the drug on an as-needed basis. The intravenous route is the fastest (onset time 2 minutes), the oral route more prolonged (up to 2–4 hours for sustained release). When a patient is on opioids, one should keep in mind that drug doses should be decreased substantially if creatinine clearance is less than 30 ml/minute per $1.73\,m^2$.

Adverse effects include nausea, dizziness, somnolence, and constipation. The first two commonly abate. With tolerance the patient needs a higher dose (or increased plasma concentration) to achieve the same pharmacological effect. Because scant information exists regarding a maximum opioid dose, many physicians increase the dose as needed and maintain a close follow-up, being especially careful that adverse effects do not incapacitate the individual being treated.

Chronic pain (cancer pain and non-cancer pain) is not always relieved by opioids. Opioid-insensitive pain can be defined as pain that does not respond to progressively increasing opioid dose. The most common causes of opioid-insensitive pain are nerve compression and nerve destruction. A useful clinical rule is that opioids may not be as effective when pain is localized in a numb area. The usual pharmacologic solutions for neuropathic pain include oral antidepressants, anticonvulsants, and local anesthetics (spinal infusions of local anesthics and opioid mixtures used for treating patients whose pain is not relieved). For some patients, adding clonidine may be beneficial when opioids are no longer effective.

As a guide in prescribing opioids for chronic non-malignant pain one should:
• Have a contract with the patient. This should cover the amount of drug that one will prescribe, the fact that the patient is not to obtain additional prescriptions (there is to be only one prescriber), and the consequences of breaking the contract.
• Monitor titration of doses, the use of short-acting opioids, the use of injectable opioids at home, and prescription of more than one opioid. The patient should be assessed at 6- to 9-week intervals.
• Avoid alcohol problems, drug problems, other treatments not tried first, and doubts.
• Aim at focusing on improved function, not pain relief, using long-acting opioids, and making prescriptions tamperproof.

Further reading

Ashburn MA, Staats PS. Management of chronic pain. *Lancet* 1999; 353: 1865–9.

Besson JM. The neurobiology of pain. *Lancet* 1999; 353: 1610–15.

Carr DB, Goudas LC. Acute pain. *Lancet* 1999; 353: 2051–8.

Cervero F, Laird JMA. Visceral pain. *Lancet* 1999; 353: 2145–8.

Chapman CR, Gavrin J. Suffering: the contributions of persistent pain. *Lancet* 1999; 353: 2233–7.

Holdcroft A, Power I. Management of pain. *BMJ* 2003; 326: 635–9.

Loeser JD, Melzack R. Pain: an overview. *Lancet* 1999; 353: 1607–9.

McQuay H. Opioids in pain management. *Lancet* 1999; 353: 2229–32.

Merkskey H, Bogduk N. *Classification of Chronic Pain*. Seattle: International Association for the Study of Pain Press; 1994, p. 210.

Nurmikko TJ, Nash TP, Wiles JR. Control of chronic pain. *BMJ* 1998; 317: 438–41.

Turk DC, Okifuji A. Assessment of patients' reporting of pain: an integrated perspective. *Lancet* 1999; 353: 1784–8.

Vanderah TW. Pathophysiology of pain. *Med Clin N Am* 2007; 91: 1–12.

Verdugo RJ, Cea JG, Campero M, Castillo JL. Pain and temperature. In: Goetz CG, editor. *Textbook of Clinical Neurology*, 2nd ed. Philadelphia: Saunders; 2003, pp. 351–69.

Chapter 171
Headache

Stephen D. Silberstein
Thomas Jefferson University, Philadelphia, PA, USA

Introduction

The International Classification of Headache Disorders (ICHD-2) divides headache into primary and secondary disorders. A primary headache disorder is one in which headache itself is the illness and no other etiology is diagnosed. Headache attributed to an identifiable structural or metabolic abnormality constitutes a secondary headache disorder.

Migraine headache

Pathogenesis and pathophysiology

Migraine aura is probably due to cortical spreading depression (CSD), a slowly spreading wave (at a rate of 2–3 mm/minute) of neuronal and glial depolarization that lasts about 1 minute. CSD develops within brain areas, such as the cerebral cortex, cerebellum, or hippocampus, after electrical or chemical stimulation. CSD is associated with a marked decrease in neuronal membrane resistance, a massive increase in extracellular K^+ and neurotransmitters, and an increase in intracellular Na^+ and Ca^{2+}. It is believed that patients with migraine have a reduced threshold for CSD. How CSD is triggered in the human cortex during a migraine attack is uncertain.

Headache probably results from activation of meningeal and blood vessel nociceptors combined with a change in central pain modulation. Trigeminal sensory neurons contain substance P, calcitonin gene-related peptide, and neurokinin A. Stimulation results in the release of substance P and calcitonin gene-related peptide from sensory C-fiber terminals and neurogenic inflammation. The neuropeptides interact with the blood vessel wall, producing dilation, plasma protein extravasation, and platelet activation. Neurogenic inflammation sensitizes nerve fibers (peripheral sensitization), which now respond to previously innocuous stimuli, such as blood vessel pulsations, causing, in part, the pain of migraine. Central sensitization (CS) of trigeminal nucleus caudalis neurons can also occur. CS may play a key role in maintaining the headache. The migraine aura can trigger headache: CSD activates trigeminovascular afferents. How does a headache begin in the absence of aura? CSD may occur in silent areas of the cortex or the cerebellum. In addition, direct activation of the trigeminal nerve can occur.

Migraine may be a result of a change in pain and sensory input processing. The aura is triggered in the hypersensitive cortex (CSD). Headache is generated by central pain facilitation and neurogenic inflammation. CS can occur, in part mediated by supraspinal facilitation. Decreased antinociceptive system activity and increased peripheral input may be present.

Epidemiology and risk factors

In the United States, 18% of women, 6% of men, and 4% of children have migraine. The disorder usually begins in the first three decades of life, and prevalence peaks in the fifth decade.

Chronic daily headache (CDH) refers to a group of disorders characterized by very frequent headaches (15 or more days a month). The major primary disorders defined by ICHD-2 are chronic migraine (CM), hemicrania continua (HC), chronic tension-type headache (CTTH), and new daily persistent headache (NDPH). Patients who have daily headaches that persist for months often have transformed migraine, and have a past history of episodic migraine that typically began in their teens or twenties. Most of these patients are women, 90% of whom have a history of migraine without aura. The headaches grow more frequent, and the associated symptoms of photophobia, phonophobia, and nausea become less severe and less frequent than during typical migraine. Patients often develop a pattern of daily, or nearly daily, headaches that phenomenologically resemble CTTH, with mild to moderate pain but with photophobia, phonophobia, or gastrointestinal features. Other features of migraine, including unilaterality and aggravation by menstruation and other trigger factors, may persist. Attacks of full-blown migraine

International Neurology: A Clinical Approach. Edited by Robert P. Lisak, Daniel D. Truong, William M. Carroll, and Roongroj Bhidayasiri. © 2009 Blackwell Publishing, ISBN: 978-1-4051-5738-4.

superimposed on a background of less severe headaches often occur. Many patients with transformed migraine overuse symptomatic medication. Stopping the overused medication frequently results in distinct headache improvement. Eighty percent of patients with transformed migraine have depression, which frequently lifts when the pattern of medication overuse and daily headache is interrupted.

Clinical features and associated disorders

The migraine attack can be divided into four phases: (1) the prodrome, which occurs hours or days before the headache; (2) the aura, which immediately precedes the headache; (3) the headache itself; and, (4) the postdrome. Migraine with aura may occur with or without the headache, but migraine without aura requires the headache for its diagnosis.

The migraine aura is a complex of focal neurologic symptoms (positive or negative phenomena) that precedes or accompanies an attack. Most aura symptoms develop over 5–20 minutes and usually last less than 60 minutes. The aura can be characterized by visual, sensory, or motor phenomena and may also involve language or brain stem disturbances.

The typical migraine headache is unilateral, throbbing, moderate to marked in severity, and aggravated by physical activity. The pain may be bilateral at the onset or start on one side and become generalized. The pain usually lasts between 4 and 72 hours in adults and 2 and 48 hours in children. The average migraineur experiences from one to three headaches a month.

The pain of migraine is accompanied by other features. Anorexia is common, nausea occurs in almost 90% of patients and vomiting occurs in about one-third. Many patients have photophobia, phonophobia, and osmophobia, and seek a dark, quiet room. Following the headache, during the postdrome phase, the patient may feel tired, "washed out," irritable, and listless, and may have impaired concentration, scalp tenderness, or mood changes. A variety of migraine clinical subtypes have been described. Attacks of migraine lasting longer than 72 hours define *status migrainosus*.

Differential diagnosis

Similar headaches may occur as a result of abnormalities of the brain, including tumors, infections, and vascular malformations. Idiopathic intracranial hypertension (IIH), low pressure headache, and intracranial neoplasms may also mimic migraine, as may hypoxia, hypoglycemia, dialysis, pheochromocytoma, and various chemicals and medications. Sinusitis or glaucoma may occasionally resemble migraine. Other primary headache disorders, such as TTH, cluster headache, and hypnic headache, should be considered.

Evaluation

Patients who have normal neurologic examinations and benign recurrent headaches that fit ICHD-2 criteria do not require brain imaging. Patients who have an abnormal neurologic examination, an atypical history, or a sudden, unexplained change in the frequency or major characteristics of their headaches should be imaged.

Management

The two strategies of migraine treatment are: (1) acute treatment, to terminate attacks, and (2) preventive treatment, to prevent future attacks. Acute treatment can be specific or non-specific. Non-specific medications (analgesics, antiemetics, anxiolytics, non-steroidal anti-inflammatory drugs (NSAIDs), steroids, neuroleptics, and opioids) are used to control the pain and associated symptoms of migraine or other pain disorders, while specific medications (ergots and triptans) control the migraine attack but are not useful for other pain disorders. Analgesics are used for mild to moderate headaches. Triptans or dihydroergotamine mesylate (DHE) are first-line drugs for severe attacks and for less severe attacks that do not adequately respond to analgesics. The sooner acute treatment is begun, the more effective it will be. Early intervention prevents escalation and may increase efficacy. Triptans can prevent the development of cutaneous allodynia (CA), and CA predicts triptans' effectiveness.

The goals of preventive treatment are to reduce the frequency, duration, and severity of attacks, improve responsiveness to acute attack treatment, improve function, and reduce disability. Preventive drug treatments include antidepressants, β-blockers, calcium channel blockers, NSAIDs, serotonin antagonists, and anticonvulsants. Preventive treatment is used because of: (1) recurring migraine that significantly interferes with the patient's daily routine despite acute treatment; (2) frequent headaches (>4 attacks/month); (3) contraindication to, failure with, overuse of, or intolerance to acute therapies; (4) frequent, very long, or uncomfortable auras; (5) patient preference; or (6) certain migraine conditions, including hemiplegic migraine, basilar migraine, migraine with prolonged aura, and migrainous infarction.

Preventive medication should be chosen based on documented efficacy, side-effect profiles, ease of use, and coexistent comorbid conditions. Medications can be divided into five major categories: (1) drugs that have been proven effective (some β-blockers, amitriptyline, topiramate, divalproex, and methysergide); (2) drugs that are probably effective (gabapentin, fluoxetine, venlafaxine, cyproheptadine, MIG-99 (feverfew), coenzyme Q10, and vitamin B_2); (3) drugs that are possibly effective; (4) drugs for which evidence is inadequate or conflicting; and (5) drugs that are probably ineffective.

Medication should be started at a low dose and increased slowly until headache severity or frequency decreases, the maximum recommended dose is reached, or adverse effects develop. When the headaches have been controlled, attempts can be made to taper and discontinue therapy. Patients should be monitored for acute medication overuse, which may result in chronic refractory headaches and withdrawal symptoms when the medication is discontinued. Some studies support the use of topiramate, tizanidine, and gabapentin for CM. Amitriptyline is perhaps the most commonly used medication, but evidence only exists for CTTH, not for CM.

Tension-type headache (TTH)

Pathogenesis and pathophysiology
TTH is not the result of sustained contraction of the pericranial muscles. The muscle ache of a TTH attack may be due to increased neuronal sensitivity and pain facilitation due to chronic or intermittent dysfunction of the monoaminergic or serotonergic function in the hypothalamus, brain stem, and spinal cord.

Epidemiology and risk factors
TTH is very common, with a lifetime prevalence of 69% in men and 88% in women. TTHs can begin at any age, but onset during adolescence or young adulthood is most common.

Clinical features and associated disorders
Episodic TTHs can be either infrequent (<1 day/month or 12 days/year) or frequent (>1 but <15 days/month or >12 but <180 days/year) The ICHD-2 requires at least 10 previous headaches, each lasting 30 minutes to 7 days (median, 12 hours), with at least two of the following characteristics: a pressing/tightening (non-pulsating) quality, mild to moderate intensity, bilateral location, and no aggravation with physical activity. In addition, the patient should not have nausea or vomiting or a combination of photophobia and phonophobia. Episodic TTH occurs less than 15 days/month, whereas CTTH occurs 15 or more days/month. The pain is a dull, achy, non-pulsatile feeling of tightness, pressure, or constriction (vise-like or hatband-like), and it is usually mild to moderate, in contrast to the moderate-to-severe pain of migraine. Most patients have bilateral pain.

Differential diagnosis
Migraine is the headache disorder that is most confused with TTH. Both can be bilateral, non-throbbing, and associated with anorexia. Migraine is more severe, often unilateral, and frequently associated with nausea. IIH, brain tumor headache, chronic sphenoid sinusitis, and cervical, ocular, and temporomandibular disorders need to be considered. What we call episodic TTH may be two

distinct disorders. The first disorder may be attacks of mild migraine. The second may be a pure TTH that is not associated with other features of migraine (nausea, photophobia, or sensitivity to movement) or with attacks of severe migraine.

Evaluation
Most patients with a long history of unchanged episodic TTHs do not require extensive evaluation if they have normal neurologic examinations and are otherwise healthy. Patients with chronic TTHs should be imaged with CT or MRI, even if their general and neurologic examinations are normal. A metabolic screen, complete blood count, electrolytes, and kidney and thyroid function studies are also appropriate.

Management
TTH patients usually self-medicate with over-the-counter analgesics. If these medications are not effective, prescription NSAIDs or combination analgesic preparations can be used. Narcotics and combination analgesics that contain sedatives should be limited, because overuse may cause dependence.

Preventive therapy should be administered when a patient has frequent headaches that produce disability or may lead to symptomatic medication overuse. Medications used for TTH prevention include antidepressants, β-blockers, and anticonvulsants. Antidepressants are the medication of first choice. An adequate trial period of at least 1–2 months must be allowed. Biofeedback therapy may improve the therapeutic benefit derived from antidepressants.

Prognosis and future perspectives
Episodic TTH usually improves with time. Some patients may, however, progress to CTTH, especially when analgesic overuse is present.

Cluster headache

Pathogenesis and pathophysiology
Cluster events are probably related to alterations in the circadian pacemaker, which may be due to hypothalamic dysfunction. Neurogenic inflammation, carotid body chemoreceptor dysfunction, central parasympathetic and sympathetic tone imbalance, and increased responsiveness to histamine have been proposed as the causes of cluster pain.

Epidemiology and risk factors
Cluster headache prevalence (0.01–1.5%) is lower than that of migraine or TTH. Prevalence is higher in men than in women and in African-American patients compared with Caucasian patients. The most common form of

cluster headache is episodic cluster. Cluster headache can begin at any age, but it generally begins in the late 20s.

Clinical features and associated disorders

Patients with cluster headache have multiple episodes of short-lived (30–90 minutes) but severe, unilateral, orbital, supraorbital, or temporal pain. At least one of the following associated symptoms must occur: conjunctival injection, lacrimation, nasal congestion, rhinorrhea, facial sweating, miosis, ptosis, or eyelid edema. Episodic cluster consists of headache periods of 1 week to 1 year, with remission periods lasting at least 1 month, whereas chronic cluster headache has either no remission periods or remissions that last less than 1 month.

The pain of a cluster attack rapidly increases (within 15 minutes) to excruciating levels. The attacks often occur at the same time each day and frequently awaken patients from sleep. The pain is deep, constant, boring, piercing, or burning in nature, located in, behind, or around the eye. It may radiate to the forehead, temples, jaws, nostrils, ears, neck, or shoulder. During an attack, patients often feel agitated or restless. Most patients have one or two cluster periods a year that last 2–3 months, with one to two attacks a day.

Differential diagnosis

This includes chronic paroxysmal hemicrania, migraine, trigeminal neuralgia, temporal arteritis, pheochromocytoma, Raeder's paratrigeminal syndrome, Tolosa–Hunt syndrome, sinusitis, and glaucoma.

Evaluation

In most cases, a careful history is all that is needed to make the diagnosis. MRI of the head is justified only in atypical cases or cases with an abnormal neurologic examination (except when the abnormality is a Horner's syndrome).

Management

Patients should avoid alcohol and nitroglycerin. Effective acute treatments include oxygen, sumatriptan, DHE, and (perhaps) topical local anesthetics. Preventive therapy includes ergotamine, calcium channel blockers, lithium, corticosteroids, divalproex, topiramate, melatonin, and capsaicin. If medical therapy fails completely, surgical intervention may be beneficial. Since cluster headache is a chronic headache disorder that may last for the patient's lifetime, the prognosis is guarded.

Idiopathic intracranial hypertension (IIH)

Pathogenesis and pathophysiology

IIH is a disorder of increased intracranial pressure of unknown cause. Some authors suggest that most patients with IIH have partial venous sinus stenosis. One explanation is that increased cerebrospinal fluid (CSF) pressure, through external compression, could account for narrowing of the venous sinuses.

Epidemiology and risk factors

IIH with papilledema occurs with a frequency of about 1 case per 100 000 per year in the general population and 19.3 cases per 100 000 per year in obese women aged 20–44. The patient with IIH is commonly a young, obese woman with chronic daily headaches, normal laboratory studies, an empty sella, and a normal neurologic examination (except for papilledema).

Clinical features and associated disorders

Headache, commonly bifrontotemporal, occurs in most, but not all, patients. The headache can be unilateral. Transient visual obscuration (visual clouding in one or both eyes lasting seconds) occurs with all forms of increased intracranial pressure with papilledema. Pulsatile tinnitus, diplopia, and visual loss can occur. Friedman and Jacobson have proposed diagnostic criteria:
- Symptoms only those of generalized intracranial hypertension or papilledema.
- Signs only those of generalized intracranial hypertension or papilledema.
- Documented elevated intracranial pressure.
- Normal CSF composition.
- MRI/MRV with no hydrocephalus, mass, or structural or vascular lesion (except for empty sella).
- Not attributable to another cause.

Differential diagnosis

IIH may be either truly *idiopathic*, with no clear identifiable cause, or *symptomatic*, a result of venous sinus occlusion, radical neck dissection, hypoparathyroidism, vitamin A intoxication, systemic lupus erythematosus, renal disease, or drug side effects (nalidixic acid, danocrine, steroid withdrawal).

Evaluation

The diagnosis of IIH is based on lumbar puncture following neuroimaging (paying attention to empty sella and sinus thrombosis). If CSF biochemical and cytological analyses are unremarkable and intracranial pressure is elevated to greater than 200 mm H2O (in non-obese subjects), IIH is the likely diagnosis.

Management

Obese patients should be encouraged to lose weight. If patients are asymptomatic and do not have visual loss, treatment is not indicated. In these cases, careful ophthalmologic follow-up is necessary. If headache is associated with visual loss or papilledema, aggressive treatment should be instituted.

The headache of IIH frequently responds to the same treatments used for migraine and TTH. If rigorous headache therapy is unsuccessful, or if there is visual loss, then a 4- to 6-week trial of furosemide or a potent carbonic anhydrase inhibitor (acetazolamide) should be given. Some physicians use topiramate because it is also a carbonic anhydrase inhibitor. High-dose steroids may be effective, but headache commonly recurs when they are withdrawn. Lumbar puncture typically relieves the headache that occurs with IIH and papilledema. Surgical treatment of IIH has been directed toward preventing visual loss secondary to papilledema, and many patients experience headache improvement with optic nerve sheath fenestration.

Prognosis and future perspectives

Most patients with IIH and papilledema can be managed successfully. The prognosis for headache control of IIH without papilledema is more guarded, although there appears to be no risk of visual deterioration.

Low pressure headache

Pathogenesis and pathophysiology

The most common cause of low pressure headache is a lumbar puncture. Spontaneous intracranial hypotension is often due to occult dural tears. Mokri believes that the disorder is primarily that of hypovolemia; hypotension is usually, but not always, present. Low CSF volume leads to brain sagging, with compression of the pituitary–hypothalamic axis and further reduction in CSF production. Occult CSF leakage may also be a major cause of low CSF volume. A history of minor trauma is often elicited.

Epidemiology and risk factors

The incidence of spontaneous or secondary intracranial hypotension is unknown. Postlumbar puncture headache is more common in women, who are affected twice as often as men, and in younger patients. An atraumatic needle reduces the risk of postlumbar puncture headache.

Clinical features and associated disorders

The headache may be frontal, occipital, or diffuse. It is accentuated by the erect position and relieved with recumbency. The pain is severe, dull, or throbbing in nature and is usually not relieved with analgesics. It is aggravated by head-shaking, coughing, straining, sneezing, and jugular compression. The longer the patient is upright, the longer it takes the headache to subside with recumbency. Physical examination is usually normal; however, mild neck stiffness and a slow pulse rate (so-called vagus pulse) may be present. Spinal fluid pressure usually ranges from 0 to 65 mm. The CSF composition is usually normal, but there may be a slight protein elevation and a few red blood cells in the fluid. Reversible Arnold–Chiari-type malformation has been reported in association with a low CSF pressure headache.

Evaluation

Diffuse pachymeningeal enhancement is the most commonly seen abnormality on head MRI. Descent of the brain is common and is manifested by descent of the cerebellar tonsils, decrease in the size of the prepontine cistern, inferior displacement of the optic chiasm, effacement of perichiasmatic cisterns, and crowding of the posterior fossa. Subdural fluid collections are usually but not always bilateral. Decrease in ventricle size is best noted by comparing a head MRI obtained after recovery with an MRI taken during the symptomatic phase. Other abnormalities include pituitary enlargement, engorged venous sinuses, and elongation of the brain stem in the antero-posterior plane.

Management

Intravenous or oral caffeine therapy is effective. If the patient continues to be symptomatic, a blood patch should be used, even if the site of the leak is unknown. If treatment is unsuccessful, one should re-evaluate the patient with radioisotope cisternography, using nasal pledgets if a cribriform plate leak is possible, or myelography to identify CSF leaks, which can be caused by very small dural tears or nerve avulsions. MRI of the spine may also identify cryptogenic leaks. If the headache of intracranial hypotension recurs, a repeat blood patch can be performed or a continuous intrathecal saline infusion attempted. A cervical or upper thoracic blood patch has been reported to be effective when lumbar blood patches fail.

Prognosis

Most patients with intracranial hypotension can be cured once the diagnosis is made. Occasionally, none of the treatments provides relief for a patient with a refractory CSF leak or a refractory low-pressure headache without apparent cause.

Other headache syndromes

Cough and exercise headache

Benign cough headache is a bilateral, throbbing headache of sudden onset, lasting less than 1 minute and precipitated by coughing in the absence of any intracranial disorder. Benign exertional headache lasts from 5 minutes to 24 hours and is produced by physical exercise without any associated systemic or intracranial disorder. Benign exertional headache starts at a younger age than benign cough headache (mean age of onset is 55 years).

MRI must be performed to rule out posterior fossa abnormalities, which can cause these headache syndromes. Symptomatic cough headache is more likely to be associated with a Chiari malformation and begin at an earlier age than benign cough headache. Symptomatic exertional headaches begin later in life and last longer than benign exertional headaches. Patients with benign cough headache often respond dramatically to indomethacin.

Benign thunderclap headache

Thunderclap headache is a sudden-onset headache that reaches maximum intensity in less than 30 seconds. It usually lasts up to several hours, with a less severe headache that lasts weeks. Attacks may be precipitated by exercise or sexual intercourse. They may be accompanied by nausea and vomiting, a variant of which has been called "crash migraine." Thunderclap headache may be accompanied by diffuse focal vasospasm in very large arteries at the circle of Willis and second and third order segments. If focal symptoms or stroke accompany the vasospasm, Call–Fleming syndrome is present. The differential diagnosis of thunderclap headache includes acute hypertensive crisis, carotid artery dissection, cerebral venous sinus thrombosis, benign (idiopathic) thunderclap headache, pituitary apoplexy, spontaneous intracranial hypotension, spontaneous retroclival hematoma, subarachnoid hemorrhage, and unruptured intracranial aneurysm.

Diagnostic evaluation includes early CT, lumbar puncture, MRI with MRA or CTA, and venography.

Further reading

Headache Classification Committee. *The International Classification of Headache Disorders*, 2nd ed. *Cephalalgia* 2004; 24: 1–160.

Lay CL, Campbell JK, Mokri B. Low cerebrospinal fluid pressure headache. In: Goadsby PJ, Silberstein SD, editors. *Headache*. Boston: Butterworth-Heinemann; 1997, pp. 355–68.

Manzoni GC, Prusinski A. Cluster headache: introduction. In: Olesen J, Tfelt-Hansen P, Welch KMA, editors. *The Headaches*. Philadelphia: Lippincott, Williams & Wilkins; 2000, pp. 675–8.

Matchar DB, Young WB, Rosenberg JA, *et al.* Evidence-based guidelines for migraine headache in the primary care setting: pharmacological management of acute attacks. *Neurology* 2000; available at http://www.aan.com

Mokri B. Headache associated with abnormalities in intracranial structure or function: low cerebrospinal fluid pressure headache. In: Silberstein SD, Lipton RB, Dalessio DJ, editors. *Wolff's Headache and Other Head Pain*. New York: Oxford University Press; 2001, pp. 417–33.

Silberstein SD. Chronic daily headache and tension-type headache. *Neurology* 1993; 43: 1644–9.

Silberstein SD. Pharmacological management of cluster headache. *CNS Drugs* 1994; 2: 199–207.

Silberstein SD. Migraine. *Lancet* 2004; 363: 381–91.

Silberstein SD, Goadsby PJ. Migraine: preventive treatment. *Cephalalgia* 2002; 22: 491–512.

Silberstein SD, McKinstry RC III. The death of idiopathic intracranial hypertension? *Neurology* 2003; 60: 1406–7.

Silberstein SD. Transformed and chronic migraine. In: Goadsby PJ, Silberstein SD, Dodick DW, editors. *Chronic Daily Headache for Clinicians*. Hamilton: BC Decker; 2005, pp. 21–56.

Chapter 172
Facial and neck pain

Kammant Phanthumchinda
Chulalongkorn University, Bangkok, Thailand

Introduction

A great deal of confusion exists as to the true etiology, mechanism, and appropriate management of facial and neck pain. Patients who are referred to a clinic with these problems may not demonstrate either recognizable structural abnormalities or a pathologic process. In general, patients who do have structural lesions need specific treatments for the underlying causes of their pain, while patients without lesions require symptomatic management and preventive measures to decrease recurrence. A thorough history and physical examination may provide clues to the correct diagnosis of most clinical syndromes and the causes may be clarified by performing the appropriate tests. The International Headache Society (IHS) defined and proposed diagnostic criteria for facial pain, cranial neuralgia, and cervicogenic headache, which can be referenced for standard diagnosis. This section will briefly summarize the important syndromes of facial and neck pain.

Facial pain

Clinicians can diagnose common facial and orofacial pain with a clearly defined pathologic process (e.g., dental pain, sinus headache) without difficulty; the most commonly undiagnosed pain conditions in this anatomical region include neuropathic and myofascial pain. The etiology and pathophysiologic mechanisms of these pain syndromes are poorly understood.

Trigeminal neuralgia
Epidemiology
The prevalence of trigeminal neuralgia is 70 per 100 000 population. This disorder affects women more commonly than men and incidence increases with age.

International Neurology: A Clinical Approach. Edited by Robert P. Lisak, Daniel D. Truong, William M. Carroll, and Roongroj Bhidayasiri. © 2009 Blackwell Publishing, ISBN: 978-1-4051-5738-4.

Pathophysiology
Although the exact mechanism is unclear, the theory of central and peripheral hypersensitivity of the trigeminal nerve has been proposed. Hypersensitivity may occur as a result of focal demyelination of the trigeminal nerve or a central demyelinating process occurring at the nerve root entry zone. The demyelination may cause epiphatic action potentials and set up a centrally mediated disinhibition of neuralgic pain.

Clinical features
Trigeminal neuralgia is characterized by short-lived episodes of neuralgic pain affecting one or more divisions of the trigeminal nerve. Patients may describe these episodes of excruciating pain as superficial, jabbing, stabbing, sharp, shooting, burning, searing, or as an electric shock sensation. The pain is usually sudden and paroxysmal, lasting from a fraction of a second to minutes. The episodes are usually separated by pain-free intervals lasting several seconds, and stimulation of the trigger area will cause no pain during these periods (referred to as refractory periods). However, pain often comes in clusters at very short intervals and aching between paroxysms may occur. The attacks are usually stereotyped in the individual patient. The episodes may occur spontaneously, but they can be triggered by a variety of non-noxious stimuli, including eating, talking, brushing the teeth, or touching a small area of nasolabial fold and/or chin (trigger area). The patient with classical trigeminal neuralgia may not allow any touch or exposure of these areas, which can differentiate this neuralgia from other facial pain conditions for which the patient may rub or massage his or her face to relieve pain. Remissions that last for months may occur. In classical trigeminal neuralgia, physical examination usually reveals no cranial neuropathy. Causes of trigeminal neuralgia include classical trigeminal neuralgia and secondary or symptomatic trigeminal neuralgia.

The cause of the classical trigeminal neuralgia is usually a neurovascular compression of the trigeminal nerve at the level of the nerve entry zone. Secondary trigeminal neuralgia is caused by other pathologic processes affecting the trigeminal nerve or trigeminal pathway, such as tumor, multiple sclerosis, aneurysm, and infection. Atypical presentations include onset under 50 years of age, bilateral symptomatology, focal neurological deficits, pain that remits, and active systemic diseases; in these cases, causes other than a vascular compression should be investigated.

Differential diagnosis of orofacial pain with neuralgic-like symptoms includes orofacial pain of dental origin and trigeminal autonomic cephalalgia. Dental evaluation for pulpitis, an infected tooth, or cracked tooth syndrome should be performed. In trigeminal autonomic cephalalgia, especially chronic paroxysmal hemicrania (CPH) and short-lasting unilateral neuralgiform headache with conjunctival injection and tearing (SUNCT), the location of pain is in the orbital-frontal area and is usually associated with autonomic features that are uncommon in classical trigeminal neuralgia. In addition, patients with CPH experience a dramatic response to indomethacin, which is frequently used as a therapeutic diagnosis. SUNCT has prominent features of lacrimation and conjunctival injection as its diagnostic clues. However, the combined syndromes of trigeminal neuralgia and trigeminal autonomic cephalalgia may coexist.

Investigations
MRI is the investigation of choice for the evaluation of trigeminal neuralgia. The technique can identify a vascular compression loop, as well as depicting other pathological processes. In patients with possible systemic diseases, appropriate diagnostic tests should be applied.

Treatment and management
Secondary or symptomatic trigeminal neuralgia should be treated according to its underlying cause. Medical treatment for a classical trigeminal neuralgia that is proposed to initiate a remission period should be started with carbarmazepine. If patients experience side effects and do not benefit from carbamazepine, alternative agents, including baclofen, diphenylhydantoin, valproic acid, or other new anticonvulsants should be considered. If the pain subsides for months, a reduction of the medication may be attempted and the therapy may be restarted if the pain recurs. When patients become intractable to medical management, surgical interventions may be considered. The common indications for surgical intervention include intolerability of the medication side effects and the patient's expectation for "cure." Microvascular decompression is the most effective and safe procedure, with a high rate of long-term remission.

Glossopharyngeal-vagoglossopharyngeal neuralgia
Epidemiology
Glossopharyngeal-vagoglossopharyngeal neuralgia is far less prevalent than trigeminal neuralgia.

Pathophysiology
The mechanism is thought to be similar to trigeminal neuralgia.

Clinical features
Neuralgic pain in glossopharyngeal neuralgia affects the area supplied by somatosensory branches of the glossopharyngeal and vagus nerves. The painful areas include the tonsil, tongue, throat, larynx, neck, angle of jaw, and external auditory meatus, which may occur in any combination. Attacks consist of abrupt, severe stabbing, shooting, knife-like, electric-shock sensations and scratching episodes similar to the trigeminal neuralgia. The pattern of attack is always paroxysmal. There is often sensation between paroxysms in the form of hard or sharp sticking or foreign body sensation or a dull, deep, continuous pain at the affected sites. Rare associated symptoms during the attack include vigorous coughing, hoarseness of voice, syncope from sick sinus syndrome, severe bradycardia, asystole, and severe hypotension. Seizures may result from cerebral hypoperfusion.

The trigger phenomena are stimulation in the pharynx such as swallowing (especially cold liquids and food with a sharp sensation of taste and smell), talking, coughing, chewing, yawning, and clearing the throat. Other tactile triggers in the external auditory meatus, lateral aspect of the neck, and pre- and postauricular area, as well as rapid head movement and ipsilateral arm elevation can precipitate the neuralgia.

Glossopharyngeal neuralgia usually has its remission and relapses. It is often bilateral (unilateral preceding, non-synchronously or simultaneously affected), with nocturnal attacks, which is different from trigeminal neuralgia. Ipsilateral glossopharyngeal and trigeminal neuralgia may occur in the same patient. Physical examination is usually normal. However, the ear on the affected side may be infected and painful. Symptomatic or secondary glossopharyngeal neuralgia is far less common than trigeminal neuralgia and the underlying pathologic processes include neoplasms, infections, ossified stylohyoid ligament (Eagle's syndrome), and multiple sclerosis. Vascular compression from ecstatic blood vessels has recently been reported as a frequent cause of glossopharyngeal neuralgia.

Investigations
MRI is the neuroimaging method of choice for identification of the pathologic processes causing secondary glossopharyngeal neuralgia. It can also demonstrate compressed and distorted ninth and tenth cranial nerves at the nerve entry zone by tortuous vertebrobasilar vessels. Skull radiography can depict ossified styloid ligament in Eagle's syndrome. In cases with secondary malignant or infectious diseases, searching for primary foci is essential.

Treatment and management

Anticonvulsants, including carbamazepine, oxcarbamazepine, diphenylhydantoin, lamotrigine, and gabapentin, as well as baclofen are usually effective in glossopharyngeal neuralgia. When medical therapy fails, rhizotomy (involving vagus and glossopharyngeal nerves) and microvascular decompression are advocated.

Neck pain and headache

Headache is strongly associated with disorder of the cervical spine only in cases with well-defined structural lesions in the craniovertebral junction and upper cervical spines (e.g., developmental anomalies or acquired lesions such as tumor, trauma, infection, and inflammatory processes). Controversy exists as to the contribution of degenerative spine and/or trivial spinal disorders to the development of various primary headache disorders, such as cervicogenic headache, migraine, and occipical neuralgia. The IHS has provided diagnostic criteria for cervicogenic headache and other headache due to cervical spine disorders. Three conditions with conflicts and contradictions are discussed below.

Occipital neuralgia
Epidemiology
No epidemiologic data are available on occipital neuralgia.

Pathophysiology
The pathophysiology is unclear; possibly, the lesion causing neuralgia may be proximal to the occipital nerve.

Clinical features
Neuralgic pain in occipital neuralgia is distributed in the areas supplied by the greater and lesser occipital nerves. The pain is usually sharp, lancinating, and electric shock-like in character. The episodes of pain are paroxysmal and may be unilateral or bilateral. Neurological examination may be normal, but patients may experience dysesthesia or diminished pain sensation in the affected area. Limitation of motion and tenderness over the nerve trunk as it crosses the superior nuchal line may be observed. In general, occipital neuralgia is not a common cause of headache and other diagnoses should be carefully considered. Unlike the C_2 root, which is more vulnerable to trauma and other pathologic processes, including nerve entrapment, meningioma, inflammatory process, and venous anomalies, occipital nerves are not usually prone to these lesions. Pain from occipital neuralgia should be differentiated from referred pain from C2–C3 joint and other referred pain from craniovertebral junction anomalies, including upper cervical spine and posterior fossa lesions. The referred pain is usually continuous without neuralgic character or impairment of sensation.

Investigations
MRI is used to exclude other causes of referred pain that can mimic occipital neuralgia. Response to anesthetic agents or nerve block of the related structure may be helpful for clarification of the precise origin of occipital pain.

Treatment and management
Studies of treatments for idiopathic occipital neuralgia are inconclusive. Carbamazepine, transcutaneous stimulation, and neck immobilization may be helpful in mild cases. In severe intractable cases, rhizotomy of the appropriate nerves may be tried.

Carotidynia
Epidemiology
The prevalence of carotidynia depends on the underlying disease (e.g., migraine-related entity, dissection of cerebral vessel, giant cell arteritis, etc.).

Pathophysiology
Stimulation of the carotid artery wall, especially at its bifurcation, produces pain at the jaw, cheek, gum, nose, eye, and teeth via sensory branches of the vagus nerve, and may be caused by various pathological processes. In migraine-related carotidynia, the pain may be produced by vascular hypersensitivity.

Clinical features
Carotidynia is a syndrome characterized by unilateral neck and/or facial pain. The pain may radiate to the ear, eye, nose, gum, cheek, jaw, or scalp. The character of the pain may be continuous and dull, with the possibility of throbbing or pounding episodes. Stabbing, burning, sharp, ice-picking-like jabs or neuralgic features may be observed. The pain is usually aggravated by head and neck movements, swallowing, coughing, sneezing, yawning, and chewing. The maximum tenderness is at the carotid bifurcation occurring along its entire length. Moreover, swelling of the overlying soft tissue may occasionally be detected.

Clues to the causes of carotidynia may be related to the natural history of pain and other associated conditions. In acute monophasic disease with or without an associated viral infection and a clinical course of less than 2 weeks, the proposed etiology is viral infection. In cases with subacute courses associated with neurological signs (e.g., Horner's syndrome), it may be associated with the dissection of the carotid artery, ruptured atherosclerotic plaque, or giant cell arteritis. In cases with recurrent or daily attacks that last hours and are associated with a throbbing headache that responds to ergotamine or methysergide, migraine may be the possible diagnosis.

Investigations

Investigation should be focused on the non-invasive diagnostic tests that are appropriate for carotid lesions (e.g., MRI angiography, carotid ultrasound). Vascular imaging can detect dissection and ruptured atherosclerotic plaque. Erythrocyte sedimentation rate (ESR), temporal artery biopsy, and a therapeutic trial with prednisolone may be appropriate for elderly individuals who are suspected of having giant cell arteritis. Systemic evaluation should include viral infection in cases with monophasic illnesses.

Treatment and management

Carotidynia is a pain syndrome in which treatment depends on the definite cause, as described above.

Cervicogenic headache

Epidemiology

Prevalence of cervicogenic headache is varied due to the heterogeneity of diagnostic criteria and controversial concept of cervicogenic headache.

Pathophysiology

Identifiable and indisputable disease or pathologic processes causing dysfunction of structure in the neck can generate and cause referred pain to the head via various neuroanatomical pathways. In cases with poorly defined lesions, the possible source of cervicogenic headache may be in the structure, including synovial joints, cervical muscles, intervertebral disc, dura of upper cervical cord, and posterior fossa, as well as vertebral and carotid arteries.

Clinical features

Sjaatad's cervicogenic headache is a syndrome or "reaction pattern" of dysfunction or disease in the neck. The syndrome is still controversial and the etiology, tissue site, and mechanism remain unclear. The main cardinal features of headache include episodic, unilateral, side-locked occipital pain associated with specific neck movement and/or posture. Headache is chronic and frequently relapses. Pain may spread forward bilaterally and evolve into persistent headache. Physical examination reveals a specific site in the upper cervical (occipito-atlas axis) region as the cervical site of pain (e.g., limitation of movement of the head or neck, flexion–extension, head tilt or reproduction of the symptom from cervical maneuver). Apart from the cardinal features, some patients may have other associated migrainous symptoms such as photophobia, phonophobia, nausea, dizziness, ipsilateral blurred vision, difficulty swallowing, or autonomic disturbance such as conjunctival injection, lacrimation, or periocular edema. However, the patient should not fulfill the IHS criteria for other primary headaches, such as migraine, tension-type headache, or trigeminal autonomic headache, and does not exhibit a dramatic response to ergotamine, triptan, or indomethacin.

Investigations

CT scan and MRI are the diagnostic tests of choice for viewing the upper cervical segment, particularly the cranio-vertebral junction and surrounding soft tissue. Neuroimaging changes will establish specific causes of cervicogenic headache when there are overt structurally visible lesions and the lesions are clinically correlated with the headache syndrome. Confirmatory evidence of the cervicogenic basis of headache by diagnostic, local anesthetic block will give clue to the location of the problem when neuroimaging fails to reveal a relevant cervical dysfunction, pathology, or disease.

Treatment and management

Treatments are controversial and therapy tends to focus on manipulation of the neck, as well as local modalities such as deep heat and physical methods. NSAIDs may be partially effective in some cases.

Further reading

Biousse V, Bousser MG. The myth of carotidynia. *Neurology* 1994; 44: 993–5.

Edmeads JG. Disorders of the neck: cervicogenic headache. In: Siberstein SD, Lipton RB, Dalessio DJ, editors. *Wolff's Headache and Other Head Pain*, 7th ed. Oxford: Oxford University Press; 2001, pp. 447–58.

Headache Classification Committee of the International Headache Society. Classification and diagnostic criteria for headache disorders, cranial neuralgia, and facial pain, 2nd ed. *Cephalalgia* 2004; 24(Suppl 1): 1–160.

Sjaastad O, Fredriken TA. Cervicogenic headache: criteria, classification and epidemiology. *Clin Exp Rheumatol* 2000; 18(2 Suppl 19): S3–6.

Zakrzewska JM, Harrison SD, editors. *Assessment and Management of Orofacial Pain. Pain Research and Clinical Management*, Vol. 14. Amsterdam: Elsevier; 2002.

Chapter 173
Fibromyalgia

Saeed Bohlega
King Faisal Specialist Hospital and Research Centre, Riyadh, Saudi Arabia

Introduction

Fibromyalgia (FM), also known as fibrositis, is a chronic and widespread musculoskeletal painful condition. It is one of the most frequent causes of non-articular rheumatism; it involves the muscles and soft tissue rather than joints. FM encompasses a spectrum of clinical features including other syndromes not involving muscles or soft tissues such as non-restorative sleep disturbances, migraine headaches, irritable bowel, diffuse pain, and memory loss.

Epidemiology

FM is highly prevalent in rheumatology clinics, pain centers, general medicine, and family practice clinics. Its prevalence is highest between ages 20 and 60 years, with the prevalence rate of 3.4% for women and 0.5% for men. Some studies found higher prevalence rates: between 4.5% and 7% in some countries such as Pakistan, Malaysia, Poland, and South Africa.

FM appears to coexist sometimes with other rheumatological disorders such as rheumatoid arthritis, osteoarthritis, and systemic lupus erythematosus. Head trauma and sleep apnea may increase the risk in men, while hypothyroidism and hyperprolactinemia are reported to increase the risk in women.

Pathogenesis

FM does not have a distinct cause or pathology; several mechanisms have been postulated to underline the diffuse lowering of nociceptive threshold. The presence of other centrally associated phenomena such as sleep disturbances and blunted stimulus response as well as the

International Neurology: A Clinical Approach. Edited by Robert P. Lisak, Daniel D. Truong, William M. Carroll, and Roongroj Bhidayasiri. © 2009 Blackwell Publishing, ISBN: 978-1-4051-5738-4.

diffuse nature of pain suggest that a central mechanism may be involved.

Several other mechanisms have been postulated including alteration of the brain concentration of regulatory neurotransmitters such as serotonin, endorphin and substance P, emotional trauma or depression, genetic familial factors, abnormal blood supply to muscles, and low level of insulin-like growth factor (IGF-1).

No microscopic, ultrastructural, biochemical, or metabolic abnormalities have been consistently demonstrated in muscle biopsy specimens from patient with FM.

Clinical features and diagnosis

Diagnostic criteria for FM are specific. According to the American College of Rheumatology (ACR) 1990 Classification Criteria diagnosis depends on a combination of:

1 Generalized pain in three or more axial and limb sites for 3 months or longer.

2 Reproducible tenderness on digital palpation in at least 11 out of the 18 prespecified sites; these bilateral areas are specified as:

  a Suboccipital muscle insertions

  b The anterior aspect of the intertransverse spaces at C5–C7

  c The upper or mid part of trapezius muscle

  d Supraspinatus muscle and the medial border of scapula

  e The costochondral junction of the second rib

  f 2 cm distal to the lateral epicodyles

  g The upper outer quadrant of the buttocks

  h The prominence of greater trochanter

  i The medial fat pad of the knee

3 Exclusion of other conditions that may cause similar pain.

These criteria have a sensitivity of 88.4% and specificity of 81%. Approximately 50% of patients complain of pain that is "all over"; the pain is frequently associated with marked stiffness, especially postexertional, and sometimes lasts all day. Additional sources of pain are headache, sore throat, and eye or pelvic pain.

Other notable features are often debilitating fatigue and disturbed sleep pattern, swelling and parasthesia of hands and feet, anxiety, panic attacks, and depression.

The hallmark finding is the presence of tender points at the above-mentioned characteristic anatomical sites, which are widely distinctive and symmetrical but generally do not produce referred pain.

Other physical findings include skin fold tenderness, reactive hyperemia, myofascial trigger points, and decreased pain threshold.

FM should be distinguished from myofascial pain (MP) conceptually and clinically. MP is a syndrome of regional muscle pain of soft tissue origin and caused by trigger points. Pressure on these axial or fascial points will evoke a transient twitch of the taut muscle band, with restricted range of motion. Pain can be alleviated by local injection into these tender points or by passively stretching the involved muscles. However, it is not uncommon that these two conditions may co-exist in the same patient.

Patients with seronegative spondyloarthropathies may also present with diffuse pain and subtle inflammatory findings. These conditions will cause back pain, morning stiffness, and disturbed sleep.

Polymyalgia rheumatica is generally seen in older individuals causing pain and stiffness of the shoulder girdle and other associated symptoms including general stiffness, weight loss, fatigue, and jaw and lingual claudication. Metabolic disorders that may be confused with FM are vitamin D deficiency, hypothyroidism and statin-induced myopathy.

Management

The reality of patients' symptoms must be acknowledged by the physician; the benign, non-deforming, and non-life-threatening nature of FM and the absence of infection should be emphasized.

A wide range of pharmacologic agents are available, but the complexity of FM and the presence of multiple symptoms will make the assessment of effective clinical trials very challenging.

Antidepressants, primarily tricyclics such as amitriptyline, cyclobenzaprine, and doxepin, are widely used and researched because they promote sleep and help depression, but they have a relatively narrow therapeutic index and their side effects (e.g., dry mouth, weight gain, and occasional daytime sedation) are limiting factors.

Selective serotonin re-uptake inhibitors (SSRIs) have better tolerability than tricyclics and play a role in improvement of mood and fatigue but do not appear to be effective in relieving FM pain. The combination of fluoxetine and amitriptyline was shown to be more effective than either agent alone or placebo.

Serotonin norepinephrine re-uptake inhibitors (SNRIs), for example, venlafaxine, milnacipran, and duloxetine, show promise in treating pain, fatigue, and sleep disturbances, with fewer side effects than tricyclics.

Many studies showed that tramadol, a weak μ-opioid receptor agonist, is effective in the treatment of FM pain. Other opioids are generally not recommended because of concern of addictive potential. Muscle relaxants, sedatives, and hypnotics have been shown to have positive results in open label trials. The new antiepileptic pregabalin has been shown to be effective for reducing many of the symptoms associated with FM, is well tolerated, and has recently been approved for treatment of FM by the United States Food and Drug Administration.

Physical therapy modalities that may be helpful include passive and active manipulation of skeletal muscles, deep heat, ultrasound, massage, and transcutaneous electrical nerve stimulation (TENS). Physical therapy is an important part of patient overall treatment and response should be used to measure the patient's progress.

Finally, the patient's psychological state and the impact of this painful condition should be addressed. Psychotherapy and relaxation therapies such as biofeedback, stress reduction, and behavioral modification will give patients significant help.

Further reading

Arshad A, Kong KO. Awareness and perceptions of fibromyalgia syndrome: a survey of Southeast Asian rheumatologists. *J Clin Rheumatol* 2007; 13(2): 59–62.

Mease P. Fibromyalgia syndrome: review of clinical presentation, pathogenesis, outcome measurements, and treatment. *J Rheumatol* 2005; 75(Suppl): 6–21.

Wolfe F, Smythe HA, Unus MB, *et al*. The American College of Rheumatology 1990 Criteria for the Classification of Fibromyalgia. Report of the Multicenter Criteria Committee. *Arthritis Rheum* 1990; 33: 160–72.

Appendix: Treatment algorithm for Parkinson's disease

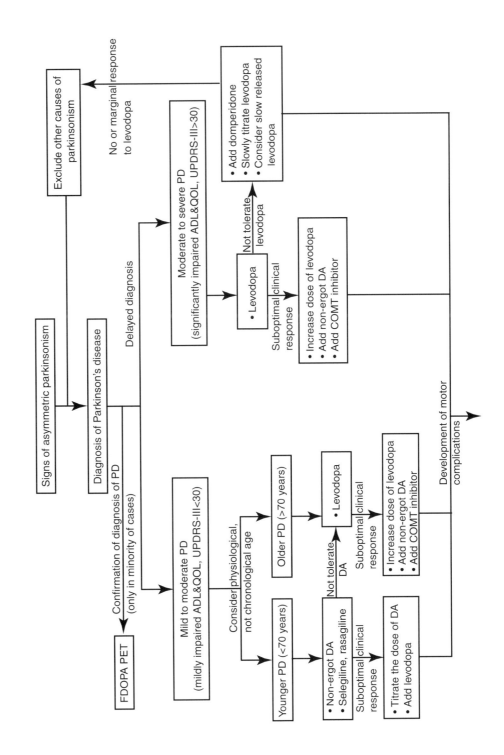

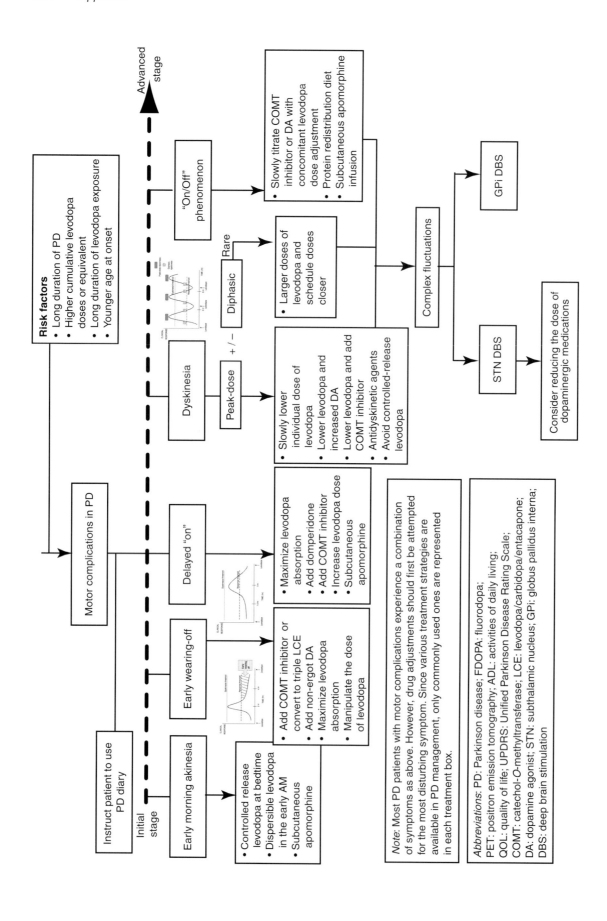

Advanced stage

Risk factors
• Long duration of PD
• Higher cumulative levodopa doses or equivalent
• Long duration of levodopa exposure
• Younger age at onset

Motor complications in PD

Instruct patient to use PD diary

Initial stage

"On/Off" phenomenon

• Slowly titrate COMT inhibitor or DA with concomitant levodopa dose adjustment
• Protein redistribution diet
• Subcutaneous apomorphine infusion

Dyskinesia

Rare

Diphasic

+ / –

Peak-dose

• Larger doses of levodopa and schedule doses closer

• Slowly lower individual dose of levodopa
• Lower levodopa and increased DA
• Lower levodopa and add COMT inhibitor
• Antidyskinetic agents
• Avoid controlled-release levodopa

Complex fluctuations

GPi DBS

STN DBS

Consider reducing the dose of dopaminergic medications

Delayed "on"

• Maximize levodopa absorption
• Add domperidone
• Add COMT inhibitor
• Increase levodopa dose
• Subcutaneous apomorphine

Early wearing-off

• Add COMT inhibitor or convert to triple LCE
• Add non-ergot DA
• Maximize levodopa absorption
• Manipulate the dose of levodopa

Early morning akinesia

• Controlled release levodopa at bedtime
• Dispersible levodopa in the early AM
• Subcutaneous apomorphine

Note: Most PD patients with motor complications experience a combination of symptoms as above. However, drug adjustments should first be attempted for the most disturbing symptom. Since various treatment strategies are available in PD management, only commonly used ones are represented in each treatment box.

Abbreviations: PD: Parkinson disease; FDOPA: fluorodopa; PET: positron emission tomography; ADL: activities of daily living; QOL: quality of life; UPDRS: Unified Parkinson Disease Rating Scale; COMT: catechol-O-methyltransferase; LCE: levodopa/carbidopa/entacapone; DA: dopamine agonist; STN: subthalamic nucleus; GPi: globus pallidus interna; DBS: deep brain stimulation

Index

α-aminolevulinic acid (ALA), 642.
　　See also porphyrias
abetalipoproteinemia, 608
abscess, 259
absence seizures, 95
Acanthamoeba species, 279
acetylcholine receptor antibody, 438
acetylcholinesterase inhibitors (AChEI), 440
acute bacterial meningitis (ABM), 238
　　antibiotics, empirical therapy for, 240*t*
　　clinical presentation, 239
　　complications, 241
　　CSF abnormalities, 240
　　diagnosis, 239
　　differential diagnosis, 240
　　　　subarachnoid hemorrhage (SAH), 240
　　　　subdural empyema, 240
　　epidemiology, 238
　　etiology, 238
　　pathology, 239
　　pathophysiology, 239
　　prevention, 241
　　prognostic signs in, 241
　　radiological investigations, 239–40
　　specific treatment, 240–41
　　steroids, role of, 241
acute demyelinating encephalomyelitis, 34
acute disseminated encephalomyelitis, 378
　　clinical features of, 381
　　laboratory findings in, 381
　　magnetic resonance imaging features of, 382
　　pathological studies of, 384
　　treatment of, 382
acute dystonic reactions (ADR), 191
acute polio, 212
　　clinical features of, 213
　　epidemiological features of, 212
　　investigations, 213–14
　　new polio cases per year, in Norway, 213*t*
　　pathophysiological features of, 212
　　treatment and management of, 214
acute retroviral syndrome, 343
acute severe vertigo, 489–90
acute tics, 192
acute viral meningitis
　　clinical features of, 308–9
　　signs and symptoms of, 309*t*
acyl-CoA dehydrogenase deficiencies, 632.
　　　　See also fatty acid oxidation disorders
adrenal leukodystrophy, 607–8
adriamycin, 530
adult-onset focal dystonias, 169–70
Aedes triseriatus, 325

age-related macular degeneration (AMD), 501
akathisia, acute, 191
ALA dehydratase deficiency porphyria, 640
albendazole, for treatment of trichinosis
　　　　infection, 300
alcohol intoxication, acute, 410–11
alcoholic myopathy, chronic, 413
alcoholic polyneuropathy, 431
Alexander's disease, 606
alkylating agent, 544
allopurinol, 639
Alpers' syndrome, 624
alpha-tocopherol, 405
alphaviruses
　　Eastern equine virus, 326
　　laboratory features and management of, 326
　　Venezuelan equine virus, 325–6
　　Western equine virus, 325
Alzheimer's disease (AD), 126, 338
　　clinical diagnosis of, 127
　　clinical features of, 126–7
　　epidemiological features of, 126
　　investigations, 127
　　pathophysiological features of, 126
　　treatment options for, 127–8
American College of Rheumatology (ACR), 45
amnesia, causes of, 121–2
amoebic disease, of CNS, 279
　　clinical features of, 280
　　epidemiological features of, 279
　　imaging and pathologic findings in, 280
　　investigations, 280
　　pathophysiological features of, 279–80
　　treatment for, 281*t*
amygdalohippocampectomy/temporal
　　　　lobectomy, 113–14
amyloid precursor protein (APP), 474
amyotrophic lateral sclerosis (ALS), 199
　　clinical features of, 200
　　epidemiological features of, 199
　　investigations, 200–201
　　pathophysiological features of, 199–200
　　treatment and management of, 201–2
anaplastic astrocytomas (AA), 506
anaplastic oligoastrocytomas, 514, 518
　　epidemiology and prognosis, 514
　　management of, 516–18
　　　　chemotherapy, 516–18
　　　　surgery and radiation therapy, 516
　　pathology and molecular biology, 515
　　prognostic factors, 514–15
　　treatment, 515
anaplastic oligodendrogliomas (AOD), 514

ancestral haplotype (AH), 474
Andersen's syndrome, 455
Angiostrongyliasis
　　causes of, 301
　　clinical features of, 302
　　epidemiology of, 301–2
Angiostrongylus cantonensis, 301
angiotensin-converting enzyme (ACE), 80
ankylosing spondylitis (AS), 83
　　clinical symptoms of, 83
　　diagnostic tests, 83
　　treatment, 84
Anopheles mosquitoes, 327
anorexia nervosa, 387
anterior poliomyelitis, acute, 426
anticardiolipin antibodies (aCL), 59
antidepressants, 680
antiepileptic drugs (AEDs), 99, 107, 642
　　broad spectrum, 110–11
　　choosing the appropriate, 111
　　classification of, 111*t*
　　narrow spectrum, 107, 110
antigen presenting cells (APC), 368
anti-GQ1b ganglioside antibodies, 256
antimalarial treatment, 288–9
anti-MuSK antibodies, 439
antineutrophilic cytoplasmic antigen
　　　　antibodies, 429
antinutrophil cytoplasmic antibodies (ANCAs), 57
antiphospholipid antibodies (aPL), 59
antiphospholipid antibody syndrome (APS), 59
　　common manifestation of, 59–60
　　diagnosis of, 60
　　management of, 60
antiphospholipid syndrome (APLS), 24
antipsychotic drugs, 130
antiretrovirals (ARVs), 354
antiretroviral toxic neuropathy (ATN), 351
antithymocyte globulin (ATG), 476
anti-U3 nucleolar ribonucleoprotein, 71
apparent diffusion coefficient (ADC), 387
Aquaporin-4 (AQP-4), 375
arbovirus prodromes, 310
Arnold–Chiari malformation, 188
aromatic *L*-amino acid decarboxylase (AADC), 592
arousal disorder (AD), 571
　　clinical course, 572
　　clinical features and differential diagnoses
　　　　of, 571–2
　　epidemiology and risk factors, 571
　　investigations, 572
　　management, 572
　　pathophysiology, 571